Medical Disorders During Pregnancy

Medical Disorders During Pregnancy

William M. Barron, M.D.
Associate Professor
Departments of Medicine and Obstetrics
    and Gynecology
University of Chicago
Chicago, Illinois

Marshall D. Lindheimer, M.D.
Professor
Departments of Medicine and Obstetrics
    and Gynecology
University of Chicago
Chicago, Illinois

Assistant Editors

John M. Davison, M.D., F.R.C.O.G.
Consultant Obstetrician and Gynaecologist
MRC Human Reproduction Group
Princess Mary Maternity Hospital
Newcastle upon Tyne, England

Jean-Pierre Grünfeld, M.D.
Professor, Department de Nephrologie
Hospital Necker
Paris, France

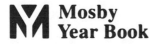
Mosby
Year Book

St. Louis   Baltimore   Boston   Chicago   London   Philadelphia   Sydney   Toronto

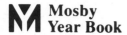
**Mosby
Year Book**

Dedicated to Publishing Excellence

Sponsoring Editor: Richard H. Lampert
Associate Managing Editor, Manuscript Services: Deborah Thorp
Production Project Coordinator: Karen Halm
Proofroom Supervisor: Barbara M. Kelly

Mosby-Year Book, Inc.
11830 Westline Industrial Drive
St. Louis, MO 63146

2 3 4 5 6 7 8 9 0 R V 95 94 93 92

Library of Congress Cataloging-in-Publication Data

Medical disorders during pregnancy / [edited by]
   William M. Barron, Marshall D. Lindheimer.
      p. cm.
   Includes bibliographical references.
   Includes index.
   ISBN 0-8151-0519-3
   1. Pregnancy, Complications of. I. Barron,
     William M. 1950— . II. Lindheimer,
     Marshall D., 1932— .
   [DNLM: 1. Pregnancy Complications. WQ 240
     M4865]
   RG571.M42   1990   91-12735
   618.3—dc20   CIP
   DNLM/DLC
   for Library of Congress

To Helen, Laurie, and Jacqueline

CONTRIBUTORS

Iris K. Aronson, M.D.
Associate Professor
Department of Dermatology
University of Illinois
Chicago, Illinois

Alfred L. Baker, M.D.
Professor, Department of Medicine
Section of Gastroenterology
University of Chicago
Chicago, Illinois

William M. Barron, M.D.
Associate Professor
Departments of Medicine and Obstetrics and
   Gynecology
University of Chicago
Chicago, Illinois

Pierre Bernades, M.D.
Professor
Division of Gastroenterology
Hôpital Beaujon
Paris, France

Kenneth M. Borrow, M.D.
Professor of Medicine and Director
Noninvasive Cardiac Imaging Laboratory
University of Chicago
Chicago, Illinois

Robert L. Brent, M.D., Ph.D.
Professor, Department of Pediatrics
Jefferson Medical College
Director of Division of Developmental Biology
Alfred I. du Pont Institute
Philadelphia, Pennsylvania

N. E. F. Cartlidge, M.D.
Consultant Neurologist
Senior Lecturer in Neurology
Newcastle Health Authority
Royal Victoria Infirmary
Newcastle upon Tyne, England

Ira J. Chasnoff, M.D.
Associate Professor
Departments of Pediatrics and Psychiatry
Director, Perinatal Center for Chemical
   Dependency
Northwestern University Medical School
Chicago, Illinois

John M. Davison, M.D., F.R.C.O.G.
Consultant Obstetrician and Gynaecologist
MRC Human Reproduction Group
Princess Mary Maternity Hospital
Newcastle upon Tyne, England

Maurice L. Druzin, M.D.
Associate Professor of Obstetrics and Gynecology
Cornell University Medical College
New York, New York

Steven G. Gabbe, M.D.
Professor and Chairman
Department of Obstetrics and Gynecology
The Ohio State University
Columbus, Ohio

Jean-Pierre Grünfeld, M.D.
Professor, Department de Nephrologie
Hopital Necker
Paris, France

Barbara Halaska, M.D.
Assistant Professor
Department of Medicine
Section of Dermatology
Loma Linda University
Loma Linda, California

Jesse B. Hall, M.D.
Associate Professor
Director, Medical Intensive Care Unit
University of Chicago
Chicago, Illinois

Mark B. Landon, M.D.
Assistant Professor
Department of Obstetrics and Gynecology
The Ohio State University
Columbus, Ohio

Roberto M. Lang, M.D.
Assistant Professor of Medicine (Cardiology)
University of Chicago
Chicago, Illinois

Richard V. Lee, M.D.
Professor of Medicine and Pediatrics
Chief, Department of Medicine
Children's Hospital of Buffalo
Buffalo, New York

Elizabeth Letsky, M.B.B.S., F.R.C.Path.
Consultant Haematologist
Queen Charlotte's Hospital for Women
London, England

Marshall D. Lindheimer, M.D.
Professor
Departments of Medicine and Obstetrics and
    Gynecology
University of Chicago
Chicago, Illinois

Michael D. Lockshin, M.D.
Director, Intramural Program
National Institutes of Arthritis and
    Musculoskeletal and Skin Diseases
Bethesda, Maryland

C. R. Madeley, M.D., F.R.C.Path.
Professor and Chairman
Department of Virology
University of Newcastle upon Tyne
Royal Victoria Infirmary
Newcastle upon Tyne, England

Robert Modigliani
Professor
Division of Gastroenterology
Hôpital Saint Lazare
Paris, France

Mark E. Molitch, M.D.
Professor of Medicine
Center for Endocrinology, Metabolism, and
    Nutrition
Northwestern University Medical School
Chicago, Illinois

Katherine E. Orr, M.B., Ch.B.
Department of Clinical Microbiology
Royal Victoria Infirmary
Newcastle upon Tyne, England

**Stephen J. Pedler, M.B., Ch.B.,
M.R.C.Path.**
Consultant Microbiologist
Department of Clinical Microbiology
Royal Victoria Infirmary
Newcastle upon Tyne, England

J. S. M. Peiris, M.D., D.Phil., M.R.C.Path.
Consultant Virologist
Royal Victoria Infirmary
Newcastle upon Tyne, England

Richard L. Schilsky, M.D.
Associate Professor of Medicine
Department of Medicine
Section of Hematology-Oncology
University of Chicago
Chicago, Illinois

Gregory A. Schmidt, M.D.
Assistant Professor
Department of Medicine
Section of Pulmonary and Critical Care
University of Chicago
Chicago, Illinois

Nada L. Stotland, M.D.
Associate Professor
Department of Psychiatry
University of Chicago
Chicago, Illinois

Stephanie F. Williams, M.D.
Assistant Professor
Department of Medicine
Section of Hematology-Oncology
University of Chicago
Chicago, Illinois

PREFACE AND GUIDELINES FOR PRESCRIBING DRUGS TO PREGNANT WOMEN

Medical disorders in pregnant women challenge clinicians. Problems may relate to diseases that antedate or arise de novo during gestation, or to maladies unique to the pregnant state. In addition, gestation alters the anatomy and physiology of most organ systems, changes that can profoundly influence the natural history of many medical disorders. Furthermore, the practitioner must deal with diseases capable of jeopardizing two patients, the mother and her fetus.

This text was written to assist all physicians who manage pregnant women with medical diseases. The editors, both internists with dual appointments in the Departments of Medicine and Obstetrics and Gynecology at the University of Chicago, are consultants to a busy urban obstetric service at the Chicago Lying-in Hospital. Our clinical experiences, research interests, and many constructive interactions with both medical and obstetric colleagues (over a period of 20 years) convinced us of the need for this text, the manner in which it is organized, and the choice of authorities who produced the 19 chapters that comprise the book.*

Training in internal medicine rarely includes significant exposure to gravid patients; hence, many internists are ill-prepared to evaluate and manage medical problems in patients who are pregnant, or in those contemplating pregnancy. This is particularly unfortunate since many women are delaying child-bearing until their 30s and 40s, and as a consequence, an increasing number of gestations are complicated by medical problems.[1, 2] Thus, one major aim of this text is to enhance the ability of the general internist and medical subspecialist to (1) render more effective consultation when called upon to examine a pregnant patient with a medical disorder and (2) provide appropriate pre-pregnancy management and counseling for women of child-bearing age who have a chronic medical disease.

Another goal of this book is to underscore the importance of cooperation and communication among physicians from different disciplines who combine their talents to manage gravidas with medical disorders. In such situations, experts managing the gestation may have limited familiarity with the complexities of a given medical problem, and medical specialists often have little understanding of the obstetric considerations. To provide optimal patient care, both physicians must familiarize themselves with the concerns of the other and agree on a plan of management, realizing that

*We also wish to cite our colleagues, Drs. John Davison and Jean-Pierre Grünfeld, who served as assistant editors, and express our thanks to the editorial personnel at Mosby-Year Book, Inc, particularly Richard Lampert, for expert guidance during the planning and preparation of this volume.

ultimate responsibility belongs to the physician charged with the delivery.

A common and problematic issue facing all who manage gravidas, or women planning pregnancy, is the use of medication. In the United States prescription drugs are extensively tested in nonpregnant populations prior to approval by the Food and Drug Administration (FDA); however, controlled trials to determine safety, efficacy, and pharmacokinetic alterations during human pregnancy are rare. The few studies available are limited in scope, often performed at the request and with the support of the pharmaceutical industry, and rarely meet the rigorous standards that good trials now require. This is unfortunate since the vast majority of drugs readily cross the placenta. Thus, there is a need for data concerning the potential short- and long-term adverse fetal effects of many medications, as well as how pregnancy alters their absorption, distribution, protein binding, and metabolism.

The FDA has put forth a scheme to categorize the potential fetal risk of drugs (Table). Unfortunately, because of the lack of data, most agents are classified in category C, which includes a statement that the drug should be given only if potential benefits justify potential risks to the fetus. However, one should bear in mind that even when medications are classified in the safer B category, data accrued are often insensitive markers of drug safety (e.g., gross morphologic abnormalities in rodent fetuses) and many more subtle effects (e.g., ability of the fetus to withstand hypoxic stress, neonatal adaptation, as well as behavioral, psychological, and intellectual development) are rarely investigated. This issue is highlighted by a recent report demonstrating that administration of aminoglycosides to pregnant rats has harmful developmental and tubular toxic effects on the fetal kidney, demonstrable only by sophisticated functional testing and histologic evaluation.[4] Studies such as the latter underscore a critical need to develop more rigorous standards for animal testing prior to exposing pregnant women to drugs. It should also be

Food and Drug Administration Pregnancy Risk Classification

Category A: Controlled studies in women fail to demonstrate a risk to the fetus in the first trimester (and there is no evidence of a risk in later trimesters), and the possibility of fetal harm appears remote.

Category B: Either animal-reproduction studies have not demonstrated a fetal risk, but there are no controlled studies in pregnant women, or animal-reproduction studies have shown an adverse effect (other than a decrease in fertility) that was not confirmed in controlled studies in women in the first trimester (and there is no evidence of a risk in later trimesters).

Category C: Either studies in animals have revealed adverse effects on the fetus (teratogenic or embryocidal effects, or other) and there are no controlled studies in women, or studies in women and animals are not available. Drugs should be given only if the potential benefit justifies the potential risk to the fetus.

Category D: There is positive evidence of human fetal risk, but the benefits from use in pregnant women may be acceptable despite the risk (e.g., if the drug is needed in a life-threatening situation, or for a serious disease for which safer drugs cannot be used or are ineffective). There will be an appropriate statement in the "warnings" section of the labeling.

Category X: Studies in animals or human beings have demonstrated fetal abnormalities, or there is evidence of fetal risk based on human experience, or both, and the risk of using the drug in pregnant women clearly outweighs any possible benefit. The drug is contraindicated in women who are or may become pregnant. There will be an appropriate statement in the "contraindications" section of the labeling.

noted that there are very few drugs in category A, a fact that highlights the paucity of human data regarding potential teratogenicity of the vast majority of therapeutic agents currently used. Thus, even drugs with an established record of safety when used in the second and third trimesters (e.g., methyldopa for hypertension) should be prescribed in the first trimester with the understanding that absolute safety has not been established.

It is also our impression that clinicians overutilize drugs in category C, interpreting this designation as evidence of safety. The danger of such an approach is exemplified by recent data concerning the use of angiotensin-converting enzyme inhibitors during pregnancy. Despite evidence in two reports associating the use of these agents with high rates of fetal death in animals[5, 6] and adverse effects in human neonates (see below), both captopril and enalapril are listed as category C in the 1990 *Physician's Desk Reference*. Although reports of adverse drug effects in animals are not always applicable to humans, such initial disturbing observations dictate that angiotensin-converting enzyme inhibitors not be used in pregnant women unless further extensive animal studies prove safety (or unless maternal health were jeopardized and no suitable alternative agent were available). In addition, an increasing experience with both captopril and enalapril in human pregnancy is being described, and it appears that both agents may cause anuric renal failure in the human fetus and/or neonate, a complication that has been fatal in several cases.[7] *Thus, we strongly caution the clinician not to view drugs in FDA category C as safe. Rather, such a classification should be interpreted as a warning that unknown adverse fetal effects may be present.* This philosophy underlies our approach to pharmacologic therapy in the pregnant patient: rely on those few drugs with a well-documented history of efficacy and safety, and avoid prescription of newer, inadequately investigated drugs.

The above should not be misinterpreted as a blanket proscription against drug use in pregnancy. In this regard, even drugs in category D (i.e., those with positive evidence of human risk) may be indicated when essential to the management of a serious medical disorder. Indeed, under such circumstance discontinuation of a required medication may jeopardize both maternal and fetal well-being. This situation is typified by the need for continuation of immunosuppressives in gravid renal allograft recipients and anti-epileptic agents in patients with seizure disorders.

With the above considerations in mind, we have asked our contributors to categorize, according to the FDA classification, those major drugs that they discuss. The reader will find this information the first time the medication is cited and/or within appropriate tables within each chapter. Further discussion of drug classification and use during pregnancy can be found in the *PDR* and several reference volumes.[8, 9] Again, we stress that the FDA classification should not be used in isolation, but rather the decision to prescribe medication to pregnant patients should be made in the context of the individual patient's disease, balancing maternal and fetal risks and benefits.

Finally, we thought it useful to provide our readers with guidance regarding gestational alterations in the normal ranges for the more commonly utilized laboratory measurements. Unfortunately, definitive data are often unavailable and in many instances are highly dependent on patient population characteristics that may vary widely. Thus, rather than prepare a table we have provided an Appendix that refers the reader to text pages where gestational alterations in normal ranges for various laboratory parameters are discussed.

WILLIAM M. BARRON, M.D.
MARSHALL D. LINDHEIMER, M.D.

1. Venutra SJ: Trends and variations in first births to older women, 1970–1986, Vital and Health Statistics, series 21, No. 47, DHHS publication No. (PHS) 89-1925. National Center for Health Statistics, Public Health Service, Hyattsville, Md, 1989.
2. Berkowitz GS, Skovron ML, Lapinski RH, and Berkowitz RL: Delayed childbearing and the outcome of pregnancy. *N Engl J Med* 1990; 322:659–664.
3. Food and Drug Administration. Prescription drug advertising: content and format for labeling of human prescription drugs. Fed Register. 1980; 44:37434–37467.
4. Mallie J-P, Coulon G, Billerey C, Faucourt A, and Morin J-P: In utero aminoglycosides-induced nephrotoxicity in rat neonates. *Kidney Int* 1988; 33:36–44.

5. Broughton Pipkin F, Symonds EM, Turner SR: The effect of captopril (SQ14,225) upon mother and fetus in the chronically cannulated ewe and in the pregnant rabbit. *J Physiol (Lond)* 1982; 323:415–422.

6. Ferris TF, Weir EK: Effect of captopril on uterine blood flow and prostaglandin E synthesis in the pregnant rabbit. *J Clin Invest* 1983; 71:809–815.

7. Rosa FW, Bosco LA, Fossum-Graham C, et al: Neonatal anuria with maternal angioten-sin-converting enzyme inhibition. *Obstet Gynecol* 1989; 74:371–374.

8. Briggs GG, Freeman RK, Yaffer SJ: *Drugs in Pregnancy and Lactation—A Reference Guide to Fetal and Neonatal Risk,* ed 2. Baltimore, Williams & Wilkins, 1986.

9. Berkowitz RI, Coustan DR, Mochizuki TK: *Handbook for Prescribing Medications During Pregnancy,* ed 2. Boston, Little, Brown and Co, 1986.

CONTENTS

CHAPTER 1

Hypertension

William M. Barron

Hypertension during pregnancy is a unique clinical problem and both evaluation and management require an approach that differs substantially from that employed in nonpregnant patients. First, the diagnostic spectrum is greater, since in addition to essential and secondary forms of chronic hypertension the patient may have a short-lived, pregnancy-specific form of hypertension, i.e., preeclampsia. The latter complication has very different maternal and fetal risks than does essential hypertension, a fact central to decisions regarding treatment. In addition, when drug therapy is considered for any hypertensive gravida, the physician must be aware not only of the benefits of such therapy to mother and fetus, but also of potential acute and long-term adverse effects on the offspring. Unfortunately, data regarding the latter are frequently lacking.

This chapter begins with a brief discussion of the course of blood pressure during normal gestation, followed by a classification of the hypertensive disorders of pregnancy. Next, various aspects of preeclampsia and eclampsia are detailed. Finally, assessment and management of the gravida with various forms of chronic hypertension are discussed. It should be noted that although the 1980s have witnessed a substantial increase in the body of literature concerning elevated blood pressure in pregnancy, this problem contin-ues to be a major worldwide cause of maternal and perinatal morbidity and mortality. Much remains to be learned about many key issues, including the pathogenesis of preeclampsia and the precise benefits of drug treatment in both preeclamptic and chronically hypertensive gravidas.

BLOOD PRESSURE IN NORMAL PREGNANCY

Measurement of Blood Pressure

There are several potential methodologic pitfalls in recording blood pressure in pregnant patients. First, there is controversy regarding the appropriate positioning of the patient, with some claiming that lateral recumbency is the preferred posture. However, if the patient's arm is kept at her right side when in left lateral recumbency, blood pressure recordings may be spuriously reduced by as much as 10–14 mm Hg.[1] Based primarily on practical considerations we recommend use of the sitting position in outpatients; lateral recumbency may be used if more convenient, especially in the hospitalized gravida; regardless of posture, care must be taken to keep the brachial artery at the level of the heart.

There is also controversy concerning determination of diastolic pressure levels; physicians in the United States focus on Korotkoff phase V (disappearance of sounds),[2] while others use phase IV (muffling).[3, 4] The latter has been recommended on the grounds that during pregnancy Korotkoff sounds may be audible to very low levels; however, this appears to occur in less than 10% of normal gravidas.[5] Furthermore, two studies[1, 6] have demonstrated that Korotkoff phase IV measurements average 10–18 mm Hg higher than intra-arterial determinations of diastolic blood pressure during both normal and hypertensive pregnancy. Also, Villar et al.[7] observed that phase IV levels averaged 12 mm Hg higher than phase V during normal gestation. Thus, it appears that phase V is a more accurate reflection of intra-arterial diastolic pressure during pregnancy, and we recommend continued use of this value; phase IV is used only when the discrepancy between muffling and disappearance of sound becomes very large.

Epidemiological Studies

Data concerning the effect of gestation on blood pressure is discordant, and virtually all available studies have some inadequacies. In 1969 MacGillivray et al.[8] reported a prospective investigation in which blood pressure was noted to be decreased early in pregnancy and reach a nadir at 16–20 weeks, at which time decrements in systolic and diastolic pressures averaged 9 and 17 mm Hg, respectively (Fig 1–1). Thereafter, blood pressure increased gradually to values that at term approached those measured post partum. In contrast, others have observed minimal or no changes in systolic pressure[9, 10] and decrements up to 12 mm Hg in diastolic blood pressure[10] during normal pregnancy.

Gestational decreases in blood pressure are accompanied by marked increases in both blood volume and cardiac output to levels ≈40% above those measured in nonpregnant populations.[11] Such changes indicate that systemic vascular resistance must also decrease significantly and this has been demonstrated using central hemodynamic monitoring and noninvasive Doppler methodology.[12, 13] An-

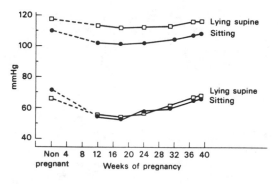

FIG 1–1.
Systolic *(upper two lines)* and diastolic *(lower two lines)* blood pressure trends during pregnancy in 226 healthy primigravidas. Original data from MacGillivray et al.[8] (From DeSwiet M: The cardiovascular system, in Hytten F, Chamberlain G (eds): *Clinical Physiology in Obstetrics.* Oxford, Blackwell Scientific Publications, 1980, pp 3–42. Used with permission.)

other characteristic cardiovascular adaptation in normal human pregnancy is marked resistance to the pressor actions of angiotensin II.

Appreciation of these physiologic alterations is important for the following reasons: (1) the anticipated fall in blood pressure in midpregnancy may influence the decision to initiate antihypertensive medication during early pregnancy in the gravida with known chronic hypertension; (2) chronic hypertension may be masked by the physiologic decrement in blood pressure if the patient is first seen in midgestation; and (3) since blood pressure normally increases during the latter stages of pregnancy, the diagnosis of preeclampsia may be erroneous if made solely on the basis of increments in pressure (see below).

Alterations in arterial pressure during pregnancy raise the question of whether the upper limits of normal differ from those in nongravid populations. Two large, prospective epidemiologic studies have demonstrated that even modest elevations in blood pressure may be associated with impaired pregnancy outcome. In one[14] fetal mortality rose abruptly when diastolic blood pressure exceeded 84 mm Hg at any stage of gestation, while in the other[15] there were increases in perinatal mortality and intrauterine growth retardation when second and third trimester mean arterial pressures exceeded 90 mm Hg (e.g., 120/75 mm Hg) and 95 mm Hg (e.g., 120/82 mm Hg), respectively. Thus, levels of blood pressure that would be considered entirely normal in nongravid women may have a significant adverse impact on pregnancy outcome. Therefore, we consider the upper limits of normal for diastolic pressure to be ≈75 mm Hg and ≈85 mm Hg during the second and third trimesters, respectively.

The cause of the hypertension appears to influence perinatal outcome more than elevated blood pressure per se. For example, hypertension alone late in pregnancy, has but a modest influence on fetal outcome; however, the combination of significant proteinuria and hypertension (i.e., preeclampsia) is associated with marked increases in both intrauterine growth retardation and perinatal mortality.[14–16]

CLASSIFICATION AND CLINICAL FEATURES

Current literature contains multiple schemes for classifying hypertension in gestation, each utilizing different nomenclature. The confusion relates in part to the difficulty in distinguishing, by clinical criteria alone, between preeclampsia, essential or secondary hypertension, chronic renal disease, and combinations thereof. This dilemma has been convincingly demonstrated by the results of several clinical-pathological correlation studies in which renal biopsy was used to determine the definitive diagnosis. Fisher and colleagues[17] reported that the clinical diagnosis of preeclampsia alone was wrong in more than 60% of multigravidas, and Katz et al.[18] failed to find renal histologic evidence of preeclampsia in 40% of gravidas with underlying renal disease who were given a clinical diagnosis of superimposed preeclampsia.

Of the numerous classifications in use[4, 19–21] we continue to prefer the approach suggested in 1972 by the Committee on Terminology of the American College of Obstetricians and Gynecologists[19] since it remains the most concise and practical (Table 1–1). (A National Institutes of Health Working Group has also recently endorsed this classification[22]).

Preeclampsia-Eclampsia

This disorder, unique to pregnancy, is characterized by hypertension, proteinuria, generalized edema, and, at times, coagulation or liver function abnormalities or both. It occurs in 5% to 10% of all pregnancies, primarily in primigravidas after the 20th gestational week and most frequently near term. Preeclampsia may progress rapidly and without warning to the convulsive phase termed *eclampsia*—one of the most dramatic and life-threatening complications of pregnancy.

TABLE 1–1.
Classification of Hypertension in Pregnancy

I. Disorder unique to pregnancy: preeclampsia-eclampsia
   Disease of 1st pregnancy, typically after 20 wk gestation
   Characterized by hypertension + proteinuria; edema not a reliable sign
   Variable degrees of ↑ uric acid, ↓ platelets and abnormal liver function tests
II. Disorders unrelated to pregnancy: chronic hypertension of whatever etiology
   Pheochromocytoma, collagen vascular disease, and/or moderate to severe renal functional impairment present most serious risks
III. Preeclampsia-eclampsia superimposed on chronic hypertension
   Diagnosis frequently incorrect; should not be based solely upon increases in blood pressure; criteria should include new onset marked proteinuria, ↑ uric acid and/or, ↓ platelets
   Associated with substantially increased risk to mother and fetus
IV. Transient or late hypertension
   Increased blood pressure near term without other evidence of preeclampsia
   Rapid resolution post partum
   Recurrent transient hypertension may be harbinger of chronic hypertension

Hypertension.—*Hypertension* is defined by most authorities as a blood pressure ≥140/90 mm Hg (but we consider diastolic pressure >85 mm Hg abnormal), or increases in systolic and/or diastolic levels of ≥30 and 15 mm Hg, respectively. The criterion of a rise in blood pressure is important, since an increase in diastolic pressure from 50 to 80 mm Hg in a young primigravida may signal serious disease. On the other hand, use of such increments may lead to "overdiagnosis," since studies cited previously[8-10] suggest that diastolic blood pressure increases ≈10 mm Hg during the third trimester in normal gestation. *Nonetheless, any significant, acute increase in blood pressure should prompt the physician to seriously consider the diagnosis of preeclampsia, since failure to recognize this disorder may endanger the life of both mother and fetus.*

Proteinuria.—The Committee on Terminology defined significant *proteinuria* as 1 g/L in a random specimen or more than 0.3 g/L in a 24-hour collection; however, no quantitative amount of protein excretion was specified as abnormal. Since total protein excretion may double in normal pregnancy, a reasonable criterion for abnormality is a level twice the upper limit of normal for nonpregnant subjects (e.g., levels above 300–500 mg/day represent pathologic proteinuria in pregnancy). In fact the Committee did not even require the presence of significant proteniuria for the clinical diagnosis of preeclampsia; however, the diagnosis is suspect in its absence.[23]

Edema.—The third major traditional criterion, *edema*, is no longer used by many authorities, since most normal gravidas develop dependent edema and this becomes generalized in ≈30%.[24, 25] Furthermore, in one large epidemiologic survey[14] neither edema nor maternal weight gain alone was associated with any adverse fetal outcome. The lack of utility of this sign is further underscored by a report in which 26 of 67 women with eclampsia had no edema.[26]

Eclamptic Seizures.—*Eclamptic seizures* are generalized motor convulsions that may be heralded by headache, apprehension, visual disturbances, right upper quadrant pain, rising blood pressure, and/or hyperreflexia. Most occur ante partum, but a substantial number also develop during labor or within 48 hours following delivery. Controversy remains about an entity known as late postpartum eclampsia, i.e., seizures occurring more than 48 hours post partum; however, in one series[27] this entity accounted for ≈10% of all cases of eclampsia. A similar syndrome characterized by postpartum hypertension, seizures, and cerebrovascular accident has been observed in more than 50 women in association with the use of bromocriptine mesylate for suppression of lactation,[28, 29] and therefore this agent is contraindicated in any postpartum patient with any hypertensive disorder. Although eclampsia is the most common major neurologic complication of preeclampsia, coma and visual disturbances, including cortical blindness and retinal detachment, may also occur.

Attempts have been made to distinguish "mild" from "severe" preeclampsia, the latter defined by systolic or diastolic pressures of 160 and 110 mm Hg or greater, respectively; the presence of heavy proteinuria; oliguria; cerebral or visual disturbances (agitation, apprehension, coma, cortical blindness); pulmonary edema; and/or cyanosis. Other evidence of severe disease includes epigastric or right upper quadrant abdominal pain, *h*emolytic anemia, *e*levated *l*iver enzymes (primarily transaminases) and *l*ow *p*latelet counts, the so-called HELLP syndrome. Another subtle sign of severity is marked hemoconcentration reflected in an increased hematocrit. It should be stressed, however, *that differentiating mild from severe preeclampsia may be dangerously misleading, for although the risks of eclampsia are greater when markers of severity are present, as many as one quarter of women with eclampsia have so-called "mild" disease and minimal elevations of blood pressure prior to the occurrence of a convulsion.*[26, 30]

Chronic Hypertension of Whatever Cause

This diagnosis rests on the presence of sustained hypertension prior to or following pregnancy. In addition, levels $\geq 140/85$ mm Hg prior to the 20th gestational week may be taken as presumptive evidence of chronic hypertension, although preeclampsia may rarely present at this early stage, especially when gestation is complicated by hydatidiform mole or nonimmune hydrops fetalis.[30]

Most women with chronically elevated blood pressure will have mild to moderate, uncomplicated essential hypertension and most will have a benign course during pregnancy, their blood pressure often falling into the normal range. One factor, however, that appears to predict a more complicated course is a failure of the normal decrease in blood pressure in midgestation (see below).[16] Poorer prognoses are also associated with certain secondary causes of hypertension, especially pheochromocytoma[31, 32] (see Chap. 4, p. 130), scleroderma,[33] periarteritis nodosa,[34] and moderate or severe renal functional impairment antedating pregnancy (see Chap. 2).

Chronic Hypertension With Superimposed Preeclampsia

This category tends to contain patients with the most severe disease, and it is in such cases that maternal complications (e.g., stroke and heart and/or renal failure) are most likely. However, as noted previously, the diagnosis of superimposed preeclampsia is difficult and often erroneous.[18] The classical criteria, increments of ≥ 30 mm Hg systolic pressure or ≥ 15 mm Hg diastolic pressure, cannot be relied on, since the blood pressure of many chronically hypertensive gravidas will increase substantially at the end of pregnancy in the absence of other evidence of preeclampsia. Therefore, it appears preferable to rely on criteria such as new onset of abundant proteinuria, hyperuricemia, thrombocytopenia, and/or elevated serum transaminase levels.

Late or Transient Hypertension

This disorder is characterized by development of hypertension alone during the latter stages of pregnancy or in the early puerperium and the subsequent return to normal blood pressure within 10 days post partum. Included in this category will be women who may have had early preeclampsia but failed to manifest other evidence of the disease as well as gravidas who have hypertension in the absence of proteinuria during two or more pregnancies and who become normotensive shortly after delivery. Such recurrent hypertension appears to be a marker for the development of chronic hypertension in much the same way that the development of gestational glucose intolerance predicts an increased risk for the occurrence of diabetes mellitus later in life.[35, 36]

PREECLAMPSIA-ECLAMPSIA

Epidemiology, Risk Factors, and Remote Prognosis

The reported incidence of hypertensive complications during pregnancy varies widely, due in part to differences in patient populations and diagnostic criteria; however, it appears that preeclampsia will develop in 2% to 10% of unselected gravidas.[15, 16, 30, 37] Factors associated with an increased risk of this disorder include nulliparity, diabetes, multiple gestation, extremes of age, hydatidiform mole, and fetal hydrops.[30] Chronic hypertension is often cited as predisposing to preeclampsia[30]; however, this may be the case only for those with moderate to marked elevations of blood pressure[38] and not for women with uncomplicated mild hypertension.[16] It has also been suggested that even mildly elevated blood pressure in the second trimester (i.e., mean arterial pressure [MAP]$>$90 mm Hg) may be a marker for the development of preeclampsia later in gestation. Although this sign is not very accurate,[36] any gravida with even mildly increased blood pressure in midpregnancy should be observed carefully for hypertensive complications as gestation progresses.

A familial tendency to preeclampsia has

been suggested and recent studies have provided evidence that the disease is heritable.[39, 40] It has been suggested that the incidence of preeclampsia is explicable on the basis of a single gene model, and Cooper et al.[39] have hypothesized that the mode of action of the involved gene may be via an effect on the interaction between uterine and placental tissue.

There has been disagreement about the remote prognosis of women who develop preeclampsia and/or eclampsia. It was once suggested that this disorder caused chronic hypertension, a notion that seems to have been refuted by more recent studies. Chesley[35] reported long-term follow-up of 267 women who survived eclampsia. In those having eclampsia in a first pregnancy, distributions of systolic and diastolic blood pressure and the prevalence of hypertension were not different from age- and race-matched controls. There was, however, a significant increase in the prevalence of chronic hypertension among women having had eclampsia as multiparas, and this appeared to account for their increased remote death rate. The authors suggested that eclampsia is neither a predictive sign of latent essential hypertension nor a cause of it, conclusions supported by the studies of Bryans (cited in references 35 and 17).

Pathologic Physiology and Morphology

An extensive review of the pathoanatomic and physiologic features of preeclampsia is beyond the scope of this chapter and only major concepts will be highlighted here. The reader is referred to several recent reviews for additional information.[41-47]

Hypertension and Vascular Reactivity

Blood pressure is extremely labile in preeclampsia and there may be reversal of the normal circadian rythm, i.e., the highest levels may be recorded at night. The underlying hemodynamic derangement is one of intense vasoconstriction and elevated systemic vascular resistance (see below). This is accompanied by markedly enhanced pressor responsiveness to endogenous vasoconstrictors[30] and augmented responses to angiotensin II may be present many weeks before the disease is recognized clinically.[48] Some suggest that changes in blood pressure and pressor responsiveness may be related to perturbations of prostaglandin biosynthesis (see below). This view is supported by a recent study in which administration of low dose aspirin (which was shown to increase the ratio of prostacyclin to thromboxane metabolites in plasma) raised the effective pressor dose of angiotensin II in gravidas who had developed sensitivity to this vasoconstrictor.[49]

Role(s) of the renin-angiotensin and sympathetic nervous systems in the pathogenesis of hypertension in preeclampsia remains unclear, but most reports suggest that preeclampsia is associated with decrements in plasma renin activity and angiotensin II levels,[47, 50] and little alteration in circulating catecholamines.[51] Nonetheless, such levels may be inappropriately increased in the presence of elevated blood pressure. Some have proposed that activation of the uteroplacental renin-angiotensin system, caused by impaired blood flow, contributes to the elevated systemic arterial pressure.[50]

Cardiovascular Hemodynamics and Volume

Studies using Swan-Ganz catheters to measure central hemodynamics in gravidas with preeclampsia have yielded conflicting data, at least in part because investigators have studied heterogeneous populations and measurements were often made after interventions such as volume loading and magnesium sulfate administration. A major exception are the studies of Wallenburg and colleagues.[1, 12] In their study of 44 untreated nulliparous women with proteinuria and preeclampsia, mean cardiac output was reduced, pulmonary capillary wedge and right atrial pressure were low to normal, and systemic vascular resistance was markedly elevated (Fig 1–2). These data are supported by the observations of some,[52, 53] but contrast with those of others[54, 55] who suggest that preeclamptic

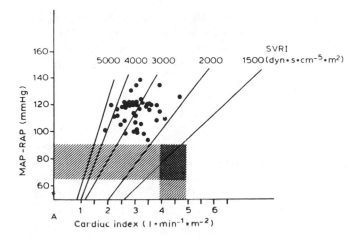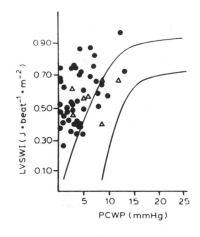

FIG 1–2.
Left, relationship between systemic perfusion pressure, cardiac index, and systemic vascular resistance index in 44 untreated nulliparous women with preeclampsia. Values for normotensive pregnant women fall within the cross-hatched area. Note that preeclamptic women have decreased cardiac output and increases in systemic arterial pressure due to markedly elevated peripheral vascular resistance. *Right,* left ventricular stroke work index plotted against pulmonary capillary wedge pressure in these same 44 patients compared to data from 7 normotensive controls *(open triangles).* Solid lines represent the normal range in nonpregnant subjects. Note that left ventricular filling pressures are lower in the hypertensive gravidas. (Modified from Wallenburg HCS: Hemodynamics in hypertensive pregnancy, in Rubin PC (ed): *Hypertension in Pregnancy,* Amsterdam, Elsevier Science Publications, 1988, pp 66–101.)

patients present with a broader spectrum of central hemodynamics in which cardiac output is typically normal to high, while pulmonary capillary wedge and central venous pressures are often normal.

Although some uncertainty remains about central blood volume in preeclampsia, decreased total circulating plasma volume is a typical feature of this disease; the magnitude of the deficit correlates roughly with the severity of the clinical disorder and with reductions in infant birthweight.[56] There is ongoing controversy as to whether intravascular volume contraction is a primary event or secondary to vasoconstriction and hypertension (i.e., pressure natriuresis). Favoring the former are observations that relative hypovolemia may occur prior to overt hypertension in preeclampsia.[57, 58] Factors leading to hypovolemia are unclear but increased vascular permeability[59] as well as decrements in plasma oncotic pressure[60] may play important roles. These alterations may also help to explain the generalized edema and expansion of the interstitial space that accompanies re-

duced intravascular volume in preeclampsia. Such changes in Starling forces may also play an important role in the pathogenesis of pulmonary edema, which occasionally complicates preeclampsia.

Renal Abnormalities

Glomerular filtration rate (GFR) and renal plasma flow decrease in preeclampsia, however, because renal hemodynamics are augmented in normal pregnancy, values may still be at or above nonpregnant levels. In this regard serum creatinine ranges from 0.4–0.8 mg/dL (35–70 μmol/L) in normal gestation and values at or above 0.9 mg/dL (≈80 μmol/L), which are observed frequently in preeclampsia, should be regarded as abnormal.[56, 61]

Decrements in renal hemodynamics may be due to vasoconstriction but also reflect glomerular intra-capillary cell swelling (often termed glomerular endotheliosis), the characteristic renal lesion of preeclampsia, which is rarely seen in other conditions. Some suggest that preeclampsia may be a cause of focal glomerular sclerosis; however, others believe the latter reflects preexisting nephrosclerosis or primary renal disease.[42, 62]

The combination of reduced intravascular volume and an ischemic renal lesion may explain the impaired ability to excrete a sodium load,[63] as well as the oliguria that is observed in some preeclamptic patients. Decreased urine volume, especially in acute clinical situations, often concerns the physician, and has led some to recommend therapeutic volume expansion.[64] However, such a maneuver, which increases the risk of pulmonary edema, is rarely necessary, as acute renal failure is a very unusual complication of preeclampsia (see the section on volume expansion therapy below).

Uric acid clearance decreases in preeclampsia and hyperuricemia may be a helpful diagnostic sign. Decrements in urate clearance may antedate alterations in glomerular filtration and the magnitude of hyperuricemia has been reported to be correlated with the degree of volume contraction, severity of the preeclamptic lesion, and fetal prognosis.[65]

Proteinuria, which may occur relatively late in preeclampsia, is nonselective. The magnitude may range from minimal to severe, and in one study preeclampsia was the most common cause of nephrotic proteinuria occurring during gestation.[17]

Hormonal Regulation of Sodium Balance and Volume

The role of volume-sensitive hormones in the sodium retention and disturbed volume regulation of preeclampsia remains unclear. Aldosterone levels are normal in midgestation in women destined to develop preeclampsia, but production, plasma concentrations, and urinary excretion are decreased when preeclampsia is clinically apparent. Plasma levels of deoxycorticosterone, another potent mineralocorticoid, have been reported to be both decreased and unchanged in preeclamptic gravidas.[61, 66]

A decrease in levels of hormone(s) with natriuretic activity could conceivably lead to pathologic sodium retention. Although plasma progesterone is unaltered in preeclampsia, it has been suggested that conversion of this natriuretic hormone at extra-adrenal sites (including the kidney) to the potent sodium-retaining steroid, deoxycorticosterone,[67] may be accelerated in patients with this disorder.[68] Urinary metabolites of vasodilator and natriuretic prostaglandins such as prostacyclin are decreased in preeclampsia and may help to explain the observed sodium retention.[46] Finally, circulating levels of atrial natriuretic peptide and its intracellular second messenger, cyclic guanosine monophosphate (cGMP), appear to be increased[69, 70] in preeclampsia despite contracted circulating volume.

Liver Dysfunction

Hepatic dysfunction which may be manifest as right upper quadrant pain (or tenderness) and/or elevated serum transaminases and bilirubin, occur in a minority of gravidas with preeclampsia or eclampsia[71]; however, its presence indicates severe disease and is an indication for delivery. The primary lesions are periportal hemorrhage and sinusoidal fibrin and fibrinogen deposition[30, 72, 73]; hemorrhage may be extensive[74] and include the subcapsular region with resultant hepatic rupture and death from exsanguination. More recently it has been suggested that hepatic microvesicular fat deposition characteristic of acute fatty liver of pregnancy is also a frequent (but often overlooked) accompaniment of preeclampsia, and that these two clinical disorders may represent manifestations of the same pathophysiological process (see Chap. 10).[75, 76]

Eclampsia and Other Neurologic Complications

Cerebral involvement is the most frequent cause of death in preeclampsia-eclampsia.[72, 77] Pathological features include cortical and subcortical hemorrhages and microinfarctions, cerebral edema, subarachnoid hemorrhage and large intracerebral hematoma. Donaldson[77] has suggested that the classic microscopic lesion, pericapillary ring hemorrhage, can be attributed to failure of precapillary arteriolar constriction to limit the pressure exerted on capillaries. Thus, the pathophysiology of eclampsia and cortical blindness is said to represent one form of hypertensive encephalopathy. However, eclampsia may occur with systolic and diastolic blood pressures less than 140 and 90 mm Hg, respectively,[72, 78] observations that cast doubt on this hypothesis. To what degree pregnancy and/or preeclampsia alter the autoregulation of cerebral blood flow is unknown.

Cranial computed tomography of eclamptic patients may demonstrate edema and/or hemorrhages but is frequently normal.[77–79] Magnetic resonance imaging may be a more sensitive method of identifying cerebral cortical edema.[80] Typical electroencephalographic abnormalities include diffuse or focal slow waves; however, paroxysmal spike activity is rarely observed unless the patient is actively convulsing.[81] Arteriography may demonstrate vasospasm, which, as noted previously, is a fundamental pathophysiologic feature of preeclampsia-eclampsia. Finally, cerebrospinal fluid examination may reveal elevated protein and varying numbers of red blood cells; however, frequently no abnormalities are observed.[77, 78]

Diagnostic tests of neurologic function in eclamptic gravidas are often normal or reveal nonspecific abnormalities and therefore, such investigation is most commonly used to identify other causes of seizures. In this regard it has been suggested that neurodiagnostic tests be restricted to evaluation of patients with focal neurologic deficits or late postpartum eclampsia.[78] Persistent abnormalities of mental status also warrant investigation.

Placental Perfusion

In normal pregnancy, implantation of the embryo is followed by migration of trophoblastic cells into the walls of the uterine spiral arteries.[82] These vessels thereby lose their muscular media and appear as passive conduits that serve to accommodate a tenfold increase in uterine blood flow. It is claimed that this process fails to occur in preeclampsia, and in combination with lesions termed "acute atherosis," produced later when hypertension is present, result in diminished placental blood flow. These events have been proposed as the cause of the intrauterine growth retardation and fetal loss associated with preeclampsia. If true, treatment of hypertension in this disorder would not be expected to prevent the basic disease process. Equally important, the influence of any therapeutic intervention on an already compromised placental perfusion must be taken into account if fetal jeopardy is to be avoided.

Immunologic Alterations

A number of immunologic abnormalities have been described in patients with preeclampsia and this has led to immunogenetic hypotheses regarding the pathogenesis of the disease.[83] For example, there appears to be a genetic predisposition to preeclampsia that is associated with HLA-DR4.[39, 40] Investigations of humoral immunity and complement suggest a number of abnormalities, including circulating antibodies directed at trophoblast, amniotic glycoprotein, and laminin (a glycoprotein component of basement membrane in trophoblast and renal glomerulus). Recently Ware and colleagues[84] reported that 7 of 43 women with severe, early onset preeclampsia had significant levels of antiphospholipid antibody and several had thrombotic complications. Whether these patients actually had preeclampsia or an antiphospholipid antibody syndrome (see Chap. 11) that merely mimics preeclampsia is unclear. It has also been suggested that preeclampsia may be an immune complex disease; however, data concerning immune complexes in the circulation and in various tissues are inconsistent. Finally, studies of cellular immune function in preeclampsia are extremely limited and the contradictory results prohibit conclusions.

Coagulation

Abnormalities of coagulation appear to

be a characteristic pathophysiologic phenomenon in preeclampsia, but controversy exists as to the extent and frequency.[85] Discrepancies in the literature likely result from differences in populations studied, as well as from variances in assay performance. It appears that standard tests of coagulation activity (e.g., prothrombin and partial thromboplastin times, fibrinogen levels) are normal in the majority of patients, even those with eclampsia.[71, 86] However, studies employing more sensitive tests, such as the ratio of factor VIII clotting activity to factor VIII-related antigen, antithrombin III, fibrinopeptide A, and soluble fibrin monomer suggest that the coagulation process is activated in the majority of gravidas with preeclampsia.[85] Also of interest is the observation that levels of antithrombin III may decrease several weeks before preeclampsia is recognized clinically. Although it has been suggested that antithrombin III levels may therefore be of value in the early recognition and differential diagnosis of preeclampsia,[85] the precise clinical utility of this test remains to be determined. In addition to evidence supporting increased generation of fibrin in preeclampsia, sensitive assays of α_2-antiplasmin suggest activation of the fibrinolytic system. The above data are consistent with observations of deposits of fibrin and fibrin-like material in many organs of patients with preeclampsia (e.g., placenta, liver, kidney).[85]

The incidence of thrombocytopenia in preeclampsia is unclear, but the majority (70% to 85%) of gravidas with eclampsia have platelet counts above 150,000/mm³ (150 10⁹/L) and levels less than 100,000/mm³ (100 10⁹/L) occur in less than 30%.[71, 86] However, when patients are followed serially with each woman acting as her own control, a relative reduction in counts may be seen more commonly, often many weeks prior to the onset of clinical disease.[87] Investigations employing more sensitive assays, i.e., platelet size, β-thromboglobulin, platelet factor IV, and platelet life span, indicate that platelet activation occurs in many, if not most, patients with preeclampsia even when circulating platelet counts are not decreased.[85]

The precise relationship of the above coagulation abnormalities to preeclampsia remains uncertain, but most believe that they are a consequence rather than a cause of the disorder. The etiology of the coagulopathy also remains obscure, but current theories suggest that vascular endothelial damage, either in the systemic or uteroplacental circulation, plays a central role in the enhanced platelet activation and fibrin generation.

Eicosanoid Metabolism

Normal pregnancy is accompanied by marked increases in the biosynthesis of prostaglandins which decrease platelet aggregation and are vasodilatory (e.g., prostacyclin and PGE_2) and in those that have opposing biologic actions (i.e., thromboxane A_2).[46] In preeclampsia, production of the former is markedly decreased while biosynthesis of thromboxane appears to be augmented. Such alterations may be causally related to much of the pathophysiology of preeclampsia, including coagulation abnormalities, increased vascular reactivity, decreased placental perfusion, and injury in the kidneys, brain, and liver. The unifying aspect of this postulate is appealing, appears to be supported by a considerable body of data, and underlies increasing enthusiasm for the use of low dose aspirin in the prevention of preeclampsia (see below).

Endothelial Cell Damage

Normal endothelium serves many important functions, including inhibition of both platelet aggregation and the coagulation cascade and modification of contractile activity of vascular smooth muscle. Morphologic and biochemical data suggest that endothelial damage is an important feature of preeclampsia, and that as a conscquence, the above biologic processes may be disrupted. Recently Roberts et al.[44] hypothesized that endothelial damage may explain many features of preeclampsia, including platelet activation, increased fibrin formation, increased vascular permeability, alterations in prostaglandin biosynthesis, and heightened vascular sensitivity. Such phenomena may in turn lead to hypertension and multiple-organ (renal, liver,

TABLE 1–2.
Differential Diagnosis of Preeclampsia and Chronic Hypertension

	Preeclampsia	Chronic Hypertension
Age	Extremes of age	More often older
Parity	Nulliparous	Multiparous
Onset	Rare before 20 wk	May have BP elevation noted before 20 wk gestation
History	Negative	Positive, often with hypertension in previous pregnancy
Fundi	Retinal edema, arteriolar spasm	May have chronic changes of arteriosclerosis
Cardiac status	Usually normal	Ventricular hypertrophy if disease is long-standing
Deep tendon reflexes	Hyperactive	Normoactive
Proteinuria	Increased	May be absent or minimal
Uric acid	Elevated	Normal
Liver function	May have right upper quadrant pain/tenderness and increased transaminases	Normal
Hematologic tests	May have variable degrees of thrombocytopenia, intravascular coagulation, and hemolytic anemia	Normal

and cerebral) dysfunction. The same authors further speculated that uterine ischemia (of uncertain etiology) leads to the release of an endothelial toxin into the circulation.[44] Evidence for the presence of such a toxin exists,[88] and Hubel and colleagues[45] have suggested that lipid peroxides, which are increased in patients with preeclampsia, may mediate endothelial injury in this disorder.

Differential Diagnosis

Distinguishing Preeclampsia From Chronic Hypertension

Optimal management of hypertension in the pregnant patient necessitates accurate diagnosis as the approach and prognosis will differ dramatically among the categories outlined in Table 1–1. Differentiation between preeclampsia and chronic hypertension is particularly important, as the former necessitates inpatient management to preempt development of eclampsia and fetal death. Table 1–2 summarizes selected differential diagnostic features that may be of help in distinguishing these two disorders. In addition, a wide variety of laboratory tests including urinary excretion of calcium,[89] serum iron and carboxyhemoglobin,[90] placental isoferritin,[91] an-

tithrombin III,[85] and plasma fibronectin[92] have been touted as valuable markers of preeclampsia. Unfortunately, most of these reports suffer from serious methodologic flaws that preclude definitive statements about the accuracy and clinical utility of such tests.

Differential Diagnosis of the HELLP Syndrome

As noted previously, preeclampsia may be complicated by *h*emolytic anemia, *e*levated *l*iver function tests, and *l*ow *p*latelet counts, a syndrome that has been given the acronym HELLP. Although preeclampsia is the most common cause of the constellation of hypertension, proteinuria, and liver and coagulation abnormalities during gestation, several other important disorders, including acute fatty liver of pregnancy (AFLP), hepatitis (see Chap. 10), thrombotic thrombocytopenic purpura (TTP) and hemolytic uremia syndrome (HUS) must also be considered. A summary of the clinical and laboratory features that may help in the differential diagnosis of these disorders is presented in Table 1–3. *The distinction between preeclampsia and fatty liver may be a particularly difficult one; however, the diagnostic process should not be prolonged since* *the primary treatment of both disorders is expeditious delivery.* In contrast, if the diagnosis of viral hepatitis is established, premature termination of the pregnancy is not mandatory, at least from a maternal standpoint. Finally, separating the HELLP syndrome from both TTP and HUS is extremely important since in the latter disorders prompt plasma exchange or pheresis, antiplatelet agents, and/or steroids may be life saving (see Chap. 8, p. 306), while such therapy is rarely necessary in patients with the HELLP syndrome.[92a]

PREVENTION OF PREECLAMPSIA

Several approaches to the prevention of preeclampsia have been proposed, including administration of diuretics, antihypertensives, calcium or magnesium supplements, and most promisingly, low dose aspirin.

Diuretics

Prophylactic administration of diuretics was actively investigated in the 1960s based on the theory that sodium retention was etiologically related to the disorder. In 1985, Collins and colleagues[93] analyzed nine prospective, randomized trials of diuretic therapy administered primarily for edema and/or rapid weight gain. When data from all studies were combined there appeared to be a significant reduction in the incidence of preeclampsia in the drug-treated compared to control groups. However, several methodologic difficulties precluded a firm conclusion. First, criteria used to establish a diagnosis of preeclampsia were varied, unreliable, and, in some series, not stated. Second, since diuretics can be expected to decrease blood pressure and reduce edema, such therapy may simply mask two of the diagnostic signs of preeclampsia without altering the presence of the underlying

TABLE 1–3.
Differential Diagnosis of Preeclampsia Complicated by Hematologic and Hepatic Involvement

	Preeclampsia	AFLP*	Viral or Drug-Induced Hepatitis	TTP*	HUS*
Symptoms					
Onset	>20 wk	>28 wk	Anytime	Anytime	Anytime
Nausea/vomiting	− or +	+ + +	+ + +	+	+ to + + +
Abdominal pain	+ to + + +	+ +	+/+ +	+	−
Signs					
Hypertension	+ to + + +	−/+	−	+	+ to + + +
Fever	−	−/+	−/+	+	−/+
Abnormal mental status	− to + + +	− to + + +	−/+	− to + + +	−/+
Liver function tests					
Bilirubin	NL to 5 × ↑	SL to 30 × ↑	5–40 × ↑	↑ indirect	↑ indirect
ALT (SGPT)	SL to 100 × ↑	SL to 20 × ↑	SL to >100 × ↑	NL to SL ↑	NL to SL ↑
Glucose	NL	NL or ↓	NL or ↓	NL	NL
Ammonia	NL	↑	NL or ↑	NL	NL
Hematology					
White blood cell count	NL to ↑	↑ ↑	NL or ↑	NL or ↑	NL or ↑
Schistocytes	+/+ +	+/+ +	−	+ + +	+ + +
Normoblasts	−	+/+ +	−	+ + +	+ + +
Platelets	30K to NL	20–150K	NL	5–100K	5–100K
Prothombin time	NL or SL ↑	NL to ↑ ↑ ↑	NL to ↑ ↑ ↑	NL	NL
Fibrinogen	NL or SL ↓	NL or ↓	↑, NL or ↓	NL	NL or SL ↓
Fibrin degradation products	NL or SL ↑	NL or ↑	NL	NL	NL or SL ↑
Antithrombin III	↓	↓	↓	NL	NL
Renal					
Creatinine	NL to 5 × ↑	NL to 10 × ↑	NL	NL to 5 × ↑	Rapid and marked ↑
Proteinuria	1 + to 4 +	1 + to 4 +	NL	0 to 4 +	0 to 4 +
Uric acid	↑	↑	NL	NL or ↑	↑

*AFLP = acute fatty liver of pregnancy; TTP = thrombotic thrombocytopenic purpura; HUS = hemolytic uremia syndrome; NL = normal; SL = slight.

disease and its adverse fetal impact. In this regard, when all nine studies were combined, rates of stillbirth and neonatal death were 1.9% in controls and 1.7% in diuretic-treated women, a nonsignificant difference.[93] Evaluation of adverse drug effects failed to reveal significant differences between treated and control groups, although careful laboratory evaluations were not performed in most studies. Of note, however, are several case reports of diuretic-induced maternal volume depletion, electrolyte imbalance, and pancreatitis, including four fatal instances of the latter, as well as neonatal thrombocytopenia and jaundice.[94-101] In addition, placental perfusion may be adversely affected by diuretic therapy.[102]

In summary, the above data fail to support a clear benefit for diuretics in the prevention of preeclampsia. In addition, although prospective trials fail to demonstrate a major adverse effect, there are rare reports of serious and sometimes fatal complications associated with such therapy. Thus, the balance of risk-benefit considerations preclude the use of prophylactic diuretic treatment during pregnancy.

Antihypertensive Drugs

Another approach is based on the premise that early treatment of hypertension may forestall appearance of other manifestations of preeclampsia. There is, however, little reason to believe this to be the case since the placental, renal, hepatic and coagulation abnormalities of preeclampsia do not appear to be a direct consequence of elevated blood pressure. While one study[103] has demonstrated a reduced incidence of proteinuria in gravidas with hypertension treated with atenolol, this report has been criticized in part because of an excessive incidence of proteinuria in the control group. Furthermore, results of several other studies fail to support this observation.[104-108]

Calcium and Magnesium

Dietary calcium deficiency has been suggested to underlie hypertension in both non-pregnant and pregnant populations.[109] In this regard, Taufield et al.[89] noted hypocalciuria in most women with pure and superimposed preeclampsia while Kawasaki et al.[110] reported that administration of 600 mg/day of supplemental calcium to normal gravidas enhanced pressor resistance to infused angiotensin. Results of randomized trials of calcium supplementation in normal pregnancy are contradictory. Two studies have failed to reveal a clinically significant beneficial effect of such therapy[109]; however, López-Jaramillo and colleagues[111] recently reported that 2 g/day of supplemental calcium significantly reduced the incidence of pregnancy-induced hypertension in a group of healthy primigravidas. It is hoped that results of a multicenter study planned for the early 1990s in the United States will help clarify this issue.

Deficiency of magnesium has also been implicated in the pathogenesis of hypertension as well as in the vasospasm that characterizes preeclampsia. However, a recently reported randomized trial failed to demonstrate any clinical benefit of oral magnesium supplementation during pregnancy.[112]

Low-Dose Aspirin

A more promising strategy for the prevention of preeclampsia involves administration of low-dose aspirin. The premise is that small amounts of aspirin (30–100 mg/day) produce a greater inhibition of thromboxane production compared to that of prostacyclin in both pregnant women and their fetuses,[49, 113-116] thus preventing or reversing the vasodilator-vasoconstrictor eicosanoid imbalance that may underlie much of the pathophysiology of preeclampsia (see above). In favor of the above hypothesis are observations by several investigators that administration of low-dose aspirin (60–100 mg/day) to gravidas with a variety of risk factors for the development of preeclampsia, significantly reduced the incidence of hypertension[116, 117] and appeared to improve fetal growth.[115, 116] It is important to note that no increase in either maternal or fetal hemorrhage could be attributed to aspirin therapy, an observation that may be explained by a relatively greater inhibition of maternal than fetal thromboxane biosynthesis.[114, 115] An important caveat, however, is that these studies involved small numbers of women carefully selected on the basis of risks for the development of hypertension. Thus, although these early results are most promising, proof of the safety and efficacy of low-dose aspirin therapy awaits the results of several multicenter trials that are ongoing at this time. *Prior to the availability of such data, low-dose aspirin should not be given routinely to otherwise healthy pregnant women.*

APPROACH TO THE TREATMENT OF HYPERTENSION IN PREGNANCY

The decision to treat elevated blood pressure during gestation is complex and controversial due in part to the relatively short duration of the problem and the need to consider a second patient, the fetus. In addition, the majority of data bearing on this issue come from nonrandomized, uncontrolled, often retrospective observations of gravidas with different types of hypertension. Current controversies in this area are underscored by an extraordinary divergence of opinion among physicians regarding the management of hypertension in pregnancy.[118] The following discussion addresses maternal and fetal benefits and risks that must be contemplated when considering antihypertensive drug therapy for the pregnant patient. The considerations raised apply, in general, to all forms of hypertension (see Table 1–1); details regarding the treatment of acutely elevated blood pressure in preeclampsia and chronic hypertension are addressed later in separate sections.

Maternal Considerations

The major risks to the pregnant patient from severe hypertension are cerebrovascular accident and cardiac decompensation. In contrast, hazards of mild to moderately elevated blood pressures, over a period of several weeks to months, are less clear. Therefore, the rationale used to treat such levels of blood

pressure in nonpregnant populations, i.e., prevention of vascular pathologic lesions that require years to develop, cannot reasonably be applied during gestation. On the other hand, treatment of mild to moderately elevated blood pressure during pregnancy may reduce the progression to severe hypertension and/or the need for hospitalization and there are some data to support this.[103, 119]

Fetal Considerations

Benefits of Treatment

Although fetal risks associated with even minimally elevated blood pressure during pregnancy appear clear,[14, 15] whether or not they can be altered by drug therapy remains to be established. In this regard Fletcher and Bulpitt[120] have reviewed five randomized controlled trials of drug therapy vs. no treatment[103–105, 121, 122] for hypertension complicating pregnancy. Although four of the five failed to demonstrate a significant reduction in perinatal mortality, the pooled relative risk of fetal or neonatal loss for all five studies showed a significant benefit favoring treatment. Of note is that in the largest trial in which the reduction in perinatal mortality was the greatest,[105] the improved outcome was due to a reduction in the incidence of midtrimester stillbirths, leading the authors to suggest that the mechanism of any potential benefit may be independent of a reduction in blood pressure per se (see discussion of methyldopa therapy below). Another potential positive effect of antihypertensive therapy is the prevention of premature delivery necessitated by severe maternal hypertension. Although early studies[105, 121] suggested that this might be the case, gestational age at delivery in more recent trials was similar in treated and untreated subjects.[103, 104]

Finally, it should be noted that many of the above-cited studies included small numbers of patients with a variety of hypertensive disorders. This major methodologic problem makes interpretation of results extremely difficult. An exception is a recently reported prospective randomized trial[108] in which antihypertensive therapy of patients with mild chronic hypertension failed to improve the course or outcome of pregnancy (see section below on treatment of chronic hypertension).

Risks of Treatment

The potential maternal and fetal benefits of antihypertensive treatment must be weighed carefully against possible adverse effects, both immediate and long-term, on the offspring. This area has been particularly poorly studied in large, partly because there are no standards for animal and/or human drug testing that include (1) effects of the agent on the fetus' ability to withstand hypoxic stress, (2) a thorough analysis of morphologic and physiologic variables in the newborn, and (3) long-term evaluation of physical as well as intellectual development.

The Food and Drug Administration has put forth a classification that theoretically permits an assessment of the risk an individual drug poses to the fetus (see Preface). Unfortunately, because of the lack of studies, most drugs have not been assigned a risk factor by the manufacturer, leading to widely different categorization by various authors. For example, Ferris[123] has classified thiazide diuretics in risk category A, while Briggs et al.[124] have assigned these agents risk factor D.

Physicians may be lulled into a false sense of security about prescribing drugs to pregnant women because of a notation in the package insert that no adverse fetal or reproductive effects have been described. These supposedly reassuring assertions are typically based on a very few studies of gross markers of drug safety, whereas many more subtle effects are not evaluated. For example, a recent study has demonstrated heretofore unrecognized in utero developmental and tubular damage consequent to administration of aminoglycosides to pregnant rats.[125] In addition, the teratogenicity of all antihypertensive drugs remains virtually unknown, since drug trials of even the best studied agents, such as methyldopa, have generally included gravidas only when they are beyond the first trimester. Since almost all drugs prescribed to pregnant women reach

the fetus[124] the above considerations serve as a reminder that therapeutic agents of any kind should be prescribed to pregnant women with the utmost caution.

One major concern specific to the use of antihypertensive drugs during pregnancy is that placental blood flow may be adversely affected. As noted previously, the uterine spiral arteries lose their muscular media in early gestation and therefore appear to behave as maximally dilated passive conduits, which has led some to suggest that placental blood is not effectively autoregulated. Data from animal studies of this issue have led to discordant conclusions.[126–129] Whether or not placental blood flow is effectively autoregulated, it is clear that uteroplacental blood flow can be influenced by several vasoconstrictors (probably by acting on the proximal uterine vasculature), and that circulating levels of endogenous pressor hormones may be markedly augmented following excessive drug induced decrements in maternal arterial pressure.

Recommendations

The above considerations have led various authorities to divergent recommendations regarding the treatment of hypertension in pregnancy. Some believe therapy should be initiated when blood pressure is >140/90 mm Hg,[123, 130] while others, reporting impressive fetal and maternal outcome statistics, withhold treatment until levels are 150–170/110 mm Hg.[16, 131, 132] It should be noted, however, that use of Korotkoff phase IV by some and phase V by others (levels that differ $\approx$12 mm Hg during pregnancy[7]) means that the above recommendations may not be as discrepant as they appear.

Our own approach is an intermediate one. In the acute inpatient setting, drug therapy is initiated when phase V diastolic blood pressure is $\approx$105 mm Hg. Our goal is to lower such levels to between 90 and 100 mm Hg, a point at which the risk of hypertension-induced cerebrovascular hemorrhage is extremely low. Nonetheless, it is important to individualize therapy; women with lower blood pressures in the second trimester should be treated earlier, since the magnitude and rate of increase may be more closely related to adverse events than the absolute level of arterial pressure.

Regarding the chronically hypertensive gravida, a National Institutes of Health Working Group has recently suggested that drug treatment be initiated when phase V diastolic blood pressure is ≥100 mm Hg,[22] an approach that appears reasonable. Important exceptions to this are gravidas with renal disease and/or diabetes in whom a more aggressive approach is taken in order to prevent further renal glomerular damage.

PREECLAMPSIA-ECLAMPSIA: GENERAL APPROACH

Ambulatory treatment has little place in the management of preeclampsia and suspicion of this disease is justification for hospitalization. We take this approach because eclamptic convulsions cannot be predicted accurately on clinical grounds and because life-threatening elevations in blood pressure may occur with alarming rapidity.

In general, if preeclampsia or severe hypertension occurs beyond the 36th gestational week, a point at which fetal pulmonary maturity has generally occurred, delivery is the therapy of choice following control of elevated blood pressure and administration of magnesium sulfate to prevent seizures (see below). Delivery is also indicated regardless of gestational age if there is evidence of advanced disease or impending eclampsia, since progression is virtually inevitable unless the uterus is evacuated. Particularly worrisome symptoms and signs include headache, blurred vision, scotomata, epigastric pain, diastolic blood pressure >110 mm Hg after 24 hours of hospitalization, clonus, rising serum creatinine levels, consumptive coagulopathy, and abnormal liver function tests (even if the latter two parameters are only mildly disturbed).

In selected cases of apparently mild disease, or when it is unclear if the patient has preeclampsia, temporizing may be indicated. Such an approach, employing hospitalization, modest bed rest, and an unrestricted diet without the use of antihypertensive agents, has been highly successful at the high risk pregnancy unit at Parkland Memorial Hospital in Dallas.[133] Although prolonged hospitalization may be criticized as unduly expensive, the costs (financial and emotional) of such antenatal management are less than those of caring for a critically ill premature infant with respiratory distress syndrome.[133] It is stressed that this approach does not apply to patients who present remote from term with markedly elevated blood pressure and profuse proteinuria, particularly when accompanied by hematologic and hepatic abnormalities. So-called "conservative management" of such patients is accompanied by an unacceptable maternal morbidity including eclampsia, abruptio placenta, renal failure, ruptured liver, and intracerebral hemorrhage.[134]

DRUG THERAPY OF ACUTE HYPERTENSION

The ideal agent for the urgent or emergent treatment of severe hypertension during pregnancy should act quickly and reliably to reduce blood pressure in a gradual manner, avoiding hypotension and baroreflex-mediated sympathetic responses, both of which may reduce placental blood flow. In addition, such a drug should act directly on the uteroplacental vasculature to reverse vasospasm induced by the hypertensive disease process and be free of adverse effects on both mother and fetus.[132] Obviously, no such agent is currently available; however, when used cautiously, several of the drugs discussed below can be used successfully in the gravida with hypertension (Table 1–4).

As noted previously, our general approach in the acute setting is to administer

TABLE 1–4.
Drug Therapy of Acute, Severe Hypertension in Pregnancy*†

Drug [FDA Class]‡	Dose/Route	Onset of Action	Adverse Effects§	Comments
Agent of choice				
Hydralazine [C]	5 mg IV/IM, then 5–10 mg every 20–40 min; or constant infusion of 0.5–10 mg/hr	IV: 10 min; IM: 10–30 min	Headache, flushing, tachycardia, nausea, vomiting	Broad experience of safety and efficacy
Second-line agents				
Labetalol [C]	20 mg IV, then 20–80 mg every 20–30 min, up to 300 mg; or constant infusion of 1–2 mg/min until desired effect, then stop or reduce to 0.5 mg/min	5–10 min	Flushing, nausea, vomiting, tingling of scalp	Limited experience in pregnancy
Diazoxide [C]	30–50 mg IV every 5–15 min	2–5 min	Inhibition of labor; hyperglycemia, fluid retention with repeated doses	Doses of 150–300 mg may cause severe hypotension; may displace phenytoin from serum protein binding sites
Nifedipine [C]	5–10 mg by mouth; repeat in 30 min if necessary, then 10–20 mg by mouth every 3–6 hr	10–15 min	Flushing, headache, tachycardia, nausea, inhibition of labor	May have synergistic interaction with MgSO₄; limited experience in pregnancy
Relative contraindication				
Nitroprusside [C]	0.5–10 µg/kg/min by constant IV infusion	Instantaneous	Cyanide toxicity, nausea, vomiting	Use only in critical care unit at low doses for briefest time feasible; may cause fetal cyanide toxicity

*IV = intravenous; IM = intramuscular.
†Indicated for acute elevation of Korotkoff Phase V diastolic blood pressure to >105 mm Hg; goal is gradual reduction to 9C–100 mm Hg. See text for details.
‡United States Food and Drug Administration Classification—see Preface for details.
§All agents may cause marked hypotension, especially in severe preeclampsia.

hypotensive agents when the phase V diastolic blood pressure is ≈105 mm Hg, aiming to gradually reduce levels to 90–100 mm Hg.

Hydralazine

This direct vasodilator, which is the most frequently used agent in the United States, to treat severe hypertension near term or in the peripartum period, has a long history of use, established effectiveness, and an acceptable side effect profile.[1, 135–138] Studies of Wallenburg and colleagues[1, 12] utilizing Swan-Ganz catheters during the intravenous administration of this drug to untreated nulliparas with preeclampsia have provided a clearer understanding of the hemodynamic effects of this agent. Diastolic pressure decreased from an average near 100 mg Hg to approximately 90 mm Hg; heart rate increased substantially, resulting in an increase in cardiac output; and pulmonary capillary wedge pressure and stroke volume actually decreased. Of concern, urinary volume decreased and most patients became oliguric. These observations, supported by the recent report of Belfort and colleagues[53] underscore the therapeutic implications of the volume contraction typically observed in preeclampsia (see above), i.e., that such gravidas, particularly those with severe disease, may be exquisitely sensitive to the hypotensive actions of vasodilators. In this regard Assali et al.[139] and Kuzniar et al.[137] reported that preeclamptics are more sensitive to the hypotensive actions of hydralazine than are gravidas with chronic hypertension, an observation that may be explained by the greater degree of volume contraction in the former. Other adverse effects of parenteral hydralazine include headache, tremulousness, nausea, and vomiting, symptoms that may confound the clinician as they are similar to those observed in gravidas with imminent eclampsia.

The effect of hydralazine on uteroplacental blood flow remains unclear, as both increased and decreased perfusion have been observed in animal and human studies.[140–146] Such divergent results may reflect variation in study design including the magnitude of the blood pressure decrement, the methodology used to determine flow as well as species differences. In assessing the impact of vasodilator therapy on placental blood flow, it is also important to recall that such drugs may evoke reflex sympathetic activation, which may then cause uteroplacental vasoconstriction.[147–149]

Fetal distress following parenteral hydralazine has been reported by several investigators.[1, 135, 136] Vink et al.[135] administered 12.5 mg of hydralazine intravenously to 33 gravidas with severe hypertension, reducing blood pressure from an average >110 mm Hg to "therapeutic levels between 70 and 90 mm Hg." This was associated with evidence of fetal distress in 19, observations indicating that the dose of hydralazine was too high and the goal diastolic blood pressure too low. Fetal distress has even been observed when diastolic pressure was lowered slowly by administering 5 mg intravenously every ten minutes until the diastolic blood pressure was below 100 mm Hg.[136]

The above-described data in combination with observations of Wallenburg[1] suggest a critical role for intravascular volume depletion in the fetal distress observed after hydralazine administration. In the latter report, parenteral hydralazine induced abnormalities in fetal heart rate tracings in 4 of 7 gravidas, which changes were reversed by infusion of 0.5–1.5 L colloid. In contrast, no fetal distress occurred in an additional 23 gravidas when volume expansion preceded vasodilator therapy (see below for discussion of volume expansion therapy).

Since volume expansion therapy cannot be accomplished safely in preeclampsia in the absence of invasive monitoring, a procedure indicated only rarely (see below), we recommend that hydralazine treatment be commenced with 5 mg, given intravenously, followed by 5 to 10 mg every 20 to 30 minutes. It is not prudent to repeat the drug more often since the time to peak effect may vary from 10 to 40 minutes.[137, 150] Alternatively, a constant intravenous infusion of the drug may be used (see Table 1–4).

Labetalol

Parenteral use of this adrenergic inhibitor, with combined beta and α_1-blocking properties, has been purported to reduce blood pressure more reliably[151, 152] and produce less headache and flushing than hydralazine,[151, 153] but others have found both drugs similarly efficacious[136, 153] and well tolerated.[136, 152] The effects of intravenous labetalol on the fetus and neonate remain unclear. In two limited studies[154, 155] no changes in uteroplacental, umbilical venous or fetal aortic blood flow, or in fetal heart rate were observed following parenteral labetalol administration. Similarly, Mabie and colleagues[136] reported no adverse fetal or neonatal effects of intravenous labetalol. Others, however, have observed fetal distress[153] and neonatal bradycardia,[152] but in these latter reports it is unclear if these were drug effects or a result of underlying maternal disease. One concern regarding the use of drugs such as labetalol is that studies in sheep indicate that intact adrenergic mechanisms appear important for fetal compensatory responses to hypoxemia.[156–159]

Nifedipine

There is little information regarding the efficacy and safety of calcium-channel blockers in hypertensive pregnancy, although a number of trials with these agents are in progress. There are, however, encouraging preliminary reports, including two uncontrolled studies, one noting effective control of acute hypertension near term or in the immediate puerperium,[160] and the other suggesting that nifedipine may increase platelet counts in preeclamptic women.[161] Even in these small series maternal side effects including headache, flushing, and nausea were frequent, although generally well tolerated.

The effect of nifedipine on placental blood flow has hardly been studied and results from normotensive and hypertensive animal models are of unclear relevance.[162, 163] In the study of Walters and Redman[160] no adverse effects on fetal heart rate tracings were observed in the 13 women who received the drug antenatally. Nifedipine has potent uterine muscle relaxant properties and it has been used successfully to treat premature labor.[164, 165] Whether use of nifedipine as an antihypertensive agent will significantly alter patterns of labor or increase postpartum uterine atony and hemorrhage remains unclear.[160, 166]

There is one caution concerning the use of calcium channel blockers in gravidas with preeclampsia receiving magnesium sulfate therapy to prevent eclamptic seizures. The latter agent may interfere with calcium-dependent excitation-contraction coupling in both smooth and skeletal muscle, and therefore produce excessive calcium channel blockade when given with an agent such as nifedipine. This may explain recent reports of severe hypotension[167] and neuromuscular blockade[168] in gravidas when nifedipine and magnesium sulfate were used simultaneously. Thus, calcium channel blockers should be administered with extreme caution to patients currently receiving magnesium sulfate or who may require such therapy in the near future. For these reasons we find little use for this agent in preeclampsia.

Diazoxide

This congener of the thiazide diuretics is a potent arteriolar vasodilator. In the past, intravenous boluses of 300 mg were recommended; however, this dose frequently caused precipitous decreases in blood pressure in both pregnant and nonpregnant patients.[169–171] Current recommendations are to administer the drug in smaller, 30–150 mg, doses every two to five minutes or by continuous infusion.[171–174] Nonetheless, doses as low as 60 mg have been reported to cause significant hypotension in pregnant patients.[173] In this respect, Dudley[174] reported results from 34 hypertensive gravidas treated with a 30 mg "minibolus" of diazoxide every one to two minutes until diastolic pressure was less than 90 mm Hg. His goal blood pressure was achieved in all subjects within 10 minutes, and in fact blood pressure decreased to 105/70 mm Hg in one subject, a level sufficiently low to jeopardize fetal well-being. Bolus injections of diazoxide in normotensive and hypertensive pregnant sheep typically reduce uterine blood flow,[175–177] the magnitude of the change being directly related to the degree of maternal blood pressure reduction. Caritis et al.,[176] however, noted that the adverse maternal and fetal hemodynamic consequence of bolus diazoxide administration could be markedly attenuated by a slow infusion protocol.[176]

Diazoxide, like other smooth muscle relaxants, may arrest labor,[169, 178, 179] an effect that can generally be overcome by the administration of oxytocin. Other adverse effects include maternal and neonatal hyperglycemia[169, 170] due to suppression of insulin release. Boulos et al.[180] observed fetal hyperglycemia and severe degeneration of pancreatic islet cells in sheep and goats subjected to repeated administration of diazoxide. Thus, it would be of interest to have long-term follow-up studies involving children whose mothers received diazoxide during gestation focusing on the incidence of diabetes or other disorders of pancreatic function; however, no such data are available. Finally, diazoxide may displace highly protein-bound drugs, such as phenytoin, from their binding sites, and thereby increase the risk of toxicity from the latter.[77]

Given the above concerns, we reserve diazoxide (in 30 to 50 mg IV doses every 5 to 15 minutes) for the exceptional patient with severe hypertension unresponsive to hydralazine and/or labetalol, a rare event in our experience.

Sodium Nitroprusside

Use of this potent vasodilator has been reported in very few pregnant women,[181, 182] usually in an emergency situation such as pulmonary edema or life-threatening hypertension unresponsive to more conventional therapy. This drug, which is metabolized to cyanide and thiocyanate, crosses the placenta (at least in pregnant sheep), thus raising concern regarding potential fetal toxicity. In this regard Naulty and colleagues[183] observed markedly elevated fetal blood cyanide levels and death in four sheep following a 60-minute infusion averaging 25 μg/kg/minute. However, in a second group receiving less than 1 μg/kg/minute there were no apparent adverse effects. These results are consistent with other observations in both animals and humans that brief infusions of relatively low doses (<4 μg/kg/minute) have not been associated with maternal or fetal blood cyanide levels in the toxic range or with clinically evident toxicity.[181, 182, 184] Nonetheless, nitroprusside should, in general, be reserved for the rare gravida with life-threatening hypertension unresponsive to more conventional therapy.

Volume Expansion Therapy in Preeclampsia

As noted previously, hemoconcentration and decrements in plasma volume are a fundamental pathophysiologic disturbance in preeclampsia, and recent studies indicate that many preeclamptic gravidas have a reduced central blood volume (see above). For this reason several investigators have studied volume expansion therapy in this disorder.[1, 12, 53, 185–190] The hemodynamic effects are quite consistent: increases in both cardiac filling pressures and cardiac output and decreases in systemic vascular resistance. The latter were frequently sufficient to result in reductions in mean arterial pressure, which in one study[186] was sustained for up to 48 hours.

While volume expansion therapy has a transient salutary hemodynamic effect, we are unaware of studies demonstrating that this reduces maternal or fetal morbidity or mortality in preeclampsia. Some have voiced concern when oliguria is present[64] and suggest that volume expansion is indicated in such situations. However, most such oliguric patients demonstrate little change in serum creatinine, a more accurate marker of kidney function, and acute renal failure is rare even in severe preeclampsia.[191] Although volume-mediated increments in cardiac output might potentially benefit the fetus, Jouppila et al.[189] failed to detect any improvement in intervillous blood flow following intravenous albumin infusion in gravidas with severe preeclampsia.

While volume expansion has not been shown to improve pregnancy outcome in preeclampsia, such therapy may increase the risk of pulmonary[192, 193] or cerebral edema,[194] particularly in the immediate puerperium. These complications may be partially explained by (1) increased vascular permeability;[59] (2) decrements in colloid oncotic pressure, which are most marked postpartum and are aggravated by crystalloid administration;[60, 195] and (3) increases in central filling pressures following delivery.[52]

Given the above balance of risks and benefits we caution against the routine use of volume expansion therapy in preeclamptic patients. Our approach, similar to that of Pritchard and colleagues,[138] is to minimize crystalloid infusions (75–125 mL/hour) in preeclamptic women during labor and following delivery until diuresis is established. In the unusual patient with preeclampsia in whom volume expansion is deemed essential (e.g., severe oliguria with worsening azotemia), right heart catheterization should be considered as a guide to therapy since central venous pressure measurements do not accurately reflect pulmonary capillary wedge pressures in patients with preeclampsia.[196] Additional indications for central hemodynamic monitoring in hypertensive gravidas are congestive heart failure and pulmonary edema of unclear etiology. The use of this technology in preeclamptic patients managed with epidural anesthesia remains controversial.[197] In this author's experience, right ventricular catheterization has rarely been required in the management of hypertensive pregnant patients.

Prevention and Treatment of Eclampsia

The most common cause of peripartum seizures is eclampsia; however, the physician should consider other potential disorders when confronted with a patient who has convulsions and is near term or in the immediate puerperium (Table 1–5). The mechanism(s) responsible for eclamptic seizures is unknown, a fact that underlies current controversies about their prevention and treatment. As noted previously, some feel that this represents one form of hypertensive encephalopathy (see above section on pathophysiology of preeclampsia). However, observations that ≈20% of gravidas have minimally elevated blood pressure shortly before convulsions occur[72, 78] indicates that control of blood pressure will not entirely prevent eclamptic convulsions.

In the United States parenteral magnesium sulfate is the drug of choice for both the prevention and treatment of eclampsia,[138] and although prospective, randomized trials comparing this drug with other agents have not been reported through 1989, maternal mortality decreased dramatically following its introduction into clinical use.[30] It should be emphasized that magnesium sulfate is not used as an antihypertensive agent since blood pressure reductions following parenteral administration are modest and transient.[198]

The use of magnesium sulfate in preeclampsia-eclampsia has become increasingly controversial[199, 200] and criticized as archaic, associated with excessive risk, and irrational on the grounds that it is not a proved anticonvulsant.[77, 200] Some believe its primary action lies at the myoneural junction, blocking the peripheral motor responses to cerebral cortical dysfunction. Borges and Gucer[201] have reported that magnesium sulfate in doses mimicking those used clinically suppresses penicillin induced seizures in several animal models; however, these results have been criticized.[202] More recently, evidence has been presented that magnesium stimulates prostacyclin synthesis in vivo[203] and in vitro,[204] raising the possibility that a salutary effect on cerebral vasospasm and/or platelet aggregation may be responsible for its apparent beneficial effects in the prevention and treatment of eclampsia.

Despite the above concerns, the excellent

TABLE 1–5.
Differential Diagnosis of Peripartum Seizures*

	Blood Pressure	Proteinuria	Fits	Timing	Cerebrospinal Fluid	Other Features
Eclampsia	Increased	+ to +++	+++	Third trimester	Early: RBCs 0–1000, protein 50 to 150 mg/dL Late: grossly bloody	Platelets normal or ↓; RBCs usually normal, occasionally fragmented; hyperuricemia
Epilepsy	Normal	Normal to +	+++	Any trimester	Normal	Low anticonvulsant levels
Subarachnoid hemorrhage	Variably increased (labile)	0 to +	+	Any trimester	Grossly bloody	
Thrombotic thrombocytopenic purpura	Normal to mildly increased	++	++	Any trimester	RBCs 0–100	Platelets ↓↓, fragmented RBCs, fever
Amniotic fluid embolus	Shock	–	+	Intrapartum	Normal	Hypoxia, cyanosis; platelets ↓↓; RBCs normal
Cerebral vein thrombosis	Mildly increased	–	++	Postpartum	Normal (early)	Headache
Water intoxication	Normal	–	++	Intrapartum	Normal	Serum Na <124 mEq/L
Pheochromocytoma	Variably increased (labile)	+	+	Any trimester	Normal	Neurofibromatosis
Toxicity of local anesthetic	Variable	–	++	Intrapartum	Normal	

*Modified from Donaldson JO: *Neurology of Pregnancy*, ed 2. Philadelphia, WB Saunders, 1989.

clinical results of Pritchard and colleagues[138] remain the standard against which other anti-eclamptic regimens must be judged. In their series of 245 cases of eclampsia there was but a single maternal mortality, this the consequence of administration of five times the recommended dose. Nonetheless, some have recommended that magnesium be abandoned in favor of anticonvulsive agents used frequently in nonpregnant patients such as diazepam, phenobarbital, and phenytoin.[77, 123, 200] Although uncontrolled studies supporting the efficacy and safety of phenytoin in preeclampsia-eclampsia have recently been published,[205, 206] there are also disturbing anecdotal reports of eclamptic seizures following administration of this agent.[205, 207, 208] In addition, available data suggest that neonatal depression is more common following maternal administration of diazepam than after magnesium sulfate.[209, 210] Assessment of the relative fetal and neonatal toxicities of phenytoin and magnesium awaits controlled prospective trials.

With the above considerations in mind, we believe that in the United States, magnesium sulfate remains the drug of choice for the prevention and/or treatment of eclamptic convulsions until large, prospective randomized trials demonstrate a clinically significant benefit for alternative agents, such as phenytoin.

CHRONIC HYPERTENSION

Evaluation

The initial history, physical examination and laboratory testing of the pregnant patient with chronic hypertension is similar to that employed in nonpregnant subjects[2, 211] and is directed at answering three questions:

1. *Does the patient have primary or secondary hypertension?* Although the vast majority of pregnant patients with elevated blood pressure will have uncomplicated essential hypertension, some will have secondary causes, including parenchymal renal disease, reno-vascular hypertension, pheochromocytoma, Cushing's syndrome, primary hyperaldosteronism, hyperthyroidism, and coarctation of the aorta. Of particular importance is the early recognition of pheochromocytoma, since maternal mortality approaches 50% when unrecognized prior to the onset of labor. Hence, suspicion of this disorder is an indication for laboratory testing (for discussion of all adrenal tumors see Chap. 4). In addition, the presence of renal insufficiency must not be overlooked, since the courses of such pregnancies are much more likely to be complicated by marked elevation of blood pressure and premature delivery (see Chap. 2).

2. *Is end-organ disease present?* Renal, cardiac and/or cerebrovascular disease is unusual in women of child-bearing age with chronic hypertension, but these complications do occur and must be identified, as they are associated with increased risk for both the pregnant patient and fetus. This may be especially true in gravidas over age 40 years in whom hypertension may have been present for more than a decade.

3. *Are there cardiovascular risk factors present in addition to elevated blood pressure, i.e., glucose intolerance, hyperlipidemia, and smoking?* (see Chaps. 3 and 6).

The minimal laboratory testing required to address the above questions (i.e., urinalysis, serum creatinine, potassium, calcium, glucose) is similar in pregnant and nonpregnant patients, with the exception that it may be worthwhile to obtain baseline determinations of platelet count, uric acid, and antithrombin III, as changes in these parameters may be helpful in distinguishing between preeclampsia and exacerbation of chronic hypertension in the gravida with rising blood pressure late in pregnancy (see Table 1–2).

Course of Blood Pressure

The blood pressure of chronically hypertensive women is variably altered by pregnancy.[16, 212] Many (40% to 50%) will experience a decrease during the second trimester, often to levels well into the normal range. This is important to recognize since, as was noted previously, the presence of chronic hypertension may be masked in the gravida seen for the first time in midtrimester; in addition, anticipation of this decrement may obviate the need for antihypertensive drugs during early pregnancy in the patient with mild to moderate essential hypertension. The blood pressure of another 35% to 50% of hypertensive patients will fail to undergo the normal second trimester decrement and that of 10% to 20% will actually increase during this time. It is in these two groups, and especially the latter, where there is the greatest risk of a severe exacerbation of hypertension during the third trimester.[16]

Maternal and Fetal Risks

Maternal risks associated with chronic hypertension include superimposed preeclampsia or eclampsia, deterioration of renal function, cerebrovascular accident, congestive heart failure, and hemorrhage secondary to placental abruption. These events are very unusual in gravidas with mild chronic hypertension,[16] and are seen most often in patients with more severe degrees of chronic blood pressure elevation.[38] Within the latter group it is the superimposition of preeclampsia that appears to produce the greatest risk.[38]

Fetal and neonatal effects of chronic hypertension in pregnancy include increased incidence of intrauterine growth retardation, prematurity, and perinatal mortality. As is the case for maternal complications, fetal jeopardy is greatest in those women with the most markedly elevated blood pressures and especially in those who develop superimposed preeclampsia.[38] In this regard, the severity of chronic hypertension seems to correlate with the risk of superimposed preeclampsia, as the latter has been reported to be 10% in gravidas with mild chronic hypertension[16] but in ≈50% of those with severe elevations of blood pressure (>170/110 mm Hg in the first trimester).[38] Such observations may explain the excellent pregnancy outcomes in mild disease

and the high incidence of prematurity, growth retardation, and perinatal mortality reported in gravidas with severe chronic hypertension.

Benefits of Antihypertensive Therapy

As noted previously, the hazards of years of chronically elevated blood pressure in nonpregnant patients differ substantially from those incurred over a period of several months during pregnancy, and thus the rationale used to treat hypertension in nonpregnant populations cannot be applied during gestation. Similarly, it would not be appropriate to use results of many trials of antihypertensive therapy in nongravid populations as a basis for treating pregnant women.

Unfortunately, there is a paucity of data concerning the benefits of drug therapy of chronic hypertension in pregnancy. The few published controlled trials (see previous section on the approach to the treatment of hypertension in pregnancy) generally contain few subjects, often enroll patients in the latter weeks of gestation and typically include a mixture of different types of hypertension (i.e., chronic hypertenson, preeclampsia, transient hypertension), methodologic flaws that make conclusions about the benefits of therapy in chronic hypertension impossible.

The recent study of Sibai et al.,[108] the only large, prospective, randomized trial of therapy for chronic hypertension in pregnancy of which we are aware, is an exception to many of the above concerns. Two hundred sixty-three gravidas with mild chronic hypertension, blood pressure averaging ≈140/91 mm Hg (phase IV being used for diastolic levels) in the first trimester were randomized to receive labetalol, methyldopa, or no treatment. The objective of drug therapy was to keep blood pressure <140/90 mm Hg. Results demonstrated similar incidences of superimposed preeclampsia, cesarean delivery, prematurity, and small-for-gestational-age infants in both drug-treated groups and the control group. Thus, as of early 1990, prospective, controlled trials have failed to demonstrate a maternal or fetal benefit of drug therapy of mild to moderate chronic hypertension in pregnancy. However, the negative results of the above study[108] may be due to the relatively mild degree of hypertension treated, since this subset of hypertension patients is that with the lowest risk of pregnancy complications. Thus, although the data of Sibai and colleagues[108] contributes importantly to our knowledge, it does not resolve the controversy regarding precisely what level of blood pressure elevation should be treated.

Risks of Drug Treatment

The potential risks of drug therapy must be carefully balanced against the possible benefits (see approach to the treatment of hypertension—fetal considerations, above). Unfortunately, there are few adequate studies concerning teratogenicity, direct fetal toxicity, effects on uteroplacental blood flow, influences on the ability of the fetus to respond to hypoxic stress, and/or impact on long-term neurobehavioral development consequent to maternal antihypertensive drug administration. As a consequence such effects are often identified only during postmarketing drug surveillance, a good of example of which concerns the angiotensin-converting enzyme inhibitors (see below). Therefore, we advise that physicians use the utmost caution in prescribing medication to pregnant women, and recommend use of those agents that have been studied the most thoroughly and/or have been in use in pregnant patients for the longest time.

Recommendations Regarding Initiation of Drug Treatment

Given the ill-defined benefits and risks of drug therapy of chronic hypertension during pregnancy it is not surprising that current literature contains a variety of disparate recommendations. For example one standard text suggests withholding therapy until levels are 150/110 mm Hg,[131] while another[123] recommends that blood pressure be kept below 140/90 mm Hg with medication. However, such discrepancies may not be as great as they appear, since authors of the former text utilize phase IV diastolic levels which, as noted previously, average 10 to 12 mm Hg above phase V values in pregnant women.[7]

The National Institutes of Health Working Group[22] has recently advised initiating drug treatment of uncomplicated chronic hypertension during pregnancy when phase V diastolic levels are ≥ 100 mm Hg (a value similar to phase IV levels of 110 mm Hg suggested by others[131]), a recommendation that we believe is reasonable. If a patient receiving antihypertensive agents is counseled prior to pregnancy or in the first trimester, we make an attempt to stop all drugs, since little is known about the teratogenicity of hypotensive agents. In addition, the hypotensive effect of early gestation will often lower blood pressure below levels requiring drug treatment. In the patient in whom continued drug therapy is deemed necessary (i.e., moderate to severe hypertension when untreated or the presence of renal disease and/or diabetes mellitus) we prefer to replace current medication with methyldopa (including discontinuation of diuretics) for reasons detailed below. An alternative strategy, endorsed by the NIH Working Group[22] is to continue the patient's current medication regimen.

Secondary Causes of Hypertension

While secondary causes are present only in a small minority of hypertensive gravidas, it is important to recognize those few with disorders such as renal parenchymal disease, renal vascular abnormalities, pheochromocytoma, Cushing's disease, primary hyperaldosteronism, and coarctation of the aorta since each presents unique diagnostic, therapeutic, and prognostic considerations. For example, gravidas with primary renal parenchymal disease and hypertension frequently experience marked elevation of blood pressure and increased rates of prematurity, intrauterine growth retardation, and perinatal mortality. This may be especially true for a number of rheumatic disorders, such as periarteritis nodosa and progressive systemic sclerosis (see Chap. 2, p. 60). Also, pheochromocytoma is associated with a maternal mortality of ≈50% when unrecognized prior to the onset of labor (for a discussion of adrenal tumors see Chap. 4, p. 124) and coarctation of the aorta is accompanied by an increased risk of aortic dissection and/or rupture during pregnancy (see Chap. 5, p. 175).

The influence of gestation on renovascular hypertension and the effects of the latter on pregnancy outcome are unclear. The literature contains only a few anecdotal reports of such patients, often selected because they had severe hypertension.[213–215] Thus, the approach to this problem must be highly individualized. If markedly elevated blood pressure is present in the first trimester, therapeutic abortion should be recommended since such pregnancies are accompanied by substantial maternal and fetal risk, and correction of the lesion is best performed when the patient is not pregnant. In those cases in which the pregnancy is continued, drug therapy is the treatment of choice. In this regard, angiotensin-converting enzyme inhibitors are frequently used with minimal risk in nonpregnant patients, however, such agents are associated with substantial fetal renal toxicity (see below). Therefore, other agents should be tried initially; however, if hypertension is unresponsive and threatens maternal well-being then administration of an angiotensin-converting enzyme inhibitor would be justifiable.[215] Finally, several uneventful pregnancies following correction of renal artery stenosis have been reported.[214]

Drug Treatment of Chronic Hypertension

Central Adrenergic Inhibitors

Methyldopa has a long history of effective use in pregnancy and has been prospectively evaluated in randomized clinical trials,[105, 108, 121] one of which included periodic evaluation of offspring to the age of 7 years[216] (Table 1–6). The most complete is that of Redman et al.[105] of 242 gravidas with diastolic blood pressures 90 to 110 mm Hg (phase IV)

randomized to receive either methyldopa or no treatment. There were nine pregnancy losses in the control group, four of which were midtrimester stillbirths, while there was only one fetal loss in the treated group. Based on these results, which were similar to those of a previous study by Leather and colleagues,[121] the authors concluded that the benefits could not be attributed to the control of hypertension per se and suggested that some as-yet-undefined action of methyldopa may have been responsible. It is of note, however, that the recently reported large, prospective trial of Sibai and colleagues[108] failed to demonstrate any reduction in midtrimester fetal losses consequent to methyldopa treatment.

Although use of methyldopa as a single agent has been criticized on the basis of limited efficacy in controlling hypertension,[123] several studies suggest otherwise. Redman and colleagues[119] reported that the frequency of severe hypertension occurring antenatally or in labor was significantly reduced by methyldopa treatment and additional reports have demonstrated that this drug is as effective as a β-blocker[217–219] or clonidine[220] for hypertension during pregnancy.

The well-documented side effect profile of methyldopa indicates that maternal adverse effects are generally mild and well tolerated.[119] Rigorous assessment of the offspring in the study of Redman et al.[105, 216, 221, 222] has provided reassuring data regarding the fetal and neonatal safety of this drug. Birth weights, neonatal complications, and progress in the first year of life were similar in methyldopa-treated and control groups,[221, 222] although in one other uncontrolled investigation neonatal tremors were associated with maternal ingestion of the drug.[223] Studies in animals[224] have demonstrated that antenatal administration of methyldopa is associated with depletion of neonatal cardiac catecholamine levels, raising the possibility that the ability of the fetus or newborn to mount an adequate cardiovascular response to stress may be impaired; however, such observations have not been reported in humans.

Long-term follow-up of offspring whose

TABLE 1–6.
Drug Therapy of Chronic Hypertension in Pregnancy*†

Drug [FDA Class]‡	Daily Dose	Adverse Effects and Comments
Agent of choice		
Methyldopa [C]	500–3000 mg in 2–4 divided doses	Safety for mother and fetus (after 1st trimester) is well documented
Second-line agents		
Hydralazine [C]	50–300 mg in 2–4 divided doses	May be ineffective when used as sole agent—best combined with methyldopa or a beta-blocker; few controlled trials but extensive experience with few serious adverse effects documented; several reports of neonatal thrombocytopenia
Beta-adrenergic inhibitors (and the combined alpha-beta blocker, labetalol)	Dependent of specific agent used	May cause fetal bradycardia and impair fetal responses to hypoxia; risk of intrauterine growth retardation remains unclear
Third-line agents		
Thiazide diuretics [D assignation in reference 124]	Dependent on agent used	Most controlled studies in normotensive gravidas; little data in hypertensive gestation; implicated in volume depletion, electrolyte imbalance, pancreatitis, and thrombocytopenia
Clonidine [C]	0.1–0.8 mg in 2 divided doses	Limited data
Nifedipine [C]	30–120 mg in 3–4 divided doses	Limited data; may inhibit labor; may have synergistic action with $MgSO_4$
Prazosin [C]	1–30 mg in 2–3 divided doses	Limited data
Contraindicated		
Angiotensin-converting enzyme inhibitors [D]	Dependent on agent used	High rates of fetal loss in animals; numerous cases of neonatal anuric acute renal failure in humans, occasionally fatal; FDA risk category C by manufacturer as of 1990, but recent data justify category D; use only when absolutely necessary to preserve maternal well-being

*Note that safety during the first trimester has not been established for any antihypertensive agent.
†Drug therapy indicated for uncomplicated chronic hypertension when phase V diastolic BP ≥100 mm Hg. Treatment at lower levels may be indicated for patients with renal disease and/or diabetes mellitus.
‡United States Food and Drug Administration Classification—see Preface for details.

mothers received methyldopa while pregnant also attests to the drug's safety. Among children of women who entered the above methyldopa trial between weeks 16 and 20, head circumference at 4[225] and 7[216] years of age was slightly but significantly less in the sons of methyldopa-treated women; however, mean intelligence quotients and performance on tests from the British Ability Scales were similar in the two groups of children.

Thus, because methyldopa has been extensively studied and has a well-documented record of safety, we believe it to be the agent of choice for the treatment of chronic hypertension during gestation.

Clonidine, another α_2-agonist, has been compared with methyldopa in a randomized, double-blind trial and there were no significant differences between the drugs in terms of efficacy or adverse effects.[220] One long-term follow-up study comparing 22 children whose mothers had received clonidine during pregnancy with matched controls found no effect of the drug on head circumference, neurological development, or school performance; however, there was some excess sleep disturbance in the clonidine group.[226] These observations led the authors to question whether this drug is a behavioral teratogen and serves as a reminder that prenatal drug administration may have subtle, remote adverse effects.

We find little use for this agent as its mechanism of action is similar to that of methyldopa, it offers no clinical advantage over the latter, and it has not been as well studied.

Vasodilators

Hydralazine has been used in pregnancy primarily as a parenteral agent in the therapy of acute, severe hypertension (see above). It has also been employed successfully in the chronic setting as a second-line agent in combination with either methyldopa or a β-blocker.[106, 218, 219, 227, 228] In a small prospective, randomized trial Rosenfeld et al.[229] found hydralazine monotherapy to be as effective as hydralazine plus pindolol; however, a much higher incidence of palpitations, dizziness, and headache was observed in subjects not receiving a β-blocker. Hydralazine appears reasonably safe for the fetus, although thrombocytopenia of uncertain etiology has been reported in a few infants whose mothers were treated with this drug.[230] We are unaware of any long-term follow-up studies on children exposed to this drug in utero. Our practice is to use oral hydralazine as a second-line agent in patients whose blood pressure is inadequately controlled on methyldopa.

β-Adrenergic Blockers

There have been numerous studies of β-blockers in animal pregnancy and their use in humans has been extensively reported.[103, 104, 106, 130, 217–219, 228, 229, 231–241] Nonetheless, the safety and precise indication for use of these antihypertensives remain unclear. These agents cross the placenta,[231, 241–244] and studies in animals have suggested potential adverse maternal and fetal effects. For instance, decreased uteroplacental blood flow[245–247] and altered fetal cardiovascular responses to hypoxia[156, 158, 159] have been observed in sheep subjected to β-adrenoreceptor blockade. Another, albeit theoretical, concern is that since β-agonists have a relaxant effect on the myometrium, β-blocking drugs might induce premature labor.[245, 246]

Initial reports of retrospective, uncontrolled observations associating maternal propranolol use with intrauterine growth retardation, neonatal respiratory depression, bradycardia, and hypoglycemia[231–233, 235, 236] were disturbing; however, more recent results of prospective randomized comparisons of atenolol[103] and metoprolol,[104, 106] each vs. no drug therapy, failed to document significant adverse maternal or fetal effects of these drugs. Modest decreases in fetal and neonatal heart rates in drug treated groups were reported;[248, 249] however, this did not appear to be associated with any significant morbidity. Further evidence of safety has been provided by a one-year follow-up study that failed to detect any adverse effect of in utero exposure to atenolol on later development.[250]

Oxprenolol, a nonselective β-blocker, (currently unavailable in the United States) has been compared with methyldopa in two randomized trials.[218, 219] Control of hypertension as well as measures of perinatal outcome were comparable with the two drugs, although Fidler et al.[218] observed more intrapartum fetal bradycardia in women treated with oxprenolol. Also of note are the studies of Gallery et al.[130, 219] in which plasma volume and birth weight were significantly greater in oxprenolol- compared to methyldopa-treated patients; however, this was not confirmed in a similar study by Fidler and colleagues.[218]

Despite the above reassuring results of controlled trials,[103, 104, 106, 217–219, 251] the data should be interpreted with caution. Each study was relatively small, and gestational age at entry was generally 29 to 33 weeks, leaving unanswered the possibility that treatment of larger numbers of patients and/or a longer duration of drug administration may reveal heretofore unrecognized adverse effects. In this regard, in a preliminary report[238] of a placebo-controlled trial in which atenolol was initiated for chronic hypertension between 12 and 24 weeks of pregnancy, a clinically significant reduction in infant and placental weights was observed in the drug treated group. These data emphasize that the safety of β-blockers in pregnancy has not been fully established, and our practice, therefore, is to use these agents only when blood pressure is not adequately controlled with methyldopa.

Labetalol, a β-blocker with some α-adrenoreceptor blocking activity, has been claimed to be superior to other agents in the treatment of hypertension in pregnancy,[240, 252] however, data from well-designed randomized trials do not support this view. Redman reported that maternal side effects and pregnancy outcome were similar in gravidas treated with labetalol or methyldopa,[253] observations consistent with the recent report of Sibai and colleagues.[108]

α-Adrenergic Blockers

Prazosin, an α_1-receptor antagonist, has been used in uncontrolled studies of chronic hypertension[254-256] and pheochromocytoma[257, 258] complicating gestation. No specific untoward effects have been identified; however, given the limited data and the lack of benefit over other more well-studied agents, there is little reason to use this drug for hypertension during pregnancy. One important exception is the gravida with pheochromocytoma in whom α-blockade with phenoxybenzamine or prazosin is extremely important (see Chap. 4, p. 130).

Calcium Channel Blockers

The use of oral nifedipine during pregnancy in circumstances other than acute hypertension has scarcely been reported,[166, 259, 260] and given the paucity of patients and the uncontrolled nature of the observations, its safety remains unclear. Furthermore, as noted previously, administration of magnesium sulfate (which is not infrequent) to the gravida receiving a calcium channel blocker may result in severe hypotension[167] and neuromuscular blockade[168] due to the synergistic actions of these two agents. For these reasons we prefer not to use nifedipine or similar agents in chronically hypertensive gravidas.

Angiotensin-Converting Enzyme (ACE) Inhibitors

Administration of captopril to gravid

sheep and rabbits is accompanied by an extraordinary fetal wastage.[261, 262] More disturbing, however, are the increasing number of reports suggesting adverse effects of converting enzyme inhibitors on human fetal and neonatal renal function.[263, 264] Recently, investigators at the United States Food and Drug Administration described a total of 14 neonates with anuric renal failure (five of whom died) following in utero exposure to either captopril or enalapril.[263] Such data led us to conclude that these drugs are contraindicated during gestation (even though listed by their manufacturer as risk category C in the 1990 *Physicians' Desk Reference*).

Diuretics and Sodium Restriction

Although there have been many trials of the effect of prophylactic diuretic treatment in pregnancy (see above section on prevention of preeclampsia), there are few data concerning the use of these agents in established hypertension. In one of the few prospective studies available, Sibai et al.[265] randomized 20 gravidas with mild to moderate chronic hypertension treated with diuretics prior to pregnancy to either continue their medication or stop treatment. Blood pressure in the two groups was similar at every stage of gestation; the addition of methyldopa was required in 2 of 10 subjects continued on diuretics and in 1 of 10 in whom the medication was stopped. Of potential importance was the observation that when diuretic therapy was discontinued, a physiologic degree of volume expansion (+52%) occurred, however, increments in volume were significantly less (+18%) in those who continued on drug treatment. Conclusions regarding the clinical importance of these observations will require much larger prospective studies, but it is of note that suboptimal plasma volume expansion in chronically hypertensive gravidas has been associated with impaired fetal growth.[266] Thus, because of the paucity of data concerning diuretic therapy of chronic hypertension during pregnancy while concerns remain about a number of adverse effects, we caution against their routine use in this disorder. (The National Institutes of Health Working Group[22] has indicated that diuretics may be continued in the chronically hypertensive patient who becomes pregnant; however, we prefer to substitute methyldopa.) The only gravidas for whom we prescribe saliuretics unhesitatingly are those with pulmonary edema and/or left ventricular failure.

We are unaware of any well-designed, prospective investigations of the benefits and risks of limiting dietary sodium in the treatment of chronic hypertension complicating gestation; however, such an approach has been anecdotally associated with severe volume depletion, azotemia, and electrolyte disturbance.[99, 100, 267] In view of such reports and the lack of documented benefit, we do not employ sodium restriction in the management of elevated blood pressure during gestation unless there is evidence of accompanying heart failure. If, however, a patient with chronic hypertension enters pregnancy on a moderately restricted sodium intake, dietary habits need not be altered.

Breast Feeding

There is a paucity of data regarding the safety of antihypertensive agents for the breast-fed infant, and the reader is referred to the volume by Briggs et al.,[124] recommendations of the Committee on Drugs of the American Academy of Pediatrics,[268] and the brief review by White[269] for details concerning specific agents. With regard to the more commonly used antihypertensive agents it has been recommended that chlorothiazide and similar diuretics be avoided, since the former has been used to suppress lactation.[268, 269] Although the Committee on Drugs considers atenolol compatible with breast feeding, this β-blocker as well as metoprolol and nadolol appear to be concentrated in breast milk. This property is not shared by propranolol, and it has therefore been suggested that if a β-blocker were indicated this agent would be the drug of choice.[269] Reports concerning hydralazine are sparse; however, the Committee on Drugs considers this agent compatible with breast

feeding. We are unaware of data concerning the use of calcium channel blockers in this context. Although angiotensin converting enzyme inhibitors, known to be excreted in breast milk,[124] were previously felt to be safe,[269], recent reports[263, 264] of adverse fetal and neonatal renal effects associated with maternal prenatal ingestion of captopril and enalapril (see above) indicate that these agents are best avoided in the breast-feeding mother. In addition, given the scarcity of data regarding all of the above mentioned drugs, breast-fed infants of mothers taking antihypertensive agents should be carefully monitored for potential adverse effects. Finally, as previously noted, postpartum hypertension, seizures, and cerebrovascular accidents have been associated with the use of bromocriptine mesylate for suppression of lactation[28, 29] and therefore this agent is contraindicated in postpartum patients with any hypertensive disorder.

REFERENCES

1. Wallenburg HCS: Hemodynamics in hypertensive pregnancy, in Rubin PC (ed): *Hypertension in Pregnancy.* Amsterdam, Elsevier Science Publications, 1988, pp 66–101.
2. Joint National Committee: The 1988 Report of the Joint National Committee on Detection, Evaluation, and Treatment of High Blood Pressure. *Arch Intern Med* 1988; 148:1023–1038.
3. Rubin PC: Hypertension in pregnancy: Clinical features, in Rubin PC (ed): *Handbook of Hypertension:* vol 10, *Hypertension in Pregnancy.* Amsterdam, Elsevier Science Publications, 1988, pp 10–15.
4. Davey DA, MacGillivray I: The classification and definition of the hypertensive disorders of pregnancy. *Am J Obstet Gynecol* 1988; 158:892–898.
5. Wichman K, Ryden G: Blood pressure and renal function during normal pregnancy. *Acta Obstet Gynecol Scand* 1986; 65:561–566.
6. Ginsburg J, Duncan S: Direct and indirect blood pressure measurement in pregnancy. *Br J Obstet Gynaecol* 1969; 76:705–710.

7. Villar J, Repke J, Markush L, et al: The measuring of blood pressure during pregnancy. *Am J Obstet Gynecol* 1989; 161:1019–1024.

8. MacGillivray M, Rose GA, Rowe B: Blood pressure survey in pregnancy. *Clin Sci* 1969; 37:395–407.

9. Christianson RE: Studies on blood pressure during pregnancy. *Am J Obstet Gynecol* 1976; 125:509–513.

10. Wilson M, Morganti AA, Zervoudakis I, et al: Blood pressure, the renin-aldosterone system and sex steroids throughout normal pregnancy. *Am J Med* 1980; 68:97–104.

11. De Swiet M: The cardiovascular system, in Hytten F, Chamberlain G (eds): *Clinical Physiology in Obstetrics*. Oxford, Blackwell Scientific Publications, 1980, pp 3–42.

12. Groenendijk R, Trimbos JBMJ, Wallenburg HCS: Hemodynamic measurements in preeclampsia: Preliminary observations. *Am J Obstet Gynecol* 1984; 150:232–236.

13. Robson SC, Hunter S, Boys RJ, et al: Serial study of factors influencing changes in cardiac output during human pregnancy. *Am J Physiol* 1989; 256:1060–1065.

14. Friedman EA, Neff RK: *Pregnancy Hypertension: A Systemic Evaluation of Clinical Diagnostic Criteria*. Littleton, Mass, PSG Publishing Co, 1977.

15. Page EW, Christianson R: The impact of mean arterial pressure in the middle trimester upon the outcome of pregnancy. *Am J Obstet Gynecol* 1976; 125:740–746.

16. Sibai BM, Ardella TN, Anderson GD: Pregnancy outcome in 211 patients with mild chronic hypertension. *Obstet Gynecol* 1983; 61:571–576.

17. Fisher KA, Luger A, Spargo BH, et al: Hypertension in pregnancy: Clinical-pathological correlations and remote prognosis. *Medicine* 1981; 60:267–276.

18. Katz AI, Davidson JM, Hayslett JP, et al: Pregnancy in women with kidney disease. *Kidney Int* 1980; 18:192–206.

19. Hughes EC. *Obstretric Gynecologic Terminology*. Philadelphia, FA Davis, 1972.

20. Nelson TR: A clinical study of preeclampsia. *Br J Obstet Gynecol* 1955; 62:48–57.

21. Management of preeclampsia. *Am Coll Obstet Gynecol* 1986; 91:1–6.

22. National High Blood Pressure Education Program Working Group: Report on High Blood Pressure in Pregnancy. Department of Health and Human Services, National Heart, Lung and Blood Institute, Bethesda, Maryland, 1990.

23. Chesley LC: Diagnosis of preeclampsia. *Obstet Gynecol* 1985; 65:423–425.

24. Thomson AM, Hytten FE, Billewicz WZ: The epidemiology of oedema during pregnancy. *Br J Obstet Gynaecol* 1967; 74:1–10.

25. Robertson EG: The natural history of oedema during pregnancy. *Br J Obstet Gynaecol* 1971; 78:520–529.

26. Sibai BM, McCubbin JH, Anderson GA, et al: Eclampsia: I. Observations from 67 recent cases. *Obstet Gynecol* 1981; 58:609–613.

27. Watson DL, Sibai BM, Shaver DC, et al: Late postpartum eclampsia: An update. *South Med J* 1983; 76:1487–1489.

28. Katz M, Kroll D, Pak I, et al: Puerperal hypertension, stroke, and seizures after suppression of lactation with bromocriptine. *Obstet Gynecol* 1985; 66:822–824.

29. Watson DL, Bhatia RK, Norman GS, et al: Bromocriptine mesylate for lactation suppression: A risk for postpartum hypertension? *Obstet Gynecol* 1989; 74:573–576.

30. Chesley LC: Blood pressure and circulation, in Chesley LC (ed): *Hypertensive Disorders in Pregnancy*. New York, Appleton-Century-Crofts, 1978, pp 119–154.

31. Mulcahy D, O'Dwyer WF, Carmody M, et al: Phaeochromocytoma presenting in pregnancy. *Ir J Med Sci* 1984; 153:389–391.

32. Burgess GE III: Alpha blockade and surgical intervention of pheochromocytoma in pregnancy. *Obstet Gynecol* 1979; 53:266–270.

33. Ballou SP, Morley JJ, Kushner I: Pregnancy and systemic sclerosis. *Arthritis Rheum* 1984; 27:295–298.

34. Owen J, Hauth JC: Polyarteritis nodosa in pregnancy: A case report and brief literature review. *Am J Obstet Gynecol* 1989; 160:606–607.

35. Chesley LC: Hypertension in pregnancy: Definitions, familial factor and remote prognosis. *Kidney Int* 1980; 18:234–240.

36. Chesley LC, Sibai BM: Clinical significance of elevated mean arterial pressure in the second trimester. *Am J Obstet Gynecol* 1988; 159:275–279.

37. Moutquin JM, Rainville C, Giroux L, et al: A prospective study of blood pressure in pregnancy: Prediction of preeclampsia. *Am J Obstet Gynecol* 1985; 151:191–196.

38. Sibai BM, Anderson GD: Pregnancy outcome of intensive therapy in severe hypertension in first trimester. *Obstet Gynecol* 1986; 67:517–522.

39. Cooper DW, Hill JA, Chesley LC, et al: Genetic control of susceptibility to eclampsia and miscarriage. *Br J Obstet Gynaecol* 1988; 95:644–653.

40. Kilpatrick DC, Gibson F, Liston WA, et al: Association between susceptibility to pre-eclampsia within families and HLA DR4. *Lancet* 1989; 1:1063–1065.

41. Rubin PC: *Handbook of Hypertension:* vol 10, *Hypertension in Pregnancy.* Amsterdam, Elsevier Science Publishers, 1988.

42. Lindheimer MD, Katz AI: Preeclampsia: Pathophysiology, diagnosis and management. *Annu Rev Med* 1989; 40:233–250.

43. De Swiet M: The physiology of normal pregnancy, in Rubin PC (ed): *Handbook of Hypertension:* vol 10, *Hypertension in Pregnancy.* Amsterdam, Elsevier Science 1988, pp 1–9.

44. Roberts JM, Taylor RN, Musci TJ, et al: Preeclampsia: An endothelial cell disorder. *Am J Obstet Gynecol* 1989; 161:1200–1204.

45. Hubel CA, Roberts JM, Taylor RN, et al: Lipid peroxidation in pregnancy: New perspectives on preeclampsia. *Am J Obstet Gynecol* 1989; 161:1025–1034.

46. Fitzgerald DJ, Fitzgerald GA: Eicosanoids in the pathogenesis of preeclampsia, in Laragh JH, Brenner BM (eds): *Hypertension: Pathophysiology, Diagnosis and Management.* New York, Raven Press, 1990, pp 1789–1807.

47. August P, Sealey JE: The renin-angiotensin system in normal and hypertensive pregnancy and in ovarian function, in Laragh JH, Brenner BM (eds): *Hypertension: Pathophysiology, Diagnosis and Management.* New York, Raven Press, 1990, pp 1761–1778.

48. Gant NF, Worley RJ, Everett RB, et al: Control of vascular responsiveness during human pregnancy. *Kidney Int* 1980; 18:253–258.

49. Spitz B, Magness RR, Cox SM, et al: Low dose aspirin: I. Effect on angiotensin II pressor responses and blood prostaglandin concentrations in pregnant women sensitive to angiotensin II. *Am J Obstet Gynecol* 1988; 159:1035–1043.

50. Broughton-Pipkin F: The renin-angiotensin system in normal and hypertensive pregnancies, in Rubin PC (ed): *Handbook of Hypertension: vol 10, Hypertension in Pregnancy.* Amsterdam, Elsevier Science Publishers, 1988, pp 118–151.

51. Pedersen EP: Autonomic nervous system and vascular reactivity in normal and hypertensive pregnancy, in Rubin PC (ed): *Handbook of Hypertension: vol 10, Hypertension in Pregnancy.* Amsterdam, Elsevier Science Publishers, 1988, pp 152–167.

52. Hankins GDV, Wendel GD Jr, Cunningham G, et al: Longitudinal evaluation of hemodynamic changes in eclampsia. *Am J Obstet Gynecol* 1984; 150:506–512.

53. Belfort M, Uys P, Dommisse J, et al: Haemodynamic changes in gestational proteinuric hypertension: The effects of rapid volume expansion and vasodilator therapy. *Br J Obstet Gynaecol* 1989; 96:634–641.

54. Cotton DB, Lee W, Huhta JC, et al: Hemodynamic profile of severe pregnancy-induced hypertension. *Am J Obstet Gynecol* 1988; 158:523–529.

55. Mabie WC, Ratts TE, Sibai BM: The central hemodynamics of severe preeclampsia. *Am J Obstet Gynecol* 1989; 161:1443–1448.

56. Chesley LC, Lindheimer MD: Renal hemodynamics and intravascular volume in normal and hypertensive pregnancy, in Rubin PC (ed): *Handbook of Hypertension: vol 10, Hypertension in Pregnancy.* Amsterdam, Elsevier Science Publishers, 1988, pp 38–65.

57. Nisell H, Hjemdahl P, Linde B: Cardiovascular responses to circulating catecholamines in normal pregnancy and in pregnancy-induced hypertension. *Clin Physiol* 1985; 5:479–493.

58. Hays PM, Cruikshank DW, Dunn LJ: Plasma volume determination in normal and preeclamptic pregnancies. *Am J Obstet Gynecol* 1985; 151:958–966.

59. Oian P, Maltau JM, Noddeland H, et al: Transcapillary fluid balance in preeclampsia. *Br J Obstet Gynaecol* 1986; 93:235–239.

60. Zinaman M, Rubin J, Lindheimer MD:

Serial plasma oncotic pressure levels and echoencephalography during and after delivery in severe pre-eclampsia. *Lancet* 1985; 1:1245–1247.

61. Lindheimer MD, Katz AI. The kidney and hypertension in pregnancy, in Brenner BM, Rector FC Jr (eds): *The Kidney,* ed 4. Philadelphia, WB Saunders Co, 1990.

62. Gaber LW, Spargo BH: Pregnancy-induced nephropathy: The significance of focal segmental glomerulosclerosis. *Am J Kidney Dis* 1987; 9:317–323.

63. Brown MA: Sodium and plasma volume regulation in normal and hypertensive pregnancy: A review of physiology and clinical implications. *Clin Exp Hypertens Pregnancy* 1988; B7:265–282.

64. Clark SL, Greenspoon JS, Aldahl D, et al: Severe preeclampsia with persistent oliguria: Management of hemodynamic subsets. *Am J Obstet Gynecol* 1986; 154:490–494.

65. Hill LM: Metabolism of uric acid in normal and toxemic pregnancy. *Mayo Clin Proc* 1978; 53:743–751.

66. Barron WM, Lindheimer MD: Renal sodium and water handling in pregnancy. *Obstet Gynecol Annu* 1984; 13:35–69.

67. Winkel CA, Simpson ER, Milewich L, et al: Deoxycorticosterone biosynthesis in human kidney: Potential for formation of a potent mineralocorticosteroid in its site of action. *Proc Natl Acad Sci* USA 1980; 77:7069–7073.

68. Winkel CA, Casey ML, Guerami A: Ratio of plasma deoxycorticosterone (DOC) levels to plasma progesterone (P) levels in pregnant women who did or did not develop pregnancy-induced hypertension, (abstract). Presented at the Society for Gynecologic Investigation 30th annual meeting, Washington, D.C., 1983, p 185.

69. Miyamoto S, Shimokawa S, Sumioki H, et al: Physiologic role of endogenous human atrial natriuretic peptide in preeclamptic pregnancies. *Am J Obstet Gynecol* 1989; 160:155–159.

70. Bond AL, August P, Druzin ML, et al: Atrial natriuretic factor in normal and hypertensive pregnancy. *Am J Obstet Gynecol* 1989; 160:1112–1116.

71. Sibai BM, Anderson GD, McCubbin JH: Eclampsia: II. Clinical significance of laboratory findings. *Obstet Gynecol* 1982; 59:153–157.

72. Sheehan HL, Lynch JB: *Pathology of Toxaemia of Pregnancy.* London, Churchill, 1973.

73. Rolfes DB, Ishak KG: Liver disease in toxemia of pregnancy. *Am J Gastroenterol* 1989; 81:1138–1144.

74. Manas KJ, Welsh JD, Rankin RA, et al: Hepatic hemorrhage without rupture in preeclampsia. *N Engl J Med* 1985; 312:424–426.

75. Minakami H, Oka N, Sato T, et al: Preeclampsia: A microvesicular fat disease of the liver? *Am J Obstet Gynecol* 1988; 159:1043–1047.

76. Riely CA, Latham PS, Romero R, et al: Acute fatty liver of pregnancy. *Ann Intern Med* 1987; 106:703–706.

77. Donaldson JO: *Neurology of Pregnancy,* ed 2. Philadelphia, WB Saunders Co, 1989.

78. Sibai BM: Eclampsia, in Rubin PC (ed): *Handbook of Hypertension: vol 10, Hypertension in Pregnancy.* Amsterdam, Elsevier Science Publishers, 1988, pp 320–340.

79. Brown CEL, Purdy P, Cunningham FG: Head computed tomographic scans in women with eclampsia. *Am J Obstet Gynecol* 1988; 159:915–920.

80. Crawford S, Varner MW, Digre KB, et al: Cranial magnetic resonance imaging in eclampsia. *Obstet Gynecol* 1987; 70:474–477.

81. Sibai BM, Spinnato JA, Watson DL, et al: Effect of magnesium sulfate on electroencephalographic findings in preeclampsia-eclampsia. *Obstet Gynecol* 1984; 64:261–266.

82. Fox H: The placenta in pregnancy hypertension, in Rubin PC (ed): *Handbook of Hypertension: vol 10, Hypertension in Pregnancy.* Amsterdam, Elsevier Science Publishers, 1988, pp 16–37.

83. El-Roeiy A, Gleicher N: The immunologic concept of pre-eclampsia, in Rubin PC (ed): *Handbook of Hypertension: vol 10, Hypertension in Pregnancy.* Amsterdam, Elsevier Science Publishers, 1988, pp 257–266.

84. Ware BD, Andres R, Digre KB, et al: The association of antiphospholipid antibodies with severe preeclampsia. *Obstet Gynecol* 1989; 73:541–545.

85. Weiner CP: Clotting alterations associated with the pre-eclampsia/eclampsia syndrome, in Rubin PC (ed): *Handbook of Hy-*

pertension: vol 10, Hypertension in Pregnancy. Amsterdam, Elsevier Science Publishers, 1988, pp 241–256.

86. Pritchard JA, Cunningham FG, Mason RA: Coagulation changes in eclampsia: Their frequency and pathogenesis. *Am J Obstet Gynecol* 1976; 124:855–864.

87. Redman CWG, Bonnar J, Beilin L: Early platelet consumption in pre-eclampsia. *Br Med J* 1978; 1:467–469.

88. Rodgers GM, Taylor RN, Roberts JM: Preeclampsia is associated with a serum factor cytotoxic to human endothelial cells. *Am J Obstet Gynecol* 1988; 159:908–914.

89. Taufield PA, Ales KL, Resnick LM, et al: Hypocalciuria in preeclampsia. *N Engl J Med* 1987; 316:715–718.

90. Entman SS, Kambam R, Bradley CA, et al: Increased levels of carboxyhemoglobin and serum iron as an indicator of increased red cell turnover in preeclampsia. *Am J Obstet Gynecol* 1987; 156:1169–1173.

91. Maymon R, Bahari C, Moroz C: Placental isoferritin: A new serum marker in toxemia of pregnancy. *Am J Obstet Gynecol* 1989; 160:681–684.

92. Ballegeer V, Spitz B, Kieckens L, et al: Predictive value of increased plasma levels of fibronectin in gestational hypertension. *Am J Obstet Gynecol* 1989; 161:432–436.

92a. Martin JN Jr, Files JC, Blake PG, et al: Plasma exchange for preeclampsia: I. Postpartum use for persistently severe pre-eclampsia-eclampsia with HELLP syndrome. *Am J Obstet Gynecol* 1990; 162:126–137.

93. Collins R, Yusuf S, Peto R: Overview of randomised trials of diuretics in pregnancy. *Br Med J* 1985; 290:17–23.

94. Chesley LC: The control of hypertension in pregnancy. *Obstet Gynecol Annu* 1981; 10:69–84.

95. Minkowitz S, Soloway HB, Hall JE, et al: Fatal hemorrhagic pancreatitis following chlorothiazide administration in pregnancy. *Obstet Gynecol* 1964; 24:337–342.

96. Miller Jr JN: Hyponatremia: A complication of the treatment of the edema of pregnancy. *Obstet Gynecol* 1960; 16:587–590.

97. Pritchard JA, Walley PJ: Severe hypokalemia due to prolonged administration of chlorothiazide during pregnancy. *Am J Obstet Gynecol* 1961; 81:1241–1244.

98. Rodriquez SUI, Leikin SL, Hiller MC: Neonatal thrombocytopenia associated with ante-partum administration of thiazide drugs. *N Engl J Med* 1964; 270:881–884.

99. Mule JG, Tatum HJ, Sawyer RE: "Nitrogenous retention" in patients with toxemia of pregnancy—an unusual complication of salt restriction. *Am J Obstet Gynecol* 1957; 74:526–537.

100. Palomaki JF, Lindheimer MD: Sodium depletion simulating deterioration in a toxemia pregnancy. *N Engl J Med* 1970; 282:88–89.

101. MacGillivray I, Hytten FE, Taggart N, et al: The effect of a sodium diuretic on total exchangeable sodium and total body water in pre-eclamptic toxaemia. *Br J Obstet Gynaecol* 1962; 69:458–462.

102. Gant NF, Madden JD, Siiteri PK, et al: The metabolic clearance rate of dehydro-isoandrosterone sulfate: III. The effect of thiazide diuretics in normal and future preeclamptic pregnancies. *Am J Obstet Gynecol* 1975; 123:159–163.

103. Rubin PC, Butters L, Clark DM, et al: Placebo-controlled trial of atenolol in treatment of pregnancy-associated hypertension. *Lancet* 1983; 1:431–434.

104. Wichman K, Ryden G, Karlberg B: A placebo controlled trial of metoprolol in the treatment of hypertension in pregnancy. *Scand J Clin Lab Invest* 1984; 44(suppl 169):90–95.

105. Redman CWG, Beilin LJ, Bonnar J, et al: Fetal outcome in trial of antihypertensive treatment in pregnancy. *Lancet* 1976; 1:753–756.

106. Hogstedt S, Lindeberg S, Axelsson O, et al: A prospective controlled trial of metoprolol-hydralazine treatment in hypertension during pregnancy. *Acta Obstet Gynecol Scand* 1985; 64:505–510.

107. Plouin PF, Breart G, Llado J, et al: A randomized comparison of early with conservative use of antihypertensive drugs in the management of pregnancy-induced hypertension. *Br J Obstet Gynaecol* 1990; 97:134–141.

108. Sibai BM, Mabie WC, Shamsa F, et al: A comparison of no medication versus methyldopa or labetalol in chronic hypertension during pregnancy. *Am J Obstet Gynecol* 1990; 162:960–967.

109. Belizan JM, Villar J, Repke J: The rela-

tionship between calcium intake and pregnancy-induced hypertension: Up-to-date evidence. *Am J Obstet Gynecol* 1988; 158:898–902.

110. Kawasaki N, Matsui K, Ito M, et al: Effect of calcium supplementation on the vascular sensitivity to angiotension II in pregnant women. *Am J Obstet Gynecol* 1985; 153:576–582.

111. López-Jaramillo P, Narvaez M, Weigel RM, et al: Calcium supplementation reduces the risk of pregnancy-induced hypertension in an Andes population. *Br J Obstet Gynaecol* 1989; 96:648–655.

112. Sibai BM, Villar MA, Bray E: Magnesium supplementation during pregnancy: A double-blind randomized controlled clinical trial. *Am J Obstet Gynecol* 1989; 161:115–119.

113. Ylikorkala O, Makila UM, Kaapa P, et al: Maternal ingestion of acetylsalicylic acid inhibits fetal and neonatal prostacyclin and thromboxane in humans. *Am J Obstet Gynecol* 1986; 155:345–349.

114. Sibai BM, Mirro R, Chesney CM, et al: Low-dose aspirin in pregnancy. *Obstet Gynecol* 1989; 74:551–557.

115. Benigni A, Gregorini G, Frusca T, et al: Effect of low-dose aspirin on fetal and maternal generation of thromboxane by platelets in women at risk for pregnancy-induced hypertension. *N Engl J Med* 1989; 321:357–362.

116. Schiff E, Peleg E, Goldenberg M, et al: The use of aspirin to prevent pregnancy-induced hypertension and lower the ratio of thromboxane A2 to prostacyclin in relatively high risk pregnancies. *N Engl J Med* 1989; 321:351–356.

117. Wallenburg HCS, Dekker GA, Makovitz JW, et al: Low-dose aspirin prevents pregnancy-induced hypertension and pre-eclampsia in angiotensin-sensitive primigravidae. *Lancet* 1986; 1:1–3.

118. Lewis PJ, Bulpitt CJ, Zuspan FP: A comparison of current British and American practice in the management of hypertension in pregnancy. *J Obstet Gynaecol* 1980; 1:78–82.

119. Redman CWG, Beilin LJ, Bonnar J: Treatment of hypertension in pregnancy with methyldopa: Blood pressure control and side effects. *Br J Obstet Gynaecol* 1977; 84:419–426.

120. Fletcher AE, Bulpitt CJ: A review of clinical trials in pregnancy hypertension, in Rubin PC (ed): *Handbook of Hypertension: vol 10, Hypertension in Pregnancy.* Amsterdam Elsevier, 1988, pp 186–201.

121. Leather HM, Baker P, Humphreys DM, et al: A controlled trial of hypotensive agents in hypertension in pregnancy. *Lancet* 1968; 2:488–490.

122. Walker JJ, Crooks A, Erwin L, et al: Labetalol in pregnancy-induced hypertension: Fetal and maternal effects, in Riley A, Symonds EM (eds): *The Investigation of Labetalol in the Management of Hypertension in Pregnancy.* Amsterdam, Excerpta Medica, 1982, pp 148–160.

123. Ferris TF: Toxemia and hypertension, in Burrow GN, Ferris TF (eds): *Medical Complications During Pregnancy,* ed 3. Philadelphia, WB Saunders Co, 1988, pp 1–33.

124. Briggs GG, Freeman RK, Yaffe SJ: *Drugs in Pregnancy and Lactation: A Reference Guide to Fetal and Neonatal Risk,* ed 2. Baltimore, Williams & Wilkins, 1986.

125. Mallie JP, Coulon G, Billerey C, et al: In utero aminoglycosides-induced nephrotoxicity in rat neonates. *Kidney Int* 1988; 33:36–44.

126. Venuto RC, Cox JW, Stein JH, et al: The effect of changes in perfusion pressure on uteroplacental blood flow in the pregnant rabbit. *J Clin Invest* 1976; 57:938–941.

127. Ladner C, Brinkman CR III, Weston P, et al: Dynamics of uterine circulation in pregnant and nonpregnant sheep. *Am J Physiol* 1970; 218:257–263.

128. deSwiet M, Hoffbrand BI: Effect of bethanidine on placental blood flow in conscious rabbits. *Am J Obstet Gynecol* 1971; 111:374–378.

129. Greiss FC Jr: Uterine pressure-flow relationships, in Moawad AH, Lindheimer MD (eds): *Uterine and Placental Blood Flow.* New York, Masson Publishing USA, 1982, pp 67–71.

130. Gallery EDM, Saunders DM, Hunyor SN, et al: Randomised comparison of methyldopa and oxprenolol for treatment of hypertension in pregnancy. *Br Med J* 1979; 1:1591–1594.

131. Cunningham FG, MacDonald PC, Gant NF: *Williams Obstetrics,* ed 18. East Norwalk, Conn, Appleton-Century-Crofts, 1989.

132. Naden RP, Redman CWG: Antihyperten-

sive drugs in pregnancy. *Clin Perinatol* 1985; 12:521–538.

133. Gant NF, Worley RJ: *Hypertension in Pregnancy: Concepts and Management*. New York, Appleton-Century-Crofts, 1980.

134. Sibai BM, Taslimi M, Abdella TN, et al: Maternal and perinatal outcome of conservative management of severe preeclampsia in midtrimester. *Am J Obstet Gynecol* 1985; 152:32–37.

135. Vink GJ, Moodley JH, Philpott RH: Effect of dihydralazine on the fetus in the treatment of maternal hypertension. *Obstet Gynecol* 1980; 55:519–522.

136. Mabie WC, Gonzalez AR, Sibai BM, et al: A comparative trial of labetalol and hydralazine in the acute management of severe hypertension complicating pregnancy. *Obstet Gynecol* 1987; 70:328–333.

137. Kuzniar J, Skret A, Piela A, et al: Hemodynamic effects of intravenous hydralazine in pregnant women with severe hypertension. *Obstet Gynecol* 1985; 66:453–458.

138. Pritchard JA, Cunningham FG, Pritchard SA: The Parkland Memorial Hospital protocol for treatment of eclampsia: Evaluation of 245 cases. *Am J Obstet Gynecol* 1984; 148:951–963.

139. Assali NS, Kaplan S, Oighenstein S, et al: Hemodynamic effects of 1-hydrazinophthalazine (Apresoline) in human pregnancy: Results of intravenous administration. *J Clin Invest* 1953; 32:922–930.

140. Lipshitz J, Ahokas RA, Reynolds SL: The effect of hydralazine on placental perfusion in the spontaneously hypertensive rat. *Am J Obstet Gynecol* 1987; 156:356–359.

141. Ring G, Krames E, Shnider SM, et al: Comparison of nitroprusside and hydralazine in hypertensive pregnant ewes. *Obstet Gynecol* 1977; 50:598–602.

142. Ladner CN, Weston PV, Brinkman CR III, et al: Effects of hydralazine on uteroplacental and fetal circulations. *Am J Obstet Gynecol* 1970; 108:375–381.

143. Suonio S, Saarikoski S, Tahvanainen K, et al: Acute effects of dihydralazine mesylate, furosemide, and metoprolol on maternal hemodynamics in pregnancy-induced hypertension. *Am J Obstet Gynecol* 1986; 155:122–125.

144. Jouppila P, Kirkinen P, Koivula A, et al: Effects of dihydralazine infusion on the fetoplacental blood flow and maternal pros-

tanoids. *Obstet Gynecol* 1985; 65:115–118.

145. Gant NF, Madden JD, Siiteri PK, et al: The metabolic clearance rate of dehydroisoandrosterone sulfate. *Am J Obstet Gynecol* 1976; 124:143–148.

146. Lunell NO, Lewander R, Nylund L, et al: Acute effect of dihydralazine on uteroplacental blood flow in hypertension during pregnancy. *Gynecol Obstet Invest* 1983; 16:274–282.

147. Girard H, Brun J-L, Muffat-Joly M: An angiographic study of the sensitivity to epinephrine of the uterine arteries of the guinea pig: A comparison with angiotensin. *Am J Obstet Gynecol* 1971; 111:687–691.

148. Wallenburg HCS, Hutchinson DL: A radioangiographic study of the effects of catecholamines on uteroplacental blood flow in the Rhesus monkey. *J Med Primatol* 1979; 8:57–65.

149. Jansson T: Responsiveness to norepinephrine of the vessels supplying the placenta of growth-retarded fetuses. *Am J Obstet Gynecol* 1988; 158:1233–1237.

150. Cotton DB, Gonik B, Dorman KF: Cardiovascular alterations in severe pregnancy-induced hypertension seen with an intravenously given hydralazine bolus. *Surg Gynecol Obstet* 1985; 161:240–244.

151. Walker JJ, Greer I, Calder AA: Treatment of acute pregnancy-related hypertension: Labetalol and hydralazine compared. *Postgrad Med J* 1983; 59:168–170.

152. Davey DA, Dommisse J, Garden A: Intravenous labetalol and intravenous dihydralazine in severe hypertension in pregnancy, in Riley A, Symonds EM (eds): *The Investigation of Labetalol in the Management of Hypertension in Pregnancy*. Amsterdam, Excerpta Medica, 1982, pp 51–61.

153. Ashe RG, Moodley J, Richards AM, et al: Comparison of labetalol and dihydrallazine in hypertensive emergencies of pregnancy. *S Afr Med J* 1987; 71:354–356.

154. Lunell NO, Nylund L, Lewander R, et al: Acute effect of an antihypertensive drug, labetalol, on uteroplacental blood flow. *Br J Obstet Gynaecol* 1982; 89:640–644.

155. Jouppila P, Kirkinen P, Koivula A, et al: Labetalol does not alter the placental and fetal blood flow or maternal prostanoids in pre-eclampsia. *Br J Obstet Gynaecol* 1986; 93:543–547.

156. Joelsson I, Barton MD: The effect of

blockade of the beta receptors of the sympathetic nervous system of the fetus. *Acta Obstet Gynecol Scand* 1969; 48(suppl 3):75–79.

157. Reuss ML, Parer JT, Harris JL, et al: Hemodynamic effects of alpha-adrenergic blockade during hypoxia in fetal sheep. *Am J Obstet Gynecol* 1982; 142:410–415.

158. Cottle MKW, Van Petten GR, van Muyden P: Maternal and fetal cardiovascular indices during fetal hypoxia due to cord compression in chronically cannulated sheep. *Am J Obstet Gynecol* 1983; 146:678–685.

159. Kjellmer I, Dagbjartsson A, Hrbek A, et al: Maternal beta-adreneceptor blockade reduces fetal tolerance to asphyxia. *Acta Obstet Gynecol Scand* 1984; 118:75–80.

160. Walters BNJ, Redman CWG: Treatment of severe pregnancy-associated hypertension with the calcium antagonist nifedipine. *Br J Obstet Gynaecol* 1984; 91:330–336.

161. Rubin PC, Butters L, McCabe R: Nifedipine and platelets in preeclampsia. *Am J Hypertens* 1988; 1:175–177.

162. Veille JC, Bissonnette JM, Hohimer AR: The effect of a calcium channel blocker (nifedipine) on uterine blood flow in the pregnant goat. *Am J Obstet Gynecol* 1986; 154:1160–1163.

163. Harake B, Gilbert RD, Ashwal S, et al: Nifedipine: Effects on fetal and maternal hemodynamics in pregnant sheep. *Am J Obstet Gynecol* 1987; 157:1003–1008.

164. Read MD, Wellby DE: The use of a calcium antagonist (nifedipine) to suppress preterm labour. *Br J Obstet Gynaecol* 1986; 93:933–937.

165. Golichowski AM, Hathaway DR, Fineberg N, et al: Tocolytic and hemodynamic effects of nifedipine in the ewe. *Am J Obstet Gynecol* 1985; 151:1134–1140.

166. Constantine G, Beevers DG, Reynolds AL, et al: Nifedipine as a second line antihypertensive drug in pregnancy. *Br J Obstet Gynaecol* 1987; 94:1136–1142.

167. Harrison GL, Moore LG: Blunted vasoreactivity in pregnant guinea pigs is not restored by meclofenamate. *Am J Obstet Gynecol* 1989; 160:258–264.

168. Snyder SW, Cardwell MS: Neuromuscular blockade with magnesium sulfate and nifedipine. *Am J Obstet Gynecol* 1989; 161:35–36.

169. Neuman J, Weiss B, Rabello Y, et al: Diazoxide for the acute control of severe hypertension complicating pregnancy: A pilot study. *Obstet Gynecol* 1979; 53:S50–S55.

170. Morris JA, Arce JJ, Hamilton CJ, et al: The management of severe preeclampsia and eclampsia with intravenous diazoxide. *Obstet Gynecol* 1977; 49:675–680.

171. Thien TH, Koene RAP, Schijf CH, et al: Infusion of diazoxide in severe hypertension during pregnancy. *Eur J Obstet Gynecol Reprod Biol* 1980; 10(6):367–374.

172. Ram CV, Kaplan NM: Individual titration of diazoxide dosage in the treatment of severe hypertension. *Am J Cardiol* 1979; 43:627–630.

173. Sankar D, Moodley J: Low-dose diazoxide in the emergency management of severe hypertension in pregnancy. *S Afr Med J* 1984; 65:279–280.

174. Dudley DKL: Minibolus diazoxide in the management of severe hypertension in pregnancy. *Am J Obstet Gynecol* 1985; 151:196–200.

175. Nuwayhid B, Brinkman CR III, Katchen B, et al: Maternal and fetal hemodynamic effects of diazoxide. *Obstet Gynecol* 1975; 46:197–203.

176. Caritis SN, Morishima HO, Stark RI, et al: The effect of diazoxide on uterine blood flow in pregnant sheep. *Obstet Gynecol* 1976; 48:464–468.

177. Wallenburg HCS, Kuijken JPJA: Effects of diazoxide on maternal and fetal circulations in normotensive and hypertensive pregnant sheep. *J Perinat Med* 1984; 12:85–95.

178. Landesman R, deSouza FJA, Coutinho EM, et al: The inhibitory effect of diazoxide in normal term labor. *Am J Obstet Gynecol* 1969; 103:430–433.

179. Morishima HO, Caritis SN, Yeh MN, et al: Prolonged infusion of diazoxide in the management of premature labor in the baboon. *Obstet Gynecol* 1976; 48:203–207.

180. Boulos BM, Davis LE, Almond CH, et al: Placental transfer of diazoxide and its hazardous effect on the newborn. *J Clin Pharmacol* 1971; 11:206–210.

181. Stempel JE, O'Grady JP, Morton MJ, et al: Use of sodium nitroprusside in compli-

cations of gestational hypertension. *Obstet Gynecol* 1982; 60:533–538.

182. Shoemaker CT, Meyers M: Sodium nitroprusside for control of severe hypertensive disease of pregnancy: A case report and discussion of potential toxicity. *Am J Obstet Gynecol* 1984; 149:171–173.

183. Naulty J, Cefalo RC, Lewis PE: Fetal toxicity of nitroprusside in the pregnant ewe. *Am J Obstet Gynecol* 1981; 139:708–711.

184. Ellis SC, Wheeler AS, James FM III, et al: Fetal and maternal effects of sodium nitroprusside used to counteract hypertension in gravid ewes. *Am J Obstet Gynecol* 1982; 143:766–770.

185. Sehgal NN, Hitt JR: Plasma volume expansion in the treatment of pre-eclampsia. *Am J Obstet Gynecol* 1980; 138:165–168.

186. Gallery EDM, Delprado W, Gyory AZ: Antihypertensive effect of plasma volume expansion in pregnancy-associated hypertension. *Aust N Z J Med* 1981; 11:20–24.

187. Gallery EDM, Mitchell MDM, Redman CWG: Fall in blood pressure in response to volume expansion in pregnancy-associated hypertension (pre-eclampsia): Why does it occur? *J Hyperten* 1984; 2:177–182.

188. Joyce JH III, Debnath KS, Baker EA: Preeclampsia—relationship of CVP and epidural analgesia. *Anesthesiology* 1979; 510:S297.

189. Jouppila P, Jouppila R, Koivula A: Albumin infusion does not alter the intervillous blood flow in severe pre-eclampsia. *Acta Obstet Gynecol Scand* 1983; 62:345–348.

190. Wasserstrum N, Kirshon B, Willis RS, et al: Quantitative hemodynamic effects of acute volume expansion in severe pre-eclampsia. *Obstet Gynecol* 1989; 73:546–550.

191. Grunfeld J-P, Pertuiset N: Acute renal failure in pregnancy: 1987. *Am J Kidney Dis* 1987; 69:359–362.

192. Sibai BM, Mabie BC, Harvey CJ, et al: Pulmonary edema in severe preeclampsia-eclampsia: Analysis of 37 consecutive cases. *Am J Obstet Gynecol* 1987; 156:1174–1179.

193. Benedetti TJ, Kates R, Williams V: Hemodynamic observations in severe preeclampsia complicated by pulmonary edema. *Am J Obstet Gynecol* 1985; 152:330–334.

194. Benedetti TJ, Quilligan EJ: Cerebral edema in severe pregnancy-induced hypertension. *Am J Obstet Gynecol* 1980; 137:860–862.

195. Gonik B, Cotton D, Spillman T, et al: Peripartum colloid osmotic pressure changes: Effects of controlled fluid management. *Am J Obstet Gynecol* 1985; 151:12–15.

196. Cotton DB, Gonik B, Dorman K, et al: Cardiovascular alterations in severe pregnancy-induced hypertension: relationship of central venous pressure to pulmonary capillary wedge pressure. *Am J Obstet Gynecol* 1985; 151:762–764.

197. Clark SL, Cotton DB: Clinical indications for pulmonary artery catheterization in the patient with severe preeclampsia. *Am J Obstet Gynecol* 1988; 158:453–458.

198. Cotton DB, Gonik B, Dorman KF: Cardiovascular alterations in severe pregnancy-induced hypertension: Acute effects of intravenous magnesium sulfate. *Am J Obstet Gynecol* 1984; 148:162–165.

199. Dinsdale HB: Does magnesium sulfate treat eclamptic seizures?. *Arch Neurol* 1989; 45:1360–1361.

200. Kaplan PW, Lesser RP, Fisher RS, et al: No, magnesium sulfate should not be used in treating eclamptic seizures. *Arch Neurol* 1988; 45:1361–1364.

201. Borges LF, Gucer G: Effect of magnesium on epileptic foci. *Epilepsia* 1978; 19:81–91.

202. Koontz WL, Reid KH: Effect of parenteral magnesium sulfate on penicillin-induced seizure foci in anesthetized cats. *Am J Obstet Gynecol* 1985; 153:96–99.

203. Watson KV, Moldow CF, Ogburn PL, et al: Magnesium sulfate: Rationale for its use in preeclampsia. *Proc Natl Acad Sci* 1986; 83:1075–1078.

204. Nadler JL, Goodson S, Rude RK: Evidence that prostacyclin mediates the vascular action of magnesium in humans. *Hypertension* 1987; 9:379–383.

205. Ryan G, Lange IR, Naugler MA: Clinical experience with phenytoin prophylaxis in severe preeclampsia. *Am J Obstet Gynecol* 1989; 161:1297–1304.

206. Slater RM, Smith WD, Patrick J, et al: Phenytoin infusion in severe pre-eclampsia. *Lancet* 1987; 1:1417–1421.

207. Tuffnel D, O'Donovan P, Lilford RJ, et al:

Phenytoin in pre-eclampsia. *Lancet* 1989; 2:273–274.

208. Sibai BM: Magnesium sulfate is the ideal anticonvulsant in preeclampsia-eclampsia. *Am J Obstet Gynecol* 1990; 162:1141–1145.

209. Cree JE, Meyer J, Hailey DM: Diazepam in labour: Its metabolism and effect on the clinical condition and thermogenesis of the newborn. *Br Med J* 1973; 4:251–255.

210. Stone SR, Pritchard JA: Effect of maternally administered magnesium sulfate on the neonate. *Obstet Gynecol* 1970; 35:574–577.

211. Kaplan NM: *Clinical Hypertension*, ed 5. Baltimore, Williams & Wilkins, 1990.

212. Chesley LC, Annitto JE: Pregnancy in the patient with hypertensive disease. *Am J Obstet Gynecol* 1947; 53:372–381.

213. Landesman R, Halpern M, Knapp RC: Renal artery lesions associated with the toxemias of pregnancy. *Obstet Gynecol* 1961; 18:645–652.

214. Sellars L, Siamopoulos K, Wilkinson R: Prognosis for pregnancy after correction of renovascular hypertension. *Nephron* 1985; 39:280–281.

215. Millar JA, Wilson PD, Morrison N: Management of severe hypertension in pregnancy by a combined drug regimen including captopril: Case report. *N Z Med J* 1983; 96:796–798.

216. Cockburn J, Moar VA, Ounsted M, et al: Final report of study on hypertension during pregnancy: The effects of specific treatment on the growth and development of the children. *Lancet* 1982; 1:647–649.

217. Livingstone I, Craswell PW, Bevan EB, et al: Propranolol in pregnancy—three year prospective study. *Clin Exp Hypertens Pregnancy* 1983; B2:341–350.

218. Fidler J, Smith V, Fayers P, et al: Randomised controlled comparative study of methyldopa and oxprenolol in treatment of hypertension in pregnancy. *Br Med J* 1983; 286:1927–1930.

219. Gallery EDM, Ross MR, Gyory AZ: Antihypertensive treatment in pregnancy: Analysis of different responses to oxprenolol and methyldopa. *Br Med J* 1985; 291:563–566.

220. Horvath JS, Phippard A, Korda A, et al: Clonidine hydrochloride—A safe and effective antihypertensive agent in pregnancy. *Obstet Gynecol* 1985; 66:634–638.

221. Mutch LMM, Moar VA, Ounsted MK, et al: Hypertension during pregnancy, with and without specific hypotensive treatment. II. The growth and development of the infant in the first year of life. *Early Hum Dev* 1977; 1(1):59–67.

222. Mutch LMM, Moar VA, Ounsted MK, et al: Hypertension during pregnancy, with and without specific hypotensive treatment. I. Perinatal factors and neonatal morbidity. *Early Hum Dev* 1977; 1(1):47–57.

223. Bodis J, Sulyok E, Ertl T, et al: Methyldopa in pregnancy hypertension and the newborn. *Lancet* 1982; 2:498–499.

224. Hoskins EJ, Friedman WF: Influence of maternal alpha-methyldopa on sympathetic innervation in the newborn rabbit heart. *Am J Obstet Gynecol* 1980; 137:496–498.

225. Ounsted MK, Moar VA, Good FJ, et al: Hypertension during pregnancy with and without specific treatment: The development of the children at the age of 4 years. *Br J Obstet Gynaecol* 1980; 87:19–24.

226. Huisjes JH, Hadders-Algra M, Touwen BCL: Is clonidine a behavioural teratogen in the human? *Early Hum Dev* 1986; 14:43–48.

227. Sandstrom B: Adrenergic beta-receptor blockers in hypertension of pregnancy. *Clin Exp Hypertens Pregnancy* 1982; 1:127–141.

228. Bott-Kanner G, Schweitzr A, Reisner SH, et al: Propranolol and hydrallazine in the management of essential hypertension in pregnancy. *Br J Obstet Gynaecol* 1980; 87:110–114.

229. Rosenfeld J, Bott-Kanner G, Boner G, et al: Treatment of hypertension during pregnancy with hydralazine monotherapy or with combined therapy with hydralazine and pindolol. *Eur J Obstet Gynecol Reprod Biol* 1986; 22:197–204.

230. Widerlov E, Karlman I, Storsater J: Hydralazine-induced neonatal thrombocytopenia. *N Engl J Med* 1980; 303:1235.

231. Cottrill CM, McAllister RG Jr, Gettes L, et al: Propranolol therapy during pregnancy, labor, and delivery: Evidence for transplacental drug transfer and impaired neonatal drug disposition. *J Pediatr* 1977; 91:812–814.

232. Gladstone GW, Hordof A, Gersony WM: Propranolol administration during preg-

nancy: Effects on the fetus. *Pediatrics* 1975; 86:962–964.

233. Lieberman BA, Stirrat GM, Cohen SL, et al: The possible adverse effect of propranolol on the fetus in pregnancies complicated by severe hypertension. *Br J Obstet Gynaecol* 1978; 85:678–683.

234. Eliahou HE, Silverberg DS, Reisin E, et al: Propranolol for the treatment of hypertension in pregnancy. *Br J Obstet Gynaecol* 1978; 85:431–436.

235. Habib A, McCarthy JS: Effects on the neonate of propranolol administered during pregnancy. *J Pediatr* 1977; 91:808–811.

236. Pruyn SC, Phelan JP, Buchanan GC: Long-term propranolol therapy in pregnancy: Maternal and fetal outcome. *Am J Obstet Gynecol* 1979; 135:485–489.

237. Sandstrom B: Antihypertensive treatment with the adrenergic beta-receptor blocker metoprolol during pregnancy. *Gynecol Obstet Invest* 1978; 9:195–204.

238. Butters L, Kennedy S, Rubin P: Atenolol and fetal weight in chronic hypertension, (abstract). *Clin Exp Hypertens Pregnancy* 1989; B8:265.

239. Rubin PC: Beta-blockers in pregnancy. *N Engl J Med* 1981; 305:1323–1326.

240. Schrier RW: Pathogenesis of sodium and water retention in high-output and low-output cardiac failure, nephrotic syndrome, cirrhosis and pregnancy (first and second parts). *N Engl J Med* 1988; 319:1065–1072;1127–1334.

241. Lardoux H, Gerard J, Blazquez G, et al: Hypertension in pregnancy: Evaluation of two beta blockers atenolol and labetalol. *Eur Heart J* 1983; 4:35–40.

242. Taylor EA, Turner P: Anti-hypertensive therapy with propranolol during pregnancy and lactation. *Postgrad Med J* 1981; 57:427–430.

243. O'Hare MF, Murnaghan GA, Russell CJ, et al: Sotalol as a hypotensive agent in pregnancy. *Br J Obstet Gynaecol* 1980; 87:814–820.

244. Melander A, Niklasson B, Ingemarsson I, et al: Transplacental passage of atenolol in man. *Eur J Clin Pharmacol* 1978; 14:93–94.

245. Barden TP, Stander RW: Myometrial and cardiovascular effects of an adrenergic blocking drug in human pregnancy. *Am J Obstet Gynecol* 1968; 101:91–99.

246. Mahon WA, Reid DWJ, Day RA: The in vivo effects of beta adrenergic stimulation and blockade on the human uterus at term. *J Pharmacol Exp Ther* 1967; 156:178–185.

247. Harbert GM Jr, Spisso KR: Effect of adrenergic blockade on dynamics of the pregnant primate uterus (*Macaca mulatta*). *Am J Obstet Gynecol* 1981; 139:767–780.

248. Rubin PC, Butters L, Clark D, et al: Obstetric aspects of the use in pregnancy-associated hypertension of the B-adrenoceptor antagonist atenolol. *Am J Obstet Gynecol* 1984; 150:389–392.

249. Wichman K: Metoprolol in the treatment of mild to moderate hypertension in pregnancy—effects on fetal heart activity. *Clin Exp Hypertens Pregnancy* 1986; B5(2):195–202.

250. Reynolds B, Butters L, Evans J, et al: First year of life after the use of atenolol in pregnancy associated hypertension. *Arch Dis Child* 1984; 59:1061–1063.

251. Williams ER, Morrissey JR: A comparison of acebutolol with methyldopa in hypertensive pregnancy. *Pharmatherapeutica* 1983; 3:487–491.

252. Michael CA, Potter JM: A comparison of labetalol with other antihypertensive drugs in the treatment of hypertensive disease of pregnancy, in Riley A, Symonds EM (eds): *The Investigation of Labetalol in the Management of Hypertension in Pregnancy.* Amsterdam, Excerpta Medica, 1982, pp 111–122.

253. Redman CWG: A controlled trial of the treatment of hypertension in pregnancy: Labetalol compared with methyldopa, in Riley A, Symonds EM (eds): *The Investigation of Labetalol in the Management of Hypertension in Pregnancy.* Amsterdam, Excerpta Medica, 1982, pp 101–110.

254. Lubbe WF, Hodge JV: Combined α- and β-adrenoceptor antagonism with prazosin and oxprenolol in control of severe hypertension in pregnancy. *N Z Med J* 1981; 94:169–172.

255. Rubin PC, Butters L, Low RA, et al: Clinical pharmacological studies with prazosin during pregnancy complicated by hypertension. *Br J Clin Pharmacol* 1983; 16:543–547.

256. Dommisse J, Davey DA, Roos PJ: Prazo-

sin and oxprenolol therapy in pregnancy hypertension. *S Afr Med J* 1983; 64:231–233.

257. Devoe LD, O'Dell BE, Castillo RA, et al: Metastatic pheochromocytoma in pregnancy and fetal biophysical assessment after maternal administration of alpha-adrenergic, beta-adrenergic, and dopamine antagonist. *Obstet Gynecol* 1986; 68(suppl):S15-S18.

258. Venuto R, Burstein P, Schneider R: Pheochromocytoma: Antepartum diagnosis and management with tumor resection in the puerperium. *Am J Obstet Gynecol* 1984; 150:431–432.

259. Ulmsten U: Treatment of normotensive and hypertensive patients with preterm labor using oral nifedipine, a calcium antagonist. *Arch Gynecol* 1984; 236:69–72.

260. Greer IA, Walker JJ, Bjornsson S, et al: Second line therapy with nifedipine in severe pregnancy induced hypertension. *Clin Exp Hypertens Pregnancy* 1989; B8:277–292.

261. Broughton Pipkin F, Symonds EM, Turner SR: The effect of captopril (SQ14,225) upon mother and fetus in the chronically cannulated ewe and in the pregnant rabbit. *J Physiol (Lond)* 1982; 323:415–422.

262. Ferris TF, Weir EK: Effect of captopril on uterine blood flow and prostaglandin E synthesis in the pregnant rabbit. *J Clin Invest* 1983; 71:809–815.

263. Rosa FW, Bosco LA, Fossum-Graham C, et al: Neonatal anuria with maternal angiotensin-converting enzyme inhibition. *Obstet Gynecol* 1989; 74:371–374.

264. Schubiger G, Flury G, Nussberger J: Enalapril for pregnancy-induced hypertension: Acute renal failure in a neonate. *Ann Intern Med* 1988; 108:215–216.

265. Sibai BM, Grossman RA, Grossman HG: Effects of diuretics on plasma volume in pregnancies with long-term hypertension. *Am J Obstet Gynecol* 1984; 150:831–835.

266. Gallery EDM, Hunyor SN, Gyory AZ: Plasma volume contraction: A significant factor in both pregnancy-associated hypertension (preeclampsia) and chronic hypertension in pregnancy. *Q J Med* 1979; 192:593–602.

267. Schewitz LJ: Hypertension and renal disease in pregnancy. *Med Clin North Am* 1971; 55:47–69.

268. Committee on Drugs of the American Academy of Pediatrics: The transfer of drugs and other chemicals into human breast milk. *Pediatrics* 1983; 72:375–383.

269. White WB: Management of hypertension during lactation. *Hypertension* 1984; 6:297–300.

CHAPTER 2

Renal Disorders

Marshall D. Lindheimer
John M. Davison

"Children of women with renal disease used to be born dangerously, or not at all—not at all, if their doctors had their way."[1] This quotation from a *Lancet* editorial reflects the pessimism concerning pregnant women with kidney disorders as it existed 30 years ago. Such attitudes were based on a poorly documented and selective literature, and led to many unnecessary pregnancy terminations. The *Lancet* editorial also signaled a change toward views which are considerably more optimistic. Current opinion, based on several large, albeit retrospective studies, which survey over 1,000 patients whose diseases were confirmed by renal biopsy, have led to the view that most women who have minimal renal dysfunction can conceive with the knowledge that over 90% of their gestations will succeed, and that pregnancy will not have adverse effects on the natural history of their disease.

This chapter reviews management, obstetric course, and renal prognosis in women with a variety of urinary tract diseases. Also discussed are acute renal failure, dialysis, and transplantation in relation to gestation.

CHANGES IN THE URINARY TRACT AND VOLUME HOMEOSTASIS DURING PREGNANCY

Anatomic Alterations

Cognizance of the normal anatomic and physiologic changes affecting the urinary system in gestation is basic to our understanding the course of renal disease in pregnancy. The following is a brief summary of these changes focusing on their relevance to clinical circumstance.

Kidney volume, weight, and size increase in gestation, renal length increasing 1 cm when measured radiographically.[2-5] More striking changes, however, occur in the collecting system where calyces, renal pelves, and ureters all dilate markedly[2, 5-7] (Fig 2-1). Dilation, observed as early as the first trimester, is more marked on the right, affects 90% of women at term, and may persist 3 to 4 months post partum.[5, 6, 8, 9] The etiology of these changes, detailed elsewhere,[5-7] has been ascribed to both humoral (e.g., progesterone, estrogens, prostaglandins) and mechanical (the enlarged

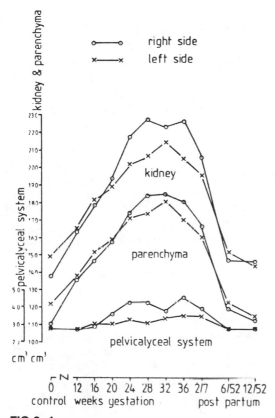

FIG 2–1.
Renal pelvicalyceal and parenchymal volumes throughout primigravid pregnancy measured by ultrasonic techniques. (Derivation of these values and their standard deviations can be found on Table IV of reference 4.) (From Cietak KA, Newton JR: *Br J Radiol* 1985; 58:405–413. Used by permission.)

uterus) factors. While ultrasonic evidence that dilation occurs before the uterus has enlarged sufficiently to become an obstructive factor favors the former view,[5, 8, 9] the bulk of the evidence supports the mechanical hypothesis. For instance, increased ureteral pressure, provoked by having third-trimester women stand or lie supine, is present above the pelvic brim, and falls rapidly when the obstructive effect of the enlarged uterus is removed by assumption of a lateral decubitus or knee-chest position, or by cesarean delivery of the fetus.[10] There are also elegant studies reported by Dure-Smith,[11] which note that ureteral dilation terminates at the level of the pelvic brim, suggesting that obstruction there is due to the uterus pressing on the ureter when it crosses the iliac artery. At this point, one may see a pyelographic filling defect termed the *iliac sign* (Fig 2–2).

The above-described anatomic changes have several clinical implications:

1. Acceptable norms of kidney size should be increased by 1 cm if estimated during pregnancy or in the immediate puerperium, and reductions in renal length noted several months post partum need not be attributed to pathologic decrements in renal parenchymal mass.

2. There may be substantial errors in the collection of timed urine volumes. This is because large quantities of urine may remain in the dilated collecting system, which, especially in hydropenic patients, results in large timing as well as collection errors. Such problems can be avoided by having the patient hydrated and positioned in lateral recumbency for 30 minutes to 1 hour prior to starting, and again before completing, a collection. Errors should thus be minimized because the same dead-space error will occur both when discarding urine prior to commencing and again when completing the collection, while production of a modest diuresis ensures that any residual urine in the urinary tract or bladder is dilute and of recent origin.

3. Urinary obstruction or stasis may explain why gravidas with symptomatic bacteriuria are more prone to develop frank pyelonephritis. There may also be a higher frequency of vesicoureteral reflux in pregnancy, which further disposes the pregnant women to symptomatic infection.[5]

4. Frank urinary tract obstruction may be difficult to diagnose during gestation. In this respect there is a "distention" syndrome in late pregnancy characterized by abdominal pain, marked hydronephrosis, and variable increases in serum creatinine levels, managed successfully by the placement of ureteral stents.[12, 13]

Functional Changes

Renal Hemodynamics

Alterations in renal hemodynamics are another striking feature of normal gestation.

Both glomerular filtration rate (GFR) and effective renal plasma flow (ERPF) increase to values 35% to 50% greater than those measured in nonpregnant women (reviewed in references 5, 14, 15). Twenty-four-hour creatinine clearances rise immediately after the first missed menstrual period, become significantly elevated by gestational week 4, and peak at levels 40% to 50% above preconception values at 9 to 11 weeks gestation. These increments are then sustained through gestational week 36, after which a decrease may occur (usually 20%, but sometimes nonpregnant levels are reached by term). Increases in GFR of a similar magnitude have also been confirmed during short-term inulin infusion studies.[5, 14, 15]

Effective renal plasma flow also increases markedly in pregnancy and is 50% to 80% above nonpregnant levels during the initial trimesters.[5, 14, 15] Near term ERPF decreases approximately 25% but is still considerably above nonpregnant values.

Reasons why renal hemodynamics increase during pregnancy are obscure, and various hypotheses are discussed by us elsewhere.[5, 16] Of interest, the stimulus appears maternal in origin,[16] and micropuncture studies in the rat demonstrate that gestational vasodilation involves even reductions in the tone of the pre- and postglomerular arterioles so that intraglomerular blood pressure is maintained constant.[5, 16, 17] If the latter is true in humans, it would suggest that 9 months of

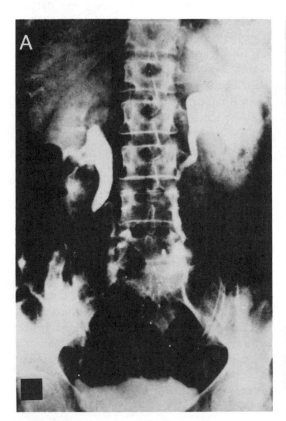 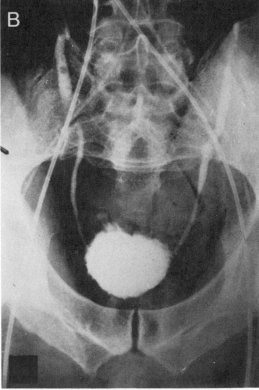

FIG 2–2.
A, intravenous pyelogram demonstrating ureteral dilation in pregnancy. There is a sharp cutoff of each ureter at the pelvic brim where it crosses the iliac artery (the "iliac sign"). **B,** the relationships of the uterus and iliac arteries at the pelvic brim demonstrated in postmortem injection studies which suggest an explanation of the iliac sign. (From Dure-Smith P: *Radiology* 1970; 96:545–550. Used by permission.)

hyperfiltration will have few, if any, adverse effects on the kidney (see below).

The increments in renal hemodynamics during pregnancy have several clinical implications:

1. Levels of creatinine and urea nitrogen decrease from a mean of 0.7 and 12 mg/dL (62 μmol/L and 4.3 mmol/L) to 0.5 and 9 mg/dL (44 μmol/L and 3.2 mmol/L), respectively, while values of 0.9 and 14 mg/dL (80 μmol/L and 5.0 mmol/L) already suggest underlying renal disease and prompt further evaluation.

2. Increases in GFR and ERPF may also explain, in part, why excretion of several solutes, including glucose, amino acids, water-soluble vitamins, and protein, increase during pregnancy. The upper limits defining normal proteinuria should be doubled during gestation, and values as high as 300 to 500 mg/24 hr are not considered abnormal.[5, 14, 16, 18]

3. Gravidas with underlying renal lesions may experience marked increments in protein excretion, which should not be misconstrued as exacerbations of their disease.

Tubular Function

There may be decrements in the tubular reabsorption of glucose which, when combined with the marked increase in this solute's filtered load, explain why many women with normal carbohydrate metabolism manifest considerable glycosuria during pregnancy.[5, 14, 16, 19, 20] The same may be true for the renal handling of several amino acids, as substantial aminoaciduria also characterizes normal gestation.[5, 14, 17, 21]

Plasma urate levels decrease in pregnancy, and levels exceeding 5 mg/dL (30 μmol/L) are abnormal. This decrement reflects both decreases in the fractional reabsorption of urate as well as increases in GFR.[5, 14, 16, 22, 23] The relevance of the above-described tubular changes are as follows:

1. Glycosuria, when present, is intermittent and bears no consistent relationship to plasma glucose levels; thus urine glucose mea-

surements are unreliable for managing diabetic gravidas (a practice rarely employed anymore in nonpregnant populations with easy access to portable capillary blood glucose meters).

2. Increased excretion of glucose and amino acids may be another reason gravidas with asymptomatic bacteriuria often develop symptomatic disease.

3. An increase in plasma urate may be an early sign of preeclampsia.

Acid-Base Regulation

Renal bicarbonate reclamation and hydrogen ion secretion appear intact during normal gestation.[5, 24-27] However, a mild alkalemia is present, blood hydrogen levels decreasing by 2 to 4 nmol/L, and arterial (or arterialized capillary) blood pH increasing to 7.42 to 7.44 units. The changes occur early in pregnancy, and are sustained until term. This alkalemia is respiratory in origin, for pregnant women normally hyperventilate and their arterial P_{CO_2} decreases from a mean of 39 torr prior to conception to 31 torr during pregnancy.[5, 25, 27] In addition, plasma bicarbonate decreases approximately 4 mEq/L and values of 18 to 22 mEq/L are normal.

Alterations in acid-base metabolism have several consequences: (1) Because P_{CO_2} is already reduced, the gravida will be at a disadvantage in defending pH in the face of acute metabolic acidosis; (2) a gravida may be hypercapnic with a P_{CO_2} considered normal in the nonpregnant state. For example, a pregnant asthmatic whose P_{CO_2} is 40 torr already has carbon dioxide retention.

Osmoregulation

Plasma osmolality (P_{osmol}) starts to decrease immediately after conception and by gestational week 10 reaches a nadir 8 to 10 mOsm/kg below that measure before pregnancy.[28] This lower level of body tonicity is maintained through term, returning to nonpregnant osmolalities by 2 weeks post partum.[29, 30] Only about 1.5 mOsm/kg of this decrement represents decreased urea nitrogen levels and most of the change is due to a decline in plasma sodium and its attendant ions. *Thus, pregnancy is characterized by a true decrease in effective osmolality.*

The above-described changes in tonicity are due to decrements in the osmotic thresholds for thirst and vasopressin (AVP) release, both of which also decrease 8 to 10 mOsm/kg in pregnancy.[29, 30] In essence, lowering the osmotic drinking threshold early in gestation stimulates increased water intake and dilution of body fluids. Because AVP release is not suppressed at the usual level of tonicity, it still circulates and water is retained. Plasma osmolality declines until it decreases below the thirst threshold (situated several milliosmoles per kilogram above that for hormone secretion) when a new steady state, with little change in water balance, ensues. Otherwise said, gravidas concentrate and dilute their urines around a P_{osmol} which is 10 mOsm/kg below that present before conception.

Other osmoregulatory changes include a substantial rise in the metabolic clearance rate (MCR) of AVP, which increases fourfold between gestational week 10 and midtrimester.[31] The rise appears to parallel the appearance of, and marked increases in, circulating levels of a placental enzyme vasopressinase (also called oxytocinase), which is a cystine aminopeptidase capable of inactivating large quantities of AVP in vitro. The MCR of 1-deamino-8-D-AVP (desmopressin acetate, DDAVP), an analogue of vasopressin that is resistant to degradation by vasopressinase, is hardly altered in gestation, suggesting that the aminopeptidase enzymes are also active in vivo.[32]

The osmoregulatory changes in pregnancy have considerable clinical relevance:

1. The necessity of maintaining a decreased P_{osmol} must be taken into account when managing women with known central diabetes inspidus (DI).[33, 34] If AVP (Pitressin) is used, a substantial increment in dose schedule may be required by midgestation. However, most patients are now managed with desmopressin, and little change in therapy will be required.

2. There is a syndrome labeled *transient diabetes insipidus of pregnancy,* which usually is present during the second half of gestation and remits post partum.[33–36] Some women with this complication appear to have had subclinical lesions of central DI, brought to the fore by the increased MCR of AVP late in gestation.[35, 36] Even more intriguing are patients in whom transient DI seems to reflect massive in vivo AVP destruction, due, perhaps, to extremely high levels, or to exaggerated effects, of vasopressinase.[37–39] These are women whose disorder, characterized by marked polyuria and polydipsia and the presence of dilute urine, is resistant to pharmacologic quantities of AVP. The patients, however, can be managed and concentrate their urine appropriately, when treated with desmopressin, which as noted, is resistant to degradation by the aminopeptidase enzyme (Fig 2–3). (See also Chap. 4.)

Volume Regulation

There are changes in both volume homeostasis and the regulation of blood pressure in normal gestation (see also Chap. 1). Most healthy women gain approximately 12.5 kg during their initial pregnancy, and 1 kg less during subsequent gestations.[5] Generations of practitioners have considered these averages as the upper limits of permissible weight gain, ignoring the fact that there is a plus and a minus to deviations about a mean. As a result, many pregnant women have been unnecessarily admonished for excessive weight gain, and their salt intake and calories, or both, restricted.

Most of the weight increase is fluid, total body water, increasing by 6 to 8 L, 4 to 6 L of which are extracellular.[5] Plasma volume increases 40% to 50% during gestation, the largest rate of increment occurring during midpregnancy, whereas increments in the interstitial space are greatest in the third trimester. There is also a gradual cumulative retention of approximately 900 mEq of sodium, distributed between the products of conception and the maternal extracellular

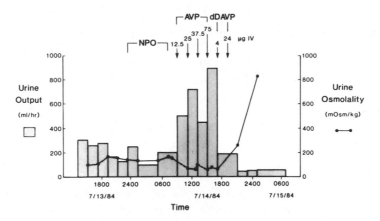

FIG 2–3.

Urinary volume and urine osmolality (U_{osmol}) on postpartum day 6 in a patient who developed diabetes insipidus in pregnancy and whose marked polyuria continued during the immediate puerperium. She was unable to concentrate her urine during fluid restriction (*NPO*) and plasma vasopressin (P_{AVP}) was undetectable despite a P_{Na} of 153 mEq/L. Large doses of AVP (Pitressin) had no effect on U_{osmol} (when theoretically P_{AVP} should have measured several thousand picograms per milliter), but U_{osmol} increased to 800 mOsm/kg when desmopressin acetate (DDAVP) was administered. The authors measured a P_{AVP} of 240 pg/mL, 30 minutes after the last AVP dose but demonstrated in elegant fashion that this radioimmunoassayable material was not bioactive and probably represented fragments. Plasma vasopressin levels at this time were manyfold those normally measured at the end of gestation. (From Durr JA, Haggard JG, Hunt JM, et al: *N Engl J Med* 1987; 316:1070–1074. Used by permission.)

space.[5] These increases in maternal intravascular and interstitial compartments produce a physiologic hypervolemia, yet the gravida's volume receptors sense these changes as normal, and when sodium restriction or diuretic therapy limits this physiologic expansion, maternal responses resemble those in salt-depleted nonpregnant subjects. This is one reason why sodium restriction has little or no place in modern prenatal care, and gravidas are now advised to salt their food to taste. In fact, some researchers believe that a liberal sodium intake is beneficial during gestation.[5, 40]

The influence of humoral changes during normal pregnancy, including activation of the renin-angiotension system, and increases in the circulating levels of several mineralocorticoids on renal sodium handling and volume regulation is incompletely understood (and also discussed further in Chap. 1). The increment in GFR means that over 10,000 additional milliequivalents of sodium must be reabsorbed by the renal tubules each day, a quantity considerably greater than the expected salt-retaining effects of high circulating levels of estrogens, aldosterone, and desoxycorticosterone.

Finally, the practical consequences of volume changes are as follows: Increments in intravascular volume and a concomitant physiologic hemodilution are positive signs when managing gravidas with underlying renal disease.[5, 16] The physiologic volume changes of pregnancy must also be taken into account when managing gravidas undergoing dialysis treatments after acute renal failure, or for end-stage renal disease.

Table 2–1 summarizes the major anatomic and functional alterations discussed in this section, once again underscoring the need to familiarize ourselves with the normal adaptations in pregnancy before we can define disease.

DETECTION OF RENAL DISEASE IN PREGNANCY

Examination of the Urine

Healthy nonpregnant women excrete considerably less than 100 mg of protein in the urine each day, but due to the relative imprecision and variability of testing methods used by hospital laboratories, proteinuria is not considered abnormal until it exceeds 150 mg/day. As noted, there is increased protein excretion during gestation and amounts up to 300 mg/day (some accept 500 mg/day) may still be normal.[18] Also, approximately 5% of healthy adolescents and young adults have postural proteinuria, which may become apparent or first be detected in pregnancy. Postural proteinuria may also appear or increase near term when gravidas tend to assume a more lordotic posture, which aggravates excretion.

There are only sporadic reports concerning the excretion of small-molecular-weight proteins or enzymuria in normal and abnormal pregnancy, and therefore these tests have little current value in gestation.[5] It is also unclear whether or not urinary albumin excretion increases in normal pregnancy.[41-43] Research in the latter area is of interest, for the detection of microalbuminuria is one of the earliest signs of renal dysfunction in diseases such as diabetes and may have predictive value vis-à-vis the occurrence of preeclampsia.[44]

There have been few attempts to quantitate the urine sediment in pregnancy. The excretion of red blood cells may increase, but whether leukocyturia also occurs is unclear.[5] One should also be aware that gross or microscopic hematuria may complicate otherwise uneventful gestations.[45] The differential diagnosis includes all causes of hematuria in nongravid patients (detailed in reference 46), but frequently no etiology is demonstrable and bleeding subsides post partum. It has been suggested that these events are due to the rupture of small veins around the dilated renal pelvis[45] and such hematuria may or may not occur in subsequent gestations. In any event, a complete investigation of the hematuria can often be deferred until after delivery, and noninvasive techniques, including ultrasound and/or magnetic resonance, are helpful in arriving at such decisions.

TABLE 2–1.
Renal Changes in Normal Pregnancy

Alteration	Manifestation	Clinical Relevance
Increased renal size	Renal length approx. 1 cm greater on roentgenograms	Postpartum decreases in size should not be mistaken for parenchymal loss
Dilation of pelves, calyces, and ureters.	Resembles hydronephrosis on ultrasound or IVP (more marked on right)	Not to be mistaken for obstructive uropathy; retained urine leads to collection errors; upper urinary tract infections are more virulent; may be responsible for "distention syndrome;" elective pyelography should be deferred to at least 12 weeks postpartum
Increased renal hemodynamics	Glomerular filtration rate and renal plasma flow increase 35%–50%	Serum creatinine and urea N values decrease during normal gestation; >0.8 mg/dL (>72 μmol/L) creatinine already suspect; protein, amino acid, and glucose excretion all increase
Changes in acid-base metabolism	Renal bicarbonate threshold decreases; progesterone stimulates respiratory center	Serum bicarbonate and P_{CO_2} are 4–5 mM/L and 10 mm Hg lower, respectively, in normal gestation; A P_{CO_2} of 40 mm Hg already represents CO_2 retention
Renal water-handling	Osmoregulation altered (osmotic thresholds for AVP release and thirst decrease; hormonal disposal rates increase)	Serum osmolality decreases 10 mOsm/L (serum Na 5 mEq/L) during normal gestation; increased metabolism of AVP may cause transient diabetes insipidus in pregnancy

IVP = intravenous pyelography; AVP = vasopressin.

Renal Function Tests

Clearance of endogenous creatinine, which is the primary way of assessing GFR in nongravid subjects, is equally useful for evaluating renal function in gravidas. The lower limit of normal for creatinine clearances measured during gestation should be 30% above that of nongravid women, which in most hospitals averages 110 to 115 mL/min. One should be aware, however, that urinary creatinine results from tubular secretion, as well as from glomerular filtration. When renal dysfunction is moderate or greater (serum creatinine >1.5 mg/dL or 133 μmol/L), a substantial proportion of the clearance may then be due to secretion, resulting in considerable overestimation of the GFR.

Acid excretion and urinary concentration and dilution are similar in gravid and nonpregnant women. Thus, tests such as ammonium chloride loading (rarely indicated in gestation) give values similar to those in nongravid women.[24, 25] Supine posture can interfere with tests of maximal urinary dilution, while lateral recumbency interferes with concentration, and it is perhaps best to perform these studies with the patient seated quietly in a comfortable chair.[28]

Renal Biopsy in Pregnancy

There are very few indications for the performance of a percutaneous renal biopsy in pregnant women.[47] In fact pregnancy was once considered a relative contraindication to the procedure due to earlier reports of excessive bleeding and other complications (reviewed in references 5, 47). This view, however, stemmed from the period when many of the biopsies were performed in hypertensive patients at a time predating our current understanding of the coagulation abnormalities which may occur in preeclamptic women. It is now evident that if the biopsy is performed in women with well-controlled blood pressure and normal coagulation indices, its morbidity is similar to that of nonpregnant patients.

Packham and Fairley[48] have recently described their experience with renal biopsy during gestation, reaffirming the relative safety of the procedure. They also suggest that pregnant women with undiagnosed hematuria and/or proteinuria should have prepartum biopsies, claiming that such a policy has important relevance for management and prognosis. We believe such indications are too broad, and recommend the procedure very infrequently during gestation. Our indications are as follows:

Biopsy should be considered when there is sudden deterioration of renal function and no obvious cause is present. This is because certain forms of rapidly progressive glomerulonephritis, when diagnosed early, may respond to aggressive treatment such as steroid pulses and perhaps plasma exchange. Another situation in which biopsy is recommended is symptomatic nephrotic syndrome occurring before 32 weeks' gestation. While some might consider a therapeutic trial of steroids in such cases, we prefer to determine beforehand whether the lesion is likely to respond to steroids, because pregnancy is itself a hypercoagulable state prone to worsening by such treatment. On the other hand, proteinuria alone in a normotensive woman with well-preserved renal function who has neither marked hypoalbuminemia nor intolerable edema would lead us to examine the patient at more frequent intervals and defer the biopsy to the postpartum period. This is because the consensus among most investigators (see below) is that prognosis is determined primarily by the level of renal function and the presence or absence of hypertension, rather than by the type of renal lesion. We take a similar position in the management of pregnancies with asymptomatic microscopic hematuria alone, when neither stone nor tumor is suggested by ultrasonography. Finally, renal biopsies should not be performed after gestational week 32 since at this stage the fetus will probably be delivered in any case, and the decision to terminate the gestation usually has to be made quickly and independent of biopsy results.[47]

URINARY TRACT INFECTION

Infections of the urinary tract, which constitute the most frequent renal problem encountered during gestation, are dealt with in detail in Chapter 13 and this subject will only be briefly discussed here. The reader is also referred to two comprehensive reviews on this topic.[49, 50]

The prevalence of asymptomatic (covert) bacteriuria ranges between 2% and 10% (which is similar to that in nonpregnant populations), but higher rates have been observed in pregnant women with sickle cell trait[51] and diabetes.[52] The natural history of covert bacteriuria in pregnancy differs from that in nongravid women; while in the latter the situation is quite benign, progression to overt cystitis or pyelonephritis occurs in up to 40% of affected gravidas. There are also claims that asymptomatic bacteriuria leads to increased incidences of anemia, hypertension, and intrauterine growth retardation (or "preterm/low-birth-weight" babies),[49, 50] but only the last-named seems supported by the data.[53] In any event, we believe that all gravidas should be screened at their initial prenatal visit, and the treatment of women with confirmed positive cultures should be guided by the antibiotic sensitivity of the isolated microorganisms (see Chap. 13). Indeed, detection and therapy of asymptomatic bacteriuria appears to prevent at least two thirds of potential antepartum pyelonephritis.[54, 55] It should be noted, however, that some authors question the sensitivity and cost-effectiveness of routine screening, suggesting that testing be limited to those women with a history of recurrent urinary tract infection,[56, 57] a view that we and the authors of Chapter 13 currently oppose.

The incidence of bacteriuria increases to about 17% immediately after delivery, but decreases again to approximately 4% by the third postpartum day.[58, 59] We do not recommend "prophylactic" treatment in such instances unless symptomatic infection supervenes. This is especially true in catheterized women, where in most instances bacteriuria will clear spontaneously.[58]

Symptomatic Urinary Tract Infections

If prenatal screening is combined with rapid treatment of covert bacteriuria the incidence of symptomatic infection should be only about 0.5%. Ten percent of these cases will occur in the first trimester while the majority will present in equal proportions at midpregnancy and during the third trimester.[49, 50, 60]

The bacteriology and virulence of various pathogens causing acute pyelonephritis are discussed in Chapter 13; over 90% of the uropathogens are aerobic gram-negative rods, usually *Escherichia coli*.[49, 50, 61] One should be aware, however, that pregnancy seems to decrease tolerance to these infections. For example, acute pyelonephritis was a cause of maternal mortality in the preantibiotic era, and more recently upper urinary tract infections in gravidas have been associated with exaggerated effects of endotoxemia, including the appearance of hypotension, respiratory distress syndrome, and a variety of hematologic, liver, and renal functional abnormalities.[50] For these reasons, acute pyelonephritis should always be treated in a hospital setting, and some authorities extend treatment regimens to 3 to 5 weeks, followed by suppressive therapy or close surveillance[61] (see also Chap. 13).

Perinephric abscess, renal carbuncle, and renal cortical abscess occur very infrequently in gestation, but should be considered in cases of occult and resistant infection. This is especially true in the puerperium when the focus on uterine and abdominal sources of infection, as well as pelvic thrombophlebitis, frequently leads physicians to overlook the above-noted unusual renal problems.

ACUTE RENAL FAILURE

The incidence of acute renal failure (ARF) complicating pregnancy was approximately 1 in 5,000 in the 1960s, but has now declined to less than 0.01%.[62–64] Similarly, maternal mortality due to this complication, at one time as high as 18%, has also declined substantially. This trend, attributed to liberalization

TABLE 2–2.
Differential Diagnosis of Oliguria

	Prerenal Failure	Acute Tubular Necrosis
History	Vomiting, diarrhea, other causes of dehydration	Dehydration, ischemic insult, ingestion of nephrotoxin; no specific history in 50% of cases
Physical examination	Decreased blood pressure, increasd pulse rate, poor skin turgor	May have signs of dehydration, but physical examination often normal
Urinalysis	Concentrated urine; few formed elements on sediment, but many hyaline casts	Isosthenuria; sediment contains renal tubular cells and pigmented casts, but may be normal
Urinary sodium	<20 mEq/L; most <10 mEq/L	≥25, usually >60 mEq/L
Urine-plasma (U/P) ratios	High	Low
Osmolality	Often ≥1.5	<1.1
Urea	≥20	≤3
Creatinine	>40	<15
Fractional sodium excretion $(U/P_{Na}/U/P_{creatinine})$	<1%	>1%
Renal failure index $(U_{Na}/U/P_{creatinine})$	<1	>1

of abortion laws, more aggressive use of potent antibiotics, and improvement of prenatal care, has not been shared by the poorer and less industrialized nations, in which such patients constitute up to 25% of referrals to dialysis centers and in which renal failure in pregnancy continues to be an important cause of maternal and fetal mortality.[62, 63]

Definitions

Acute renal failure is characterized by a sudden decrease in renal function and frequently by oliguria. However, in approximately 20% of the cases urine volume is maintained, a condition termed *nonoliguric acute renal failure*. Commonly accepted values for what constitutes a "rapid" rise in creatinine levels or definition of oliguria are increments in plasma creatinine of at least 0.5 mg/dL/day (44 µmol/L/day) and a reduction of urinary volume to below 400 mL/24 hr.[65]

Etiology

Conditions which precipitate the above-described dramatic deterioration in function may be "prerenal" (causing kidney hypoperfusion), renal parenchymal, or "postrenal"

(obstructive) in origin, and include renal ischemia, nephrotoxins, obstructive uropathy, and intrinsic renal disease (e.g., acute nephritis and hemolytic-uremic syndromes).[65]

Diagnosis

Causes of ARF include rapidly reversible and specifically treatable entites such as hypoperfusion and obstruction, conditions which should be differentiated from the more common acute tubular necrosis. Diagnosis, often apparent from clinical circumstances as well as a careful history and physical examination, may be difficult because all these diseases lead to an identical syndrome characterized by deteriorating renal function. In such circumstances, solute composition, tonicity, and microscopic examination of the urine may be helpful (Table 2–2). For example, presence in the urine of few formed elements or of hyaline casts only suggests prerenal azotemia or postrenal obstruction; brownish pigmented casts and increased quantities of tubular cells, tubular necrosis; red blood cells and casts, nephritis or a vascular inflammatory disease; and clumps of leukocytes or their presence in casts, acute infectious pyelonephritis. On the other hand, acute tubular necrosis may present with minimal urinary findings. Absolute anuria is characteristic of cortical necrosis and has been described with obstruction of the ureters by the enlarged uterus (see below).

Urine osmolality (U_{osmol}), specific gravity, as well as urinary levels of sodium, creatinine, and urea also aid in differentiating the causes of ARF.[65] Tonicity (U_{osmol} or specific gravity) is usually high in prerenal failure, while isosthenuria suggests tubular necrosis. Urine-to-plasma (U/P) concentrative ratios further aid in establishing a diagnosis; U/P osmolality, urea, and creatinine often measure below 1.1, 3.0, and 15, respectively, in acute tubular necrosis, while the ratios often exceed 20 for urea and 40 for creatinine when prerenal failure is present.

Prerenal failure is further characterized by avid sodium reabsorption, concentration of this solute decreasing to below 10 mEq/L in random samples. On the other hand, reabsorptive capacity is impaired in tubular necrosis so that urinary sodium levels are at least 25 mEq/L. A more precise way of ascertaining the capacity of the renal tubule to handle sodium is to calculate fractional sodium excretion ($U/P_{Na}/U/P_{creatinine}$) or its index ($U_{Na}/U/P_{creatinine}$). In prerenal failure these indices rarely exceed a value of 1. One should be aware, however, that the diagnostic approach described above may be less useful if the patient is being volume-expanded with saline or with an osmotic agent, has recently received a loop diuretic, or is manifesting non-oliguric renal failure.

Acute Renal Failure in Obstetrics

The frequency distribution of ARF in pregnancy was once bimodal. An initial peak occurred early in gestation and constituted most of the cases due to septic abortion, while a second peak occurred between gestation week 35 and the puerperium, mainly resulting from placental abruption, bleeding, and preeclampsia (reviewed in reference 63). In countries with liberalized abortion laws, the initial peak has virtually disappeared and this is the primary reason why the incidence of

renal failure and maternal mortality has declined markedly in these nations.[62, 63, 66] Still, women presenting with ARF in gestation may have a guarded prognosis, for currently a larger proportion of the cases are the result of more serious disorders such as acute cortical necrosis and a disease peculiar to gestation termed *idiopathic postpartum renal failure*.

Septic Abortion

(see Chap. 13). Septic abortions, especially those infected with clostridia, may result in a striking, life-threatening syndrome.[62, 63] Onset may be sudden, from hours to 2 days after the attempted abortion. The disease is characterized by an abrupt rise in temperature (40°C or above), and the presence of myalgia, vomiting, and diarrhea, which may be bloody. Muscular pain is most intense in the proximal limbs, thorax, and abdomen. The clinical picture may be confused with intraabdominal inflammatory disease, especially when a history of provoked abortion is denied or not sought. Vaginal bleeding may be absent, and clostridia organisms difficult to culture or to detect in the smear. The situation is further confounded by the normal presence of clostridia in the female genital tract. Once signs and symptoms develop, hypotension, dyspnea, and progression to shock occur rapidly. Furthermore, the patient is often jaundiced, and may have a peculiar bronze color due to the association of jaundice with cutaneous vasodilation, cyanosis, and pallor.

Characteristic laboratory findings include severe anemia with markedly elevated bilirubin levels (due to hemolysis), evidence of disseminated intravascular coagulation, a striking leukocytosis ($\geq 25,000/mm^3$), and thrombocytopenia ($\leq 50,000 mm^3$). Hypocalcemia of sufficient severity to provoke tetany has been described, and an abdominal x-ray may demonstrate air in the uterus or abdomen due to gas-forming organisms and/or perforation.

Death occurs in hours in a small percentage of the women while most respond to antibiotic treatment and volume replacement, leaving a patient whose renal failure must be managed. The clinical cause of the latter complication is usually that of acute tubular necrosis in general, but on occasion the more ominous cortical necrosis may occur. The oliguric phase in women with tubular necrosis due to septic abortion may be prolonged to 3 or more weeks, and anuria may occur in this period. In fact, just when one worries that the patient has underlying cortical rather than tubular necrosis is when the diuretic phase often begins.

Management.—The initial phase of treatment requires vigorous supportive therapy and antibiotics (see Chap. 13). Use of antitoxin, hyperbaric oxygen, and exchange transfusion in the treatment of clostridial infections remains controversial. In addition, major disagreements exist on the role of surgical intervention. Some consider the uterus to be a huge culture medium for bacterial growth and toxin formation, resistant to treatment, and recommend rapid removal of this organ, believing such an aggressive approach is crucial if the mother is to survive.[67] Others note that modern-day antibiotic therapy suffices, and that surgery in these critically ill women may be too risky and counterproductive.[68] Data supporting both the radical and conservative approaches are sparse.[63, 66, 68]

Other Causes of Tubular Necrosis in Pregnancy

Volume depletion is the precipitating cause of acute tubular necroses complicating hyperemesis gravidarum, or when severe vomiting occurs with pyelonephritis.[62, 63] It has also been suggested that the vasculature of gravidas is more sensitive to endotoxin, explaining why pregnant women appear to have a greater propensity to develop renal failure from pyelonephritis than do nonpregnant subjects.[69]

Uterine hemorrhage is another major cause of renal failure in late gestation and the immediate puerperium. Antepartum bleeding may be difficult to diagnose, or underestimated, when most of the blood loss remains behind the placenta ("concealed hemorrhage"), and suspicion of this requires rapid ultrasonic studies. Uterine hemorrhage most often leads to tubular necrosis, but especially when associated with abruption can cause cortical necrosis (see below).

Preeclampsia, characterized by generalized vasoconstriction, is a major cause of renal dysfunction in gestation. However, the reduction in GFR is usually mild (approximately 30%),[15] but on rare occasions, especially when the disease is neglected and accompanied by a marked coagulopathy, preeclampsia may progress to acute tubular and even cortical necrosis.[62, 63, 70–72]

Renal Cortical Necrosis

Cortical necrosis, characterized by tissue death throughout the cortex, with sparing of the medullary portions of the kidney is fortunately a rare cause of ARF, but when it occurs is more apt to be associated with pregnancy.[62–64, 71–74] Its incidence, too, has declined markedly in the industrialized nations. For instance, statistics from the National Maternity Hospital in Dublin demonstrate a decrease from 1 in 10,000 during 1961–1970, to less than 1 in 80,000 in the next decade.[64]

Cortical necrosis is most common late in gestation, most frequently after abruption and less commonly following prolonged intrauterine death or as a consequence of preeclampsia. Abruptio placentae should always be considered when ARF develops suddenly, between the 26th and 30th gestational week, as 45% of the patients in one series had concealed hemorrhage.[74]

Although cortical necrosis may involve the entire renal cortex with resultant irreversible renal failure, it is the incomplete or "patchy" variety that occurs more often in pregnancy (Fig 2–4).[74] The latter condition is characterized by an initial episode of severe oliguria and even anuria, lasting longer than uncomplicated tubular necrosis. This is followed by a variable return of function, a stable period of moderate renal insufficiency, which in some cases progresses years later to end-stage disease.[62, 63]

Why pregnant women are more susceptible to develop cortical necrosis than non-pregnant patients is obscure. Many of the women are older multiparas who have preexisting nephrosclerosis, suggesting their kidneys are more "vulnerable" to the inciting factor(s) (ischemia or coagulation). Of interest, the Sanarelli-Shwartzman reaction can be more easily produced in pregnant animals than in nongravid controls.[75]

Acute Renal Failure Specific to Pregnancy

There are two unusual forms of acute renal failure peculiar to pregnancy. One is a complication of *acute fatty liver,* a disease characterized by jaundice and severe hepatic dysfunction in the third trimester or the early puerperium[2, 62, 63, 76] (see also Chap 10). The earliest manifestations of acute fatty liver are nausea and vomiting, important clues that are frequently overlooked and considered functional because the patient is pregnant. Laboratory investigation often reveals evidence of disseminated intravascular coagulation, including decrements in antithrombin III.[3, 62, 63, 76–78] Serum urate levels may be elevated out of proportion to the degree of renal dysfunction, and hyperuricemia may precede the clinical onset of the disease. Ultrasonography and computed tomography may also aid in the diagnosis.[63] Since this disease is uncommon, it may be misdiagnosed as septicemia or as preeclampsia complicated by

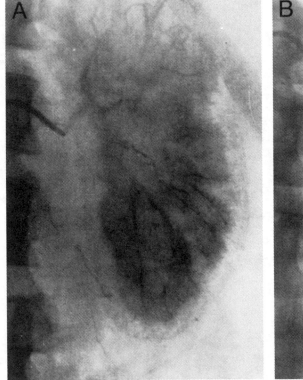 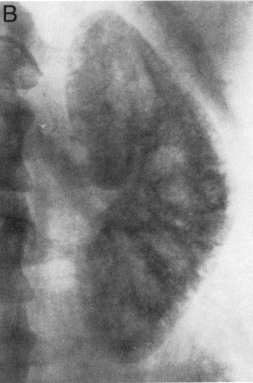

FIG 2–4.
A, selective renal arteriogram in total cortical necrosis. Cortical nephrogram is totally absent. The outer edge of the cortex is poorly outlined and separated from the inner layer by a clear nonvascularized area. **B,** selective renal arteriogram demonstrating partial ("patchy") cortical necrosis. Note the nonhomogeneous cortical nephrogram with alternating clear and densely striped perfused areas. An appreciable amount of the inner cortex was also spared. The patient had a partial recovery. (From Kleinknecht D, Grünfeld JP, Gomez PC, et al: *Kidney Int* 1973; 4:390–400. Used by permission.)

liver involvement—and some suggest that fatty liver and preeclampsia coexist frequently.[62, 63, 77]

The cause of acute fatty liver of pregnancy is unknown, although in the past tetracycline toxicity has been implicated in several instances.[63] Reversible urea cycle enzyme abnormalities resembling those seen in Reye's syndrome have also been described, and it has been suggested that this condition may be an adult form of Reye's syndrome provoked by the metabolic stress of pregnancy.[62, 63, 79, 80] Against this, however, is that women surviving acute fatty liver of pregnancy have had subsequent uneventful gestations.[62, 63]

The hepatic lesion is characterized by deposition of fat microdroplets within the hepatocytes. Inflammation and necrosis are usually absent, but there are exceptions,[77, 80] and some cases of acute fatty liver may be misdiagnosed as hepatitis. Such errors can be avoided by studying freshly frozen tissue, using special fat stains.

The incidence of ARF in women with fatty liver of pregnancy, once as high as 60%,[62, 63] is considerably less today. This may be due to earlier recognition of the disease followed by rapid intervention to end the pregnancy.[63, 77] The renal lesion is mild, as kidney structure may be within normal limits or abnormalities may be limited to fatty vacuolization and other nonspecific changes of the tubule cells.[63] The cause of the renal failure is obscure and may be due to hemodynamic factors, as in the "hepatorenal syndrome," or perhaps to a consequence of the coagulopathy. The mortality rate for mother and fetus, once quoted as surpassing 70% to 75%,[63] probably reflected an older literature selective of patients with poorest outcome. Currently the prognosis is improving with survival exceeding 80% to 90%. This is because milder forms of the disease are being recognized.[63, 76, 77]

The second condition, known as *idiopathic postpartum renal failure,* is characterized by the onset of renal failure in the puerperium after an uneventful gestation. This disease is for-tunately rare; fewer than 200 cases have been identified from its delineation in the 1960s through 1990. This condition goes by a variety of names such as *postpartum malignant nephrosclerosis, accelerated nephrosclerosis and postpartum acute renal failure in normotensive women, irreversible postpartum intravascular coagulation with acute renal failure,* and *postpartum hemolytic uremic syndrome*[62, 63] (reference 63 contains approximately 50 citations).

Idiopathic postpartum renal failure may occur between 1 day and several weeks after delivery. A typical patient presents with oliguria, or at times anuria, rapidly progressing azotemia, and often with evidence of microangiopathic hemolytic anemia or a consumption coagulopathy. Blood pressure on admission varies from normal or only minimally elevated to severe accelerated hypertension. Some patients exhibit extrarenal manifestations involving the cardiovascular system (cardiac dilation and congestive heart failure) and central nervous system symptoms (lethargy, convulsion), which appear disproportionate to the degree of uremia, hypertension, or volume overload present.

The cause of this syndrome is unknown. Suggestions include a viral illness prior to the onset of the disease, retained placental fragments, or drugs such as ergotamine compounds, oxytocic agents, or oral contraceptives prescribed shortly after delivery.[62, 63] Several patients have manifest hypocomplementemia, suggesting a possible immunologic cause, and deficiencies in prostaglandin production, and antithrombin III levels akin to those described in the hemolytic-uremic syndrome have been ascribed to idiopathic postpartum renal failure as well.[62, 63]

The pathophysiology of postpartum renal failure has been compared to that of thrombotic thrombocytopenic purpura as well as to other diseases characterized by disseminated intravascular coagulation such as the adult hemolytic-uremic syndrome. This disease has also been compared to the generalized Sanarelli-Shwartzman reaction, which as noted above develops more readily in pregnant animals.[75]

The renal pathologic findings, detailed elsewhere,[62, 63] differ substantially in various reports but fall into two general categories: (1) changes in the glomerular capillaries resembling those seen in the hemolytic-uremic syndrome, and (2) arteriolar lesions reminiscent of malignant nephrosclerosis or scleroderma. Some believe that glomerular lesions suggesting thrombotic microangiopathy are more apt to be noted in specimens obtained soon after the disease begins, while those resembling accelerated nephrosclerosis are seen in biopsy material taken later in the course. An increased incidence of postbiopsy bleeding has also been reported.[62]

The prognosis of this disease is guarded. Most women have either succumbed, required chronic dialysis, or have survived with severely reduced renal function, and only a few have recovered. Of interest is a patient reported to have a mild form of "postpartum hemolytic syndrome," whose disease occurred in two successive gestations.[81]

Treatment is aimed primarily at reduction of the high blood pressure, when present, and general supportive measures used for all patients with ARF. In the past, bilateral nephrectomy was used as a lifesaving measure in a few women with accelerated hypertension unresponsive to treatment. This should be unnecessary today when potent vasodilators, converting enzyme inhibitors, and calcium channel blocking agents are available.

Some have claimed that the early use of anticoagulant therapy such as heparin and fibrinolytic agents may reverse the renal failure (reviewed in reference 63), but data thus far have not been convincing, and it should be kept in mind that such drugs are not harmless. In view of the possible contributing role of retained placental fragments, dilatation and curettage should be considered for women in whom the syndrome occurs close to delivery. Other regimens, including antiplatelet therapy (which may be of use in a possible variant of postpartum renal failure linked to circulating lupus anticoagulants[82]), infusion of blood products, including concentrates of an-

tithrombin III, or plasma exchange, have been advocated on the basis of their alleged success in patients with thrombotic thrombocytopenia purpura or in the adult hemolytic-uremic syndrome.[63, 83] Several of these patients have received kidney allografts and most have done well after transplantation.[63]

Miscellaneous Causes of Acute Renal Failure

Acute renal failure has occurred after intraamniotic saline administration, after amniotic fluid embolism, and following illnesses or accidents unrelated to the gestation, such as drug ingestion, bacterial endocarditis, and incompatible blood transfusions.[63] Sudden renal failure during pregnancy has also complicated sarcoidosis,[84] various nephritides or collagen disorders, and can also be due to obstructive uropathy related to the enlarged uterus.[7, 62, 63, 85–91] Most of the last-named problem has been in women with solitary kidneys, but there have also been instances of bilateral obstruction.[85–87, 89–91] These cases may be managed conservatively by placement of intraureteral stents under local anesthesia.[13, 91–93] Finally, some gravidas with underlying renal disease and good or adequate renal function are more susceptible to develop acute tubular necrosis, especially when their gestation is complicated by superimposed preeclampsia or other causes of increased blood pressure.

Guidelines for Managing Acute Renal Failure in Pregnancy

Management of ARF in pregnancy or the puerperium is, in general, the same as in nonpregnant subjects,[94] but certain points pertinent to antepartum or intrapartum ARF deserve emphasis. Since uterine hemorrhage late in pregnancy may be concealed and the blood loss underestimated, blood should be replaced early and the patients may even be slightly overtransfused in order to forestall the development of acute tubular or cortical necrosis. Both peritoneal dialysis and hemodialysis have been widely used in patients with obstetric renal failure.[63, 95–97] The former is preferred because it causes more gradual changes in fluid and solute levels, and is less likely to be associated with precipitous hypotension and/or premature uterine contractions.[96] If hemodialysis is the mode utilized, the above problems can be minimized by daily treatment for shorter time periods, avoiding high-flux technology. Finally, as urea, creatinine, and probably other metabolites (or toxins) that accumulate in uremia cross the placenta, dialysis should be undertaken early, with the aim of maintaining the blood urea nitrogen below 50 mg/dL (20 mmol/L), if possible. Thus, the advantages of early dialysis that have been enumerated for nonpregnant patients become even more important for pregnant subjects and make the argument for prophylactic dialysis compelling.

Prognosis for survival is considerably better in obstetric ARF than in patients whose disease is due to surgical or medical causes, and as noted earlier, maternal mortality has declined sharply in the past two decades. Prognosis for the fetus, in contrast, is worse than that for the mother, and many pregnancies end in abortion or stillbirth.[63] However, here too the outlook is improving dramatically, as increasing fetal survival is being reported. Finally, there are few data concerning the effects of ARF on subsequent maternal reproductive performance, but it appears that once the patient has recovered she should have no difficulty conceiving or carrying a gestation to term.

CHRONIC RENAL DISEASE

As noted in the introductory paragraph to this chapter, parenchymal renal disease, of any severity, was once considered a virtual contraindication for pregnancy,[1] a view now radically altered as a result of several studies reported after 1980.[98–103] The results of these last-named investigations, which survey large numbers of patients (albeit retrospectively), virtually all of whom have a tissue diagnosis

confirming their nephropathy, have led to the following guidelines for counseling women with chronic renal disease who wish to conceive, and for managing their gestation (Table 2–3).

Overview

As renal disease progresses and function declines, the ability to sustain a viable pregnancy decreases. Normotensive women whose underlying lesions are associated with intact or only mildly decreased and stable renal function at conception usually do well, and pregnancy does not appear to affect adversely the course of their disease. This statement, true for most patients, must be tempered somewhat in certain nephropathies which appear to be more sensitive to intercurrent gestation, such as lupus nephropathy and perhaps membranoproliferative glomerulonephritis, and does not apply for women who have scleroderma and periarteritis nodosa, for whom pregnancy should be emphatically discouraged. However, authorities disagree as to whether or not gestation influences adversely the natural history of three specific entities—IgA nephropathy, focal segmental glomerulosclerosis, and reflux nephropathy[5, 99–111]—differences of opinion which have remained unresolved through 1990. The presence of hypertension prior to conception increases the incidence of both maternal and fetal complications, but even in these patients the outlook for a successful pregnancy has improved dramatically.[112]

Prognosis becomes poorer if renal function is moderately impaired (serum creatinine ≥1.5 to 3.0 mg/dL or 133 to 275 μmol/L). While fetal outcome seems good in this group, a substantial proportion (about one third) of such patients appear to experience renal functional deterioration during gestation, accelerated progression of the underlying disease after delivery, and the appearance of late-pregnancy hypertension, which is often severe and difficult to control.[5, 113]

Women with severe renal dysfunction (serum creatinine levels ≥3 mg/dL or ≥275

TABLE 2–3.
Chronic Renal Disease and Pregnancy

Renal Disease	Effects
Chronic glomerulonephritis and focal glomerular sclerosis (FGS)	There may be an increased incidence of high blood pressure late in gestation, but usually no adverse effect if renal function is preserved and hypertension absent prior to gestation; some disagree, believing that coagulation changes in pregnancy exacerbate these diseases, especially IgA nephropathy, FGS, and membranoproliferative glomerulonephritis
Systemic lupus erythematosus	Expect more problems than most glomerular diseases, but prognosis most favorable if disease is in remission 6 or more months prior to conception
Periarteritis nodosa and scleroderma	Fetal prognosis is poor; associated with maternal deaths; reactivation of quiescent scleroderma can occur during pregnancy and post partum; therapeutic abortion should be considered
Diabetic nephropathy	Pregnancy does not accelerate functional loss; increased frequency of covert bacteriuria; high incidence of heavy proteinuria and hypertension late in gestation
Chronic pyelonephritis (infectious tubulointerstitial disease)	Bacteriuria in pregnancy may lead to acute exacerbations, but otherwise well tolerated
Polycystic disease	Functional impairment and hypertension usually minimal in childbearing years, and not affected by pregnancy
Urolithiasis	Ureteral dilation and stasis do not seem to affect natural history, but infections can be more frequent; stents have been successfully placed during gestation
Permanent urinary diversion	There may be other malformations of the urogenital tract; urinary tract infection common during pregnancy, and renal function may undergo reversible decrease; no significant obstructive problem, but caesarean section may be necessary for abnormal presentation.

μmol/L) are often infertile.[114] This is especially true with end-stage renal disease, but exceptions to this statement occur, especially in women managed with chronic ambulatory peritoneal dialysis, as the latter are more apt to experience return of ovulatory cycles.[115] When conception does occur the success rate is low, i.e., below 25% in patients receiving dialysis who conceive,[95–97] and maternal morbidity is increased, two compelling reasons to discourage pregnancy in such patients.

Finally, one must reemphasize that this overview of the natural history of kidney disease and of fetal outcome in women with renal lesions is based primarily on retrospective data, most of which describe patients with mild functional impairments. Confirmation of the above views and a more definitive perspective especially in regard to women with moderate renal dysfunction, requires large prospective trials.

Pathophysiology

Renal Function

Women with intact or mildly decreased renal function usually manifest gestationally induced increases in their GFR and ERPF (measured either serially as 24-hour creatinine clearance or during short-term infusion studies utilizing inulin and *p*-aminohippurate), often similar to those seen in normal gravidas.[98] Similar increments in renal hemodynamics occur during gestation in women with a single kidney and in transplant recipients,[5, 18] although in those two groups GFR is already substantially increased prior to conception owing to compensatory morphologic and functional hypertrophy. These examples of functional gestational increments, however, seem to be restricted to patients with only mild dysfunction, for although data are sparse, GFR does not appear to increase in pregnancy when preconception creatinine levels exceed 1.4 mg/dL (124 μmol/L), and as stated, accelerated loss in function may occur in some of these women.[113]

Proteinuria

Urinary protein excretion, which usually doubles in normal pregnancy, may increase markedly in pregnant women with underlying parenchymal renal disease. In one series[98] comprising 121 gestations, development of, or increase in, abnormal proteinuria was common, occurring in nearly half of all pregnancies, and was severe (≥3 g/day) in 39 of the 57 proteinuric women, leading frequently to nephrotic edema. Appearance of "heavy proteinuria" was observed in virtually every type of renal disease with the exception of chronic interstitial nephritis, and appeared for the first time during gestation in a substantial number of women. Of importance is that even such degrees of protein loss were usually well tolerated, having little, if any, influence on the subsequent course of the renal disease, and fetal salvage was good.

Hypertension

The effect of pregnancy on blood pressure in women with preexisting renal disease is more difficult to assess. In the series described above, which comprised 89 women with preserved renal function prior to conception,[98] significant hypertension occurred in 23% of the pregnancies, but blood pressure had been elevated prior to gestation in approximately half of these cases. Increments in pressure usually occurred late in gestation, when it was difficult to distinguish superimposed preeclampsia and underlying parenchymal disease. Some authors believe certain diseases, such as IgA nephropathy, have a greater propensity to manifest gestational hypertension.[112] Finally, changes in vascular reactivity appear to occur much more frequently in gravidas with moderate or severe renal insufficiency, as worsening of hypertension, often to severe levels, occurred in 9 of 23 pregnant patients with moderate renal insufficiency reported by Hou et al.[113]

Specific Diseases

Acute and Chronic Glomerulonephritis

Acute poststreptococcal glomerulonephritis complicating pregnancy is unusual, but when it occurs may mimic preeclampsia.[51] In the few instances where documentation of the diagnosis appears to be correct, recovery of maternal renal function was complete and the gestation usually succeeded.[5, 116] Gestation in women with a history of acute glomerulonephritis with full recovery is uneventful.[5]

Similarly, women with *chronic glomerulonephritis* (a term which encompasses many morphologically and presumably distinct entities) seem to do well vis-à-vis both gestation and renal prognosis when function is preserved and hypertension absent.[5, 98–103] There is evidence of transient transfer of nephritic factor from mother to fetus in women with membranoproliferative glomerulonephritis.[117] This is also one entity where some suggest that pregnancy accelerates the decline in renal function,[104] and others report a high incidence of preeclampsia (especially in women whose renal lesion is of the dense intramembranous deposit variety[5]).

IgA Nephropathy.—As noted, the course of gestation in women with IgA nephropathy is disputed. One group persistently notes substantial and occasionally irreversible declines in renal function when women with this disease conceive.[103, 106, 110, 111] They also stress the appearance of de novo hypertension, which may not remit post partum, as well as increased fetal loss. Others, however, find that the natural history of this disease and pregnancy outcome follow the generalization that both prognoses are excellent when hypertension is absent before conception, and GFR is well preserved.[99–102]

Hereditary Nephritis.—This disease may become clinically manifest for the first time during pregnancy[5] and there is an interesting report of two sisters with the disorder each of whom developed rapidly progressive crescentic glomerulonephritis associated with pregnancy.[118] Still, most gestations are uneventful, especially in women with the benign variety of the disease characterized by thinning of the glomerular basement membrane alone. Finally, there is a variant of hereditary nephritis associated with thrombocytopenia or thrombocytopathy, in which gestation may be complicated by bleeding problems, especially at delivery.[5]

Focal Segmental Glomerulosclerosis

This is another disease whose natural history remains disputed, perhaps because the disorder may have variable etiologies. Again, one group[103, 106] noted hypertension, often severe, in three fourths of their patients which persisted post partum in almost 20% of the women. There were also the anticipated increments in proteinuria in most patients, and functional deterioration, at times not reversed by delivery, in 45% of the women. Increased fetal losses were also described.[99] Others[107] dispute these data, again noting success when function is preserved and hypertension absent. However, the total reported experience with this disease is sparse, and obviously the contested issues described above require considerably more data if meaningful conclusions are to be drawn.

Collagen Disorders

These diseases are detailed in Chapter 11, and the following generalizations summarize our views. The outlook for gravidas with lupus nephropathy but preserved renal function is complex. Clearly, exacerbations of this systemic disease or its initial presentation occur during pregnancy and/or the puerperium, and while a number of recent reports[119–123] seem to have clarified views on the course of lupus nephropathy during gestation, one must always remember that the disease is characterized by an unpredictable course regardless of pregnancy. Still, it appears that if the disease is in remission for 6 months prior to conception, and renal function is preserved, the pregnancy and functional outlook are good, albeit poorer than for most other glomerular diseases. Presence of disease activity in the 6

months preceding or at conception leads to a more guarded prognosis. A view suggesting that exacerbations are more apt to occur in the puerperium,[124] so that steroid therapy should be enhanced at that time, does not seem to have been confirmed in a carefully performed case-control study.[125] Maternal management, including use of pulsed steroids and chemotherapy, as well as fetal outcome and its relation to circulating cardiolipins and anticoagulants, and transmission of the disease to fetus or neonate, are discussed further in Chapter 11.

Whereas prognosis for gravidas with systemic lupus is debated, the disease is usually sufficiently benign to allow conception in women who so desire. In contrast, the outcome of pregnancy in patients with renal involvement due to periarteritis nodosa and scleroderma is extremely poor, often related to the associated hypertension, which is frequently malignant.[5] Not only is the fetal prognosis poor, but many of the cases described in the literature, albeit selective, ended with a maternal death.[5] For these reasons we counsel against conception in these last two entities, and suggest termination when the disease is present in the first trimester.

Diabetes

Diabetes is discussed in Chapter 3. There are several studies which focus on pregnancy in gravidas with overt diabetic nephropathy.[126–129] Renal and fetal prognoses are very good when kidney function is well preserved, almost 95% of the gestations ending successfully. However, nephrotic-range proteinuria and hypertension complicate the third trimester of over two thirds of these women and gestation is usually terminated before gestational week 37. Of interest is the appearance de novo during gestation of hypothyroidism in a significant number of nephrotic diabetics.[130]

Tubulointerstitial Disease and Reflux Nephropathy

Most tubulointerstitial disease is infectious in nature and pregnancy outcome relates to patients' functional status prior to conception.[5] One series[131] suggests that such patients are more prone to hypertension in pregnancy, but another study[98] suggests that prognosis and gestational outcome are better than in women with glomerular disease. Renal tuberculosis does not seem to be affected by gestation.[5]

Polycystic kidney disease may remain undetected in pregnancy, but careful questioning for family history of renal problems and the judicious use of ultrasonography facilitate earlier detection.[5, 132] These patients do have a greater propensity to develop preeclampsia,[133] but the general prognosis is good when function is preserved.

Reflux nephropathy, a disease which begins during childhood, is present in a substantial number of women of childbearing age. Some[105] believe pregnancy adversely influences the course of this disease, but careful review of the data reveals that patients who do poorly are those who had hypertension and moderate renal insufficiency prior to conception.[107, 108] These patients require special care during gestation, including frequent urine cultures and prompt treatment when signs of urinary tract infection occur.

Stone Disease

Urolithiasis has a prevalence between 0.03 and 0.35 in pregnant women who live in the Western Hemisphere. Most stones contain calcium salts and some are infectious in origin (reviewed in references 5 and 134). The older literature stressed the dramatic complications that occur when obstructive uropathy or infection supervenes, but more recent studies suggest that pregnancy has little influence on the course of urolithiasis, although women with renal calculi may have an increased incidence of both urinary tract infection and perhaps spontaneous abortion as well as premature labor.[134–139] The above synopsis relates primarily to women with calcium oxalate stones and the same is probably true for the less common stone disease, cystinuria.[140] In the latter disorder it is important to ensure hydration in early pregnancy, when women

are frequently nauseous, and although experience is limited, no unique adverse effects of *d*-penicillamine (FDA category D) on either gravida or fetus has been established.

One note of caution, however: Virtually all the series summarized above focus on women whose calculi are mainly of the "non-infectious" variety and little is known of the natural history during gestation of the more serious struvite stones. In any event, urinary tract infection in the presence of nephrolithiasis requires prompt and prolonged treatment (3–5 weeks), followed by suppressive therapy through the immediate puerperium, since the calculus may represent a nidus of infection resistant to sterilization.

Renal calculi are among the more common causes of abdominal pain (of nonobstetric origin) requiring hospitalization during gestation[5, 134] and when complications suggest the need for surgical intervention, pregnancy should not be a deterrent to pyelographic x-ray examination. If the stone obstructs the ureter, surgery may be necessary, and in this respect approximately 30% of patients described in the literature have undergone an operative procedure such as open lithotomy and percutaneous nephrostomy.[134, 141, 142] Also, rigid ureteroscopy (direct vision) performed under general anesthesia has been utilized early in gestation.[142] More recently, however, a less invasive technique, the placement of a stent, has made it possible to manage gravidas through gestation, deferring more definitive surgical procedures to the postpartum period.[92, 142]

MANAGEMENT OF CHRONIC RENAL DISEASE IN PREGNANCY

When counseling patients with chronic renal disease on the advisability of conception or whether to continue a gestation already in progress, neither answers nor decisions come simply! Patient expectation is high, and the desire for motherhood often so strong as to tempt the sympathetic clinician to take unwarranted risks. Furthermore, patients conceive against advice, or refuse termination for religious or emotional reasons, in which case the clinicians must be ready to manage a difficult gestation and be prepared for serious complications.

We recommend that pregnancy not be undertaken if serum creatinine exceeds 1.4 mg/dL (124 μmol/L), but some permit gestation in women with pre-conception levels up to 2 mg/dL (177 μmol/L), especially in women with a single kidney, and individuals with primary interstitial disease. In all instances diastolic blood pressure (Korotkoff phase V) prior to conception should be 90 mm Hg or less.

Pregnant women with renal disease are best managed at a tertiary care center under the coordinated care of a fetal-maternal medicine specialist and a general internist or nephrologist. Initial laboratory tests should include a *database,* which helps in the early detection of renal functional loss as well as the onset of superimposed preeclampsia. Thus, besides the usual prenatal screening tests, the following renal parameters should be sought:

1. Serum creatinine (and/or its timed clearance) and electrolyte concentrations. These values monitor renal function as well as osmolar, potassium, and acid-base homeostasis.
2. Serum albumin and cholesterol levels (important in regard to nephrotic manifestations).
3. Urine analysis and screening bacterial culture; 24-hour protein excretion.
4. Uric acid levels, oxaloacetic and pyruvate transaminases, lactic dehydrogenase, and platelet count (tests which aid in detecting superimposed preeclampsia) should be determined.

We suggest biweekly visits until gestational week 32, after which the patient should be seen weekly. Renal parameters should be tested every 4 to 5 weeks, unless more frequent evaluations become necessary. Fetal surveillance is best started early (e.g., 30–32 weeks), especially in nephrotic gravidas, as these women are already oligemic and further intravascular volume depletion may impair uteroplacental perfusion. Furthermore, since blood pressure normally declines during pregnancy, saliuretic therapy could conceivably precipitate circulatory collapse or thromboembolic episodes. This recommendation, however, is relative, because we have observed occasional patients whose kidneys were retaining salt so avidly that diuretics had to be used cautiously. Some authorities recommend the use of prophylactic anticoagulation (i.e., mini-dose heparin) in nephrotic gravidas, but there are no data to prove the efficacy of such treatment.

Dietary Counseling

High-protein diets were advocated in the past for patients with nephrotic proteinuria, especially during gestation when anabolic requirements increase. In 1990, nephrologists are treating most patients with renal disease (with or without nephrotic syndrome) with protein-restricted diets. The theoretical reasons for this are as follows: Increased glomerular filtration accelerates the progression of renal disease because the combination of hyperfiltration and increased intraglomerular capillary pressure in residual (intact) nephrons of patients (or of individuals with a single kidney following uninephrectomy) causes glomerulosclerosis and leads to progressive loss of GFR.[143, 144] Protein restriction protects the kidney by preventing glomerular hyperfiltration and decreasing intraglomerular capillary pressure and, paradoxically, may increase plasma albumin in severely nephrotic patients, due to decreased urinary protein loss and perhaps to decrements in the albumin catabolic rate.[143, 145]

Should protein be restricted in gravidas with renal dysfunction, a policy already suggested by one author?[146] We caution against this view, and recommend that such therapeutic regimens be avoided in pregnancy until more is known regarding fetal outcome, especially brain development, first from studies in animal models and then in carefully conducted clinical trials. Also of interest are preliminary data noting that protein loading does not affect adversely pregnant rats that were uninephrectomized or had experimental glomerular disease.[17, 147] Finally, concerning "hyperfiltration," three groups of investigators[102, 107, 148] compared the remote renal prognosis of patients with renal disorders who had undergone pregnancies with that of women who never conceived (in a case-control fashion). Few if any adverse effects of gestation have been noted. These data, however, are sparse, and obviously more studies are required.

Course of Gestation

Glomerular filtration rate and blood pressure are the two parameters that determine the course of the gestation. Evidence of renal functional deterioration or the appearance (or rapid worsening) of hypertension is best evaluated in hospital, and failure to reverse these events is grounds for termination of the pregnancy. Since plasma creatinine determinations may be quite variable in some laboratories, decisions should not be made until the direction and rate of change are very clear from repeat tests. It is important to remember that a decrement in creatinine clearance of 15% to 20% may occur normally near term, and that increased proteinuria in the absence of hypertension need not cause alarm. Such changes therefore do not suggest a need for hospitalization.

Gravidas with preexisting renal disease or essential hypertension may be more susceptible than control populations to superimposed preeclampsia, which frequently occurs in midpregnancy or early in the third trimester. Superimposed preeclampsia, however, may be difficult to differentiate from aggravation of the underlying disease, especially in women with glomerular disease who are prone to hypertension and proteinuria. In any event, when these situations occur, the patient should be hospitalized and treated as if she had superimposed preeclampsia, a prudent

policy considering the potentially explosive and dangerous nature of this disorder (see Chap. 1).

RENAL TRANSPLANTATION

The first gravida with a renal allograft delivered over 30 years ago and probably over 3,000 gestations have occurred since then.[149] We believe such gestations must be managed in a multidisciplinary fashion at a tertiary care center by an obstetric specialist and a nephrologist. The reader is referred to several reviews and editorials[150-155] which complement the following brief synopsis.

Transplantation usually reverses the abnormal reproductive function associated with end-stage renal disease; menses and ovulation resume and such women can readily conceive.[156, 157] In fact, it appears that as many as 1 in every 50 women of childbearing age with a functional renal transplant becomes pregnant, often because they are unaware that they may be fertile.[152, 156] This suggests a failure on our part to inform these patients properly. Said otherwise, it is important that all allograft recipients of childbearing age be informed that they *may* be able to conceive and receive appropriate contraceptive counseling.

Davison,[152] in a survey of the literature through 1986, documented 1,569 gestations in 1,009 renal allograft recipients (many more were probably never reported). Data were often incomplete, but it appeared that the mean interval between transplantation and conception was 40 months, with a range which included one instance of transplanting a recipient already pregnant through women whose allografts had been present for as long as 13 years. Twenty-two percent of these gestations were terminated "therapeutically" and 16% ended in spontaneous abortions (an incidence similar to normal women who conceive) and the incidence of ectopic pregnancy was about 0.5%. Thus just over 60% of these gestations continued beyond the first trimester, and 92% ended successfully. Kidney prognosis and pregnancy outcome seemed to parallel the dictum for pregnancy in women with renal disease in general; that is, the better the renal function prior to conception, the more satisfactory the results; and prognosis was best when the transplanted kidney came from a living donor (however, this occurred in only 20% of the pregnancies).[151, 152]

While the majority of those gestations continuing beyond the first trimester succeeded, there were many maternal and fetal problems. Complications included ectopic pregnancies, steroid-induced hyperglycemia, leukopenia, septicemia, uterine rupture, allograft rejection, and maternal death,[158–160] as well as prematurity, respiratory distress syndrome, intrauterine growth retardation, congenital anomalies, hypoadrenalism, hepatic insufficiency, thrombocytopenia, and serious infection in the fetus.[151–153] Of interest, too, is that hypertension complicated 30% of the pregnancies, and in such situations plasma uric acid levels and urinary protein excretion were not useful markers for either the onset or severity of preeclampsia, as both indices could be substantially above the norm at any stage of gestation in otherwise uncomplicated pregnancies in allograft recipients.

Many women with renal allografts experienced increases in renal hemodynamics during gestation, but most values were below those observed in normal gestation. In addition, functional declines occurred in 15% of the pregnancies, most frequently in the patients with the poorest prepregnancy levels.[18, 152] Most, but not all, of these declines were transient in nature and occurred in late pregnancy. Unfortunately, there are little data comparing the natural history of renal function in allograft recipients who undergo pregnancy to those who do not, but one small investigation suggests there are no differences.[161] This is our view too, but there are dissenting opinions suggesting that gestation may compromise the life span of the transplanted kidney (see reference 162 and accompanying editorials[154, 155]).

Finally, there is evidence that pregnant diabetics with renal allografts fare much worse than their nondiabetic counterparts.[163] The outlook may be considerably better when women who have received a pancreas as well as a kidney allograft conceive.[164]

Management Guidelines

Counseling and Early Pregnancy Assessment

When discussing conception with transplant recipients one must review a number of problems in addition to the pregnancy prognosis alone. Stress is already a factor in the everyday lives of these patients who continually receive steroids and other immunosuppressive agents, and who always have a "baseline of uncertainty." These include some harsh realities which relate to maternal prospects of survival, including the threat of rejection, risk of infection, and increased incidence of remote neoplastic and cardiovascular disorders.[150, 152, 165–167]

Although allograft recipients have been conceiving since the 1950s there have been no formal efforts to establish guidelines or criteria for pre-conception counseling. Individual centers have their own recommendations; ours are summarized in Table 2–4. The rea-

TABLE 2–4.
Pre-conception Guidelines* for Renal Allograft Recipients

---

1. Patients with transplants should wait 2 yr before attempting conception and be in good health (some permit 1 yr if graft is from living donor)
2. Stable renal function with plasma creatinine ≤2 mg/dL (177 μmol/L) and preferably <1.5 mg/dL (133 μmol/L); no evidence of rejection; no or minimal proteinuria; absence of pelvicalyceal distention on recent urogram
3. Absent or easily managed hypertension (see Chap. 1 for antihypertensive drugs used in pregnancy)
4. Drug therapy reduced to maintenance levels: prednisone ≤15 mg/day, azathioprine ≤2 mg/kg/day†; a safe dosage for cyclosporine has not been established due to limited experience (try to avoid its use [e.g., by substituting azathioprine] or maintain dosage at ≤5 mg/kg/day)

*Failure to meet guidelines should be considered as relative proscriptions.
†Data suggest congenital anomalies occur when dosage is >2.2 mg/kg/day.[168]

son we recommend a wait of 2 years post-transplant is that if graft function is well maintained at 24 months, there is a high probability that this good function will be sustained over the next 5 years.

One should also note that most of the recommendations in Table 2–4 are relative, and are derived from data which predate the current widespread use of cyclosporine. As of 1990, however, experience with pregnancy in women receiving this immunosuppressive drug was too sporadic and fragmentary to permit firm conclusions.[152, 153, 169–173] Of concern, however, are the following: Cyclosporine causes both decreases in GFR, hypertension, and rarely a hemolytic-uremic-type syndrome. Thus it may hinder the anticipated renal adaptation in gestation, and gravidas seem to have a greater propensity to thrombocytopenic coagulopathies than nonpregnant women. Also disturbing is a report of growth retardation, often severe, in 9 of 16 offspring of women with allografts who received cyclosporine during their gestations.[174] Thus we currently prefer that women planning to conceive not use cyclosporine or receive low doses (quoted anecdotally as less than 5 mg/kg daily).

Antenatal Management

In general, these women should be managed in a manner similar to that outlined for all women with underlying parenchymal kidney disease. In addition, it is wise to screen for asymptomatic bacteriuria at more frequent intervals (e.g., every 8–10 weeks). Liver function tests, calcium and phosphate levels, as well as white blood counts, should be checked at 6-weekly intervals. This is because the liver of gravidas may be more sensitive to the hepatotoxic actions of azathioprine and decreasing white counts are predictive of neutropenia and thrombocytopenia in the newborn (both problems managed by decreasing the dose[150, 152, 175]). Monitoring calcium and phosphate levels is especially important. First, some women will have had a partial parathyroidectomy in the past, while others may manifest tertiary hyperparathyroidism. Also,

as these women ingest steroids, it is best to screen for glucose intolerance both at mid-pregnancy and again in the early third trimester.

The "high-risk" nature of these gestations requires close prenatal and perinatal care, and for obvious reasons all pelvic examinations in transplant recipients should be performed with strict aseptic technique. While obstructed labor due to the position of the graft has occurred, this is very unusual for the transplanted kidney, is in the false pelvis, and is not apt to obstruct the birth canal. Cesarean sections should therefore be performed for obstetric reasons only. One valid cause, in this respect, is that transplant patients may have pelvic osteodystrophy related to their previous renal failure or prolonged steroid therapy.[150–152] Finally, the pediatric team should be alerted at time of delivery as many of these infants are born preterm, and there is a suggestion of an increased incidence of adrenocortical insufficiency and overwhelming neonatal infection in the newborn.[150–152] Steroids are secreted in breast milk, but not in sufficient quantity to affect the infant at the usual therapeutic doses. Metabolites of both azathioprine and cyclosporine appear in breast milk. Their levels are minimal, but in the absence of definitive data we discourage breast-feeding.[150–152, 169, 176, 177]

Maternal Follow-up

There are few guidelines concerning contraception in allograft recipients. Intrauterine contraceptive devices may aggravate menstrual problems, and obscure signs and symptoms of abnormalities in early pregnancy. The increased long-term risk of pelvic infection in an immunosuppressed patient is also worrisome, as insertion or replacement of these devices is normally associated with bacteremia in at least 1 in 10 women. Furthermore, the efficacy of intrauterine contraceptive devices may be reduced because of the immunosuppressive and anti-inflammatory agents these patients ingest.[150, 152, 178] Finally, oral contraceptives may cause or aggravate hypertension and thromboembolism, and may produce subtle changes in the immune system. Use of the "mini-dose" pill seems to have decreased these problems, but these drugs are yet to be systematically tested in a transplant population. Still, many use the low-dose estrogen pills combined with careful surveillance, the alternative being barrier methods which have a considerable failure rate.

Acknowledgments

We thank Mrs. Barbara Youpel for her excellent secretarial assistance. Much of our own work cited in this review was made possible by generous grants from the The National Institutes of Health, The Medical Research Council of Great Britain, The American Heart Association, and the Mother's Aid Research Fund of Lying-In Hospital.

REFERENCES

1. Pregnancy and renal disease (editorial). *Lancet* 1975; 2:801–802.
2. Bailey RR, Rolleston GL: Kidney length and ureteric dilatation in the puerperium. *J Obstet Gynaecol Br Commw* 1971; 78:55–61.
3. Sheehan HL, Lynch JP: *Pathology of Toxaemia of Pregnancy.* Baltimore, Williams & Wilkins Co, 1973.
4. Cietak KA, Newton JR: Serial quantitative maternal nephrosonography in pregnancy. *Br J Radiol* 1985; 58:405–413.
5. Lindheimer MD, Katz AI: The kidney and hypertension in pregnancy, in Brenner BM, Rector FC Jr (eds): *The Kidney,* ed 4. Philadelphia, WB Saunders Co, in press 1990.
6. Kaupilla A, Satuli R, Vourinen P: Ureteric dilatation and renal cortical index after normal preeclamptic pregnancies. *Acta Obstet Gynecol Scand* 1972; 51:147–153.
7. Rasmussen PE, Nielsen FR: Hydronephrosis during pregnancy: A literature survey. *Eur J Obstet Gynecol Reprod Biol* 1988; 27:249–259.
8. Fried AM, Woodring JH, Thompson DS: Hydronephrosis in pregnancy. A prospective sequential study of course of dilatation. *J Ultrasound Med* 1983; 2:255–259.
9. Cietak KA, Newton JR: Serial qualitative nephrosonography in pregnancy. *Br J Radiol* 1985; 58:399–404.
10. Rubi RA, Sala NL: Ureteral function in pregnant women III. Effect of different positions and of fetal delivery upon ureteral tonus. *Am J Obstet Gynecol* 1968; 101:230–237.
11. Dure-Smith P: Pregnancy dilatation of the urinary tract. The iliac sign and its significance. *Radiology* 1970; 96:545–550.
12. Myers SJ, Lee RV, Munschauer RW: Dilatation and nontraumatic rupture of the urinary tract during pregnancy. A review. *Obstet Gynecol* 1985; 66:809–815.
13. Nielsen FR, Rasmussen PE: Hydronephrosis during pregnancy: Four cases of hydronephrosis causing symptoms during pregnancy. *Eur J Obstet Gynecol Reprod Biol* 1988; 27:245–248.
14. Dunlop W, Davison JM: Renal haemodynamics and tubular function in human pregnancy. *Clin Obstet Gynaecol* 1987; 1:769–787.
15. Chesley LC, Lindheimer MD: Renal hemodynamics and intravascular volume in normal and hypertensive pregnancy, in Rubin PC (ed): *Handbook of Hypertension, Vol, 10: Hypertension in Pregnancy.* Amsterdam, Elsevier Science Publishers, 1988, pp 38–65.
16. Baylis C, Davison J: The urinary system, in Hytten F, Chamberlain G (eds): *Clinical Physiology in Obstetrics.* ed 2. Oxford, Blackwell Scientific Publishers, in press 1990.
17. Baylis C: Glomerular filtration and volume regulation in gravid animal models. *Clin Obstet Gynaecol* 1987; 1:789–813.
18. Davison JM: The effect of pregnancy on kidney function in renal allograft recipients. *Kidney Int* 1985; 27:74–79.
19. Davison JM, Lovedale C: The excretion of glucose during normal pregnancy and after delivery. *J Obstet Gynaecol Br Commw* 1974; 81:30–34.
20. Davison JM, Hytten FE: The effect of pregnancy on the renal handling of glucose. *J Obstet Gynaecol Br Commw* 1974; 82:374–381.
21. Hytten FE, Cheyne GA: The aminoaciduria of pregnancy. *J Obstet Gynaecol Br Commw* 1972; 79:424–432.
22. Semple PF, Carswell W, Boyle JA: Serial studies of the renal clearance of urate and inulin during pregnancy and after the puerperium in normal women. *Clin Sci Mol Med* 1974; 47:559–565.

23. Dunlop W, Davison JM: The effect of normal pregnancy upon the renal handling of uric acid. *Br J Obstet Gynaecol* 1977; 84:13–21.

24. Assali NS, Herzig D, Singh BP: Renal response to ammonium chloride acidosis in normal and toxemic pregnancies. *J Appl Physiol* 1955; 7:367–374.

25. Lim VS, Katz AI, Lindheimer MD: Acid base regulation in pregnancy. *Am J Physiol* 1976; 231:1764–1770.

26. Gallery EDM, Györy AZ: Urinary concentration, acid excretion, and acid-base status in normal pregnancy. Alterations in pregnancy-associated hypertension. *Am J Obstet Gynecol* 1979; 135:27–36.

27. Lyons HA, Antonio R: The sensitivity of the respiratory center in pregnancy and after administration of progesterone. *Trans Assoc Am Physicians* 1959; 72:173–180.

28. Davison JM, Vallotton MB, Lindheimer MD. Plasma osmolality and urinary concentration and dilution during and after pregnancy. Evidence that lateral recumbency inhibits maximal concentrating ability. *Br J Obstet Gynaecol* 1981; 88:472–479.

29. Davison JM, Shiells EA, Philips PR, et al: Serial evaluation of vasopressin release and thirst in human pregnancy. Role of human chorionic gonadotrophin in gestation. *J Clin Invest* 1988; 81:798–806.

30. Lindheimer MD, Barron WM, Davison JM: Osmoregulation of thirst and vasopressin release in pregnancy. *Am J Physiol* 1989; 257:F159–F169.

31. Davison JM, Shiells EA, Barron WM, et al: Changes in the metabolic clearance of vasopressin and in plasma vasopressinase throughout human pregnancy. *J Clin Invest* 1989; 83:1313–1316.

32. Davison JM, Shiells EA, Philips PR, et al: Metabolic clearance rates (MCR) of arginine vasopressin (dDAVP) and 1-deamino-8-D-AVP (dDAVP) in human pregnancy (P): Evidence that placental enzymes increase MCRs of AVP in gestation (abstract). *Clin Res* 1989; 37:596A.

33. Barron WM: Water metabolism and vasopressin secretion during pregnancy. *Clin Obstet Gynaecol* 1987; 1:853–871.

34. Durr JA: Diabetes insipidus syndromes of pregnancy, in Cowley AW Jr, Liard J-F, Ausiello DA (eds): *Vasopressin: Cellular and Integrative Functions.* New York, Raven Press, 1988, pp 257–263.

35. Baylis PH, Thompson C, Burd J, et al: Recurrent pregnancy-induced polyuria and thirst due to hypothalamic diabetes insipidus: An investigation into possible mechanisms responsible for polyuria. *Clin Endocrinol* 1986; 24:459–466.

36. Hughs JM, Barron WM, Vance MC: Recurrent diabetes insipidus associated with pregnancy. Pathophysiology and therapy. *Obstet Gynecol* 1989; 73:462–464.

37. Barron WM, Cohen LH, Ulland LA, et al: Transient vasopressin resistant diabetes insipidus of pregnancy. *N Engl J Med* 1984; 310:442–444.

38. Durr JA, Hoggard JG, Hunt JM, et al: Diabetes insipidus in pregnancy associated with abnormally high circulating vasopressinase *N Engl J Med* 1987; 316:1070–1074.

39. Shah SV, Thakur V: Vasopressinase and diabetes insipidus of pregnancy. *Ann Intern Med* 1988; 109:435–436.

40. Robinson M: Salt in pregnancy. *Lancet* 1958; 1:178–181.

41. Lopez-Espinosa, Dhar H, Humphrey S, et al: Urinary albumin excretion in pregnancy. *Br J Obstet Gynaecol* 1986; 93:176–181.

42. Wright A, Steele P, Bennett JR, et al: The urinary excretion of albumin in normal pregnancy. *Br J Obstet Gynaecol* 1987; 94:408–412.

43. Mogensen CE, Klebe JG (ed): Microalbuminuria and diabetic pregnancy, in Mogensen CE (ed): *The Kidney and Hypertension in Diabetes Mellitus.* Boston, Martinus Nijhoff, 1988, pp 223–229.

44. Rodrigues MH, Masak DI, Mestman J, et al: Calcium/Creatinine ratio and microalbuminuria in the prediction of preeclampsia. *Am J Obstet Gynecol* 1988; 159:1452–1455.

45. Danielli L, Korchazak L, Beyar H, et al: Recurrent hematuria during multiple pregnancies. *Obstet Gynecol* 1987; 69:446–448.

46. Coe FL: Clinical and laboratory assessment in the patient with renal disease, in Brenner BM, Rector FC Jr (eds): *The Kidney,* ed 3. Philadelphia, WB Saunders Co, 1986, pp 703–734.

47. Lindheimer MD, Davison JM: Renal biopsy in pregnancy. "To b . . . or not to b . . .?" *Br J Obstet Gynaecol* 1987; 94:932–934.

48. Packham D, Fairley KF: Renal biopsy: Indications and complications in pregnancy. *Br J Obstet Gynaecol* 1987; 94:935–939.

49. McFadyen IR: Urinary tract infection in

pregnancy, in Andreucci VE (ed): *The Kidney in Pregnancy.* Boston, Martinus Nijhoff, 1986, pp 205–229.

50. Cunningham FG: Urinary tract infections complicating pregnancy. *Clin Obstet Gynaecol* 1987; 1:891–908.

51. Whalley PJ, Martin FG, Pritchard JA: Sickle cell trait and urinary tract infection during pregnancy. *JAMA* 1964; 189:903–906.

52. Bruns W, Weuffen W, Godel E, et al: Frequency of urinary tract infection in diabetic gravidas (in German). *Z Gesamte Inn Med* 1968; 23:520–523.

53. Romero R, Oyarzun E, Mazor M, et al: Meta-anaylsis of relationship between asymptomatic bacteriuria and preterm delivery/low birthweight. *Obstet Gynecol* 1989; 72:576–582.

54. Whalley PJ: Bacteruria of pregnancy. *Amer J Obstet Gynecol* 1967; 97:723–738.

55. Harris RE: The significance of eradication of bacteriuria during pregnancy. *Obstet Gynecol* 1979; 53:71–73.

56. Editorial: Urinary tract infection during pregnancy. *Lancet* 1985; 2:190–192.

57. Campbell-Brown M, McFadyen IR, Seal DV, et al: Is screening for bacteriuria in pregnancy worthwhile? *Br Med J* 1987; 294:1579–1582.

58. Marraro RV, Harris RE: Incidence of resolution of spontaneous bacteriuria. *Am J Obstet Gynecol* 1977; 128:722–723.

59. Eng J, Torkidsen EM, Christiansen A: Bacteriuria in the puerperium: An evaluation of methods for collecting urine. *Am J Obstet Gynecol* 1978; 131:739–742.

60. Gilstrap LC, Cunningham FG, Whalley PJ: Acute pyelonephritis in pregnancy. An anterospective study. *Obstet Gynecol* 1981; 57:409–413.

61. Lenke RR, Vandorstan JP, Schifrin BS: Pyelonephritis in pregnancy. A prospective randomized trial to prevent recurrent disease evaluating suppressive therapy with nitrofurantoin and close surveillance. *Am J Obstet Gynecol* 1983; 146:953–957.

62. Pertuiset N, Grunfeld JP: Acute renal failure in pregnancy. *Clin Obstet Gynaecol* 1987; 1:873–890.

63. Lindheimer MD, Katz AI, Ganavel D, et al: Acute renal failure in pregnancy, in Brenner BM, Lazarus JM (eds): *Acute Renal Failure,* ed 2. New York, Churchill Livingstone, 1988, pp 597–620.

64. Madias NE, Donohoe JF, Harrington JT: Postischemic acute renal failure, in Brenner BM, Lazarus JM (eds): *Acute Renal Failure,* ed 2. New York, Churchill Livingstone, 1988, pp 251–278.

65. Brezis M, Rosen S, Epstein FH: Acute renal failure, in Brenner BM, Rector FC Jr (eds): *The Kidney,* ed 3. Philadelphia, WB Saunders Co, 1986, pp 735–799.

66. Turney JH, Ellis CM, Parson FM: Obstetric acute renal failure: 1956–1987. *Br J Obstet Gynaecol* 1989; 96:679–687.

67. Bartlett RH, Yahia C: Management of septic abortion with renal failure: Report of five consecutive cases with five survivors. *N Engl J Med* 1969; 281:747–775.

68. Hawkins OF, Sevitt LH, Fairbrother DF, et al: Management of chemical septic abortion with renal failure. Use of a conservative regimen. *N Engl J Med* 1975; 292:722–725.

69. Whalley PJ, Cunningham FG, Martin FG: Transient renal dysfunction associated with acute pyelonephritis of pregnancy. *Obstet Gynecol* 1975; 46:174–177.

70. Stratta P, Canavese C, Dolgiani M, et al: Pregnancy-related acute renal failure. *Clin Nephrol* 1988; 32:14–20.

71. Chugh KS, Singhal PC, Kher VK, et al: Spectrum of acute cortical necroses in Indian patients. *Am J Med Sci* 1983; 286:10–20.

72. Sheehan HL, Moore HC: *Renal Cortical Necroses and the Kidney of Concealed Accidental Hemorrhage.* Springfield, Ill, Charles C Thomas, 1953.

73. Williams TF: Renal cortical necrosis, renal infarction, and hypertension due to renal disease, in Strauss MB, Welt LG (eds): *Diseases of The Kidney.* Boston, Little, Brown & Co, 1963, pp 526–539.

74. Kleinknecht D, Grünfeld JP, Gomez PC, et al: Diagnostic procedures and long-term prognosis in bilateral renal cortical necroses. *Kidney Int* 1973; 4:390–400.

75. Conger JD, Falk S, Guggenheim SJ: Glomerular dynamics and morphologic changes in the generalized Shwartzman reaction in postpartum rats. *J Clin Invest* 1981; 67:1334–1344.

76. Kaplan ML: Acute fatty liver in pregnancy. *N Engl J Med* 1985; 313:367–370.

77. Reily CA, Latham PS, Romero R, et al: Acute fatty liver of pregnancy. A reassessment based on observations in 9 patients.

Ann Intern Med 1987; 106:703–706.

78. Liebman HA, McGehee WG, Patch MJ, et al: Severe depression of antithrombin III associated with disseminated intravascular coagulation in women with fatty liver of pregnancy. *Ann Intern Med* 1983; 98:330–333.

79. Weber FL, Snodgrass PJ, Powell DE, et al: Abnormalities of hepatic mitochondrial urea-cycle enzyme activities in acute fatty liver of pregnancy. *J Lab Clin Med* 1979; 94:27–41.

80. Rolfes DB, Ishak KG: Acute fatty liver of pregnancy: A clinicopathologic study of 35 cases. *Hepatology* 1985; 5:1149–1158.

81. Gomperts ED, Sessel L, DuPlesses V, et al: Recurrent postpartum haemolytic uraemic syndrome. *Lancet* 1978; 1:48.

82. Kincaid-Smith P, Fairley KF, Kloss M: Lupus anticoagulant associated with thrombotic microangiopathy and pregnancy related renal failure. *Q J Med* 1988; 69:795–815.

83. Brandt P, Jespersen J, Gregersen G: Postpartum haemolytic uraemic syndrome successfully treated with antithrombin III. *Br Med J* 1980; 280:449 [also published in *Nephron* 1981; 27:15–18].

84. Warren GV, Sprague SM, Corwin HC: Sarcoidosis presenting as acute renal failure in pregnancy. *Am J Kidney Dis* 1988; 12:161–163.

85. O'Shaughnessy R, Weprin SA, Zuspan FP: Obstructive renal failure by an overdistended uterus. *Obstet Gynecol* 1980; 55:247–259.

86. Hamilton DV, Kelly MB, Pryor JS: Polyhydramnios and acute renal failure. *Postgrad Med J* 1980; 56:798–799.

87. Homans DC, Blake DG, Harrington JT, et al: Acute renal failure caused by ureteral obstruction by a gravid uterus. *JAMA* 1981; 246:1230–1231.

88. Maizels M, Victor TA, Garnett J, et al: Matrix obstruction of a solitary kidney during pregnancy. *Urology* 1982; 20:305–308.

89. Lewis GJ, Chatterjee SF, Rowse AD: Acute renal failure presenting in pregnancy secondary to idiopathic hydronephrosis. *Br Med J* 1985; 290:1250–1251.

90. Weiss Z, Shalev E, Zuckerman H, et al: Obstructive renal failure and pleural effusion caused by the gravid uterus. *Acta Obstet Gynecol Scand* 1986; 65:187–189.

91. Eika B, Skajaa K: Acute renal failure due to bilateral ureteral obstruction by the pregnant uterus. *Urol Int* 1988; 43:315–317.

92. Loughlin KR, Bailey RB: Internal ureteral stents for conservative management of ureteral calculi during pregnancy. *N Engl J Med* 1986; 315:1647–1649.

93. Lowes JJ, Mackenzie JC, Abrams PH, et al: Acute renal failure and acute hydronephrosis in pregnancy: Use of double J stent. *J R Soc Med* 1987; 80:524–525.

94. Brenner BM, Lazarus (eds): *Acute Renal Failure*, ed 2. New York, Churchill Livingstone, 1988, pp 743–874.

95. Hou S: Peritoneal dialysis and haemodialysis in pregnancy. *Clin Obstet Gynaecol* 1987; 1:1009–1025.

96. Redraw M, Cherem L, Elliott J, et al: Dialysis and management of pregnant patients with renal insufficiency. *Medicine* 1988; 67:199–208.

97. Yasin SY, Beydoun SM: Hemodialysis in pregnancy. *Obstet Gynecol Surv* 1988; 43:655–668.

98. Katz AI, Davison JM, Hayslett JP, et al: Pregnancy in women with kidney disease. *Kidney Int* 1980; 18:192–206.

99. Surian M, Imbasciati E, Bonfi G, et al: Glomerular disease and pregnancy. A study of 123 pregnancies in patients with primary and secondary glomerular diseases. *Nephron* 1984; 36:101–105.

100. Abe S, Amagasacki Y, Konishi K, et al: The influence of antecedent renal disease on pregnancy. *Am J Obstet Gynecol* 1985; 153:508–514.

101. Jungers P, Forget D, Henry-Amer M, et al: Chronic kidney disease and pregnancy. *Adv Nephrol* 1986; 15:103–141.

102. Barcelo P, Lopez-Lillo J, Cabero L, et al: Successful pregnancy in primary glomerular disease. *Kidney Int* 1986; 30:914–919.

103. Packam DK, North RA, Fairly KF, et al: Primary glomerulonephritis and pregnancy. *Q J Med* 1989; 266:537–553 [see also: Pregnancy and glomerulonephritis (editorial). *Lancet* 1989; 2:253–254].

104. Rovatti E, Perrino ML, Barbiano de-Belgioso G, et al: Pregnancy and course of primary glomerulonephritis. *Contrib Nephrol* 1984; 37:182–189.

105. Becker GJ, Ihle BV, Fairley KF, et al: Effect of pregnancy on moderate renal failure in reflux nephropathy. *Br Med J* 1986; 292:796–798.

106. Kincaid-Smith P, Fairley KF: Renal disease in pregnancy. Three controversial areas. Mesangial IgA nephropathy, focal glomerular sclerosis (focal and segmental hyalinosis and sclerosis), and reflux nephropathy. *Am J Kidney Dis* 1987; 9:328–333.

107. Junger P, Forget D, Houllier P, et al: Pregnancy in lgA nephropathy, reflux nephropathy and focal glomerular sclerosis. *Am J Kidney Dis* 1987; 9:334–338.

108. Junger P, Houllier P, Forget D: Reflux nephropathy and pregnancy. *Clin Obstet Gynaecol* 1987; 1:953–969.

109. Packham DK, North RA, Fairley KF, et al: Pregnancy in women with primary focal and segmental hyalinosis and sclerosis. *Clin Nephrol* 1988; 29:185–192.

110. Packham DK, North RA, Fairley KF, et al: lgA glomerulonephritis and pregnancy. *Clin Nephrol* 1988; 30:15–21.

111. Packham DK, Fairley KF, Ihle BV, et al: Histological features of lgA glomerulonephritis as predictors of pregnancy outcome. *Clin Nephrol* 1988; 30:22–26.

112. Packham DK, Fairley KF, Whitworth JA, et al: Comparison of pregnancy outcome between normotensive and hypertensive women with primary glomerulonephritis. *Clin Exp Hypertens* 1988; B(6):387–400.

113. Hou SH, Grossman SD, Madias N: Pregnancy in women with renal disease and moderate renal insufficiency. *Am J Med* 1985; 78:185–194.

114. Lim, VS: Reproductive endocrinology in uremia. *Clin Obstet Gynaecol* 1987; 1:997–1010.

115. Galler M, Spinowitz B, Charytan C, et al: Reproductive function in dialysis patients. CAPD vs hemodialysis. *Periton Dial Bull* 1983; 3(suppl 1):30S.

116. Singson E, Fisher KF, Lindheimer MD: Acute glomerulonephritis in pregnancy. *Am J Obstet Gynecol* 1980; 137:857–858.

117. Davis AE, Armour MA, Alper CA, et al: Transfer of C_3 nephritic factor from mother to fetus. *N Engl J Med* 1977; 297:144–145.

118. Harris JP, Rakowski TA, Argy WP, et al: Alport's syndrome presenting as crescentric glomerulonephritis. A report of two siblings. *Clin Nephrol* 1978; 10:245–249.

119. Hayslett JP, Lynn RI: Effect of pregnancy in patients with lupus nephropathy. *Kidney Int* 1980; 18:207–220.

120. Hauser MT, Fish AJ, Tagatz GE, et al: Systemic lupus erythematosus in pregnancy. *Am J Obstet Gynecol* 1980; 138:409–413.

121. Fine LG, Barnett EV, Danovitch GM, et al: Systemic lupus erythematosus in pregnancy. *Ann Intern Med* 1981; 94:667–677.

122. Imbasciati E, Surian M, Bottino S, et al: Lupus nephropathy and pregnancy. A study of 26 pregnancies in patients with systemic lupus erythematosus and nephritis. *Nephron* 1984; 36:46–51.

123. Bobrie G, Liote F, Houllier P, et al: Pregnancy in lupus nephritis and related disorders. *Am J Kidney Dis* 1987; 9:337–343.

124. Lupus nephritis and pregnancy (editorial). *Lancet* 1989; 2:82–83.

125. Lockshin MD, Reinitz E, Druzin NL, et al: Case control prospective study demonstrating absence of lupus exacerbation during or after pregnancy. *Am J Med* 1984; 77:893–898.

126. Kitzmiller JL, Brown ER, Phillippe M, et al: Diabetic nephropathy and prenatal outcome. *Am J Obstet Gynecol* 1981; 141:741–751.

127. Jovanovic R, Jovanovic L: Obstetric management when normologycemia is maintained in diabetic pregnant women with vascular compromise. *Am J Obstet Gynecol* 1984; 149:617–623.

128. Grenfell A, Brudenell JM, Doddridge RMC, et al: Pregnancy in diabetic women who have proteinuria. *Q J Med* 1986; 59:379–386.

129. Reece EA, Coustan DR, Hayslett JP, et al: Diabetic nephropathy. Pregnancy performance and fetal-maternal outcome. *Am J Obstet Gynecol* 1988; 159:56–66.

130. Jovanovic-Peterson L, Peterson CM: De-novo clinical hypothyroidism in pregnancy complicated by type I diabetes, sub-clinical hypothyroidism, and proteinuria: A new syndrome. *Am J Obstet Gynecol* 1988; 159:442–446.

131. Klockars M, Saarikoski S, Ikonen E, et al: Pregnancy in patients with renal disease. *Acta Med Scand* 1980; 207:207–214.

132. Mitcheson HD, Williams G, Castro JE: Clinical aspects of polycystic disease and the kidneys. *Br Med J* 1977; 1:1196–1198.

133. Milutinovic J, Agoda LY, Phillips LA, et al: Fertility and pregnancy complications in women with autosomal dominant polycystic disease. *Obstet Gynecol* 1983; 61:566–570.

134. Maikrantz P, Coe FL, Parks JH, et al: Nephrolithiases and gestation. *Clin Obstet Gynaecol* 1987; 1:909–919.

135. Coe FL, Park JH, Lindheimer MD: Neph-

rolithiasis during pregnancy. *N Engl J Med* 1978; 298:324–326.

136. Jones WA, Correa RJ, Ansell JS: Urolithiasis associated with pregnancy. *J Urol* 1978; 122:333–351.

137. Lattanzi DR, Cook WA: Urinary calculi in pregnancy. *Obstet Gynecol* 1980; 56:462–466.

138. Drago JR, Rohner TJ Jr, Chez RA: Management of urinary calculi in pregnancy. *Urology* 1982; 20:578–581.

139. Perrault JP, Paquin JM, Faucher R, et al: Urinary calculi in pregnancy. *Can J Surg* 1982; 25:453–454.

140. Gregory MC, Mansell MA: Pregnancy and cystinuria. *Lancet* 1983; 2:1958–1960.

141. Horowitz E, Schmidt JD: Renal calculi in pregnancy. *Clin Obstet Gynecol* 1985; 28:324–338.

142. Rodriguez PN, Klein AS: Management of urolithiasis during pregnancy. *Surg Gynecol Obstet* 1988, 166:103–106.

143. Harris RC, Meyer T, Brenner BM: Nephron adaptation to renal injury, in Brenner BM, Rector FC Jr (eds): *The Kidney,* ed 3. Philadelphia, WB Saunders Co, 1986, pp 1553–1585.

144. Anderson S: Progression of chronic renal disease: Role of systemic and glomerular hypertension. *Am J Kidney Dis* 1989; 6(suppl 1):8–12.

145. Mitch WE: The influence of the diet on the progression of renal insufficiency. *Annu Rev Med* 1984; 35:249–264.

146. Ferris T: Pregnancy and chronic renal diseases. *Kidney* 1986; 19:1–4.

147. Baylis C: Renal disease in gravid animals. *Am J Kidney Dis* 1987; 9:350–353.

148. Davison JM: The effect of pregnancy on long term renal function in women with chronic renal disease and single kidneys (abstract). *Clin Exp Hypertens* 1989; B(8):226.

149. Murray JE, Reid DE, Harrison JH, et al: Successful pregnancies after human renal transplantation. *N Engl J Med* 1963; 269:341–343.

150. Davison JM, Lindheimer MD: Pregnancy in women with renal allografts. *Semin Nephrol* 1984; 4:240–251.

151. Penn I: Pregnancy following renal transplantation, in Andreucci VE (ed): *The Kidney in Pregnancy.* Boston, Martinus Nijhoff, 1986, pp 195–204.

152. Davison JM: Pregnancy in renal allograft

recipients: Prognosis and management. *Clin Obstet Gynaecol* 1987; 1:1027–1045.

153. Hou S: Pregnancy in organ transplant recipients. *Med Clin North Am* 1989; 73:667–683.

154. Gallery EDM: Pregnancy in women with renal transplants. *Int J Artif Organs* 1989; 12:141–143.

155. Davison JM, Lindheimer MD: Pregnancy and renal transplantation: Look before you leap. *Int J Artif Organs* 1989; 12:144–146.

156. Markatz IR, Schwartz GH, David S, et al: Resumption of female reproductive function following renal transplantation. *JAMA* 1971; 216:1749–1754.

157. Whitiker RH, Hamilton D: Effect of transplantation on nonrenal effects of renal failure. *Br Med J* 1982; 284:221–222.

158. Rifle G, Traeger J: Pregnancy after renal transplantation: An international survey. *Transplant Proc* 1975; 7:723–728.

159. Rudolph JE, Schweizer RT, Bar SA: Pregnancy in renal transplant patients. *Transplantation* 1979; 27:26–29.

160. Penn I, Makowski EL, Harris P: Parenthood following renal transplantation. *Kidney Int* 1980; 18:221–233.

161. Whetham JCG, Cardelle C, Harding M: Effect of pregnancy on graft function and graft survival. *Am J Obstet Gynecol* 1983; 145(2) 193–197.

162. O'Connell PJ, Caterson RJ, Stewart JH, et al: Problems associated with pregnancy in renal allograft recipients. *Int J Artif Organs* 1989; 12:147–152.

163. Ogburn PL, Kitzmiller JC, Hare JW, et al: Pregnancy following renal transplantation in class T diabetes mellitus. *JAMA* 1986; 255:911–915.

164. Tyden U, Bratterstrom E, Bjorkman et al: Pregnancy after combined pancreas-kidney transplantation. *Diabetes* 1989; 39(suppl 1):43–45.

165. Hoover R, Fraumeni JR: Risk of cancer in renal transplant recipients. *Lancet* 1973; 2:55–57.

166. Morris PJ: Renal transplantation: Indications, outcome complications and results, in Schrier RW, Gottschalk CW (eds): *Diseases of The Kidney,* ed 4. Boston, Little, Brown & Co, 1988, pp 3211–3234.

167. Alloub MI, Barr BBB, McLaren KM, et al: Human papilloma virus infection and cervical intraepithelial neoplasia in women

with renal allografts. *Br Med J* 1989; 298:153–156.

168. Registration Committee of the European Dialysis and Transplant Association: Successful pregnancies in women treated by dialyses and kidney transplantation. *Br J Obstet Gynaecol* 1980; 87:839–845.

169. Lewis GJ, Lamont CA, Lee HA, et al: Successful pregnancy in a renal transplant recipient taking cyclosporine A. *Br Med J* 1983; 286:603.

170. Flechner SM, Katz AR, VanBuren C, et al: The presence of cyclosporine in body tissues and fluids during pregnancy. *Am J Kidney Dis* 1985; 5:60–63.

171. Duggan CJ, Boyce ES, Caterson RJ, et al: Successful pregnancy in a renal transplant recipient taking cyclosporine A. *Aust N Z J Med* 1986; 16:813–814.

172. Derfler K, Schaller A, Harold L, et al: Successful outcome of a complicated pregnancy in a renal transplant recipient taking cyclosporine A. *Clin Nephrol* 1988; 29:96–102.

173. Beisenbach G, Grafinger P, Keinser W, et al: Successful outcome of high risk pregnancy within 1 year following kidney transplantation with cyclosporin as the immunosuppressive agent. *Schweiz Med Wochenschr* 1988; 118:929–934.

174. Pickerell MD, Sawers R, Michael J: Pregnancy after renal transplantation: Severe intrauterine growth retardation during treatment with cyclosporine. *Br Med J* 1988; 296:825.

175. Davison JM, Dellagrammatikas H, Parkin JM: Maternal azathioprine therapy and depressed haemopoiesis in babies of renal allograft patients. *Br J Obstet Gynaecol* 1985; 92:233–239.

176. Fagerholm MI, Coulam CB, Moyer TP: Breast feeding after renal transplantation: 6-Mercaptopurine content of human breast milk: *Surg Forum* 1980; 31:447–450.

177. Coulam CB, Moyer TP, Jiang NS, et al: Breast feeding after renal transplantation. *Transplant Proc* 1982; 14:605–609.

178. Murray S, Hickey J, Houang E: Significant bacteremia associated with replacement of intrauterine contraceptive device. *Am J Obstet Gynecol* 1987; 156:698–699.

CHAPTER 3

Diabetes Mellitus

Mark B. Landon
Steven G. Gabbe

The discovery of insulin in 1921 remains the most significant advancement in the treatment of the pregnancy complicated by diabetes mellitus. Before the discovery of insulin, pregnancy in the diabetic woman was uncommon and was accompanied by high maternal and fetal mortality. Through improved understanding of the pathophysiology of diabetes in pregnancy as well as the development of techniques to prevent complications, fetal and neonatal mortality have fallen from approximately 65% before the discovery of insulin to 2% to 5% at the present time (Fig 3–1). If optimal care is provided for the diabetic woman, the perinatal mortality rate, excluding major congenital malformations, is equivalent to that observed in normal pregnancies.

Controversy still exists regarding the management of pregnancy complicated by diabetes. While the benefit of careful regulation of maternal glucose levels is generally well accepted, the level of glycemic control necessary to optimize perinatal outcome remains a controversial issue. A better understanding of factors that contribute to the significant neonatal morbidity observed in the infant of the diabetic mother (IDM) may resolve this question.

There is also continued controversy concerning methods for the assessment of antepartum fetal well-being and the timing and mode of delivery. The diagnosis of gestational diabetes mellitus (GDM) along with its implications has also come under great scrutiny in recent years. Before considering these issues, we begin by first reviewing carbohydrate metabolism and some aspects of the pathophysiology of diabetes in pregnancy.

MATERNAL METABOLISM AND THE PATHOPHYSIOLOGY OF DIABETES IN PREGNANCY

During pregnancy, maternal metabolism adjusts to provide adequate nutrition for both the mother and the growing fetoplacental unit. Early in pregnancy, glucose homeostasis is altered by increasing levels of estrogen and progesterone which lead to beta cell hyperplasia and an increased insulin response to a glucose load.[1] The heightened peripheral utilization of glucose causes a 10% reduction in maternal fasting glucose levels by the end of the first trimester. Thus, insulin-requiring diabetics commonly experience periods of hypoglycemia in early pregnancy. The fall in maternal glucose levels results in a decline in fasting insulin concentrations leading to a marked starvation ketosis. Fasting blood levels of beta-hydroxybutyrate and acetoacetate are severalfold higher in pregnancy. Compensatory mechanisms to offset this state of

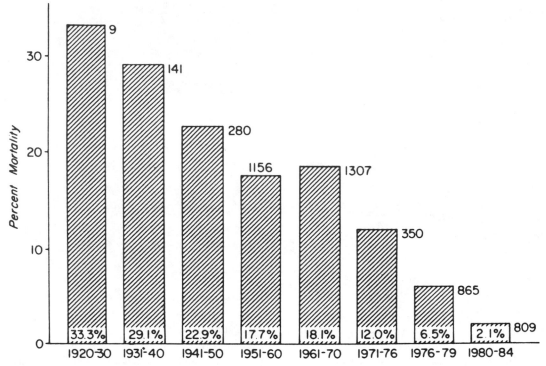

FIG 3–1.
Perinatal mortality in pregnancies complicated by insulin-dependent diabetes mellitus, classes B through R. Number at the top of column indicates total number of cases in each time period. (Adapted from Gabbe SG: Management of diabetes in pregnancy. Six decades of experience, in Pitkin RM, Zlatnik FJ (eds): *Year Book of Obstetrics and Gynecology, 1980.* Chicago, Year Book Medical Publishers, Inc., 1980, p 37. Used by permission.)

"accelerated starvation" include increased protein catabolism and accelerated gluconeogenesis from amino acid precursors, particularly alanine.[2]

Despite the above processes, early and midpregnancy are periods of maternal anabolism marked by increasing maternal protein and fat stores. The relative hyperinsulinemia observed early in pregnancy serves to promote lipogenesis and decrease lipolysis. Glucagon levels are relatively suppressed in normal pregnant women following meals, resulting in more prolonged hyperglycemia and hyperinsulinemia after feeding. This period of "facilitated anabolism" may offset the accelerated starvation of the fasting state.[2]

During the second half of pregnancy rising levels of human placental lactogen (hPL) and other "contrainsulin" hormones synthesized by the placenta modify maternal utilization of glucose and amino acids. The blood glucose response to an oral or intravenous carbohydrate load is greater than in the non-pregnant state (Fig 3–2). The actions of hPL are responsible, in part, for the "diabetogenic state" of pregnancy characterized by an exaggerated rate and amount of insulin release associated with a decreased sensitivity to insulin at the cellular level.[3] Insulin resistance in the liver allows mobilization of hepatic stores of glycogen and increased hepatic glucose production. Other hormones which appear to modify this response include elevated levels of prolactin, estrogen, and progesterone.[4, 5] The primary action of hPL, stimulation of lipolysis with release of free fatty acids from maternal adipose tissue, spares glucose, one of the most important fuels for fetal growth. Insulin receptors on circulating monocytes are not reduced during late pregnancy, suggesting that insulin resistance may be related primarily to postreceptor events.[6]

Maintenance of normal glucose homeostasis during pregnancy is achieved by a compensatory increase in plasma insulin levels. In normal pregnancies, maternal beta cell hyperplasia yields a 30% increase in basal insulin production at term. In addition, the insulin response to a challenge of oral or intravenous glucose in the last trimester is nearly twice that observed in the nonpregnant state.[7] The increased insulin requirement seen during the last trimester of pregnancy in women with diabetes is roughly equivalent to the endogenous increase noted in normal gestation. If a pregnant patient has borderline pancreatic reserve, her endogenous insulin pro-

duction may be inadequate, and thus diabetes will then be revealed for the first time. Unlike known insulin-requiring patients, gestational diabetics with limited beta cell reserve and presumed insulin resistance may require large doses of insulin.[8]

The placenta not only produces hormones which alter maternal metabolism but also controls the transport of nutrients to the fetal compartment. Substrate supply to the fetus depends upon the specific modes of transfer. Glucose transport across the placenta occurs by carrier-mediated facilitated diffusion. Therefore, glucose levels in the fetus are directly proportional to maternal plasma

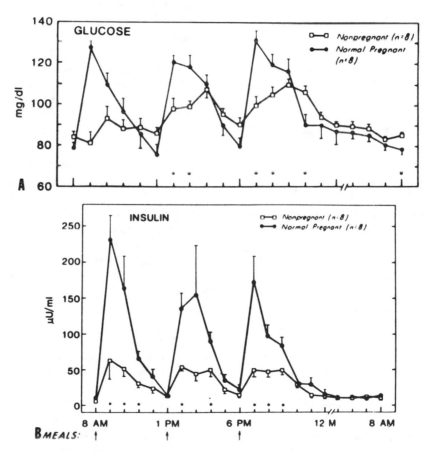

FIG 3–2.
Mean (± SEM) values for (**A**) glucose and (**B**) insulin at intervals of 1 hour from 8:00 A.M. to midnight and 2 hours thereafter in eight nonpregnant and eight normal pregnant women in the third trimester. Mealtimes are indicated by *arrows* along the abscissa. Pregnant women demonstrate a greater amplitude in plasma glucose excursions after meals. The increased postprandial insulin secretion is apparent. (From Phelps RL, Metzger BE, Freinkel N: *Am J Obstet Gynecol* 1981, 140:730. Used by permission.)

glucose concentrations. Glucose is the primary fuel utilized by the fetus for protein and fat synthesis. The degree of placental transfer of glucose and other fuels is also affected by placental metabolism. In the sheep model, the placenta uses approximately one half of the glucose delivered to the uterus to support its own metabolic processes.[9] Further modification of the transfer of carbohydrate may be influenced by placental insulin receptors. The placenta is essentially impermeable to protein hormones such as insulin, glucagon, growth hormone, and hPL.[10] Although maternal insulin does not cross the placenta, it may enhance placental glucose transport by affecting the glucose carrier.[10] In addition to glucose transfer, many amino acids are actively transported across the placenta to the fetal compartment. This process contributes to the maternal hypoaminoacidemia observed in the fasting state. Keto acids appear to diffuse freely across the placenta and may serve as a fetal fuel during periods of maternal starvation.[10]

Fetal glucose levels are normally maintained within narrow limits because maternal carbohydrate homeostasis is so well regulated. During pregnancy in the insulin-dependent diabetic woman, periods of hyperglycemia lead to fetal hyperglycemia. Persistent elevations of glucose and perhaps amino acids may then stimulate the fetal pancreas resulting in beta cell hyperplasia and fetal hyperinsulinemia.[11]

PERINATAL MORBIDITY AND MORTALITY

Fetal Death

In the past, sudden and unexplained stillbirth occurred in 10% to 30% of pregnancies complicated by insulin-dependent diabetes.[12] Although relatively uncommon today, such losses still plague the pregnancies of patients who do not receive optimal care. Stillbirths have been most often observed after the 36th week of pregnancy, in patients with vascular disease, poor glycemic control, hydramnios, fetal macrosomia, or preeclampsia. In an effort to prevent intrauterine deaths, a strategy of scheduled preterm deliveries was established. While this empiric approach reduced the number of stillbirths, errors in estimation of fetal size and gestational age as well as the functional immaturity characteristic of the IDM contributed to many neonatal deaths from hyaline membrane disease.

The precise cause of the excessive stillbirth rate in pregnancies complicated by diabetes mellitus remains unknown. Yet, it has become evident that, when maternal glucose levels are maintained within physiologic limits, sudden intrauterine deaths rarely occur. Because extramedullary hematopoiesis is frequently observed in stillborn IDMs, chronic intrauterine hypoxia has been cited as a likely cause of these intrauterine fetal deaths. Maternal diabetes may produce alterations in red blood cell oxygen release and placental blood flow.[9] While there is little evidence that red blood cell oxygen release is impaired in well-regulated pregnant diabetic women, in poorly controlled patients a shift to the left may occur in the oxyhemoglobin dissociation curve. This change, which may be most marked in patients recovering from diabetic ketoacidosis, results in increasing hemoglobin oxygen affinity, and therefore reduced red cell oxygen delivery at the tissue level.

Reduced uterine blood flow is thought to contribute to the increased incidence of intrauterine growth retardation observed in the pregnancies complicated by diabetic vasculopathy. Investigations using radioactive tracers have also suggested a relationship between poor maternal control and reduced uteroplacental blood flow.[13] Ketoacidosis and preeclampsia, two factors known to be associated with an increased incidence of intrauterine deaths, may further reduce uterine blood flow. In diabetic ketoacidosis, hypovolemia and hypotension due to dehydration may reduce flow through the intervillous space, while in preeclampsia narrowing and vasospasm of spiral arterioles may result.

Alterations in maternal and, in turn, fetal carbohydrate metabolism may also contribute to intrauterine asphyxia.[14–16] In normally

TABLE 3–1.
Factors Which May Reduce Fetal Oxygenation in
Pregnancies Complicated by Diabetes Mellitus*

Maternal
  1. Alterations in oxyhemoglobin dissociation curve
  2. Ketoacidosis
Placental
  1. Reduced uteroplacental blood flow
     a. Hyperglycemia
     b. Ketoacidosis
     c. Preeclampsia
  2. Reduced oxygen transfer
     a. Increased diffusion distance
Fetal
  1. Hyperglycemia
  2. Hyperinsulinemia
  3. Ketonemia
*Adapted from Madsen H. *Dan Med Bull* 1986; 33:64–74.

oxygenated fetal lambs, hyperglycemia produces a small increase in lactate but little change in pH. However, when hyperglycemia is produced in slightly hypoxic lambs, a marked rise in lactate is noted and resulting acidosis develops.[16] There is considerable evidence linking hyperinsulinemia and fetal hypoxia. Hyperinsulinemia induced in fetal lambs by an infusion of exogenous insulin produces an increase in oxygen consumption and a decrease in arterial oxygen content.[17, 18] Hypoxemia may occur as a result of increased oxygen extraction by fetal tissues without a corresponding increase in oxygen delivery. Using a sheep model, Miodovnik and coworkers have shown that an increase in fetal ketoacid levels may also reduce oxygenation.[19] Infusion of beta-hydroxybutyrate led to a rise in fetal lactate levels and a fall in pH. Thus, hyperinsulinemia in the fetus of the diabetic mother may increase fetal metabolic rate and oxygen requirements in the face of several factors such as hyperglycemia, ketoacidosis, preeclampsia, and maternal vasculopathy which can reduce placental blood flow and fetal oxygenation (Table 3–1).

Congenital Malformations

With the reduction in intrauterine deaths and a marked decrease in neonatal mortality related to hyaline membrane disease and traumatic delivery, congenital malformations have emerged as the most important cause of perinatal loss in pregnancies complicated by insulin-dependent diabetes mellitus (IDDM). In the past, these anomalies were responsible for approximately 10% of all perinatal deaths. At present, however, malformations account for 30% to 50% of perinatal mortality.[12] Neonatal deaths now exceed stillbirths in pregnancies complicated by IDDM and fatal congenital malformations account for this changing pattern.

Most studies have documented a two- to fourfold increase in major malformations in infants of insulin-dependent diabetic mothers. In one published prospective analysis, Simpson and colleagues observed an 8.5% incidence of major anomalies in the insulin-dependent diabetic population, while the malformation rate in a small group of concurrently gathered control subjects was 2.4%.[20] Similar figures were obtained in the recently completed Diabetes in Early Pregnancy Study in the United States.[21] The incidence of major anomalies was 2.1% in 389 control patients and 9.0% in 279 insulin-dependent diabetic women. In general, the incidence of major malformations in worldwide studies of offspring of insulin-dependent diabetic mothers has ranged from 5% to 10%.

The profile of a woman most likely to produce an infant with a congenital anomaly would include a patient with poor periconceptional control, longstanding diabetes (onset before age 20 years), and vasculopathy.[22] The significance of confounding risk factors for malformations such as family history is difficult to interpret. Genetic susceptibility to the teratogenic influences of diabetes may be involved. While Koppe and Smoremberg-Schoorl[23] have suggested that certain maternal HLA types may be more often associated with anomalies, data presented by Simpson et al.[20] failed to reveal a specific HLA pattern that conferred an increased risk. A higher malformation rate has not been demonstrated in women who develop gestational diabetes or in infants of diabetic fathers, thus emphasizing the importance of the intrauterine environment as a contributing factor.[24]

The insult which causes malformations in the infants of diabetic mothers impacts on most organ systems and occurs before the seventh week of gestation.[25] The congenital defect thought to be the most characteristic of diabetic embryopathy is sacral agenesis or caudal dysplasia, an anomaly found 200 to 400 times more often in offspring of diabetic women.[26] Central nervous system malformations, particularly anencephaly, open spina bifida, and possibly holoprosencephaly, are increased tenfold.[22] Cardiac anomalies, especially ventricular septal defects and complex lesions such as transposition of the great vessels, are increased fivefold (Table 3–2).

Maternal hyperglycemia has been proposed by most investigators as the primary metabolic factor responsible for abnormal embryogenesis, but hyperketonemia and hypoglycemia have also been suggested.[27] Over 20 years ago, studies in alloxan-induced diabetic rats confirmed that a critical period of organogenesis existed during which teratogenic effects produced by maternal diabetes were likely to occur and that these effects could be offset by treatment with insulin.[28, 29] More recently, Baker et al. demonstrated two types of lumbar and/or sacral malformations, a fusion defect and an ossification defect, anomalies analogous to those occurring in the infant of a diabetic mother when streptozotocin was used to induce diabetes in pregnant rats on day 6 of gestation, a critical period for fusion of the neural tube in the lumbosacral area.[30] These malformations were observed in 17% of the rat fetuses. When diabetes was induced after day 6, the incidence of lumbosacral malformations was not increased. Furthermore, these investigators were able to eliminate the lumbosacral defects when insulin therapy was used to produce normal maternal serum glucose concentrations. Baker and colleagues[30] confirmed that the quality of maternal diabetes control was critical because dams treated with insulin that were allowed to maintain moderately elevated glucose levels delivered fetuses with an 8.6% incidence of lumbosacral defects.

Whole-embryo culture techniques have substantiated the teratogenic effects of elevated glucose concentrations and contributed new insights about other potential teratogens. Cockroft and Coppola[31] found that rat embryos cultured in high concentrations of D-glucose (12–15 mg/mL) exhibited neural tube defects. In contrast, Sadler and Horton[27] found that insulin had no teratogenic potential in mouse embryos exposed to insulin concentrations 500 times normal. Whole-embryo cultures have also revealed the possible synergistic effect of ketones in producing diabetic embryopathy. In mouse embryos, beta-hydroxybutyrate will delay neural tube closure and retard fetal growth.[32] Hypoglycemia has also been cited as a teratogenic factor using this model. Exposure to glucose concentrations ranging from 30% to 50% of normal maternal blood sugar levels for as little as 12 hours significantly affected rodent embryo neuralation.[33] A final teratogenic factor, somatomedin inhibitors, has also been identified in whole-embryo culture studies.[34]

Several mechanisms have been proposed by which the teratogenic factors discussed above produce malformations. Freinkel et al.[11]

TABLE 3–2.
Congenital Malformations in Infants of Diabetic Mothers

Cardiovascular
Transposition of the great vessels
Ventricular septal defect
Atrial septal defect
Hypoplastic left ventricle
Situs inversus
Anomalies of the aorta
Central nervous system
Anencephaly
Encephalocele
Meningomyelocele
Microcephaly
Skeletal
Caudal regression syndrome
Spina bifida
Genitourinary
Absent kidneys (Potter's syndrome)
Polycystic kidneys
Double ureter
Gastrointestinal
Tracheoesophageal fistula
Bowel artesia
Imperforate anus

have suggested that anomalies might arise from inhibition of glycolysis, the key energy-producing process during embryogenesis. They found that D-mannose added to the culture medium of rat embryos inhibited glycolysis and produced growth retardation and derangements of neural tube closure. The effects of mannose could be offset by adding more glucose to the medium to increase glycolytic activity or by increasing atmospheric oxygen to enhance oxidative metabolism. Freinkel and colleagues[11] stressed the sensitivity of normal embryogenesis to alterations in these key energy-producing pathways, a process they labeled "fuel-mediated" teratogenesis. Goldman et al.[35] have suggested that the mechanism responsible for the increased incidence of neural tube defects in embryo cultures in hyperglycemic medium may involve a functional deficiency of arachidonic acid, since supplementation with arachidonic acid or *myo*-inositol will reduce the frequency of neural tube defects in this experimental model. Indomethacin reversed the protection provided by myoinositol. Pinter[36] and Reece[37] and co-workers have confirmed these studies and demonstrated that the hyperglycemia-induced alterations in neural tube closure include disordered cells, decreased mitoses, and increased differentiation and cell processes, changes indicative of premature maturation.

Macrosomia

Excessive growth may predispose the fetus of the diabetic mother to shoulder dystocia, traumatic birth injury, and asphyxia. Newborn adiposity may also be associated with a significant risk for obesity in later life.[38] For these reasons, the pathogenesis, diagnosis, and prevention of macrosomia in the infant of diabetic mothers have become areas of great interest in perinatal medicine.

While some have defined macrosomia as a birth weight in excess of 4,000 to 5,000 g, others prefer categorizing infants as large-for-gestational-age (LGA, a birth weight above the 90th percentile) using population-specific growth curves. According to these definitions,

macrosomia has been observed in as many as 50% of pregnancies complicated by gestational diabetes mellitus, and 40% of insulin-dependent diabetic pregnancies.[39, 40] Delivery of an infant weighing greater than 4,500 g occurs *10 times* more often in diabetic women when compared to a nondiabetic control population.[41]

Fetal macrosomia in the infants of diabetic mothers is reflected by increased adiposity, muscle mass, and organomegaly (Fig 3–3). The disproportionate increase in the size of the trunk and shoulders when compared to the head may contribute to the likelihood of a difficult vaginal delivery.[42] An increase in total body fat in the infants of diabetic mothers has been supported by direct measurements as well as assessment of subcutaneous stores using skin-fold thickness measurements.[43, 44] Brans and colleagues[43] performed anthropometric measurements in a large series of infants of diabetic mothers and noted that 67% had increased skin-fold thickness when compared to controls.[43] Enzi et al.[44] performed gluteal fat biopsies in 25 of such infants, demonstrating fat cell hypertrophy secondary to an increase in the triglyceride content of the adipocytes. The amount of subcutaneous fat present in the infant may be an indication of the quality of diabetic control achieved during gestation.[45] In the study of Enzi et al.,[44] maternal blood glucose levels, as well as neonatal immunoreactive insulin levels measured in cord blood, were significantly correlated with fat cell weight.

The concept that maternal hyperglycemia leading to fetal hyperglycemia and hyperinsulinemia results in excessive fetal growth and adiposity was first advanced by the Danish internist Pedersen.[46] Several autopsy studies have confirmed the existence of pancreatic islet hyperplasia in the infants of diabetic mothers.[47, 48] Increased beta cell mass may be identified as early as the second trimester.[49] Using a rhesus monkey model, Susa and Schwartz[50] have confirmed the central role of excess insulin in accelerated fetal growth. Subcutaneous minipumps were implanted in monkeys during the third trimester to provide

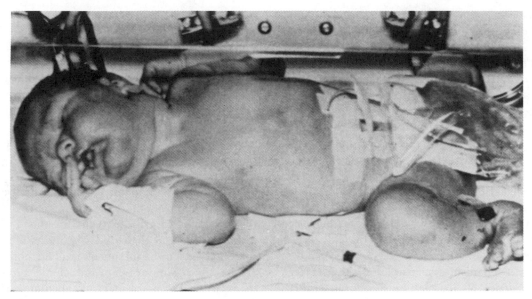

FIG 3–3.
Macrosomic infant of a diabetic mother. The large-for-gestational-age infant may complicate up to 50% of diabetic pregnancies.

a constant infusion of insulin. To assess the independent effect of fetal hyperinsulinemia, maternal and fetal glucose levels were maintained within the normal range. Increased body weight and organomegaly of the liver, heart, and placenta in the infused monkeys resembled the features characteristic of human macrosomic infants of diabetic mothers.[50] Further evidence supporting the Pedersen hypothesis has come from studies of amniotic fluid and cord blood insulin and C peptide levels. Both are increased in the amniotic fluid of insulin-treated diabetic women at term.[51] Elevated amniotic fluid insulin levels are observed in LGA infants of insulin-dependent diabetic mothers as well as those of women with gestational diabetes mellitus.[51–53] Persson and colleagues[54] have also confirmed a positive relationship between maternal blood glucose and amniotic fluid C peptide in pregnancies complicated by IDDM and GDM.[54] Cord blood levels of C peptide are also increased in the infant of the diabetic mother.[55] In addition to glucose, other substrates can modify the fetal insulin secretory response. Of the major nutrients, it is likely that amino acids are important regulators of fetal insulin secretion.[56]

The results of several clinical series have validated the Pedersen hypothesis inasmuch as good maternal glycemic control has been associated with a decline in the incidence of macrosomia. In a series of 260 insulin-dependent women achieving fasting plasma glucose levels between 109 and 140 mg/dL (6.0 and 7.8 mmol/L), Gabbe et al.[57] observed 58 (22%) macrosomic infants. Kitzmiller et al.[58] reported that 11% of 134 women achieving fasting levels between 105 and 121 mg/dL (5.8 and 6.7 mmol/L) were delivered of an infant with a birth weight in excess of 4,000 g. Several reports have demonstrated a reduction in the rate of macrosomia when more physiologic control is achieved. Roversi et al.[59] instituted a program of "maximally tolerated" insulin administration and observed macrosomia in only 6% of cases, while Jovanovic and co-workers[60] eliminated macrosomia in 52 women who achieved a mean glucose level of 80 to 87 mg/dL (4.4 to 4.8 mmol/L) throughout gestation. It has also been reported that the incidence of macrosomia in pregnancies complicated by diabetes mellitus does not increase significantly until mean glucose values approach 130 mg/dL (7.2 mmol/L).[61] Differences in methodology employed in the assessment of glycemic control may explain in part some of the disparate findings cited above. In a recent study using daily capillary glucose values obtained during the second and third trimesters in insulin-dependent patients, only 9% of infants of women with mean capillary glucose values less than 110 mg/dL (6.1 mmol/L) were found to be LGAs compared with 34% of infants of women with less optimal control.[62]

Hypoglycemia

Neonatal hypoglycemia, a blood glucose below 40 mg/dL (2.2 mmol/L) during the first 12 hours of life, results from a rapid fall in plasma glucose concentration following clamping of the umbilical cord. The degree of hypoglycemia may be influenced by at least two factors: (1) maternal glucose control during the latter half of pregnancy, and (2) maternal glycemic control during labor and delivery. Maternal blood glucose levels greater than 90 mg/dL (5.0 mmol/L) during delivery have been found to increase significantly the frequency of neonatal hypoglycemia.[63] Presumably, prior poor maternal glucose control can result in fetal beta cell hyperplasia leading to exaggerated insulin release following delivery. Infants of diabetic mothers exhibiting hypoglycemia have elevated cord C peptide and free insulin levels at birth and an exaggerated pancreatic response to glucose loading.[55, 64, 65]

Although Karlsson and Kjellmer[66] were unable to correlate maternal blood glucose control with the incidence of hypoglycemia, few cases of neonatal hypoglycemia have been noted in several recent series in which physiologic maternal glucose levels have been maintained.[66] Jovanovic et al.[60] reported only one case of hypoglycemia in the offspring of diabetic women whose mean blood glucose was less than 87 mg/dL (4.8 mmol/L). Similarly, Roversi et al.[59] found that only 35 of 240 (15%) infants became hypoglycemic after birth.

Respiratory Distress Syndrome (RDS)

The precise mechanism by which maternal diabetes affects pulmonary development remains unknown. Experimental animal studies have focused primarily on the effects of hyperglycemia and hyperinsulinemia on pulmonary surfactant biosynthesis. An extensive review of the literature confirms that both of these factors are involved in delayed pulmonary maturation in the infant of a diabetic mother.[67] In vitro studies have documented that insulin can interfere with substrate availability for surfactant biosynthesis.[68, 69] Smith[70] has postulated that insulin interferes with the normal timing of glucocorticoid-induced pulmonary maturation in the fetus. Apparently, cortisol acts on pulmonary fibroblasts to induce synthesis of fibroblast-pneumocyte factor, which then acts on type II cells to stimulate phospholipid synthesis.[71] Carlson et al.[72] have shown that insulin blocks cortisol action at the level of the fibroblast by reducing the production of fibroblast-pneumocyte factor. An alternative explanation for insulin's antagonism of cortisol-induced lung lecithin synthesis has been proposed by Rooney et al.[73] In their study of cultures of fetal rat lung cells, dexamethasone-induced stimulation of choline phosphate cytidyltransferase was prevented by insulin administration. This important enzyme is involved in the pathway which eventually converts phosphatidic acid to phosphatidylglycerol (PG).

Clinical studies investigating the effect of maternal diabetes on fetal lung maturation have produced conflicting data. In a series of 805 IDMs delivered over a 10-year period, Robert and co-workers[74] found the corrected risk for RDS to be nearly six times that of mothers without diabetes mellitus. With the introduction of protocols which have emphasized glucose control and antepartum surveillance until lung maturity has been established, RDS has become a less common occurrence in the infant of a diabetic mother. Several studies agree that in well-controlled

TABLE 3–3.
Modified White Classification of Pregnant Diabetic Women*

Class	Diabetes Onset Age (yr)		Duration (yr)	Vascular Disease	Insulin Need
Gestational diabetes					
A$_1$	Any		Any	0	0
A$_2$	Any		Any	0	+
Pregestational diabetes					
B	20		<10	0	+
C	10–19	or	10–19	0	+
D	10	or	20	+	+
F	Any		Any	+	+
R	Any		Any	+	+
T	Any		Any	+	+
H	Any		Any	+	+

*Modified from White P: *Am J Med* 1949; 7:609–616.

diabetic women delivered at term, the risk of RDS is no higher than that observed in the general population.[75, 76] In recent studies which have emphasized rigorous maternal glycemic control, RDS has been virtually eliminated.[60, 77]

Calcium and Magnesium Metabolism

Neonatal hypocalcemia, serum levels below 7 mg/dL (1.75 mmol/L), occurs at an increased rate in the infant of a diabetic mother, when one controls for predisposing factors such as prematurity and birth asphyxia.[78] Hypocalcemia in the infant of a diabetic mother has been associated with a failure to increase parathyroid hormone synthesis following birth.[79, 80] Decreased serum magnesium levels have also been documented in pregnant diabetic women as well as their infants. A recent study described reduced amniotic fluid magnesium concentrations in insulin-dependent diabetics.[81] These findings may be explained by a fall in fetal urinary magnesium excretion which would accompany a relative magnesium-deficient state. Magnesium deficiency may then paradoxically inhibit fetal parathyroid hormone secretion.

Hyperbilirubinemia and Polycythemia

Hyperbilirubinemia is frequently observed in the infant of a diabetic mother. Neonatal jaundice has been reported in as many as 53% of pregnancies complicated by IDDM and 38% of pregnancies with GDM.[82, 83] Although several mechanisms have been proposed to explain these clinical findings, the pathogenesis of hyperbilirubinemia remains uncertain. In the past, jaundice observed in the infant of a diabetic mother was often attributed to prematurity. Several studies which have carefully analyzed morbidity according to gestational age, however, have rejected this concept.[84–86]

While severe hyperbilirubinemia may be observed independent of polycythemia, a common pathway for these complications most likely involves increased red blood cell production stimulated by increased erythropoietin in the infant of a diabetic mother. Presumably, the major stimulus for red cell production is a state of relative hypoxia in utero as described previously. While cord erythropoietin levels are generally normal in IDMs whose mothers demonstrate good glycemic control during gestation, Shannon et al.[87] and Ylinen et al.[88] found that hemoglobin A$_{1c}$ values in late pregnancy were significantly elevated in mothers of hyperbilirubinemic infants.

MATERNAL CLASSIFICATION AND RISK ASSESSMENT

Counseling a pregnant patient involves formulating a plan of management that requires assessment of both maternal and fetal risk. Priscilla White pointed out that the age of onset of diabetes, its duration, and the severity of complicating vascular disease influence perinatal outcome. She developed a classification scheme which has experienced wide application.[89] Use of the updated White classification system has allowed physicians to focus on those patients who are at greater risk during pregnancy (Table 3–3).

Gestational diabetes mellitus is a form of latent diabetes in which the diabetogenic stress of pregnancy reveals glucose intolerance for the first time. Following pregnancy, carbohydrate metabolism can be expected to return to normal in the marjority of cases. The term *gestational diabetes* fails to specify if the therapy for the patient includes diet alone or insulin. This distinction is most important because those patients who are normoglycemic in the fasting state have a significantly lower perinatal mortality rate. They do not appear to have an increased incidence of intrauterine death.[90]

Class A_1 gestational diabetes mellitus includes those patients who, during pregnancy, have demonstrated carbohydrate intolerance during a 100-g 3-hour glucose tolerance test (GTT); however, their fasting and 2-hour postprandial glucose levels are less than 105 mg/dL (5.8 mmol/L) and 120 mg/dL (6.6 mmol/L), respectively. These patients are generally managed by dietary regulation alone. If the fasting value of the GTT is elevated ($\geq$105 mg/dL [5.8 mmol/L]), and/or postprandial glucose levels exceed 120 mg/dL (6.6 mmol/L), patients are designated as class A_2. Insulin is most often required for these women. Gestational diabetics who go on to receive insulin therapy (class A_2) have been noted to have poorer outcomes than those controlled by diet alone. It is likely that many of these women have glucose intolerance antedating pregnancy.

Pregestational diabetic women patients requiring insulin are designated by the letters B, C, D, R, and F, and T. Class B patients are those whose onset of disease is after age 20. They have had diabetes less than 10 years and have no vascular complications.

Class C diabetes includes patients with onset of their disease between the ages of 10 and 19 years. Vascular disease is not present.

Class D includes women with disease of 20 years' duration or greater, or whose onset occurred before age 10, or who have benign retinopathy. This includes microaneurysms, exudates, and venous dilatation.

Class F describes the 5% to 10% of patients with underlying renal disease. This includes those with reduced creatinine clearance and/or proteinuria of at least 400 mg in 24 hours measured during the first trimester. Several factors present prior to 20 weeks' gestation appear to be predictive of poor perinatal outcome in these women (e.g., perinatal death or birth weight less than 1,100 g). These include:

1. Proteinuria greater than 3.0 g/24 hr
2. Serum creatinine greater than 1.5 mg/dL (130 μmol/L)
3. Anemia with hematocrit less than 25%
4. Hypertension (mean arterial pressure >107 mm Hg)

Nephropathy (See also Chap. 2)

In a series of 27 class F women, if any one of the factors listed above was present early in gestation, over half of the pregnancies resulted in perinatal deaths or infants weighing less than 1,100 g.[91] In contrast, when no risk factors were present, over 90% experienced a successful perinatal outcome.

Several studies have failed to demonstrate a permanent worsening of diabetic renal disease as a result of pregnancy.[92, 93] Kitzmiller and colleagues[92] reviewed 35 pregnancies complicated by diabetic nephropathy. Proteinuria increased in 69% and hypertension developed in 73%. Following delivery, proteinuria declined in 65% of cases. In only two patients did protein excretion increase after gestation. Changes in creatinine clearance during pregnancy are variable in class F patients. Kitzmiller,[94] in reviewing 44 patients from the literature, noted that about one third of women had an expected rise in creatinine clearance during gestation, compared to one third who had a decline of more than 15% by the third trimester. Of interest, most patients with severe reduction in creatinine clearance (<60 mL/min) measured during the first trimester did not demonstrate a further reduction in clearance during pregnancy.[93] However, a decline in renal function was evident in 20% to 30% of cases. Several authors have confirmed that any deterioration of renal function after pregnancy is consistent with the natural course of diabetic nephropathy and is not related to pregnancy per se.[95]

With improved survival of diabetic patients following renal transplantation, a small group of kidney recipients have now achieved pregnancy (class T). In one report nine cases of pregnancy complicated by diabetes and prior renal transplantation were described.[96] Prednisone and azathioprine were administered throughout gestation and there were no episodes of renal allograft rejection. A single maternal death and two fetal deaths did occur in patients with preexisting peripheral vascular disease, and superimposed preeclampsia occurred in six patients. All seven surviving infants were delivered prior to term, with fetal compromise evident in six of these cases. Most recently, improved results have been described in women who underwent combined renal and pancreatic transplant prior to gestation (see Chap 2).

Retinopathy

Class R diabetes designates patients with proliferative retinopathy. There is no difference in the prevalence of retinopathy in women who have or have not been pregnant.[97] However, retinopathy may worsen significantly during pregnancy in spite of the major advances that have been made in diagnosis and treatment. Laser photocoagulation therapy during pregnancy with careful follow-up has helped maintain many pregnancies to a gestational age at which neonatal survival is likely. In a large series of 172 patients, background retinopathy was present in 40 cases with proliferative changes noted in 11. Only 1 patient developed proliferative retinopathy during pregnancy.[98]

A review of the literature by Kitzmiller et al.[99] confirms the observation that progression to proliferative retinopathy during pregnancy rarely occurs in women with background retinopathy or those without any eyeground changes. Of the 561 women in these two categories, only 17 (3.0%) developed neovascularization during gestation.[99] In contrast, 23 of 26 (88.5%) with untreated proliferative disease experienced worsening retinopathy during pregnancy.

Moloney and Drury[100] have reported that pregnancy may increase the prevalence of some background changes. These authors noted a characteristic increase in streak-blob hemorrhages and soft exudates which often resolve between examinations. Retinopathy progressed despite strict metabolic control. Phelps and colleagues[101] have related worsening retinal disease to levels of plasma glucose at the first prenatal visit as well as to the magnitude of improvement in glycemia during early pregnancy. Chang and colleagues[102] have also reported the development of proliferative changes with rapid normalization of glucose control. Whether improved control contributes to a deterioration of background retinopathy remains uncertain. Fortunately, most patients who require laser photocoagulation will respond to this therapy and therefore should be promptly treated. However, those women who demonstrate severe florid disc neovascularization that is unresponsive to laser therapy during early pregnancy may be at great risk for deterioration of their vision. Termination of pregnancy should be considered in this group of patients.

In addition to background and proliferative eye disease, Sinclair and colleagues[103] have described vasoocclusive lesions associated with the development of macular edema during pregnancy. Cystic macular edema is most often found in patients with proteinuric nephropathy and hypertensive disease leading to retinal edema. Macular capillary permeability is a feature of this process. The degree of macular edema is directly related to the fall in plasma oncotic pressure present in these women. In the series of Sinclair et al.,[103] seven women with minimal or no retinopathy before becoming pregnant developed severe macular edema associated with pre-proliferative or proliferative retinopathy during the course of their pregnancies. Although proliferation was controlled with photocoagulation, the macular edema worsened until delivery in all cases and was often aggravated by photocoagulation. Macular edema and retinopathy both regressed after delivery in some patients but persisted in others, resulting in significant visual loss.[103]

Coronary Artery Disease

Class H diabetes refers to the presence of diabetes of any duration associated with ischemic myocardial disease. There is evidence that the small number of women who have coronary artery disease are at an increased risk for mortality during gestation.[104] This is especially true of women with previous myocardial infarction or infarction during pregnancy where mortality rates exceed 50%.[105] While there are a few reports of successful pregnancies following myocardial infarction in diabetic women, cardiac status should be carefully assessed during early gestation or preferably prior to pregnancy. If electrocardiographic abnormalities are encountered, echocardiography may be employed to assess ventricular function, or modified stress testing may be undertaken. (See also Chap. 5.)

DETECTION OF DIABETES IN PREGNANCY

It has been estimated that diabetes mellitus complicates 2% to 3% of all pregnancies, and 90% of these cases represent women with gestational diabetes mellitus (GDM). This is a state restricted to pregnant women whose impaired glucose tolerance is first discovered during pregnancy. Patients with GDM represent a group with significant risk for developing glucose intolerance later in life. O'Sullivan has reported that up to 60% of these patients will become diabetic in the 16 years following pregnancy.[106] More recently, Metzger and colleagues[107] have reported that 23% of GDM women treated with diet alone

will be overtly diabetic when evaluated within 1 year of delivery. According to these data, 95% of patients with marked fasting hyperglycemia (>130 mg/dL [7.2 mmol/L]) during pregnancy develop diabetes at 1-year follow-up.[107]

As mentioned earlier, the diabetogenic stress of pregnancy is most often encountered during late gestation and is most often recognized in the fed state. In the majority of cases, patients with GDM will demonstrate a normal fasting glucose value. Therefore, some challenge of glucose tolerance must be undertaken to detect carbohydrate intolerance. In the past, physicians would assess glucose tolerance in patients thought to be at increased risk for GDM. This group included a patient with a family history of diabetes, unexplained stillbirth, malformed infant, or macrosomia. Obesity, hypertension, glycosuria, and maternal age over 25 to 30 were other indications for screening.

It is of interest that over half of all patients who exhibit an abnormal oral glucose tolerance test (OGTT) lack the risk factors mentioned above. Furthermore, it does not seem advisable to look for GDM after an adverse outcome has occurred.[108] Coustan and colleagues[109] have reported that in a series of 6,214 women, when using historical risk factors and an arbitrary age cutoff of 30 years for screening, 35% of cases of GDM would be missed. It has therefore been recommended that *all* pregnant women be screened between 24 and 28 weeks by administering a 50-g oral glucose load followed by a glucose determination 1 hour later.[110] The 50-g glucose challenge may be administered early in gestation to women with significant risk factors for GDM such as morbid obesity, history of a macrosomic stillbirth, or a strong family history of diabetes.

The 50-g glucose challenge may be performed in the fasting or fed state, although Coustan and colleagues[111] suggest that sensitivity is improved if the test is performed fasting. A plasma value between 135 and 140 mg/dL (7.5 and 7.8 mmol/L) is commonly used as a threshold for performing a 3-hour

OGTT. Using a portable reflectance meter, capillary value cutoffs can be established which are generally higher than plasma determinations. In addition to adhering to guidelines concerning calibration and quality control, an appropriate threshold for screening should be established by comparing reflectance meter values to laboratory determinations.[112] Few false-negative results are obtained when the 50-g screening test is performed at 24 to 28 weeks' gestation. One can expect approximately 15% of patients with an abnormal screening value to have an abnormal 3-hour OGTT. Patients whose 1-hour screening value exceeds 190 mg/dL (10.5 mmol/L) rarely exhibit a normal OGTT.[113] In these women, it is preferable to check a fasting blood glucose level before administering a 100-g carbohydrate load. If the fasting glucose is 100 mg/dL or greater, the patient is treated as a gestational diabetic.

The OGTT rather than the intravenous test is favored because it is probably more physiologic and assesses the gastrointestinal factors involved in insulin secretion. The oral test also appears to be more sensitive and has been well standardized. The criteria for establishing the diagnosis of gestational diabetes are listed in Table 3–4. The patient must have a normal fasting value and two abnormal postprandial glucose determinations to be designated as class A_1. In a patient who demonstrates a normal OGTT despite significant risk factors, including obesity, advanced maternal age, or a previous history of GDM, a repeat test may be performed at 32 to 34 weeks' gestation.[114]

TABLE 3–4.
Detection of Gestational Diabetes

	Plasma Level	
	(mg/dL)	(mmol/L)
Screening Test—50 g		
1 hr	140	7.8
*Diagnostic test—100 g oral glucose tolerance test**		
Fasting	105	5.8
1 hr	190	10.5
2 hr	165	9.2
3 hr	145	8.0

*Diagnosis of gestational diabetes is made when any two values are met or exceeded.

The criteria used to establish the diagnosis of GDM are based on the data of O'Sullivan et al.[115] which examined the likelihood of subsequent development of overt diabetes mellitus. As these criteria are unrelated to pregnancy outcome, there remains a need to better define the level of glycemia that poses a risk for fetal and neonatal complications such as macrosomia. Tallarigo et al.[116] have suggested that subtle degrees of maternal hyperglycemia, levels below those which would classify an individual as a gestational diabetic, can have a detrimental effect on perinatal outcome. In the study of Tallarigo et al., women with a 2-hour plasma glucose value between 120 and 165 mg/dL (6.7 and 9.2 mmol/L) during a 3-hour OGTT were more likely to have a macroscomic infant than women with lower 2-hour values. Women with an abnormal 50-g screening value and normal 3-hour OGTT may also be more likely to produce a large infant when controlling for factors such as obesity.[117] However, other retrospective studies continue to support the use of the criteria of O'Sullivan et al. in defining a group of pregnancies at risk for abnormal outcome.[118]

TREATMENT OF THE INSULIN-DEPENDENT PATIENT

Self-glucose monitoring combined with aggressive insulin therapy has made the maintenance of maternal normoglycemia (levels of 60–120 mg/dL [3.3–6.7 mmol/L]) a therapeutic reality.[119] Patients should monitor their glucose control using glucose-oxidase-impregnated reagent strips and a reflectance meter. Glucose determinations are made in the fasting state and before lunch, dinner, and bedtime (Table 3–5). Postprandial values and determinations at 2 to 3 A.M. may also be helpful. Urine glucose determinations are not helpful as they do not reflect blood glucose values, especially during pregnancy when the renal threshold for glucose elimination may be lowered and glucosuria is frequent in patients with normal carbohydrate tolerance.

TABLE 3–5.
Target Plasma Glucose Levels in Pregnancy

Time	mg/dL	mmol/L
Before breakfast	60–90	3.3–5.0
Before lunch, supper, bedtime snack	60–105	3.3–5.8
2 hr after meals	≤120	≤6.7
2 A.M.–6 A.M.	>60	>3.3

During pregnancy, most insulin-dependent patients will require multiple insulin injections. A combination of intermediate-acting and regular insulin both before breakfast and at dinnertime is a commonly employed regimen. As a general rule, the amount of intermediate-acting insulin taken in the morning will exceed that of regular insulin by a 2:1 ratio. Patients often receive two thirds of their total insulin dose at breakfast and the remaining third at suppertime. Our preferred regimen is to administer separate injections of regular insulin at dinnertime and intermediate-acting insulin at bedtime to reduce nocturnal hypoglycemia. (see Fig 3–4). Although oral hypoglycemia agents have been employed in pregnancy, we do not treat either pregestational or GDM patients with these

medications. The sulfonylureas cross the placenta and may result in fetal β cell stimulation.

Diet therapy is critical to successful regulation of maternal diabetes. Most patients do well on a program consisting of three meals and several snacks. There is, however, a great deal of variation among patients who work shifts and maintain less normal hours. Dietary composition should be 50% to 60% carbohydrate, 20% protein, and 25% to 30% fat with less than 10% saturated fats, up to 10% polyunsaturated fatty acids, and the remainder derived from monounsaturated sources.[120]

Caloric intake is established based on prepregnancy weight and weight gain during gestation. Patients should consume approximately 35 kcal/kg ideal body weight. Obese women may be managed with an intake as low as 1,600 kcal/day. However, weight reduction is not advised. If ketonuria develops, the caloric content of the diet may be increased.

In spite of multiple insulin and dietary adjustments, there remains a small group of patients who may require continuous insulin infusion pump therapy to maintain adequate control. The initiation of this treatment will

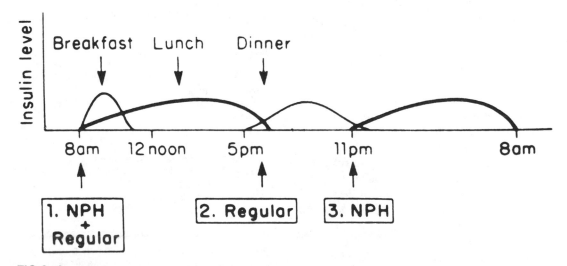

FIG 3–4.
Schematic diagram of serum insulin levels achieved with our preferred multiple-injection regimen of NPH and regular insulins. (From Jovanovic L, Peterson CM: Modern management of diabetes in pregnancy, in Jovanovic L, Peterson CM, Fuhrmann K (eds): *Diabetes and Pregnancy. Teratology, Toxicity, and Treatment.* New York, Praeger, 1986, p 306. Used by permission.)

usually require hospitalization. A basal infusion rate of regular insulin is established which is approximately 1 unit/hr. Bolus infusions are then given with meals and possibly snacks. Patients are taught to adjust their basal infusion rate and meal boluses based on frequent blood glucose determinations. Pump therapy demands close observation in order to prevent periods of hyper- and hypoglycemia.

Utilizing continuous insulin infusion therapy, glucose values may become normalized with minimal amplitude of daily excursions in a select group of pregnant diabetics. Episodes of hypoglycemia are usually secondary to errors in dose selection or failure to adhere to the required diet.[119] The risk of nocturnal hypoglycemia is markedly increased in the pregnant state, and ketoacidosis has been observed in association with pump failure or maternal infection. Therefore, great care should be taken in selecting candidates for continuous infusion therapy. While this technique may be valuable for a small group of pregnant women with diabetes mellitus, it has not been demonstrated to be superior to multiple injection regimens. Coustan and colleagues[121] randomized 22 pregnant women to intensive conventional therapy with multiple injections versus pump therapy. There were no differences between the two treatment groups with respect to outpatient mean glucose levels, glycosylated hemoglobin levels, or glycemic excursions.[121] In our experience over the past decade, we found it necessary to institute pump therapy to achieve good glycemic control in only one patient. However, we have chosen to maintain women who have demonstrated good control using continuous infusion devices prior to pregnancy on this therapy throughout gestation.

Most patients with IDDM are followed with outpatient visits at 1- or 2-week intervals. At each visit, control is assessed and adjustments in insulin dosage are made. However, the patient should be instructed to call at any time if periods of hypoglycemia (<50 mg/dL [<2.8 mmol/L]) or hyperglycemia (>200 mg/dL [>11.1 mmol/L]) occur. Daily phone contact may be required, particularly in early pregnancy, to arrive at a stable insulin regimen (Table 3–6).

Ketoacidosis

With the implementation of antenatal care programs stressing strict metabolic control of blood glucose levels for insulin-dependent women, diabetic ketoacidosis has fortunately become a less common occurrence. Diabetic ketoacidosis does frequently occur in newly diagnosed diabetics and the hormonal milieu of pregnancy may become the background for this phenomenon. As pregnancy is a state of relative insulin resistance marked by enhanced lipolysis and ketogenesis, diabetic ketoacidosis may develop in a pregnant woman with glucose levels barely exceeding 200 mg/dL (11.1 mmol/L). The biochemical definition of diabetic ketoacidosis in pregnancy may be modified from the nonpregnant state to include a plasma glucose in excess of 200 mg/dL (11.1 mmol/L), plasma HCO_3^- less than 15 mEq/L, and a pH value less than 7.30. Serum acetone is positive at a 1:2 dilution.

TABLE 3–6.
Management of the Pregestational Diabetic Pregnancy

Initial visit
  Counsel patient regarding need for excellent glycemic control and review methods for self–blood glucose monitoring
  Counsel patient regarding the risk for fetal malformations and neonatal morbidity
  Dietary assessment
  Laboratory baseline data
    1. Glycosylated hemoglobin level
    2. 24 hr urine collection for creatinine clearance, protein excretion
    3. Electrocardiogram
    4. Ophthalmologic consultation
Follow-up visits
  Review glucose values and adjust insulin dosage
  Review obstetrician's plan for anomaly screening including maternal serum alpha fetoprotein screening, ultrasonography, and fetal echocardiography
  Repeat renal function tests and opthalmologic evaluation at a minimum each trimester

Early recognition of signs and symptoms of diabetic ketoacidosis will improve both maternal and fetal outcome. As in the nonpregnant state, clinical signs of volume depletion follow the symptoms of hyperglycemia, which include polydipsia and polyuria. Malaise, headache, nausea, and vomiting are common complaints. Occasionally, diabetic ketoacidosis may present in an undiagnosed diabetic woman receiving β-mimetic agents to arrest preterm labor. Because of the risk of hyperglycemia and diabetic ketoacidosis in insulin-dependent women receiving intravenous medications such as ritodrine, magnesium sulfate has become the preferred tocolytic for cases of preterm labor in these women.

Once the diagnosis of diabetic ketoacidosis is established and the patient is stabilized, she should be transported to a facility where tertiary care in both perinatology and neonatology is available. Therapy hinges on the meticulous correction of metabolic and fluid abnormalities. An attempt at treatment of any underlying cause for ketoacidosis, such as infection, should be instituted as well. The general management of diabetic ketoacidosis in pregnancy is outlined in Table 3–7. Diabetic ketoacidosis does represent a substantial risk for fetal compromise. Fetal monitoring is therefore recommended in cases where the gestational age indicates a reasonable chance for survival. In situations where delivery is considered for fetal distress, it should only be accomplished if the maternal condition is stable enough to allow for delivery. However, successful fetal resuscitation will often accompany correction of maternal acidosis. Every effort should therefore be made to correct the maternal condition before intervening prematurely on behalf of the fetus.

Fetal Evaluation

During the third trimester, when the risk of sudden intrauterine death increases, an outpatient program of fetal surveillance is initiated. Maternal assessment of fetal activity may also be a helpful screening technique. The improved understanding of the impor-

TABLE 3–7.
Management of Diabetic Ketoacidosis During Pregnancy

1. Laboratory Assessment
   Obtain arterial blood gases to document degree of acidosis present; measure glucose, ketones, electrolytes, at 1–2-hr intervals
2. Insulin
   Low-dose, intravenous
   Loading dose: 0.2–0.4 unit/kg
   Maintenance: 2.0–10.0 units/hr
3. Fluids
   Isotonic NaCl
   Total replacement in first 12 hr = 4–6 L
   1.0 L in first hr
   500–1,000 mL/hr for 2–4 hr
   250 mL/hr until 80% replaced
4. Glucose
   Begin 5% D/NS when plasma level reaches 250 mg/dL (14 mmol/L)
5. Potassium
   If initially normal or reduced, an infusion rate up to 15–20 mEq/hr may be required
   If elevated, wait until levels decline into the normal range, then add to intravenous solution in a concentration of 20–30 mEq/L
6. Bicarbonate
   Add one ampule (44 mEq) to 1 L of 0.45% NS if pH is <7.10

tance of maternal control in relation to fetal outcome has played a major role in reducing perinatal mortality in diabetic pregnancies. Therefore, antepartum fetal monitoring tests have been used primarily to reassure the obstetrician and avoid unnecessary premature intervention. These techniques have few false-negative results, and in a patient who is well controlled and exhibits no vasculopathy or significant hypertension, reassuring antepartum testing allows the fetus to benefit from further maturation in utero.

The nonstress test (NST), the preferred screening method to assess antepartum fetal well-being in the patient with diabetes mellitus, evaluates the presence of accelerations of the baseline fetal heart rate.[122] A reactive NST exhibits at least two accelerations of the fetal heart rate of 15 beats per minute amplitude and 15 seconds' duration in a 20-minute period of monitoring. If the NST is nonreactive, a contractions stress test or bio-physical profile is then performed. Heart rate monitoring is begun early in the third trimester, usually by 32 weeks' gestation. Barrett et al.[123] documented six antepartum deaths in 425 patients having weekly tests, a significantly greater fetal death rate than in other high-risk pregnancies. Other studies have also demonstrated an increased fetal death rate compared with other high-risk pregnancies within 1 week of a reactive NST.[124] Such data confirms that if the NST is to be used as the primary method of antepartum heart rate testing, we suggest it be done at least twice-weekly once the patient reaches 32 weeks' gestation. In patients with vascular disease or poor control, in whom the incidence of abnormal tests and intrauterine deaths is greater, testing is performed more frequently.[125]

Recently, we have found that Doppler studies of the umbilical artery may also be predictive of fetal outcome in diabetic pregnancies complicated by vascular disease.[126] Elevated placental resistance as evidence by an increased systolic-diastolic ratio is associated with fetal growth retardation and pre-eclampsia in these high-risk patients.[126] In contrast, well-controlled patients without vascular disease rarely demonstrate abnormal fetal umbilical artery waveforms.

It is important to include not only the results of antepartum fetal testing but to recognize all the clinical features involving mother and fetus before a decision is made to intervene for suspected fetal distress, especially if this decision may result in a preterm delivery. In reviewing six series involving 777 diabetic patients, an abnormal test of fetal condition led to delivery 4% of the time.[122] It appears that outpatient testing protocols work well in insulin-dependent patients. Whether such testing is required for all patients with insulin-dependent diabetes mellitus remains controversial. Certainly those women whose diabetes is poorly controlled, who have hypertension, or who have significant vasculopathy that may be associated with fetal growth retardation require a program of antepartum fetal surveillance.

Ultrasound is an extremely valuable tool in evaluating fetal growth, estimating fetal weight, and detecting hydramnios and malformations. A determination of maternal serum alpha fetoprotein (MSAFP) at 16 weeks' gestation should be employed in association with a detailed ultrasound study at 18 weeks in an attempt to detect neural tube defects and other anomalies. Normal values of MSAFP for diabetic women are lower than in the nondiabetic population.[127] Nevertheless, a lower threshold for the upper limit of normal (1.5 multiples or the median) may be preferable in pregnancies complicated by diabetes mellitus because the frequency of spina bifida and other major malformations is increased in this population. Fetal echocardiography is performed at 20 to 22 weeks' gestation for the investigation of possible cardiac anomalies.

Ultrasound examinations may then be repeated at 4 to 6-week intervals to assess fetal growth. The detection of fetal macrosomia, the leading risk factor for shoulder dystocia, is important in the selection of patients who are best delivered by cesarean section. Sonographic measurements of the fetal abdominal circumference have proved most helpful in predicting fetal macrosomia.[128] The abdomen is likely to be large because of increased glycogen deposition in the fetal liver. Using serial sonographic examinations, accelerated abdominal growth can be identified by 32 weeks' gestation.[129]

Timing and Mode of Delivery

Delivery should be delayed until fetal maturation has taken place, provided that the patient's diabetes is well controlled and that antepartum surveillance remains normal. In our practice, elective induction of labor is often planned at 38 to 40 weeks in well-controlled patients without vascular disease. Before elective delivery, prior to 39 weeks' gestation, an amniocentesis may be performed to document fetal pulmonary naturity. Although the value of the lecithin-sphingomyelin (L/S) ratio has been questioned in pregnancies complicated by diabetes mellitus, as mentioned earlier, many series report a low incidence of respiratory distress syndrome (RDS) with a mature ratio of 2.0 or greater.[76]

The presence of the acidic phospholipid phosphatidylglycerol (PG) is the final marker of fetal pulmonary maturation. Several authors have suggested that hyperinsulinemia may be associated with delayed appearance of PG and an increased incidence of RDS. Landon et al.[62] have correlated the appearance of PG in amniotic fluid with maternal glycemic control during gestation. RDS may occur in the IDM with a mature L/S ratio but absent PG. Caution should be used, therefore, in planning the delivery of patients with an L/S ratio of 2.0 and absent PG. Most important, the clinician must be familiar with the laboratory analysis of amniotic fluid in his or her institution and the neonatal outcome for the IDM at various L/S ratios in the presence or absence of PG.

When antepartum testing suggests fetal compromise, delivery must be considered. If amniotic fluid analysis yields a mature L/S ratio, delivery should be accomplished promptly. In the presence of an immature L/S ratio, the decision to proceed with delivery should be based on confirmation of deteriorating fetal condition by several abnormal tests. For example, if the NST as well as the CST indicates fetal compromise, delivery is indicated. Finally, there remain several maternal indications for delivery including preeclampsia, worsening renal function, or deteriorating vision secondary to proliferative retinopathy.

The route of delivery for the diabetic patient remains controversial. Cousins,[130] in reviewing over 1,600 (White class B, C, D, R) patients in the literature between 1965–1985, noted a cesarean section rate of approximately 45%. This figure is likely to represent the practice trends of most obstetricians and perinatologists.[131] Delivery by cesarean section is usually favored when fetal distress is suggested by antepartum heart rate monitoring. If a patient reaches 38 weeks' gestation with a mature fetal lung profile and is at sig-

nificant risk for intrauterine demise because of poor control or a history of a prior stillbirth, an elective delivery is scheduled. Elective cesarean section is performed if the cervix is not favorable for induction or if the infant is believed to be macrosomic.

During labor, continuous fetal heart rate monitoring is mandatory. Labor is allowed to progress as long as normal rates of cervical dilatation and descent are documented. Despite attempts to select patients with obvious fetal macrosomia for delivery by elective cesarean section, arrest of dilatation or descent should alert the physician to the possibility of cephalopelvic disproportion. About 25% of macrosomic infants ($\geq$4000 g) delivered after a prolonged second stage will have shoulder dystocia.[132] Acker et al.[133] have reported that the overall risk for shoulder dystocia in the IDM is greater for the macrosomic than for the normal infant. In their series of diabetic women, the risk for shoulder dystocia with a fetal weight greater than 4,000 g was approximately 30%. It follows that a patient who demonstrates a significant protracted labor or failure of descent is best delivered by cesarean section.

Glucoregulation During Labor and Delivery

As neonatal hypoglycemia is in part related to maternal glucose levels during labor, it is important to maintain maternal plasma glucose levels at approximately 100 mg/dL (5.6 mmol/L). The patient is given nothing by mouth after midnight of the evening before induction of elective cesarean section. The usual bedtime dose of insulin is administered. Upon arrival to labor and delivery, early in the morning, the patient's capillary glucose level is assessed with a bedside reflectance meter. Continuous infusions of both insulin and glucose are then administered based on maternal glucose levels. Ten units of regular insulin may be added to 1,000 mL of solution containing 5% dextrose. An infusion rate of 100 to 125 mL/hr (1 unit/hr) will, in most cases, result in good glucose control. Insulin may also be infused from a syringe pump at a dose of 0.25 to 2.0 units/hr, and adjusted to maintain normal glucose values.[134] Jovanovic and Peterson[135] have noted that well-controlled patients will often be euglycemic once active labor begins.[135] In such patients, when glucose falls below 70 mg/dL (3.9 mmol/L), the infusion is changed from saline to 5% dextrose at a rate of 2.5 mg/kg/min. Glucose levels are recorded hourly and the infusion rate is adjusted accordingly. Regular insulin is administered if glucose values exceed 140 mg/dL (7.8 mmol/L). This commonly occurs during the second stage of labor with increased catecholamine secretion.

When cesarean section is to be performed, it should be scheduled for early morning. This simplifies intrapartum glucose control and allows the neonatal team to prepare for the care of the newborn. The patient is given nothing by mouth and her usual morning insulin dose is withheld. If surgery is not performed early in the day, one third of the patient's intermediate-acting dose of insulin may be administered. Epidural anesthesia is preferred as it allows the anesthesiologist to detect early signs of hypoglycemia. Following surgery, glucose levels are monitored every 2 hours and an intravenous solution of 5% dextrose is administered.

After delivery, insulin requirements are usually significantly lower than were pregnancy or prepregnancy needs. The objective of "tight control" used in the antepartum period is relaxed, and glucose values of 150 to 200 mg/dL (8.3 to 11.1 mmol/L) are acceptable. Patients delivered vaginally, who are able to eat a regular diet, are given one half of their prepregnancy dose of NPH insulin on the morning of the first postpartum day. Frequent glucose determinations are used to guide insulin dosage. If the patient has been given supplemental regular insulin in addition to the morning NPH insulin dose, the amount of NPH insulin given on the following morning is increased in an amount equal to two thirds of the additional regular insulin. Most patients are stabilized on this regimen within a few days after delivery.

Women with diabetes are encouraged to breast-feed. The additional 500 kcal required daily are given as approximately 100 g of carbohydrate and 20 g of protein.[120] The insulin dose may be somewhat lower in lactating diabetic women. Hypoglycemia appears to be common in the first week following delivery and immediately after nursing.

MANAGEMENT OF THE PATIENT WITH GESTATIONAL DIABETES

Women with gestational diabetes mellitus (GDM) generally do not need hospitalization for dietary instruction and management. Once the diagnosis is established, patients are begun on a dietary program of 2,000 to 2,500 kcal daily.[136] Obese women with GDM may be managed on as little as 1,700 to 1,800 kcal/day with less weight gain and no apparent reduction in fetal size.[137]

The single most important therapeutic intervention in pregnancy complicated by GDM is the careful monitoring of maternal glucose levels throughout the third trimester. Fasting and 2-hour postprandial glucose levels are monitored at least weekly. Some advocate self-glucose monitoring to better ascertain the level of glycemic control achieved by diet therapy.[8, 138] If the fasting plasma glucose level exceeds 105 mg/dL (5.8 mmol/L) and/or postprandial values are greater than 120 mg/dL (6.7 mmol/L), therapy with human insulin is begun (Table 3–8).

TABLE 3–8.
Management of Gestational Diabetic Pregnancy

Initial visit
  Review results of diagnostic 3-hr oral glucose
    tolerance test
  Counsel patient regarding diagnosis
    Risks to pregnancy
    Risks for diabetes mellitus later in life
  Institute appropriate diet or insulin therapy
  Review plan for assessment of blood glucose
    control
Follow-up visits
  Review blood glucose data
  Institute insulin therapy if significant fasting or
    postprandial hyperglycemia occurs

Other authors have proposed that a repetitive fasting blood glucose of 95 mg/dL (5.3 mmol/L) or greater requires insulin to reduce the frequency of macrosomia.[139] Coustan and Imrah[140] have reported that "prophylactic" insulin given to patients who would normally be treated by diet alone may reduce the frequency of macrosomia, cesarean section, and birth trauma. It has been suggested that insulin may reduce subtle degrees of postprandial hyperglycemia which can promote excessive fetal growth.[140] Alternatively, insulin may regulate maternal levels of other fetal insulin secretagogues such as branched chain amino acids. In contrast to the study of Coustan and Imrah, Persson and co-workers[141] performed a prospective randomized study concerning "prophylactic insulin" therapy. These authors noted similar rates of macrosomia and skin-fold thickness among diet and diet-plus-insulin-treated GDM women.[141] *Until larger prospective randomized studies indicate the benefit of prophylactic insulin, such therapy should be reserved for women who demonstrate significant fasting or postprandial hyperglycemia.*

Patients with GDM who are well controlled are at low risk for intrauterine death. However, gestational diabetics requiring insulin undergo fetal testing in a manner similar to uncomplicated insulin-dependent patients.[90] Antepartum fetal heart rate testing prior to term has been recommended in three groups of patients with GDM: (1) those who require insulin; (2) those with hypertension; and (3) those who have a history of prior stillbirth. Maternal assessment of fetal activity is begun at 28 weeks. Gestational diabetics may be safely managed until 40 weeks as long as fasting and postprandial glucose values remain normal. At 40 weeks, fetal surveillance is begun with nonstress testing. As with overt diabetic patients, ultrasound is employed to identify macrosomia and help select the safest route of delivery.

Counseling the IDDM Woman

Anomalies of the cardiac, renal, and central nervous systems arise during the first 7 weeks of gestation, a time when it is most unusual for patients to seek prenatal care. Therefore, the management and counseling of women with diabetes in the reproductive age group should begin prior to conception. Unfortunately, it has been estimated that less than 20% of diabetic women in the United States seek prepregnancy care.[131]

Molsted-Pedersen[142] has demonstrated a reduced rate of major congenital malformation in patients optimally managed before conception in hospitals with special diabetes clinics. The rate of malformations fell from 19.4% to 8.5% in class D and F patients who attended a prepregnancy clinic. In East Germany, Fuhrmann et al.[143] found that intensive treatment begun prior to conception in 307 diabetic women reduced the malformation rate to 1%. Nearly 90% of women in this study maintained mean glucose levels less than 100 mg/dL (5.6 mmol/L). In contrast, the incidence of anomalies in the offspring of 593 diabetic women who registered for care after 8 weeks' gestation was 8.0% (47/593). Only 20% of those women had mean daily glucose levels of less than 100 mg/dL (5.6 mmol/L). Most recently, Mills et al.[21] have reported that diabetic women registered prior to pregnancy had fewer infants with anomalies when compared to late registrants (4.9% vs. 9.0%). While the incidence of 4.9% remains higher than that in a normal control population (2%), normalization of glycemia was not established in the early-entry group.

Glycosylated hemoglobin levels obtained during the first trimester may be used to counsel diabetic women regarding the risk for an anomalous infant. In a retrospective study at the Joslin Clinic, Miller and colleagues[144] observed that elevated hemoglobin A_{1c} concentrations early in pregnancy correlated with an increased incidence of malformations. In 58 patients with elevated glycosylated hemoglobin levels, 13 (22%) malformed infants were noted. Their findings have been confirmed by Ylinen et al.[83] who measured glycosylated hemoglobin before the 15th week of gestation in 142 pregnancies. In pregnancies complicated by fetal malformations, mean values were significantly higher than in pregnancies without malformations. In the subgroup of patients with glycosylated hemoglobin values greater than 10% (normal <8%), fetal malformations were present in 6 of 17 cases. Overall, the risk of a major fetal anomaly may be as high as 1 in 4 or 1 in 5 when the glycosylated hemoglobin level is several percent above normal values. In contrast to the studies cited above is the recent report of Mills et al.[21] in which malformation rates in infants of diabetic mothers were not correlated with first-trimester maternal glycosylated hemoglobin levels. The authors suggested that more sensitive measures are needed to identify teratogenic mechanisms or that not all malformations can be prevented by good glycemic control. Regardless of the glycosylated hemoglobin value obtained, all patients require a careful program of surveillance, as outlined earlier, to detect fetal malformations. The risk for spontaneous abortion also appears to be increased with marked elevations in glycosylated hemoglobin. However, for diabetic women in good control, there appears to be no greater likelihood for miscarriage.[145]

With the increasing evidence that poor control is responsible for the congenital malformations seen in pregnancies complicated by diabetes, it is apparent that pre-conception counseling involving the patient and her family should be instituted. Physicians who care for young women with diabetes must be aware of the importance of such counseling. At this time, the nonpregnant patient may learn techniques for self-glucose monitoring as well as the need for proper dietary management. Questions may be answered regarding risk factors for complications and the plan for general management of diabetes in pregnancy. Planning for pregnancy should optimally be accomplished over several months. Glycosylated hemoglobin measurements are performed to aid in the timing of conception. The patient should attempt to achieve a glycosylated hemoglobin level within 2 SD of the mean for the reference laboratory.[146]

Contraception

There is no evidence that diabetes mellitus impairs fertility. Family planning is thus an important consideration for the diabetic woman. A careful history and complete gynecologic examination and counseling are required before selecting a method of contraception. Barrier methods continue to be a safe and inexpensive method of birth control. The diaphragm, used correctly with a spermicide, has a failure rate of less than 10%. Because there are no inherent risks to the diaphragm and other barrier methods, these have become the preferred interim method of contraception of insulin-dependent diabetic women.

Combined oral contraceptives (OCs) are the most effective reversible method of contraception with failure rates generally less than 1%. There is, however, continued controversy regarding their use in the diabetic woman. The serious side effects of pill use, including thrombemobolic disease and myocardial infarction, may be increased in diabetic women using combined OCs. In a retrospective study, Steel and Duncan[147] observed five cardiovascular complications in 136 diabetic women using primary low-dose pills. Three patients had cerebrovascular accidents, one had a myocardial infarction, and one an axillary vein thrombosis. Several other women exhibited rapid progression of retinopathy. Other than that study, there are limited data concerning the safety of the combined OC pill in diabetic women. Most physicians, therefore, refrain from using OCs in diabetic women and encourage other forms of contraception. For those who prescribe low-dose OCs to diabetic women, their use should be restricted to patients without vascular complications or additional risk factors such as a strong family history of myocardial disease.

Women using the OCs may demonstrate increased resistance to insulin as a result of a diminished concentration of insulin receptors.[148] Despite the fact that carbohydrate metabolism may be affected by the progestin component of the pill, disturbances in diabetic control are actually uncommon with its use. In Steel and Duncan's study,[149] 81% of patients using the pill did not require a change in insulin dose.[149] Triphasic OCs may also be used safely in former GDM women without other risk factors. Skouby et al.[150] have demonstrated that normal glucose tolerance and lipid levels can be expected in nonobese former GDM women followed after 6 months of therapy.[150] After the completion of childbearing, permanent sterilization including tubal ligation and vasectomy should be discussed with the patient as well as her partner.

CONCLUSION

The risk of mortality for the offspring of the diabetic mother has been reduced substantially during the past several decades. A further reduction in neonatal mortality from severe congenital anomalies remains an important goal for the future. Prepregnancy counseling stressing the importance of euglycemia at the time of early embryonic development may decrease the incidence of fetal malformations. Further investigation is required to define the precise role that glucose and other factors play in this process.

Neonatal morbidity continues to be a significant problem in the infant of the diabetic mother. At present, it appears that improving maternal diabetic control can greatly reduce much of this morbidity.

REFERENCES

1. Kalkhoff RK, Kissebah AH, Kim H-J: Carbohydrate and lipid metabolism during normal pregnancy: Relationship to gestational hormone action, in Merkatz IR, Adam PAF (eds): *The Diabetic Pregnancy: A Perinatal Perspective.* New York, Grune & Stratton, Inc, 1979, pp 3–21.
2. Freinkel N, Phelps RL, Metzger BE: Intermediary metabolism during normal pregnancy, in Sutherland HW, Stowers JM (eds): *Carbohydrate Metabolism in Pregnancy and the Newborn.* New York, Springer-Verlag, 1978, pp 1–31.
3. Spellacy WH: Human placental lactogen (HPL)—The review of a protein hormone important to obstetrics and gynecology. *South Med J* 1969; 62:1054–1057.
4. Costrini NV, Kalkhoff RK: Relative effects of pregnancy, estradiol and progesterone on plasma insulin and pancreatic islet secretion. *J Clin Invest* 1971; 50:992–999.
5. Yen SSC: Endocrine regulation of metabolic homeostasis during pregnancy. *Clin Obstet Gynecol* 1973; 16:130–147.
6. Puavilon G, Drobny EC, Domont LA, et al: Insulin receptors and insulin resistance in human pregnancy: Evidence for a postreceptor defect in insulin action. *J Clin Endocrinol Metab* 1982; 54:247–253.
7. Cousins L, Rigg L, Hollingsworth D, et al: The 24 hour excursion and diurnal rhythm of glucose, insulin, and C-peptide in normal pregnancy. *Am J Obstet Gynecol* 1980; 136:483–488.
8. Langer O, Anyaegbunam A, Brustman L, et al: Gestational diabetes: Insulin requirements in pregnancy. *Am J Obstet Gynecol* 1987; 157:669–675.
9. Madsen H: Fetal oxygenation in diabetic pregnancy. *Dan Med Bull* 1986; 33:64–74.
10. Hay WW, Sparks JW: Placental, fetal, and neonatal carbohydrate metabolism. *Clin Obstet Gynecol* 1985; 28:473–485.
11. Freinkel N, Lewis NJ, Akazama S, et al: The honeybee syndrome—implications of the teratogenicity of mannose in rat-embryo culture. *N Engl J Med* 1984; 310:223–230.
12. Gabbe SG: Management of diabetes in pregnancy: Six decades of experience, in Pitkin RM, Zlatnik F (eds): *Year Book of Obstetrics and Gynecology, 1980.* Chicago, Year Book Medical Publishers, Inc, 1980, pp 37–217.
13. Nyland L, Lunell N-O, Lewander B, et al: Uteroplacental blood flow in diabetic pregnancy: Measurements with indium 113m and a computer-linked gamma camera. *Am J Obstet Gynecol* 1982; 144:298–302.
14. Kitzmiller JL, Phillippe M: Hyperglycemia, hypoxia, and fetal acidosis in Rhesus monkeys. Presented at 28th Annual Meeting of the Society for Gynecologic Investigation, St. Louis, March 1981.

15. Phillips AF, Dubin JW, Matty PJ, et al: Arterial hypoxemia and hyperinsulinemia in the chronically hyperglycemic fetal lamb. *Pediatr Res* 1982; 16:653–658.

16. Shelley JH, Bassett JM, Milner RD: Control of carbohydrate metabolism in the fetus and newborn. *Br Med Bull* 1975; 31:37–43.

17. Carson BS, Philipps AF, Simmons MA, et al: Effects of a sustained insulin infusion upon glucose uptake and oxygenation of the ovine fetus. *Pediatr Res* 1980; 14:147–152.

18. Quissel BJ, Bonds DR, Krell LS, et al: The effects of chronic fetal insulin infusion upon fetal oxygenation. *Clin Res* 1980; 28:125A.

19. Miodovnik M, Lavin JP, Harrington D, et al: Effect of maternal ketoacidemia on the pregnant ewe and fetus. *Am J Obstet Gynecol* 1982; 144:585–593.

20. Simpson JL, Elias S, Martin AO, et al: Diabetes in pregnancy, Northwestern University Series (1977–1981). I. Prospective study of anomalies in offspring of mothers with diabetes mellitus. *Am J Obstet Gynecol* 1983; 146:263–270.

21. Mills JL, Knopp RH, Simpson JL, et al: Lack of relation of increased malformation rates in infants of diabetic mothers to glycemic control during organogenesis. *N Engl J Med* 1988; 318:671–676.

22. Reece EA, Hobbins JC: Diabetic embryopathy: Pathogenesis, prenatal diagnosis and prevention. *Obstet Gynecol Surv* 1986; 41:325–335.

23. Koppe J, Smoremberg-Schoorl M: Diabetes, congenital malformations and HLA types, in Lsten E, Band H, Frus-Hansen B (eds): *Intensive Care in the Newborn*, vol 4. Masson Publishing, Newark, 1983, pp 15–28.

24. Mills J: Malformations in infants of diabetic mothers. *Teratology* 1982; 25:385–394.

25. Mills JL, Baker L, Goldman AS: Malformations in infants of diabetic mothers occur before the seventh gestational week. Implications for treatment. *Diabetes* 1979; 28:292–293.

26. Kucera J: Rate and type of congenital anomalies among offspring of diabetic women. *J Reprod Med* 1971; 7:73–82.

27. Sadler TW, Horton WE Jr: Mechanisms of diabetes-induced congenital malformations are studied in mammalian embryo culture, in Jovanovic L, Peterson CM, Fuhrmann K (eds): *Diabetes in Pregnancy. Teratology, Toxicity and Treatment.* New York, Praeger, 1986, pp 51–71.

28. Watanabe G, Ingalls TH: Congenital malformations in the offspring of alloxan-diabetic mice. *Diabetes* 1963; 12:66–72.

29. Horii K, Watanabe G, Ingalls TH: Experimental diabetes in pregnant mice. Prevention of congenital malformations in offspring by insulin. *Diabetes* 1966; 15:194–204.

30. Baker L, Egler JM, Klein SH, et al: Meticulous control of diabetes during organogenesis prevents congenital lumbosacral defects in rats. *Diabetes* 1981: 30:955–959.

31. Cockroft DL, Coppola PT: Teratogenic effects of excess glucose on head-fold rat embryos in culture. *Teratology* 1977; 16:141–146.

32. Horton WE Jr, Sadler TW: Effects of maternal diabetes on early embryogenesis: Alterations in morphogenesis produced by the ketone body, beta-hydroxybutyrate. *Diabetes* 1983; 32:610–616.

33. Sadler TW, Hunter ES: Hypoglycemia: How little is too much for the embryo? *Am J Obstet Gynecol* 1987; 157:190–193.

34. Cockroft DL, Freinkel LN, Phillips LS, et al: Metabolic factors organogenesis in diabetic pregnancy. *Clin Res* 1981; 29:557A.

35. Goldman AS, Baker L, Piddington R, et al: Hyperglycemia-induced teratogenesis is mediated by a functional deficiency of arachidonic acid. *Proc Natl Acad Sci USA* 1985; 82:8227–8231.

36. Pinter E, Reece EA: Arachidonic acid prevents hyperglycemia-associated yolk sac damage and embryopathy. *Am J Obstet Gynecol* 1986; 155:691–702.

37. Pinter E, Reece EA, Leranth CZ, et al: Yolk sac failure in embryopathy due to hyperglycemia: Ultrastructural analysis of yolk sac differentiation associated with embryopathy in rat conceptuses under hyperglycemic conditions. *Teratology* 1986; 33:73–84.

38. Pettit DJ, Baird HR, Aleck KA, et al: Excessive obesity in offspring of Pima Indian women with diabetes during pregnancy. *N Engl J Med* 1983; 308:242–245.

39. Lavin JP, Lovelace DR, Miodovnik M, et al: Clinical experience with one hundred seven diabetic pregnancies. *Am J Obstet Gynecol* 1983; 147:742–752.

40. Sepe SJ, Connell FA, Geiss LA, et al: Gestational diabetes: Incidence, maternal characteristics, and perinatal outcome. *Diabetes* 1985; 34 (suppl 2):13–16.

41. Spellacy WN, Miller S, Winegar A, et al: Macrosomia-maternal characteristics and infant complications. *Obstet Gynecol* 1985; 66:158–161.

42. Modanlou HD, Komatsu G, Dorchester W, et al: Large-for-gestational age neonates: Anthropometric reasons for shoulder dystocia. *Obstet Gynecol* 1982; 60:417–423.

43. Brans YW, Shannon DL, Hunter MA: Maternal diabetes and neonatal macrosomia. II. Neonatal anthropometric measurements. *Early Hum Dev* 1983; 8:297–305.

44. Enzi G, Inelman EM, Caretta F, et al: Development of adipose tissue in newborns of gestational diabetic and insulin-dependent diabetic mothers. *Diabetes* 1980; 29:100–104.

45. Whitelaw A: Subcutaneous fat in newborn infants of diabetic mothers: An indication of quality of diabetic control. *Lancet* 1977; 1:15–18.

46. Pedersen J: Weight and length at birth of infants of diabetic mothers. *Acta Endocrinol* 1954; 16:330–342.

47. Driscoll SG, Benirschke K, Curtis GW: Neonatal deaths among infants of diabetic mothers. *Am J Dis Child* 1960; 100:818–835.

48. Naeye RL: Infants of diabetic mothers: A quantitative morphologic study. *Pediatrics* 1965; 35:980–988.

49. Reiher H, Fuhrmann K, Noack S, et al: Age-dependent insulin secretion of the endocrine pancreas in vitro from fetuses of diabetic and nondiabetic patients. *Diabetes Care* 1983; 6:446–451.

50. Susa JB, Schwartz R: Effects of hyperinsulinema in the primate fetus. *Diabetes* 1985; 34:36–41.

51. Falluca F, Gargiulo P, Troili F, et al: Amniotic fluid insulin, C peptide concentrations, and fetal morbidity in infants of diabetic mothers. *Am J Obstet Gynecol* 1985; 153:534–540.

52. Lin CC, River P, Moawad AH, et al: Prenatal assessment of fetal outcome by amniotic fluid C-peptide levels in pregnant diabetic women. *Am J Obstet Gynecol* 1981; 141:671–676.

53. Weiss PAM, Hofman H, Winter R, et al: Gestational diabetes and screening during pregnancy. *Obstet Gynecol* 1984; 63:776–780.

54. Persson B, Pschera H, Lunell NO, et al: Amino acid concentration in maternal plasma and amniotic fluid in relation to fetal insulin secretion during the last trimester of pregnancy in gestational and type I diabetic women and women with small-for-gestational age infants. *Am J Perinatol* 1986; 3:98–103.

55. Sosenko IR, Kitzmiller JL, Loo SW, et al: The infant of the diabetic mother—correlation of increased cord C-peptide levels with macrosomia and hypoglycemia. *N Engl J Med* 1979; 301:859–862.

56. Milner RD, Hill DH: Fetal growth control: The role of insulin and related peptides. *Clin Endocrinol* 1984; 21:415–433.

57. Gabbe SG, Mestman JH, Freeman RK, et al: Management and outcome of pregnancy in diabetes mellitus, Classes B-R. *Am J Obstet Gynecol* 1977; 129:723–732.

58. Kitzmiller JL, Cloherty JP, Younger MD, et al: Diabetic pregnancy and perinatal morbidity. *Am J Obstet Gynecol* 1978; 131:560–580.

59. Roversi GD, Gardiulo M, Nicolini U, et al: A new approach to the treatment of diabetic pregnant women. *Am J Obstet Gynecol* 1979; 135:567–576.

60. Jovanovic L, Druzin M, Peterson CM: Effect of euglycemia on the outcome of pregnancy in insulin-dependent diabetic women as compared with normal control subjects. *Am J Med* 1981; 71:921–927.

61. Willman SP, Leveno KJ, Guziek DS, et al: Glucose threshold for macrosomia in pregnancy complicated by diabetes. *Am J Obstet Gynecol* 1986; 154:470–475.

62. Landon MB, Gabbe SG, Piana R, et al: Neonatal morbidity in pregnancy complicated by diabetes mellitus: Predictive value of maternal glycemic profiles. *Am J Obstet Gynecol* 1987; 156:1089–1095.

63. Soler NG, Soler SM, Malins JM: Neonatal morbidity among infants of diabetic mothers. *Diabetes Care* 1978; 1:340–350.

64. Kuhl C, Anderson GE, Hertel J, et al: Metabolic events in infants of diabetic mothers during first 24 hours after birth. *Acta Paediatr Scand* 1982; 71:19–25.

65. Phelps RL, Freinkel N, Rubenstein AH, et al: Carbohydrate metabolism in pregnancy. XV. Plasma C-peptide during intravenous glucose tolerance in neonates from normal and insulin-treated diabetic mothers. *J Clin*

Endocrinol Metab 1978; 46:61–68.

66. Karlsson K, Kjellmer I: The outcome of diabetic pregnancies in relation to the mother's blood sugar level. *Am J Obstet Gynecol* 1972; 112:213–220.

67. Bourbon JR, Farrell PM: Fetal lung development in the diabetic pregnancy. *Pediatr Res* 1985; 19:253–267.

68. Engle M, Langan SM, Saunders RL: The effects of insulin and hyperglycemia on surfactant phospholipid biosynthesis in organotypic cultures of type II pneumocytes. *Biochim Biophys Acta* 1983; 753:6–13.

69. Smith BT, Giroud CJP, Robert M, et al: Insulin antagonism of cortisol action on lecithin synthesis by cultures fetal lung cells. *J Pediatr* 1975; 87:953–955.

70. Smith BT: Pulmonary surfactant during fetal development and neonatal adaptation: Hormonal control, in Robertson B, Van Golde LMB, Batenbrug JJ (eds): *Pulmonary Surfactant*. Amsterdam, Elsevier Scientific Publishers, 1984, pp 357–381.

71. Post M, Barsoumian A, Smith BT: The cellular mechanisms of glucocorticoid acceleration of fetal lung maturation. *J Biol Chem* 1986; 261:2179–2184.

72. Carlson KS, Smith BT, Post M: Insulin acts on the fibroblast to inhibit glucocorticoid stimulation of lung maturation. *J Appl Physiol* 1984; 57:1577–1579.

73. Rooney SA, Ingleson LD, Wilson CM, et al: Insulin antagonism of dexamethasone induced stimulation of choline phosphate cytidyltransferase in fetal rat lung in organ culture. *Lung* 1980; 158:151–155.

74. Robert MF, Neff RK, Hubbell JP, et al: Association between maternal diabetes and the respiratory distress syndrome in the newborn. *N Engl J Med* 1976; 294:357–360.

75. Dudley DKL, Black DM: Reliability of lecithin/sphingomyelin ratios in diabetic pregnancy. *Obstet Gynecol* 1985; 66:521–524.

76. Gabbe SG, Lowensohn RI, Mestman JH, et al: Lecithin/sphingomyelin ratio in pregnancies complicated by diabetes mellitus. *Am J Obstet Gynecol* 1977; 128:577–760.

77. Coustan DR, Berkowitz RL, Hobbins JC: Tight metabolic control of overt diabetes in pregnancy. *Am J Med* 1980; 68:845–852.

78. Tsang RC, Kleinman LI, Sutherland JM, et al: Hypocalcemia in infants of diabetic mothers. *J Pediatr* 1972; 80:384–395.

79. Cruikshank DP, Pitkin RM, Reynolds WA, et al: Altered maternal calcium homeostasis in diabetic pregnancy. *J Clin Endocrinol Metab* 1980; 50:264–267.

80. Tsang RC, Chen I-W, Friedman MA, et al: Parathyroid function in infants of diabetic mothers. *J Pediatr* 1975; 86:399–404.

81. Mimouni F, Miodovnik M, Tsang RC, et al: Decreased amniotic fluid magnesium concentration in diabetic pregnancy. *Obstet Gynecol* 1987; 69:12–14.

82. Widness JA, Cowett RM, Coustan DR, et al: Neonatal morbidities in infants of mothers with glucose intolerance in pregnancy. *Diabetes* 1985: 34 (suppl 2):61–65.

83. Ylinen K, Aula P, Staman U-H, et al: Risk of minor and major fetal malformation in diabetes with high haemoglobin A_1 values in early pregnancy. *Br Med J* 1984; 289:345–346.

84. Gabbe SG, Lowensohn RI, Wu PY, et al: Current patterns of neonatal morbidity and mortality in infants of diabetic mothers. *Diabetes Care* 1978; 1:335–339.

85. Lemons JA, Vargas P, Delaney JJ: Infant of the diabetic mother: Review of 225 cases. *Obstet Gynecol* 1981; 57:187–192.

86. Stevenson DK, Bartoletti AL, Ostrander CR, et al: Pulmonary excretion of carbon monoxide in the human infant as an index of bilirubin production. II. Infants of diabetic mothers. *J Pediatr* 1979; 94:956–958.

87. Shannon K, Davis JC, Kitzmiller JL, et al: Erythropoiesis in infants of diabetic mothers. *Pediatr Res* 1986; 20:161–165.

88. Ylinen K, Raivio K, Teramo K: Haemoglobin A_{1c} predicts the perinatal outcome in insulin-dependent diabetic pregnancies. *Br J Obstet Gynaecol* 1981; 88:961–967.

89. White P: Pregnancy complicating diabetes. *Am J Med* 1949; 7:609–616.

90. Landon MB, Gabbe SG: Antepartum surveillance in gestational diabetes. *Diabetes* 1985; 34 (suppl 2): 50–54.

91. Main EK, Main DM, Landon MB, et al: Factors predicting perinatal outcome in pregnancies complicated by diabetic nephropathy (Class F). Presented at Sixth Annual Meeting, Society of Perinatal Obstetricians, San Antonio, Texas, February 1986.

92. Kitzmiller JL, Brown ER, Phillippe M, et al: Diabetic nephropathy and perinatal out-

come. *Am J Obstet Gynecol* 1981; 141:741–751.

93. Reece EA, Coustan DR, Hayslett JP, et al: Diabetic nephropathy: Pregnancy performance and fetomaternal outcome. *Am J Obstet Gynecol* 1988; 159:56–66.

94. Kitzmiller JL: Diabetic nephropathy, in Reece EA, Coustan DR (eds): *Diabetes Mellitus in Pregnancy. Principles and Practice.* New York, Churchill Livingston, Inc, 1988, pp 489–513.

95. Hayslett JP, Reece EA: Effect of diabetic nephropathy on pregnancy. *Am J Kidney Dis* 1987; 9:344–349.

96. Ogburn PL Jr, Kitzmiller JL, Hare JW, et al: Pregnancy following renal transplantation in Class T diabetes mellitus. *JAMA* 1986; 255:911–915.

97. Carstensen LL, Frost-Lansen K, Fulgeberg S, et al: Does pregnancy influence the prognosis of uncomplicated insulin-dependent diabetes? *Diabetes Care* 1982; 5:1–5.

98. Horvat M, Maclear H, Goldberg L, et al: Diabetic retinopathy in pregnancy: A 12 year prospective study. *Br J Ophthalmol* 1980; 64:398–403.

99. Kitzmiller JL, Gavin LA, Gin GD, et al: Managing diabetes and pregnancy. *Curr Probl Obstet Gynecol Fertil* 1988; 11:113–167.

100. Moloney JBM, Drury MI: The effect of pregnancy on the natural course of diabetic retinopathy. *Am J Ophthalmol* 1982; 93:745–756.

101. Phelps RL, Sakol P, Metzger BE, et al: Changes in diabetic retinopathy during pregnancy, correlations with regulation of hyperglycemia. *Arch Ophthalmol* 1986; 104:1806–1810.

102. Chang S, Fuhrmann M, and the Diabetes in Early Pregnancy Study Group: Pregnancy, retinopathy, normoglycemia: A preliminary analysis. *Diabetes* 1985; 34(suppl):3A.

103. Sinclair SH, Nesler C, Foxman B, et al: Macular edema and pregnancy in insulin-dependent diabetes. *Am J Ophthalmol* 1984; 97:154–167.

104. Silfen SL, Wapner RJ, Gabbe SG: Maternal outcome in Class H diabetes mellitus. *Obstet Gynecol* 1980; 55:749–751.

105. Hare JW: Maternal complications, in Hare JW (ed): *Diabetes Complicating Pregnancy. The Joslin Clinic Method.* New York, Alan R Liss, Inc, 1989, pp 95–96.

106. O'Sullivan JB: Body weight and subse-quent diabetes mellitus. *JAMA* 1982; 248:949–952.

107. Metzger BE, Bybee DE, Freinkel N, et al: Gestational diabetes mellitus. Correlations between the phenotypic and genotypic characteristics of the mother and abnormal glucose tolerance during the first year postpartum. *Diabetes* 1985; 34 (suppl 2):111–115.

108. Coustan DR, Carpenter MW: Detection and treatment of gestational diabetes. *Clin Obstet Gynecol* 1985; 28:507–515.

109. Coustan DR, Nelson C, Carpenter MW, et al: Maternal age and screening for gestational diabetes: A population based study. *Obstet Gynecol* 1989; 73:557–561.

110. Freinkel N, Beard R, Haddin D, et al: Summary and Recommendations of the Second International Workshop-Conference on Gestational Diabetes. *Diabetes* 1985; 34 (suppl 2):123–126.

111. Coustan DR, Widness JA, Carpenter MW, et al: Should the fifty-gram, one-hour plasma glucose screening test be administered in the fasting or fed state? *Am J Obstet Gynecol* 1986; 154:1031–1035.

112. Landon MB, Cembrowski G, Gabbe SG: Capillary blood glucose screening for gestational diabetes: A preliminary investigation. *Am J Obstet Gynecol* 1986; 155:717–721.

113. Carpenter MW, Coustan DR: Criteria for screening tests for gestational diabetes. *Am J Obstet Gynecol* 1982; 144:768–773.

114. Jovanovic L, Peterson CM: Screening for gestational diabetes, optimum timing and criteria for retesting. *Diabetes* 1985; 34 (suppl 2): 21–23.

115. O'Sullivan JB, Mahan CM, Boston AB: Criteria for the oral glucose tolerance test in pregnancy. *Diabetes* 1964; 13:278–285.

116. Tallarigo L, Giampietro O, Penno G, et al: Relation of glucose tolerance to complications of pregnancy in nondiabetic women. *N Engl J Med* 1986; 315:989–992.

117. Leikin EL, Jenkins JH, Pomerantz GA, et al: Abnormal glucose screening tests in pregnancy: A risk factor for fetal macrosomia. *Obstet Gynecol* 1987; 69:570–573.

118. Weiner CP: Effect of varying degrees of "normal" glucose metabolism on maternal and perinatal outcome. *Am J Obstet Gynecol* 1988; 159:862–870.

119. Landon MB, Gabbe SG: Glucose monitoring and insulin administration in the preg-

nant diabetic patient. *Clin Obstet Gynecol* 1985; 28:496–506.

120. Hollingsworth D, Ney DM: Dietary management of diabetes during pregnancy, in Reese EA, Coustan DR (eds): *Diabetes Mellitus in Pregnancy*. New York, Churchill Livingston, Inc, 1988, pp 285–311.

121. Coustan DR, Reece EA, Sherwin RS, et al: A randomized clinical trial of the insulin pump vs intensive conventional therapy in diabetic pregnancies. *JAMA* 1986; 255:631–636.

122. Gabbe SG: Antepartum fetal surveillance in the pregnancy complicated by diabetes mellitus, in Gabbe SG, Oh W (eds.): *Infant of the Diabetic Mother*. Columbus, Ohio, Ross Laboratories, 1987, pp 86–95.

123. Barrett JM, Salyer SL, Boehm FH: The non-stress test: An evaluation of 1000 patients. *Am J Obstet Gynecol* 1981; 141:153–157.

124. Miller JM Jr: Antepartum fetal heart rate testing in diabetic pregnancy (Class B–F). Presented at Third Annual Meeting, Society of Perinatal Obstetricians, San Antonio, Texas, January 1983.

125. Teramo K, Ammala P, Ylinen K, et al: Pathologic fetal heart rate associated with poor metabolic control in diabetic pregnancies. *Obstet Gynecol* 1983; 61:559–565.

126. Landon MB, Gabbe SG, Burner JP, et al: Doppler umbilical artery velocimetry in pregnancy complicated by insulin-dependent diabetes mellitus. *Obstet Gynecol* 1989; 73:961–965.

127. Milunsky A, Alpert E, Kitzmiller JL, et al: Prenatal diagnosis of neural tube defects VIII. The importance of serum alpha-fetoprotein screening in diabetic pregnant women. *Am J Obstet Gynecol* 1982; 142:1030–1032.

128. Mintz MC, Landon MB: Sonographic diagnosis of fetal growth disorders. *Clin Obstet Gynecol* 1988; 31:44–52.

129. Landon MB, Mintz MC, Gabbe SG: Sonographic evaluation of fetal abdominal growth: Predictor of the large-for-gestational-age infant in pregnancies complicated by diabetes mellitus. *Am J Obstet Gynecol* 1989; 160:115–121.

130. Cousins L: Pregnancy complications among diabetic women: Review 1965–1985. *Obstet Gynecol Surv* 1987; 42:140–149.

131. Gabbe SG, Landon MB: Management of diabetes mellitus in pregnancy. Survey of maternal-fetal subspecialists in the United States, in Sutherland H (ed): *Carbohydrate Metabolism in Pregnancy and the Newborn*. New York, Springer-Verlag 1989.

132. Benedetti TJ, Gabbe SG: Shoulder dystocia: A complication of fetal macrosomia and prolonged second stage of labor with midpelvic delivery. *Obstet Gynecol* 1978; 52:526–529.

133. Acker DB, Sachs BP, Friedman EA: Risk factors for shoulder dystocia. *Obstet Gynecol* 1985; 66:762–768.

134. West TE, Lowy C: Control of blood glucose during labor in diabetic women with combined glucose and low dose insulin infusion. *Br Med J* 1977; 1:1252–1254.

135. Jovanovic L, Peterson CM: Management of the pregnant, insulin-dependent diabetic woman. *Diabetes Care* 1980; 3:63–68.

136. Gabbe SG, Mestman JA, Freeman RK, et al: Management and outcome of Class A diabetes mellitus. *Am J Obstet Gynecol* 1977; 116:895–900.

137. Algert S, Shragg P, Hollingsworth DR: Moderate caloric restriction in obese women with gestational diabetes. *Obstet Gynecol* 1985; 65:487–491.

138. Goldberg J, Franklin B, Lasser L, et al: Gestational diabetes: Impact of home glucose monitoring on neonatal birth weight. *Am J Obstet Gynecol* 1986; 154:546–550.

139. Langer O, Mazze RM: The relationship between large-for-gestational age infants and glycemic control in women with gestational diabetes. *Am J Obstet Gynecol* 1988; 159:1478–1483.

140. Coustan DR, Imrah J: Prophylactic insulin treatment of gestational diabetes reduces the incidence of macrosomia, operative delivery, and birth trauma. *Am J Obstet Gynecol* 1984; 150:836–842.

141. Persson B, Stangenberg M, Hasson U, et al: Gestational diabetes mellitus: Comparative evaluation of two treatment regimens, diet versus insulin and diet. *Diabetes* 1985; 34(suppl 2): 101–105.

142. Molsted-Pedersen L: Pregnancy and diabetes. A survey. *Acta Endocrinol* 1980; 94(suppl 234):13–19.

143. Fuhrmann K, Reiher H, Semmler K, et al: Prevention of congenital malformations in infants of insulin-dependent diabetic mothers. *Diabetes Care* 1983; 6:219–223.

144. Miller E, Hare JW, Cloherty JP, et al: Ele-

vated maternal HGA₁ in early pregnancy and major congenital anomalies in infants of diabetic mothers. *N Engl J Med* 1981; 304:1331–1334.

145. Mills J, Simpson JL, Driscoll SG, et al: Incidence of spontaneous abortion among normal and insulin-dependent diabetic women whose pregnancies were identified within 21 days of conception. *N Engl J Med* 1988; 319:1617–1623.

146. Freinkel N: Diabetic embryopathy and fuel-mediated organ teratogenesis: Lessons from animal models. *Horm Metab Res* 1988; 20:463–475.

147. Steel JM, Duncan LJP: Serious complica-tions of oral contraception in insulin-dependent diabetes. *Contraception* 1978; 17:291–295.

148. DePiaro R, Forte F, Bertoli A, et al: Changes in insulin receptors during oral contraception. *J Clin Endocrinol Metab* 1981; 52:29–33.

149. Steel JM, Duncan LJP: The effect of oral contraceptives on insulin requirements in diabetic. *Br J Fam Plann* 1978; 3:77.

150. Skouby S, Kuhl C Molsted-Pederson L, et al: Triphasic oral contraception: Metabolic effects in normal women and those with previous gestational diabetes. *Am J Obstet Gynecol* 1985; 153:495–500.

CHAPTER 4

Pituitary, Thyroid, Adrenal, and Parathyroid Disorders

Mark E. Molitch

PITUITARY

Normal Pituitary Physiology During Pregnancy

The six anterior pituitary hormones are controlled by hypothalamic release and inhibitory factors and feedback from target organ hormones. Excessive and insufficient secretion of these pituitary hormones may affect fertility and the normal course of pregnancy. Conversely, the pregnancy itself alters normal pituitary function and may even promote the growth of some types of pituitary tumors.

The normal pituitary enlarges during pregnancy, predominantly due to hyperplasia of the prolactin (PRL)-producing lactotroph cells.[1] Estrogens produced by the placenta stimulate lactotroph DNA synthesis and mitotic activity, PRL messenger RNA (mRNA) levels and PRL synthesis.[2–5] Progesterone has also been shown to stimulate PRL secretion.[6, 7] During pregnancy there is a progressive rise in serum prolactin levels[8, 9] with a parallel increase in the size and number of lactotroph cells.[1, 10, 11] This stimulatory effect of pregnancy on the pituitary has important implications for the patient with a preexisting prolactinoma who desires pregnancy. It has also been hypothesized that this growth causes the pituitary to outgrow its blood supply in some patients, and may be a contributing fac-

tor in the development of postpartum infarction (Sheehan's syndrome; see below)

In the second half of pregnancy, pituitary growth hormone (GH) secretion falls and a GH variant made by the placenta increases in the circulation.[12] The physiologic significance of this change in the source of circulating GH is not known.

Pituitary Tumors

Pituitary tumors are characterized by the hormones that they make and can be divided by size into microadenomas with diameters less than 10 mm and macroadenomas with diameters greater than 10 mm. The latter group is also subclassified radiologically as to whether there is extrasellar extension, local invasion, or compression of the optic chiasm. Visual defects from chiasmal compression are best characterized by formal Goldmann perimetry testing. The size of the tumor and visual involvement are important when considering the efficacy and adverse effects of the various treatment modalities as well as the effects of pregnancy on the tumor.

Pituitary function is usually normal outside of the hormone oversecretion in patients with microadenomas. Varying degrees of hypopituitarism may be present in patients with macroadenomas because of compression of the hypothalamus or pituitary stalk, and pitui-

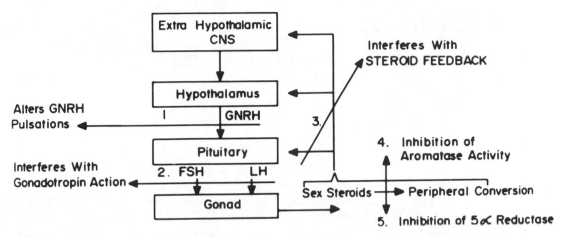

FIG 4–1.
How hyperprolactinemia produces hypogonadism. Schematic presentation of sites where hyperprolactinemia interferes with the reproductive system and sex steroid action. GNRH = gonadotropin releasing hormone; FSH = follicle-stimulating hormone; LH = luteinizing hormone. (From Odell WD: Prolactin-producing tumors (prolactinomas), in Odell WD, Nelson D (eds): *Pituitary Tumors.* Mt Kisco, NY, Futura Publishing Co, Inc, 1984, p 159, as modified by Malarkey WB. Effects of hyperprolactinemia on other endocrine systems, in Olefsky JM, Robbins RJ (eds): *Prolactinomas.* New York, Churchill Livingstone, Inc, 1986, p 21. Used by permission.)

tary function should be assessed prior to pregnancy in all such patients.

Prolactinomas

Hyperprolactinemia has been found in some series to be the cause of infertility in about one third of women presenting with this problem.[13–15] Hyperprolactinemia impairs the hypothalamic-pituitary-ovarian axis at several levels (Fig 4–1), the primary site of inhibition being at the hypothalamic level.[16, 17] The differential diagnosis of the causes of hyperprolactinemia is extensive (Table 4–1).[18] Prolactinomas account for more than 50% of cases and the diagnosis is made by radiologic means (high-resolution computed tomography [CT] or magnetic resonance imaging [MRI]) once secondary causes, such as

TABLE 4–1.
Differential Diagnosis of Hyperprolactinemia

Pituitary disease	Neurogenic	Medications
Prolactinomas	Chest wall lesions	Phenothiazines
Acromegaly	Spinal cord lesions	Butyrophenones
"Empty sella syndrome"	Breast stimulation	Monoamine oxidase
Lymphocytic hypophysitis		inhibitors
Cushing's disease	Other	Tricyclic antidepressants
Pituitary stalk section	Pregnancy	Reserpine
	Hypothyroidism	Methyldopa
Hypothalamic disease	Renal failure	Metoclopramide
Craniopharyngioma	Cirrhosis	Amoxapine
Meningiomas	Pseudocyesis	Verapamil
Dysgerminomas		
Nonsecreting pituitary		
tumors		
Other tumors		
Sarcoidosis		
Eosinophilic granulomas		
Neuraxis irradiation		
Vascular		

TABLE 4–2.
Effect of Pregnancy on Prolactinomas*

Tumor Type	Prior Therapy	No.	Symptomatic Enlargement[†]	Asymptomatic Enlargement[‡]
Microadenomas	None	246	4	11
Macroadenomas	None	45	7	4
Macroadenomas	Yes	46	2	0

*Adapted from Molitch ME: *N Engl J Med* 1985; 312:1364–1370.
[†]Requiring intervention—surgery or bromocriptine
[‡]Determined by postpartum CT scanning

hypothyroidism, medications, renal insufficiency, and hypothalamic disease, have been excluded. When no tumor is visualized after exclusion of these secondary causes, the patient is said to have idiopathic hyperprolactinemia. In any circumstance, a hyperprolactinemic woman is almost always infertile.

Two therapeutic approaches are now available to correct hyperprolactinemia and infertility: transsphenoidal selective adenoma resection and bromocriptine. Whereas the former is reserved for patients with tumors, the latter has been used for both groups of patients. For the patient with a prolactinoma, this choice of therapy may have important consequences for the course of the pregnancy.

Transsphenoidal surgery is successful initially in restoring PRL levels to normal in 60% to 80% of patients with microadenomas and in 25% to 40% of those with macroadenomas, although there is a recurrence rate of about 20% to 25% for the hyperprolactinemia.[18, 19] With return of the hyperprolactinemia, there is usually a recurrence of infertility and such patients may then need bromocriptine to restore fertility. Transsphenoidal surgery rarely causes hypopituitarism when done for microadenomas, but may cause this complication more commonly when done for macroadenomas.

Dopamine is the predominant hypothalamic PRL inhibiting factor. Bromocriptine is a long-acting dopamine receptor agonist, acting directly on the pituitary and possibly on hypothalamic dopaminergic pathways. Many studies have shown that bromocriptine reduces elevated PRL levels and restores ovulatory menses in 80% to 90% of women.[18, 19] Mechanical contraception is used until the first two or three cycles have occurred, so that an intermenstrual interval can be established. In this way, a woman will know when she has missed a menstrual period and a pregnancy test can be performed quickly. Thus, bromocriptine will have been given for only about 3 to 4 weeks of the gestation. In addition to its efficacy in lowering PRL levels, bromocriptine has been documented to reduce the size of PRL-secreting macroadenomas by at least 50% in over 50% of patients.[19, 20] In some cases, tumors may reexpand once the bromocriptine is stopped, especially if therapy has been of less than 1 year's duration. Bromocriptine is generally well tolerated, the side effects of nausea, vomiting, and orthostatic hypotension being lessened by low starting doses and gradual increments.[18–20] Pergolide is also now available and is a dopamine agonist similarly effective in reducing PRL levels. However, there is little safety experience regarding its use during the first several weeks of gestation and generally is tried only when bromocriptine is found to be ineffective.

Effects of Pregnancy on Prolactinoma Growth.—As noted above, the hormonal milieu of pregnancy is stimulatory to pituitary lactotrophs. In women with prolactinomas, this may result in significant tumor enlargement during gestation. In a survey of 16 series of patients reported in the literature,[21] symptomatic tumor enlargement was found to have occurred during pregnancy in 4 of 246 women with PRL-secreting microadenomas who had been treated only with bromocriptine (Table 4–2). In 2 of these women severe headaches had developed and in the other 2 visual field defects developed. None required surgery. Eleven of these women had asymptomatic tumor enlargement as documented by CT scanning post partum. These series included 45 women with macroadenomas who became pregnant; 7 (15.5%) developed symptomatic tumor enlargement and 4 (8.9%) developed asymptomatic tumor enlargement. In these same series, 46 women with macroadenomas had been treated with irradiation or surgery before pregnancy; only 2 of the 46 (4.3%) had symptomatic tumor enlargement and none had asymptomatic tumor enlargement during gestation. About 25% to 50% of the cases of symptomatic tumor enlargement required surgery before it was known that bromocriptine could reduce tumor size. More recently, however, bromocriptine has been used successfully during pregnancy to reduce symptomatic tumor enlargement in many cases.[21]

Effects of Hyperprolactinemia and Treatment on Pregnancy.—Once ovulation and fertilization occur, there appear to be no further effects of hyperprolactinemia on the development of the fetus and the course of pregnancy. When bromocriptine is taken for only the first few weeks of gestation, it has not been found to cause any increase in spontaneous abortions, ectopic pregnancies, trophoblastic disease, multiple pregnancies, or congenital malformations[21, 22] (Table 4–3). Bromocriptine, however, has been given throughout pregnancy to only a limited number of women. In 114 such pregnancies, there was reported only 1 malformation (talipes),[22] not an unexpected frequency. Bromocriptine crosses the placenta,[23] however, and it is not recommended that it be used for longer than necessary during pregnancy. The effects of transsphenoidal surgery during gestation are not known specifically but would not be expected to be significantly different from the effects of other types of surgery.

Management.—*Prepregnancy Counseling.*—The risks of surgery vs. medical therapy must be explained in detail to each patient. For the patient with a microadenoma, bromocriptine use is clearly safe for the fetus when stopped early in gestation and the risk to the mother of tumor enlargement is very small. Transsphenoidal surgery is certainly an acceptable alternative. For the patient with a macroadenoma that is intrasellar or with only inferior extension, the risk of bromocriptine treatment again appears to be quite small. However, when the tumor is very large or

TABLE 4–3.
Effect of Bromocriptine on Pregnancy*

	Bromocriptine		Normal Population %
	n	%	
Pregnancies	6,239	100.0	100.0
Spontaneous abortion	620	9.9	10–15
Terminations	75	1.25	
Ectopic	31	0.5	0.5–1.0
Hydatidiform moles	11	0.2	0.05–0.7
Deliveries (known duration)	4,139	100.0	100.0
At term (>38 wk)	3,620	87.5	85
Preterm (<38 wk)	519	12.5	15
Deliveries (known outcome)	5,120	100.0	100.0
Single births	5,031	98.3	98.7
Multiple births	89	1.7	1.3
Babies (known details)	5,213	100.0	100.0
Normal	5,030	96.5	95.0
With malformations	93	1.8	3–4
With perinatal disorders	90	1.7	>2

*Adapted from Krupp P, Monka C, Richter K: *Program of the Second World Congress of Gynecology and Obstetrics*, Rio de Janeiro, 1988, p 9.

extends to the optic chiasm or into the cavernous sinus, the risk of significant tumor enlargement is considerably greater. The decision must then be individualized for each patient as to the following possibilities: (1) preoperative surgical debulking, (2) very intensive monitoring of bromocriptine, or (3) continuous bromocriptine treatment. The safety of continuous bromocriptine is certainly not established. On the other hand, should pregnancy be discovered after the first few weeks of gestation, the data that exist are reassuring and would not justify therapeutic abortion.

Antenatal Management.—Patients with microadenomas should be seen each trimester and assessed for symptoms such as headaches or visual problems. Patients with macroadenomas should be seen monthly for such assessments. Prolactin levels do not always rise during pregnancy in women with prolactinomas, as they do in normal women, nor do they always rise with pregnancy-induced tumor enlargement.[24] Therefore, periodic checking of PRL levels is of no benefit. A CT or MRI scan of the sella should be done in all patients prior to conception to assess tumor size but need not be repeated during the pregnancy unless there is clinical suspicion of tumor enlargement. Visual field testing should also be done as a baseline and repeated each trimester in patients with macroadenomas. Visual field testing need only be done in patients with microadenomas when clinically indicated.

When there is evidence of tumor enlargement during pregnancy, bromocriptine therapy should be reinstituted immediately and the dose increased as rapidly as is tolerated. Such therapy must be very closely monitored and transsphenoidal surgery or delivery (if the pregnancy is far enough advanced) should be performed if there is no response to bromocriptine.[21]

Postpartum Management.—CT or MRI scans should be performed post partum to detect the presence of any asymptomatic tumor enlargement. When such enlargement occurs, repeat scans at 6- to 12-month intervals are warranted. A trial of bromocriptine to shrink the enlarged tumor is certainly also indicated. It is common, however, for PRL levels post partum to fall to levels considerably lower than ante partum.[25] Thus, bromocriptine rather than surgery may be the best therapy post partum to treat persistent hyperprolactinemia. Of course, reinstitution of bromocriptine will lower PRL levels to normal and inhibit lactation.

Breast-Feeding.—Although suckling stimulates PRL secretion in normal women for the first few weeks to months post partum,[8] there are no data to suggest that breast-feeding can cause tumor growth. Thus, there seems to be no reason to discourage nursing in women with microadenomas. Women with macroadenomas can also be encouraged to nurse, but they should be followed closely for the unlikely possibility of tumor enlargement. Although there have been a number of case reports of women having seizures or strokes who were using bromocriptine to prevent postpartum lactation, the precise relationship of these complications to the use of bromocriptine remains unclear.[26]

Contraception.—Withholding bromocriptine and allowing a woman to remain anovulatory may be the most efficacious mode of contraception. However, such women are hypoestrogenemic and predisposed to osteoporosis,[27] so that this form of contraception is not recommended. The estrogens in oral contraceptives can increase PRL levels modestly in normal women[28] and estrogens clearly can stimulate normal lactotrophs (see above). Although oral contraceptives cannot be implicated in the pathogenesis of prolactinomas[29] it would seem prudent to avoid their use in women with known prolactinomas to avoid any possible stimulatory effect. Estrogen use has been implicated in the pathogenesis of a prolactinoma in a male-to-female transsexual.[30] Using oral contraceptives along with bromocriptine may prevent tumor stimulation and one short-term study indicates that this may be safe.[31] However, such women should be followed very carefully. Barrier means of contraception appear to be safest.

Acromegaly

Reports of pregnancies in acromegalic patients are uncommon,[23, 32–34] perhaps because of the fact that about 40% of such patients are hyperprolactinemic.[35] Indeed, correction of the hyperprolactinemia with bromocriptine may be necessary to permit ovulation and conception in these patients.[23, 34] The GH-secreting tumors of acromegaly usually arise de novo within the pituitary. Rarely, acromegaly may be due to a GH releasing hormone secreting tumor of pancreatic or carcinoid origin that produces pituitary somatotroph cell hyperplasia rather than true tumor formation.[35, 36]

The acral enlargement and other features of acromegaly are well known. Much of these effects are mediated by the GH-induced increase in the levels of somatomedin C (also known as insulin-like growth factor I or IGF-I).[35, 36] Untreated acromegaly carries a two-fold increased mortality risk, primarily from cardiovascular, cerebrovascular, and respiratory causes.[37, 38]

Standard treatment consists of transsphenoidal selective removal of the GH-secreting adenoma. True "cures" are less common than in patients with prolactinomas, ranging from 25% to 50% of various series, and depend upon the criteria of cure that are used.[35] Irradiation can cause a fall in GH to an acceptable range (<5 ng/mL[5 μg/L]) in 42% to 44% of patients by 5 years and in 60% by 10 years.[39] However, this is accompanied by a risk of hypopituitarism, loss of gonadotropin function occurring in about 50% of patients by 10 years following irradiation. Bromocriptine has also been used for the treatment of acromegaly[40] but it is not nearly as effective as it is for prolactinomas. Recently, a long-acting parenteral, somatostatin agonist, octreotide (Sandostatin), has been found to be quite effective in lowering GH levels and treating acromegaly in nonpreg-

nant subjects.[35] Medical therapy is usually given to patients not cured by surgery and who are awaiting the permanent effects of irradiation.

Effects of Pregnancy on Acromegaly.—In patients who have combined GH- and PRL-secreting tumors, the stimulatory effects of the hormonal milieu of pregnancy could, in theory, cause tumor enlargement; no such occurrences have been reported, however. Thus, patients with acromegaly should all have PRL levels ascertained before considering pregnancy and those with PRL elevations should be treated as prolactinoma patients with respect to the potential hazard of tumor growth (see above).

Effects of Acromegaly and Treatment on Pregnancy.—Certain complications of acromegaly could have potentially harmful effects on the mother and fetus. Carbohydrate intolerance has been found in up to 50% and overt diabetes in 10% to 20% of patients with acromegaly.[35] The GH-induced insulin resistance could potentially be additive to that of pregnancy, leading to an increased risk of gestational diabetes.

Hypertension is present in 25% to 35% of patients and salt retention also occurs. Cardiac disease is also present in about one third of patients and there may be a specific cardiomyopathy associated with acromegaly. Coronary artery disease may also be increased.[35]

As noted above for prolactinomas, bromocriptine is well tolerated by mother and fetus. The same considerations should be used when this drug is used for patients with acromegaly as discussed above for patients with prolactinomas. Through 1989, there were no data documenting the safety of octreotide during pregnancy (Louis Boyaji, Ph.D., Sandoz Pharmaceuticals Corp., personal communication) and it should not be used during pregnancy.

Management.—The complications of acromegaly and decreased pituitary function should be assessed prior to pregnancy. In those patients with PRL oversecretion, caution is needed regarding pregnancy-induced tumor enlargement, as for prolactinomas (see above).

Cushing's Disease

Adrenocorticotropic hormone (ACTH)–secreting pituitary tumors are discussed below in the section on adrenal disease. The issues regarding the mass effects of such tumors are similar to those for all pituitary tumors discussed above.

Thyrotropin-Secreting Tumors

Thyrotropin-secreting tumors can occur because of longstanding primary hypothyroidism with resultant thyrotroph hyperplasia and eventual tumor formation. Clinically, such patients present with primary hypothyroidism. Thyrotropin-secreting tumors may also present de novo, causing hyperthyroidism.[41] We are unaware of any case reports of pregnancies occurring in patients with thyrotropin-secreting tumors. The issues regarding the mass effects of such tumors are similar to those for all pituitary tumors. It would not be expected that pregnancy would have any influence on tumor size. The specific problems regarding hypo- and hyperthyroidism are discussed below in the section on thyroid disease.

Gonadotroph Cell Tumors

These tumors secrete intact gonadotropins and/or their subunits and are more common in men.[42] Characteristically, follicle-stimulating hormone (FSH) levels are higher than are luteinizing hormone (LH) levels. The tumors usually are quite large and generally present because of mass effects. We are also unaware of any reports of pregnancies occurring in patients with gonadotroph cell tumors. The issues regarding the mass effects of such tumors are similar to those for all pituitary tumors. It would not be expected that pregnancy would have any influence on tumor size.

Nonsecreting Tumors

These tumors appear to be functionless,

although some produce glycoprotein subunits and other peptides of unknown clinical significance.[43] The tumors usually are quite large and generally present because of mass effects. The issues regarding the mass effects of such tumors are similar to those for all pituitary tumors. It would not be expected that pregnancy would have any influence on tumor size.

Hypopituitarism

Chronic Hypopituitarism

Hypopituitarism can occur from a variety of causes, including tumors, trauma, infiltrative disease, and vascular disease. The most common form of trauma is prior neurosurgery. Hormone deficits can be partial or complete and loss of gonadotropin secretion is common. Therefore, induction of ovulation may be difficult and is usually done by an experienced reproductive endocrinologist. Thus pregnancy will be planned.

In adult women the only hormone replacement to be considered are thyroid hormones and adrenal hormones, which are discussed below in the sections on hypothyroidism and adrenal insufficiency.

In patients with congenital short stature of varying etiologies, there may be difficulties with the pregnancy, labor, and delivery simply from cephalopelvic disproportion. Early cesarean section may be necessary because of a reduced cardiopulmonary state associated with the expanding uterine size.[44] There is a high incidence of fetal wastage unassociated with obstetric problems, possibly related to the basic genetic defects.[44]

Sheehan's Syndrome

Sheehan's syndrome refers to the development of pituitary necrosis within a few hours of delivery.[45] The degree of necrosis dictates the subsequent course of the patient. Although it is commonly thought that patients with this syndrome usually present months to years later with a history of failure of postpartum lactation, failure to resume menses, fatigue, and cold intolerance, it should be rec-

TABLE 4–4.
Symptoms and Signs of Sheehan's Syndrome

Acute Form	Chronic Form
Hypotension	Lightheadedness
Tachycardia	Fatigue
Failure to lactate	Failure to lactate
Hypoglycemia	Persistent amenorrhea
Failure to regrow shaved pubic hair	Decreased body hair
	Dry skin
Extreme fatigue	Loss of libido
Nausea and vomiting	Nausea and vomiting
	Cold intolerance

ognized that there is a much more acute, potentially lethal form, as 25% of women dying within 30 days of delivery have evidence of pituitary infarction. In this acute form, usually less than 10% of normal pituitary tissue remains.[46]

The pathogenesis of Sheehan's syndrome is still not fully understood. In almost all cases there is antecedent hypotension and usually shock, most commonly due to obstetric hemorrhage. In a series of 332 autopsies of patients who died within 35 days of delivery, there was a 38% chance that a massive or large pituitary necrosis would be found following serious postpartum hemorrhage or retained placenta with shock.[47] The primary event causing the necrosis is pituitary ischemia. Sheehan's opinion is that the ischemia is caused by occlusive spasm of the arteries that supply the anterior lobe directly and of those that supply the stalk and thus provide the source of the hypothalamic-pituitary portal circulation.[47] The size of the necrosis depends on the severity, duration, and distribution of the spasm.[47] No other theories have come forth to dispute Sheehan's hypothesis that the primary lesion is occlusive vascular spasm, although the roles of estrogen and pregnancy-induced pituitary enlargement have also been implicated.[48] Pituitary necrosis may also occur in patients with diabetes mellitus,[49] but whether there is an increased frequency of postpartum necrosis in women with diabetes is not known.

Acute Form.—In the acute form of Sheehan's syndrome, patients may present with persistent hypotension, tachycardia, failure to lactate, and hypoglycemia (Table 4–4). Although such patients were described by Sheehan,[46] there have been few cases described with modern methods of hormone testing and treatment; Lakhdar et al.[50] described two cases with symptomatic hypopituitarism in whom testing performed 3 to 4 weeks post partum confirmed the diagnosis and they stressed the potentially lethal nature of this disorder.

Diagnosis.—Diagnosis and treatment should be done on an emergency basis in all patients with obstetric hemorrhage and a prolonged course of hypotension not responsive to appropriate blood product replacement (Table 4–5). Blood should be obtained for ACTH, cortisol, thyroxine (T_4), triiodothy-

TABLE 4–5.
Hormonal Evaluation and Treatment of Sheehan's Syndrome*

Evaluation
Hormone	
ACTH	Measure basal cortisol and ACTH levels
	Insulin tolerance test (0.1–0.15 unit/kg of regular insulin IV), with assessment of cortisol and ACTH at 0, 30, 60, 90, 120 min
TSH	Measure basal TSH, T_4, T_3RU levels
PRL	Measure basal PRL levels
LH/FSH	Measure basal LH, FSH, and estradiol levels
GH	Measure GH levels during insulin tolerance test

Treatment
1. Give normal saline with 5%–10% dextrose for volume expansion after blood loss corrected
2. Give equivalent of 100 mg of hydrocortisone IV as a bolus followed by additional 100 mg q8h for first 24 hr and then taper
3. Replace thyroid hormone and estrogens after evaluation demonstrates need
4. Observe for the development of polyuria after glucocorticoid replacement; if polyuria develops, test for the presence of diabetes insipidus (see Table 4–6)

*ACTH = adrenocorticotropic hormone; TSH = thyroid-stimulating hormone; T_4 = thyroxine; T_3RU = triiodothyronine resin uptake; PRL = prolactin; LH = luteinizing hormone; FSH = follicle-stimulating hormone; GH = growth hormone.

ronine (T_3), PRL, and GH basally. ACTH and cortisol levels should both be low basally but an ACTH (cosyntropin, Cortrosyn) stimulation test will be normal, as the adrenal glands have not yet atrophied. Stimulation with metyrapone is dangerous, as it may precipitate a worsened adrenal crisis by eliminating any adrenal reserve left. Thyroxine levels may not yet be decreased because of the 7-day half-life of T_4; T_3 levels will likely be low but that may also be due to the euthyroid sick syndrome (see below). PRL levels, normally five- to tenfold elevated in the puerperium, and GH levels will likely be quite low.

Treatment.—Treatment should be begun after blood is obtained for these tests but before the return of results. Initial treatment is with the equivalent of 100 mg of hydrocortisone intravenously (IV) as a bolus followed by an additional 200 mg within the first 24 hours (see below under Adrenal Insufficiency for additional details and further management). Saline with 5% to 10% dextrose is used for volume expansion after blood loss has been corrected. Once the patient has recovered, additional testing can be done to assess the need for other hormone replacement, as in the patient who presents with the more usual, chronic form of Sheehan's syndrome. Such testing often will include measuring the ACTH, cortisol, and GH responses to insulin-induced hypoglycemia.

Chronic Form.—Patients with the chronic form have lesser degrees of pituitary infarction[46] and present from weeks to years following delivery. The degree of hormone deficiency determines the clinical presentation (see Table 4–4). In these chronic cases, amenorrhea and loss of libido are common but many women cycle normally and subsequent spontaneous pregnancies have been reported.[50, 51] Cold intolerance, dry skin, and other symptoms may occur that are compatible with hypothyroidism. There is frequently a history of failure to lactate postpartum and some breast atrophy. Fatigue, loss of axillary and pubic

hair, nausea, vomiting, abdominal pain, and diarrhea may suggest adrenal insufficiency. In formal testing, blood glucose levels usually fail to return to normal during an insulin tolerance test and basal and peak cortisol, ACTH, PRL, and GH levels are usually low.[52–54] Basal T_4 levels are usually low and the thyroid-stimulating hormone (TSH) response to TSH releasing hormone (TRH) is usually low.[52–54] The LH and FSH responses to gonadotropin releasing hormone (GnRH) usually are also low.[52–54] Because of the nonspecificity of TRH and GnRH stimulation tests,[48] the only tests that are needed are measurements of the cortisol and ACTH responses to hypoglycemia, and basal PRL, T_4, TSH, LH, FSH, and estradiol levels. GH assessment is not necessary in adults but, if done, should only be done after estrogen replacement.

Three studies have also looked at posterior pituitary function in patients with chronic Sheehan's syndrome. In one series of 20 patients, 8 had remembered transient polyuria and polydipsia following their episodes of shock, only to have these symptoms recur later after replacement therapy with cortisol and T_4.[54] All 20 patients demonstrated decreased responses of urine vasopressin levels and urine concentrating abilities after osmolar loads, even after cortisol and T_4 replacement[54]; none were significantly symptomatic. However, Jialal et al.[53] observed that 3 of 16 patients with Sheehan's syndrome had partial diabetes insipidus as documented by dehydration testing. Two of these patients complained of nocturia but only one was truly symptomatic with polyuria and polydipsia. In the third series,[55] 4 of 12 women had had a history of transient polyuria post partum, but were asymptomatic at the time of testing. All 12 had normal serum osmolalities when studied, but their plasma vasopressin levels were lower than normal basally and in response to hypertonic saline. The diabetes insipidus appears to be due to vascular occlusion with resultant atrophy and scarring of the neurohypophysis[56] and lesions in the supraventricular and paraventricular nuclei.[57] Thus, overnight dehydration testing[58] should also be performed in patients with Sheehan's syndrome.

Lymphocytic Hypophysitis

Lymphocytic hypophysitis is characterized by massive infiltration of the pituitary by lymphocytes and plasma cells with destruction of the normal parenchyma. The disorder is thought to have an autoimmune basis. Most cases occur in association with pregnancy and women present during pregnancy or post partum either with symptoms of varying degrees of hypopituitarism or symptoms related to the mass lesion, such as headaches or visual field defects. Mild hyperprolactinemia and diabetes insipidus may also be found. On CT or MRI scan a sellar mass is found which may extend in an extrasellar fashion and may cause visual field defects. The condition is usually confused with that of a pituitary tumor and, in fact, cannot be distinguished from a tumor except by biopsy. By virtue of the hypopituitarism it produces, lymphocytic hypophysitis can also be confused clinically with Sheehan's syndrome except that there is no history of obstetric hemorrhage.[59–63]

The diagnosis of lymphocytic hypophysitis should be entertained in women with symptoms of hypopituitarism and/or mass lesions of the sella during pregnancy or post partum, especially in the absence of a history of obstetric hemorrhage. An evaluation of pituitary function is warranted as well as a CT or MRI scan. If PRL levels are only modestly elevated (<150 ng/mL [<150 μg/L]) in the presence of a large mass, the diagnosis is unlikely to be an enlarging prolactinoma and more likely to be hypophysitis or a nonsecreting tumor. Hormone replacement therapy should be instituted promptly when hypopituitarism is determined to be present. Unless there are visual field defects, uncontrollable headaches, or radiologic evidence of progressive enlargement of the sellar mass, rapid surgical intervention is not warranted, as some women may undergo a spontaneous regression of the mass[64, 65] and return of pituitary function.[62]

Diabetes Insipidus

Normal Regulation of Water Balance

Water balance is controlled by a combination of the regulated secretion of vasopressin and thirst. Vasopressin acts on the distal tubule to alter permeability, permitting water reabsorption without solute reabsorption. Tenfold higher concentrations of vasopressin in blood are necessary to activate the receptors on the vasculature that result in vasoconstriction and blood pressure elevation. Thus, under normal physiologic circumstances, vasopressin does not play a significant role in blood pressure regulation. In the event of severe blood volume loss, such as hemorrhage, however, levels of vasopressin are achieved that can raise blood pressure.

The primary regulator of vasopressin secretion is the osmolality of the plasma, sensed by the osmoreceptors. As plasma osmolality rises, vasopressin is secreted in direct proportion, as little as a 1% change in osmolality resulting in a significant change in vasopressin levels. This increase in vasopressin results in increased water permeability of the distal tubule and increased water reabsorption with a more concentrated urine. The osmotic threshold for vasopressin release in nonpregnant subjects is a plasma tonicity of about 280 to 285 mOsm/kg with a normal range of 275 to 290 mOsm/kg. Thirst is generally stimulated at a plasma osmolality level several milliosmoles per kilogram above that for vasopressin release, a level near where maximum concentration of urine will already have been achieved. The intensity of the thirst sensation increases with increasing plasma osmolality. Although in the normal individual thirst is rarely activated by plasma osmolality, its importance cannot be denied. Managing patients with diabetes insipidus (see below) is not terribly difficult as long as thirst mechanisms are intact; management of the unconscious patient with diabetes insipidus is exceedingly difficult, however.[66]

Alterations in Water Balance During Pregnancy

In pregnancy there is a lowering of the

"osmostat," the set-point for serum osmolality, by about 10 mOsm/kg (see Chap. 2, p. 45). The decline in plasma osmolality begins by the time of the first missed menstrual period and gradually increases until the 10th week of gestation, after which there is little further change.[67] Pregnant women experience thirst and release vasopressin at lower levels of serum osmolality than do nonpregnant individuals to maintain this lower osmolality. A water load will suppress vasopressin secretion appropriately, resulting in dilute urine and excretion of this water load, thereby maintaining this lower osmolality.[68] This reset osmostat results in a lowering of the serum sodium by about 4 to 5 mEq/mL.[67] When a patient presents with polyuria and polydipsia, the finding of lower-than-expected serum sodium levels should not, therefore, exclude the diagnosis of diabetes insipidus.[69] Testing in a pregnant woman should be performed in the sitting position, as the lateral recumbent position results in an inhibition of maximal urinary concentrating ability (Table 4–6).[67] (See also Chap. 2, p. 45.)

Alterations in Vasopressin Metabolism During Pregnancy

The placenta produces vasopressinase, an enzyme that inactivates vasopressin rapidly. Vasopressinase levels increase 1000-fold between the 4th and 38th weeks of gestation. How much this increase in vasopressinase activity contributes to the threefold increased clearance of endogenous vasopressin during pregnancy is not clear, however.[68, 69] This increased metabolism of vasopressin makes determination of plasma vasopressin levels very difficult during pregnancy when performing diagnostic evaluations.[68, 69]

Management of Chronic Diabetes Insipidus During Pregnancy

Diabetes insipidus (DI) may be divided etiologically into central and nephrogenic causes. In the former, there is loss of vasopressin secretion and in the latter there is failure of vasopressin to act normally to effect urinary concentration.

TABLE 4–6.
Protocol for Assessing Diabetes Insipidus (DI) in Pregnancy*

Procedure
1. Weigh patient at beginning of test (usually 9–10 P.M. if mild polyuria or 7 A.M. if severe polyuria.
2. Complete fluid deprivation overnight or until 3% of body weight is lost.
3. Measure urine specific gravities hourly beginning at 6 A.M. or when 3% of body weight is lost (save urine specimens for osmolality measurements). During the period of these collections, women should be sitting and not lying down.
4. When specific gravities are constant for two or preferably three consecutive specimens, obtain plasma for osmolality measurement.
5. After plasma and last urine specimens are obtained, administer 5 µg of desmopressin IV.
6. Measure hourly urine specific gravities (and later osmolalities) for next 3 hr.

Interpretation
1. At end of dehydration period in normal pregnant women, plasma osmolality averages 278 ±3 mOsm/kg and urinary osmolality averages 835 ±144 mOsm/kg.
2. Only patients with central DI will have a rise in urinary osmolality >9% in response to vasopressin.
3. Patients with nephrogenic DI may have a significant rise in urinary osmolality, but this is usually small and not to a level greater than plasma osmolality.
4. If patients respond to the desmopressin in this test, the test can be repeated using aqueous vasopressin to determine the role of vasopressinase in causing the DI to become manifest.

*Modified from Miller M, Dalakos T, Moses AM, et al: *Ann Intern Med* 1970; 73: 721–729; and Davison JM, Vallotton MB, Lindheimer MD: *Br J Obstet Gynaecol* 1981; 88: 472–479.

Central DI may be due to tumors, such as pituitary adenomas with suprasellar extension; hypothalamic tumors or metastases to the hypothalamus; infiltrative disease, such as histiocytosis X or sarcoidosis; trauma, such as neurosurgery or automobile accidents; or it may be idiopathic.[70] In the majority of such cases there is a worsening of the DI during pregnancy,[69, 71] likely due to the increased clearance of vasopressin by the increased levels of vasopressinase. Thus, mild cases treated with either increased fluids or chlorpropamide will likely experience considerable worsening. Chlorpropamide should always be stopped when pregnancy is contemplated or discovered, to avoid hypoglycemia in the fetus, because it readily crosses the placenta. Rarely, asymptomatic women will experience symptomatic DI only during pregnancy.[72] Women being treated with vasopressin tannate (Pitressin Tannate) in oil or with lysine vasopressin spray may also experience such worsening. The vasopressin analogue DDAVP (desmopressin acetate) is not affected by vasopressinase and a number of women have been treated quite satisfactorily with this medication.[69] In one case, however, desmopressin requirements increased threefold during the course of the pregnancy.[73] There is minimal if any transference of desmopressin into breast milk[74] and its use is not a contraindication to breast-feeding.[69]

In patients with idiopathic DI, oxytocin levels have been reported to be normal and labor has had spontaneous onset and proceeded smoothly.[75, 76] Although in some cases labor has not progressed normally and uterine atony has been noted,[74, 77, 78] such cases have not been documented with oxytocin levels. In patients with tumor, trauma, or infiltrative disease as causes of their DI, it is possible that the oxytocinergic pathways could also be affected. In such patients, it would be reasonable to be alert for the possibility of oxytocin deficiency with resultant poor progress of labor and uterine atony.

Congenital nephrogenic DI is a rare disorder that predominantly affects males. As in the nonpregnant state, treatment is with thiazide diuretics.[69]

Development of New Diabetes Insipidus During Pregnancy

Diabetes insipidus may develop during pregnancy for a number of reasons. Partial DI may actually predate the pregnancy but not be symptomatic.[72] Only when the clearance of vasopressin is increased does it become manifest clinically. Patients who have had transient DI related to neurosurgery or other forms of trauma and who are asymptomatic carriers in families with hereditary DI are at particular risk and should be followed

closely for the development of DI during pregnancy.

Transient vasopressin-resistant forms of DI occurring sporadically during one pregnancy but not recurring in another have been reported.[69, 79] Some of these cases respond to desmopressin and some do not.[69, 80] All become asymptomatic by several weeks following delivery.[69, 79, 80] Regardless of the cause, vasopressinase may be playing a substantial role in these cases and the prompt use of desmopressin is indicated.

As discussed above, DI that develops initially post partum is probably due to Sheehan's syndrome, especially if there is a history of obstetric hemorrhage. Occasionally the DI only becomes manifest after glucocorticoid replacement,[69] owing to the requirement of the distal tubule for glucocorticoids for the generation of free water.

THYROID

Changes in Normal Thyroid Physiology During Pregnancy

A number of changes occur in the thyroid and the measurement of thyroid hormones during pregnancy. The renal clearance of iodine is increased because of the increased glomerular filtration rate that occurs with pregnancy. When iodine intake is marginal, this increased loss results in iodine deficiency.[81] The iodine in iodized salt and prenatal vitamins usually prevents iodine deficiency. Excessive iodine ingestion is to be avoided, because it crosses the placenta and may cause neonatal goiter (see below).

It is widely believed that a goiter commonly develops during pregnancy. This belief stems from noncontrolled early observations and other studies, such as one in Scotland in which goiters were found in 70% of 184 pregnant women but in only 37% of nonpregnant controls.[82] It appears, however, that most such studies were done in iodine-deficient regions. In iodine-replete regions, there is no increase in the frequency of goiters during pregnancy.[83–85] Of 309 pregnant adolescents evaluated by Long et al.,[85] 2 had Graves' disease and were hyperthyroid, 3 had Hashimoto's thyroiditis, 1 being hyperthyroid, and 4 had subacute thyroiditis, 1 being hyperthyroid. The other 9 with goiters were thought to have simple nontoxic goiters. The presence of a goiter in iodine-replete areas, therefore, indicates significant disease in about 50% of patients and should always be evaluated.

The fetal thyroid and the fetal hypothalamic-pituitary-thyroid axis develop independently of maternal thyroid status. At 11 to 12 weeks of gestation, the fetal thyroid begins to concentrate iodine. The placenta is freely permeable to iodine and to medications used to treat hyperthyroidism, such as propylthiouracil (PTU), methimazole, and propranolol; T_3 and TSH cross the placenta only minimally.[86] Thyroxine crosses the placenta in somewhat larger amounts and, late in gestation, is able to ameliorate the effects of hypothyroidism in infants with congenital hypothyroidism due to enzyme defects or agenesis of the thyroid.[87]

Bioassayable thyroid-stimulating activity in serum is increased in the midtrimester, possibly due to intrinsic thyroid-stimulating activity of human chorionic gonadotropin (hCG).[88] There is also a human chorionic thyrotropin made by the placenta but it actually has little thyroid-stimulating activity and probably plays no physiologic role.[88]

Alteration of Thyroid Function Tests During Pregnancy

Basal Metabolic Rate

The basal metabolic rate (BMR) is increased by about 20% to 25% during pregnancy, attributable to the contribution of the placenta and fetus.[89] This test is rarely done at present.

Thyroid Hormone Levels

Thyroxine is the major thyroid hormone in the circulation and is about 85% bound to thyroxine-binding globulin (TBG) and about 15% bound to thyroxine-binding prealbumin, less than 1% being unbound or "free." The increased estrogens of the placenta stimulate increased production of TBG, resulting in an increase in bound T_4 measurements, beginning by 4 to 6 weeks of gestation (Fig 4–2).[88] The amount of binding of hormone to TBG may be estimated using the resin uptake, which decreases as TBG increases. The metabolic activity of the hormones correlates best with the free hormone levels. Free T_4 levels may be estimated indirectly using the resin uptake to compensate for the increase in TBG and the total T_4 levels (frequently referred to as the *free T_4 index*) or they may be measured directly by equilibrium dialysis. The latter is more accurate but more difficult to perform. When there is any question, the free T_4 measurements by dialysis should be performed. Free T_4 levels are usually normal during pregnancy, although they may be minimally elevated over nonpregnant levels while still in the normal range.[88] Harada et al[88] have postulated that these slightly elevated free T_4 levels may be due to the stimulating activity of the high levels of hCG. T_4 turnover is normal despite the elevated total T_4 levels and in the

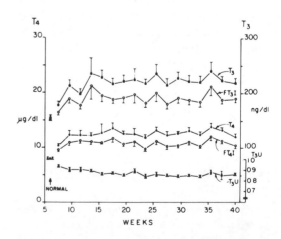

FIG 4–2.
Serum thyroxine (T_4), serum triiodothyronine (T_3), T_3 uptake (T_3U), free T_4 index (FT_4I), and free T_3 index (FT_3I) at various weeks of pregnancy ($\pm$ SE). *Left,* nonpregnant control values. Serum T_4, T_3, FT_4I, and FT_3I were significantly elevated and T_3U was reduced throughout pregnancy. (From Harada A, Hershman JM, Reed AW, et al: *J Clin Endocrinol Metab* 1979; 48:793–797. Used by permission.)

patient receiving T_4 replacement there is no need to increase the dose during pregnancy.[90] T_3 is bound to TBG with somewhat less affinity than is T_4 but the same increase in total T_3 measurements is seen as with T_4 during pregnancy.[88] TSH levels are minimally decreased during pregnancy, possibly due to the increased free T_4 levels.[88]

Hyperthryodism

Etiology

Hyperthyroidism occurs in about 2 of every 1,000 pregnancies.[91] About 95% of such cases of hyperthyroidism are due to Graves' disease, an autoimmune disorder associated with circulating thyroid stimulating immunoglobulins. Often, preexisting Graves' disease ameliorates during pregnancy, as do other autoimmune disorders, perhaps due to the alterations in immune mechanisms that occur with pregnancy.[92] The clinical improvement in such patients usually occurs in the second half of pregnancy and parallels a fall in the titer of the stimulatory immunoglobulins.[92] On the other hand, Graves' disease sometimes presents during pregnancy and Graves' disease that had been in remission may relapse during pregnancy.[91] Other causes of hyperthyroidism include toxic solitary nodules, toxic multinodular goiter, Hashimoto's thyroiditis, and trophoblastic disease.

Diagnosis

Because of the hyperdynamic state of pregnancy, the clinical diagnosis of hyperthyroidism may prove difficult. The features of tachycardia, warm skin, systolic flow murmurs, and heat intolerance, are common to both. Even the finding of a goiter may not be specific. Weight loss, a marked tachycardia, eye signs, and a bruit over the thyroid are more suggestive of hyperthyroidism.[91] Infiltrative dermopathy or ophthalmopathy are specific for Graves' disease but do not indicate the degree of hyperthyroidism.

Confirmation of the diagnosis is made by measuring free T_4 and T_3 levels in blood. Early in the disease and especially in patients with toxic solitary nodules, T_3 only may be elevated ("T_3 toxicosis"). Because of the elevation of TBG in blood (see above) it is common for total T_4 and T_3 to be elevated and free hormone levels must be assessed. If the free T_4 index that has been calculated by the laboratory from the total T_4 and the resin uptake is not elevated despite a strong clinical suspicion, then a free T_4 done by dialysis should be performed. TSH levels are suppressed to below the level of sensitivity of the assay with older assays and below normal with the newer, ultrasensitive assays.

Scanning or uptakes with radioactive tracers such as iodine 131 or technetium 99 should be avoided to prevent exposure to the developing fetus. The fetal thyroid is 20 to 50 times more avid for iodine than the maternal thyroid.[92] However, the tracer dose used in these studies is so small that it is not sufficient to cause concern[93] and does not justify a therapeutic abortion in the event of inadvertent administration to someone not known to be pregnant (See also Chap. 18).

Effect of Hyperthyroidism on Pregnancy

Untreated hyperthyroidism clearly has an adverse consequence on fetal outcome. Among 19 cases of untreated hyperthyroidism reported by Montoro and Mestman,[94] there were 15 premature deliveries, 5 perinatal deaths, and 5 cases of serious neonatal morbidity. Maternal weight loss may be particularly deleterious as it is more likely to lead to a small-for-gestational-age baby.[91] Given these concerns, virtually all cases should be treated during pregnancy.

Management of Hyperthryoidism During Pregnancy

Medical Therapy.—Medical therapy is the treatment of choice for hyperthyroidism during pregnancy (Table 4–7). The thionamide derivatives, propylthiouracil (PTU) and methimazole, are equally efficacious, although PTU has the theoretical advantage in that it partially inhibits the conversion of T_4 to T_3. The primary mode of action of these

TABLE 4–7.
Drugs Useful in the Treatment of Hyperthyroidism*

Name	Mode of Action	Usual Dose	Side Effects	Indication	Precautions with Pregnancy (FDA Risk Category)†
Propylthiouracil	Inhibition of thyroid hormone synthesis	50–150 mg q8h po	Rash, fever, agranulocytosis, sore throat	All hyperthyroidism	Crosses placenta Use lowest dose (D)‡
Methimazole	Inhibition of thyroid hormone synthesis	5–20 mg q8h po	Rash, fever, agranulocytosis, sore throat	All hyperthyroidism	Crosses placenta Use lowest dose (D)‡
Propranolol	Decreases adrenergic signs & symptoms	10–80 mg q6–8h po 1–10 mg q6–8h IV	Bronchospasm, CHF	Symptomatic relief of adrenergic symptoms Thyroid storm	Crosses placenta ?Neonatal bradycardia, hypoglycemia, growth retardation (C)
Iodide SSKI NaI	Inhibits thyroid hormone release	1–2 drops q8h po 1 g q8h IV	Rash, sialadenitis, conjunctivitis	Thyroid storm, preparation for thyroidectomy	Crosses placenta Goiter, hypothyroidism (D)
Glucocorticoids	Inhibit thyroid hormone release	2 mg q6h × 4	None	Thyroid storm	Cross placenta (B)
Reserpine	Decreases adrenergic signs & symptoms by depleting catecholamines; sedation	1–5 mg q4–6h IM	Sedation, postural hypotension	Thyroid storm	Crosses placenta Neonatal nasal congestion and respiratory secretions; cyanosis; anorexia (D)
Guanethidine	Decreases adrenergic signs & symptoms	1 mg/kg/day q12h po	Postural hypotension, diarrhea	Thyroid storm	Unknown (C)
Diltiazem	Decreases adrenergic signs & symptoms; calcium channel blocker	30–60 mg q6h po	AV block, bradycardia, edema, headache, rash	Symptomatic relief of adrenergic symptoms ?Thyroid storm	Crosses placenta High concentrations in breast milk—nursing contraindicated (C)
Phenobarbital	Sedation, increases T$_4$ catabolism	30–60 mg q6–8h po	Sedation	Thyroid storm	Crosses placenta May cause dependence, decreased clotting factors, respiratory depression (D)

*SS = saturated solution; CHF = congestive heart failure; AV = atrioventricular
†See Preface for description of FDA Risk Classification.
‡Although these agents are class D, the risks of untreated hyperthyroidism to mother and fetus warrant their use during pregnancy.

drugs is to inhibit thyroid hormone synthesis by blocking the incorporation of iodine into tyrosine and the coupling of the iodotyrosines.[95] As a result of this block in synthesis, stored hormone gradually leaks out over several weeks and hormone levels return to normal over 4 to 8 weeks. The most severe side effect is agranulocytosis, which occurs in approximately 0.2% of patients and is more common with higher doses and in elderly patients.[96] Patients should be warned that if a fever or sore throat develops, they should cease taking the drug immediately and telephone their physician so that a white blood cell count (WBC) with differential can be done. Obviously, most occurrences of a sore throat and fever will be due to a viral infection, but in all cases a WBC should be checked immediately. A WBC with differential should also be done before starting these drugs to serve as a baseline, as the WBC tends to be a little low in hyperthyroidism per se.[95] However, routine WBCs are unnecessary, as the agranulocytosis may develop at any time in the first few weeks of therapy with no warning. A transient, benign leukopenia (WBC <4,000/mm³ [4 10⁹/L]) may occur in up to 12% of treated adults.[95] Other uncommon side effects include rash, cholestatic jaundice, hepatitis, arthralgias, vasculitis, nausea, and pruritus.[94] Although there has been some suggestion that infants exposed to methimazole may have an increased chance of developing a congenital scalp lesion known as aplasia cutis,[97, 98] further analyses of large numbers of offspring have failed to support this suggestion.[99, 100] Thus there is no clear benefit of preferring one antithyroid drug to the other.

The usual starting dose of PTU is 300 to 450 mg/day and of methimazole is 30 to 45 mg/day; both are given in divided doses every 8 hours. After the first 4 to 6 weeks of therapy, the dose can often be lowered considerably.[95] The dose of PTU or methimazole should be the lowest that will maintain thyroid hormone levels in the upper normal to minimally elevated range.[101] These drugs cross the placenta and these lower doses will prevent unnecessary fetal exposure. Even doses of PTU as low

as 100 to 200 mg/day may cause mild, transient fetal hypothyroidism.[102] An earlier practice of using higher doses of antithyroid drugs plus supplementing with thyroid hormone has been abandoned, as it is now known that thyroid hormones cross the placenta in only small quantities and such combined therapy will yield a euthyroid mother at the expense of a hypothyroid infant. A neonatal goiter may sometimes be apparent at delivery but this is not clearly related to the dose of PTU or methimazole. In fact, some women who have required very high doses of antithyroid drugs do not end up with children with goiters. These goiters usually reflect fetal hypothyroidism[95] and hormone levels in these infants must be checked immediately. The goiters that occur are modest in size and do not interfere with respiration. Goiters due to inadvertent iodide administration may be quite large and may interfere with respiration (see below). Long-term follow-up of children exposed in utero to PTU has shown no ill effects with respect to physical or intellectual development.[103]

β-Adrenergic receptor blocking drugs may be useful in the patient with severe hyperthyroidism and those with marked tachycardia (rates >120/min) or tachyarrhythmias. β-Blockers also cross the placenta. Some early reports suggested that such use was associated with neonatal bradycardia and hypoglycemia[104, 105] but other reports noted no ill effects.[106, 107] In an extensive review of the literature on the use of β-blockers for all indications during pregnancy, Rubin[108] concluded that these medications were relatively safe. More recently, Fox et al.[109] noted cardiorespiratory depression, hypoglycemia, and growth retardation in the infant of a mother who had taken naldolol, which is less protein-bound than propranolol, perhaps giving higher fetal levels. Unlike the thionamides, β-blockers do not reduce the increased BMR and protein catabolism that occur during hyperthyroidism. Therefore, they should not be used as the sole medical therapy for hyperthyroidism and, in fact, patients have gone into thyroid storm during labor when their sole therapy has been β-blockade.[110] I reserve propranolol for those patients who are severely symptomatic or who have tachyarrhythmias or for patients who are in thyroid storm (see below). When such drugs are used near term, the infants should be checked for hypoglycemia and bradycardia. Usually the outcome is quite good for such infants.[108] (See also Chap. 1, p. 28.)

Iodides cross the placenta quite readily and can cause fetal hypothyroidism and large goiters.[111] They should be used only for a short time to aid in the preparation of patients for surgery or for the rare case of thyroid storm.

Although lithium carbonate (FDA Class D) has been used to decrease thyroid hormone release in nonpregnant women with hyperthyroidism, it is teratogenic when given in the first trimester and may cause neonatal lithium intoxication and goiters when given near term.[112] In general, its use is best avoided during pregnancy, even during thyroid storm, unless toxic reactions to the many other antithyroid drugs preclude their use.

Surgery.—Surgery is generally an effective means of treating hyperthyroidism.[113] Patients should be prepared medically prior to surgery to prevent thyroid storm (see below). Standard doses of thionamides should be used to effect euthyroidism over a period of 4 to 6 weeks and propranolol, 40 to 80 mg/day, and iodides (one or two drops per day of a saturated solution of potassium iodide) should be given for 7 to 14 days to decrease gland vascularity.

Radioactive Iodine.—Radioactive iodine can cross the placenta and permanently ablate the gland of the fetus as well as that of the mother. Therapeutic doses of radioactive iodine are, therefore, *absolutely contraindicated* during pregnancy. A pregnancy test should be performed before such treatment in all women at risk for being pregnant.

Choice of Therapy.—Surgery of all types in which anesthesia is given is associated with an increase in the spontaneous abortion rate. This rate increased about 1.5-fold, from 5.1% to 8.0%, with surgery in the first trimester and 5.0-fold, from 1.4% to 6.9%, with surgery in the second trimester.[114] Thyroid surgery, in general, carries with it a 1% to 2% risk of permanent damage to the recurrent laryngeal nerve and a 1% to 2% risk of permanent hypoparathyroidism. Few series have compared the outcomes of medical vs. surgical treatment for hyperthyroidism during pregnancy and the results from any one center are for small numbers of patients.[113, 115] In a retrospective review of the literature, Pekonen and Lamberg[116] found that of 318 women treated with antithyroid drugs during pregnancy, 80% had normal term deliveries, 6% had premature deliveries, 10% aborted, and 4% had perinatal infant deaths. Of 288 women undergoing thyroidectomy, 91% had normal term deliveries, 1% had premature deliveries, 4% aborted, and 4% had perinatal infant deaths. Most of these operations were performed in the second trimester and prior first-trimester abortions were necessarily excluded. The authors' overall conclusion was that there was no apparent advantage to either form of therapy.

In nonpregnant patients, the general tendency in the United States has been to use radioactive iodine rather than surgery for the long term treatment of hyperthyroidism, primarily because of the increased morbidity and mortality of the latter. Surgery during pregnancy may pose an increased risk to the fetus. For all of these reasons, I favor medical therapy for hyperthyroidism during pregnancy, as have others.[86, 88, 90, 117, 118] Surgery is reserved for those patients who do not respond well to medication or who develop an intolerance for the medication (rash, allergy, agranulocytosis, etc.). Following delivery, the patient can continue on medication, be operated on, or receive radioactive iodine. Hyperthyroidism may be exacerbated in the days following delivery, possibly because the pregnancy has an ameliorating effect on the disease which then is lost.

Thyroid Storm

Thyroid storm is a medical emergency

TABLE 4–8.
Management of Thyroid Storm*

1. Clinical findings: fever, tachycardia, restlessness, stupor, vomiting, hypotension
2. Laboratory findings: elevated T_4, T_3, T_3RU, free T_4; suppressed TSH*
3. Drug therapy
   a. Propylthiouracil 600–800 mg po stat; then 150–200 mg po q4–6h (if NPO use methimazole rectal suppositories [see text])
   b. SSKI 2–5 drops q8h po or NaI 0.5–1.0 g IV g8h, STARTING 1–2 HR AFTER PROPYLTHIOURACIL
   c. Dexamethasone 2 mg q6h × 4 doses
   d. Propranolol 20–80 mg po or 1–10 mg IV q4h
      i. If severe bronchospasm, then:
         (a) Reserpine 1–5 mg IM q4–6h
         (b) Guanethidine 1 g/kg po q12h
         (c) Diltiazem 60 mg po q4–6h
   e. Phenobarbital 30–60 ng q6–8h prn
4. Supportive Therapy
   a. Fluids
   b. Calories
   c. Oxygen
   d. Vitamins: vitamin B complex, vitamin C, thiamine
   e. Antipyretics: salicylates, cooling blanket, iced gavage
   f. Digoxin, if necessary
5. Treat any underlying illness

*For abbreviations see footnote, Table 4–5.

and still carries an appreciable mortality for mother and fetus (Table 4–8). Most commonly, it is precipitated in an undiagnosed patient by stress, such as an infection, or in the case of the pregnant patient, by labor or caesarian section or other surgery.[117]

Fever is invariably present and is progressive. The fever of thyroid storm usually begins a few hours following surgery or delivery; fever starting 24 to 48 hours later is more likely due to other causes, such as atelectasis.[119] A tachycardia out of proportion to the fever is present; atrial fibrillation with a rapid ventricular response may also be present. Although the blood pressure is usually normal, showing an increased pulse pressure, shock may ensue with prolonged duration.[120] Mental status is frequently altered, ranging from extreme restlessness and nervousness to confusion, psychosis, seizures, and coma.[120, 121]

Severe diarrhea, nausea, vomiting, abdominal pain, and jaundice may also be present.[120, 121] If the patient has a large goiter, exophthalmos, or a known history of hyperthyroidism, the diagnosis of thyroid storm may not be difficult. However, in a patient without these obvious findings, it may be difficult to establish the diagnosis of thyroid storm on the basis of the above clinical manifestations. Unfortunately, the clinical assessment is the only tool available under these circumstances, as the necessity for speed in therapy precludes waiting for laboratory confirmation. Nonetheless, blood should be obtained for serum T_3, T_4, T_3 resin uptake, and free T_4 measurements before commencing therapy.[122]

Propylthiouracil should be given in high doses with an initial dose of 600 to 1,000 mg and subsequent doses of 150 to 200 mg every 6 hours orally or via nasogastric tube to block further synthesis of thyroid hormone. In the event that a postoperative ileus precludes the administration of a thionamide, it should be made into an absorbable rectal suppository form. Methimazole (1,200 mg) is dissolved in 12 mL of water to which is added a mixture of two drops of sorbitan monooleate (Span 80) in 52 mL of cocoa butter warmed to 37°C. The entire mixture is stirred to form a water-oil emulsion, poured into 2.6-mL suppository molds, and cooled.[123] Nabil et al.[123] have found that equivalent serum levels are achieved with the same dose of methimazole given orally or as a rectal suppository in this fashion.

One to 2 hours following the initial PTU dose, a saturated solution of potassium iodide (SSKI), two to five drops orally, or sodium iodide, 0.5 to 1.0 g IV every 8 hours, should be given to block thyroid hormone release.[124] Dexamethasone, 2 mg every 6 hours for four doses, should also be given to decrease hormone release and peripheral conversion of T_4 to T_3.[125] Although continuation of steroids has been recommended until the severe toxic state has resolved,[121] there are no data to document that this is efficacious. Finally, propranolol 20 to 80 mg orally every 4 to 6 hours or 1 to 10 mg IV over 5 to 10 minutes every 2 to 4 hours, should be administered to reduce adrenergic "overactivity."[126] In the event that β-blockers cannot be used because of bronchospasm, reserpine, 1 to 5 mg intramuscularly (IM) every 4 to 6 hours, or guanethidine, 1 mg/kg of body weight orally every 12 hours, can be given.[127, 128] Unlike propranolol, these agents have a delay of several hours before their effects are apparent clinically. Recently, diltiazem has been shown to have antiadrenergic effects similar to β-blockers in patients with hyperthyroidism.[129] Its use in thyroid storm has not been documented, however.

In addition to high-dose PTU, iodides, steroids, and β-blockers, these patients require considerable supportive care and should be managed in an intensive care unit with constant cardiac monitoring. Because of the excessive sweating and fever, insensible fluid losses are often great and careful fluid and electrolyte repletion is necessary. Glucose should be provided to meet immediate caloric needs, and if the patient is unable to eat for more than 24 hours, amino acid supplements should be employed to achieve nitrogen balance. Total parenteral nutrition should be considered because of the excessive caloric requirements of the hyperthyroid state. Thiamine, vitamin B complex, and vitamin C should be provided in liberal amounts since subclinical deficits may be present.[121] The body temperature should be reduced using a cooling blanket and iced saline gavage (if the patient can be fed thus). The use of salicylates is controversial. Larsen[130] has shown that salicylates result in a displacement of T_3 and T_4 from binding proteins, resulting in substantial increase in the free hormone concentration in blood. In addition, aspirin is also known to be calorigenic itself.[131] Although acetaminophen might therefore be theoretically the more desirable antipyretic, no untoward effects from the use of aspirin have been reported,[132] and either acetaminophen or aspirin would appear to be satisfactory in this regard. Sedation is often indicated for extreme restlessness. Barbiturates, owing to their effects in lowering thyroid hormones by increasing their catabolism, appear to be the drugs of choice.[133] Phenobarbital, 30 to 60 mg every 6 to 8 hours,

has been employed for this purpose. Short-term acute use of barbiturates should pose no harm to the fetus. When reserpine is used as the "antiadrenergic" agent, its sedating effect obviates the use of other agents. Oxygen should be administered to help support the increased oxygen demands of the hyperthyroid tissues.[122]

Hyperthyroidism and Hyperemesis Gravidarum

Nausea and vomiting may occasionally be the predominant presenting symptom in patients with hyperthyroidism. When this occurs during pregnancy it may present as hyperemesis gravidarum.[134, 135] In one series of patients with hyperemesis gravidarum 2 of 39 patients were found to be thyrotoxic.[136] However, elevated free T_4 and T_3 levels may be found transiently in up to one third of subjects presenting with hyperemesis gravidarum,[137] so that a careful evaluation of thyroid function (see above) and close follow-up are indicated in all such patients.

Graves' Disease and Thyroid Function in the Neonate

Fetal and neonatal hypothyroidism may occur from passage of thionamides across the placenta (see above). Fetal and neonatal bradycardia and the presence of a goiter may indicate hypothyroidism, but other physical signs may be lacking.[138] Iodide use during pregnancy may be associated with a massive goiter.[111, 112] Cord blood should be obtained for measurement of T_4 and TSH. These levels should be repeated 3 days later, as transient hypothyroidism due to thionamide passage across the placenta is usually gone by then.[101]

About 10% of neonates may develop transient hyperthyroidism, due to passage across the placenta of thyroid-stimulating immunoglobulins[139] and, possibly, thyrotropin-binding inhibitory immunoglobulins.[140] Because of the great variability in the measurements of such immunoglobulins in the various commercial assays, the utility of such measurements as predictors of hyperthyroidism is low. The finding of a high titer of such immunoglobulins in the blood of an infant is highly predictive of the development of hyperthyroidism, but the absence of such titers does not mean the infant will not develop hyperthyroidism.

The hyperthyroidism may be manifest in utero by increased fetal heart rate and the infant may present with tachycardia, irritability, exophthalmos, goiter, jaundice, frontal bossing with cranial synostosis, heart failure, and hepatosplenomegaly, although most infants are not overtly hyperthyroid.[141] Occasionally, the hyperthyroidism is masked initially because of suppression of thyroid hormone synthesis by thionamides that have crossed the placenta, and the infant only becomes hyperthyroid after discharge from the hospital. Thus the infant should be carefully examined and T_4 and T_3 measurements should be done on cord blood and again at 1 to 2 weeks if there is any question of hyperthyroidism at that time. It has been suggested that intrauterine fetal hyperthyroidism could be treated by increasing maternal thionamide dosage, titrating the dose to the fetal heart rate.[141] Such treatment has not been subjected to controlled clinical trials, however.

Hyperthyroidism and Breast-Feeding

Radioiodine treatment is contraindicated during breast-feeding because of passage of the isotope into milk. Scanning should be avoided but the doses are very small and the amount found in the milk is small. In a report of an infant who breast-fed 4 hours after the mother had received ^{99m}Tc, the exposure to the thyroid was 300 mrad, to the upper large intestine 180 mrad, and to other organs considerably less.[142] The total dose received by the infant was 82.5 μCi. However, it was estimated that a feeding at 30 minutes after the isotope was given would result in the ingestion of 728 μCi. These authors suggest that at least 48 hours elapse after scanning before resumption of breast-feeding and that formula be substituted in the interim.

Both methimazole and PTU appear in breast milk. However, the amounts are small and should not affect neonatal thyroid function,[143-146] although checking thyroid function in breast-feeding infants is still recommended.[146] Infants could also develop idiosyncratic reactions to these drugs, which may not be dose-dependent. No cases of jaundice, rash, or agranulocytosis in such infants have been reported, however.[146]

Hyperthyroidism Associated With Trophoblastic Neoplasms

Biochemical hyperthyroidism is found in over 50% of patients with trophoblastic disease, either benign hydatidiform mole or choriocarcinoma, but clinical hyperthyroidism is present in only 20% to 50% of these cases.[147-149] It is not clear why such women are usually asymptomatic, but it may relate to the relatively short duration of disease.[148] However, severe hyperthyroidism and even thyroid storm have been reported.[149] The hyperthyroidism abates with evacuation of the neoplasm or chemotherapy with actinomycin D.[148, 149] Human chorionic gonadotropin is structurally related to TSH and has thyroid-stimulating ability.[148] Most evidence now suggests that hCG, or some variant, that is present in very high quantities in patients with trophoblastic neoplasms, is the causative agent in trophoblastic hyperthyroidism.[148, 149]

Hypothyroidism

Etiology

Hypothyroidism most commonly arises because of a primary thyroid problem; uncommonly it is secondary to pituitary or hypothalamic disease. Primary thyroid disease usually is due to destruction of thyroid tissue, either by autoimmune disease or via radioactive iodine therapy or surgery. Rarely, there may be iodine deficiency or congenital defects in thyroid hormone synthesis. There is also a rare syndrome of generalized resistance to thyroid hormones in which thyroid hormone levels and TSH are elevated but the body remains hypothyroid (Refetoff's syndrome).

Diagnosis

Clinically, patients may experience fatigue, hair loss, dry skin, constipation, cold intolerance, eyelid edema, weight gain, and a hoarse voice, findings similar to those in non-pregnant patients.[150, 151] A goiter may or may not be present. T_4 and T_3 levels may be low or in the normal range but, when corrected for the increase in TBG, are low. TSH levels are elevated in all but those cases associated with hypopituitarism.[150, 151]

In cases associated with additional illness, such as pyelonephritis, patients may experience the euthyroid sick syndrome. Illness or malnutrition (even a few days of postoperative, calorically inadequate IV fluid intake) causes a decrease in deiodination of the outer ring, resulting in decreased serum T_3 levels.[152] Total T_4 levels may also be low, due to accelerated metabolism of T_4, a decrease in thyroid T_4 release, and a decrease in thyroid-binding prealbumin and TBG. Thus, these laboratory values may cause confusion with hypothyroidism. Of importance, in this syndrome, the free T_4 and TSH levels are normal.[122]

Effects of Hypothyroidism on Pregnancy

Early studies suggested that hypothyroid women had a higher incidence of abortions, stillbirths, prematurity, and congenital anomalies.[86] One study found essentially a normal pregnancy outcome in 11 pregnancies in 9 women with hypothyroidism; in 4 the diagnosis was made at the end of the first trimester and in the rest it was made after the 24th week of gestation.[150] However, in a second series of 16 pregnancies in 14 women, there appeared to be an excess of complications, including preeclampsia, abruptio placentae, stillbirths, anemia, postpartum hemorrhage, and cardiac dysfunction.[151] In these women T_4 replacement had been started in 13 of the 16 pregnancies at various points in the gestation.

In general, mild to moderately hypothyroid patients tolerate stress, such as labor and delivery and other surgery, quite well.[153, 154] However, sedatives and analgesics need to be administered cautiously because of their slow

metabolism. Because of the prolonged effects of these drugs and the general anesthesia that may be used, and because of the depressed hypoxic and ventilatory drives of these patients, they may need to be intubated and ventilated with a respirator for a prolonged period. These patients may also have a decreased ability to clear free water and may develop hyponatremia. Postoperative ileus may also be prolonged.[122]

Management of Hypothyroidism

Patients documented to be hypothyroid should be brought up to full replacement dose relatively quickly. Therapy should be carried out using levothyroxine exclusively. It was formerly thought that T_3 was primarily secreted by the thyroid and that thyroid medication containing T_3 (e.g., dessicated thyroid) was necessary for proper hormone replacement. It is now clear that about 80% of circulating T_3 is derived from the peripheral deiodination of T_4, and normal T_4 and T_3 levels have been found with pure levothyroxine therapy in doses of 0.1 to 0.2 mg daily. In fact, therapy with T_4 and T_3 combinations and dessicated thyroid have been found to result in a greater incidence of hyperthyroid side effects, resulting in normal T_4 levels but usually elevated T_3 levels when compared to therapy with levothyroxine alone.[155] Because virtually all women in this age range will have normal coronary arteries, they can be started on 0.1 mg/day, which is increased by 0.025- to 0.05-mg increments at 2-week intervals until the TSH level and the free T_4 index are normal. Levothyroxine is 79.9% absorbed in the fasting state and 59.6% absorbed when taken with meals.[156] Because of this, when patients are unable to take medications orally I usually recommend giving about half to two thirds of the usual dose IV. If the patient is to have nothing by mouth for only 2 to 3 days, then such parenteral therapy is not necessary because of the 7-day half-life of the drug.

In patients with known, chronic hypothyroidism who have been stabilized on an appropriate dose of T_4, the dose does not

need to be altered during pregnancy, as the rate of turnover of T_4 is not altered by the pregnancy.[89]

Myxedema Coma

Myxedema coma is extremely rare in pregnant patients because it usually occurs in older patients and such severe hypothyroidism usually results in anovulation and infertility. However, it is a true medical emergency with a 20% mortality even when treated properly. It is usually seen in a patient in whom hypothyroidism had not been diagnosed and who had become comatose as a result of hyponatremia, excessive sedation, infection, hypoxia, or anesthesia. Clinical features suggestive of myxedema coma include hypothermia, bradycardia, delayed return of or absent deep tendon reflexes, impaired consciousness, and other general evidence of hypothyroidism. Patients may have hyponatremia, hypoglycemia, hypoxia, and hypercapnia.[122]

After appropriate blood tests have been obtained, therapy should begin immediately with supportive care to correct the metabolic abnormalities and with thyroid hormone administration. Central warming via heated air or oxygen may be useful. An IV dose of 0.5 mg of levothyroxine is usually recommended initially and results in repletion of the total T_4 pool. This is followed by daily doses of 0.05 mg. Some improvement is usually seen by 6 to 12 hours and clear-cut improvement should be seen within 24 hours.[122]

Postpartum Thyroiditis

Postpartum, subacute lymphocytic thyroiditis occurs in 5% to 10% of women.[91, 157, 158] Characteristically, the syndrome consists of transient hyperthyroidism associated with a low radioactive iodine uptake that occurs about 6 to 12 weeks post partum, followed by transient hypothyroidism associated with a goiter and high titers of antithyroid microsomal antibodies that generally resolves spontaneously by about 6 to 9 months post partum (Table 4–9).[86, 91] The hyperthyroid phase may

be asymptomatic, but many patients complain of fatigue, shoulder stiffness, increased appetite, sweating, and nervousness.[157] Goiter is present in about 50% of patients in the hyperthyroid phase. The hyperthyroidism always resolves and may go on to hypothyroidism.

Hypothyroidism may occur with or without preceding hyperthyroidism; about 80% of patients resolve spontaneously but 20% develop persistent hypothyroidism. The titer of antimicrosomal antibodies appears to be predictive, higher titers tending to be associated with persistent hypothyroidism.[158] The hypothyroid phase may also be asymptomatic but may cause fatigue, lack of initiative, weight gain, and depression.[159] It is likely that a significant number of women with "postpartum depression" actually have thyroiditis, and thyroid function tests should be obtained in all such women.

TABLE 4–9.
Features of Postpartum Thyroiditis

Hyperthyroid phase
 Occurs about 6–12 wk post partum
 Symptoms: fatigue, shoulder stiffness, increased appetite, sweating, nervousness
 Goiter present in 50%
 Usually high titers of antithyroid microsomal antibodies
 Low radioactive iodine uptake
 Resolves spontaneously in several weeks, usually to go on to hypothyroid phase
 Thionamides ineffective; use β-blockers if symptomatic relief needed
Hypothyroid phase
 May or may not have preceding hyperthyroid phase
 Symptoms: fatigue, lack of initiative, weight gain, depression (may be confused with postpartum depression)
 About 80% resolve spontaneously
 20% go on to permanent hypothyroidism—those with very high titers of antithyroid microsomal antibodies
 If treated with T_4, take off every 6 months × 2 to see if underlying condition has resolved spontaneously

Management

The laboratory evaluation for postpartum thyroiditis includes measurement of T_4, T_3 resin uptake, T_3, and TSH. Because of the changing course, these measurements may need to be repeated at 4- to 8-week intervals. Treatment should be reserved for symptomatic cases, as most resolve spontaneously. Women in whom the hyperthyroidism becomes significantly symptomatic should have a radioactive iodine uptake test to differentiate the condition from Graves' disease, which has developed during this period. Thionamide antithyroid drugs are not effective in postpartum thyroiditis and β-blockers are indicated for symptomatic relief. For postpartum hypothyroidism that is symptomatic, treatment with levothyroxine, as above, is indicated. However, as this disorder is usually transient, patients should be taken off therapy after 6 months, and again at least one more time 6 months later for a period of 6 weeks, to be retested.[158] Patients with very high antimicrosomal antibody titers should be followed carefully for the development of persistent hypothyroidism.[158]

Thyroid Nodules and Cancer

Diagnostic Evaluation

Most goiters that develop during pregnancy are diffuse. The development of a solitary nodule is more suggestive of malignancy, although only about 10% of these are malignant. A history of prior head and neck irradiation greatly increases this risk, however.[160] Of cancers found in this age group, about 65% are papillary, 30% are follicular, 3% are medullary, 1% are anaplastic, and 1% are other types, such as metastatic disease to the thyroid or lymphoma.[161] The 20-year survival rates, assuming such tumors are diagnosed and resected, are 99% for papillary, 98% for follicular, and 50% for medullary, with less than a 10% one-year survival rate for anaplastic carcinoma.[161] For these carcinomas, a wait of 6 to 9 months before definitive surgery would not be expected to materially alter these long-term survival rates, except possibly for medullary and anaplastic carcinoma.[161]

Because almost all of these malignancies have decreased uptake on radioisotopic scanning, this is usually the first procedure performed to evaluate a nodule. However, these procedures should not be done during pregnancy (see above). Fine-needle aspiration certainly could be done during the pregnancy and it has excellent sensitivity and specificity. A finding of "benign" lowers the expected malignancy rate from the initial 10% down to 1%.[161] A finding of "malignant" raises the expected malignancy rate from the initial "a priori" 10% to 88%. However, a finding of "suspicious" or "indeterminate" only changes the rate from 10% to 17%.[161]

Management

A solitary nodule first found during pregnancy should probably be aspirated. Because waiting until after delivery for surgery will not alter the prognosis, except possibly for medullary and anaplastic carcinoma, surgery in general ought to be deferred until then. Regardless of the finding, again with the exception of medullary and anaplastic carcinoma, all such patients ought to have their thyroid glands suppressed with exogenous levothyroxine. For benign lesions, thyroxine will help to prevent further growth. For papillary and follicular carcincomas, thyroxine will also retard growth,[162] making the delay for surgery to the postpartum period even less of a problem. The aim of levothyroxine therapy is to suppress TSH levels below normal in patients with suspicious lesions and also in patients with previously treated thyroid cancer. If the thyroid aspiration shows medullary or anaplastic carcinoma, surgery should proceed forthwith. Pregnancy itself appears to have no effect on the prognosis of thyroid cancer.[163]

ADRENAL CORTEX

Changes in Adrenal Physiology During Pregnancy

Cortisol levels increase progressively over the course of gestation, resulting in a two- to threefold increase by term.[164] Most of the elevation of cortisol levels is due to the estrogen-

induced increase in cortisol-binding globulin (CBG) levels[165, 166] but the biologically active "free" fraction is elevated as well.[166, 167] This is reflected in an elevated urinary free cortisol level.[168] The increased CBG results in a prolonged cortisol half-life in plasma, but the cortisol production rate is also increased.[167] Urinary 17-hydroxycorticosteroid levels are decreased, however, due to a decrease in the excretion of cortisol tetrahydro metabolites.[169, 170] Cortisol can cross the placenta and the major direction of transfer is from mother to fetus.[171]

ACTH levels have been variously reported as being normal,[172] suppressed,[164] and elevated[173] early in gestation. During the pregnancy, there is a progressive rise, followed by a final surge of ACTH and cortisol levels during labor.[164, 172] ACTH does not cross the placenta[174] but is manufactured by the placenta, as is corticotropin releasing hormone (CRH). The relationship of placental ACTH and CRH to maternal adrenal function is unknown.

Cushing's Syndrome

Differential Diagnosis and Evaluation

Cushing's syndrome refers to the state of hypercortisolism that is due to a variety of causes. The most common type is that due to a pituitary tumor secreting ACTH, causing bilateral adrenal hyperplasia. This type is referred to as *Cushing's disease*. There is a subtype of Cushing's disease referred to as *adrenonodular hyperplasia*, in which macroscopic nodules are found and ACTH levels are variable. It is likely that this variant arises from pituitary oversecretion of ACTH and then progresses to have autonomous adrenal function.[175] ACTH produced ectopically by a nonpituitary neoplasm is the next most common type. The most common tumor type is oat cell carcinoma of the lung, but many other types can cause this. Adrenal carcinoma is the next most common type and adrenal adenoma is the most uncommon. Ectopic production of CRH has been reported but is exceedingly rare. In addition to these endogenous causes, corticosteroid therapy must also be included in the differential diagnosis.

Just under 70 cases of Cushing's syndrome and pregnancy have been reported.[176, 177, 177a] Although the distribution of cases discussed above is the usual one, in pregnancy this does not appear to hold true. Less than 50% of the cases reported to 1990[176, 177, 177a] had pituitary adenomas, a like number had adrenal adenomas, and seven had adrenal carcinomas. We are aware of but one report of pregnancy associated with the ectopic ACTH syndrome.[177a]

Clinically, there are a few specific features that distinguish some of the above syndromes. The typical features of Cushing's syndrome are well known.[175] In patients with the ectopic ACTH syndrome, the tumors are usually rapidly growing and add the features of tumor cachexia so that weight gain and the typical centripetal fat distribution are rarely seen. Hyperpigmentation due to the melanocyte-stimulating properties of the ACTH and lipotropin is common with the ectopic ACTH syndrome. Muscle weakness and severe hypokalemia are also characteristic of the ectopic ACTH syndrome. It is likely that the catabolic effects that occur when the tumors are malignant are sufficient to interfere with pregnancy. However, there are a number of benign or very slowly progressive neoplasms, such as carcinoids or medullary carcinoma of the thyroid, associated with ectopic ACTH secretion that do not cause systemic catabolism and which could be associated with normal fertility. Because of altered enzymatic pathways in adrenal carcinomas, there is usually a disproportionate elevation of adrenal androgens resulting in virilization.

Diagnosis of Cushing's syndrome during pregnancy may be difficult. Both may be associated with weight gain in a central distribution, fatigue, edema, emotional upset, glucose intolerance, and hypertension. The striae associated with the weight gain and increased abdominal girth are usually white in normal pregnancy and red or purple in Cushing's. Hirsutism and acne may point to excessive androgen production.

The laboratory evaluation of Cushing's syndrome during pregnancy is not straightforward. The overnight dexamethasone test usually demonstrates inadequate suppression during gestation.[178] Standard dexamethasone testing for 2 days at low dose (0.5 mg q6h × 8) and high dose (2 mg q6h × 8) appears to give reliable results, however. In pregnant patients with Cushing's disease, plasma cortisol levels are suppressed minimally with 2 days of low-dose dexamethasone but are suppressed quite well with the high dose.[177] Plasma cortisol levels in patients with adrenal adenomas are not suppressed with the high dose of dexamethasone.[178–182] Because of the altered urinary free cortisol and 17-hydroxysteroid measurements, these are of uncertain validity when evaluating patients for Cushing's syndrome. There are little data concerning ACTH levels in these patients. ACTH levels may not be elevated in patients with Cushing's disease[175] and have been reported to be relatively low and normal in two patients with this disorder during pregnancy.[176, 183] However, similar ACTH levels were recently reported in a patient with an adrenal adenoma.[177] There has been no experience reported with more recently used techniques such as CRH stimulation testing or petrosal venous sinus sampling.[175]

When biochemical evidence points to the presence of Cushing's syndrome and to a pituitary or adrenal origin, radiologic imaging becomes necessary. Often an adrenal mass will be visible on ultrasound.[184] Usually, however, CT or MRI scanning of the pituitary or adrenal will be necessary.[175, 184] With the techniques and equipment available in 1990, CT and MRI appeared to be about equal in detecting adrenal masses. Because MRI may be safer during pregnancy, it may be the technique of choice for localizing the mass. Most adrenal lesions are unilateral, so that localization is important.

Effects of Cushing's Syndrome on Pregnancy

Cushing's syndrome is associated with a high fetal mortality and increased prematurity. There is a 25% fetal mortality, equally distributed between spontaneous abortion, stillbirth, and early neonatal death due to extreme prematurity.[176] Bevan et al.[176] point out that the fetal loss rate is probably even higher because several of the patients had had spontaneous abortions before the diagnosis had been made. Premature labor occurs in over 50% of cases, regardless of etiology.[176] The passage of cortisol across the placenta occasionally causes suppression of the fetal adrenals.[185] This appears to be uncommon but the neonate should be tested for this potential problem and administered steroids until the results of the evaluation are known.

Maternal complications may also occur. Hypertension develops in almost 90% of patients.[186, 177a] Severe preeclampsia may supervene and myopathy is common.[176] Postoperative wound infection and dehiscence are common following cesarean section.[176]

The course of Cushing's syndrome may be influenced by the pregnancy. In some patients, there appears to be an amelioration of Cushing's[187] but in others there appears to be an exacerbation.[188]

Management of Cushing's Syndrome During Pregnancy

Bevan et al.[176] performed a careful analysis of maternal and fetal outcome depending upon whether surgery for the cause of the Cushing's syndrome was performed before or after delivery. They noted a fetal loss in one (9%) and premature labor in 2 (20%) of the 11 women treated during pregnancy and fetal loss in 8 (31%) and premature labor in 12 (48%) of the 26 women in whom treatment was delayed.

Medical therapy for Cushing's syndrome is not very effective, in general.[175, 189] Metyrapone has been used in two pregnant patients—one with an adrenal carcinoma[180] and another with an adrenal adenoma.[179] In the former, this resulted in a greatly increased amount of 11-deoxycortisone and aldosterone and a significant worsening of hypertension, but in the latter there was substantial clinical improvement. Urinary estriol levels decreased with metyrapone treatment due to blockade of C19 hydroxylation.[179]

Surgical removal of an adrenal adenoma via the posterior approach can be done safely even into the early third trimester and has been done many times.[176] Because of the rather high incidence of adrenal carcinomas among adrenal masses and the poor prognosis of adrenal carcinomas, early surgery may offer additional benefit to the mother. Recently, transsphenoidal resection of a pituitary ACTH-secreting adenoma was done successfully at 22 weeks' gestation.[177] As discussed above, transsphenoidal surgery has been done for an expanding prolactinoma many times during pregnancies with no untoward consequences. While any surgery has risk to the mother and fetus, it appears that with Cushing's syndrome the risk of not operating is considerably higher than proceeding with surgery.

Adrenal Insufficiency

Adrenal insufficiency most commonly arises because of autoimmune destruction of the adrenals. Adrenal insufficiency caused by infiltrative diseases, such as tuberculosis, fungal diseases, and metastatic cancer, is much less common. This disorder may also occur in association with other autoimmune endocrine disorders, such as thyroiditis, as part of a multiple endocrine gland insufficiency syndrome. Rarely, bilateral adrenal hemorrhage may occur in association with surgery. This usually presents as an acute adrenal crisis that is manifested by fever, abdominal or flank pain, vomiting, confusion, and hypotension.[190] Adrenal hemorrhage may also occur in association with anticoagulant use.[191] Adrenal insufficiency is very uncommon during pregnancy.[192]

Diagnosis

Patients commonly present with fatigue, anorexia, nausea, vomiting, weight loss, depression, and nonspecific abdominal pain.[192] Obviously, it may be difficult to sort out the features of fatigue, nausea, and vomiting dur-

TABLE 4–10.

Diagnostic and Therapeutic Protocol for Adrenal Insufficiency

1. Clinical presentation: hyperpigmentation, apathy, lethargy, weakness, weight loss, nausea, diarrhea, abdominal pain, hypotension, fever
2. Draw blood for cortisol (serum) and ACTH (heparinized on ice), electrolytes, BUN, creatinine
3. Give dexamethasone 4 mg IV
4. Administer COsyntropin (synthetic$_{1-24}$ ACTH), 1 ampule (0.25 mg) IM or IV
5. Draw blood for cortisol measurement 30–60 min after administration of COsyntropin
6. Administer hydrocortisone 100 mg IM or IV q8h for 24 hr and then taper
7. Administer 2–5 L of 5% dextrose in 0.9% saline over first 24 hr to correct fluid deficit
8. If COsyntropin stimulation test and ACTH level substantiate hypoadrenalism, further detailed testing should be carried out when patient is stable

ing the first trimester, but persistence of these symptoms should at least trigger a screening diagnostic evaluation (Table 4–10). Patients with normal pituitaries respond by increasing ACTH and lipotropin secretion, resulting in increased pigmentation in skin creases and mucous membranes. On examination, patients will usually display evidence of orthostatic hypotension. Mild cases may go undetected during pregnancy, only to go into adrenal crisis with the stress of labor or other illness, such as a urinary tract infection or dehydration from excessive sun exposure.[192, 193] In some cases, severe adrenal insufficiency may not develop until the postpartum period, possibly due to maintenance of maternal cortisol levels by fetal adrenal production.[194] Maternal adrenal insufficiency has been associated with intrauterine growth retardation in some cases.[193, 194]

Laboratory features of adrenal insufficiency include hyperkalemia, due to aldosterone deficiency; hyponatremia, due to an inability to excrete free water by the kidney; azotemia; eosinophilia; and lymphocytosis. Fasting hypoglycemia may also be present. If the signs, symptoms, and laboratory database suggest adrenal insufficiency, then diagnostic and therapeutic procedures should be carried out quickly and simultaneously (see Table 4—10).

Blood should be obtained for serum cortisol and ACTH measurements. The cortisol level should be inappropriately low for the length of gestation and ACTH levels will be elevated if the disease is primary and not secondary adrenal insufficiency. A stimulation test with COsyntropin (synthetic$_{1-24}$ ACTH) 25 μg should be performed immediately after obtaining the above baseline measurements, without waiting for the results. The second cortisol level obtained 60 minutes later should show an inadequate increment (i.e., less than a doubling of the basal levels and/or an increase to >18 μg/dL (500 nmol/L) in nonpregnant individuals; normal values have not been established for pregnant women).

Treatment

Chronic Treatment During Pregnancy.—In previously diagnosed adrenal insufficiency, women will have been stabilized on a dose of glucocorticoid, usually hydrocortisone, 20 mg in the morning and 10 mg in the evening, cortisone acetate, 25 mg in the morning and 12.5 mg in the evening, or prednisone, 2.5 to 5.0 mg in the morning and 2.5 mg in the evening. Because of the known increased cortisol production rate during pregnancy[167] this dose theoretically ought to be increased. However, this does not seem to be necessary in practice.[138, 195] Patients often require mineralocorticoid replacement, usually in the form of fludrocortisone acetate (Florinef) 0.05 to 0.1 mg daily.

Increased Steroid Requirements during Labor and Stress.—Additional glucocorticoids are needed for stress, such as labor and delivery (Table 4–11). Because normal individuals secrete 100 to 300 mg of cortisol per 24 hours in the face of severe stress, I recommend giving 300 mg/day on the day of surgery or in the face of severe stress such as overwhelming infection. Thus 100 mg of hydrocortisone can be given IM as labor begins, 100 mg can be given by IV infusion over the course of the labor and delivery, and 100 mg

can be given IM on the evening of the delivery. Assuming that the delivery is uneventful, the dose can be decreased by 50% each day. If the postpartum course is not smooth, then the rate of tapering should be slower. Hydrocortisone in large doses has enough mineralocorticoid activity that additional therapy with fludrocortisone or deoxycorticosterone acetate is not necessary until the dose of hydrocortisone is less than 100 mg/day. In addition, adequate hydration with saline must be maintained.[122]

Treatment of Acute Adrenal Insufficiency.—The patient that presents with what appears to be an acute adrenal crisis is essentially treated in the same fashion as the woman going into labor and delivery. However, prompt rehydration with saline is very important. If the patient had not been diagnosed previously, it is important to obtain proper baseline blood samples of cortisol and ACTH before giving the steroids.

Treatment of Patients Receiving Pharmacologic Doses of Steroids.—Patients who have received greater than physiologic replacement doses of glucocorticoids as anti-inflammatory therapy should be consid-

TABLE 4–11.
Glucocorticoid Therapy for Labor, Surgery or Other Severe Stress in Patients With Adrenal Insufficiency

1. Hydrocortisone* 100 mg IM/IV on call to operating room or at onset of labor
2. Hydrocortisone 100 mg IV over course of surgery or labor; repeat q8h if labor is prolonged
3. Hydrocortisone 100 mg IM/IV in recovery room
4. Hydrocortisone 50 mg IM q8H postoperative or postpartum day 1†
5. Hydrocortisone 25–50 mg po or IM q8h postoperative or postpartum day 2†
6. Hydrocortisone 25 mg po or IM q8–12h postoperative or postpartum day 3
   Fludrocortisone* 0.1 mg po daily
7. Hydrocortisone 20 mg po A.M. and 10 mg po P.M. (or equivalent in other preparation)
   Fludrocortisone 0.1 mg po daily thereafter

*Hydrocortisone sodium succinate; fludrocortisone acetate.
†For major procedures, unstable course, or supervening infection, the higher dosage figures should be used with slower tapering

ered to be adrenally insufficient for up to 9 months after having stopped such treatment.[196] Such patients should be treated with stress doses of steroids during labor and delivery as above. These patients are also subject to the postoperative difficulties that patients with endogenous Cushing's syndrome may have, including the development of transient adrenal insufficiency in the neonate (see above). Although there has been some suggestion that there is an increased risk of cleft palate in infants born of mothers who had received pharmacologic doses of steroids before the 14th week of gestation,[197] this risk is less than 1% and it is difficult to know whether there is truly a cause-and-effect relationship. A review of the literature by Turner et al.[198] in 1980 suggests that steroid use during pregnancy is quite safe. Prednisone but not prednisolone appears to cross the placenta readily.[199] Suppression of neonatal adrenal function in offspring of women taking prednisone during pregnancy is very uncommon, however.[200] Glucocorticoids may also pass to the neonate in breast milk, but the amounts (0.14% of the maternal blood levels) are not sufficient to alter neonatal adrenal function, even with large maternal doses of prednisone.[201]

Congenital Adrenal Hyperplasias

There are a number of enzyme defects in the biosynthetic pathways of cortisol synthesis that result in decreased cortisol synthesis, a resulting increase in ACTH levels, and a building up of precursors. About 90% to 95% of patients have a partial or complete block in the 21-hydroxylase enzyme which is necessary for the conversion of 17-hydroxyprogesterone to 11-deoxycorticosterone. In this form there is increased synthesis of adrenal androgenic precursors that may result in virilization of the female.[202] In most patients treatment with glucocorticoids and mineralocorticoids results in normal growth and development, although menarche is often delayed.[203] In one series of women desiring pregnancy, the fertility rate was 64%.[203] Of the 15 pregnancies reported in this group, 2

were electively terminated and there were 1 first-trimester abortion; two spontaneous midtrimester abortions; 1 infant born alive with multiple skeletal anomalies and a meningomyelocele, who died of sepsis at 2 weeks of age; 1 infant born at 7 months; and 8 full-term deliveries. In all of the full-term pregnancies, cesarean section was required because of cephalopelvic disproportion. Glucocorticoid replacement doses were not altered during these pregnancies except for an increase during labor and delivery.

Adequate suppression of adrenal androgens during the pregnancy is important, because the excessive androgens may virilize the fetus. Monitoring of urinary 17-ketosteroids or serum androgens is important in this regard. Excessive doses of steroids, on the other hand, may suppress the fetal adrenal and result in neonatal adrenal insufficiency. Recently, suppression of fetal androgen production to prevent virilization of an affected fetus has been successfully achieved by giving 1.5 mg/day of dexamethasone to the mother beginning at 5 weeks gestation.[204] As yet, such attempts should still be considered experimental, however.

Primary Hyperaldosteronism

Primary hyperaldosteronism consists of the excessive secretion of aldosterone by an adrenal adenoma or by bilateral adrenal hyperplasia; surgery is performed only for unilateral adenomas. The characteristic features are hypertension in association with marked hypokalemia, which may be especially aggravated by diuretic treatment. The hypokalemia may partially inhibit insulin secretion and potentially could aggravate glucose intolerance during pregnancy. Elevation of plasma aldosterone levels is accompanied by suppression of plasma renin activity.

The disorder is quite uncommon and has been reported in pregnant women rarely.[205, 206] In the nonpregnant individual, treatment consists of medical therapy with spironolactone, an aldosterone antagonist, or surgery, in the case of an adenoma. Spironolactone can cross the placenta, however. As spironolactone is a potent antiandrogen, it may cause abnormal development of genitalia[207] and thus is contraindicated during pregnancy. If the hypertension responds to other agents acceptable during pregnancy, then surgery may be deferred to the postpartum period. If the hypertension cannot be controlled, then surgery may be necessary.

Hyporeninemic Hypoaldosteronism

This disorder is most commonly seen in patients with diabetes who have modest degrees of renal insufficiency (serum creatinine 1.5–2.5 mg/dL [130–220 μmol/L]).[208] The aspect of this disorder of most concern is the hyperkalemia, which may occasionally be life-threatening. Treatment consists of mineralocorticoids in normotensive patients and diuretics in hypertensive patients. The proper balance of these two classes of drugs in the pregnant patient has not been established.

PHEOCHROMOCYTOMA

Presentation

Pheochromocytomas have been found in up to 0.1% of hypertensive patients in some series and malignant pheochromocytomas make up between 1% and 10% of these patients.[209] The clinical features and diagnostic tests have been well described, but certain features are worth reemphasizing. Many patients do not have paroxysmal hypertension associated with headaches but rather have sustained hypertension. Some patients may have episodes that are very infrequent and therefore the first suspicion of the pheochromocytoma may occur with a blood pressure rise during the induction of anesthesia or during labor or surgery. Failure to recognize this possibility may result in death of the patient.[210] On the other hand, extraadrenal tumors, which make up about 10% of cases, may provoke paroxysmal symptoms after particular activities. A frequent site is the organ of Zuckerkandl, located at the bifurcation of the aorta. The following case is illustrative:

A 27-year-old woman presented to the emergency room at 34 weeks of gestation with severe headaches and a blood pressure of 240/130 mm Hg and was diagnosed as being preeclamptic. Despite no other evidence of preeclampsia, the patient was delivered by cesarean section under spinal anesthesia with gradual resolution of her hypertension. A large, retrouterine "fibroid," found at the time of her cesarean section, was scheduled for elective resection 2 months later. Although normotensive on admission to the operating room for removal of the fibroid, upon induction of anesthesia her blood pressure increased to 200/140 mm Hg and she developed pulmonary edema and cardiac arrest ensued. She was resuscitated and eventually recovered from acute renal failure, heart failure requiring intraaortic balloon assistance, a pneumothorax, heparin-induced thrombocytopenia, and gastrointestinal bleeding. Upon further evaluation for suspected pheochromocytoma, she was found to have greatly elevated urinary and blood norepinephrine levels. An MRI scan showed normal adrenal glands and an 8-cm retrouterine fibroid or mass adjacent to the uterus (Fig 4–3,A). A radioisotopic metaiodobenzylguanidine (MIBG) scan localized catecholamine production to the mass (Fig 4–3,B). After preoperative preparation with phenoxybenzamine and metyrosine, a large pheochromocytoma was successfully removed from its retrouterine site at the organ of Zuckerkandl.

Pheochromocytomas may be familial and a careful family history is important. Bilateral pheochromocytomas are more common in the familial variety. Medullary carcinoma of the thyroid occurs in many of these familial cases, an association known as multiple endocrine adenomatosis, type II, or Sipple's syndrome. Coexistent hyperparathyroidism is also common. Many patients will have a marfanoid habitus and some may have multiple mucosal neuromas.[211]

Diagnosis

The diagnosis is primarily biochemical and has been presented in detail elsewhere.[212] Twenty-four-hour urinary collections should

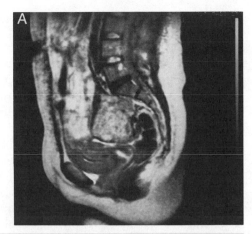

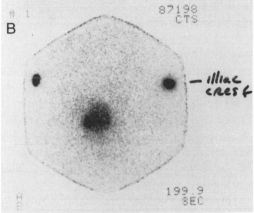

FIG 4–3.
A, magnetic resonance imaging scan (0.5T) demonstrating 7- × 8- × 7-cm lobulated mass anterior to the upper sacrum and superior and posterior to the uterus. **B**, ^{131}I-metaiodobenzylguanidine (MIBG) scan showing uptake in the retrouterine mass at 72 hours. At surgery this mass was confirmed to be a pheochromocytoma.

show elevated levels of norepinephrine or epinephrine or one of their metabolites, such as normetanephrine, metanephrine, and vanillylmandelic acid (VMA). Because of the episodic secretion of some tumors, timed urine specimens with onset of the collection at the time of a symptomatic episode can be quite useful. Plasma epinephrine and norepinephrine are also useful, especially if drawn during a symptomatic episode.[212] Extraadrenal pheochromocytomas characteristically have elevations of norepinephrine and not epinephrine, because high cortisol levels are necessary for the full activity of the enzyme phenylethan-

olamine-*N*-methyltransferase which methylates norepinephrine to epinephrine. Stimulation tests using clonidine, glucagon, or betazole hydrochloride (Histalog) have not proved to be of additional benefit in my experience.

Once the diagnosis is made biochemically, then efforts should be made to localize the tumor. Both CT and MRI scanning are excellent in detecting the presence of tumors (see Fig 4–3,A). More recently, ^{131}I-MIBG scanning has proved to be quite useful in localizing tumors (see Fig 4–3,B).[212] However, it should be noted that false-negatives occur with this technique. Isotopic scanning is, in general, contraindicated during pregnancy. However, if the clinical and biochemical suspicions are so strong and the tumor cannot be localized by other techniques, then this scan may be indicated, because of the significant risks to mother and fetus from not operating immediately (see below).

Special Considerations During Pregnancy

A key consideration in pheochromocytomas occurring during pregnancy is to differentiate them from preeclampsia. Careful evaluation may reveal the absence of proteinuria, edema, or hyperuricemia. Urinary catecholamines have been reported to be modestly elevated during preeclampsia and eclampsia,[213] so the biochemical differentiation may be difficult.

The maternal mortality rate from undiagnosed pheochromocytomas is about 50%; this rate has been reported to decrease to 11% if the diagnosis is made ante partum.[214, 215] The fetal loss rate is similar, even if the diagnosis is made during pregnancy.[215] Catecholamines cross the placenta only minimally[216] and therefore the fetus appears to be unaffected by the high maternal levels. However, there may be some element of hypoxia due to vasoconstriction of the uterine vascular bed.[217]

Management

Once the diagnosis is made, chronic α-adrenergic blockade should be achieved with phenoxybenzamine, given in a dose of 10 to 30 mg two to four times daily with meals (Table 4–12). Side effects may be limiting and include sedation, nasal congestion, nausea, vomiting, diarrhea, orthostatic hypotension, and fatigue. There have been no reports of teratogenicity with α-blockers and the fetus appears to tolerate these medications well.[217, 218] Should treatment with phenoxybenzamine not result in satisfactory lowering

TABLE 4–12.
Drugs Used in the Management of Pheochromocytoma in Pregnancy

Hypertensive emergencies
1. Phentolamine (Regitine) (C)*
    a. Given in 1–5-mg boluses IV at 1 mg/min
    b. Low-dose IV drip: 10 μg/mL (5 mg in 500 mL 5% D/W)
    c. High-dose IV drip: 80 μg/mL (40 mg in 500 mL 5% D/W)
2. Sodium nitroprusside† (Nipride) (C): light-sensitive; shield with aluminum foil; stable in solution for only 4 hr; risk of maternal and fetal cyanide toxicity
    a. Low-dose IV drip: 100 μg/mL (50 mg in 500 mL 5% D/W)
    b. High-dose IV drip: 500 μg/mL (250 mg in 500 mL 5% D/W)
3. Norepinephrine bitartrate (Levophed): for *phentolamine-induced hypotension*
    a. Low-dose IV drip: 4 μg/mL (4 mL in 1,000 mL 5% D/W)
    b. High-dose IV drip: 64 μg/mL (64 mL in 1,000 mL 5% D/W)

Arrhythmias
1. Lidocaine (Xylocaine) (B)
    a. Given in 50–100-mg boluses IV at 25–50 mg/min
    b. IV drip: 1 mg/mL (1 g in 1,000 mL 5% D/W)
2. Propranolol hydrochloride (Inderal) (C)
    a. Given in 0.25–5.0-mg boluses IV at maximum rate of 1 mg/min

Chronic management
1. Phenoxybenzamine hydrochloride (Dibenzyline) (C): 10-mg capsules
    a. Usual dose: 10–20 mg 3–4 times/day
2. Propranolol (C): tablets containing 10, 20, 40, 60, 80 mg
    a. Usual dose: 10–40 mg q4–6h N.B. Only to be used after α-blockade established
3. Metyrosine (Demser) (C): 250-mg tablets
    a. Usual dose: 250–1,000 mg q6h

*Letters in parentheses refer to FDA risk category.
†Avoid prolonged use as there is risk of fetal cyanide toxicity.

of the blood pressure, metyrosine, a substance which interferes with catecholamine synthesis, may prove useful in doses of 1 to 4 g daily in divided doses.[212] Metyrosine has been used in one pregnant patient with a pheochromocytoma with no apparent ill effects on the fetus.[218] Because of its effects on interrupting normal catecholamine synthesis it cannot be judged to be free of adverse effects on the fetus based on this one case, however. Nonetheless, because of the potential lethal nature of an uncontrolled pheochromocytoma, the use of metyrosine in this circumstance can certainly be justified. A normal blood pressure should be achieved for at least 1 to 2 weeks prior to any surgery to allow reexpansion of the contracted vasculature, thereby preventing postoperative hypotension.[212]

Because the hypertension is mediated by α-adrenergic mechanisms, β-blockers should never be used without prior α-blockade (or nitroprusside) because worsening of the hypertension may result. If arrhythmias or severe tachycardia is a problem, propranolol can be added in doses of 10 to 40 mg four times a day.

Hypertensive emergencies, should they occur, may be treated with phentolamine as an IV bolus of 1 to 5 mg or as a continuous IV infusion (see Table 4–12). Alternatively, nitroprusside may be used; however, prolonged use should be avoided since fetal cyanide toxicity may ensue. Rarely, tachyphylaxis to these agents may occur and emergency surgery may be necessary. Arrhythmias may be managed with lidocaine or β-blockers, after α-blockade has been established.[122]

When the patient is medically stabilized, surgery to remove the tumor should be considered. There are no definitive data to judge the best time of surgery for the pheochromocytoma. Fudge et al.[219] and Schenker and Granat[215] have recommended surgery for the tumor before 24 weeks of gestation, realizing that surgery could result in premature labor, and have recommended prolonged medical therapy after 24 weeks until fetal viability, at which point combined cesarean section and exploration for the pheochromocytoma could be done.[214, 220, 221] A common-sense approach might be to determine the site of the tumor and how well the patient responds to medical therapy. A tumor at the organ of Zuckerkandl might be expected to become progressively more difficult to manage as the uterus continues to enlarge. The patient who is monitored closely and who responds well to medical therapy might well be coaxed along until fetal viability. Any patient difficult to control should be operated on sooner.

The intraoperative and postoperative management of patients with pheochromocytomas is beyond the scope of this chapter and is discussed elsewhere.[122, 215, 221]

CALCIUM

Changes in Calcium Metabolism During Pregnancy

About 25 to 30 g of calcium is transferred from mother to fetus during gestation, about 300 mg/day being transferred in the third trimester.[222] In addition to the net transfer from the mother to the fetus of calcium, there is a net loss of calcium into the urine because of the increased glomerular filtration.[223] A number of changes in maternal calcium homeostasis occur during pregnancy that prevent the mother from going into markedly negative calcium balance.

The primary adaptational event appears to be an increase in parathyroid hormone (PTH) levels due to these calcium losses.[224] The increased PTH levels then stimulate the conversion of 25-hydroxyvitamin D to 1,25-dihydroxyvitamin D, the biologically active metabolite of vitamin D.[225, 226] Although the kidney is the predominant site of this 1-hydroxylation step, a significant amount of 1-hydroxylation of 25-hydroxyvitamin D also occurs in the placenta.[226] Levels of vitamin D-binding protein also increase during gestation but it appears that both the bound and free fractions of 1,25-dihydroxyvitamin D increase.[225] The increased levels of 1,25-dihydroxyvitamin D stimulate increased levels of intestinal calcium-binding protein and cal-

cium absorption.[222] The efficiency of gastrointestinal calcium absorption, i.e., the amount absorbed related to the amount ingested, actually increases. Pitkin et al.[224] have referred to pregnancy as a state of "physiologic hyperparathyroidism." It is likely that those women who have very poor calcium intakes during gestation could develop significant negative calcium balance despite these adaptative changes and thus an intake of at least 1,200 to 1,600 mg/day has been recommended.[227]

Serum calcium levels in the fetus are greater than those in the mother, suggesting an active transport of calcium in the placenta.[226] PTH and calcitonin do not cross the placenta, however.[222] 25-Hydroxyvitamin D readily crosses the placenta but 1,25-dihydroxyvitamin D crosses less well.[226] The fetal hypercalcemia appears to suppress the fetal parathyroids[222] so that at birth the neonate is relatively hypoparathyroid and the elevated calcium levels present in cord blood fall to a nadir that usually occurs at 24 to 48 hours of age. Generally, there is a quick recovery of the parathyroid glands in the neonate, unless there are confounding factors, such as maternal diabetes mellitus, preterm birth, or birth hypoxia.[222]

Hypercalcemia

Presentation

Most patients found to be hypercalcemic are asymptomatic, the condition being discovered on routine screening with a multichannel autoanalyzer. It is uncommon now for patients to present because of renal calculi, peptic ulcer disease, bone disease, or mental dysfunction. This is especially true of women in the reproductive age. Rarely, the diagnosis in the mother is made only after an evaluation is done because of hypocalcemia in the neonate.[228]

Differential Diagnosis

A variety of conditions may be associated with hypercalcemia, and hypercalcemia itself is very common, being present in 0.1% to 0.6% of the population.[229, 230] A careful in-

TABLE 4–13.
Causes of Hypercalcemia*

Common	Uncommon
Hyperparathyroidism	Sarcoidosis
Cancer (solid)	Diuretic phase of acute
With osseous	tubular necrosis
metastases	Immobilization (in ado-
Without osseous	lescent or patient with
metastases	Paget's disease)
Secreting PTH-like	Addison's disease
peptide	Myxedema
Secreting PGE_2	Leukemia/lymphoma
Secreting other	Other granulomatous
peptides?	diseases (tuberculosis,
Hyperthyroidism	coccidiodomycosis,
Thiazide diuretics	berylliosis,
Multiple myeloma	blastomycosis)
Vitamin D toxicity	Milk-alkali syndrome
Estrogen (antiestrogen)	Idiopathic (associated
therapy of breast	with supravalvular aor-
cancer	tic stenosis in
	children)

*PTH = parathyroid hormone; PGE_2 = prostaglandin E_2.

vestigation should always be performed, but the great majority of women in this age group will be found to have hyperparathyroidism (Table 4–13). Many causes can be ascertained by a careful history and physical examination and routine laboratory screening. The list of causes can be essentially broken down into hyperparathyroidism, in which serum PTH levels are elevated, and the rest. Thus PTH levels are critical in the evaluation of these patients. Although PTH levels may not be absolutely elevated in hyperparathyroidism, the levels will be relatively elevated for the degree of hypercalcemia. It is now known that the peptide which causes hypercalcemia in most patients with malignancies is similar but not identical to PTH,[231] and generally it is not detected on routine PTH assays. Further evaluation of these other causes of hypercalcemia is beyond the scope of this discussion and the subject is reviewed elsewhere.[231]

Effect of Hypercalcemia and Hyperparathyroidism on Pregnancy

Although somewhat under 100 cases of hyperparathyroidism occurring in pregnant women have been reported in the literature, it is likely that this is due to considerable bias in that asymptomatic patients are often either not diagnosed or not reported. Hypercalcemia can affect both mother and fetus. Rarely, women may develop severe hypercalcemia ("hypercalcemic crisis"), presenting with rapidly progressive anorexia, nausea, vomiting, weakness, fatigue, dehydration, and stupor. This condition may be fatal[232] and demands emergency treatment (see below). Another less common but severe complication is acute pancreatitis.[233] More common clinical findings include hypertension, nausea, and vomiting. The vomiting may be mistaken for hyperemesis gravidarum.[234] Patients with persistent vomiting must be hydrated rapidly to avoid a worsening of the hypercalcemia from dehydration. In general, pregnancy has an ameliorating affect on the hypercalcemia due to a shunting of calcium from mother to fetus. This may lead to a dramatic worsening and even hypercalcemic crisis post partum when such shunting is lost.[232, 234, 235]

Ludwig[236] first called attention to the rather disastrous consequences hyperparathyroidism can have upon the fetus. In that early series of 39 pregnancies, there were 8 stillbirths, 2 spontaneous abortions, and 5 premature deliveries plus an 18% incidence (7/39) of neonatal tetany. More recent series have confirmed a persistent 15% to 25% risk of severe hypocalcemia with or without tetany, but the risks of stillbirth and neonatal deaths have declined to about 2% each, the risk of premature delivery has declined to about 10%, and the risk of spontaneous abortion remains low at 8%.[232, 234, 237]

The neonatal hypocalcemia is due to the placental transfer of the elevated calcium levels with suppression of the fetal parathyroid glands. At delivery, the calcium transfer stops but the involuted parathyroid glands cannot maintain adequate calcium levels. Generally the hypocalcemia is transient, lasting up to 3 to 5 months, and can be managed with calcium and vitamin D supplements.[232, 234] In some infants the hypocalcemia develops only after several months, at a time of conversion from breast-feeding to cow's milk or formula with their higher phosphate content.[234] Of greater concern is the rare development of permanent hypoparathyroidism in a few offspring. In one case, the hypoparathyroidism was part of the DiGeorge syndrome, i.e., it was associated with thymic aplasia.[232] This raises the possibility of early directed teratogenicity of the hypercalcemia on the embryologic development of the third and fourth branchial clefts.

Management of Primary Hyperparathyroidism During Pregnancy

Because of the potential hazards to mother and child, all patients with known primary hyperparathyroidism should be operated on prior to conception. The major difficulties arise, of course, when the diagnosis is made during gestation. Recently, Mansberger and Mansberger[238] reviewed the literature regarding the outcome of surgery vs. expectant therapy for this condition. Of 12 patients operated on since 1975, there was 1 fetal death (in a mother with a calcium of 19 mg/dL (4.74 mmol/L), in severe hypercalcemic crisis with pancreatitis undergoing emergency neck exploration) and no other instances of fetal complications. Mother and fetus, in general, appear to tolerate parathyroidectomy quite well. Of 15 patients treated either expectantly or with oral phosphates, there were no fetal deaths but 6 instances of neonatal hypocalcemia. Oral phosphate (Fleet's phosphosoda, 15–50 mL/day in divided doses) has been used to control hypercalcemia quite well during pregnancy and appears to prevent neonatal hypocalcemia.[239, 240] Although surgery has been recommended rather uniformly unless the patient is diagnosed late in gestation,[232, 234, 237, 238] perhaps a reasonable course would be to reserve surgery for those who do not achieve stable calcium levels with oral phosphate. The experience of several of the patients treated only with phosphate suggests that such patients also do well.[239, 240] Thus close follow-up is necessary for such patients, monitoring calcium levels every 2 to 4 weeks.

Even should hypocalemia develop in the neonate, this can generally be easily treated.

Emergency Treatment of Severe Hypercalcemia

In the severely hypercalcemic patient (calcium ≥14.0 mg/dL [3.49 mmol/L]) or in the obtunded patient, the first step in emergency therapy is adequate rehydration with saline: 4 to 10 L/24 hours are given and furosemide may be added to further increase calcium excretion.[241] It is necessary for the intravascular volume to stay on the "full" side and a central venous pressure catheter may be helpful. Urinary potassium and magnesium must be measured and their losses replaced.[122] Although mithramycin (plicamycin; FDA Class X) is the next agent of choice,[242] its safety in pregnancy has not been established. Calcitonin (FDA Class B) is probably safe and is moderately effective.[243] Glucocorticoids are particularly useful for the hypercalcemia associated with sarcoidosis, multiple myeloma, and vitamin D toxicity,[231] and are safe in pregnancy (see above). A number of other treatment modalities that have been used for hypercalcemia, such as the bisphosphonates, IV phosphate, and gallium nitrate,[231] have not been used in pregnant patients and their safety in this setting has not been established. Patients who do not respond readily to the above modalities are candidates for emergency surgery.

Hypocalcemia

The most common cause of hypocalcemia is hypoparathyroidism. Vitamin D deficiency and other causes are extremely uncommon. Hypoparathyroidism is usually secondary to surgery performed for hyperparathyroidism or thyroid disease. Idiopathic, autoimmune, and infiltrative causes are quite rare. Chronic therapy includes calcium supplementation, 1 to 4 g/day, and 1,25-dihydroxyvitamin D, 0.5 to 2.5 μg/day. Thiazide diuretics are also commonly used to decrease calcium excretion.[122]

Patients who are not well controlled may

experience muscle cramps, carpopedal spasm, and even tetany. Paresthesias in the hands and feet may occur. Other less common problems include seizures, choreiform movements, parkinsonian-like rigidity, anxiety, agitation, delirium, cataracts, and raised intracranial pressure.[122]

Effects of Hypoparathyroidism and Hypocalcemia on Pregnancy

Maternal hypocalcemia results in inadequate amounts of calcium being transferred to the fetus with subsequent fetal hypocalcemia. This fetal hypocalcemia stimulates the fetal parathyroids and this may cause generalized skeletal demineralization, subperiosteal resorption, and even osteitis fibrosa cystica.[244] Similar findings have been found in a baby of a mother with pseudohypoparathyroidism.[245]

Treatment of Hypoparathyroidism During Pregnancy

Because of the continued drain of calcium from the mother by the fetus, an increased dose of calcium and vitamin D may be necessary to keep maternal calcium levels normal. The dose of 1,25-dihydroxyvitamin D may need to be increased as much as four- to sixfold over the course of gestation.[246, 247] Dose adjustments are made on the basis of keeping serum calcium levels in the normal range. The fetus can tolerate large changes in 1,25-dihydroxyvitamin D dosage well. In one reported case of a woman receiving 1,25-dihydroxyvitamin D in a dose of 17 to 36 μg/day because of hereditary insensitivity to 1,25-dihydroxyvitamin D, there was considerable transplacental passage of this compound, resulting in 20-fold elevated levels in cord blood. Despite such levels, the neonate was only minimally hypercalcemic transiently and showed no other abnormalities.[248] As with hypoparathyroidism treatment outside of pregnancy, 1,25-dihydroxyvitamin D is preferable to vitamin D_3 itself because of its rapidity of onset and offset of action, thereby allowing more precise modulation of serum calcium levels.

In one woman with hypoparathyroidism, 1,25-dihydroxyvitamin D requirements fell dramatically during lactation.[249] It is tempting to speculate that this phenomenon may be related to the production of a PTH-like peptide made by mammary epithelium and that it is the same peptide implicated in the humoral hypercalcemia of malignancy.[250] This may also be the reason why some babies with neonatal hypocalcemia from maternal hyperparathyroidism become more hypocalcemic upon transfer from breast to cow's milk or formula.

OBESITY

Maternal Risks Associated With Obesity

Obesity only begins to affect overall mortality rates when weight exceeds 120% of the average body weight for a given height.[251] Obese people have an increased likelihood of having hypertension, diabetes mellitus, hypertriglyceridemia, and coronary artery disease.[252, 253] Operative wound infections and dehiscence and postoperative thromboembolic disease are also more common.[254]

In patients with morbid obesity (>100 lb [45 kg] overweight or >200% of ideal body weight), respiratory impairment may be a major source of morbidity and takes three forms. The first is directly due to increased chest wall and abdominal fat and consists of a reduction in lung and chest wall compliance. This results in the closure of small peripheral lung units, an increased energy cost of breathing with decreased respiratory muscle efficiency, hypoventilation of dependent lobes, and a reduction in vital capacity and functional residual capacity.[255, 256] The closure of peripheral lung units results in ventilation-perfusion mismatching and large anatomic shunts.[254] In an ambulatory setting, these patients do not retain carbon dioxide,[255, 256] but they may be slightly hypoxic, especially when supine.[257] After abdominal surgery, such as a cesarean section, massively obese patients have a further reduction in arterial oxygen pressure (PaO_2) with the nadir appearing on the second postoperative day.[257]

A much smaller group of massively obese patients have hypoventilation, hypercapnea, hypoxia, somnolence, and markedly reduced lung compliance—a constellation of findings that has been referred to as the pickwickian syndrome.[253, 255] Finally, some patients with obesity develop upper airway obstruction when asleep (or when given sedation) and become hypoxic and even apneic.[258, 259]

As could be predicted, the above concerns have important implications for the obese woman who becomes pregnant, and several series reporting data in obese pregnant women have been published. In women in the top 5th percentile (>90 kg at term), hypertension was found to be fourfold elevated and gestational diabetes was increased by 50%.[260] In two other series, women weighing more than 150% of ideal body weight and a two- to eightfold increase in hypertension and a four- to eightfold increase in gestational diabetes.[261, 262] In these series, there were slight increases in the complication rates in some other categories as well, including thrombophlebitis, preeclampsia, urinary tract infections, and wound/episiotomy infections.[260–262] Although an increased respiratory complication rate due to the further influence of the expanding uterine contents on an already impaired respiratory apparatus would be expected, this was not found in these series.[260–262] The cesarean section rate was increased in these women in one series[262] but not in the other two.[260, 261] Thus, the obese woman should be screened periodically for gestational diabetes and monitored carefully for the development of hypertension, urinary tract infections, and preeclampsia. For the obese woman with a complicated delivery who may remain at bed rest for an extended period, prophylactic subcutaneous heparin may be indicated. In the massively obese woman, care must be taken to prevent respiratory compromise as well.

The fetal complication rates are also increased due to maternal obesity. Birth weights are increased and this is not due to the associated gestational diabetes.[260–262] Follow-up of these infants shows that at 12 months the infants of obese mothers weigh significantly more than infants of nonobese mothers.[261] There is also increased shoulder dystocia, meconium, and late decelerations during labor.[262] Although Garbaciak et al.[262] found an increase in perinatal mortality due to obesity, this was not found in the other two series.[260, 262] The above data are compatible with data from earlier series reviewed by Edwards et al.[261] and Kliegman and Gross.[263]

Management of Weight Gain in the Morbidly Obese Woman During Pregnancy

It has been estimated that the usual increase in calories required during pregnancy is between 40,000 and 80,000.[263] The normal, non-obese woman usually gains little during the first trimester, then gains, on average, 0.36 kg/week between weeks 13 and 18, 0.45 kg/week between weeks 18 and 28, and finally 0.36 kg/week between week 28 and term.[263] Of the recommended 9- to 13.5-kg weight gain during pregnancy, about 3.6 kg is actually maternal fat.[263] Many obese women resist diets that cause them to gain the recommended amount of weight, 10% to 40% gaining less than 5.4 kg during gestation.[263] This may not be harmful, however, as the birth weights of term infants of obese mothers who actually lose weight are greater than the birth weights of infants of normal-weight mothers who gain the recommended amount of weight.[263] Thus, obese mothers may be able to mobilize nutrient stores and transmit nutrients to the fetus better than normal-weight women, because the latter would generally have infants with intrauterine growth retardation with inadequate weight gain. Because of these findings, a weight gain of 4.5 to 9.0 kg for obese women has been recommended, although careful attention to fetal growth by serial ultrasound measurements is necessary.[263] Strenuous efforts may be necessary to prevent excessive weight gain, as such weight gain will only exacerbate the risks of gestational diabetes and hypertension and will result in more permanent weight gain as well.

REFERENCES

1. Goluboff LG, Ezrin C: Effect of pregnancy on the somatotroph and the prolactin cell of the human adenohypophysis. *J Clin Endocrinol Metab* 1969; 29:1533–1538.
2. Vician L, Shupnik MA, Gorski J: Effects of estrogen on primary ovine pituitary cell cultures: Stimulation of prolactin secretion, synthesis, and preprolactin messenger ribonucleic acid activity. *Endocrinology* 1979; 104:736–743.
3. Shupnik MA, Baxter LA, French LR, et al: In vivo effects of estrogen on ovine pituitaries: Prolactin and growth hormone biosynthesis and messenger ribonucleic acid translation. *Endocrinology* 1979; 104:729–735.
4. West B, Dannies PS: Effects of estradiol on prolactin production and dihydroergocryptine-induced inhibition of prolactin production in primary cultures of rat pituitary cells. *Endocrinology* 1980; 106:1108–1113.
5. Maurer RA: Relationship between estradiol, ergocryptine, and thyroid hormone: Effects on prolactin synthesis and prolactin messenger ribonucleic acid levels. *Endocrinology* 1982; 110:1515–1520.
6. Rakoff JS, Yen SSC: Progesterone induced acute release of prolactin in estrogen primed ovariectomized women. *J Clin Endocrinol Metab* 1978; 47:918–921.
7. Bohnet HG, Naber NG, del Pozo E, et al: Effects of synthetic gestagens on serum prolactin and growth hormone secretion in amenorrheic patients. *Arch Gynecol* 1978; 226:233–240.
8. Tyson JE, Hwang P, Guyda H, et al: Studies of prolactin secretion in human pregnancy. *Am J Obstet Gynecol* 1972; 113:14–21.
9. Rigg LA, Lein A, Yen SSC: Pattern of increase in circulating prolactin levels during human gestation. *Am J Obstet Gynecol* 1977; 129:454–456.
10. Pasteels JL, Gausset P, Danguy A, et al: Morphology of the lactotropes and somatotropes of man and rhesus monkeys. *J Clin Endocrinol Metab* 1972; 34:959–967.
11. Asa SL, Penz G, Kovacs K, et al: Prolactin cells in the human pituitary: a quantitative immunocytochemical analysis. *Arch Pathol Lab Med* 1982; 106:360–363.
12. Frankenne F, Closset J, Gomez F, et al: The physiology of growth hormones (GHs) in pregnant women and partial characterization of the placental GH variant. *J Clin Endocrinol Metab* 1988; 66:1171–1180.
13. Moore DM, Buckingham MS, Singh MM, et al: Serum-prolactin in female infertility. *Lancet* 1978; 2:1243–1245.
14. Skrabanek P, McDonald D, de Valera E, et al: Plasma prolactin in amenorrhoea, infertility, and other disorders: A retrospective study of 608 patients. *Ir J Med Sci* 1980; 149:236–245.
15. Kredentser JV, Hoskins CF, Scott JZ: Hyperprolactinemia: A significant factor in female infertility. *Am J Obstet Gynecol* 1981; 139:264–267.
16. Evans WS, Cronin MJ, Thorner MO: Hypogonadism in hyperprolactinema: proposed mechanisms, in Ganong WF, Martini L (eds): *Frontiers in Neuroendocrinology*, vol 7. New York, Raven Press, 1982, pp 77–122.
17. McNeilly AS: Prolactin and ovarian function, in Muller EE, MacLeod RM (eds): *Neuroendocrine Perspectives*, vol 3. New York, Elsevier Science Publishers, 1984, pp 279–316.
18. Molitch ME: Management of prolactinomas. *Annu Rev Med* 1989; 40:225–232.
19. Vance ML, Thorner MO: Prolactinomas, in Molitch ME (ed): Pituitary tumors: Diagnosis and management. *Endocrinol Metab Clin North Am* 1987; 16:731–753.
20. Molitch ME, Elton RL, Blackwell RE, et al: Bromocriptine as primary therapy for prolactin-secreting macroadenomas: Results of a prospective multicenter study. *J Clin Endocrinol Metab* 1985; 60:698–705.
21. Molitch ME: Pregnancy and the hyperprolactinemic woman. *N Engl J Med* 1985; 312:1364–1370.
22. Krupp P, Monka C, Richter K: The safety aspects of infertility treatments. Program of the Second World Congress of Gynecology and Obstetrics, Rio de Janeiro, 1988, p 9.
23. Bigazzi M, Ronga R, Lancranjan I, et al: A pregnancy in an acromegalic woman during bromocriptine treatment: Effects on growth hormone and prolactin in the maternal, fetal, and amniotic compartments. *J Clin Endocrinol Metab* 1979; 48:9–12.

24. Divers WA, Yen SSC: Prolactin-producing microadenomas in pregnancy. *Obstet Gynecol* 1983; 62:425–429.

25. Rjosk NK, Fahlbusch R, von Werder K: Influence of pregnancies on prolactinomas. *Acta Endocrinol* 1982; 100:337–346.

26. Rothman KJ, Funch DP, Dreyer NA: Bromocriptine and puerperal seizures. *Epidemiology* 1990, in press.

27. Klibanski S, Biller BMK, Rosenthal DL, et al: Effects of prolactin and estrogen deficiency in amenorrheic bone loss. *J Clin Endocrinol Metab* 1988; 67:124–130.

28. Abu-Fadil S, DeVane G, Siler TM, et al: Effects of oral contraceptive steroids on pituitary prolactin secretion. *Contraception* 1976; 13:79–85.

29. Molitch ME: Clinical features and epidemiology of prolactinomas in women, in Olefsky JM, Robbins RJ (eds): *Prolactinomas* New York, Churchill Livingstone, Inc, 1986, pp 67–95.

30. Gooren LJG, Assies J, Asscheman H, et al: Estrogen-induced prolactinoma in a man. *J Clin Endocrinol Metab* 1988; 66:444–446.

31. Moult PJA, Dacie JE, Rees LH, et al: Oral contraception in patients with hyperprolactinaemia. *Br Med J* 1982; 284:868.

32. Abelove WA, Rupp JJ, Paschkis KE: Acromegaly and pregnancy. *J Clin Endocrinol* 1954; 14:32–44.

33. Finkler RS: Acromegaly and pregnancy, case report. *J Clin Endocrinol* 1954; 14:1245–1246.

34. Luboshitzky R, Dickstein G, Barzilai D: Bromocriptine-induced pregnancy in an acromegalic patient. *JAMA* 1980; 244:584–586.

35. Molitch ME: Acromegaly, in Collu R, Brown GM, Van Loon GR (eds): *Clinical Neuroendocrinology*. Boston, Blackwell Scientific Publications, Inc, 1988, pp 189–227.

36. Baumann G: Acromegaly, in Molitch ME (ed): Pituitary tumors: Diagnosis and management. *Endocrinol Metab Clin North Am* 1987; 16:685–703.

37. Wright AD, Hill DM, Lowy C, et al: Mortality in acromegaly. *Q J Med (NS)* 1970; 153:1–16.

38. Alexander L, Appleton D, Hall R, et al: Epidemiology of acromegaly in the Newcastle region. *Clin Endocrinol* 1980; 12:71–79.

39. Eastman RC, Gorden P, Roth J: Conventional supervoltage irradiation is an effective treatment for acromegaly. *J Clin Endocrinol Metab* 1979; 48:931–940.

40. Moses AC, Molitch ME, Sawin CT, et al: Bromocriptine therapy in acromegaly: Use in patients resistant to conventional therapy and effect on serum levels of somatomedin C. *J Clin Endocrinol Metab* 1982; 53:752–758.

41. Smallridge RC: Thyrotropin-secreting pituitary tumors, in Molitch ME (ed): Pituitary tumors: Diagnosis and management. *Endocrinol Metab Clin North Am* 1987; 16:765–792.

42. Snyder PJ: Gonadotroph cell pituitary adnomas, in Molitch ME (ed): Pituitary tumors: Diagnosis and management. *Endocrinol Metab Clin North Am* 1987; 16:755–764.

43. Klibanski A: Nonsecreting pituitary tumors, in Molitch ME (ed): Pituitary tumors: Diagnosis and management. *Endocrinol Metab Clin North Am* 1987; 16:793–804.

44. Tyson JE, Barnes AC, McKusick VA, et al: Obstetric and gynecologic considerations of dwarfism. *Am J Obstet Gynecol* 1970; 108:688–703.

45. Sheehan HL: Post-partum necrosis of the anterior pituitary. *J Pathol Bacteriol* 1937; 45:189–214.

46. Sheehan HL: Simmonds's disease due to post-partum necrosis of the anterior pituitary. *Q J Med (NS)* 1939; 32:277–309.

47. Sheehan HL, Davis JC: Pituitary necrosis. *Br Med Bull* 1968; 24:59–70.

48. Martin JB, Reichlin S: *Clinical Neuroendocrinology,* ed 2. Philadelphia, FA Davis Co, 1987.

49. Sheehan HL, Summers VK: The syndrome of hypopituitarism. *Q J Med (NS)* 1949; 72:319–362.

50. Lakhdar AA, McLaren EH, Davda NS, et al: Pituitary failure from Sheehan's syndrome in the puerperium. Two case reports. *Br J Obstet Gynaecol* 1987; 94:998–999.

51. Bowers JH, Jubiz W: Pregnancy in a patient with hormone deficiency. *Arch Intern Med* 1974; 133:312–314.

52. Shahmanesh M, Ali Z, Pourmand M, et al: Pituitary function tests in Sheehan's syndrome. *Clin Endocrinol* 1980; 12:303–311.

53. Jialial I, Naidoo C, Norman RJ, et al: Pituitary function in Sheehan's syndrome. *Obstet Gynecol* 1984; 63:15–19.

54. Bakiri F, Benmiloud M, Vallotton MB: Arginine-vasopressin in postpartum panhypopituitarism: Urinary excretion and kidney response to osmolar load. *J Clin Endocrinol Metab* 1984; 58:511–515.

55. Iwasaki Y, Oiso Y, Yamauchi K, et al: Neurohypophyseal function in postpartum hypopituitarism: Impaired plasma vasopressin response to osmotic stimuli. *J Clin Endocrinol Metab* 1989; 68:560–565.

56. Sheehan HL: The neurohypophysis in post-partum hypopituitarism. *J Pathol Bacteriol* 1963; 85:145–169.

57. Whitehead R: The hypothalamus in postpartum hypopituitarism. *J Pathol Bacteriol* 1963; 86:55–67.

58. Miller M, Dalakos T, Moses AM, et al: Recognition of partial defects in antidiuretic hormone secretion. *Ann Intern Med* 1970; 73:721–729.

59. Quencer RM: Lymphocytic adenohypophysitis: Autoimmune disorder of the pituitary gland. *AJNR* 1980; 1:343–345.

60. Asa SL, Bilbao JM, Kovacs K, et al: Lymphocytic hypophysitis of pregnancy resulting in hypopituitarism: A distinct clinicopathologic entity. *Ann Intern Med* 1981; 95:166–171.

61. McGrail KM, Beyerl BD, Black P, et al: Lymphocytic adenohypophysitis of pregnancy with complete recovery. *Neurosurgery* 1987; 20:791–793.

62. McDermott MW, Griesdale DE, Berry K, et al: Lymphocytic adenohypophysitis. *Can J Neurol Sci* 1988; 15:38–43.

63. Cosman F, Post KD, Holub DA, et al: Lymphocytic adenohypophysitis. Report of 3 new cases and review of the literature. *Medicine* 1989; 68:240–256.

64. Zeller JR, Cerletty JM, Rabinovitch RA, et al: Spontaneous regression of a postpartum pituitary mass demonstrated by computed tomography. *Arch Intern Med* 1982; 142:373–374.

65. Leiba S, Schindel B, Weinstein R, et al: Spontaneous postpartum regression of pituitary mass with return of function. *JAMA* 1986; 255:230–232.

66. Molitch ME: The pituitary gland, in Philipp EE, Setchell ME (eds): *Scientific Foundations of Obstetrics and Gynecology,* ed 11. London, Heinemann Medical Books, in press.

67. Davison JM, Vallotton MB, Lindheimer MD: Plasma osmolality and urinary concentration and dilution during and after pregnancy: Evidence that lateral recumbency inhibits maximal urinary concentrating ability. *Br J Obstet Gynaecol* 1981; 88:472–479.

68. Lindheimer MD, Barron WM, Davison JM: Osmoregulation of thirst and vasopressin release in pregnancy. *Am J Physiol* 1989; 257:F159–F169.

69. Durr JA: Diabetes insipidus in pregnancy. *Am J Kidney Dis* 1987; 9:276–283.

70. Verbalis JG, Robinson AG, Moses AM: Postoperative and post-traumatic diabetes insipidus. *Front Horm Res* 1985; 13:247–265.

71. Hime MC, Richardson JA: Diabetes insipidus and pregnancy case report, incidence and review of literature. *Obstet Gynecol Surv* 1978; 33:375–379.

72. Hughes JM, Barron WM, Vance ML: Recurrent diabetes insipidus associated with pregnancy: pathophysiology and therapy. *Obstet Gynecol* 1989; 73:462–464.

73. Campbell JW: Diabetes insipidus and complicated pregnancy. *JAMA* 1980; 243:1744–1746.

74. Burrow GN, Wassenaar W, Robertson GL, et al: DDAVP treatment of diabetes insipidus during pregnancy and post-partum period. *Acta Endocrinol* 1981; 97:23–25.

75. Hawker RW, North WG, Colbert IC, et al: Oxytocin blood levels in two cases of diabetes insipidus. *Br J Obstet Gynaecol* 1987; 74:430–431.

76. Shangold MM, Freeman R, Kumaresan P, et al: Plasma oxytocin concentrations in a pregnant woman with total vasopressin deficiency. *Obstet Gynecol* 1983; 61:662–667.

77. Blotner H, Kunkel: Diabetes insipidus and pregnancy. *N Engl J Med* 1942; 227:287–292.

78. Maranon G: Diabetes insipidus and uterine atony (a case observed over a period of 26 years). *Br Med J* 1947; 15:769–771.

79. Barron WM, Cohen LH, Ulland LA, et al: Transient vasopressin-resistant diabetes insipidus of pregnancy. *N Engl J Med* 1984; 310:442–444.

80. Shah SV, Thakur V: Vasopressinase and diabetes insipidus of pregnancy. *Ann Intern Med* 1988; 109:435–436.

81. Feely J: The physiology of thyroid function in pregnancy. *Postgrad Med J* 1979; 55:336–339.

82. Crooks J, Aboul-Khair SA, Turnbull AC, et al: The incidence of goitre during pregnancy. *Lancet* 1964; 2:334–336.

83. Crooks J, Tulloch MI, Turnbull AC, et al: Comparative incidence of goiter in pregnancy in Iceland and Scotland. *Lancet* 1967; 2:625–627.

84. Levy RP, Newman DM, Rejai LS, et al: The myth of goiter in pregnancy. *Am J Obstet Gynecol* 1980; 137:701–703.

85. Long TJ, Felice ME, Hollingsworth DR: Goiter in pregnant teenagers. *Am J Obstet Gynecol* 1985; 152:670–674.

86. Thomas R, Reid RL: Thyroid disease and reproductive dysfunction: A review. *Obstet Gynecol* 1987; 70:789–798.

87. Vulsma T, Gons MH, deVijlder JJM: Maternal-fetal transfer of thyroxine in congenital hypothyroidism due to a total organification defect or thyroid agenesis. *N Engl J Med* 1989; 321:13–16.

88. Harada K, Hershman JM, Reed AW, et al: Comparison of thyroid stimulators and thyroid hormone concentrations in the sera of pregnant women. *J Clin Endocrinol Metab* 1979; 48:793–797.

89. Komins JI, Snyder PJ, Schwarz RH: Hyperthyroidism in pregnancy. *Obstet Gynecol Surv* 1975; 30:527–539.

90. Dowling JT, Appleton WG, Nicoloff JT: Thyroxine turnover during human pregnancy. *J Clin Endocrinol* 1967; 27:1749–1750.

91. Van der Spuy ZM, Jacobs HS: Management of endocrine disorders in pregnancy. Part 1—Thyroid and parathyroid disease. *Postgrad Med J* 1984; 60:245–252.

92. Salvi M, How J: Pregnancy and autoimmune disorders. *Endocrinol Metab Clin North Am* 1987; 16:431–445.

93. Burrow GN: Thyroid diseases, in Burrow GN, Ferris TF (eds): *Medical Complications During Pregnancy,* ed 3. Philadelphia, WB Saunders Co, 1988, pp 224–253.

94. Montoro M, Mestman JH: Graves' disease and pregnancy. *N Engl J Med* 1981; 305:48.

95. Cooper DS: Antithyroid drugs. *N Engl J Med* 1984; 311:1353–1362.

96. Cooper DS, Goldminz D, Levin AA, et al: Agranulocytosis associated with antithyroid drugs: Effects of patient age and drug dose. *Ann Intern Med* 1983; 98:26–29.

97. Milham S Jr., Elledge W: Maternal methimazole and congenital defects in children. *Teratology* 1972; 5:125–126.

98. Mujtaba Q, Burrow GN: Treatment of hyperthyroidism in pregnancy with propylthiouracil and methimazole. *Obstet Gynecol* 1975; 46:282–286.

99. Momotani N, Ito K, Hamada N, et al: Maternal hyperthyroidism and congenital malformation in the offspring. *Clin Endocrinol* 1984; 20:695–700.

100. Van Dijke CP, Heydendael RJ, De Kleine MJ: Methimazole, carbimazole, and congenital skin defects. *Ann Intern Med* 1987; 106:60–61.

101. Momotani N, Noh J, Oyanagi H, et al: Antithyroid drug therapy for Graves' disease during pregnancy. *N Engl J Med* 1986; 315:24–28.

102. Cheron RG, Kaplan MM, Larsen PR, et al: Neonatal thyroid function after propylthiouracil therapy for maternal Graves' disease. *N Engl J Med* 1981; 304:525–528.

103. Burrow GN, Klatskin EH, Genel M: Intellectual development in children whose mothers received propylthiouracil during pregnancy. *Yale J Biol Med* 1978; 51:151–156.

104. Gladstone GR, Hordof A, Gersony WM: Propranolol administration during pregnancy: Effects on the fetus. *J Pediatr* 1975; 86:962–964.

105. Habib A, McCarthy JS: Effects on the neonate of propranolol administered during pregnancy. *J Pediatr* 1977; 91:808–811.

106. Bullock JL, Harris RE, Young R: Treatment of thyrotoxicosis during pregnancy with propranolol. *Am J Obstet Gynecol* 1975; 121:242–245.

107. Cottrill CM, McAllister RG, Gettes L, et al: Propranolol therapy during pregnancy, labor, and delivery: Evidence for transplacental drug transfer and impaired neonatal drug disposition. *J Pediatr* 1977; 91:812–814.

108. Rubin PC: Beta-blockers in pregnancy. *N Engl J Med* 1981; 305:1323–1326.

109. Fox RE, Marx C, Stark AR: Neonatal effects of maternal nadolol therapy. *Am J Obstet Gynecol* 1985; 152:1045–1046.

110. Eriksson M, Rubenfeld S, Garber AJ, et al: Propranolol does not prevent thyroid storm. *N Engl J Med* 1977; 296:263–264.

111. Senior B, Chernoff HL: Iodide goiter in the newborn. *Pediatrics* 1971; 47:510–515.

112. Linden S, Rich CL: The use of lithium during pregnancy and lactation. *J Clin Psychiatry* 1983; 44:358–361.

113. Stice RC, Grant CS, Gharib H, et al: The management of Graves' disease during pregnancy. *Surg Gynecol Obstet* 1984; 158:157–160.

114. Brodsky JB, Cohen EN, Brown BW, et al: Surgery during pregnancy and fetal outcome. *Am J Obstet Gynecol* 1980; 138:1165–1167.

115. Worley RJ, Crosby WM: Hyperthyroidism during pregnancy. *Am J Obstet Gynecol* 1974; 119:150–155.

116. Pekonen F, Lamberg B-A: Thyrotoxicosis during pregnancy. *Ann Chir Gynaecol* 1978; 67:165–173.

117. Burrow GN: Current concepts: The management of thyrotoxicosis in pregnancy. *N Engl J Med* 1985; 313:562–566.

118. Edwards OM: The management of thyroid disease in pregnancy. *Postgrad Med J* 1979; 55:340–342.

119. Nelson NC, Becker WF: Thyroid crisis. Diagnosis and treatment. *Ann Surg* 1969; 170:263–273.

120. Rosenberg, IN: Thyroid storm. *Pharmacol Ther C* 1976; 1:423–429.

121. Wartofsky L: Thyrotoxic storm, in Ingbar SH, Braverman LE (eds): *The Thyroid,* ed 5. Philadelphia, JB Lippincott Co, 1986, p 974.

122. Molitch ME: Endocrinology, in Molitch ME (ed): *Management of Medical Problems in Surgical Patients.* Philadelphia, FA Davis Co, 1982, pp 151–218.

123. Nabil N, Miner DJ, Amatruda JM: Methimazole: An alternative route of administration. *J Clin Endocrinol Metab* 1982; 54:180–181.

124. Ingbar SH: The thyroid gland, in Wilson JD, Foster DW (eds): *Textbook of Endocrinology,* ed 7. Philadelphia, WB Saunders Co, 1985, pp 682–815.

125. Williams DE, Chopra IJ, Orgiazzi J, et al: Acute effects of corticosteroids on thyroid activity in Graves' disease. *J Clin Endocrinol Metab* 1975; 41:354–361.

126. Grossman W, Robin NI, Johnson LW, et al: Effects of beta blockade on the peripheral manifestations of thyrotoxicosis. *Ann Intern Med* 1971; 74:875–879.

127. Mazzaferri EL, Skillman TG: Thyroid storm. *Arch Intern Med* 1969; 124:684–690.

128. Dillon PT, Baba J, Meloni CR, et al: Reserpine in thyrotoxic crises. *N Engl J Med* 1970; 283:1020–1024.

129. Roti E, Montermini M, Roti S, et al: The effect of diltiazem, a calcium channel-blocking drug, on cardiac rate and rhythm in hyperthyroid patients. *Arch Intern Med* 1988; 148:1919–1921.

130. Larsen PR: Salicylate-induced increases in free triiodothyronine in human serum. *J Clin Invest* 1972; 51:1125–1134.

131. Hoch FR: Synergism between calorigenic effects: L-thyroxine and 2,4 dinitrophenol or sodium salicylate in euthyroid rats. *Endocrinology* 1965; 76:335–341.

132. Newmark SR, Himathongkam T, Shane JM: Hyperthyroid crisis. *JAMA* 1974; 230:592–593; 1975; 233:508–509 (letters).

133. Cavalieri RR, Sung LC, Becker CE: Effects of phenobarbital on thyroxine and triiodothyronine kinetics in Graves' disease. *J Clin Endocrinol Metab* 1973; 37:308–316.

134. Dozeman R, Kaiser FE, Cass O, et al: Hyperthyroidism appearing as hyperemesis gravidarum. *Arch Intern Med* 1983; 143:2202–2203.

135. Jeffcoate WJ, Bain C: Recurrent pregnancy-induced thyrotoxicosis presenting as hyperemesis gravidarum. Case report. *Br J Obstet Gynaecol* 1985; 92:413–415.

136. Lao TT, Chin RKH, Chang AMZ: The outcome of hyperemetic pregnancies complicated by transient hyperthyroidism. *Aust NZ J Obstet Gynaecol* 1987; 27:99–101.

137. Swaminathan R, Chin RK, Lao TTH, et al: Thyroid function in hyperemesis gravidarum. *Acta Endocrinol* 1989; 120:155–160.

138. Hollingsworth DR: Endocrine disorders of pregnancy, in Creasy RK, Resnik R (eds): *Maternal-Fetal Medicine: Principles and Practice,* ed 2. Philadelphia, WB Saunders Co, 1989, 989–1031.

139. Munro DS, Dirmikis SM, Humphries H, et al: The role of thyroid stimulating im-

munoglobulins of Graves' disease in neonatal thyrotoxicosis. *Br J Obstet Gynaecol* 1978; 85:837–843.

140. Matsuura N, Fujieda K, Yasuhiro I, et al: TSH-receptor antibodies in mothers with Graves' disease and outcome in their offspring. *Lancet* 1988; 1:14–18.

141. Cove DH, Johnston P: Fetal hyperthyroidism: Experience of treatment in four siblings. *Lancet* 1985; 1:430–432.

142. Rumble WF, Aamodt RL, Jones AE, et al: Case reports: Accidental ingestion of Tc-99m in breast milk by a 10-week old child. *J Nucl Med* 1978; 19:913–915.

143. Low LCK, Lang J, Alexander WD: Excretion of carbimazole and propylthiouracil in breast milk. *Lancet* 1979; 2:1011.

144. Kampmann JP, Johansen K, Hansen JM, et al: Propylthiouracil in human milk. *Lancet* 1980; 1:736–737.

145. Lamberg BA, Ikonen E, Osterlund K, et al: Antithyroid treatment of maternal hyperthyroidism during lactation. *Clin Endocrinol* 1984; 21:81–87.

146. Cooper DS: Antithyroid drugs: To breastfeed or not to breast-feed. *Am J Obstet Gynecol* 1987; 157:234–235.

147. Higgins HP, Hershman JM, Kenimer JG, et al: The thyrotoxicosis of hydatidiform mole. *Ann Intern Med* 1975; 83:307–311.

148. Hershman JM: Hyperthyroidism caused by trophoblastic tumors. *Thyroid Today* 1981; 4:1–5.

149. Rajatanavin R, Chailurkit LO, Srisupandit S, et al: Trophoblastic hyperthyroidism: Clinical and biochemical features of five cases. *Am J Med* 1988; 85:237–241.

150. Montoro M, Collea JV, Frasier SD, et al: Successful outcome of pregnancy in women with hypothyroidism. *Ann Intern Med* 1981; 94:31–34.

151. Davis LE, Leveno KJ, Cunningham FG: Hypothyroidism complicating pregnancy. *Obstet Gynecol* 1988; 72:108–112.

152. Richmand D, Molitch ME, O'Donnell TF: Altered thyroid hormone levels in bacterial sepsis: The role of nutritional adequacy. *Metabolism* 1980; 29:936–942.

153. Weinberg AD, Brennan MD, Gorman CA, et al: Outcome of anesthesia and surgery in hypothyroid patients. *Arch Intern Med* 1983; 143:893–897.

154. Ladenson PW, Levin AN, Ridgway EC, et al: Complications of surgery in hypothyroid patients. *Am J Med* 1984; 77:261–266.

155. Jackson IMD, Cobb WE: Why does anyone still use desicated thyroid USP? *Am J Med* 1978; 64:284–288.

156. Wenzel KW, Kirschsieper HE: Aspects of the absorption of oral *l*-thyroxine in normal man. *Metabolism* 1977; 26:1–8.

157. Amino N, Mori H, Iwatani Y, et al: High prevalence of transient postpartum thyrotoxicosis and hypothyroidism. *N Engl J Med* 1982; 306:849–852.

158. Nikolai TF, Turney SL, Roberts RC: Postpartum lymphocytic thyroiditis: Prevalence, clinical course, and long-term follow-up. *Arch Intern Med* 1987; 147:221–224.

159. Jansson R, Dahlberg PA, Karlsson A: Postpartum thyroid dysfunction. *Scand J Clin Lab Invest* 1984; 44:371–375.

160. Schneider AB, Shore-Freedman E, Ryo UY, et al: Radiation-induced tumors of the head and neck following childhood irradiation. *Medicine* 1985; 64:1–15.

161. Molitch ME, Beck JR, Dreisman M, et al: The cold thyroid nodule: An analysis of diagnostic and therapeutic options. *Endocr Rev* 1984; 5:185–199.

162. Mazzaferri EL: Papillary and follicular thyroid cancer: A selective approach to diagnosis and treatment. *Annu Rev Med* 1981; 32:73–91.

163. Hill CS Jr., Clark RL, Wolf M: The effect of subsequent pregnancy on patients with thyroid carcinoma. *Surg Gynecol Obstet* 1966; 122:1219–1222.

164. Carr BR, Parker CR Jr, Madden JD, et al: Maternal plasma adrenocorticotropin and cortisol relationships throughout human pregnancy. *Am J Obstet Gynecol* 1981; 139:416–422.

165. DeMoor P, Steeno O, Brosens I, et al: Data on transcortin activity in human plasma as studied by gel filtration. *J Clin Endocrinol* 1966; 26:71–78.

166. Doe RP, Dickinson P, Zinneman HH, et al: Elevated nonprotein-bound cortisol (NPC) in pregnancy, during estrogen administration and in carcinoma of the prostate. *J Clin Endocrinol* 1969; 29:757–766.

167. Nolten WE, Lindheimer MD, Rueckert PA, et al: Diurnal patterns and regulation

of cortisol secretion in pregnancy. *J Clin Endocrinol Metab* 1980; 51:466–472.

168. Murphy BE: Clinical evaluation of urinary cortisol determinations by competitive protein-binding radioassay. *J Clin Endocrinol* 1968; 28:343–348.

169. Cohen M, Stiefel M, Reddy WJ, et al: The secretion and disposition of cortisol during pregnancy. *J Clin Endocrinol* 1958; 18:1076–1092.

170. Migeon CJ, Kenny FM, Taylor FH: Cortisol production rate. VIII. Pregnancy. *J Clin Endocrinol* 1968; 28:661–666.

171. Beitins IZ, Bayard F, Anges IG, et al: The metabolic clearance rate, blood production, interconversion and transplacental passage of cortisol and cortisone in pregnancy near term. *Pediatr Res* 1973; 7:509–519.

172. Rees LH, Burke CW, Chard T, et al: Possible placental origin of ACTH in normal human pregnancy. *Nature* 1975; 254:620–622.

173. Genazzani AR, Felber JP, Fioretti P: Immunoreactice ACTH, immunoreactive human chorionic somatomammotrophin (HCS) and 11-OH steroids plasma levels in normal and pathological pregnancies. *Acta Endocrinol* 1977; 83:800–810.

174. Allen JP, Cook DM, Kendall JW, et al: Maternal-fetal ACTH relationship in man. *J Clin Endocrinol Metab* 1973; 37:230–234.

175. Aron DC, Findling JW, Tyrrell JB: Cushing's disease, in Molitch ME (ed): Pituitary tumors: Diagnosis and management. *Endocrinol Metab Clin North Am* 1987; 16:705–730.

176. Bevan JS, Gough MH, Gillmer MDG, et al: Cushing's syndrome in pregnancy: The timing of definitive treatment. *Clin Endocrinol* 1987; 27:225–233.

177. Casson IF, Davis JC, Jeffreys RV, et al: Successful management of Cushing's disease during pregnancy by transsphenoidal adenectomy. *Clin Endocrinol* 1987; 27:423–428.

177a. Aron DC, Schnall AM, Sheeler LR: Cushing's syndrome and pregnancy. *Am J Obstet Gynecol* 1990; 162:244–252.

178. Streeten DHP, Stevenson CT, Dalakos TG, et al: The diagnosis of hypercortisolism. Biochemical criteria differentiating patients from lean and obese normal subjects and from females on oral contraceptives. *J Clin Endocrinol* 1969; 29:1191–1211.

179. Gormley MJJ, Hadden DR, Kennedy TL, et al: Cushing's syndrome in pregnancy—treatment with metyrapone. *Clin Endocrinol* 1982; 16:283–293.

180. Connell JMC, Cordiner J, Davies DL, et al: Pregnancy complicated by Cushing's syndrome: Potential hazard of metyrapone therapy. Case report. *Br J Obstet Gynaecol* 1985; 92:1192–1195.

181. Koerten JM, Morales WJ, Washington SR, et al: Cushing's syndrome in pregnancy: A case report and literature review. *Am J Obstet Gynecol* 1986; 154:626–628.

182. Barasch E, Sztern M, Spinrad S, et al: Pregnancy and Cushing's syndrome: Example of endocrine interaction. *Isr J Med Sci* 1988; 24:101–104.

183. Semple CG, McEwan H, Teasdale GM, et al: Recurrence of Cushing's disease in pregnancy. Case report. *Br J Obstet Gynaecol* 1985; 92:295–298.

184. Abrams HL, Siegelman SS, Adams DF, et al: Computed tomography versus ultrasound of the adrenal gland: A prospective study. *Radiology* 1982; 143:121–128.

185. Kreines K, DeVaux WD: Neonatal adrenal insufficiency associated with maternal Cushing's syndrome. *Pediatrics* 1971; 47:516–519.

186. Mazor M, Leiberman JR, Korenblum R, et al: Pregnancy complicated by Cushing's syndrome. *Arch Gynecol Obstet* 1987; 241:191–193.

187. Lee R, Rapoport A: Cushing's syndrome with amelioration during pregnancy. *JAMA* 1972; 221:392–396.

188. Liu L, Jaffe R, Borowski GD, et al: Exacerbation of Cushing's disease during pregnancy. *Am J Obstet Gynecol* 1983; 145:110–111.

189. Schteingart DE: Cushing's syndrome. *Endocrinol Metab Clin North Am* 1989; 18:311–338.

190. Xarli VP, Steele AA, Davis PJ, et al: Adrenal hemorrhage in the adult. *Medicine* 1978; 57:211–221.

191. Portnay GI, Vagenakis AG, Braverman LE, et al: Anticoagulant therapy and acute adrenal insufficiency. *Ann Intern Med* 1974; 81:115.

192. Brent F: Addison's disease and pregnancy.

Am J Surg 1950; 79:645–652.

193. O'Shaughnessy RW, Hackett KJ: Maternal Addison's disease and fetal growth retardation. *J Reprod Med* 1984; 29:752–756.

194. Drucker D, Shumak S, Angel A: Schmidt's syndrome presenting with intrauterine growth retardation and postpartum Addisonian crisis. *Am J Obstet Gynecol* 1984; 149:229–230.

195. Van der Spuy ZM, Jacobs HS: Management of endocrine disorders in pregnancy. Part II—Pituitary, ovarian and adrenal disease. *Postgrad Med J* 1984; 60:312–320.

196. Graber AL, Ney RL, Nicholson WE, et al: Natural history of pituitary-adrenal recovery following long-term suppression with corticosteroids. *J Clin Endocrinol Metab* 1965; 25:11–16.

197. Bongiovanni AM, McPadden AJ: Steroids during pregnancy and possible fetal consequences. *Fertil Steril* 1960; 11:181–186.

198. Turner ES, Greenberger PA, Patterson R: Management of the pregnant asthmatic patient. *Ann Intern Med* 1980; 93:905–918.

199. Beitins IZ, Bayard F, Ances IG, et al: The transplacental passage of prednisone and prednisolone in pregnancy near term. *J Pediatr* 1972; 81:936–945.

200. Kenny FM, Preeyasombat C, Spaulding JS, et al: Cortisol production rate: IV. Infants born of steroid-treated mothers and of diabetic mothers. Infants with trisomy syndrome and with anencaphaly. *Pediatrics* 1966; 37:960–966.

201. McKenzie SA, Selly JA, Agnew JE: Secretion of prednisolone into breast milk. *Arch Dis Child* 1975; 50:894–896.

202. Speroff L: The adrenogenital syndrome and its obstetrical aspects. *Obstet Gynecol Surv* 1965; 20:185–214.

203. Klingensmith GJ, Garcia SC, Jones HW Jr., et al: Glucocorticoid treatment of girls with congenital adrenal hyperplasia: Effects on height, sexual maturation, and fertility. *J Pediatr* 1977; 90:996–1004.

204. Pang S, Pollack MS, Marshall RN, et al: Prenatal treatment of congenital adrenal hyperplasia due to 21-hydroxylase deficiency. *N Engl J Med* 1990; 322:111–115.

205. Aoi W, Doi Y, Tasaki S, et al: Primary aldosteronism during peripartum period. *Jpn Heart J* 1978; 19:946–978.

206. Logering FK, Derkx FMH, Wallenburg HCS: Primary aldosteronism in pregnancy. *Am J Obstet Gynecol* 1986; 155:986–988.

207. Tremblay RR: Treatment of hirsutism with spironolactone. *Clin Endocrinol Metab* 1986; 15:363–371.

208. DeFronzo RA: Hyperkalemia and hyporeninemic hypoaldosteronism. *Kidney Int* 1980; 17:118–134.

209. Manger WM, Gifford RW Jr: *Pheochromocytoma.* New York, Springer-Verlag, 1977.

210. Cross DA, Meyer JS: Postoperative deaths due to unsuspected pheochromocytoma. *South Med J* 1977; 70:1320.

211. Valk TW, Frager MS, Gross MD et al: Spectrum of pheochromocytoma in multiple endocrine neoplasia. *Ann Intern Med* 1981; 94:762–767.

212. Shapiro B, Fig LM: Management of pheochromocytoma. *Endocrinol Metab Clinics North Am* 1989; 16:443–481.

213. Zuspan FP: Adrenal gland and sympathetic nervous system response in eclampsia. *Am J Obstet Gynecol* 1972; 114:304–311.

214. Schenker JG, Chowers I: Pheochromocytoma and pregnancy. *Obstet Gynecol Surv* 1971; 26:739–747.

215. Schenker JG, Granat M: Phaeochromocytoma and pregnancy—an updated appraisal. *Aust NZ J Obstet Gynaecol* 1902; 22:1–10.

216. Thiery M, Deromy RMJ, van Kets HE, et al: Pheochromocytoma in pregnancy. *Am J Obstet Gynecol* 1967; 97:21–29.

217. Griffith MI, Felts JH, James FM, et al: Successful control of pheochromocytoma in pregnancy. *JAMA* 1974; 229:437–439.

218. Devoe LD, O'Dell BE, Castillo RA, et al: Metastatic pheochromocytoma in pregnancy and fetal biophysical assessment after maternal administration of alpha-adrenergic, beta-adrenergic, and dopamine antagonists. *Obstet Gynecol* 1986; 68:155–185.

219. Fudge TL, McKinnon WMP, Geary WL: Current surgical management of pheochromocytoma during pregnancy. *Arch Surg* 1980; 115:1224–1225.

220. Leak D, Carroll JJ, Robinson DC, et al: Management of pheochromocytoma during pregnancy. *Can Med Assoc J* 1977; 116:371–375.

221. Burgess III: Alpha blockade and surgical

intervention of pheochromocytoma in pregnancy. *Obstet Gynecol* 1979; 53:266–270.

222. Pitkin RM: Calcium metabolism in pregnancy and the perinatal period: A review. *Am J Obstet Gynecol* 1985; 151:99–109.

223. Maikranz P, Holley JL, Parks JH, et al: Gestational hypercalciuria causes pathological urine calcium oxalate supersaturations. *Kidney Int* 1989; 36:108–113.

224. Pitkin RM, Reynolds WA, Williams GA, et al: Calcium metabolism in normal pregnancy. A longitudinal study. *Am J Obstet Gynecol* 1979; 133:781–787.

225. Bouillon R, van Assche FA, van Baelen H, et al: Influence of the vitamin D-binding protein on the serum concentration of 1,25-dihydroxyvitamin D_3. Significance of the free 1,25-dihydroxyvitamin D_3 concentration. *J Clin Invest* 1981; 67:589–596.

226. Gray TK, Lowe W, Lester GE: Vitamin D and pregnancy: the maternal-fetal metabolism of vitamin D. *Endocr Rev* 1981; 2:264–274.

227. Rush D, Johnstone FD, King JC: Nutrition and pregnancy, in Burrow GN, Ferris TF (eds): *Medical Complications During Pregnancy,* ed 3. Philadelphia, WB Saunders Co, 1988, pp 117–135.

228. Salem R, Taylor S: Hyperparathyroidism in pregnancy. *Br J Surg* 1979; 66:648–650.

229. Boonstra CE, Jackson CE: Serum calcium survey for hyperparathyroidism. Results in 50,000 clinical patients. *Am J Clin Pathol* 1971; 55:523–526.

230. Christensson T, Hellstrom K, Wengle B: Hypercalcemia and primary hyperparathyroidism. *Arch Intern Med* 1977; 136:1138–1142.

231. Bilezikian JP: Etiologies and therapy of hypercalcemia. *Endocrinol Metab Clin North Am* 1989; 18:389–414.

232. Croom RD, Thomas CG: Primary hyperparathyroidism during pregnancy. *Surgery* 1984; 96:1109–1117.

233. Rajala B, Abbasi RA, Hutchinson HT, et al: Acute pancreatitis and primary hyperparathyroidism in pregnancy: Treatment of hypercalcemia with magnesium sulfate. *Obstet Gynecol* 1987; 70:460–462.

234. Shangold MM, Dor N, Welt SI, et al: Hyperparathyroidism and pregnancy: A review. *Obstet Gynecol Surv* 1982; 37:217–228.

235. Matthias GSH, Helliwell TR, Williams A: Postpartum hyperparathyroid crisis. Case report. *Br J Obstet Gynaecol* 1987; 94:807–810.

236. Ludwig GD: Hyperparathyroidism in relation to pregnancy. *N Engl J Med* 1962; 267:637–642.

237. Delmonico FL, Neel RM, Cosimi AB, et al: Hyperparathyroidism during pregnancy. *Am J Surg* 1976; 131:328–337.

238. Mansberger JA, Mansberger AR Jr: Hyperparathyroidism and pregnancy. Case report and therapy update. *J Med Assoc Ga* 1988; 77:309–312.

239. Montoro MN, Collea JV, Mestman JH: Management of hyperparathyroidism in pregnancy with oral phosphate therapy. *Obstet Gynecol* 1980; 55:431–434.

240. Patterson R: Hyperparathyroidism in pregnancy. *Obstet Gynecol* 1987; 70:457–460.

241. Suki WN, Yium JJ, von Minden M, et al: Acute treatment of hypercalcemia with furosemide. *N Engl J Med* 1970; 283:836–840.

242. Ralston SH, Gardner MD, Dryburgh FJ, et al: Comparison of aminodyroxypropylidene diphosphonate, mithramycin, and corticosteroids/calcitonin in treatment of cancer-associated hypercalcaemia. *Lancet* 1985; 2:907–910.

243. Wisneski LA, Croom WP, Silva OL, et al: Salmon calcitonin in hypercalcemia. *Clin Pharmacol Ther* 1978; 24:219–222.

244. Aceto T Jr, Batt RE, Bruck E, et al: Intrauterine hyperparathyroidism: A complication of untreated maternal hypoparathyroidism. *J Clin Endocrinol Metab* 1966; 26:487–492.

245. Glass EJ, Barr DGD: Transient neonatal hyperparathyroidism secondary to maternal pseudohypoparathyroidism. *Arch Dis Child* 1981; 56:565–568.

246. Sadeghi-Nejad A, Wolfsdorf JI, Senior B: Hypoparathyroidism and pregnancy treatment with calcitriol. *JAMA* 1980; 243:254–255.

247. Salle BL, Berthezene F, Glorieux FH, et al: Hypoparathyroidism during pregnancy: treatment with calcitriol. *J Clin Endocrinol Metab* 1981; 52:810–813.

248. Marx SJ, Swart EG Jr, Hamstra AJ, et al: Normal intrauterine development of the

fetus of a woman receiving extraordinarily high doses of 1,25-dihydroxyvitamin D. *J Clin Endocrinol Metab* 1980; 51:1138–1142.

249. Cundy T, Haining SA, Guilland-Cumming DF, et al: Remission of hypoparathyroidism during lactation: Evidence for a physiological role for prolactin in the regulation of vitamin D metabolism. *Clin Endocrinol* 1987; 26:667–674.

250. Thiede MA, Rodan GA: Expression of a calcium-mobilizing parathyroid hormone-like peptide in lactating mammary tissue. *Science* 1988; 242:278–280.

251. National Institutes of Health Consensus Development Conference Statement: Health implications of obesity. *Ann Intern Med* 1985; 103:147–151.

252. Bray GA: *The Obese Patient*. Philadelphia, WB Saunders Co, 1976.

253. Messerli FH: Cardiovascular effects of obesity and hypertension. *Lancet* 1982; 2:1165–1168.

254. Pasulka PS, Bistrian BR, Benotti PN, et al: The risks of surgery in obese patients. *Ann Intern Med* 1986; 104:540–546.

255. Rochester DF, Enson Y: Current concepts in the pathogenesis of the obesity hypoventilation syndrome. *Am J Med* 1974; 57:402–420.

256. Vaughan RW, Conahan TJ III: Cardio-

pulmonary consequences of morbid obesity. *Life Sci* 1980; 26:2119–2127.

257. Vaughan RW, Engelhardt RC, Wise L: Postoperative hypoxemia in obese patients. *Ann Surg* 1976; 180:877–882.

258. Walsh RE, Michaelson ED, Harkleroad LE, et al: Upper airway obstruction in obese patients with sleep disturbance and somnolence. *Ann Intern Med* 1972; 76:185–192.

259. Kryger M, Quesney LF, Holder D, et al: The sleep deprivation syndrome of the obese patient. A problem of periodic nocturnal upper airway obstruction. *Am J Med* 1974; 56:531–539.

260. Calandra C, Abell DA, Beischer NA: Maternal obesity in pregnancy. *Obstet Gynecol* 1981; 57:8–12.

261. Edwards LE, Dickes WF, Alton IR, et al: Pregnancy in the massively obese: Course, outcome, and obesity prognosis of the infant. *Am J Obstet Gynecol* 1978; 131:479–483.

262. Garbaciak JA, Richter M, Miller S, et al: Maternal weight and pregnancy complications. *Am J Obstet Gynecol* 1985; 152:238–245.

263. Kliegman RM, Gross T: Perinatal problems of the obese mother and her infant. *Obstet Gynecol* 1985; 66:299–306.

CHAPTER 5

Heart Disease

Roberto M. Lang

Kenneth M. Borow

The maternal cardiovascular system undergoes extensive changes during pregnancy. While these result in an increased hemodynamic burden for healthy women, they are especially important in women with underlying cardiac disease.[1-3] In recent years the relative frequency of rheumatic and congenital heart disease in women of childbearing age has undergone a significant change.[4, 5] Although the incidence of rheumatic heart disease has declined, the number of patients with congenital heart disease who have had corrective surgery and are now reaching childbearing age has increased.[6]

HEMODYNAMIC CHANGES DURING PREGNANCY

In order to understand the importance of cardiac disease during pregnancy, it is necessary to be familiar with the normal cardiovascular physiology of pregnancy. The hemodynamic changes associated with pregnancy have been ascribed to numerous factors including (a) the low resistance shunt created by the placenta, (b) decreased resistance in the peripheral vasculature created by the vasodilatory hormones, and (c) water and sodium retention.[1-3, 7, 8] The net result is a complex interaction between ventricular heart rate,

contractile state, preload, and afterload that can result in highly variable effects on overall left ventricular performance (Table 5–1).

Cardiorespiratory Physical Examination

Upon auscultation, the first heart sound is increased in intensity and is often widely split[1, 9, 10] (Fig 5–1). After the first 30 weeks of pregnancy, there is a tendency for a decrease in the splitting interval between aortic and pulmonic components of the second heart sound with inspiration. By the 20th week, 84% of women with normal pregnancies have a third heart sound.[9] Two types of innocent systolic murmurs can be heard in healthy pregnant women: (a) a pulmonary midsystolic murmur loudest at the left upper sternal border which is present in up to 96% of pregnant women and represents audible vibrations caused by right ventricular ejection of blood into the pulmonary trunk, and (b) a supraclavicular systolic murmur which originates in the brachiocephalic arteries at their point of branching from the aortic arch. The most common continuous murmur is the suprasternal or upper sternal venous hum which promptly vanishes with compression of the ipsilateral deep jugular vein. Another continuous murmur sometimes heard is the systolic mammary souffle murmur which is best heard

TABLE 5–1.

Definitions of the Determinants of Left Ventricular
Performance

Contractility:
  Chemical and mechanical processes within the
    myocardium that lead to force generation and fi-
    ber shortening
Preload:
  Maximal force exerted on myocardial fibers at end
    diastole approximated by left ventricular end-dia-
    stolic dimension or volume
Afterload:
  Force opposing left ventricular fiber shortening dur-
    ing ventricular systole (i.e., force opposing ejec-
    tion of blood from the ventricle)

over the breasts late in pregnancy and in the
postpartum period in lactating women. This
murmur is loudest over the second or third
left or right intercostal spaces bilaterally.[11]
On occasion, only a systolic component is audible. The hyperdynamic state associated with
pregnancy also alters the physical signs of
heart disease. In mitral and aortic stenosis
this leads to amplification of murmurs that
might not have been heard before pregnancy.
On the other hand, murmurs associated with
mitral and aortic regurgitation may become
less noticeable during pregnancy due to the

fall in systemic vascular resistance that occurs, at least in part, due to the placenta.[12]

Pedal edema is a normal occurrence in
pregnancy, occurring in 50% to 80% of
healthy gravid women.[1, 7, 13] The frequency of
pedal edema increases with maternal age, especially after the age of 30. Dependent edema
is probably a natural consequence of the increase in body water and total exchangeable
sodium in addition to partial inferior vena
caval compression caused by the gravid uterus.
In general, asymptomatic normotensive gravidas require no drug treatment and pedal
edema improves with rest in lateral recumbency and elevation of the feet.

Cardiac Output

The most important change in cardiovascular hemodynamics during pregnancy is
a 30% to 50% increase in cardiac output above
the resting nonpregnancy values.[1–3, 14–16] This
increase in cardiac output, which begins early
in pregnancy, reaches its peak by the midportion of the second trimester and thereafter
remains relatively constant throughout the rest
of pregnancy[14–16] (Fig 5–2).

Investigators previously reported decre-

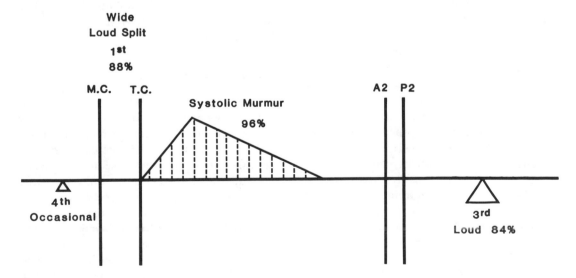

FIG 5–1.
Auscultatory findings during pregnancy. (From Cutforth R, MacDonald CB: *Am Heart J* 1966; 71:741–747. Used
with permission.)

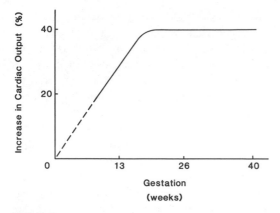

FIG 5–2.
Changes in cardiac output during pregnancy. Note that cardiac output is considerably increased by the end of the first trimester, and the increase is maintained until term. (From DeSwiet M: The cardiovascular system, in Hytten FE, Chamberlain GVP (eds): *Clinical Physiology in Obstetrics.* Oxford, England Blackwell Scientific Publications, 1980, pp 3–42. Used with permission.)

ments in cardiac output starting at about the 28th gestational week, but these declines are currently considered to have been posturally induced.[3] Some investigators, however, continue to report a fall in cardiac output near term.[2] In general, cardiac output values are higher when the pregnant woman is in a left lateral rather than supine position. This is especially true during the latter part of pregnancy due to compression of the inferior vena cava by the uterus when the patient is in the supine position.[17, 18] The resultant decrease in systemic venous return can reduce cardiac output by 25% to 30%. In less than 10% of pregnant women (i.e., those with a strong tendency toward vasovagal reactions) the interference of both arterial and venous flow with the patient in the supine position may lead to a decrease in heart rate and blood pressures with consequent lightheadedness, nausea, and dizziness or even syncope. This "supine hypotensive syndrome of pregnancy" is promptly relieved when the supine position is abandoned[19, 20] and the uterus moves anterolaterally relative to the inferior vena cava.[19, 20]

The changes in cardiac output begin very early in pregnancy, occurring in parallel with changes in body temperature, fat storage, res-

piration, and osmolality. The early increase in cardiac output apparently results from increases in heart rate and ventricular performance together with a reduction in peripheral vascular resistance.[14, 16] Heart rate increases further during the second trimester during which left atrial and left ventricular end-diastolic dimensions increase, thereby suggesting an increase in venous return.[16]

Recently, the advent of echocardiography in conjunction with Doppler ultrasound has provided a unique noninvasive technique for reproducible accurate and serial measurements of cardiac output during pregnancy.[14, 16] If this method is applied systematically and the sources of error understood, there seems little doubt that this technique will become increasingly useful in clinical obstetric practice, not only in the investigation of normal cardiovascular adaptations but also in the assessment of hemodynamic changes in patients with cardiac disease and hypertension.

Heart Rate

Heart rate rises during pregnancy with a mean increase of about 10% to 20% relative to prepregnancy values. At term, mean heart rate generally varies from 80 to 90 beats per minute[2, 3, 21, 22] (Fig 5–3). The pulse is fastest in the sitting position.

Systemic Blood Pressure

Most studies have shown a slight fall in systolic blood pressure in association with a considerable decrease in diastolic blood pressure (see also Chap. 1).[1, 3, 22, 23] These changes are associated with a decrease in mean aortic pressure and widening of the pulse pressure. Systemic vascular resistance falls during pregnancy reflecting the increased cardiac output, the decreased mean aortic pressure, and in mid- and late gestation, the creation of a low-resistance circulation in the gravid uterus.[16] It is also likely that these changes in systemic vascular resistance are coupled to hormonal activity. Women whose systemic

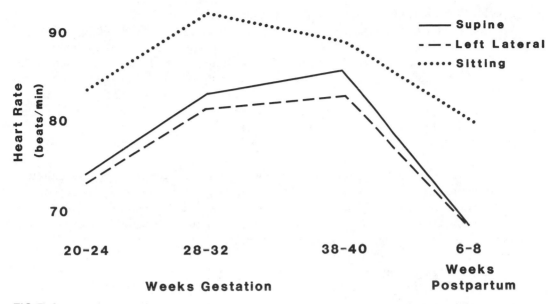

FIG 5–3.
The effects of gestational age and maternal posture on maternal heart rate. (From Lund CJ, Donovan JC: *Am J Obstet Gynecol* 1967; 98:393–403. Used with permission.)

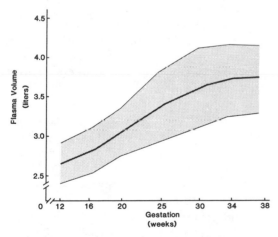

FIG 5–4.
Mean (±SD) plasma volume in normal pregnancy. (From Pirani BBK, Campbell DM, MacGillivary I: *J Obstet Gynaecol Br Commw* 1973; 80:884. Used with permission.)

blood pressure fails to fall during early gestation or whose diastolic levels remain about 70 mm Hg are thought to be more prone to develop systemic hypertension in the third trimester.

Blood Volume

Plasma volume increments start in the first trimester, accelerate in the second trimester, and peak near gestational week 32 at a level 40% above prepregnant values.[24, 25] Thereafter, blood volume remains stable until term. The increase in volume results in part from a 20% to 40% increase in the number of erythrocytes, but a larger factor is the expansion of plasma volume, which increases by 50% by week 32 (Fig 5–4).[24] The difference in red cell and plasma volume changes accounts for the relative anemia seen in normal pregnancy. The extent to which blood volume increases appears to be proportional to the size of the products of conception.

Left Ventricular Contractility

Whether the hormonal changes that occur during pregnancy augment myocardial contractility remains to date conjectural. Assessment of left ventricular (LV) contractility during pregnancy has resulted in conflicting data mainly due to the fact that the commonly used ejection phase indices (e.g., cardiac output, ejection fraction) are highly dependent upon LV loading conditions. These load-dependent indices reflect overall LV performance which is the net result of the interplay between preload, afterload, heart rate, and LV contractility.[14, 16, 26]

During pregnancy, the combination of decreased afterload, increased preload, and augmented heart rate results in increased overall LV performance (e.g., cardiac output) (Fig 5–5). Echocardiographic studies performed serially during pregnancy show an increase in the velocity of LV circumferential fiber shortening while systolic time intervals show a decrease in the preejection period and an increase in the LV ejection time.[27, 28] These latter findings are consistent with augmented LV stroke volume and increased ventricular preload as well as a possible increase in LV contractile state.

Response to Exercise

Exercise has numerous effects on the pregnant woman, the developing fetus, and the placenta. The normal exercise-induced fall in systemic vascular resistance still occurs; however, its magnitude may be somewhat blunted.[29] Light-to-moderate exercise during uncomplicated pregnancy provokes an appropriate increase in cardiac output and ox-

ygen consumption.[30] However, the cardiac output for any given level of exercise is increased during pregnancy compared with the prepregnant state. The relative increase in cardiac output exceeds that of the oxygen consumption and thus the arteriovenous oxygen difference at each work load is lower during pregnancy.[31]

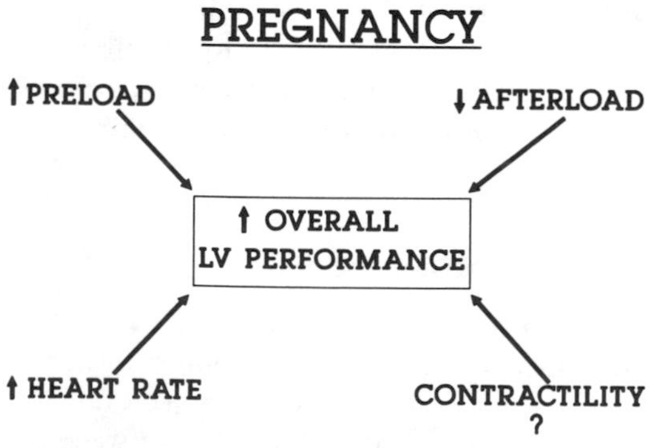

It is not clear whether any of these hemodynamic changes are detrimental to the mother and/or fetus, but they suggest that maternal cardiac reserve is lowered during pregnancy and that shunting of blood flow away from the pregnant uterus may occur during and after exercise.[32]

Effects of Labor and Delivery

During vaginal delivery in a lightly sedated patient it has been reported that 300 to 500 cc of blood are squeezed out of the uterus and into the maternal circulation during each uterine contraction, resulting in an effective "autotransfusion."[33–37] This leads to a 15% to 20% increase in cardiac output and a 10% increase in mean systemic arterial pressure (Fig 5–6). Reflex bradycardia due to baroreceptor stimulation may occur.[1, 21, 33–37] This acute preload stress is well tolerated by the normal heart but may represent the deciding physiologic stress in a diseased heart that has become increasingly compromised during pregnancy and labor.

Maternal pain and anxiety may result in increased sympathetic stimulation with a rise in blood pressure and heart rate during the second stage of labor. Maternal blood loss from a vaginal delivery is usually 300 to 400 mL while a cesarean section may result in a 500- to 800-mL loss. Cesarean sections are often performed in order to avoid the cyclic hemodynamic alterations associated with labor. Nevertheless, it should be kept in mind that maternal hemodynamics during cesarean section are affected by the type of anesthesia employed.[38, 39] Abrupt reduction in preload may be seen following institution of spinal anesthesia (with concomitant sympathetic blockade) in a patient not hydrated ade-

PREGNANCY

↑ PRELOAD   ↓ AFTERLOAD

┌─────────────────┐
│   ↑ OVERALL   │
│ LV PERFORMANCE │
└─────────────────┘

↑ HEART RATE   CONTRACTILITY
                              ?

FIG 5–5.
Effect of loading conditions on overall left ventricular (LV) performance.

quately prior to the procedure. Epidural anesthesia, however, if instituted slowly and with proper prehydration, can provide quite stable hemodynamics. General anesthesia may be the technique of choice in patients with severe preload-dependent lesions. However, general anesthesia may result in myocardial depression and/or hypertension during intubation and extubation if anesthesia is inadequate. The potent volatile anesthetic agents may also cause myocardial depression.

Postpartum Hemodynamics

In the immediate postdelivery period, cardiac output may increase as much as 10% to 20% above predelivery levels due to the relief of inferior vena caval compression by the gravid uterus.[34, 36, 37, 40] At this time a relative bradycardia is common. Subsequently, resting cardiac output progressively falls to baseline levels. By 4 to 6 weeks after delivery, maternal hemodynamics have returned to their pregravid values.

Noninvasive Cardiac Tests

Most diagnostic cardiac testing performed during pregnancy should utilize noninvasive techniques that do not require ionizing radiation. Nuclear studies have little place in the diagnosis of pregnant patients with valvular or coronary heart disease. When necessary, right heart catheterization can be successfully performed without fluoroscopy using a flow-directed catheter. Chest roentgenogram films should not be ordered routinely and, if necessary, should be performed with adequate shielding of the pelvic area. Still, such tests should not be withheld when necessary to decide therapy for seriously ill patients. In such instances fetal radiation can usually be kept below acceptable limits (see Chap. 18) and risk-benefit considerations favor expeditious maternal evaluation and treatment.

On the electrocardiogram (ECG), atrial and ventricular premature beats are relatively frequent.[41] A small rightward deviation of av-

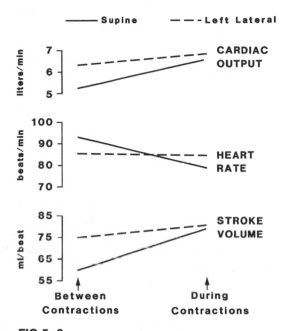

FIG 5–6.
The influence of uterine contractions on cardiac output, heart rate, and left ventricular stroke volume in supine and left lateral positions. With the pregnant woman in the left lateral position, stroke volume and cardiac output are maintained between contractions and changes during contractions are minimized. (From Lund CJ, Donovan JC: *Am J Obstet Gynecol* 1967; 98:393–403. Used with permission.)

erage mean QRS axis is recorded in the first trimester and a small leftward deviation in the third trimester due to progressive elevation of the left hemidiaphragm. A leftward deviation of the mean T axis is also noted.[41] Nonspecific ST-T wave changes may be present. Holter monitoring is useful when arrhythmias are suspected.

Since echocardiography can be used repeatedly during pregnancy with no risk to the fetus, it provides an excellent opportunity to noninvasively follow cardiac hemodynamics during pregnancy. An increase in LV end-diastolic volume and internal dimension is generally noted during pregnancy.[22, 42] In general, the heart appears mildly volume-overloaded and hyperkinetic during the latter half of gestation.[22] Echocardiography is a useful technique for the assessment of cardiovascular lesions during pregnancy, especially in the diagnosis and management of multiple lesions such as mitral and aortic stenosis and regurgitation, mitral valve prolapse, obstructive cardiomyopathy, tetralogy of Fallot, and Ebstein's anomaly of the tricuspid valve. In Marfan's syndrome, the extent of aortic root dilatation and the propensity for rupture can be predicted by echocardiography. Associated cardiac lesions in both Marfan's syndrome and coarctation of the aorta can also be diagnosed. Recently, the advent of Doppler echocardiography, with its ability to quantitate cardiac output as well as measurements of valvular gradients and areas, cardiac shunts, and the extent of valvular regurgitation has further decreased the need for invasive studies in pregnant patients (Fig 5–7).[14–16]

Pre-Conception Counseling

Maternal mortality varies directly with functional class. The expectant mother's cardiac reserve is inherently limited by the combination of heart disease and the additional circulatory demands imposed by pregnancy. Table 5–2 describes the New York Heart Association (NYHA) functional classification while Table 5–3 describes the maternal and fetal outcome according to functional class and cardiovascular disorder.

Women with serious correctable lesions should undergo repair before they become pregnant. For patients with conditions as potentially dangerous as Eisenmenger's syn-

AORTIC FLOW VELOCITY INTEGRAL

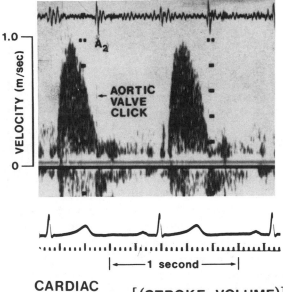

CROSS-SECTIONAL AREA OF PROXIMAL AORTA

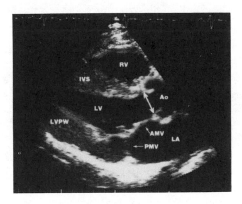

$$\text{CARDIAC OUTPUT} = [(\text{STROKE VOLUME})](\text{HR})$$
$$= [(\text{MEAN FLOW VELOCITY})(\text{EJECTION TIME})(\text{CSA})](\text{HR})$$
$$[(\text{FLOW VELOCITY INTEGRAL})(\text{CSA})](\text{HR})$$

FIG 5–7.
Doppler-determined cardiac output is obtained as the product of flow velocity integral times cross-sectional area (CSA) of the proximal aorta.

TABLE 5–2.
New York Heart Association Functional Classification

I. Patients with cardiac disease but without resulting limitations of physical activity.

II. Patients with cardiac disease resulting in slight limitation of physical activity. They are comfortable at rest. Ordinary physical activity results in fatigue, palpitation, dyspnea, or anginal pain.

III. Patients with cardiac disease resulting in marked limitation of physical activity. Less than ordinary physical activity causes fatigue, palpitation, dyspnea, or anginal pain.

IV. Patients with cardiac disease resulting in inability to carry out any physical activity without discomfort.

drome, primary pulmonary hypertension, Marfan's syndrome with aortic root involvement, or NYHA functional class III or IV disease of any etiology, pregnancy is contraindicated.[43–45]

Choice of Delivery and Anesthetic Management

For most patients with heart disease complicating pregnancy, assisted vaginal delivery with outlet forceps still remains the delivery method of choice. Cesarean section is usually only reserved for obstetric indications.[38]

Epidural anesthesia reduces maternal pain and anxiety, thereby avoiding the rise in blood pressure, heart rate, and cardiac output seen during the second stage of labor. In addition, due to its vasodilator action, epidural anesthesia results in reduced systemic vascular resistance, reflecting its peripheral vasodilator effect. The latter appears to be of benefit in conditions such as congestive heart failure and mitral and aortic regurgitation. However, in conditions in which a decrease in systemic vascular resistance is not well tolerated (e.g., pulmonary hypertension, obstructive cardiomyopathy, and aortic stenosis) epidural anesthesia may be both harmful and dangerous.[38, 46]

The risk of cardiovascular complications associated with cesarean section has decreased over the past decade due to improved surgical techniques and more knowledgeable

manipulation of cardiac loading conditions using pharmacologic therapy and anesthetic manipulation. Further refinement of treatment has been possible through the use of flow-directed Swan-Ganz catheters and direct measurements of intraarterial blood pressures. Cesarean section can be safely performed with either lumbar epidural, or general anesthesia provided the anesthesiologist is armed with the necessary hemodynamic information and a thorough understanding of the effect of a given anesthetic agent on the patient's specific cardiac lesion. Spinal anesthesia is generally associated with considerable hemodynamic imbalance and should therefore be avoided in pregnant patients with severe cardiac disease. Inhalational agents with negative inotropic effects may be beneficial in conditions such as obstructive car-

TABLE 5–3.
Relationship Between Cardiovascular Disorders and Maternal and Fetal Mortality*

Pregnancy Well Tolerated	Pregnancy Poorly Tolerated
NYHA class I and II[†] (maternal and fetal mortality, nil)	NYHA class III and IV[†] (maternal mortality, 0.4% & 7% respectively; fetal mortality, 30%)
Valvular regurgitation: mitral regurgitation, aortic regurgitation	Valvular stenosis: mitral stenosis, aortic stenosis
Left-to-right shunt (without pulmonary hypertension): atrial septal defect, ventricular septal defect, persistent ductus arteriosus	Right-to-left shunt: Eisenmenger's syndrome
Idiopathic hypertrophic subaortic stenosis	Primary pulmonary hypertension
	Marfan's syndrome
	Acute myocardial infarction

*From Rutherford JD: *Choices Cardiol* 1987; 2:176–179. Used by permission.
†NYHA = New York Heart Association. See Table 5–2.

diomyopathy, coarctation of the aorta, or Marfan's syndrome. In contrast, these agents may be dangerous in patients with severely dilated cardiomyopathies, aortic stenosis, and hemodynamically important mitral or aortic regurgitation.[38, 46]

TYPES OF HEART DISEASE IN WOMEN OF CHILDBEARING AGE

Acquired Heart Disease

The decline in maternal mortality in countries with well-developed maternity services is directly attributable to the decreased number of deaths resulting from hemorrhage, infection, and hypertensive disorders.[4, 47, 48] In contrast, the contribution of heart disease to maternal mortality remains relatively unchanged and heart disease continues to be a leading cause of maternal death in Ireland, Great Britain, and the United States. Published estimates of the frequency of heart disease in pregnancy vary from 0.9% to 3.7%. In a recent series of pregnancies complicated by maternal heart disease at the National Maternity Hospital, Dublin, Ireland, 83.5% were of rheumatic origin, 13.4% were congenital, and the remaining 3.1% were a miscellaneous group which included cases of cor pulmonale and coronary artery disease.[4]

Despite the declining incidence of active rheumatic fever in the United States, it still remains a problem throughout much of the world and is still the most common cause of severe heart disease encountered in pregnancy.

Mitral Stenosis

Mitral stenosis accounts for 90% of the rheumatic valvular lesions noted during pregnancy.[47–49] This valvular lesion, which impedes blood flow from the left atrium to the left ventricle, presents a particularly challenging set of problems since the increasing blood volume, cardiac output, and heart rate accompanying pregnancy increase pulmonary venous pressure and may lead to symptoms of congestive heart failure. The latter are most likely to occur in the third trimester, during labor, or following delivery.[48] The vast majority of cases of LV inflow tract obstruction seen in adults are due to rheumatic mitral stenosis. Left atrial (LA) myxoma and parachute mitral valve are rare causes of obstruction to LV filling.

In the mitral valve of a patient with an initial episode of acute rheumatic carditis, small nodules form along the closure line of the leaflets. The most common finding on physical examination at this time is mitral regurgitation. With the healing process or repeated episodes of rheumatic carditis, rheumatic mitral stenosis can occur. This is characterized by leaflet thickening, calcified commissural fusion, shortening of the chordae tendineae, and ablation of the interchordal spaces. The net result is obstruction to LV inflow at the leaflet and subleaflet levels.

The predominant symptoms of uncomplicated mitral stenosis are due to pulmonary venous hypertension and reflect the need for high LA-to-LV pressure gradients to maintain adequate transmitral blood flow. As LA and pulmonary venous pressures rise, there is usually a passive, obligatory increase in mean pulmonary arterial pressure to ensure blood flow across the pulmonary vascular bed. However, in some patients with mitral stenosis, pulmonary artery pressure increases out of proportion to the rise in LA and pulmonary venous pressures. This reactive pulmonary hypertension can lead to right ventricular (RV) dilatation and dysfunction in association with functional tricuspid regurgitation. Symptoms of right heart failure may supersede those of pulmonary venous hypertension in these patients.[50]

The most common symptom of mitral stenosis is dyspnea, initially on exertion and eventually at rest. The normal mitral valve cross-sectional area is in excess of 4 cm². In general, exercise is well tolerated when the area of the mitral valve orifice is narrowed to 2.5 cm². With narrowing to 1.5 to 2.5 cm², moderately severe exercise may precipitate dyspnea. Further reduction in orifice size will usually be associated with progressive disa-

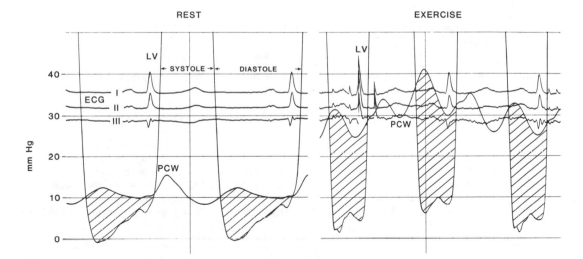

REST   EXERCISE

FIG 5–8.

Simultaneous left ventricular (*LV*) and pulmonary capillary wedge (*PCW*) pressure recordings in a patient with mitral-stenosis. Before exercise there is a mean diastolic gradient of 5 mm Hg (*shaded area*) between the LV and PCW pressures. Immediately after exercise the mean diastolic pressure gradient increased to over 18 mm Hg. (From Feldman TE: *IMJ* 1987; 76:628–633. Used by permission.)

bility. Usually when the mitral orifice is diminished to a critical valve area of 1.0 cm², even mild exercise causes dyspnea. Not uncommonly, because of adaptation in life styles from active to sedentary modes with progression of the disease, symptoms are often difficult to quantify and do not always reflect the severity of the mitral valve orifice narrowing.[50]

A major advance in the assessment of mitral valve stenosis was Gorlin's derivation in 1951 of the hydraulic equation for calculating the orifice area of stenotic valves.[51] Considerable insight into the pathophysiology of mitral valve area narrowing can be obtained by examining this formula:

$$\text{Mitral valve area} = \frac{\text{cardiac output/diastolic seconds per minute}}{\text{(constant)} \sqrt{\text{mean diastolic gradient}}}$$

$$\text{Mean diastolic gradient} = \left[\frac{\text{cardiac output/diastolic seconds per minute}}{\text{(constant) (mitral valve area)}}\right]^2$$

Given a fixed mitral valve area, the formula shows how variations in cardiac output and diastolic filling time (i.e., heart rate) affect the mean transmitral gradient. Conditions that increase cardiac output or shorten the diastolic filling period (e.g., exercise, fever, excitement, tachyarrhythmias) will raise the mean diastolic mitral gradient, thereby significantly elevating the LA pressure which may lead to pulmonary capillary engorgement and dyspnea. Figure 5–8 demonstrates how dynamic exercise can dramatically increase the mean diastolic as well as instantaneous gradients in a patient with mitral valve stenosis.

Due to the "normal" physiologic changes that occur during pregnancy (e.g., increased cardiac output, heart rate, and blood volume in association with reduced systemic and pulmonary vascular resistances), a seemingly well-compensated patient with mitral stenosis may decompensate and suddenly experience symptoms (Table 5–4). Since cardiac output and heart rate rise during the course of pregnancy, it is not surprising that LA and pulmonary venous hypertension are common in mitral stenosis. Symptoms occur in as many as 25% of patients with mitral stenosis during pregnancy. Symptoms of pulmonary congestion are frequently apparent by the midportion of the second trimester. Worsening of symptoms is common at the time of labor and delivery.

TABLE 5–4.
Mitral Stenosis in Pregnancy: Physiologic Changes and Management*

Relevant Hemodynamic Change in Pregnancy	Result	Time of Greatest Risk	Management
↑ Cardiac output ↑ Heart rate ↑ Blood volume ↓ Pulmonary vascular resistance	↑ Pulmonary capillary pressure	>12 wk (when hemo-dynamic changes become significant)	Throughout pregnancy should be followed with echocardiography and quantitative Doppler imaging Rheumatic fever and endocarditis prophylaxis Limit demands for cardiac output based on symptoms
Obstruction of inferior vena cava by uterus Blood loss at delivery	↓ Venous return ↓ LA filling ↓ LV filling ↓ Cardiac output	Late in pregnancy when supine (labor, delivery, surgery) and post partum	Heart rate control/atrial fibrillation Elective induction of labor/Swan-Ganz catheter During delivery blood losses should be replaced "mL for mL"

*LA = left atrial; LV = left ventricular.

Management (see Table 5–4).—The management of the patient with rheumatic mitral stenosis should include both rheumatic fever (Table 5–5) and endocarditis prophylaxis (Tables 5–6, 5–7).[52–55] If hemodynamically important mitral stenosis is diagnosed prior to pregnancy, either balloon valvuloplasty or mitral valve surgery should be considered.[56–58] Throughout pregnancy the patient should be followed with echocardiographic imaging and quantitative Doppler studies (Fig 5–9).[59, 60] These techniques provide accurate noninvasive evaluation of the anatomy of the mitral valve apparatus and LA size as well as assessment of the transmitral diastolic gradient and valve area.[60]

Should symptoms of pulmonary congestion develop in the patient with mitral stenosis who is in normal sinus rhythm, attempts should be made to restrict physical activity and sodium ingestion. In addition, treatment with a β-blocking agent (e.g., atenolol) during both sinus rhythm and atrial fibrillation may be helpful by blunting the heart rate response to exercise and anxiety.[61] This, in turn, may allow for a longer diastolic filling period per beat, thereby improving transmitral flow. In a recent study performed during pregnancy, treatment with atenolol and furosemide in patients in normal sinus rhythm with hemodynamically significant mitral stenosis resulted in increased exercise tolerance in association

TABLE 5–5.
Secondary Prevention of Rheumatic Fever (Prevention of Recurrent Attacks)*

Agent	Dose	Mode
Penicillin G benzathine	1 million units	IM every 4 wk†
	or	
Penicillin V	250 mg twice daily	Oral
	or	
Sulfadiazine‡	0.5 g once daily for patients <60 lb 1.0 g once daily for patients >60 lb	Oral
For individuals allergic to penicillin and sulfadiazine:		
Erythromycin	250 mg twice daily	Oral

*From Dajani AS, Bisno AL, Chung KJ, et al: *Circulation* 1988; 78:1082–1086. Used by permission.
†In high-risk situations, administration every 3 weeks is advised.
‡Prophylaxis with sulfonamides (i.e., sulfadiazine) is contraindicated in late pregnancy because of transplacental passage and competition with bilirubin for neonatal albumin-binding sites.

TABLE 5–6.
Cardiac Conditions for Which Endocarditis Prophylaxis Is and Is Not Recommended*

Endocarditis prophylaxis recommended
  Prosthetic cardiac valves (including biosynthetic valves)
  Most congenital cardiac malformations
  Surgically constructed systemic-pulmonary shunts
  Rheumatic and other acquired valvular dysfunction
  Idiopathic hypertrophic subaortic stenosis
  Previous history of bacterial endocarditis
  Mitral valve prolapse with insufficiency†

Endocarditis prophylaxis not recommended
  Isolated secundum atrial septal defect
  Secundum atrial septal defect repaired without a patch ≥6 mo earlier
  Persistent ductus arteriosus ligated and divided ≥6 mo earlier
  Postoperatively after coronary artery bypass graft surgery

*Adapted from Shulman ST, Amren DP, Bisno AL, et al: *Circulation* 1984; 70:1123A–1127A.
†Definitive data to provide guidance in management of patients with mitral valve prolapse are particularly limited. In general, such patients are clearly at low risk for development of endocarditis, but the risk-benefit ratio of prophylaxis in mitral valve prolapse is uncertain.

with an excellent outcome for both mother and baby; fetal wastage was only 4%.[61]

The onset of atrial fibrillation in the patient with mitral stenosis has important hemodynamic consequences due to the resultant increased heart rate (i.e., decreased diastolic filling time) and the loss of atrial contribution to LV filling. If atrial fibrillation occurs suddenly it can lead to pulmonary congestion and pulmonary edema. In these cases, intravenous verapamil (5–10 mg IV) should be given or electrocardioversion should be attempted promptly. The latter has been performed successfully during pregnancy without apparent adverse fetal effect. Nevertheless, it is recommended that fetal heart rate monitoring be instituted prior to attempted electrocardioversion. Chronic oral digoxin or β-blockade will usually ensure a reasonably slow ventricular response rate should atrial fibrillation recur. Another complication of atrial fibrillation is the tendency of emboli to develop.[62] Thrombi may form in the left atrium and fragments may be shed into the systemic arterial circulation. Atrial fibrillation in the presence of mitral valve disease constitutes one of the most common indications for anticoagulation during pregnancy. (See Anticoagulants later in this chapter.)

Closed mitral commissurotomy has been performed successfully during pregnancy.[57, 58] The procedure is usually well tolerated and maternal mortality has been reported to be less than 2%. However, fetal mortality has been approximately 10% in some series while no untoward effects were reported in others. The long-term results of closed mitral valvotomy performed during pregnancy were identical to those operations carried out in nonpregnant women. Nevertheless, it is not recommended that this procedure be undertaken unless the maternal condition deteriorates rapidly to class III or IV. The mitral valve also has been successfully replaced during pregnancy.[56] This operation entails the use of a pump oxygenator and extracorporeal circulation and has a higher risk of maternal and fetal mortality when compared to mitral valvotomy.[38, 63] If valve replacement is deemed

TABLE 5–7.
American Heart Association Recommendations for Prophylaxis of Endocarditis in Patients at Risk During Obstetric and Gynecologic Procedures*

Standard regimen

	Ampicillin, 2.0 g IM or 1.5 g IV plus gentamicin 1.5 mg/kg IM or IV, given 0.5–1.0 hr before procedure; one follow-up dose may be given 8 hr later

Special regimens

Oral regimen for minor or repetitive procedures in low-risk patients	Amoxicillin, 3.0 g orally 1 hr before and 1.5 g 6 hr later
Penicillin-allergic patients	Vancomycin, 1.0 g IV slowly over 1 hr, plus gentamicin 1.5 mg/kg IM or IV given 1 hr before procedure; may be repeated once 8–12 hr later

*From Shulman ST, Amren DP, Bisno AL, et al: *Circulation* 1984; 70:1123A–1127A. Used by permission.

necessary during pregnancy, consideration should be given to a biologic valve rather than a mechanical valve because of the difficulties associated with management of anticoagulants during pregnancy.[64] Since only a few surgeons are currently adequately trained in performing closed commissurotomies in the United States, a potential alternative therapeutic procedure for patients in their third trimester of pregnancy (when fetal organogenesis is completed) might be balloon valvuloplasty.

Since labor and delivery present an additional burden to the maternal cardiovascular system, carefully planned management of labor and delivery in the woman with mitral stenosis is considered essential.[65] For example, in patients with mitral stenosis, the

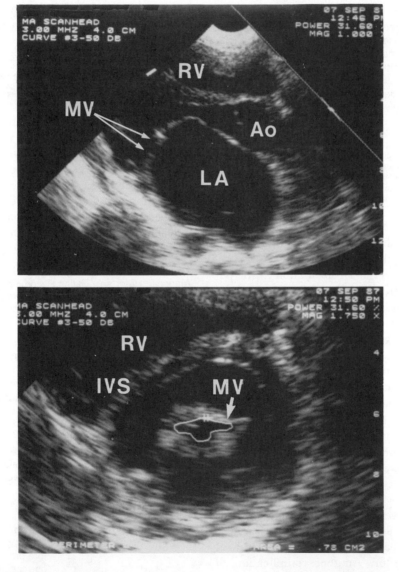

FIG 5–9.
Top panel, early diastolic frame from a two-dimensional echocardiogram of a stenotic mitral valve. Note doming of the anterior mitral valve leaflet and enlargement of the left atrium. *Bottom panel,* short-axis examination provides the opportunity for two-dimensional measurement of the mitral valve area. Planimetry resulted in a mitral valve area of 0.75 cm². See text for explanation.

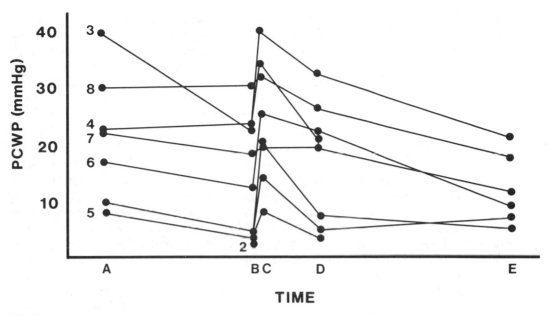

FIG 5–10.
Intrapartum alterations in pulmonary capillary wedge pressure (*PCWP*) in eight patients with mitral stenosis. *A*, first-stage labor; *B*, second-stage labor, 15 to 30 minutes before delivery; *C*, 5 to 15 minutes post partum; *D*, 4 to 6 hours post partum; *E*, 18 to 24 hours post partum. (From Clark SL, Phelan JP, Greenspoon J: *Am J Obstet Gynecol* 1985; 152:984–988. Used by permission.)

hemodynamic changes associated with the late second stage of labor and the initial 15 post-partum minutes result in an increase in pulmonary capillary wedge pressure (Fig 5–10). Ueland and Hansen[37] have shown that in normal pregnancies an increase in cardiac output of up to 45% can occur during the second stage of labor with an additional 15% increase during contractions. Such changes seem to be largely on the basis of sympathetic-mediated increases in heart rate as well as increased stroke volume during contractions. The early postpartum period in particular appears to be hemodynamically hazardous since cardiac output can increase up to 65%.[34, 36, 37, 40] This increase is felt to be due to postpartum volume shifts secondary to the release of inferior vena caval obstruction by the gravid uterus and the sudden decrease in vascular capacitance associated with the loss of the low-resistance circulation in the placenta.[17] The postpartum decrease in plasma colloidal osmotic pressure that accompanies normal pregnancy appears to also contribute to the development of pulmonary congestion.[66]

Successful hemodynamic management of the woman with mitral stenosis requires the physician to anticipate rather than to merely respond to cardiovascular events. Elective induction of labor is often indicated. In these cases, careful consultation between the obstetrician, anesthesiologist, and internist/cardiologist is essential. At the time of labor, effective anesthesia should minimize pain and anxiety and thereby decrease the hemodynamic burden on the heart. A bedside ECG monitor should be used to assess the presence of rhythm disturbances. Tachycardia of any etiology (including labor, pain, or anxiety) leads to shortened ventricular filling time and a possible fall in cardiac output leading to systemic hypotension. This may be reduced by the use of epidural anesthesia to eliminate the pain and tachycardia accompanying uterine contractions. If moderate mitral stenosis is present, hemodynamic data acquired using a thermodilution Swan-Ganz catheter are frequently useful in decision making regarding fluid management. If the patient becomes hypotensive secondary to the anesthetic agent, treatment with large amounts of volume expanders should be performed with caution. In these cases, hemodynamic data, including cardiac output and pulmonary capillary wedge pressures, are essential for optimal patient care. Since pulmonary edema is the major danger in patients with mitral stenosis, care must be taken to avoid volume overloading. During delivery, blood losses should be replaced "milliliter for milliliter." Not uncommonly, women with moderate to severe mitral stenosis will have pulmonary artery hypertension and pulmonary edema for the first 24 to 48 hours post partum even when diligent care is provided. Interestingly, the patient with pulmonary edema and hypoxemia during labor and delivery is frequently asymptomatic by 4 to 6 weeks post partum.

Mitral Regurgitation

Unlike mitral stenosis, which is usually rheumatic in origin, mitral regurgitation has multiple etiologies.[67, 68] Echocardiography is a clinically useful tool for determining the etiology of mitral regurgitation by showing evidence of either rheumatic deformity of the valve, mitral valve prolapse, vegetative endocarditis, or ruptured chordae tendineae.[69] In patients with LV dilatation due to dilated cardiomyopathy, worsening of spatial disorientation of the papillary muscles may occur resulting in mitral regurgitation. Patients with asymmetric septal hypertrophy frequently also exhibit mitral insufficiency.[70] Patients with mitral regurgitation often remain asymptomatic for many years. This valvular lesion is usually well tolerated during pregnancy because of the fall in systemic valvular resistance which may actually result in a decrease in the severity of the valvular incompetence. In general, symptoms of congestive heart failure due to mitral regurgitation in the pregnant woman are rare and valve replacement is almost never indicated. Prophylaxis against bacterial endocarditis is usually recommended.

Valvular Aortic Stenosis

Hemodynamically important valvular aortic stenosis is uncommon in women of childbearing age. It may be due to rheumatic inflammation, in which case it is invariably associated with mitral valve deformity, or it may be congenital.[71, 72] Mild to moderately severe valvular aortic stenosis is usually well tolerated during pregnancy. This is not necessarily the case in severe aortic stenosis. The critical hemodynamic problem in severe valvular aortic stenosis is fixed cardiac output in response to cardiovascular stress. In these cases, exertional activity as well as factors leading to diminished venous return can diminish cardiac output. Any reduction is preload resulting from blood loss, sympathetic blockade from regional anesthesia, or vena caval occlusion in association with the supine position may result in cardiac and cerebral hypoperfusion as well as compromised uterine blood flow. In the older literature, cases of hemodynamically severe aortic stenosis have been associated with maternal mortalities as high as 17% and fetal mortality as high as 32%.[71, 72] With the current noninvasive techniques, which allow for earlier diagnosis and physiologic assessment of the severity of disease, these high mortality rates would probably be lower.

Evaluation and Management.—Management of pregnancy complicated by aortic stenosis requires accurate assessment of the severity of the disease. Unlike mitral stenosis, clinical symptoms appear very late in the course of the disease. Currently, intracardiac pressure gradients can be accurately assessed noninvasively by Doppler echocardiography.[73] Pressure gradients can be calculated using the formula $PG = 4V^2$, where PG is the peak instantaneous pressure gradient across the deformed aortic valve and V is the maximal velocity of blood flow across the valve (Fig 5–11). Because pressure gradients are flow-dependent, gradient alone may provide misleading information about the severity of the valve narrowing, particularly during pregnancy when cardiac output is increased. In this setting, calculation of the aortic valve area using the continuity equation provides a

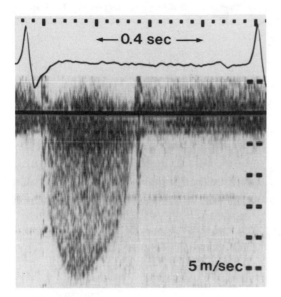

$$V_{MAX} = 5.3 \text{ m/sec}$$

$$PG_{MAX} = 112 \text{ mmHg}$$

$$PG_{MEAN} = 75 \text{ mmHg}$$

FIG 5–11.
Continuous-wave Doppler echocardiographic recording from a patient with aortic stenosis. Continuous-wave Doppler has been shown in several recent reports to be accurate in the quantitation of transvalvular aortic gradients. Using the modified Bernoulli equation, one can calculate the peak instantaneous transvalvular (PG_{MAX}) = gradient = $4(V_{MAX})^2$. Alternatively, the area under the Doppler-determined instantaneous gradient curve can be planimetered and divided by the ejection time to give the mean gradient (PG_{MEAN}). V_{MAX} = peak Doppler velocity.

more accurate index of the severity of the valvular stenosis (Fig 5–12).[73]

Reduced activity is the mainstay of the antepartum management of the patient with moderately severe valvular aortic stenosis. Preload must be maintained for the left ventricle to generate an adequate cardiac output. Filling pressures should be monitored during labor and delivery using a Swan-Ganz catheter. Critical aortic stenosis creates a narrow window for appropriate fluid loading. Small decreases in preload due to blood loss or anesthesia may result in decreased cardiac output and hypotension.[72] On the other hand, small

increases in intravascular volume in a stiff hypertrophied left ventricle may produce dramatic increases in filling pressures resulting in pulmonary edema. The goal of hemodynamic monitoring, therefore, should be to maintain LV filling pressures within this narrow therapeutic window. Epidural anesthesia should not be used in patients with severe aortic stenosis because of potential significant decreases in LV preload and afterload.[38, 72] Effective anesthesia can prevent the tachycardia associated with the pain of labor. During labor the lateral decubitus position should be assured. The first stage of labor is usually managed according to usual obstetric standards with special concern that the patient may be highly susceptible to supine hypotension. The second stage should be managed with minimal pushing; operative assistance should be given when adequate station is achieved. The third state should be managed aggressively to avoid potential hemorrhage. As noted previously for the patient with mitral

CONTINUITY EQUATION

$$(A_{LVOT})(FVI_{LVOT}) = (AVA)(FVI_{AV})$$

$$(A_{LVOT})\left[\frac{FVI_{LVOT}}{FVI_{AV}}\right] = AVA$$

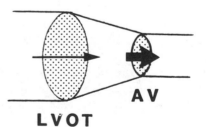

FIG 5–12.
Use of the continuity equation for calculating aortic valve area (*AVA*). The continuity principle states that flow through the left ventricular outflow tract (*LVOT*) is equal to flow through the aortic valve (*AV*). The ratio of the flow velocity integrals (*FVI*) times the LVOT area (*A*) yields the AVA.

stenosis, immediate postpartum filling pressures may rise requiring a diuretic.[72]

If critical aortic stenosis is diagnosed prior to pregnancy, surgical correction should be recommended. In most cases a commissurotomy will suffice.[64, 74] If a prosthetic valve is required, a heterograft may avoid the need for long-term anticoagulation. As with mitral stenosis, the maternal risks for valve replacement and surgical valvotomy are relatively low, but fetal mortality with cardiopulmonary bypass surgery has been reported to be as high as 9.5%.[72] Recently, Angel et al.[75] described the use of percutaneous balloon aortic valvuloplasty in pregnancy as an alternative method to operative intervention in pregnant patients with severe aortic stenosis.[75] The radiation exposure to the fetus was primarily via transdiaphragmatic scatter and was calculated to be approximately 1 rad, which is not associated with a statistically significant increase in the absolute risk of gross congenital malformation (See Chap. 18 for risks of diagnostic imaging). Prophylaxis against bacterial endocarditis is also indicated.

Aortic Regurgitation

This lesion is more common than aortic stenosis in women of childbearing age. It may be the result of a congenital abnormality of the valve, or the valve may be damaged by rheumatic fever, endocarditis, or a systemic vasculitis such as rheumatoid arthritis or systemic lupus erythematosus. When due to rheumatic fever, it is almost invariably associated with mitral valve disease. Aortic regurgitation may also result from dilatation of the aortic root. As a result of the valvular incompetence, a portion of the LV output returns to the ventricle during diastole. To compensate, the left ventricle dilates and the stroke volume increases.[76] Like mitral regurgitation, aortic insufficiency is usually well tolerated during pregnancy. The severity of aortic regurgitation may actually decrease during pregnancy due to the fall in systemic vascular resistance.[1-3, 22, 23] If pulmonary congestion develops, restriction of physical activity and sodium ingestion are essential. Antibiotic pro-

phylaxis during labor and delivery are usually advised.[52-55] When aortic regurgitation results from active endocarditis, early surgery should be considered if the infection is not rapidly controlled or if progressive hemodynamic deterioration occurs.

Prevention of Recurrent Rheumatic Fever

Prevention of both initial and recurrent attacks of acute rheumatic fever (see Table 5–5) depends on control of group A β-hemolytic streptococcal upper respiratory tract infections including tonsillopharyngitis and associated conditions such as otitis, sinusitis, and mastoiditis. The current recommendations reflect the quite low incidence of rheumatic fever in most areas of the United States.[52] These recommendations do not apply to certain areas of the United States where sharp increases in occurrence of rheumatic fever have been noticed recently or to regions of the world that continue to have a high incidence of rheumatic fever.

Rheumatic fever prophylaxis should be continued during pregnancy for all patients with suspected rheumatic heart disease. Patients who have had rheumatic carditis are at a relatively high risk for recurrence of carditis and are likely to sustain serious cardiac involvement with each recurrence. Therefore, patients who have had rheumatic carditis should receive long-term antibiotic prophylaxis well into adulthood and perhaps for life. Prophylaxis should continue even after valve surgery (including prosthetic valve replacement) because these patients remain at risk for recurrence of rheumatic fever.

An injection of 1.2 million units of intramuscular penicillin G benzathine (every 4 weeks), oral penicillin V (250 mg twice daily), or oral sulfadiazine (1.0 g daily for patients >60 lb) are the recommended methods for prevention of recurrent rheumatic fever. For patients allergic to penicillin or sulfadiazine, erythromycin (250 mg twice daily) is suggested (see Table 5–5). Long-acting penicillin is of particular value in patients with a high risk of rheumatic fever recurrence. Prophylaxis with sulfonamides is best avoided in late pregnancy because of transplacental passage and competition with bilirubin for neonatal albumin-binding sites. Data comparing sulfadiazine with other sulfonamides are not available. When advising patients on the method of choice for prevention of rheumatic fever, it should be considered that, even with optimal compliance, the risk of recurrence is higher in those receiving oral prophylaxis when compared to those receiving penicillin G benzathine.[52]

Prosthetic Valves

Pregnancy may be hazardous in patients with mechanical prosthetic heart valves, primarily because administration of an oral *anticoagulant* may be harmful to the fetus (see Anticoagulants below); however, failure to undergo such treatment exposes the mother to an increased risk of embolic complications. Anticoagulation regimens are less well established in pregnant than in nonpregnant patients because neither the safety of oral anticoagulant therapy during pregnancy nor the efficacy of heparin therapy for prophylaxis of systemic embolism are established.[77] Until controlled trials comparing adjusted-dose subcutaneous heparin with warfarin are performed, strict guidelines cannot be provided. One recommended approach is to use heparin throughout gestation administered every 12 hours by subcutaneous injection in doses adjusted to keep the midinterval partial thromboplastin time at 1.5 times the control. An alternative is to use heparin until the 13th week, change to warfarin (to keep the prothrombin time 1.5 to 2.0 times control) until the middle of the third trimester and then restart heparin until delivery.[77-80] When pregnancy is well planned, subcutaneous heparin should be substituted prior to conception. Heparin can be terminated at the onset of labor and reinstituted shortly (12–24 hr) after delivery.

The difficulties associated with anticoagulant therapy raise the issue of use of tissue valves in women of childbearing age, as such valves are generally nonthrombogenic.[64, 74, 77-79,81, 82] If the left atrium is not significantly enlarged and the patient is in normal sinus rhythm, anticoagulant treatment may not be necessary with the exception of the initial 3 postoperative months. The use of a bioprosthesis, however, does not necessarily eliminate the need for anticoagulation since the coexistence of low cardiac output, previous embolic accidents, atrial thrombus, large LA size, and atrial fibrillation are considered valid indications for anticoagulation in patients with biologic valves.[74] However, it should be remembered that in children and young adults, the rate of calcification and leaflet degeneration of bioprosthetic valves is higher than in adults.[64, 02, 03] Pregnancy may also favor calcification of porcine heterografts leading to early bioprosthetic failure. Nevertheless, Bortolotti et al. suggest that pregnancy in patients with a porcine bioprosthesis is well tolerated and successfully carried out in most cases.[61] In their series, no embolic episodes were noted despite (1) the lack of anticoagulant therapy and (2) the hypercoagulable state of pregnancy.

Because of the potentially harmful effects of aspirin (e.g., intracranial hemorrhage in premature infants), it has been recommended that pregnant women with bioprostheses who are in sinus rhythm not be treated with antiplatelet agents.[84] The data on the benefit-risk balance of the use of aspirin in pregnant patients with bioprosthetic valves and atrial fibrillation is, however, not conclusive. Some authors are inclined to use platelet antiaggregants in this situation because the potential threat of thromboembolism in this type of patient seems more important than the potential harmful fetal effect of aspirin. Alternatively, adjusted-dose subcutaneous heparin can be administered throughout pregnancy. Although this approach avoids fetal abnormalities and is likely to be efficacious, it exposes the mother to a small risk of heparin-induced osteoporosis.

In summary, when selecting a prosthetic valve for the woman who wishes to have children, consideration should be given to the important teratogenic effect that oral anticoagulants may have upon the fetus.[85-90]

Tissue valves allow a normal pregnancy and delivery independent of the atrial rhythm. Although limited durability of bioprostheses is a well-known fact, it is generally believed that women contemplating pregnancy should have their pathologic valves replaced with tissue valves despite the fact that they will be at risk of another operation in the future.[64, 74, 82, 83, 85-90]

Ischemic Heart Disease

Ischemic heart disease is uncommon in obstetric practice with an estimated incidence of myocardial infarction of 1 in 10,000.[91-96] This extremely small incidence of coronary atherosclerosis in women of childbearing age is likely to rise in the future mainly due to the modern trend toward delaying marriage and pregnancy, along with the increasing prevalence of coronary artery disease in women.[94] Epidemiologically, the major cornary risk factors for coronary atherosclerosis are hypercholesterolemia, smoking, diabetes,[94] and hypertension. Oral contraceptives have been thought to constitute another important risk factor. Mann et al.[97] have reported that the risk of myocardial infarction is 2.7 times greater in women between 30 and 39 years of age taking oral contraceptives and 5.7 times greater in women 40 to 49.[98] However, more recently Mishell found no evidence to suggest an increase in the risks of cardiovascular diseases among past healthy and nonsmoking users of oral contraceptives (even with prolonged use) containing less than 50 μg of estrogen.

Myocardial infarction in the *postpartum period* is a very rare occurrence.[93, 95] This "postpartum" infarct appears to differ in several respects from the more frequently reported acute myocardial infarction occurring during pregnancy. Acute myocardial infarction in the postpartum period occurs mostly in primiparous women in their mid-twenties, usually within 1 to 2 weeks of delivery. More than half of these patients had preeclampsia requiring hypotensive therapy during delivery. Case reports suggest that coronary arterial thromboembolism or spasm may be the sub-

strate for the ischemic event.[93, 99-101] In contrast, patients with myocardial infarction occurring during pregnancy tend to be older and multiparous. Although angiographic confirmation is seldom available, atherosclerosis is presumed to be the cause of most acute infarcts during pregnancy.

Management.—Proper management of coronary disease is predicated on an accurate clinical diagnosis. Echocardiography is a noninvasive test that can be safely performed during pregnancy and is of value to assess ventricular regional wall motion and thickening abnormalities. If indicated, a submaximal exercise stress test can be performed. Radionuclide studies may detect perfusion defects related to abnormal coronary flow as well as wall motion abnormalities. Fetal exposure following a thallium 201 myocardial perfusion scan has been estimated at 780 mrad, a dose well below the threshold considered necessary to produce gross congenital malformations[102] (see Chap. 18 for a discussion of diagnostic imaging). In rare cases of refractory angina pectoris (not well controlled under maximal medical therapy), cardiac catheterization may be necessary for diagnostic purposes prior to possible angioplasty or coronary artery bypass surgery.[103] In these cases, the brachial artery approach is preferable with concomitant lead shielding of the abdomen and careful monitoring of fetal radiation exposure.[103]

Pharmacologic therapy of symptomatic coronary artery disease during pregnancy does not differ substantially from the approach used in nonpregnant patients.[104] Because nitrates produce venous dilatation they may lead to significant hypotension, particularly in the standing position. There are numerous reports of the use of β-blockers during pregnancy, primarily for hypertension. Although many attest to their safety, some concerns remain about the possibility that these agents may produce intrauterine growth retardation when begun early in pregnancy. The experience with calcium channel blockers in human gestation is much more limited; however, we are unaware of any serious adverse fetal effects of this class of drug. (See Chap. 1 for a more detailed discussion of both β-adreno-receptor and calcium channel blocking agents.) Despite the lack of definitive studies on the safety of both β-adrenoceptor and calcium channel blocking agents in human pregnancy, the potential benefits of such treatment outweigh the risks in the gravida with symptomatic coronary artery disease.[104]

The repeated documentation of successful pregnancy following myocardial infarction or coronary artery bypass suggests that it does not necessarily require termination of the pregnancy.[105, 106] If coronary artery disease becomes clinically manifest during pregnancy, it usually presents as an acute myocardial infarction rather than angina pectoris. Usually, a previous small myocardial infarction is well tolerated by mother and fetus. The greatest mortality occurs when the infarction occurs during the last months of pregnancy and during labor. In general, for most pregnant patients with ischemic heart disease, a vaginal delivery is preferable; a cesarean section is only indicated for obstetric reasons. However, a full obstetric, medical, surgical, and anesthesiologic team should be available in the event of complications.[95] Regarding the management of these patients during labor and delivery, particular attention should be paid to maintaining the balance between myocardial oxygen supply and demand, utilizing the following measures: (1) continuation of daily cardiac medications (e.g., nitrates, calcium channel blockers, and β-blockers); (2) inhalation of supplemental oxygen; (3) avoidance of aortocaval compression; (4) early institution of lumbar epidural block since it results in near complete pain relief and alleviates the cardiovascular, respiratory, metabolic, and hormonal stress responses to uterine contractions; (5) monitoring of ECG and of arterial pressure by noninvasive means; and (6) monitoring of intravascular fluid status using a thermodilution catheter is recommended for unstable patients (i.e., refractory angina pectoris, recent cardiovascular ischemic events, etc.).[95]

Peripartum Cardiomyopathy

Peripartum cardiomyopathy is a relatively uncommon form of heart disease affecting women in their reproductive years.[107–110] Epidemiologic studies estimate that peripartum cardiomyopathy has an incidence between 1 in 4,000 and 1 in 15,000 gestations.[107–111] Demakis[112] and Rahimtoola and co-workers[113] have suggested the following criteria for the diagnosis of peripartum or postpartum cardiomyopathy: (1) development of heart failure in the last month of pregnancy or within the first 5 postpartum months, (2) absence of another determinable etiology for the cardiac failure, and (3) absence of heart disease prior to the last month of pregnancy (Fig 5–13). Epidemiologic studies reveal that in the United States this disease predominates in older black multiparous women and is more frequently encountered in patients with pregnancy-induced hypertension (i.e., preeclampsia) or with twin pregnancies.[107–113]

There is no consensus regarding the pathogenesis of the ventricular dysfunction in peripartum cardiomyopathy despite claims that viral cardiomyopathy may play a role in some patients.[114, 115] Recent observations of a rise in antimyosin antibodies in a patient with peripartum cardiomyopathy have raised the additional possibility that this entity may have an autoimmune etiology.[116] Many other causative mechanisms have been invoked including nutritional deficiencies, hormonal imbalance, and excessive salt intake, particularly in Nigerian patients.[107, 110] In the absence of specific clinical or laboratory findings, some authors have questioned whether peripartum cardiomyopathy is indeed a distinct entity. Moreover, Cunningham et al.[110] recently concluded that in most women with peripartum heart failure of obscure etiology, underlying chronic diseases such as anemia, preeclampsia, infection, etc. can be identified. Heart

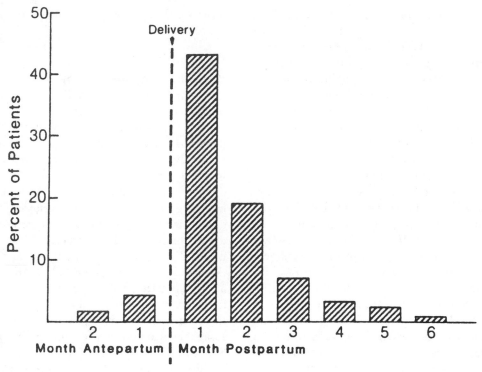

FIG 5–13.
Onset of peripartum cardiomyopathy in relation to time of delivery. (From Homans DC: *N Engl J Med* 1985; 312:1432–1437. Used by permission.)

failure in these women ensues when the cardiovascular demands of normal pregnancy are amplified further by common pregnancy complications superimposed upon underlying conditions that cause ventricular hypertrophy. The chief support for the existence of peripartum cardiomyopathy as a distinct entity is epidemiologic data suggesting a clustering of cardiomyopathic cases in the peripartum period.[107] However, this clustering does not completely prove that this condition represents a distinct entity since, in fact, it may reflect exacerbation of underlying heart failure due to the hemodynamic stress of pregnancy, or possibly a predisposition of pregnant women to acquire cardiomyopathy secondary to other currently unknown mechanisms.[107]

Women with peripartum cardiomyopathy usually present with fatigue, dyspnea on exertion, and edema. Other symptoms include embolic phenomena, chest pain, hemoptysis, and cough.[107, 108, 111–113, 117, 118] Physical examination usually demonstrates elevated

jugular venous pressure, pulmonary rales, cardiomegaly, S3 gallop, murmurs of mitral and/or tricuspid regurgitation, and peripheral edema. The ECG in dilated cardiomyopathy initially may show nothing more than nonspecific ST-T wave abnormalities, but occasionally Q wave "infarct" patterns are present. Echocardiography with Doppler evaluation and color flow imaging identify the morphologic and physiologic aspects of peripartum cardiomyopathy. Typically, internal end-diastolic ventricular dimensions are increased and there is diminished ventricular wall motion (Fig 5–14). Two-dimensional imaging should also be used to search for endocardial thrombi, which are most likely to lodge at the apex of the left ventricle.

Once the diagnosis of peripartum cardiomyopathy is made, conservative medical therapy should be started as early as possible. Therapy consists of the treatment of heart failure and its complications. (1) Digitalis should be administered cautiously since these patients may be very sensitive to this drug and may develop arrhythmias. (2) Dietary sodium restriction and diuretics are usually required. Care should be taken to avoid hypokalemia, which could further increase the sensitivity to digitalis. (3) Vasodilator therapy (e.g., nitrates, hydralazine, and prazosin) have a definite place in the treatment of these patients since they have been demonstrated to improve cardiac output and reduce LV filling pressures. Angiotensin converting enzyme inhibitors should not be used during pregnancy because of their reported adverse effects on fetal and neonatal renal function (see Chap. 1, p. 29). (4) Because of the high incidence of thromboembolic events in peripartum cardiomyopathy, anticoagulant therapy is usually recommended. Recently, orthotopic cardiac transplantation has been successfully performed in a group of patients with peripartum cardiomyopathy and end-stage heart failure.

The prognosis of this disorder varies in different parts of the world. In the United States mortality rates are reported to range from 25% to 50%.[107–110, 118–120] The long-term prognosis is usually poor if cardiomegaly persists for 6 months or more after institution of conventional treatment. One interesting feature of peripartum cardiomyopathy is its tendency to recur with subsequent pregnancies. For this reason we believe that in these patients, subsequent pregnancies should be discouraged, even in patients in whom heart size returns to normal within the first year of the initial cardiomyopathic episode. To date, it is still unclear whether recurrence during a second pregnancy represents an exacerbation of persisting subclinical heart failure or the reactivation of an underlying disease process. Should heart failure recur during pregnancy, the effect of early pregnancy termination on cardiac function remains unclear; neverthe-

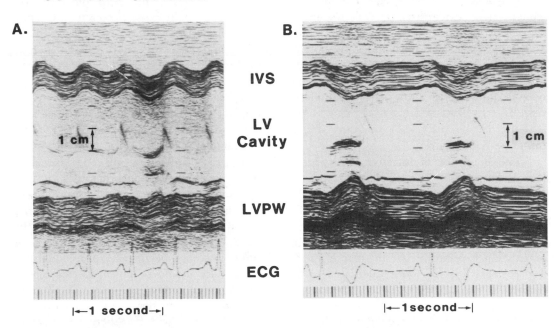

FIG 5–14.
A, M-mode echocardiogram from a 28-year-old woman with peripartum cardiomyopathy. Left ventricular (*LV*) systolic performance is markedly depressed. Note the lack of systolic thickening of the posterior wall. The patient demonstrates sinus tachycardia with a resting heart rate of 122 beats/min. *B,* M-mode echocardiogram from the same patient repeated 4 weeks after delivery. LV systolic performance is significantly improved. This is associated with a good long-term prognosis. Note the much slower heart rate in association with improved ventricular function. *IVS* = interventricular septum; *LVPW* = left ventricular posterior wall; *ECG* = electrocardiogram.

less, abortion has often been recommended in this situation. Fetal prognosis is believed to correlate best with the timing of presentation of maternal heart failure and is reported to be better when maternal heart failure develops in the postpartum period and worse when heart failure develops during the third trimester.

Currently there are no data to support prohibition of breast-feeding since improvement of ventricular function has been noted despite its continuation. Finally, oral contraceptives should be avoided in patients with cardiomyopathy because of their association with thromboembolic events.

Pericardial Disease

There are only a limited number of publications describing acute and constrictive pericarditis occurring during pregnancy.[121] Acute pericarditis during pregnancy usually runs a benign course. Symptoms generally respond to aspirin, but at times steroids are required and have been used successfully.[122] Constrictive pericarditis during pregnancy should be managed medically if symptoms and hemodynamic abnormalities are not severe. If constrictive pericarditis appears to be hemodynamically severe, pericardiectomy has been performed with a low maternal and fetal risk.[123]

Infective Endocarditis

The incidence of infective endocarditis (see Tables 5–6, 5–7) after obstetric and gynecologic procedures is low and decreasing. Seaworth and Durack[124] calculated that for all deliveries the incidence varies from 0.03 to 0.14/1,000. In the subgroup of patients with preexisting cardiac disease the rate of infective endocarditis has been calculated to be between 5.5 to 9.0/1,000. Among the factors responsible for this favorable trend are (1) a decreasing incidence of rheumatic heart disease, (2) legalization of abortion, and (3) decreased incidence and improved management of obstetric and gynecologic infections in the antibiotic era.

Present standards of care require that prophylactic antibiotics be used for procedures that cause significant bacteremia in patients with heart lesions that are highly susceptible to endocarditis (see Table 5–6).[54, 55, 124, 125] Whereas the frequency and characteristics of bacteremia after dental procedures have been well studied, there have been very few reports regarding the incidence of bacteremia after obstetric and gynecologic events.[126, 127] Positive blood cultures occur in less than 5% of patients after uncomplicated vaginal delivery.[126, 127] No evidence currently exists for bacteremia after cesarean section. While recognizing that the data in the literature are scanty, the rate of bacteremia expected after normal delivery and cesarean section is too low to justify the routine use of antibiotic prophylaxis.[55] Thus, the decision whether to give antibiotics for endocarditis prophylaxis in obstetric or gynecologic settings should be individualized.[124] Two risk factors should be considered: (1) the underlying cardiac lesion and (2) the obstetric procedure that might cause bacteremia. Certain cardiac lesions appear to carry a relatively higher risk (see Table 5–6). These include prosthetic valves, ventricular septal defects, persistent ductus arteriosus, acquired rheumatic heart disease, previous infective endocarditis, cyanotic congenital heart disease, and mitral valve prolapse when associated with a murmur of mitral regurgitation.[54, 55, 128] Obstetric procedures which may be associated with bacteremia include premature rupture of the membranes associated with prolonged labor, a prolonged third stage of labor, and manual removal of the placenta.[124] If both the cardiac lesion and the obstetric procedure seem to pose significant risks, prophylaxis for endocarditis should be given. If only one of the risk factors poses significant risk, prophylaxis should be considered optional. However, because patients with prosthetic heart valves and those with surgically constructed systemic-pulmonary shunts appear to be at especially high risk for infective endocarditis, it may be prudent to administer prophylactic antibiotics to such individuals even for low-risk procedures such as uncomplicated vaginal delivery.[55] The number of antibiotics actually shown to be safe for use in pregnancy is small. Fortunately, as noted in Table 5–7, current regimens include only a few doses of a penicillin derivative and an aminoglycoside and such therapy does not appear to pose a significant risk to fetal well-being.[56, 129]

Heart Transplantation

As the number and survival time of heart transplant recipients continues to increase, their quality of life, including sexuality and childbearing, have become important medical issues.[130] During the past few years, heart and heart-lung transplantation have emerged as reliable therapeutic alternatives in the treatment of end-stage congestive heart failure and irreversible primary pulmonary hypertension.[131, 132] Survival rates after heart transplantation currently average 80% at 1 year, 65% at 2 years, and 60% at 5 years.[133]

Currently, there is only limited information regarding reproductive histories of female patients undergoing heart or heart-lung transplantation because (a) this procedure has been generally limited to patients with severe coronary artery disease or other forms of nonischemic cardiomyopathy which are not typically seen in women of reproductive age, and (b) most heart transplantation centers recommend tubal ligations for heart recipients of reproductive age.[130] Reasons for the "sterilization policy" are based on the potential reduced longevity of the prospective mother as well as the concern regarding the teratogenicity of the immunosuppressive drugs. Thus, it is not surprising that, to date, very few cases of successful pregnancy after heart transplantation have been reported in the literature.[134, 135]

Most of the information to guide counseling in women who have successfully undergone cardiac transplantation is extrapolated from pregnancies in kidney allograft recipients[130, 136–138] (see also Chap. 2, p. 63.) Several issues appear to be pertinent: (1) Immunosuppressive medications do not appear

to adversely affect fertility. (2) No predominant developmental abnormalities have been described in the offspring of female patients taking conventional immunosuppressants. Preliminary data on cyclosporine suggest the same.[139] (3) Breast-feeding should be discouraged to avoid any potential risk to the neonate. (4) Gynecologic cancer is more prevalent in immunosuppressed patients; therefore, all female transplant recipients receiving conventional immunosuppressive therapy should undergo frequent surveillance for cervical carcinoma.

In summary, pregnancy after cardiac transplantation appears to be a realistic possibility. It is important that heart recipients considering pregnancy have normal cardiac performance with no evidence of rejection on endomyocardial biopsy.

Congenital Heart Disease

The advances in medical and surgical management of patients with congenital cardiac abnormalites have increased the number of women with congenital cardiac abnormalities that reach the childbearing years. The impact and outcome of pregnancy in these mothers as well as the impact of the mother's heart condition on fetal development have been matters of recent concern. Much of our current knowledge derives from prospective studies performed by Whittemore and co-workers[140, 141] who followed the outcome of pregnancies in young women with various congenital heart defects.

The various types of congenital malformations can be divided into three groups: (1) volume overload or left-to-right shunts (e.g., atrial or ventricular septal defects, persistent ductus arteriosus), (2) pressure overload (e.g., aortic and pulmonary stenosis, coarctation of the aorta, hypertrophic subaortic stenosis), and (3) cyanotic lesions or right-to-left shunts (e.g., tetralogy of Fallot or Eisenmenger's syndrome).

Volume Overload Lesions

One of the major determinants of the

magnitude of a left-to-right shunt is the ratio of pulmonary to systemic vascular resistance. During pregnancy the resistances on both systemic circulations fall to a similar degree, resulting in no significant change in the degree of shunting. There is no excessive amount of prematurity or dysmaturity in the offspring of mothers with volume overload lesions. Approximately 4% of infants have concordant defects and close to 10% have other forms of congenital abnormalities covering a wide spectrum of abnormalities.[140–145] Left-to-right shunting can occur at various levels, including the (a) interatrial septum, (b) interventricular septum, and (c) great vessels.

Atrial Septal Defect.—Atrial septal defects (ASDs) account for 7% of all congenital heart disease and 30% of congenital heart disease in adults, second only to bicuspid aortic valve.[146, 147] Atrial septal defects can be divided into three anatomic types. The most common is the ostium secundum defect, which accounts for approximately 70% of all ASDs. It is located in the region of the fossa ovalis and may be either single or have a fenestrated appearance. Secundum ASD is three times as common in females as in males and is particularly common in the hereditary disease known as Holt-Oram syndrome. Approximatley 20% to 30% of patients with secundum ASD will have associated findings suggestive of a myxomatous abnormality of the mitral valve. Mitral valve prolapse is not uncommon in these patients. The second type of ASD is the sinus venosus defect, which accounts for approximately 15% of ASDs. This defect is located in the upper portion of the interatrial septum near the orifice of the superior vena cava. This defect is often associated with partial anomalous pulmonary venous drainage. The third type of defect is the ostium primum ASD, which accounts for about 15% of ASDs. It results from a defect in the lower portion of the atrial septum, the area of the ostium primum or atrioventricular (AV) canal septum. This defect is often associated with a "cleft" or maldeveloped anterior mitral valve leaflet as well as rudimentary chordae tendineae attached to the upper rim of the ventricular septum.

Blood flow through the ASD occurs primarily during early and late ventricular systole, early ventricular diastole, and atrial systole. The magnitude of the left-to-right shunt depends on the size of the defect, the relationship of the right-to-left ventricular compliance, and indirectly on the ratio of the pulmonary to systemic vascular resistance. The net result in an uncomplicated ASD is volume overload and enlargement of the right atrium and right ventricle without dilatation of the left-sided chambers. The augmented blood volume associated with pregnancy poses a significant additional volume load on the right ventricle and increases pulmonary flow. Since the right ventricle is normally more compliant than the left ventricle, blood flows preferentially into the right chambers of the heart.[146, 147]

ASD is the most common maternal congenital lesion noted. Not infrequently, it is first diagnosed during pregnancy when a murmur is elicited.[146–149] Most women with an uncomplicated secundum ASD endure the hemodynamic challenge of pregnancy without difficulty, even when pulmonary blood flow is several times higher than the aortic blood flow.[140, 141] The pulmonary artery pressure remains normal mainly due to the physiologic adaptation of the pulmonary system. Congestive heart failure rarely develops and when it occurs it should be treated in the conventional manner with digoxin and diuretics. Persistent refractory congestive heart failure may necessitate surgical repair.

Prophylaxis for bacterial endocarditis is generally considered unnecessary before or after repair of an uncomplicated secundum ASD, unless a patch is used. However, associated lesions, such as mitral valve prolapse or cleft mitral or tricuspid valve, may require prophylaxis. Rare patients, especially those with pulmonary artery hypertension, may experience paradoxical emboli following delivery. Paroxysmal supraventricular tachycardias, sometimes persisting post partum, have been reported.

Marked elevation of the pulmonary vascular resistance is associated with high maternal death rates, especially at the time of delivery.[140, 141] This risk does not diminish until after the first postpartum week. Pregnancy should therefore be avoided by patients with ASD and pulmonary artery hypertension. If early termination of pregnancy in this setting is not possible, close monitoring of the patient is required throughout the pregnancy. The risk of thromboembolism in cyanotic patients with ASD is an absolute contraindication to the use of oral contraceptives. Intrauterine devices are relatively contraindicated due to the risk of infection. Tubal ligation may be considered, and injectable Deprovera has been used on an experimental basis.[150] The offspring of a parent with an ASD has a 2% to 3% chance of having a similar congenital defect.[151] In most cases, ASDs should be closed in nonpregnant women when there is a left-to-right shunt with a pulmonary-to-systemic blood flow ratio greater than 1.5:1.0, unless serious associated diseases (e.g., severe pulmonary artery hypertension) are present.[146–148]

Ventricular Septal Defect.—Ventricular septal defect (VSD) is the most common congenital cardiac anomaly seen at birth, accounting for 30% of malformations.[152] In adult patients, it follows bicuspid aortic valve, ASD, and pulmonic stenosis in frequency of appearance, and is slightly more common than persistent ductus arteriosus. The usual major reason for finding a VSD in adult patients is lack of diagnosis at an earlier time. The etiology of VSD is probably multifactorial with genetic and environmental components. The number of reported cases of VSD has risen substantially in the United States over the past 10 years; the reason for this increase is unknown.

The most common form of VSD occurs in the membranous septum, inferior to the crista supraventricularis. This type accounts for 75% of all VSDs. Muscular defects account for 10% of defects. They may be located anywhere in the muscular septum, but when single are usually found in the posterior portion. Less common are defects beneath the pulmonic valve located just above the crista supraventricularis; these constitute approximately 5% of all VSDs. Pulmonic and aortic valvular tissue are contiguous through these supracristal defects. These defects are generally small, but may result in progressive aortic regurgitation due to prolapse of an aortic leaflet into the defect.

Persistent common AV canal, or endocardial cushion defect, differs from VSD in that, in addition to deficiency of the membranous and posterior basal muscular ventricular septum, there is an associated ostium primum defect of the interatrial septum. These defects are often large and occupy the posterior ventricular septum near the junction of the mitral and tricuspid valve annuli and the lower interatrial septum. Atrioventricular canal defects occur most frequently in patients with trisomy 21. These defects result from failure of the AV endocardial cushions to fuse. The anterior mitral and septal tricuspid valve leaflets are frequently cleft, and there are abnormal chordal attachments to the rim of the ventricular septum. Lesions most frequently associated with VSD include ASD, persistent ductus arteriosus, mitral regurgitation, right aortic arch, L-transposition of the great arteries, and double outlet right ventricle.

The functional significance of a VSD depends on its size and on the status of the pulmonary vascular bed.[153] A small, restrictive defect permits only a small left-to-right shunt with normal RV and pulmonary artery pressures while large defects allow both ventricles to function as a single chamber with equal systemic and pulmonary artery pressures. Congestive heart failure and pulmonary hypertension do not ordinarily develop when the defect is less than 1.25 cm². The ratio of pulmonary to systemic blood flow defines the magnitude of the shunt, and depends on the relationship between pulmonary and systemic vascular resistance. As pulmonary resistance rises the left-to-right shunt decreases and left atrial and ventricular end-diastolic pressures fall. Pulmonary artery diastolic pressure rises, eventually equaling the aortic diastolic pressure. This occurs only with large defects, at least one-half to two-thirds the aortic diameter.

Pregnancy is well tolerated among women with small to moderate left-to-right shunts and only moderate pulmonary hypertension (peak pulmonary artery pressure <50 mm Hg). Patients with large left-to-right shunts may develop LV failure. Those with pulmonary artery hypertension may have further increases in pulmonary artery pressure. Eisenmenger's syndrome, which consists of pulmonary hypertension at the systemic level due to high pulmonary vascular resistance with reversal or bidirectional shunts at the aortopulmonary, ventricular, or atrial level, is associated with up to 50% mortality. Pregnancy is contraindicated in these patients.[140–142, 148] Close monitoring is necessary when early termination of the pregnancy is not possible in patients with marked elevation of the pulmonary artery resistance. The risk of thromboembolism in those with cyanosis is a contraindication to the use of oral contraceptives. Intrauterine devices are relatively contraindicated due to the risk of infection.

In adult patients with right-to-left shunts the presence of LV failure should suggest the presence of associated heart disease, such as coronary artery disease, cardiomyopathy, an additional congenital lesion, aortic insufficiency, or infective endocarditis.

Bacterial endocarditis represents a significant cause of mortality for patients with VSD that would otherwise have an uncomplicated course.[152, 154] Endocarditis prophylaxis should be given to all patients with VSD. The risk of endocarditis is markedly diminished following VSD repair, but remains high in those with residual defects. There are no reported cases of bacterial endocarditis following spontaneous closure of VSD.

Persistent Ductus Arteriosus.—The persistent ductus arteriosus (PDA) extends from the aortic isthmus near the origin of the left subclavian artery to the left pulmonary artery just distal to the pulmonary artery branch bifurcation. The physiologic consequences of a persistent ductus arteriosus are determined by the caliber of the ductal lumen and by the ratio of the pulmonary to systemic vascular resistance. In the case of a large PDA, blood flows through the ductus into the lungs throughout the cardiac cycle reflecting the persistent pressure gradient that exists between the aorta and the pulmonary artery. The net result is increased pulmonary blood flow and enlargement of the pulmonary arteries, left atrium, left ventricle, and ascending aorta.

This defect has become a rare finding in pregnancy since virtually all PDA cases are diagnosed and surgically corrected in early childhood. Most patients with PDA tolerate pregnancy without major difficulties and require no treatment other than prophylaxis against infectious endocarditis; however, occasionally patients may develop congestive heart failure during pregnancy. If pulmonary hypertension and shunt reversal occur, maternal and fetal complications are common.[140, 141]

Pressure Overload Lesions

In patients with fixed outflow tract obstruction, valvular gradients across stenotic lesions can be expected to increase during pregnancy due to the augmented stroke volume. Most patients with pressure overload lesions tolerate pregnancy fairly well. The increased preload associated with pregnancy is beneficial to maintain forward output; during late pregnancy, as preload becomes positional, forward flow can be substantially decreased in the supine position. In severe aortic stenosis, coronary perfusion is critical to maintain ventricular performance, and reductions of aortic diastolic pressure due to decreased peripheral vascular resistance is not well tolerated. Mothers with outflow obstruction have the highest incidence of cardiac abnormalities in their offspring; approximately 30% of infants and young children have been noted to have congenital abnormalities. Interestingly, approximately one half of the defects will be concordant with the maternal cardiac abnormality.[140–142]

Congenital Aortic Valve Disease.— The most common form of congenital valvular aortic stenosis is the bicuspid aortic valve. Unlike rheumatic valvular aortic stenosis, this type of aortic valve disease is usually not associated with mitral valve abnormality. Women with mild to moderate aortic valve stenosis tolerate pregnancy without significant difficulty. In severe aortic stenosis, cardiac reserve is limited, and syncope, especially during exercise, may first appear during gestation. In all cases, abrupt or vigorous dynamic exercise as well as isometric exercise should be avoided.

Pulmonary Stenosis.— Valvular pulmonary stenosis is a relatively common congenital cardiac defect with equal occurrence among males and females.[155, 156] The additional load on the heart during pregnancy in patients with pulmonic stenosis is tolerated fairly well as indicated by the study of Mendelson where heart failure was noted only in 5 out of 59 cases.[157] With today's improvements in medical therapy, the incidence of heart failure should be even smaller. The need for antibiotic prophylaxis remains controversial.

Coarctation of the Aorta.— Coarctation of the aorta is a focal narrowing of the distal aortic arch due to an abnormality of the media. In infants, the lesion forms opposite or proximal to the ductus arteriosus. In adults, the lesion usually appears distal to the ligamentum arteriosum. The obstruction to flow through the aorta results in hypertension proximal to the lesion with LV hypertrophy and relative hypotension and delayed pulses distal to the lesion. Prominent collateral formation is common.

Coarctation of the aorta is one of the causes of surgically correctable hypertension. While it may cause LV failure in infancy, adult patients with this anomaly are usually asymptomatic and are frequently discovered during a search for the etiology of hypertension. Coarctation of the aorta may be associated with a bicuspid aortic valve, hypoplastic aortic arch, endocardial fibroelastosis, VSD, PDA, or Turner's syndrome.[158–160]

Coarctation of the aorta may result in aortic dissection, heart failure, and premature atherosclerosis; intracranial hemorrhage may result from aneurysm formation in the circle of Willis. Endocarditis may occur at the site of coarctation, the aortic or mitral valve.

Medical management of the pregnant woman with coarctation can be challenging.[158, 160] Most pregnancies with coarctation of the aorta are uncomplicated and infants are normal. Due to the increased cardiac output associated with the second and third trimester of pregnancy, patients with unrepaired coarctation of the aorta may experience a significant increase in systolic blood pressure. In many cases, antihypertensive therapy may be required. Systemic blood pressure may also become particularly elevated during labor, delivery, and the immediate postpartum period. Hydralazine and/or nitroprusside infusion may be warranted at these times. Recent data have shown that nitroprusside readily crosses the placenta[161, 162] and close monitoring including serial determinations of maternal serum cyanide levels is indicated in the rare case where nitroprusside is deemed necessary.

In a small fraction of pregnant women with coarctation of the aorta, aortic dissection or rupture occurs during pregnancy.[158] However, it is likely that in these cases intrinsic disease of the ascending aorta characterized by cystic medial necrosis was present prior to pregnancy.[163] Fortunately, in modern obstetric practice this complication is so rare in women with unrepaired coarctation of the aorta that there seems to be little rationale for elective coarctation repair during pregnancy. The only indications for corrective surgery during pregnancy appear to be severe uncontrolled hypertension and congestive heart failure. Because the majority of aortic ruptures have been documented to occur prior to labor, vaginal delivery is recommended.

The bacteremia that infrequently accompanies labor rarely results in endocarditis or endarteritis in pregnant patients with coarctation.

Fetal mortality approaches 15% in some series while intrauterine growth retardation occurs frequently, presumably secondary to a significant reduction in placental blood flow.[158-160] The offspring of patients with coarctation of the aorta have a 2% chance of bearing children with similar congential defects.[151] After pregnancy, elective surgical correction should be recommended. Surgical correction of the defect does not, however, ensure that the blood pressure will return to normal.

In summary, each patient should be managed individually with regard to associated cardiac defects, the severity of hypertension, previous obstetric history, presence of congestive heart failure, and functional class. The current inability to identify or predict the woman with associated aortic wall abnormality remains a disturbing factor.

Hypertrophic Obstructive Cadiomyopathy.—Hypertrophic cardiomyopathy is a primary disorder of heart muscle characterized by symmetric (i.e., concentric) or asymmetric LV and/or RV hypertrophy of unknown cause in the absence of systemic hypertension or other identifiable causes of ventricular hypertrophy.[164]

At present, there are only speculations regarding the etiology of hypertrophic cardiomyopathy. Neither the cause of myocardial fiber disarray, the predominant histopathologic disorder, nor the cause of asymmetric septal hypertrophy, the predominant anatomic abnormality, has been established. It has been suggested that a supersensitivity to catecholamines may lead to a failure of regression of fetal myocardial fiber disarray and septal hypertrophy. In addition, in myocardial tissue obtained from patients with hypertrophic cardiomyopathy, an alteration of nonhistone nuclear proteins which are known to affect gene expression has been demonstrated, suggesting a genetically determined etiology.

Hypertrophic cardiomyopathy appears in both sporadic and familial forms, in which autosomal dominance is the usual form of inheritance.[165] In an echocardiographic study of the families of 70 cases of hypertrophic cardiomyopathy, Maron et al.[166] found that this condition was familial in 55% and sporadic in 45%. Autosomal dominant transmission was most common, occurring in 76% of familial cases, with the remainder transmitted via an autosomal recessive or autosomal dominant trait with variable gene expression.[166]

The characteristic pressure gradient encountered in hypertrophic cardiomyopathy is the obstructive pressure gradient across the LV outflow tract. It is related to systolic apposition of the mitral valve leaflets and submitral valve apparatus against the interventricular septum causing obstruction to forward flow from the LV cavity to the subaortic region. This gradient increases with decreased preload and afterload and augmented inotropic state.[164]

Among the common symptoms are dyspnea, angina, presyncope, and syncope. Dyspnea, the most common symptom, appears to be related to abnormalities in LV chamber compliance resulting in elevations of LV end-diastolic and pulmonary venous pressures. Angina appears to be due to myocardial ischemia secondary to the combination of LV outflow tract obstruction and diminished myocardial blood flow. The latter is related to diminished coronary vasodilator reserve capacity. Presyncope and syncope appear to be related to stimulation of intraventricular baroreceptors which results in reflex sympathetic withdrawal and peripheral vasodilation, or may be due to the inability to increase cardiac output with exertion due to either outflow obstruction or impaired diastolic filling. Syncope due to peripheral vasodilation is particularly ominous because it worsens the outflow obstruction.

Doppler echocardiography is the standard clinical tool used to diagnose hypertrophic cardiomyopathy. This technique, which is widely available and safe, allows direct visualization and quantification of the presence and extent of ventricular hypertrophy and dynamic outflow obstruction.

In general, patients with hypertrophic obstructive cardiomyopathy do well during pregnancy but are at higher risk than normal during the time of delivery. The severity of the LV outflow tract obstruction is determined mainly by the interplay between LV preload, systemic vascular resistance, and contractile state.[70, 167–170] During early to mid-pregnancy, the increase in cardiac output and subsequent increase in end-diastolic dimension may reduce the LV outflow obstruction. On the other hand, the falling systemic vascular resistance counteracts the potentially beneficial effects of increased preload. In pregnancy, reduction in preload in the supine position caused by partial inferior vena caval compression may increase LV outflow obstruction. During labor multiple variables interact. Performance of a Valsalva maneuver at the time of uterine contraction increases LV outflow obstruction by decreasing end-diastolic dimension (i.e., a measure of preload). This is counterbalanced by the rise in central blood volume and LV end-diastolic size that occurs during uterine contractions. The time of maximal risk is during delivery when acute blood loss can result in a marked decrease in LV chamber size and an acute increase in the severity of LV outflow tract obstruction.

Management of the pregnant patient with hypertrophic obstructive cardiomyopathy should include the following: (1) avoidance of digitalis or sympathomimetic medications since they can increase the severity of dynamic obstruction; (2) assumption of the lateral decubitus rather than the supine position when possible, thus avoiding decreases in LV preload; (3) avoidance of excessive diuresis or drugs that decrease preload and/or systemic vascular resistance. Of note, oxytocin does not seem to be contraindicated and may, in fact, lessen LV outflow obstruction. Most pregnant patients with hypertrophic obstructive cardiomyopathy tolerate pregnancy and a vaginal delivery relatively well. They should be well hydrated at the time of delivery. A Swan-Ganz catheter may be helpful in maintaining appropriate LV filling pressure and volume while providing information regarding impending pulmonary edema. Cesarean section should be reserved only for obstetric indications. Antibiotic prophylaxis to prevent vegetative endocarditis is indicated when mitral or aortic regurgitation is present.

Cyanotic Lesions

In patients with cyanotic congenital heart disease who survive to adulthood, a decrease in peripheral vascular resistance leads to an increase in right-to-left shunting with exacerbation of cyanosis. Decreased oxygenation leads to impaired fetal development. In Eisenmenger's syndrome as well as in primary pulmonary hypertension, the fall in peripheral vascular resistance (particularly when associated with the reduction in preload that may occur with postural changes or blood loss during delivery) may lead to hypotension as the right ventricle becomes incapable of ejecting blood across the high-resistance pulmonary arteriolar circuit. In addition, it has been suggested that widespread thrombosis of the small vessels in the pulmonary arterial system further aggravates pulmonary artery hypertension.[171]

In pregnancies continuing past the 20th week, prematurity and dysmaturity of the infants are common; in Whittemore's experience 32% have been premature by dates and 68% have been small-for-gestational-age. In these premature and dysmature babies, respiratory distress is often less of a problem than hypoglycemia.[140, 141] After corrective surgery, the infants have been normal in size and gestational age. In this group, the incidence of cardiac abnormalities similar to those of the mother has been reported to be less frequent than in the other two groups.[44, 140–145]

Tetralogy of Fallot.—In classic tetralogy of Fallot, a large VSD (malalignment type) is associated with infundibular pulmonic stenosis, RV hypertrophy, and an overriding aorta. This congential defect is the most common form of cyanotic congenital heart disease occurring in pregnancy.[172, 1732] Patients who have not undergone surgical correction or in whom only palliative approaches have been performed are at increased risk. Although congestive heart failure is rare, cerebrovascular accidents and brain abscesses may occur.

In patients with unrepaired tetralogy of Fallot, the magnitude of the right-to-left shunt through the VSD varies inversely with the systemic vascular resistance. The falling systemic vascular resistance during pregnancy explains the tendency for increased right-to-left shunting and a fall in systemic arterial saturation. This is associated with deeper cyanosis and rising hematocrits. As in other forms of cyanotic heart disease, children are small at birth and fetal wastage is increased.[172–174] There is increased mortality and morbidity for the mother. Poor prognostic signs include (a) hematocrit greater than 60%, (b) peripheral oxygen saturation of less than 80%, (c) RV pressure at or near systemic levels, and (d) recurrent syncopal episodes. Under such circumstances gestation is contraindicated. In contrast, pregnancy is not particularly hazardous if the patient is acyanotic following surgical repair.[173] This is particularly true when patients with severe pulmonary incompetence or persistent RV outflow tract obstruction are excluded. Nevertheless, it is important to monitor for ventricular arrhythmias during pregnancy, labor, and delivery in patients with repaired tetralogy of Fallot.

Ebstein's Anomaly of the Tricuspid Valve.—Ebstein's anomaly of the tricuspid valve comprises a wide variety of anatomic derangements. The principal abnormality is downward displacement of a malformed tricuspid valve into an underdeveloped right ventricle with reduced pumping capacity. The presence of a portion of the right ventricle between the AV groove and the downward displaced origin of the septal and posterior leaflets of the tricuspid valve results in a direct communication between the right atrium and the "atrialized" right ventricle. The degree of hemodynamic compromise to RV function depends on the amount of RV tissue above the tricuspid valve as well as the extent of adherence of the valve tissue to the RV wall. Tricuspid regurgitation, a problem frequently encountered with Ebstein's anomaly, further compromises effective RV output. Many patients with Ebstein's anomaly have a concomitant interatrial communication (ASD or patent foramen ovale) that allows right-to-left shunting of blood. Cyanosis may occur in adult patients with this malformation, becoming worse with exercise, fatigue, or exposure to cold.

Many patients with Ebstein's anomaly reach adult reproductive age, although their functional status will vary according to the adequacy of RV function and the status of the interatrial shunt.[175] When a woman with Ebstein's anomaly becomes pregnant, worsened RV failure may occur secondary to increased central blood volume and cardiac output. In addition, increased right-to-left shunting could become evident for the first time or increase if previously present due to the reduction in systemic vascular resistance which occurs especially during the third trimester of pregnancy. The fetus can therefore become chronically or transiently hypoxic and at risk for inadequate fetal growth and/or death. Frequently, supraventricular tachyarrhythmias have been noted during pregnancy with this condition.

In summary, according to previous studies, it appears that mothers who have mild Ebstein's anomaly and are acyanotic may successfully complete a normal pregnancy.[175] In contrast, mothers that experience cyanosis should be counseled to avoid pregnancy. Those cyanotic patients who choose to continue a gestation should be considered extremely high-risk patients. In this latter group, pulmonary pressures should be monitored at the time of delivery. Large intravascular volume changes such as the autotransfusion induced by uterine contractions and relief of inferior vena caval obstructions may aggravate the shunt at the atrial level or worsen right-sided failure.

Eisenmenger's Complex.—The term *Eisenmenger's complex* is used specifically to refer to the anatomicophysiologic combination of a VSD, pulmonary vascular disease, and right-to-left shunting of blood. The more general term, *Eisenmenger's syndrome,* is used to describe any communication between the systemic and pulmonary circulations that produces pulmonary vascular disease of such severity that bidirectional or predominantly right-to-left shunting occurs. Most of these patients become cyanotic in adolescence or early adult life. The cyanosis along with the digital clubbing and polycythemia are generally progressive. Death often occurs suddenly, although symptomatic arrhythmias do not usually pose a problem until late in the natural history of the disease. Symptoms of heart failure are common in adults with Eisenmenger's syndrome. In general, chest pain, syncopal attacks, and hemoptysis are considered ominous prognostic signs. The combination of two-dimensional echocardiographic imaging with contrast and Doppler techniques permits not only the detection of pulmonary artery hypertension, but correct diagnosis of the underlying cause (e.g., VSD).

Patients with Eisenmenger's syndrome should be advised against pregnancy since it is associated with a maternal mortality approaching 50%.[176, 177] If patients are seen in the first trimester, they should be advised against the extreme danger of continuing with the pregnancy. If early termination of pregnancy is not possible, close fetal and maternal monitoring as well as judicious medical care is required throughout the prenatal period. Maternal and fetal risk become maximal during labor, delivery, and the immediate postpartum period. The reason for this increased mortality is unknown, although it has been proposed that marked changes in shunt flow and pulmonary hemodynamics, with or without in situ pulmonary thrombi, may be responsible. Uterine contractions, especially when associated with the application of forceps, may have an adverse effect on pulmonary and systemic hemodynamics. The latter was studied by Midwall et al. who demonstrated that uterine contractions were associated with a decrease in the ratio of pulmonary to systemic blood flow.[177] Serial arterial blood gas determinations may be useful in detecting changes in shunt flow associated with an acute increase in pulmonary vascular resistance or a sudden fall in systemic vascular resistance. Increased maternal risk extends at least several days into the postpartum period.

Combined heart-lung transplantation is potentially the only curative therapy for patients with Eisenmenger's syndrome.[178] This technique has the major advantage of removing all of the diseased cardiopulmonary tissue and replacing it with anatomically, physiologically, and immunologically matched organs.

Pulmonary Artery Hypertension.—Severe pulmonary artery hypertension in pregnancy has a maternal mortality approaching 50%.[178, 179] The pulmonary artery hypertension may be primary or secondary in etiology. Common causes of secondary pulmonary artery hypertension include prolonged left-to-right shunting, recurrent pulmonary emboli, or drug abuse. Significant pulmonary artery hypertension is a contraindication to pregnancy. Fetal mortality exceeds 40% even when the mother survives the pregnancy.[177, 179] Should pregnancy occur in a patient with pulmonary hypertension, therapeutic abortion is warranted. If termination is not feasible, treatment should include (a) strict limitation of physical activity, (b) avoidance of the supine position in late pregnancy, (c) careful monitoring of blood loss at delivery, and (d) monitoring of pulmonary artery pressures using a Swan-Ganz catheter at the time of labor and delivery.

Developmental Defects

Mitral Valve Prolapse.—Mitral valve prolapse is very common, especially in females of whom 4% to 6% appear to have this syndrome.[180] This syndrome is characterized by an abnormal prolapse of one or both leaflets of the mitral valve from the left ventricle into the left atrium during systole; it may be either primary or secondary or associated with a wide variety of disorders such as ostium secundum ASD, Marfan's syndrome, Ebstein's anomaly of the tricuspid valve, and hypertrophic cardiomyopathy.

The etiology of this syndrome is unknown; the basic abnormality is that the mitral valve apparatus is redundant and larger than appropriate relative to the size of the mitral valve orifice. The clinical picture can range from a benign course to one associated with mitral regurgitation and complex arrhythmias. Most patients are asymptomatic, and the diagnosis usually is an incidental physical or echocardiographic finding. If symptoms are present, the patient classically tends to be anxious with complaints of palpitations, dyspnea on exertion, atypical chest pain, syncope, and panic attacks. The cause of the chest pain is unknown, although it has been speculated that it is due to tension on the papillary muscles as the valve prolapses.[180]

Mitral valve prolapse is the most common cardiac abnormality in the population of pregnant women.[181] Diagnostic difficulties may arise if the patient is seen for the first time during gestation. This is due to the hemodynamic changes inherent to pregnancy which can modify or abolish the characteristic midsystolic click and late systolic murmur.[182] The effect of pregnancy on the midsystolic click and murmur of the mitral valve prolapse can be explained when considering the hypervolemia of pregnancy, which may favorably realign the mitral valve apparatus by increasing LV end-diastolic volume and by lengthening the long axis of the left ventricle. Symptoms related to mitral valve prolapse are usually less obvious during pregnancy.

Most patients tolerate pregnancy very well and cardiac complications are extremely rare.[183] The incidence of spontaneous abortion or premature delivery is no higher than in women without an apparent cardiac disorder. The frequency of intrapartum complications also is not significantly greater among patients with mitral valve prolapse when compared to those with no cardiac disorder. Most infants delivered from women with mitral valve prolapse are appropriately sized and delivered without complications. Echocardiography is a clinically useful noninvasive tool for diagnosing mitral valve prolapse.[180] The issue of antibiotic prophylaxis in patients with mitral valve prolapse is not settled. One study concluded that antibiotics are not needed for routine vaginal delivery and cesarean section in many patients with heart disease.[127] Antibiotics should, however, be given for any complicated delivery. For other than routine vaginal delivery, most authors agree that prophylaxis should be given to women with mitral valve prolapse if a mitral regurgitation murmur is present on physical examination, but not for isolated clicks.[55] There may be a familial incidence of mitral valve prolapse, and autosomal dominant inheritance has been demonstrated in certain studies. Examination of other family members is sometimes recommended. Otherwise, genetic counseling is not recommended. The routine use of propranolol during pregnancy is controversial since some studies have suggested potential adverse maternal and fetal effects.[184] However, more recent results of prospective randomized comparisons of atenolol and metoprolol, each versus no drug therapy, failed to document significant adverse maternal or fetal effects of these drugs.[185, 186] (See Chap. 1, p. 28, for a more detailed discussion of the use of β-blockers in pregnancy.)

Aortic Dissection and Marfan's Syndrome.—In most cases, the patient with aortic dissection presents with severe chest pain which is usually ripping or stabbing in nature. In general, the location of the pain varies according to the site of the dissection: anterior thorax with proximal dissections and interscapular with distal aortic involvement. The physical findings are often sufficient to allow the diagnosis to be made with reasonable assurance. Diminution or loss of principal pulses in conjunction with recent onset of aortic regurgitation are important clues for the diagnosis of proximal aortic dissection. The differential diagnosis of patients with aortic dissection includes myocardial infarction, pneumothorax, acute aortic valve rupture, and pulmonary embolism.[187] In pregnant women the differential diagnosis should also include rupture of the uterus and abruptio placentae.

A commonly used classification system for aortic dissection is that of De Bakey and colleagues who recognized three types: Types I and II both originate in the ascending aorta. A type I dissection extends beyond the ascending aorta, whereas a type II dissection is confined to it. Type III dissections originate in the descending thoracic aorta distal to the origin of the left subclavian artery.

Although dissections predominate in males, with a male-to-female ratio of 3:1, there is a clear association between aortic dissection and pregnancy.[187, 188] To date, it is still unclear why half of all dissections in women under the age of 40 years occur during pregnancy, usually in the third trimester. In nonpregnant individuals, hypertension is a major predisposing factor; however, it is only seen in 25% of those cases occurring during pregnancy. A hormonal factor has been implicated; however, women who use birth control pills have not been found to have an increased incidence of dissection.[187] Malformation of the aorta and Marfan's syndrome seem to account for most of the aortic dissections occurring during pregnancy.

Marfan's syndrome is a rare disorder of connective tissue which is inherited as an autosomal dominant trait with a high degree of penetrance.[189, 190] The predominant clinical manifestations occur in the skeletal, ocular, pulmonary, and cardiovascular systems. Aortic dilatation is generally present even in childhood and may result in three major complications: aortic dissection, aortic rupture, and aortic regurgitation. In patients with Marfan's syndrome, aortic dissection is caused by the sudden development of a tear in the aortic intima through which blood surges, separating the intima from the adventitia. Controversy still exists whether the initial event is a rupture of the intima with secondary dissection into the media or hemorrhage within a diseased media followed by disruption of subjacent intima and subsequent propagation of the dissection through the tear.[187] Nearly all patients with Marfan's syndrome also have myxomatous changes involving the aortic and/or mitral valves. When considering Marfan's syndrome, it is important to remember that women with no marfanoid appearance may still have all the cardiovascular findings of this syndrome.[189–191] Pregnancy greatly increases the risk of aortic dissection and rupture in these patients.[192] Structural alterations in the aortic wall during gestation, perhaps due to the high levels of estrogen in conjunction with the inherent abnormality of the aortic media (i.e., cystic medionecrosis), appear to predispose to aneurysm formation or dissection. The risk of cardiovascular complications, which have been reported to occur in as much as 50% of the cases, may occur at any time during pregnancy, labor, and early puerperium, but the most stressful period on the aorta seems to be during the third trimester.

Women affected by Marfan's syndrome are confronted by two problems when considering pregnancy.[190, 192] The first is a 50% risk that offspring will inherit the syndrome; the second concerns the apparently increased risk of aortic rupture during pregnancy. There is no contraindication to pregnancy in those women with Marfan's syndrome without cardiovascular manifestations. Serial echocardiographic examinations are usually recommended to diagnose any changes in aortic diameter early in the course of pregnancy. In contrast, women with pre-conceptional dilatation of the aortic root should avoid pregnancy. If dilatation of the aorta exceeds 4 cm, interruption of pregnancy should be recommended.

Noninvasive imaging techniques, especially echocardiography, computed tomographic (CT) scanning, and magnetic resonance imaging (MRI), have been widely used in the initial evaluation of aortic dissection.[43, 191] Aortic angiography still remains the definitive method for confirming the diagnosis of aortic dissection with a diagnostic accuracy of 95% to 99%. If a diagnosis of a type I or II dissection is made, the patient should be taken immediately for surgical repair of the aorta. In contrast, if the repair is distal to the origin of the left subclavian artery, medical management is the treatment of choice.[187] In all cases of dissection, initial medical treatment is aimed at halting the progression of the dissecting hematoma by reducing both systolic blood pressure and the velocity of LV ejection. Medical therapy usually includes intravenous β-adrenergic blockade and sodium nitroprusside infusion. Since surgery has been reported to be successful, the approach to aortic dissection during pregnancy should be identical to that occurring in the nonpregnant state.

THE USE OF CARDIOVASCULAR DRUGS IN PREGNANCY

As previously stated, no medication should be used during pregnancy unless there is clear justification.

Anticoagulants

Pregnancy is associated with a hypercoagulable state characterized by elevated levels of coagulation factors II, VII, VIII, and X, increased plasma fibrinogen, and augmented platelet adhesiveness. Other factors which may predispose to intravascular thrombosis in pregnancy include alterations in venous blood flow in the lower extremities and decreased plasma fibrinolytic activity. Anticoagulant therapy during pregnancy is problematic because both heparin and oral anticoagulants can potentially produce adverse maternal and fetal effects.[77]

The indications for anticoagulation in pregnancy are similar to those of the nonpregnant state and include (1) deep venous thrombosis, (2) pulmonary emboli, (3) recurrent emboli as a result of valvular heart disease, and (4) prevention of thrombosis and/or emboli in patients with arrhythmias, pros-

thetic heart valves, and congestive heart failure. Comments here will focus on cardiac sources of thromboembolism and the reader is referred to Chap. 6 for a detailed discussion of the treatment of venous thromboembolism.

Patients with artificial heart valves usually require long-term anticoagulant therapy to prevent thromboembolism. This is particularly true during pregnancy when, as mentioned above, there is a hypercoagulable state and the mother is at increased risk for systemic embolization and death. Pregnancy in these patients poses a serious challenge since the administration of coumarinics, the most commonly used agents in nonpregnant patients, results in an increased incidence of fetal death and birth defects.[193, 194]

Oral anticoagulants, such as warfarin sodium (Coumadin; FDA class D), cross the placental barrier, exposing the fetus to potential teratogenic effects. Fetal exposure to coumarinics during the first trimester of pregnancy (more specifically when embryonic exposure occurs between the sixth and ninth week of gestation) may cause a constellation of malformations known as "warfarin embryopathy." The most common features of this syndrome are nasal hypoplasia, saddle nose, and stippled epiphysis. The incidence varies in different series from 7.9% to 16%.[193, 194] In addition, studies have shown a high rate of spontaneous abortion ranging between 29% and 44%. When warfarin is administered during the second and third trimester, fetal risk persists despite the fact that organogenesis is reasonably complete. This is particularly true when warfarin is used by mothers near term and at the time of delivery. Problems include stillbirths and live offspring with severe hemorrhagic complications secondary to birth trauma.

Because of the teratogenic effect and increased abortion rates associated with the use of warfarin during the first trimester, heparin (FDA Class C) (which is a large molecule that does not cross the placenta) is the anticoagulant of choice during this period.[77] One uncontrolled study[194] suggested that administration of heparin during gestation was associated with adverse outcomes in approximately one third of such pregnancies; however, this may have been the result of coexisting medical conditions rather than the anticoagulant treatment. This possibility is supported by the recently reported retrospective cohort investigation of Ginsberg et al.[195] which demonstrated that maternal heparin therapy appears to be quite safe for the fetus.

Although the use of heparin lessens the jeopardy of fetal teratogenicity, the pregnant woman is exposed to the risks of hemorrhage and osteoporosis.[77, 196] Most of the approximately 20 cases of osteoporosis reported in patients on long-term heparin therapy have occurred in gravid women receiving at least 20,000 units/day for more than 6 months.[77] The ideal dose of heparin for pregnant patients with artificial heart valves requires further investigation. Iturbe-Alesio et al. described three cases of thrombosis of a mechanical valve prosthesis during pregnancy while on a fixed dose of 5,000 units of subcutaneous heparin, thereby demonstrating that at this dose heparin does not appear to give adequate protection against thromboembolic complications in patients with artificial mechanical heart valves.[78] This appears to be particularly true for patients with tilting-disk valves in either the mitral or aortic positions. Lee et al.[80] used adjusted subcutaneous heparin for thromboembolism prophylaxis during 18 pregnancies in 16 women with an artificial heart valve.[80] Oral warfarin was replaced by subcutaneous heparin as soon as pregnancy was confirmed. The dosage of heparin was adjusted to maintain a partial thromboplastin time at 1.5 times the control value and treatment was administered during the first trimester and the last 3 weeks of gestation. Warfarin was used between the 13th and 37th week. Using this regimen there were no maternal thromboembolic complications and none of the liveborn infants showed congenital malformations. However, there were nine spontaneous abortions (five occurring in the first 12 weeks) that were probably related to warfarin exposure at the beginning of pregnancy. These data suggest that whenever possible pre-conception replacement of warfarin by heparin should be considered. Prior to delivery *intravenous* heparin appears to be the administration route of choice.

Because of the lack of large controlled trials documenting the efficacy of heparin, definitive recommendations for anticoagulant therapy of pregnant women with artificial heart valves cannot be given. It is, however, extremely important that all women of childbearing age be counseled about this issue prior to pregnancy so that a rational strategy can be implemented. Ginsberg and Hirsch[77] have suggested two alternatives for the treatment of the gravida with an artificial valve: (1) Substitute heparin for warfarin prior to pregnancy, if possible, or before the sixth gestational week, and continue this treatment throughout pregnancy. Heparin is administered every 12 hours by subcutaneous injection in a dose adjusted to keep the midinterval partial thromboplastin time 1.5 times the control. (2) Use adjusted-dose heparin until the 13th gestational week, change to warfarin until the middle of the third trimester, and then restart heparin therapy until delivery. It should be kept in mind that with the latter approach fetopathic effects due to warfarin (e.g., central nervous system abnormalities) are still possible. Following discontinuation of heparin for delivery, it may be restarted within a few hours of an uncomplicated vaginal delivery or 24 hours after cesarean section.

Antiplatelet agents, such as aspirin (FDA Class C when used in 1st and 2nd trimester; Class D when used in 3rd trimester) and dipyridamole (FDA Class C) have been advocated as an alternative to heparin in pregnant women with mechanical valve prosthesis. However, the study of Salazar et al.[79] indicates that antiplatelet agents do not provide adequate protection against thromboembolism in pregnant women with mitral or aortic valve prosthesis.

Finally, heparin is not secreted into breast milk and can be safely administered to the lactating patient. Current data also suggest that treatment of a nursing mother with warfarin does not appear to produce an anticoagulant effect in the breast-fed infant.[77]

β-Blockers

There have been numerous studies of β-blockers (FDA Classes B and C depending on specific agent) in animal pregnancy and their use in humans has been extensively reported. Nonetheless, the safety and precise indications for the use of these agents in pregnant women remain unclear. Initial reports of retrospective, uncontrolled observations associating maternal propranolol use with intrauterine growth retardation, neonatal respiratory depression, bradycardia, and hypoglycemia were disturbing[184, 185, 197]; however, more recent results of prospective randomized comparisons of atenolol and metoprolol, each versus no drug therapy, failed to document significant adverse maternal or fetal effects of these drugs.[186, 198, 199]

Despite the above reassuring results of controlled trials the data should be interpreted with caution. In this regard, in a preliminary report of a placebo-controlled trial in which atenolol was initiated for chronic hypertension between 12 and 24 weeks of pregnancy, a clinically significant reduction in infant and placental weights was observed in the drug-treated group.[200] These data emphasize that the safety of β-blockers in pregnancy has not been fully established. Nonetheless, in the gravida with clear indications for β-adrenoceptor therapy, such as symptomatic mitral valve prolapse, supraventricular tachyarrythmias, and ischemic heart disease, we believe such therapy should not be withheld (see Chap. 1, p. 28, for a more detailed discussion of the use of β-blockers).

Diuretics

Maternal complications of diuretics (FDA Class C) include pancreatitis, volume contraction and alkalosis, decreased carbohydrate tolerance, hypokalemia, hyponatremia, and hyperuricemia.[201] Bleeding diathesis and hyponatremia have been reported in the neonate. Thus, there are few unequivocal indications for diuretic use in pregnancy. The only patients for whom saliuretics can be prescribed unhesitatingly are gravidas with heart failure, particularly when sodium restriction has been unsuccessful[201] (see Chap. 1, p. 29, for a detailed discussion of these agents.).

Cardiac Glycosides and Other Positive Inotropic Agents

Digoxin (FDA Class C) is the most widely used of all the various digitalis preparations. Indications for its use in gestation are similar to those in nonpregnant patients. Delayed gastric emptying, which may occur during pregnancy or delivery, may retard its absorption.[202] Digoxin's volume of distribution is significantly increased during pregnancy. Because the drug is only 20% to 25% bound to proteins, decreases in albumin levels during pregnancy do not greatly affect its serum concentration. Pregnancy is associated with significant increases of digoxin-like substances that may interfere with the digoxin radioimmunoassay, seriously affecting the technique's reliability as a monitoring tool of serum levels during pregnancy.[203] Transplacental passage of digoxin has been extensively documented. The latter property has been used for the in utero treatment of fetal tachyarrhythmias. When digoxin is used in combination with other antiarrhythmic agents during pregnancy, precautions regarding drug interactions apply as in nongravid patients. Digoxin is secreted in breast milk.[202, 204] The total amount of digoxin ingested by the infant, however, is approximately 1% of the recommended daily pediatric dose; no adverse effects have been observed in newborns. Reports of untoward digoxin side effects during gestation are rare. In theory, digoxin could shorten the duration of labor because of its positive inotropic effect on the myometrium. Intravenous infusions of moderate to high doses of dopamine, dobutamine, and norepinephrine (all FDA Class C) may jeopardize the fetus because of decreased uterine blood flow, however, they should not be withheld if felt essential to maternal therapy. In addition, these drugs may stimulate uterine contractions.[205–207]

Antiarrhythmic Drug Therapy in Pregnancy

Cardiac rhythm disturbances may develop in otherwise healthy pregnant women, but frequently are associated with underlying acquired or congenital heart disease. Benign atrial and ventricular premature beats are common in normal pregnancies and do not require antiarrhythmic therapy. Some patients with paroxysmal atrial tachycardia, Wolff-Parkinson-White syndrome, or both, are prone to have more frequent arrhythmic episodes during pregnancy. Atrial fibrillation and flutter are common in pregnant women with underlying heart disease and can, in some cases, be avoided by prophylactic administration of digoxin. In general, acute management of arrhythmias in pregnancy is very similar to that of the nonpregnant state. Direct-current cardioversion is thought to be safe in pregnancy (see below). Indications for anticoagulation prior to direct-current conversion are similar to the nonpregnant state, although warfarin should be avoided as discussed previously.

The pregnant woman with cardiac arrhythmias constitutes a concern and challenge for the physician since arrhythmias-related hemodynamic alterations may jeopardize the mother and harm the fetus by decreasing uterine blood flow. The decision regarding the necessity of antiarrhythmic therapy should be based upon the nature and severity of the maternal or fetal arrhythmia, balancing the benefit of successful therapy against the potential risk of adverse effects to both mother and fetus.

Although the pharmacologic principles and antiarrhythmic drug therapy in pregnant and nonpregnant patients are similar, several additional considerations apply during pregnancy.[208, 209] First, during pregnancy reduced mobility of the gastrointestinal tract may reduce the rate and extent of absorption of certain drugs. Second, the expansion of the maternal intra- and extravascular volume may affect the drug's volume of distribution, implying that the acute administration of a single drug dose may likely result in lower serum concentration in pregnant versus nonpregnant women. Third, as plasma volume increases progressively during pregnancy, plasma protein concentration tends to fall and may, in part, account for the considerable reduction in the extent of drug protein binding during pregnancy. This will result in decreased total drug concentration, increased tissue-to-plasma distribution, and, for some drugs, increased drug clearance from the body. Thus, the therapeutic concentration of a drug needed to obtain a pharmacologic effect may be diminished. Fourth, pregnancy's hormone-mediated effects on hepatic drug metabolism and the fetoplacental unit may also influence the activity of a variety of drugs.

The effect of maternal drug therapy on the fetus may result in fetal toxicity since in most antiarrhythmic drugs successful transfer across the placenta has been documented. The rapid transplacental transfer of antiarrhythmic therapy has been used successfully for the in utero treatment of fetal tachyarrhythmias. Since most antiarrhythmic agents are also secreted in breast milk, this route may also become potentially toxic for the newborn.

Antiarrhythmic Agents

Little information is available on the use of quinidine, procainamide, lidocaine, disopyramide, or any of the newer antiarrhythmic agents during pregnancy (Table 5–8).

Since quinidine is 60% to 80% bound to protein, hypoalbuminemia during pregnancy may increase the unbound readily available fraction.[202, 205, 207] Transplacental passage of quinidine has been demonstrated. At therapeutic blood levels, quinidine can decrease oxytocic activity; however, at toxic doses, premature labor may occur. Other side effects include fetal thrombocytopenia and damage to the eighth cranial nerve. Quinidine is se-

TABLE 5–8.
Safety and Adverse Effects of Antiarrhythmic Drugs During Pregnancy

Drug	Pregnancy-Related Adverse Effects	FDA Class*
Digoxin	No adverse effects established	C
Quinidine	Toxic doses may induce premature labor	C
Procainamide	Unknown	C
Disopyramide	May initiate uterine contraction	C
Lidocaine	Appears safe	B
Mexiletine	Unknown	C
Amiodarone	Unknown	C
Verapamil	Unknown	C
β-Blockers	Safety remains unclear; may cause intrauterine growth retardation and compromise fetal response to hypoxic stress; see text for details.	C

*See Preface for description of FDA (Food and Drug Administration) risk classification.

creted in breast milk in quantities that are well below the pediatric daily recommended dose.[210]

Procainamide appears to be a safe antiarrhythmic agent for use during pregnancy; no teratogenic reports have been reported to date.[202, 205, 207] However, because of the limited data available, it should be used as a second-line drug during pregnancy, after digoxin and quinidine. Lidocaine's use as an antiarrhythmic agent during pregnancy has been rarely reported. Lidocaine may produce central nervous system side effects in both the mother and the fetus. In a study of 57 pregnant women given lidocaine for caudal, epidural, cervical, or pudendal block, half of the infants with drug levels above 2.5 g/mL had low Apgar scores.[211] It thus appears that the use of lidocaine during pregnancy is safe as long as the maternal levels are kept within the low to midrange and the fetal acid-base status is normal (lidocaine is a weak base and may be trapped in the slightly acidic environment of the amniotic fluid).

The experience with mexiletine, a new class 1b antiarrhythmic drug structurally re-

lated to lidocaine, is limited.[212] Disopyramide should be used only in refractory cases because there is only limited experience with its use.[213] Moreover, disopyramide has been found in human breast milk in concentrations similar to those found in blood and has been reported to initiate uterine contractions.[213]

There are several reports describing the use of amiodarone during pregnancy for either maternal or fetal rhythm disturbances (transplacental passage concentrations reach 10%–25% of maternal levels).[214] Maternal indications were both supraventricular and ventricular tachyarrhythmias. Fetal indications were also tachyarrhythmias. Maternal amiodarone toxicity is similar to that in nonpregnant patients. Transient bradycardia and mild QT prolongation have been reported with its use during pregnancy. No other adverse or teratogenic effects have been described. Hypotension, heart block, bradycardia resistant to atropine, and junctional rhythm abnormalities have been described in patients receiving amiodarone treatment at the time of epidural or general anesthesia.

Verapamil has been used for various indications during pregnancy. In Europe it has been used experimentally (1) as part of an intravenous tocolytic mixture to treat premature labor and (2) in the treatment of pregnancy-induced hypertension.[215, 216] It also has been used as an antiarrhythmic agent for both the fetal and maternal tachyarrhythmias. Verapamil increases serum digoxin concentrations due to lowered renal clearance; therefore, when combining these two drugs, reduction of digoxin dosage is mandatory. Maternal adverse effects are similar to those seen in the nonpregnant state and no teratogenic effects have been reported. Verapamil therapy is compatible with breast-feeding.

Tocolytic Therapy

Because uterine contraction can be inhibited by stimulation of β₂-receptors, non-catechol adrenergic agonists such as ritodrine hydrochloride, terbutaline, and isoxsuprine have been used to suppress premature contractions. These drugs can result in potent cardiac-positive chronotropic and inotropic effects and should therefore be used with caution in patients with latent or manifest heart disease.[217, 218] Pulmonary edema and cardiac ischemia during and shortly after discontinuation of treatment have been reported.[219] The association of tocolytic therapy with pulmonary edema appears to be unique to the pregnant state, because this complication has not been reported when similar drugs have been used at high dosages to treat asthma. The major criteria for diagnosis of pulmonary edema associated with tocolytic therapy are (1) recent (<24 hours) or current use; (2) dyspnea occurring before delivery in less than 12 hours post partum in women who deliver despite tocolytic use; (3) a chest roentgenogram showing unilateral or bilateral alveolar infiltrates; (4) evidence of hemodilution (decreased hematocrit or hypokalemia); and (5) rapid clinical response (<24 hours) to treatment with diuretics and oxygen.[219] (See Chap. 7, p. 254, for a more detailed discussion of tocolytic-induced pulmonary edema.)

Vasodilator Therapy

Use of the potent vasodilator sodium nitroprusside has been reported in very few pregnant women,[161, 162, 220, 221] usually in an emergent situation such as pulmonary edema or life-threatening hypertension unresponsive to more conventional therapy. This drug, which is metabolized to cyanide and thiocyanate, crosses the placenta (at least in pregnant sheep), thus raising concern regarding potential fetal toxicity. In this regard Naulty et al. observed markedly elevated fetal blood cyanide levels and death in four sheep following a 60-minute infusion averaging 25 μg/kg/min.[161] However, in a second group receiving less than 1 μg/kg/min, there were no apparent adverse effects. These results are consistent with other observations (in both animals and humans) that brief infusions of relatively low doses (<4 μg/kg/min) have not been associated with maternal or fetal blood cyanide levels in the toxic range or with clinically evident toxicity.[220–222] Nonetheless, because of this concern, nitroprusside remains a drug of last resort during pregnancy. The effect of nitroprusside on uteroplacental blood flow remains unclear, since observations in normotensive and hypertensive sheep have yielded conflicting results.[161, 220–222]

Captopril, enalapril, and lisinopril are currently used as antihypertensive agents. Observations in two species of animals and humans suggest that the administration of captopril is associated with an increase in perinatal mortality. No controlled trials of the use of captopril or other angiotensin converting enzyme inhibitors in human pregnancy have been published to date; however, reports of anuric renal failure, including several fatalities, in human neonates exposed to the drug in utero lead us to conclude that these drugs are contraindicated during gestation.[223]

Hydralazine has been used in pregnancy, primarily as a parenteral agent in the therapy of acute, severe hypertension occurring near term or during labor and delivery. It has also been employed successfully in the chronic setting as a second-line agent in combination with either methyldopa or a β-blocker. Hydralazine appears to be reasonably safe for the fetus, although there are anectodal reports of fetal distress and thrombocytopenia in a few infants whose mothers were treated with this drug.[224–226] Nonetheless, if vasodilator therapy is indicated in a pregnant patient, hydralazine appears to be the agent of choice.

Prazosin, an α1-receptor antagonist, has been used in uncontrolled studies of chronic hypertension and pheochromocytoma complicating gestation. No specific untoward effects have been identified; however, given the limited data currently available, there is little reason to currently use this drug in pregnancy.[227]

Direct-Current Cardioversion

Use of direct-current cardioversion during pregnancy has been performed repeatedly.[228, 229] Energies as high as 100 watt-seconds were used. Gestation and delivery were normal in all cases. Fetal heart rate monitoring revealed no apparent effect on the fetus.

Acknowledgments

We wish to thank Claudia Korcarz, D.V.M., Dorothy J. Douglas, Valerie L. Thorn, and Pam Tolocka for their assistance in the preparation of this manuscript. We also thank David P. James and Alex Neumann for graphic support.

REFERENCES

1. Elkayam U, Gleicher N: Cardiovascular physiology of pregnancy, in Elkayam U, Gleicher N (eds): *Cardiac Problems in Pregnancy.* New York, Alan R. Liss, Inc, 1982, pp 5–26.

2. Metcalfe J, Ueland K: Maternal cardiovascular adjustments to pregnancy. *Prog Cardiovasc Dis* 1974; 16:363–374.

3. DeSwiet M: The cardiovascular system, in Hytten FE, Chamberlain GVP (eds): *Clinical Physiology in Obstetrics.* Oxford, Blackwell Scientific Publications, 1980, pp 3–42.

4. Sugrue D, Blake S, MacDonald D, et al: Pregnancy complicated by maternal heart disease at the National Maternity Hospital, Dublin, Ireland, 1969 to 1978. *Am J Obstet Gynecol* 1981; 139:1–6.

5. McFaul PB, Dornan JC, Lamki H, et al: Pregnancy complicated by maternal heart disease: A review of 519 women, *Br J Obstet Gynaecol* 1988; 95:861–867.

6. Engle MA, Perloff JK: Symposium on postoperative congential heart disease in adults. *Am J Cardiol* 1982; 50:541–656.

7. Barron WM, Lindheimer MD: Renal sodium and water handling in pregnancy. *Obstet Gynecol Annu* 1984; 13:35–69.

8. Schrier RW: Pathogenesis of sodium and water retention in high-output and low-output cardiac failure, nephrotic syndrome, cirrhosis and pregnancy. *N Engl J Med* 1988; 319:1065–1072, 1127–1134.

9. Cutforth R, MacDonald CB: Heart sounds and murmurs in pregnancy. *Am Heart J* 1966; 71:741–747.

10. Proctor HW: Alteration of the cardiac physical examination in normal pregnancy. *Clin Obstet Gynecol* 1975; 18:51–63.

11. Tabatznik B, Randall TW, Hersch C: The mammary souffle of pregnancy and lactation. *Circulation* 1960; 22:1069–1073.

12. Marcus FI, Ewy FA, O'Rourke RA, et al: The effect of pregnancy on murmurs of mitral and aortic regurgitation. *Circulation* 1970; 41:795–805.

13. Robertson EG: The natural history of oedema during pregnancy. *J Obstet Gynaecol Br Commw* 1971; 78:520–529.

14. Robson S, Hunter S, Boys RJ, et al: Serial study of factors influencing changes in cardiac output during human pregnancy. *Am J Physiol* 1989; 256:H1060–H1065.

15. Lee W, Rokey R, Cotton DB: Noninvasive maternal stroke volume and cardiac output determinations by pulsed Doppler echocardiography. *Am J Obstet Gynecol* 1988; 158:505–510.

16. Robson SC, Dunlop W, Moore M, et al: Combined Doppler and echocardiographic measurement of cardiac output: Theory and application in pregnancy. *Br J Obstet Gynaecol* 1987; 94:1014–1027.

17. Kerr MG: The mechanic effects of the gravid uterus in late pregnancy. *J Obstet Gynaecol Br Commw* 1965; 72:513–529.

18. Quilligan EJ, Tyler C: Postural effects on the cardiovascular status in pregnancy: A comparison of the lateral and supine postures. *Am J Obstet Gynecol* 1978; 130:194–198.

19. Holmes F: Incidence of the supine hypotensive syndrome in late pregnancy. A clinical study in 500 subjects. *J Obstet Gynaecol Br Emp* 1960; 67:254–258.

20. McRoberts WA: Postural shock in pregnancy. *Am J Obstet Gynecol* 1951; 62:627–631.

21. Ueland K, Novy M, Peterson EN, et al: Maternal cardiovascular dynamics. *Am J Obstet Gynecol* 1969; 104:856–864.

22. Katz R, Karliner JS, Resnik R: Effects of a natural volume overload state (pregnancy) on left ventricular performance in normal human subjects. *Circulation* 1978; 58:434–441.

23. Christianson RE: Studies on blood pressure during pregnancy. I. Influence of parity and age. *Am J Obstet Gynecol* 1976; 125:509–513.

24. Pirani BBK, Campbell DM, MacGillivray I: Plasma volume in normal first pregnancy. *J Obstet Gynaecol Br Commw* 1973; 80:884.

25. Brown MA: Sodium and plasma volume regulation in normal and hypertensive pregnancy: A review of physiology and clinical implication. *Clin Exp Hypertens [B]* 1988; 137:265–282.

26. Lang RM, Briller RA, Neumann A, et al: Assessment of global and regional left ventricular mechanics: Applications to myocardial ischemia, in Kerber RE (ed): *Echocardiography in Coronary Artery Disease.* Futura Publishing Co, 1988, pp 1–37.

27. Rubler S, Damani PM, Pinto ER: Cardiac size and performance during pregnancy estimated with echocardiography. *Am J Cardiol* 1977; 40:534–540.

28. Lim YL, Walters WAW: Systolic time intervals in normotensive and hypertensive human pregnancy. *Am J Obstet Gynecol* 1976; 126:26–32.

29. Lotgering FK, Gilbert RD, Longo LD: Maternal and fetal responses to exercise during pregnancy. *Physiol Rev* 1985; 65:1–36.

30. Artal R, Platt LD, Sperling M, et al: Exercise in pregnancy. I. Maternal cardiovascular and metabolic responses in normal pregnancy. *Am J Obstet Gynecol* 1981; 140:123–127.

31. Guzman CA, Caplan R: Cardiorespiratory response to exercise during pregnancy. *Am J Obstet Gynecol* 1970; 108:600–605.

32. Naeye TL, Peters EC: Working during pregnancy: Effects on the fetus. *Pediatrics* 1982; 69:724–727.

33. Barron WM: The pregnant surgical patient. Medical evaluation and management. *Ann Intern Med* 1984; 101:683–691.

34. Adams JQ, Alexander AM: Alterations in cardiovascular physiology during labor. *Am J Obstet Gynecol* 1958; 12:542–549.

35. Bieniarz J, Crottogini JJ, Curuchet E, et al: Autocaval compression by the uterus in late human pregnancy. *Am J Obstet Gynecol* 1968; 100:203–217.

36. Henricks CH, Quilligan EJ: Cardiac output during labor. *Am J Obstet Gynecol* 1956; 71:953–972.

37. Ueland K, Hansen JM: Maternal cardiovascular dynamics. III. Labor and delivery under local and caudal analgesia. *Am J Obstet Gynecol* 1969; 103:8–18.

38. Mangano DT: Anesthesia of the pregnant cardiac patient, in Shneider SM, Levinson G (eds): *Anesthesia for Obstetrics.* Baltimore, Williams & Wilkins Co, 1987, pp 345–379.

39. Robson S, Hunter S, Boys R, et al: Changes in cardiac output during epidural anesthesia for Caesarean section. *Anaesthesia* 1989; 44:475–479.

40. Walters WAW, MacGregor WG, Hills M: Cardiac output at rest during pregnancy and the puerperium. *Clin Sci* 1966; 30:1–11.

41. Carruth JE, Mirvis SB, Brogan DR, et al: The electrocardiogram in normal pregnancy. *Chest* 1981; 102:1075–1078.

42. Rubler S, Damani PM, Pinto ER: Cardiac size and performance during pregnancy estimated with echocardiography. *Am J Cardiol* 1977; 40:534–540.

43. Spangler RD, Nora JJ, Lortscher RH, et al: Echocardiography in Marfan's syndrome. *Chest* 1976; 69:72–78.

44. Jacoby WJ Jr: Pregnancy with tetralogy and pentalogy of Fallot. *Am J Cardiol* 1964; 14:866–873.

45. Jones AM, Howitt G: Eisenmenger's syndrome in pregnancy. *Br Med J* 1965; 2:1627–1631.

46. Pedersen H, Finster M: Anesthetic risk in the pregnant patient. *Anesthesiology* 1979; 51:439–451.

47. Szekely P, Turner R, Snaith L: Pregnancy and the changing pattern of rheumatic heart disease. *Br Heart J* 1973; 35:1293–1303.

48. Chesley LC: Severe rheumatic cardiac disease and pregnancy: The ultimate prognosis. *Am J Obstet Gynecol* 1979; 136:552–558.

49. Metcalfe J, Ueland K: Rheumatic heart disease in pregnancy. *Clin Obstet Gynecol* 1968; 11:1010–1025.

50. Bentivoglio Y, Goldberg M: Assessment of ventricular inflow and outflow obstruction, in Bentivoglio Y, Goldberg M (eds): *Cardia Catheterization Data to Hemodynamics Parameters.* Philadelphia, FA Davis Co, 1988, pp 122–152.

51. Gorlin R: Hydraulic formula for calculation of the area of the stenotic mitral

valve, other cardiac valves and central circulatory shunts. *Am Heart J* 1951; 41:1.

52. Dajani AS, Bisno AL, Chung KJ, et al: Prevention of rheumatic fever: A statement for health professionals by the Committee on Rheumatic Fever, Endocarditis, and Kawasaki Disease of the Council on Cardiovascular Disease in the Young, the American Heart Association. Special report. *Circulation* 1988; 78:1082–1086.

53. Byron MA: Prescribing in pregnancy: Treatment of rheumatic disease. *Br Med J* 1987; 294:236–238.

54. Kaye D: Prophylaxis for infective endocarditis: An update. *Ann Intern Med* 1986; 104:419–423.

55. Shulman ST, Amren DP, Bisno AL, et al: Prevention of bacterial endocarditis. A statement for health professionals by the Committee on Rheumatic Fever and Infective Endocarditis of the Council on Cardiovascular Disease in the Young. *Circulation* 1984; 70:1123–1127A.

56. Miller M, Buchanan N, Cane RD, et al: Two mitral valve replacements during the course of a single pregnancy. *Intensive Care Med* 1978; 4:41–42.

57. Vosloo S, Reichard B: The feasibility of closed mitral valvotomy in pregnancy. *J Thorac Cardiovasc Surg* 1987; 93:675–679.

58. El-Maraghy M, Abou Senna I, El-Tehewy F, et al: Mitral valvotomy in pregnancy. *Am J Obstet Gynecol* 1983; 145:708–710.

59. Henry WL, Griffith JM, Michaelis LL, et al: Measurement of mitral orifice area in patients with mitral valve disease by real-time two dimensional echocardiography. *Circulation* 1975; 51:827–831.

60. Richards KL: Doppler echocardiography quantification of stenotic valvular lesions. *Echocardiography* 1987; 4:289–303.

61. Berk MR, England MJ, Marcus RH, et al: Significant mitral stenosis during pregnancy treated with atenolol: Maternal and fetal outcome. *Circulation* 1986; 74:452A.

62. Matsuzaki M, Tomay Y, Suetsugu M, et al: Analysis of blood velocity and thrombogenesis in left atrial appendage by transesophageal two-dimensional echocardiography. *J Am Coll Cardiol* 1987; 9:212A.

63. Estafanous G, Buckley S: Management of anesthesia for open heart surgery during pregnancy. *Cleve Clin Q* 1976; 43:121–124.

64. Bortolotti U, Milano A, Mazzucco A, et al: Pregnancy in patients with porcine valve bioprosthesis. *Am J Cardiol* 1982; 50:1051–1054.

65. Clark SL, Phelan JP, Greenspoon J, et al: Labor and delivery in the presence of mitral stenosis: Central hemodynamic observations. *Am J Obstet Gynecol* 1985; 152:984–988.

66. Barron WM, Murphy MB, Lindheimer MD: Management of hypertension during pregnancy, in Laragh JH, Brenner BM (eds): *Hypertension: Pathophysiology, Diagnosis, and Management*. New York, Raven Press, 1990, pp 1809–1827.

67. Castillo RA, Llado I, Adamsons K: Ruptured chordae tendineae complicating pregnancy. *J Reprod Med* 1987; 32:137–139.

68. Caves PK, Paneth M: Acute mitral regurgitation in pregnancy due to ruptured chordae tendineae. *Br Heart J* 1972; 34:541–544.

69. Blumlein S, Bouchard A, Schiller NB, et al: Quantitation of mitral regurgitation by Doppler echocardiography. *Circulation* 1986; 74:306–314.

70. Kolabash A, Ruiz D, Lewis R: Idiopathic hypertrophic subaortic stenosis in pregnancy. *Ann Med* 1975; 82:791–794.

71. Arias F, Pineda J: Aortic stenosis and pregnancy. *J Reprod Med* 1978; 20:229–232.

72. Easterling TR, Chadwick HS, Otto CM, et al: Aortic stenosis in pregnancy. *Obstet Gynecol* 1988; 72:113–118.

73. Oh JK, Taliercio CP, Holmes DR, et al: Prediction of the severity of aortic stenosis by Doppler aortic valve area determination: Prospective Doppler-catheterization correlation in 100 patients. *J Am Coll Cardiol* 1988; 11:1227–1234.

74. Casanegra P, Aviles G, Maturana G, et al: Cardiovascular management of pregnant women with a heart valve prosthesis. *Am J Cardiol* 1975; 36:802–806.

75. Angel JL, Chapman C, Knuppel RA, et al: Percutaneous balloon aortic valvuloplasty in pregnancy. *Obstet Gynecol* 1988; 72:438–440.

76. Borow KM: Surgical outcome in chronic aortic regurgitation: A physiologic framework for assessing preoperative predictors. *J Am Coll Cardiol* 1987; 5:1165–1170.

77. Ginsberg JS, Hirsch J: Anticoagulants during pregnancy. *Annu Rev Med* 1989; 40:79–86.

78. Iturbe-Alessio I, Fonseca M, Mutchinik O, et al: Risks of anticoagulant therapy in pregnant women with artificial heart valves. *N Engl J Med* 1986; 315:1390–1393.

79. Salazar E, Zajarias A, Guiterrez N, et al: The problem of cardiac valve prostheses, anticoagulants and pregnancy. *Circulation* 1984; 70:I169–I177.

80. Lee PK, Wang R, Chow JF, et al: Combined use of warfarin and adjusted subcutaneous heparin during pregnancy in patients with an artificial heart valve. *J Am Coll Cardiol* 1986; 8:221–224.

81. Ibarra-Perez C, Arevalo-Toledo N, Alvarez-de la Cadena O, et al: The course of pregnancy in patients with artificial heart valves. *Am J Med* 1976; 61:504–512.

82. Nunez L, Larrea J, Gil-Aguado M, et al: Pregnancy in 20 patients with bioprosthetic valve replacement. *Chest* 1983; 84:26–28.

83. Milano A, Bortolotti U, Talenti E, et al: Calcific degeneration as the main cause of porcine bioprosthetic valve failure. *Am J Cardiol* 1984; 53:1066–1070.

84. Nunez L, Aguado G, Celemin D, et al: Aspirin or Coumadin as the drug of choice for porcine bioprothesis in valve replacement. *Ann Thorac Surg* 1982; 33:354–358.

85. Oakley C: Valve prosthesis and pregnancy. *Br Heart J* 1987; 58:303–305.

86. Beadle E, Luepker R, Williams R: Pregnancy in a patient with porcine valve xenografts. *Am Heart J* 1979; 98:510–512.

87. Lutz D, Noller K, Spittell J, et al: Pregnancy and complications following cardiac valve prostheses. *Am J Obstet Gynecol* 1978; 131:460–468.

88. Guidozzi F: Pregnancy in patients with prosthetic cardiac valves. *S Afr Med J* 1984; 65:961–963.

89. Buxbaum A, Aygen M, Shahin W, et al: Pregnancy in patients with prosthetic heart valves. *Chest* 1971; 59:639–642.

90. Harrison E, Roschke EJ: Pregnancy in patients with cardiac valve prostheses. *Clin Obstet Gynecol* 1975; 18:107–122.

91. Ginz B: Myocardial infarction in pregnancy. *J Obstet Gynecol* 1970; 77:610–615.

92. Sasse L, Wagner R, Murray FE: Transmural myocardial infarction during pregnancy. *Am J Cardiol* 1975; 35:448–452.

93. Beary J, Summer W, Bulkley B: Postpartum acute myocardial infarction: A rare occurrence of uncertain etiology. *Am J Cardiol* 1979; 43:158.

94. Reece EA, Egan JFX, Coustan DR, et al: Coronary artery disease in diabetic pregnancies. *Am J Obstet Gynecol* 1986; 154:150–151.

95. Lamb MA: Myocardial infarction during pregnancy: A team challenge. *Heart Lung* 1987; 16:658–661.

96. Hankins GDV, Wendel GD Jr, Leveno KF, et al: Myocardial infarction during pregnancy: A review. *Obstet Gynecol* 1985; 65:139–146.

97. Mann JI, Vessey MP, Thorogood M, et al: Myocardial infarction in young women with special reference to oral contraceptive practice. *Br Med J* 1975; 2:241–245.

98. Mishell DR: Use of oral contraceptives in women of older reproductive age. *Am J Obstet Gynecol* 1988; 158:1652–1657.

99. Glancy DL, Marcus ML, Epstein SE: Myocardial infarction in young women with normal coronary arteriograms. *Circulation* 1971; 44:495–502.

100. Husani MH: Myocardial infarction during pregnancy. *Postgrad Med J* 1971; 47:660–665.

101. Henion WA, Hilal A, Mathew PK, et al: Postpartum myocardial infarction. *NY State J Med* 1982; 82:57–66.

102. Goldman ME, Meller J: Coronary artery disease in pregnancy, in Elkayam U, Gleicher N (eds): *Cardiac Problems in Pregnancy*, New York, Alan R. Liss, Inc, 1982, pp 142–151.

103. Majdan JF, Walinsky P, Cowchock SF, et al: Coronary artery bypass surgery during pregnancy. *Am J Cardiol* 1983; 52:1145–1146.

104. Metcalfe J, McAnulty JH, Ueland K: *Heart Disease in Pregnancy*, ed 2. Boston, Little, Brown & Co, 1986, pp 300–303.

105. Rosenlund RC, Marx GF: Anesthetic management of a parturient with prior myocardial infarction and coronary artery bypass graft. *Can J Anesth* 1988; 35:515–517.

106. Chestnut DH, Zlatnik FJ, Pitkin RM, et al: Pregnancy in a patient with a history of

myocardial infarction and coronary artery bypass grafting. *Am J Obstet Gynecol* 1986; 155:372–373.

107. Homans DC: Peripartum cardiomyopathy. *N Engl J Med* 1985; 312:1432–1437.

108. O'Connell JB, Constanzo-Nordin MR, Subramanian R, et al: Peripartum cardiomyopathy: Clinical, hemodynamic, histologic, and prognostic characteristics. *J Am Coll Cardiol* 1986; 8:52–56.

109. Carvalho A, Brandao A, Martinez EE, et al: Prognosis in peripartum cardiomyopathy. *Am J Cardiol* 1989; 64:540–542.

110. Cunningham FG, Pritchard JA, Hankins GDV, et al: Peripartum heart failure: Idiopathic cardiomyopathy or compounding cardiovascular events? *Obstet Gynecol* 1986; 67:157–167.

111. Julian DG, Szekely P: Peripartum cardiomyopathy. *Prog Cardiovasc Dis* 1985; 27:223–240.

112. Demakis J, Rahimtoola SH: Peripartum cardiomyopathy. *Circulation* 1971; 44:964–968.

113. Demakis J, Rahimtoola SH, Sutton G, et al: Natural course of peripartum cardiomyopathy. *Circulation* 1971; 44:1053–1061.

114. Melvin KR, Richardson PJ, Olsen EGJ, et al: Peripartum cardiomyopathy due to myocarditis. *N Engl J Med* 1982; 307:731–734.

115. Sainani GS, Dekote MP, Ras CP: Heart disease caused by coxsackie virus B infection. *Br Heart J* 1975; 37:819–823.

116. Kossman CE: Peripartum cardiomyopathy. *J Tenn Med Assoc* 1984; 77:29–33.

117. Weitz C, Spence M: Peripartal cardiomyopathy. *Obstet Gynecol* 1983; 62:555–575.

118. Veille JC: Peripartum cardiomyopathies: A review. *Am J Obstet Gynecol* 1984; 148:805–818.

119. James TN: Myocarditis and cardiomyopathy. *N Engl J Med* 1983; 308:39–41.

120. Cepin D, James F, Carabello B: Left ventricular function in peripartum cardiomyopathy. *Chest* 1983; 83:701–704.

121. Krausz Y, Naparstek E, Eliakim M: Idiopathic pericarditis and pregnancy. *Aust NZ J Obstet Gynaecol* 1978; 18:86–89.

122. Fowler NO, Manitsas GT: Infectious pericarditis. *Prog Cardiovasc Dis* 1973; 16:323–336.

123. Richardson PM, Le Roux BT, Rogers MA, et al: Pericardiectomy in pregnancy. *Thorax* 1970; 25:627–630.

124. Seaworth BJ, Durack DT: Infective endocarditis in obstetric and gynecologic practice. *Am J Obstet Gynecol* 1986; 154:180–188.

125. Bisno AL: Antimicrobial prophylaxis for infective endocarditis. *Hosp Pract,* March, 1989; 24:209–226.

126. Dommisse J: Infective endocarditis in pregnancy. A report of three cases. *S Afr Med J* 1988; 73:186–187.

127. Sugrue D, Blake S, Troy P, et al: Antibiotic prophylaxis against infective endocarditis after normal delivery—is it necessary? *Br Heart J* 1980; 44:499–502.

128. Clemens JD, Horwitz RI, Jaffe CC, et al: A controlled evaluation of the risk of bacterial endocarditis in persons with mitral-valve prolapse. *N Engl J Med* 1982; 307:776.

129. Schwarz RH, Crombleholme WR: Antibiotics in pregnancy. *South Med J* 1979; 73:1315.

130. Kossoy LR, Herbert CM III, Colston WA: Management of heart transplant recipients: Guidelines for the obstetrician-gynecologist. *Am J Obstet Gynecol* 1988; 159:490–499.

131. Schroeder JS, Hunt SA: Cardiac transplantation: Where are we? *N Engl J Med* 1986; 315:961–963.

132. Jamieson SW, Ogumarke HO: Cardiopulmonary transplantation. *Surg Clin North Am* 1986; 66:491–501.

133. Solis E, Kaye MP: The registry of the International Society of Heart Transplantation: Third official report. *J Heart Transplant* 1986; 5:2–5.

134. Key TC, Resnik R, Dittrich HC, et al: Successful pregnancy after cardiac transplantation. *Am J Obstet Gynecol* 1989; 160:367–371.

135. Lowenstein BR, Vain NW, Perrone SV, et al: Successful pregnancy and vaginal delivery after heart transplantation. *Am J Obstet Gynecol* 1988; 158:589–590.

136. Lau JR, Scott JR: Pregnancy following renal transplantation. *Clin Obstet Gynecol* 1985; 28:339–350.

137. Davison JM: Renal transplantation and pregnancy. *Am J Kidney Dis* 1987; 9:374–380.

138. Davison JM: Pregnancy in renal allograft recipients: Prognosis and management. *Clin Obstet Gynaecol* 1987; 1:1027–1045.

139. Mason RJ, Thomson AW, Whiting PH, et al: Cyclosporin induced fetotoxicity in the rat. *Transplantation* 1985; 39:9–12.

140. Whittemore R, Hobbins J, Engle MA: Pregnancy and its outcome in woman with and without surgical treatment of congenital heart disease. *Am J Cardiol* 1982; 50:641–651.

141. Whittemore R: Congenital heart disease: Its impact on pregnancy. *Hosp Pract,* Dec 1983, vol 18, pp 65–74.

142. Rose V, Gold RJM, Chir B, et al: A possible increase in the incidence of congenital heart defects among the offspring of affected parents. *Am Coll Cardiol* 1985; 6:376–382.

143. Shime J, Mocarski JM, Hastings D, et al: Congenital heart disease in pregnancy: Short- and long-term implications. *Am J Obstet Gynecol* 1987; 156:313–322.

144. Insley J: The heritability of congenital heart disease. *Br Med J* 1987; 294:662–663.

145. Allan LD, Crawford DC, Chita SK, et al: Familial recurrence of congenital heart disease in a prospective series of mothers referred for fetal echocardiography. *Am J Cardiol* 1986; 58:334–337.

146. Feldman T, Borow KM: Atrial septal defects in adults—Diagnosis and management. *Cardiovasc Med* 1986; 11:19–26.

147. Feldman T, Borow KM: Atrial septal defects in adults. Symptoms, signs and natural history. *Cardiovasc Med* 1985; 11:31–40.

148. Borow KM, Braunwald E: Congenital heart disease in the adult, in Braunwald E (ed): *Heart Disease—A Textbook of Cardiovascular Medicine,* ed 3. Philadelphia, WB Saunders Co, 1988, pp 976–1008.

149. Andersen M, Lyngborg K, Moller I, et al: The natural history of small atrial septal defects: Longterm follow-up with serial heart catheterizations. *Am Heart J* 1976; 92:302–307.

150. McAnulty JH, Metcalfe J, Ueland K: General guidelines in the management of cardiac disease. *Clin Obstet Gynecol* 1981; 24:773.

151. Nora JJ, Nora AH: The evolution of specific genetic and environmental counseling in congenital heart diseases. *Circulation* 1978; 57:205–213.

152. Weidman WH, DuShane JW, Ellison RC: Clinical course in adults with ventricular septal defect. *Circulation* 1977; 56:178.

153. Nakazawa M, Takao A, Shimizu T, et al: Afterload reduction treatment for large ventricular septal defect dependence of hemodynamic effects of hydralazin on pretreatment systemic blood flow. *Br Heart J* 1983; 49:461.

154. Corone P, Doyon F, Gaudeau S, et al: Natural history of ventricular septal defect: A study involving 790 cases. *Circulation* 1977; 55:908.

155. Feldman T, Borow KM: Congenital pulmonic stenosis in the adult. *J Cardiovasc Med* 1984; 9:711–719.

156. Johnson LW, Grossman W, Dalen JE, et al: Pulmonic stenosis in the adult. Long term follow-up results. *N Engl J Med* 1972; 287:1159–1163.

157. Mendelson CL: *Cardiac Disease in Pregnancy* Philadelphia, FA Davis Co, 1960, pp 132–135.

158. Deal K, Wooley CF: Coarctation of the aorta and pregnancy. *Ann Intern Med* 1973; 78:706–710.

159. Etheridge MJ: Heart disease and pregnancy. *Med J Aust* 1968; 2:1172–1174.

160. Barash PG, Hobbins JC, Hook R, et al: Management of coarctation of the aorta during pregnancy. *J Thorac Cardiovasc Surg* 1975; 69:781–784.

161. Naulty J, Cefalo RC, Lewis PE: Fetal toxicity of nitroprusside in the pregnant ewe. *Am J Obstet Gynecol* 1981; 139:708–711.

162. Shoemaker CT, Meyers M: Sodium nitroprusside for control of severe hypertensive disease of pregnancy: A case report and discussion of potential toxicity. *Am J Obstet Gynecol* 1984; 149:171–173.

163. Mor-Yosef S, Younis J, Granat M, et al: Marfan's syndrome in pregnancy. *Obstet Gynecol Surv* 1988; 43:382–385.

164. Sasson Z, Rakowski H, Wigle ED: Hypertrophic cardiomyopathy. *Cardiol Clin* 1988; 6:233–288.

165. Braunwald E, Morrow AG, Cornell WP: Idiopathic hypertrophic subaortic stenosis. *Am J Med* 1960; 29:924–945.

166. Maron BJ, Nichols PF, Pickle LW: Patterns of inheritance in hypertrophic cardiomyopathy: Assessment by M-mode and two-dimensional echocardiography. *Am J Cardiol* 1984; 53:1087–1094.

167. McKenna W, Deanfield J, Faruqui A, et al: Prognosis in hypertrophic cardiomyopathy: Role of age and clinical, electrocar-

diographic and hemodynamic features. *Am J Cardiol* 1981; 47:532–538.

168. Oakley CM VIII: Hypertrophic cardiomyopathy and pregnancy, in Elkayam U, Gleicher E (eds): *Cardiac Problems in Pregnancy.* New York, Alan R Liss, Inc, 1982, pp 105–114.

169. Oakley CDG, McGarry K, Limb DG, et al: Management of pregnancy in patients with hypertrophic cardiomyopathy. *Br Med J* 1979; 1:1749–1750.

170. Turner GM, Oakley CM, Dixon HG: Management of pregnancy complicated by hypertrophic obstructive cardiomyopathy. *Br Med J* 1968; 4:281–284.

171. Sullivan JM, Ramathan KB: Management of medical problems in pregnancy. Severe cardiac disease. *N Engl J Med* 1985; 313:304–313.

172. Loh TF, Tan NC: Fallot's tetralogy and pregnancy. A report of a successful pregnancy after a complete correction. *Med J Aust* 1971; 2:141–145.

173. Ralstin JH, Dunn M: Pregnancies after surgical connection of tetralogy of Fallot. *JAMA* 1976; 235:2627–2628.

174. Hibbard LT: Maternal mortality due to cardiac disease. *Clin Obstet Gynecol* 1975; 18:27–36.

175. Waickman LA, Skorton D, Warner M, et al: Ebstein's anomaly and pregnancy. *Am J Cardiol* 1984; 53:357–358.

176. Coffer FD: Eisenmenger's complex and pregnancy. *Obstet Gynecol* 1967; 29:235–240.

177. Midwall J, Jaffin H, Herman MV, et al: Shunt flow and pulmonary hemodynamics during labor and delivery in the Eisenmenger syndrome. *Am J Cardiol* 1978; 42:299–303.

178. McGregor CGA, Jamieson SW, Baldwin JC, et al: Combined heart-lung transplantation for end-stage Eisenmenger's syndrome. *J Thorac Cardiovasc Surg* 1986; 91:443.

179. Neilson G, Galea EG, Blunt A: Eisenmenger's syndrome and pregnancy. *Med J Aust* 1971; 1:431–439.

180. Devereux RB, Kramer-Fox R, Kligfield P: Mitral valve prolapse: Causes, clinical manifestations and management. *Ann Intern Med* 1989; 111:305–317.

181. Rayburn W, Fontana M: Mitral valve prolapse and pregnancy. *Am J Obstet Gynecol* 1981; 141:9.

182. Haas JM: The effect of pregnancy on the midsistolic click and murmur of the prolapsing posterior leaflet of the mitral valve. *Am Heart J* 1976; 92:407–408.

183. Rayburn WF: Mitral valve prolapse in pregnancy, in Elkayam U, Gleicher E (eds): *Cardiac Problems in Pregnancy.* New York, Alan R Liss Inc, 1982, pp 191–196.

184. Pryn SC, Phelan JP, Buchanan GC: Long-term propranolol therapy in pregnancy: Maternal and fetal outcome. *Am J Obstet Gynecol* 1979; 135:485–489.

185. Rubin PC: Beta-blockers in pregnancy. *N Engl J Med* 1981; 305:1323–1326.

186. Wichman K: Metoprolol in the treatment of mild to moderate hypertension in pregnancy—effects on fetal heart activity. *Clin Exp Hypertens [B]* 1986; 5:195–202.

187. DeSanctis RW, Doroghazi RM, Austen WG, et al: Aortic dissection. *N Engl J Med* 1987; 317:1060–1067.

188. Hume M, Krosnick G: Dissecting aneurysm in pregnancy associated with aortic insufficiency. *N Engl J Med* 1963; 268:174–178.

189. Novell HA, Asher Jr LA, Lev M: Marfan's syndrome associated with pregnancy. *Am J Obstet Gynecol* 1958; 75:802–812.

190. Elias S, Berkowitz RL: The Marfan syndrome and pregnancy. *Obstet Gynecol* 1976; 47:358–361.

191. Super M: Diagnosing Marfan syndrome. *Br Med J* 1988; 296:1347.

192. Pyeritz RE: Maternal and fetal complications of pregnancy in the Marfan syndrome. *Am J Med* 1981; 71:784–789.

193. Lietman PS: Congenital malformations associated with the administration of oral anticoagulants during pregnancy. *J Pediatr* 1975; 86:459–462.

194. Hall JG, Pauli RM, Wilson KM: Maternal and fetal sequelae of anticoagulation during pregnancy. *Am J Med* 1980; 68:122–140.

195. Ginsberg JS, Kowalchuk G, Hirsh J, et al: Heparin therapy during pregnancy. Risks to the fetus and mother. *Arch Intern Med* 1989; 149:2233–2364.

196. Howell R, Fidler J, Letsky E, et al: The risks of antenatal subcutaneous heparin prophylaxis: A controlled trial. *Br J Obstet Gynaecol* 1983; 90:1124–1128.

197. Lieberman BA, Stirrat GM, Cohen SL, et al: The possible adverse effects of propranolol on the fetus in pregnancies complicated by severe hypertension. *Br J Obstet Gynaecol* 1978; 85:678–683.

198. Rubin PC, Butters L, Clark DM, et al: Placebo controlled trial of atenolol in the treatment of pregnancy associated hypertension. *Lancet* 1983; 1:431–434.

199. Hogstedt S, Lindberg S, Axelsson O, et al: A prospective controlled trial of metoprolol-hydralazine treatment in hypertension during pregnancy. *Acta Obstet Gynecol Scand* 1985; 64:505–510.

200. Butters L, Kennedy S, Rubin P: Atenolol and fetal weight in chronic hypertension (abstract). *Clin Exp Hypertens Pregnancy* 1989; B8:468.

201. Lindheimer MD, Katz AI: Sodium and diuretics in pregnancy. *N Engl J Med* 1973; 288:891–894.

202. Widerhorn J, Nathan R, Elkayam U: Antiarrhythmic drugs during pregnancy. *Cardiology* 1988; 104–118.

203. Graves SW, Valdes JR, Brown BA, et al: Endogenous digoxin-substance in human pregnancies. *J Clin Endocrinol Metab* 1984; 58:748–751.

204. Johnston WD, Elkayam U: Cardiac glycosides and pregnancy, in Elkayam U, Gleicher E (eds): *Cardiac Problems in Pregnancy*. New York, Alan R Liss Inc, 1982, pp 281–288.

205. Rotmensch H, Lessind J, Donchin Y: Clinical pharmacology of antiarrhythmic drugs in the pregnant patient, in Elkayam U, Gleicher E (eds): *Cardiac Problems in Pregnancy*. New York, Alan R Liss Inc, 1982, pp 227–243.

206. Allan LD, Crawford DC, Anderson RH, et al: Evaluation and treatment of fetal arrhythmias. *Clin Cardiol* 1984; 7:467–473.

207. Widerhorn J, Rubin J, Frishman W, et al: Cardiovascular drugs in pregnancy. *Cardiol Clin* 1987; 5:651–674.

208. Mitani GM, Steinberg I, Lien EJ, et al: The pharmacokinetics of antiarrhythmic agents in pregnancy and lactation. *Clin Pharmacokinet* 1987; 12:253–291.

209. Ralston DH: Perinatal pharmacology, in Shnider SM, Levinson G (eds.): *Anesthesia for Obstetrics*. Baltimore, Williams & Wilkins, 1987; pp 50–58.

210. Spinnato JA, Shaver DC, Flinn GS, et al: Fetal supraventricular tachycardia: In utero therapy with digoxin and quinidine. *Obstet Gynecol* 1984; 64:730–735.

211. Shnider SM, Way EL: Plasma levels of lidocaine (Xylocaine) in mother and newborn following obstetrical conduction anesthesia: Clinical applications. *Anesthesiology* 1968; 29:951–958.

212. Timmis AD, Jackson G, Holt DW: Mexiletine for control of ventricular dysrhythmias in pregnancy. *Lancet* 1980; 2:647–648.

213. Tadmor OP, Keren A, Rosenak D, et al: The effect of disopyramide on uterine contractions during pregnancy. *Am J Obstet Gynecol* 1990; 162:482–486.

214. McKenna W, Harris L, Rowland E, et al: Amiodarone therapy during pregnancy. *Am J Cardiol* 1983; 51:1231–1233.

215. Klein V, Repke JT: Supraventricular tachycardia in pregnancy: Cardioversion with verapamil. *Obstet Gynecol* 1984; 63:16S–18S.

216. Miller MR, Withers R, Bhamra R, et al: Verapamil and breast feeding. *Eur Clin Pharmacol* 1986; 30:125–126.

217. Niels NH, Lauersen MD: Tocolytic drugs and the cardiac patient, in Elkayam U, Gleicher E (eds): *Cardiac Problems in Pregnancy*. New York, Alan R Liss, Inc, 1982, pp 273–280.

218. Hosenpud JD, Morton MJ, O'Grady JP: Cardiac stimulation during ritodrine hydrochloride tocolytic therapy. *Obstet Gynecol* 1983; 62:52–58.

219. Pisani RJ, Rosenow EC: Pulmonary edema associated with tocolytic therapy. *Ann Intern Med* 1989; 110:714–718.

220. Stempel JE, O'Grady JP, Morton MJ, et al: Use of sodium nitroprusside in complications of gestational hypertension. *Obstet Gynecol* 1982; 60:533–538.

221. Donchin Y, Amirav B, Sahar A, et al: Sodium nitroprusside for aneurysm surgery during pregnancy. Report of a case. *Br J Anaesth* 1978; 50:849–851.

222. Ellis SC, Wheeler AS, James FM III, et al: Fetal and maternal effects of sodium nitroprusside used to counteract hypertension in gravid ewes. *Am J Obstet Gynecol* 1982; 143:766–770.

223. Rosa FW, Bosco LA, Graham CF, et al: Neonatal anuria with maternal angioten-

sin-converting enzyme inhibition. *Obstet Gynecol* 1989; 74:371–374.

224. Vink GJ, Moodley JH, Philpott RH: Effect of dihydralazine on the fetus in the treatment of maternal hypertension. *Obstet Gynecol* 1980; 55:519–522.

225. Kuzniar J, Skret A, Piela A, et al: Hemodynamic effects of intravenous hydralazine in pregnant women with severe hypertension. *Obstet Gynecol* 1985; 66:453–458.

226. Mabie WC, Gonzalez AR, Sibai BM, et al: A comparative trial of labetalol and hydralazine in the acute management of severe hypertension complicating pregnancy. *Obstet Gynecol* 1987; 70:328–333.

227. Rubin PC, Butters L, Low RA, et al: Clinical pharmacological studies with prazosin during pregnancy complicated by hypertension. *Br J Clin Pharmacol* 1983; 16:543–547.

228. Schroeder JS, Harrison DC: Repeated cardioversion during pregnancy. *Am J Cardiol* 1971; 27:445–446.

229. Lee RV, Rodgers BD, White LM, et al: Cardiopulmonary resuscitation of pregnant women. *Am J Med* 1986; 81:311–318.

CHAPTER 6

Pulmonary Disease

Gregory A. Schmidt
Jesse B. Hall

The normal physiologic adaptations of pregnancy may stress the efficiency of many body functions. This is especially true of the respiratory system which sustains a marked increase in work load. It is testimony to the remarkable reserve of pulmonary function in the normal woman that respiratory insufficiency is quite rare. Nevertheless, pregnancy can tip the balance toward deterioration when underlying lung disease is present. In addition, many biochemical and hormonal changes of pregnancy may influence the natural history of lung disease, compounding the impact on the respiratory system.

This chapter begins with an overview of the physiologic changes of normal pregnancy and is followed by a discussion of an easily avoided pulmonary problem with great impact on health: cigarette smoking. The remaining sections focus on pulmonary diseases, noting how each is influenced by gestation, the effect of illness on the pregnancy, and finally, recommendations for management. This chapter also includes a discussion of the detection and management of deep venous thrombosis and pulmonary embolism complicating pregnancy.

PHYSIOLOGIC CHANGES IN THE RESPIRATORY SYSTEM IN PREGNANCY

Oxygen consumption is increased 20% to 30% because of fetal and placental needs, as well as for maternal requirements due to increased cardiac output and work of breathing.[1, 2] Despite this increment in oxygen consumption, arterial oxygen pressure (Po_2) is maintained at nearly normal levels of above 90 mm Hg by virtue of augmented ventilation. Mild hypoxemia can be induced in up to one fourth of gravidas by the supine position, however, and the alveolar-to-arterial oxygen gradient is often slightly abnormal.[3, 4] Therefore, *when arterial blood gas analysis is indicated in pregnancy, the sample should be drawn with the woman in the seated position,* if possible. Small decrements in Po_2 are of little significance due to the flatness of the oxyhemoglobin dissociation curve, since arterial blood remains almost fully saturated even when the Po_2 is near 60 mm Hg (Table 6–1).

The increased consumption of oxygen is associated with production of more carbon dioxide, and thus a greater need for alveolar

TABLE 6–1.

Typical Arterial Blood Gas Values in Pregnancy*

	P_{O_2}	P_{CO_2}	pH	$P_A - Pa_{O_2}$	S_{O_2}
Nonpregnant	98	40	7.40	2	98%
Term pregnancy, seated	101	28	7.45	14	98%
Term pregnancy, supine	95	28	7.45	20	97%

*$P_A - Pa_{O_2}$ is the difference between the predicted alveolar P_{O_2} and the measured arterial P_{O_2}, assuming a respiratory quotient of 0.8. Normally this is less than 10 mm Hg. S_{O_2} is the saturation of hemoglobin with oxygen.

ventilation. Actually, alveolar ventilation rises beyond the need to excrete carbon dioxide so that carbon dioxide pressure (P_{CO_2}) is maintained at a partial pressure near 30 mm Hg throughout much of pregnancy.[5, 6] Tidal volume (TV) is increased by about 40% over baseline values.[7] Since respiratory rate is unchanged at 16/min, the increment in TV accounts for the increased minute ventilation of pregnancy. This is believed due to increases in circulating progesterone which affects the respiratory center.[8] Maternal pH however, is only slightly alkalemic, ranging between 7.40 and 7.45 due to renal compensation, with serum bicarbonate decreasing to 18 to 21 mEq/L[6, 9] (see Table 6–1).

The volume of air remaining in the lungs at the end of a passive exhalation is termed the *functional residual capacity* (FRC). This resting volume occurs where inward recoil of the lungs balances the outward recoil of the chest wall. The "chest wall," to the pulmonologist, includes not just the thoracic cage, but the diaphragm as well. Since the diaphragm is coupled to the abdomen, any increase in abdominal pressure is transmitted to the chest wall. In pregnancy, the increase in abdominal pressure due to the enlarged uterus results in less tendency for the chest wall to recoil outward. Since inward recoil of the lung is unchanged, a new balance is reached in which inward pull still equals outward recoil, but at a lower lung volume. This prediction, that functional residual capacity will decrease during gestation, has been confirmed many times.[10–14] This lower-than-normal FRC is clinically relevant since there is less air, and therefore less oxygen, in the lungs at the end of a passive exhalation. Combined with the

increase in oxygen consumption of pregnancy, this leaves the pregnant woman (and her fetus) more vulnerable to hypoxia in the event of apnea. Endotracheal intubation is one setting in which this vulnerability to hypoxia is important.[15]

The volume which can be exhaled from the reduced FRC, called the *expiratory reserve volume* (ERV), is also expected to be less, simply due to the fact that the starting volume (FRC) is less. This prediction too has been consistently confirmed in pregnancy.[10–14] Although FRC is lower in pregnancy, the volume which can be inhaled from FRC, termed *inspiratory capacity* (IC), is enhanced so that total lung capacity (TLC) is maintained. This increment in inspiratory capacity may be due to a mechanical advantage accruing to the inspiratory muscles at high lung volume[14] (Fig 6–1).

Closing capacity (CC) is the lung volume at which airways in dependent areas of lung close, and therefore cease to ventilate. Bevan et al. observed CC to be elevated,[16] as did Garrard and colleagues.[17] This change, in combination with the reduction in FRC, might result in airway closure even during tidal breathing. Alveoli served by these closed airways would be poorly ventilated, yet perfused, thereby contributing to hypoxemia.[16, 17] Other investigators have failed to confirm these findings, stating that CC is not altered in pregnancy.[12, 13] Still another also failed to find an increase in CC, but noted that the decrement in FRC was marked enough in the supine position that airway closure during tidal breathing occurred in one half of subjects.[3] Either of these explanations for airway closure, increased CC or greatly lowered FRC,

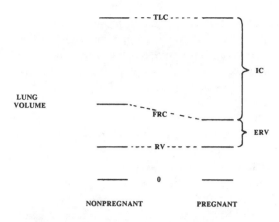

FIG 6–1.
Pulmonary function tests in pregnancy. The most notable change in pulmonary mechanics during pregnancy is the fall in functional residual capacity (FRC). The inspiratory capacity (IC) increases so that total lung capacity (TLC) is unchanged. RV = residual volume; ERV = expiratory reserve volume.

can account for the widened alveolar-to-arterial oxygen gradient, and for its worsening in the supine position.

The function of large airways does not appear to be altered in pregnancy, despite increases in levels of many hormones known to affect smooth muscle. Forced expiratory volume in 1 second (FEV_1), the ratio of FEV_1 to forced vital capacity (FEV_1 %), and specific airways conductance are no different from first trimester through term when compared with postpartum values.[10, 11, 13, 18] Flow volume loops are also unaffected by pregnancy—further evidence for normal airway function.[13]

DYSPNEA OF PREGNANCY

Before discussing pulmonary diseases per se, it is important to acknowledge that dyspnea is a frequent symptom in normal pregnancy. Women often complain of dyspnea in the first trimester, long before any mechanical effect of the enlarging uterus could be expected. By midterm, about half of women will notice dyspnea at rest.[19] The number experiencing dyspnea increases to a maximum between 28 and 31 weeks. Cugell et al.[10] were

unable to correlate breathlessness with any single mechanical parameter of pulmonary function. The two most likely explanations for the dyspnea of pregnancy are that (1) it is related to the hyperventilation of pregnancy or (2) it is a consequence of the change in conformation of the thorax that accompanies pregnancy. Any explanation must take into account that impairment of breathing by the gravid uterus is not a satisfactory explanation since many women are breathless before the uterus is of significant size.

Data supporting the view that hyperventilation of pregnancy causes the dyspnea include the increased TV that is characteristic of pregnancy, which must result from increased pressure generation by the respiratory muscles. Since respiratory rate is unchanged, this excess pressure generation results in an increased work of breathing. It is reasonable to propose that a woman could sense this increased work of breathing. In fact, dyspnea during gestation correlates with the decrement in PCO_2 from the baseline nonpregnant state,[20] and such decreases should be proportional to the rise in work of breathing. Since the fall in PCO_2 occurs in the first months of pregnancy,[21] this mechanism is in accord with the known time course of dyspnea.

Alternatively, the dyspnea of pregnancy could be the consequence of a change in thoracic shape. A review of the older literature reveals that the chest wall changes shape during pregnancy.[22] Chest x-rays have been performed throughout pregnancy, and again post partum. The angle between the xiphoid process and points 7 cm from it along the border of each costal margin, termed the *subcostal angle*, was measured from the chest x-ray. This value increased progressively from 68.5 degrees to 103.5 degrees at term, returning to 68 degrees after delivery. This increase in angle occurred before mechanical pressure from the uterus could have been implicated. The authors proposed that a hormonal effect of "relaxin," implicated in the increased mobility of the symphysis pubis, might be the explanation.[22] This change in shape of the thorax should affect the functional anatomy of the respiratory muscles, and could put them at a mechanical disadvantage. In this formulation the degree of respiratory system displacement resulting from a given neural output to the respiratory muscles would be inappropriately small. A similar hypothesis has recently been advanced to explain dyspnea associated with large pleural effusions. Of course, these two explanations for the dyspnea of pregnancy—progesterone effect and change in thoracic shape—are not mutually exclusive, and could even be additive.

CIGARETTE SMOKING

Since the release of the first Surgeon General's report on cigarette smoking in 1964 the proportion of people who smoke cigarettes has steadily fallen. However, while the percentage decline among adult male smokers has been 21.4%, the decline in women has been only 5.8%. Much of the antismoking press targets the rise of lung cancer and coronary artery disease in women. The greatest tragedy, however, may be the damaging effects of cigarette smoking on pregnancy and on the smoking mother's children. At the beginning of their pregnancy, more than one third of women under the age of 25, and one fourth of women over 25 are cigarette smokers.[23] Therefore smoking potentially impacts on the health of 1 million babies in the United States each year.[24]

There is incontrovertible evidence from numerous studies throughout the world that maternal smoking directly affects the outcome of both the pregnancy and the child. Smoking leads to a dose-related increase in the incidence of bleeding during pregnancy, abruptio placentae, placenta previa, and premature and prolonged rupture of membranes.[25, 26] Tubal pregnancy is also associated with maternal cigarette smoking.[27]

The fetus is profoundly affected by maternal smoking. Perinatal mortality, prematurity, and low birth weight are all directly attributable to cigarettes.[25, 28–30] Smoking 10 to 20 cigarettes per day throughout pregnancy reduces birth weight approximately 200 g.[31] Kleinman and colleagues estimate that if all pregnant women stopped smoking, fetal and infant deaths could be reduced by approximately 10%.[30] Oster et al.[32] have calculated the neonatal health care cost attributable to maternal smoking. Their conservative estimate, including only the increased cost of neonatal intensive care services, was that smoking adds $272 million per year to the nation's health care burden.

The true test of the importance of smoking on fetal outcome is whether cessation of smoking leads to improvement. In many series that showed lower birth weights in infants of smokers, offspring of ex-smokers were of normal weight.[33, 34] Macarthur and Knox[35] compared birth weights in women who stopped smoking at various times during pregnancy. They found that infants of mothers who stopped smoking before the 16th week of gestation weighed the same as infants of nonsmoking mothers. Babies born to mothers who stopped smoking, but after the 16th week, were intermediate in weight. Most relevant to clinical practice is the demonstration that antismoking assistance provided to pregnant women is effective in reducing maternal smoking and in improving birth weight.[36]

Clinicians and women smokers must understand that the single most effective intervention for improving the outcome of pregnancy is cessation of smoking. Ninety percent of smokers would like to quit. Nevertheless, stopping is difficult and recidivism is common. Physicians can be of tremendous assistance and support (Table 6–2). They should act as role models by not smoking and should encourage discontinuation of smoking by emphasizing the advantages of quitting. The highest immediate quit rates result from behavior modification, drug therapy, educational and commercial programs, hypnosis, acupuncture, and multiple risk factor reduction programs.[37] In the long term, the most successful programs depend heavily on education and emphasize health enhancement. Gum containing nicotine is contraindicated

TABLE 6–2.
Strategy for Encouraging Cessation of
Cigarette Smoking

1. Identify smokers
2. Counsel all smokers identified
3. Act as a nonsmoking role model
4. Encourage the *benefits* of stopping
5. Refer for intervention

in pregnancy, and falls into FDA pregnancy category X (See Preface for discussion of FDA classification.).

The successful intervention trial reported by Sexton and Hebel[36] used encouragement and assistance to stop smoking through information, support, practical guidance, and behavioral strategies, and demonstrates that antismoking intervention is feasible to conduct and accepted by women. Counseling of all pregnant smokers should include a substantial effort to achieve smoking cessation.

ASTHMA

Asthma is the commonest pulmonary problem in pregnancy, affecting approximately 1% of gravidas.[9, 38] This disease is characterized by hyperreactive airways leading to episodes of bronchoconstriction, interspersed with periods of normality. The exact cause is unknown but attacks may be precipitated by exercise, medications, allergens, infection, nonspecific irritants, and emotional upset. Asthma is often associated with a personal or family history of hay fever or eczema.

Exacerbations of asthma are marked by the clinical triad of cough, dyspnea, and wheezing, the onset of which may be explosive or subtly progressive over weeks. Attacks in pregnancy range from mildly annoying to life-threatening for both mother and fetus.[39] The physical examination reveals diffuse expiratory wheezing, but is unreliable for assessing disease severity. Spirometry, a reliable and reproducible method of quantitating airway obstruction, is needed to assess the course of disease and the effects of therapy. Typically, the FEV_1 is reduced out of proportion to the

fall in FVC, leading to a low $FEV_1\%$. Between exacerbations these spirometric values return to normal. Chest radiography reveals hyperinflation and peribronchial cuffing. Arterial blood gases demonstrate variable degrees of hypoxemia and a reduction in PCO_2. Life-threatening disease may result in an elevation of PCO_2 as a prelude to respiratory failure. *Since the PCO_2 in pregnancy is expected to be about 30 mm Hg, any value in the mid-30s or higher associated with severe dyspnea and wheezing should alert the clinician to the gravity of the situation*

Effect of Pregnancy on Asthma

Pregnancy often affects the course of asthma, but in different ways in different women. Analysis of 366 pregnancies in which patient status was serially assessed with auscultation, spirometry, and diary cards demonstrated that asthma worsened in 35%, improved in 28%, and was unchanged in 33%.[38] There was also a significant concordance in the course of asthma in 34 women observed through successive pregnancies. The above data are similar to prior retrospective studies and to other recent prospective surveys, as well as to clinicians' subjective sense of the effect of pregnancy on asthma.[40–42]

Since asthma is a generally unpredictable disease it is possible that the above-described changes are merely random fluctuations. In this respect the concordance noted in repeat gestations as well as a consistent return to prepregnancy disease activity by 3 months post partum suggests a specific effect of pregnancy on asthma.[38] Some disagree, however, having noted marked variability in the course of asthma over successive pregnancies in the same women. The latter authorities believe that pregnancy per se does not affect asthma[43]; however it seems more likely that these are simply exceptions to a general rule.

A number of hypotheses have been advanced to explain the apparent effect of pregnancy on asthma. Serum cortisol increases in pregnancy and this steroid might explain improvement in some patients. Progesterone, which increases markedly during gestation, relaxes smooth muscle and could lead to reduction in bronchial tone. Another possibility includes the attenuation of cell mediated immunity of pregnancy. On the other hand, prostaglandins E_1, E_2, and $F_{2\alpha}$ are found in amniotic fluid and have potent effects on smooth muscle. Intravenous infusions of prostaglandins E_2 and $F_{2\alpha}$, given for termination of pregnancy, have provoked increases in bronchial smooth muscle tone.[44] Leukotrienes may also mediate changes in airway tone during pregnancy. Changes in no one of these theoretically important mediators can explain why asthma worsens in some women, while improving in others. It may be that the relative amounts of bronchoconstrictors versus bronchodilators in a given woman dictates the net effect on airways. On the other hand, different women may exhibit differential sensitivities to various mediators, leading to different net effects. One may even speculate that there are yet undiscovered factors.

Effect of Asthma on Pregnancy

The effect of asthma on the outcome of pregnancy has been evaluated by several investigators. Increases in prematurity, low birth weight, and perinatal death were reported in the early literature.[45, 46] In one, a twofold increase in complications of hyperemesis, vaginal hemorrhage, or preeclampsia was reported.[46] Gordon et al.[45] correlated fetal mortality with severe maternal asthma, noting that the highest risk was in babies born to Black mothers living under depressed socioeconomic circumstances. Treatment for asthma has improved and more recent studies have failed to confirm a substantial effect on fetal outcome unless asthma is poorly controlled.[47, 48] For instance, Fitzsimons and colleagues[49] surveyed 56 pregnancies in women with severe asthma dependent on oral or inhaled steroids, noting low birth weight and small-for-gestational-age infants only when pregnancy was complicated by status asthmaticus. In the most recent series, fetal or neonatal mortality, incidence of congenital malformations, Apgar scores, incidence of

preterm birth, and birth weight were similar to those of nonasthmatic gravidas.[38, 40] These data and the historical trend suggest that effective therapy and avoidance of status asthmaticus are associated with an excellent fetal outcome. Rather than making a priority of discontinuing medications in the pregnant asthmatic, the clinician should instead seek to maintain control of disease.

Prepregnancy counseling should aim to reassure the asthmatic woman that in all likelihood, she and her infant will have a good outcome. Since the course in prior pregnancies often, but not always, predicts the course for subsequent ones, the history is useful. Previous worsening during pregnancy should lead to increased surveillance, patient education, and possibly more aggressive drug treatment rather than to a recommendation against pregnancy. The history of a benign course is reassuring, but not necessarily indicative that a subsequent pregnancy will be uncomplicated.

Management

When a woman with asthma becomes pregnant, the treatment approach is essentially unchanged, with a few added subtleties. The goal in pregnancy is to control asthma and prevent episodes of status asthmaticus, thereby avoiding fetal hypoxemia. While it is generally good practice to avoid medicines, especially in the first trimester, *symptomatic asthma should be treated. Similarly, an asthmatic who requires medication for control should not have therapy discontinued simply because she becomes pregnant.* Since a woman's asthma might improve during the pregnancy, her physician should remain alert to the possibility to taper or discontinue medicines. On the other hand, if symptoms worsen, one should not hesitate to escalate therapy since this is essential for the well-being of mother and fetus (Fig 6–2).

All asthmatics require careful clinical monitoring during pregnancy. The physical examination is an unreliable indicator of the degree of obstruction. The patient may be surprisingly unreliable in assessing the severity of disease, or have difficulty distinguishing asthma from the normal dyspnea of pregnancy. Chest radiographs are unhelpful and arterial blood gases too invasive for routine use. Spirometry, with serial measurement of parameters of obstruction (especially the FEV_1), is a reliable tool for routine clinical assessment, is safe and inexpensive, and should be routinely obtained in all patients with moderate or severe asthma. Alternatively, a simple handheld peak flowmeter can be used for serial assessment of severity of obstruction.

Most drugs used to treat asthma are thought to be safe in pregnancy. Although it is not usually possible to definitively establish

the safety of these drugs in pregnancy, most are considered safe on the basis of extensive experience or by extrapolation from the safety of similar drugs (Table 6–3).

Theophylline and related drugs are considered safe and have not been associated with fetal malformations.[50, 51] This group of drugs crosses the placenta and can cause transient nervousness and tachycardia in the neonate.[52] The effect of pregnancy on the pharmacokinetics of theophylline has not been conclusively established, some claiming a reduced clearance in the third trimester,[53, 54] and others failing to confirm this.[55] Therefore, while no specific recommendation for dose reduc-

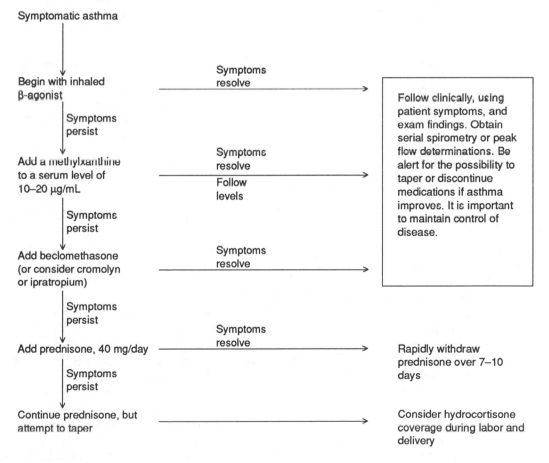

FIG 6–2.
Goals of outpatient treatment in asthma include the control of disease and the prevention of status asthmaticus. If asthma improves during pregnancy the physician may be able to safely withdraw medications. However, one should not hesitate to escalate therapy, if needed.

TABLE 6–3.
Drugs Used in the Treatment of Asthma

Class	Examples	Dose	FDA Category*	Comment
β-agonist				
Inhaled	Terbutaline	2–3 puffs q4–6h	B	Drugs of choice in mild asthma
	Albuterol		C	
	Metaproterenol		C	
Injected	Terbutaline	0.25 mL SC	B	Use only when inhaled drugs have failed
Methylxanthine	Theophylline	400–1200 mg/day	C	May require dose reduction in the third trimester, or with concomitant medications, e.g., erythromycin
	Aminophylline	in divided doses po to a serum level of 10–20 μg/mL	C	
Cromolyn	Cromolyn	2 puffs q6h	B	Especially useful for exercise-induced asthma
Anticholinergic	Ipratropium bromide	2 puffs q6h	B	Only mildly effective in asthma
Corticosteroid				
Inhaled	Beclomethasone dipropionate	2 puffs, 3–4 times daily	C	Beclomethasone is the preferred drug in this class; the mouth should be rinsed after inhalation
	Flunisolide	2 puffs, twice daily	C	
	Triamcinolone acetonide	2 puffs, 3–4 times daily	D	
Oral	Prednisone Prednisolone	Variable	B	Use only in refractory asthma; potentially teratogenic (cleft palate in rabbits); however, extensive experience in humans suggests minimal fetal risk

*See Preface for description of FDA risk classification.

tion can be made, it is prudent to check frequent theophylline levels, and be especially surveillant in the third trimester. The usual starting dose of theophylline is 200 mg of a long-acting preparation taken twice daily. The dosage should be gradually increased until therapeutic blood levels (10–20 μg/mL [55–110 μmol/L]) are reached.

Theophylline appears in breast milk with a milk-to-plasma ratio of 0.7, and is at peak concentration 2 hours following the peak plasma level.[56] Breast-feeding before the mother takes the drug decreases neonatal exposure. Excessive irritability in the infant may indicate theophylline toxicity.

Inhaled β-agonists are considered the drugs of first choice for the treatment of asthma in pregnancy.[57] These drugs are more potent bronchodilators than the theophyllines, and are less systemically absorbed. Theophylline,

however, has the virtue of an extensive safety record in pregnancy, and may be particularly useful for the control of nocturnal asthma.

A recent prospective study of inhaled β-agonists in 259 pregnancies, largely using metaproterenol, showed no change in perinatal mortality, congenital malformations, preterm births, low-birth-weight infants, small-for-gestational-age infants, mean birth weight, Apgar scores, or labor and delivery complications.[58] Terbutaline is the only inhaled β-agonist rated in pregnancy category B (FDA classification).[59] Although less data regarding safety are available for albuterol and metaproterenol, these inhaled agents are probably safe and are used interchangeably with terbutaline in pregnancy. The standard dose is two puffs every 4 to 6 hours.

Inhaled β-agonists are as effective as injected drugs, making them the preferred treatment even in the nonpregnant patient. Terbutaline does not impair uterine blood flow, as does epinephrine. Epinephrine has been implicated in a slight increase in congenital malformations when given in the first 4 months of gestation.[51] Parenteral injections of β-agonists should be administered only when inhaled agents have proved ineffective, and then terbutaline, 0.25 mg subcutaneously (SC), is preferred. There seems little role for oral β-agonists which have more adverse systemic effects and are no more effective than inhaled drugs.

Ipratropium bromide (category B) is an inhaled anticholinergic bronchodilator, effective in chronic obstructive lung disease and less so in asthma. Cromolyn sodium has no bronchodilator properties but is effective as a prophylactic agent when inhaled. It may be particularly useful in the prevention of exercise-induced bronchospasm. The FDA pregnancy category is also B, and the results of a single study suggest that cromolyn may be safe when used throughout pregnancy.[60]

Considerable controversy surrounds the use of corticosteroids, both inhaled and oral, for the treatment of asthma in pregnancy. Beclomethasone dipropionate (category C), an inhaled steroid, is teratogenic in rodents, but these findings were based on very high doses.[59] Since the inhaled preparation is only minimally absorbed, fetal toxicity, as well as neonatal adrenal insufficiency, is unlikely.[61] In fact, no adverse effects, including congenital malformations, were noted in three reports comprising 94 pregnancies.[48, 49, 62] Since there is less available information for triamcinolone acetonide (category D), and flunisolide (category C), beclomethasone is the inhaled steroid of choice. After inhalation of all corticosteroids, the mouth should be rinsed thoroughly to reduce the likelihood of developing oral candidiasis.

There is concern about the use of oral corticosteroids based primarily on an increased incidence of cleft palate in the offspring of rabbits. Also, a study in 1968 reported unexpected stillbirths and fetal distress in women receiving prednisolone, but this was

not confirmed in subsequent studies. Schatz et al.[47] examined 71 infants born to 55 women treated with a mean dose of 8.2 mg prednisone per day, noting a small excess in premature births but no increase in congenital malformations. There were no adverse effects attributed to steroids in two additional reports.[49, 63] Concern about the potential teratogenicity of steroids continues, and while it is reasonable to seek new data, it is also evident that *benefits from controlling severe asthma outweigh potential risks to the fetus*.

Drugs containing iodides or barbiturates are not indicated for the treatment of asthma, particularly in pregnancy.

Fortunately, life-threatening asthma requiring mechanical ventilation is unusual during pregnancy. It has been described, however, and successful outcomes for mother and infant have been recorded.[39] There are several anecdotal claims of benefit from lung lavage, including the use of solutions containing β-agonists, but there seems little reason to attribute recovery to the lavage.[39, 64.] Termination of pregnancy has been advocated for life-threatening status asthmaticus, and in one report two women experienced dramatic subsequent improvement in clinical status.[65] However, since epidural anesthesia, as well as inhalation with halothane, has been demonstrated to be effective in severe asthma, it is difficult to attribute resolution of bronchospasm to the termination per se rather than to one of these interventions or to concurrent conventional therapy. Thus, unless delivery is deemed in the infant's best interest because of maternal instability, we believe it quite unlikely that the mother will specifically benefit from termination, and do not recommend it.

Delivery is unlikely to be complicated by asthma. Although minute ventilation increases from a baseline of 6 L/min to as much as 20 L/min,[66] asthma tends to be quiescent during labor. For example, Schatz and colleagues[38] observed asthma symptoms in only 10% of 366 asthmatic pregnancies, and only two patients required intravenous (IV) theophylline.[38] This interesting observation might be related to high levels of catecholamines or cortisol during labor.

A history of prolonged maternal oral steroid use in the year prior to delivery should prompt coverage with hydrocortisone during labor. Hydrocortisone, 100 mg intramuscularly (IM) every 8 hours or IV every 6 hours, should be given until after delivery. There is also a potential risk of fetal adrenal insufficiency, and cases of fetal adrenal atrophy have been documented.[67] However, such events are extremely rare.[9]

CYSTIC FIBROSIS

Cystic fibrosis, the commonest lethal genetic disorder in whites, affects 1 in 2,000 births. The incidence in blacks is far lower, affecting approximately 1 in 17,000 infants. It is a generalized disorder of exocrine glands, most notably leading to pulmonary involvement and pancreatic insufficiency. The fundamental disorder will probably soon be discovered but no specific therapy or cure is yet available. The pathophysiologic abnormalities result from obstruction of glands or their ducts by abnormally viscous secretions.

The most severe manifestation of cystic fibrosis is bronchiectasis. Obstruction of airways promotes infection which leads to tissue damage. Progressive destruction of airways compounds obstruction, leading to further infection and a relentless cycle ending in pulmonary insufficiency. The disease is characterized by frequent exacerbations with infection by *Pseudomonas aeruginosa, Staphylococcus aureus,* and *Haemophilus influenzae.* Eventually, nearly all patients will harbor the mucoid form of *Pseudomonas,* which becomes impossible to eradicate.

Cystic fibrosis is no longer a disease confined to children. The median survival is now in excess of 26 years and 80% of patients reach age 20. Abnormal development of the vas deferens, epididymis, and seminal vesicles leads to decreased fertility, with more than 95% of men being aspermic. Women with this disease also exhibit diminished fertility due to thick cervical mucus, and fewer than 1 in

5 is capable of becoming pregnant.[68] Nevertheless, nearly 200 pregnancies in women with cystic fibrosis have been reported, one of which was facilitated by artificial insemination.[69] Therefore, issues of contraception, pregnancy, and delivery are becoming increasingly important.

Effect of Pregnancy on Cystic Fibrosis

The effect of pregnancy on mothers with cystic fibrosis ranges from insignificant to lethal. Serial pulmonary function testing has revealed that in contrast to normal pregnant women, residual volume rises and tidal volume fails to increase.[70] While normal women respond to the increased oxygen demand of pregnancy with an augmented cardiac output, patients with cystic fibrosis often have right heart failure due to lung disease (cor pulmonale) which can limit cardiac output. In affected women, oxygenation would be expected to deteriorate, or right heart pressures to worsen, during pregnancy. Thus in one national survey, 9 of 71 women (13%) with cystic fibrosis developed congestive heart failure during pregnancy.[71] In addition, women who developed dyspnea and cyanosis had a significant increase in maternal mortality as well as in perinatal mortality.

One large survey describes the mortality for 129 pregnancies in 84 women. Fifteen (18%) died within 24 months of delivery, 10 (12%) dying within 6 months. Cohen and colleagues[71] compared this with an expected 1-year mortality of 10% to 11% for 20-year-old women with cystic fibrosis based on data from 1966 to 1972.[72, 73] They therefore concluded that "mortality rates did not exceed those expected for cystic fibrosis women of the same age." However, this survey collected data for pregnancies occurring in 1975 and 1976. Improvement in therapy since the late 1960s should have led to improved survival for the later women. More importantly, women with cystic fibrosis who are willing and able to become pregnant are likely to have a higher performance status than those who are unwilling or unable. If so, Cohen et al. may have inadvertently selected a group expected to have much better survival than their historical comparison group. Two methods for classifying patients with cystic fibrosis according to severity of disease are in use. These include the calculation of Shwachman-Kulczycki[74] and Taussig scores,[75] each of which uses clinical and radiologic criteria to assign a score ranging from 0 to 100. A final score over 90 predicts an excellent outcome over the next several years. A score of less than 50 points indicates a high likelihood of subsequent mortality. A study of women with prepregnancy prognostic scores comparable to a group of nonpregnant controls, treated contemporaneously, would allow a more confident conclusion that the burden of pregnancy is not associated with increased maternal death.

Of interest is a survey of 11 pregnancies in eight women in which maternal outcome was related to prepregnancy performance status.[76] Women in group 1, whose overall condition returned to the pregravid level, had Shwachman-Kulczycki scores[74] over 74, and percent weight for height over 88%. Women in group 2 were those who deteriorated during pregnancy and did not return to pregravid levels. These women had prepregnancy Shwachman-Kulczycki scores less than 66, and percent weight for height less than 84%. Thus objective prepregnancy assessment is useful in predicting the effect of pregnancy and both Cohen[71] and Palmer[76] and their respective colleagues suggest that those with low scores should be advised not to become pregnant.

In summary, pregnancy most likely presents a real risk to the woman with cystic fibrosis, especially when the prepregnancy performance status is less than optimal. While the decision to become pregnant is ultimately the woman's, the physician should discourage pregnancy in those with Shwachman-Kulczycki or Taussig scores less than approximately 80.

Effect of Cystic Fibrosis on Pregnancy

Maternal disease clearly affects the fetus and neonate. While the incidence of spontaneous abortion does not appear to be increased, both preterm births and neonatal deaths are.[71, 76] Cyanosis, dyspnea, and insufficient maternal weight gain are predictors of prematurity and perinatal death.

An additional concern regarding the fetus is the effect of medications administered during maternal exacerbations. Cohen et al. noted that 65% of women were given antibiotic therapy during pregnancy, many with aminoglycosides[71]; however, no congenital anomalies were noted.

Another problem is the delivery of an infant who will have cystic fibrosis. Since the gene frequency is estimated at 1 in 20 in the white population, 2.5% of births to women with cystic fibrosis should produce a child with cystic fibrosis, and three such infants have been reported. Furthermore, all children will be carriers of the gene.

Management

Management of pregnancy in a woman with cystic fibrosis begins with prepregnancy counseling. Since there are important health consequences for mother and fetus, and since many women with the disease can conceive, contraception should be advised until pregnancy is desired. Moreover, the potential mother must consider the impact of her reduced exercise tolerance and her shortened life span on her offspring. There is one report suggesting that oral contraceptives might lead to deterioration of pulmonary status,[77] but more recently no significant deterioration was found in clinical status or pulmonary function in 10 women on a combination oral contraceptive followed with serial pulmonary function tests for 6 months.[78]

Since Taussig and Shwachman-Kulczycki scores below 80 are associated with poorer fetal outcome and with maternal mortality, patients with poor scores should be counseled against attempting pregnancy. Those with scores over 80 should be reassured that maternal and fetal outcomes are close to normal. Nevertheless, these women should be followed closely during pregnancy with serial pulmonary function testing, arterial blood gases, and clinical examinations for evidence of congestive heart failure.

Respiratory management includes routine postural drainage, bronchodilators, and maintenance of hydration. Aerobic exercise may be important for achieving optimal clearance of bronchial secretions. Clinical exacerbations with cough, increased sputum, dyspnea, and cyanosis should be treated as in the nonpregnant patient with oral or parenteral antibiotics, based on results of sputum cultures. Staphylococcus should be treated with a pencillinase-resistant penicillin or cephalosporin. Ampicillin or carbenicillin are effective for *H. influenzae*. Parenteral therapy is usually necessary when the infecting agent is *P. aeruginosa*. An aminoglycoside plus ticarcillin, carbenicillin, or azlocillin is usually effective. Alternatively, ceftazidime can be used, or possibly oral ciprofloxacin.[79] Nebulized antibiotics are an interesting approach to the problem of chronic infection, but trials of nebulized aminoglycosides have failed to demonstrate convincing benefit. Intermittent positive pressure breathing treatments are ineffective and can be complicated by pneumothorax.

Although pulmonary insufficiency is the dominant manifestation of cystic fibrosis, the clinician must be alert for other complications of the disease. Pancreatic insufficiency with malabsorption, malnutrition, and vitamin deficiency may supervene. Inadequate weight gain predicts prematurity and stillbirth.[71] Serial assessment of caloric intake may be useful.[80] A high protein, low fat diet with supplementation of vitamins A, D, and E should be recommended. Enzyme replacement with oral pancreatic enzymes is safe and effective. Hyperalimentation should be considered if other measures fail.[81] Other complications of cystic fibrosis include the development of diabetes, and hemorrhage due to vitamin K deficiency.

There is little information on which to base recommendations for treatment of cor pulmonale. Continuous oxygen may prevent fetal hypoxia and relieve maternal pulmonary hypertension, thereby improving right ventricular function. Diuretics can lessen congestion and edema but their use may worsen cardiac output. Digitalis is not clearly beneficial in right heart failure and can be dangerous in the setting of hypoxemia. Since there is a substantial risk of maternal mortality, elective abortion should be considered if this complication of chronic obstructive lung disease develops.

Since the risk of producing a child with cystic fibrosis is at least 1 in 40, several methods of intrauterine detection of cystic fibrosis have been developed. Methylumbelliferyl-guanidinobenzoate (MUGB) can be used to detect a deficiency in serine proteases in the amniotic fluid in the midtrimester.[82] In addition, polyacrylamide isoelectric focusing and column filtration of amniotic fluid have been described.[82]

Breast-feeding appears to be safe. An early report of high breast milk sodium in mothers with cystic fibrosis is thought to have been based on an error in data collection.[83] Regulation of sodium transport in breast milk is not analogous to that in sweat glands and saliva, and sodium concentration, as well as protein content in breast milk, is normal.[83]

SARCOIDOSIS

Sarcoidosis is a multisystem granulomatous disease of unknown etiology typically presenting with bilateral hilar lymphadenopathy and pulmonary infiltrates, occasionally with skin or eye lesions. It is an uncommon disease, affecting 30 patients per 100,000 in the United States. However, because it is predominantly a disease of young adults and exhibits a female preponderance, it is not rare among pregnant women. Most authors have found sarcoidosis associated with 0.05% of pregnancies. Blacks are affected at a rate tenfold that of whites.

Respiratory complaints, especially dyspnea and cough, are the presenting symptoms in about one half of all patients with sarcoidosis. One fourth have nonspecific initial manifestations such as fever, weight loss, or anorexia. A small fraction will first complain of skin lesions, eye disease, or neurologic abnormalities. One fifth of patients are discovered incidentally when a chest x-ray is obtained for an unrelated reason. The course of disease can sometimes be predicted by the pace of onset. Many patients have an insidious onset of disease followed by progressive, unrelenting pulmonary fibrosis. Others have a more acute onset associated with erythema nodosum, followed by spontaneous resolution. Most frequently, sarcoidosis pursues a benign course with eventual complete spontaneous remission.

Effect of Pregnancy on Sarcoidosis

Since sarcoidosis is characterized by spontaneous remissions and exacerbations, ascertaining the effect of pregnancy on the course of disease is difficult. Maycock et al.[84] felt that sarcoidosis improved in pregnancy but 50% of their patients experienced a flare in the puerperium. Reisfeld et al.[85] were unconvinced that pregnancy exerted any effect. Scadding's description of outcome based on chest x-ray abnormalities before pregnancy is often cited.[86] In 11 pregnancies carried to term, 3 women with initially clear lungs remained normal; 3 who had resolving disease continued to resolve; 2 with parenchymal scarring had no change; and 3 with widespread infiltrates had clearing of disease during pregnancy, then recurrences post partum. O'Leary[87] noted improvement in 5 of 27 pregnancies; however, in 11 instances steroids had been given. Fried[88] reported improvement in 4 of 13 pregnancies; however, more recently Agha et al.[89] found no consistent effect, with deterioration in 3 of 18 women and improvement in 6. Given the variable natural history of sarcoidosis, it is difficult to separate spontaneous improvement from an effect of pregnancy with any certainty. Overall, most authors feel that there is slight improvement in the disease, or at least stability in the ma-

jority of patients. This has been attributed to the well-established increase in corticosteroids during pregnancy. Although several patients with sarcoidosis have died during pregnancy, successful outcomes have been described even when pulmonary disease is severe.[85, 90]

Effect of Sarcoidosis on Pregnancy

There has been no systematic study of the impact of sarcoidosis on the outcome of pregnancy. Since there is no clear ill effect of sarcoidosis on the fetus or the pregnancy, and since the prognosis for the mother is generally excellent, prospective parents should not be counseled against pregnancy. Similarly, maternal sarcoidosis should not be an indication for elective abortion. Serial pulmonary function testing in cases of severe involvement is probably warranted. Determination of angiotensin converting enzyme levels may not be useful during pregnancy since Erksine et al.[91] have described a patient in whom a substantial increase in enzyme activity was not associated with a flare of disease. Sarcoid granulomas can synthesize vitamin D, which occasionally causes hypercalcemia. A case of postpartum hypercalcemic sarcoidosis has been reported.[92] Therefore it seems prudent to avoid the use of vitamin preparations containing vitamin D in pregnant women with sarcoidosis.

Management

The clearest indication for treatment of sarcoidosis with corticosteroids is eye involvement since ocular sarcoidosis can lead to loss of vision and treatment is effective. Severe constitutional complaints of fever, sweats, and weight loss will also respond as will the rare patient with hypercalcemic sarcoid. Progressive impairment in pulmonary function testing is an additional indication for steroids, although a long-term benefit to the mother is not certain. Life-threatening extrapulmonary involvement such as cardiac or neurologic sarcoid is usually treated in nonpregnant patients, but a beneficial effect of steroids is not convincing.

At the time of delivery, if corticosteroids have been given in the prior year for sarcoidosis, coverage with parenteral hydrocortisone, 100 mg every 8 hours IM or every 6 hours IV, should be given to prevent maternal adrenal insufficiency.

MISCELLANEOUS OBSTRUCTIVE AND RESTRICTIVE DISEASES

There is little information from which to determine the degree of pulmonary function impairment which should mandate the avoidance of pregnancy. Clearly the risk to the mother becomes substantial as the FEV_1 approaches 1 L. Nevertheless, one patient with alpha-1-antiprotease deficiency and an FEV_1 of less than 1.3 L (and measured at 0.9 L in the 15th gestational week) had an essentially uneventful pregnancy and delivered a healthy baby.[93] A woman with severe pulmonary fibrosis due to hard metal inhalation, with an FEV_1 of 1.3 L, was given oxygen for use during exercise, and also had an uncomplicated pregnancy.[94] Finally, a woman with severe restriction secondary to kyphoscoliosis, with an FEV_1 less than 1 L successfully carried her pregnancy to term with the use of nighttime nasal positive pressure ventilation.[95]

Obviously, if a woman with severe pulmonary impairment due to restrictive or obstructive lung disease desires to become pregnant, she should be aware of the potential risk to her own health. If she elects to carry a pregnancy to term she should receive careful, serial, clinical assessment and determination of spirometry. In carefully selected patients, the use of mechanical ventilatory support, especially with nasal positive pressure ventilation, may be considered to prevent overt respiratory failure.

TUBERCULOSIS

Tuberculosis is acquired through the inhalation of the tubercle bacillus. The organism causes pulmonary infection, inciting a granulomatous reaction. It can disseminate through the body, involving bone, meninges, adrenal glands, and the genitourinary system. Typically, primary infection is controlled but the organism persists intracellularly, sometimes for many years. Most clinical tuberculosis in adults is reactivation tuberculosis, resulting from recrudescent infection, rather than reinfection. Host factors, such as decreased immunity due to malnutrition, concurrent disease, or immunosuppressive drugs, play a large role in determining reactivation. Tuberculosis has become an uncommon disease since the advent of accurate diagnostic tests and effective drug therapy. However, it is not a rare disease, particularly in large urban centers, among the economically disadvantaged, in immigrants from the Third World, and now in patients with the acquired immunodeficiency syndrome (AIDS).

In most patients, reactivation occurs in the lung. Clinical manifestations include cough, sputum production, fevers, night sweats, and weight loss, although patients may be asymptomatic. Tuberculin skin test positivity indicates infection, past or present, or immunization with bacille Calmette-Guérin (BCG). The physical examination can reveal rales or signs of consolidation, and there often is evidence of weight loss. Chest radiography shows an infiltrate which most commonly involves the apex, often with cavitation. Many other patterns are possible, including lung nodules, lymphadenopathy, or pleural effusion. Smoldering tuberculous endometritis in pregnancy, and tuberculous mastitis are particularly important because of the likelihood of transmission to the fetus.[96] In active pulmonary tuberculosis, acid-fast bacilli are usually demonstrable in expectorated sputum. Less commonly, the diagnosis is made from pleural or cerebrospinal fluid, or from bone marrow, liver, or transbronchial lung biopsy.

In the nonpregnant patient treatment with some combination of isoniazid (INH), rifampin, ethambutol, and pyrazinamide is usually curative. Most treatment failures are due to noncompliance rather than to ineffective therapy. Isoniazid resistance is relatively uncommon except among Asian immigrants, but is an additional cause of treatment failure.

Effect of Pregnancy on Tuberculosis

The effect of pregnancy on the natural history of tuberculosis has intrigued physicians for thousands of years. Up until a hundred years ago, pregnancy was thought to bring improvement to the course of disease. Then medical opinion shifted and pregnancy was thought to so adversely affect the course of tuberculous disease that therapeutic abortion was mandated. In the middle of this century Hedvall[97] concluded that pregnancy had no significant effect either way on the course of tuberculosis. Antituberculous chemotherapy is just as effective in pregnant women as in their nonpregnant counterparts.[9, 98] Therefore, the age-old controversy has faded into unimportance.

Effect of Tuberculosis on Pregnancy

The effect of tuberculosis on the outcome of pregnancy is even less clear. The fetus can potentially become infected via the placenta or by aspiration of amniotic fluid. The organism has been isolated from the placenta as well as from stillborn infants. While some groups of investigators have concluded that the pregnancy is not altered by the mother's disease,[99] two recent reports include data which suggest a detrimental impact on the fetus. Bjerkedal et al.[100] noted a remarkable increase in the incidence of miscarriage, to about nine times that of controls. In addition, they observed an increase in the occurrence of vaginal hemorrhage, preeclampsia, and difficult labor, but no difference was noted in prematurity, congenital malformations, or low birth weight. In a series reported from National Jewish Hospital in Denver,[101] there was a striking rate of complications whether disease was drug-resistant or drug-sensitive. Of 27 pregnancies reviewed, there were 2 spontaneous abortions, and 2 infants developed positive tuberculin skin tests, 1 pulmo-

nary tuberculosis, 1 miliary tuberculosis, and 2 tuberculous meningitis. Only 4 of these affected infants survived. These results can be criticized, however, in that most of the diseased women were socioeconomically disadvantaged, and therefore more likely to have complicated pregnancies independent of tuberculosis. Nevertheless, the possibility remains that these outcomes represent a detrimental effect of maternal tuberculosis or its treatment.

The effect on the infant of a mother with tuberculosis is more clearly known. Although congenital infection occurs, neonatal acquisition by postpartum maternal contact is the usual means of transmission. If the infant of a tuberculous mother is not given prophylaxis, the risk of developing active disease may be as high as 50%.[102] In both congenital and neonatal infection diagnosis is difficult, leading to a 50% mortality, although prompt diagnosis and therapy yield an excellent result.[96]

Management

Prenatal chest radiographs have been advocated in the past with the hope of detecting and treating active tuberculosis before a complication could develop. With the low rate of endemic tuberculosis, however, this examination has a very low yield. Although 17% to 60% of pregnant women with active tuberculosis are asymptomatic, routine chest x-rays are no longer indicated.[96]

A better approach is to administer a tuberculin skin test early in pregnancy unless the mother has had a positive test in the past. Despite the depression of cell-mediated immunity in pregnancy, tuberculin skin tests are known to be valid. Testing of pregnant women, retested post partum (with each patient serving as her own control), has shown no effect of gestation on the results of the tuberculin test.[103] A chest x-ray is necessary only (1) in recent converters (since the risk of developing active disease is especially high in the first 2 years following conversion), (2) in those with positive skin tests and unknown time of conversion (since they may be recent converters), or (3) when symptoms or signs suggest tuberculosis (whatever the result of the skin test).

In women with positive skin tests in whom active disease has been excluded, prophylaxis with isoniazid should generally be withheld until after delivery. The risk of development of active disease is generally small and if it develops, diagnosis and treatment should be prompt. Therefore, although isoniazid is thought to be safe in pregnancy, the slight residual uncertainty outweighs the small potential benefit of prophylaxis. The single exception to this rule of deferring isoniazid until after delivery is the woman who is known to have been recently (past 2 years) infected. In such a case the risk of development of active disease is high enough that prophylaxis should be given. Even then, isoniazid should not be given in the first trimester.[104] Prophylaxis consists of isoniazid 300 mg orally once daily for 12 months although there is evidence that 6 months of therapy is as effective.

There is substantial experience with the first-line antituberculous drugs in pregnancy (Table 6–4). Isoniazid crosses the placenta, but appears not to be teratogenic, even when given in early pregnancy.[105, 106] Since there is some evidence from one series of a slight increased risk of malformations, isoniazid should be given only for active disease, or for recently infected women.[51] Pyridoxine (vitamin B_6) should always be given with isoniazid to lessen the likelihood of neurotoxicity. The standard dose is 50 mg of pyridoxine by mouth each day.

Active tuberculous disease requires prompt treatment. Untreated disease represents a far greater hazard to a woman and her fetus than does antituberculous therapy.[104] Since effective and safe therapy is available, active tuberculosis is not an indication for abortion. Initial treatment consists of isoniazid, 300 mg/day with rifampin, 600 mg/day, both given orally. Pyridoxine, 50 mg/day, should be prescribed routinely.

Rifampin, like isoniazid, crosses the placenta, but no adverse fetal effects have been described.[107] Ethambutol appears to be safe, based on a large experience, despite its well-established teratogenic effect in animals.[108] Para-aminosalicylic acid is uncommonly used for treatment of tuberculosis, but appears to be safe in pregnancy.[101]

Several drugs are known to cause problems in pregnancy. Streptomycin causes fetal ototoxicity when given at any time during the

TABLE 6–4.
Antituberculous Drugs in Pregnancy

Drug	Dose	FDA Category	Comment
Standard therapy			
Isoniazid (INH)	300 mg/day po for 9 mo	C	Add pyridoxine 50 mg/day
Rifampin	600 mg/day po for 9 mo	C	Turns secretions yellow
Use only for drug resistance or treatment failure			
Ethambutol	15 mg/kg/day po, added only when isoniazid resistance is suspected	B	Rarely, can affect visual acuity
Para-aminosalicylic acid	4 g 3 times daily po	C	Limited experience; appears safe for fetus
Ethionamide	250 mg twice daily po	C	Teratogenic in rats and rabbits
Cycloserine	250 mg twice daily po	C	Safety not established; follow blood levels
Streptomycin	1 g IM each day, initially	D	Fetal ototoxicity precludes use in pregnancy
Kanamycin		D	
Capreomycin			
Pyrazinamide	15–30 mg/kg po daily	C	Safety not established

gestation. In a series of 206 pregnancies in which streptomycin was used, 35 infants were abnormal, 34 with eighth nerve damage.[96] The related drugs capreomycin and kanamycin should be avoided for the same reason. Ethionamide is teratogenic in rabbits and rats.[109] Little is known about cycloserine and pyrazinamide. These drugs should therefore be avoided in pregnancy although drug resistance may mandate their use for the mother's benefit. Therapeutic abortion may then be considered.[101]

In nonpregnant patients a 6-month course of isoniazid, rifampin, and pyrazinamide is now known to be effective therapy for active tuberculosis. Since pyrazinamide is not used in pregnancy, this "short-course" treatment plan is not available to pregnant women. Treatment with isoniazid and rifampin must continue for 9 months. After 2 months of daily therapy, twice-weekly treatment with isoniazid 900 mg and rifampin 600 mg may be given for convenience.[104] If isoniazid resistance is suspected, ethambutol, 15 to 25 mg/kg/day by mouth, is added to the regimen, as in the nonpregnant patient. When the organism sensitivity is known, and isoniazid resistance is excluded, ethambutol can be stopped.

A high index of suspicion should be maintained for evidence of neonatal tuberculosis. If the mother has been on effective therapy and her sputum cultures have reverted to negative, this risk is small. There is no need to isolate the infant from the mother as long as the mother has been on effective chemotherapy for at least 2 weeks. Similarly, there is no contraindication to breast-feeding. Small concentrations of antituberculous drugs are secreted in breast milk, but do not produce toxicity in the infant.[104]

The amounts of drug ingested during nursing are, however, also ineffective in preventing or treating disease in the infant.[110] If treatment of the mother has begun in the 2 weeks prior to delivery, or if active maternal disease is present at delivery, prophylaxis of the infant is routinely indicated. If the mother's disease is isoniazid-sensitive, the infant should receive prophylaxis with isoniazid 10 to 20 mg/kg/day. When the infant is given prophylaxis, concomitant breast-feeding should be avoided since the addition of the isoniazid in breast milk to the infant's prophylactic dose of isoniazid may lead to toxicity.

An alternative method of prophylaxis, and the preferred method when the mother's organism is isoniazid-resistant, or daily drug therapy is thought to be impractical, is to administer BCG to the infant, one half of the adult dose. If maternal disease is well controlled at the time of delivery, neither of these methods of prophylaxis is routinely given. Skin testing of the infant at birth, then at 3-month intervals, should be adequate surveillance.[96]

Although antituberculous drugs are generally thought to be safe in pregnancy, a woman under treatment should be advised to avoid becoming pregnant until after the course of treatment is complete. To avoid the unlikely possibility of an adverse drug effect contraception should be routinely advised. It is extremely important that the patient and physician are aware that the efficacy of oral contraceptives is impaired by concurrent administration of rifampin. Numerous pregnancies have been described in women taking rifampin while using oral contraceptives. A barrier method should be prescribed in addition to, or in place of, oral contraception.

FUNGAL PNEUMONIA

The three most important systemic fungal diseases of normal human hosts are histoplasmosis, coccidioidomycosis, and blastomycosis. Histoplasmosis is caused by *Histoplasma capsulatum,* an organism that thrives in soil, particularly in areas contaminated with the excreta of birds and bats. Nearly 50 million Americans are estimated to have been infected with histoplasmosis. It is endemic in the Ohio and Mississippi river valleys of the United States, and although uncommon outside of North America, scattered cases have been reported from around the globe. *Coccid-*

ioides immitis, the causative organism of coccidioidomycosis, is found in the soil of semiarid regions, and is seen only in the Western Hemisphere. It is particularly common in the southwestern United States and northern Mexico, although sporadic cases are seen in Central and South America. Blastomycosis, caused by *Blastomyces dermatitidis,* is chiefly seen in the southeastern and midwestern United States, but cases have been reported from Canada (near the Great Lakes), Central America, Africa, and the Middle East.

Each of these diseases infects the host through the lungs, after which dissemination to the rest of the body is possible. In most instances, especially for histoplasmosis and coccidioidomycosis, infection is mild and self-limited. There is typically cough and fever, followed by gradual clinical resolution. Coccidioidomycosis may be accompanied by erythema nodosum and headache. The clinical course of blastomycosis is less well defined than the other two fungal infections, but recent evidence suggests that it, too, is often minimally symptomatic. In each case, a granulomatous reaction characterizes the body's response in the lung. Failure of the host to control the primary infection can result in dissemination to skin, bone, meninges, or other sites.

Diagnosis usually rests on isolation of the organism from sputum, body fluids, or tissue specimens. Serologic tests are often helpful in histoplasmosis or coccidioidomycosis. Skin tests are of no value in any of the fungal pneumonias.

Effect of Pregnancy on Fungal Infections

Histoplasmosis is not thought to be more common or severe in pregnancy.[111] Blastomycosis is seen only rarely.[112] Disseminated blastomycosis has been successfully treated in pregnancy, with a good outcome for mother and infant.[113] One case of intrauterine transmission has been described, but infection of the newborn may have occurred at delivery since the mother's urine was infected.[114]

Only coccidioidomycosis seems to behave differently in pregnancy, with a greater tendency to dissemination and progressive, even fatal, disease. Numerous reports attest to the severity of coccidioidomycosis in pregnancy.[115, 116] Smale and Waechter[115] reviewed cases in Kern County, California in the 1960s and concluded that disseminated coccidioidomycosis was the leading cause of maternal death in that area. Pappagianis[117] noted that the risk of dissemination increases progressively with each trimester and estimated that a pregnant woman with symptomatic infection has a 10% chance of dissemination, with a consequent 90% mortality.[117] This perception has recently been challenged. Catanzaro[112] believes that pregnancy is only a minor risk factor for severe disease, based on his informal survey of experienced practitioners and academicians in endemic areas. In a recent survey (1988) of 47,120 pregnancies in an endemic area, only 10 cases were discovered, 9 women having no underlying disease.[118] Seven women were diagnosed in the first or second trimester, and all recovered, 4 without therapy. Three were diagnosed in the first 10 days post partum, 1 recovering without therapy, and 2 developing meningitis and chronic disease. Eight healthy infants were delivered and 2 elective abortions were performed, both unrelated to the diagnosis of coccidioidomycosis. The incidence and severity of infection in this study were much less than in previously published reports; however, the authors concluded that women who acquire the disease late in pregnancy are at risk for severe, disseminated disease.[118] In summary, although the magnitude of risk of severe coccidioidomycosis in pregnancy is uncertain, it clearly is a more serious disease than in the nonpregnant host. Moreover, the risk of dissemination increases in the last months of pregnancy.

This increased risk has been attributed to the depression of cell-mediated immunity of pregnancy. However, the lack of a similar increase in severity of the other fungal infections, as well as many other infectious diseases, is puzzling. Drutz et al.[119] have made the fascinating discovery that growth of *C.*

immitis in vitro is stimulated by levels of progesterone and estradiol-17β that are achievable in vivo in the sera of pregnant women. In addition, saturable binding for progesterone and estrogen has been demonstrated in the cytosol of *C. immitis,* implying the presence of a cytosol-binding protein.[120] These findings seem to provide a pathophysiologic underpinning for the observed course of coccidioidomycosis in pregnancy.

Women who have been previously infected by *C. immitis* can harbor the infecting organism. Nevertheless, there appears to be no risk of activation of previously healed disease in pregnancy so that prior infection does not contraindicate pregnancy nor mandate special monitoring.

Treatment

Treatment of histoplasmosis, blastomycosis, and coccidioidomycosis in pregnancy depends on the pace of disease. Most patients will recover spontaneously, even without therapy. Therefore, acute but nonprogressive disease should not be treated. This is now considered to be accurate advice, even for blastomycosis. Disseminated disease is an indication for therapy with amphotericin B. Evidence of dissemination may consist of the development of ulcerating skin lesions, osteomyelitis, meningitis, multiple pulmonary nodules, hepatosplenomegaly, or diffuse lymphadenopathy. Amphotericin B crosses the placenta and can be found in the fetal circulation and amniotic fluid. The concentration in fetal blood is approximately one-third that in the maternal circulation.[121] There is little experience from which to conclude safety of amphotericin for the fetus, but among the reported treated patients, no adverse fetal outcomes have been described.[112, 113, 121] After a test dose, amphotericin B is typically given in a dose of 50 mg/day IV, to a total dose of 2 g.

Ketoconazole is also effective for the treatment of each of these fungal diseases[118] and is classified in pregnancy category C. Adverse affects on the human fetus have not been described. The initial dose is 400 mg orally per day, increasing to 800 mg if there is no response to the lower dose.

BACTERIAL PNEUMONIA

Earlier this century, pneumonia was an important cause of maternal mortality and premature delivery. The incidence of pneumonia was noted to be higher than in the general population, ranging from 0.1% of pregnancies to as high as 0.84%.[122] Little data are available from the modern era, but Benedetti et al. found pneumonia complicating only 0.04% of pregnancies.[123] There were no maternal deaths and prematurity was strikingly less common than in prior series.

The organisms seem to parallel those causing pneumonia in the general population, with *Streptococcus pneumoniae, H influenzae,* and *Mycoplasma pneumoniae* at the top of the list.[122, 123] Legionella pneumonia is now known to be an important cause of community-acquired pneumonia, occasionally rivaling pneumococcal pneumonia in frequency. Although clinical legionella pneumonia typically affects adults over the age of 60, and is more often hospital-acquired than community-acquired, cases in pregnancy have been described.[124]

Diagnosis of pneumonia demands a high index of suspicion in women with respiratory complaints, since many pneumonias follow more common viral upper respiratory illnesses. Worsening of symptoms, protracted fever, physical examination findings of consolidation, or systemic toxicity should prompt radiologic examination.

Treatment of bacterial pneumonia includes oxygen to prevent maternal and fetal hypoxemia. In the usual pregnant patient with community-acquired pneumonia, empiric therapy should probably begin with erythromycin, 1 g IV, every 6 hours, since most common organisms will be treated effectively with this regimen. Antibiotic therapy should then be tailored based on the results of cultures, or other diagnostic studies. Penicillin and ampicillin are reasonable alternatives, and safe for the fetus, but will not cover legionella. If gram-negative pneumonia is suspected, ceftriaxone is a good choice.

The efficacy and safety of pneumococcal vaccine in pregnant patients are unknown. Limited evidence suggests that there should be no detrimental effect on the fetus.[125] Therefore, when indicated for an underlying chronic disease such as cystic fibrosis, sickle cell anemia, asthma, or asplenia, pregnancy should probably not be a contraindication to the administration of pneumococcal vaccine.

VIRAL PNEUMONIAS

Influenza

Influenza, a respiratory infection caused by an RNA virus, is transmitted by aerosol, and typically spread from person to person, affecting large numbers of susceptible persons in characteristic epidemic patterns. Outbreaks typically occur in late autumn or early spring. Clinical manifestations include fever and chills with prominent systemic complaints of headache and myalgias. An initially nonproductive cough becomes productive of purulent sputum. The chest x-ray occasionally shows patchy infiltrates. During community outbreaks a clinical diagnosis can be reliably made in a patient with a febrile tracheobronchitis. Serologic tests are available to confirm the diagnosis. Bacterial superinfection with pneumococcus, hemophilus, or staphylococcus is common. Treatment is usually symptomatic although amantidine has a therapeutic effect if given in the first 48 hours of infection with influenza A.

The effect of pregnancy on the course of influenza has been evaluated by many investigators. During the pandemics of 1918–1919 and 1957–1958, pregnancy was associated with increased mortality. This has not been seen since that time, however.[126] The Centers for Disease Control considers influenza vaccine safe for use in pregnancy and recommends its use when indicated for underlying chronic disease such as diabetes, renal failure, or asthma.[126] Since there is no clear increase

in severity of influenza in pregnancy, the vaccine should no longer be routinely given to all pregnant women.

The effect of influenza on the pregnancy is less clear. The virus has been documented to traverse the placenta. Some evidence supports a teratogenic role for maternal influenza infection, with reports of increased risk of cleft lip and central nervous system abnormalities. No such relationships were observed in other studies and there is no congenital syndrome typical of maternal influenza. MacKenzie and Houghton reviewed all of the available evidence and concluded that there was no relationship between influenza and congenital malformations, nor to abortions, stillbirths, prematurity, or an increase in malignant disease in offspring.[127]

Treatment of influenza in pregnant women, as in most other patients, is symptomatic. Amantidine falls into pregnancy category C, and may be effective if given early in the clinical course, but is rarely indicated since influenza is nearly always self-limited. There has been a case report of severe influenza pneumonia in pregnancy successfully treated with amantadine and ribavirin.[128] The clinician should remain vigilant for bacterial superinfection which would require antibiotic therapy.

Varicella

Varicella infection in adults is uncommon since at least 75% of the adult population is immune. However, it is more likely to lead to varicella pneumonia in adults, and thereby more likely to cause death. Maternal chickenpox has rarely disseminated to cause varicella pneumonia. This disease seems to be more common as well as more severe in pregnancy, although there are no convincing data. Maternal mortality may be as high as 45% in varicella pneumonia.[129]

Although indications for the use of acyclovir in pregnancy remain to be established, there is virtual unanimity that maternal varicella pneumonia is one such indication. Although detectable in cord blood and amniotic fluid, acyclovir appears to be safe in pregnancy.[130] Although the optimal dose of acyclovir for varicella pneumonia in pregnancy has not been established, 7.5 mg/kg given IV every 8 hours has been recommended.[130]

Infection in any trimester is associated with congenital anomalies. In addition, if the onset of maternal disease has been within 7 days of delivery, the infant is at substantial risk of neonatal varicella. Infants at risk should be given varicella immune globulin, 1.25 mL IM.[131] Unfortunately, this gives incomplete protection, as demonstrated in a recent prospective trial, even when the dose of varicella immune globulin is doubled.[132]

ASPIRATION PNEUMONITIS

Several physiologic changes in pregnancy may compromise the normal protection of the respiratory epithelium from gastric acid. Gastric emptying is delayed, lower esophageal sphincter tone is reduced, intraabdominal pressure is elevated, and sedatives may blunt protective reflexes. Aspiration of gastric acid causes damage to the lung, resulting in chemical pneumonitis. The spectrum of disease ranges from asymptomatic, minor chest x-ray infiltrates to fulminating adult respiratory distress syndrome (ARDS). Mendelson[133] identified 66 women in a group of 43,000 whose pregnancies were complicated by this syndrome. Acid aspiration accounts for a substantial proportion of obstetric anesthetic complications and is an important contributor to maternal mortality.

The clinical course may begin abruptly or progress insidiously, and is marked by cough, sputum production, fever, bronchospasm, hypoxemia, and chest x-ray infiltrates. There can be spontaneous resolution of chemical inflammation, or bacterial infection may ensue, resulting in aspiration pneumonia or lung abscess. The degree of lung damage is related to the volume of aspirate, the presence of particulate matter, and most importantly, its pH.

Treatment begins with prevention. Women in labor should have limited oral intake and should be given nothing by mouth before cesarean section. Antacids should routinely be given before induction of anesthesia to reduce intragastric pH. This is best done by using a dilute solution of sodium citrate and citric acid (commercially available as Bicitra—Willen Drug Co.). Magnesium trisilicate is now avoided due to its particulate nature. There has been experience with H_2-blockers in Europe, and in one study the combined use of IM cimetidine, 200 mg, and sodium citrate was effective in raising gastric pH, nearly always to above 4.[134] During endotracheal intubation, cricoid pressure should be applied in case of regurgitation of gastric acid.

Management of the chemical pneumonitis of aspiration is virtually identical in pregnant and nonpregnant patients. Therapy is supportive, beginning with suctioning of the trachea and prevention of recurrent aspiration. Oxygen should be given to prevent hypoxemia. Mechanical ventilation and the use of positive end-expiratory pressure (PEEP) may be necessary in severe cases (see Chap. 7, Critical Illness in Pregnancy). In a witnessed aspiration, many physicians administer high-dose corticosteroids, for example, methylprednisolone sodium succinate (Solu-Medrol), 30 mg/kg as a one-time bolus, although there is no convincing experimental or clinical evidence to support a benefit. Once the aspiration is established, corticosteroids have no role and may be detrimental.

Antibiotics are of no use in the treatment of this chemical lesion. Bacterial superinfection, which complicates 25% to 45% of aspirations, should be treated with antibiotics. Most infections complicating aspiration in the previously healthy person are caused by anaerobes. Penicillin, 2.5 million units every 6 hours, is the drug of choice for empiric therapy. Antibiotics should be adjusted on the basis of culture results when available.

PERIPARTUM PLEURAL EFFUSION

Hughson et al.[135] reviewed the chest radiographs of 112 women studied post partum, with the striking finding of detectable pleural fluid in 51 (46%). This prompted a prospective study of 30 additional patients, all x-rayed within 24 hours of vaginal delivery. Pleural effusions were found in 20 (67%) by careful examination of the posteroanterior and lateral films.[135] Ten of these patients agreed to have lateral decubitus films, which confirmed the effusion in 7. Of the 71 patients in the combined series who had detectable pleural fluid, 66 (93%) had small effusions. However, 5 (7%) were classified as having moderate-sized effusions, defined as a pleural stripe greater than 3 mm. Hughson and colleagues[135] hypothesized that the volume overload and decreased colloid oncotic pressure of pregnancy, possibly compounded by a decrease in lymphatic drainage of the pleural space due to the Valsalva maneuver during labor, led to the accumulation of fluid.

In fact, this study confirmed a much earlier radiographic series in which pleural effusions were detected approximately 1 week post partum.[136] Hessen[136] found definite fluid in 21 (23%) of 92 women and probable fluid in another 13. Parker[137] has argued that these effusions may well be present ante partum, but since chest x-rays are avoided in pregnancy, effusions would go undetected. This seems probable since the hemodynamic factors likely to lead to pleural fluid accumulation are present well before delivery. The postulate that intrapartum Valsalva maneuvers may impair lymphatic clearance from the pleural space seems to ignore the relatively minor contribution of the lymphatics in the maintenance of a dry pleural space. The normal pleural lymph flow is only 20 mL/hr, so that even prolonged Valsalva maneuvers should result in little pleural accumulation. A recent study casts doubt on the high frequency of peripartum pleural fluid. Udeshi et al.[138] studied 50 women with ultrasound, finding pleural fluid in only one patient who also had pulmonary edema.

A practical approach, in light of the conflicting data, is to accept small, asymptomatic pleural effusions as an accompaniment of pregnancy and delivery. Large effusions, those associated with symptoms, or effusions in a clinical setting suggesting intrathoracic disease should prompt an investigation of their etiology, usually including thoracentesis.

PULMONARY EMBOLISM

The annual incidence of pulmonary embolism in the United States has been estimated at 650,000. Since approximately 30% of these patients die, pulmonary embolism is one of the leading causes of death. More than 90% of patients with pulmonary embolism have an identifiable risk factor such as malignancy, surgery, trauma, obesity, venous stasis, immobilization, prior venous thromboembolism, or pregnancy. The pathophysiology in most patients begins with clot formation in an intramuscular sinus of a leg vein, related to stasis, venous injury, or a hypercoagulable state. In some fraction of patients this clot propagates to form a proximal deep venous thrombus. This proximal extension provides the source for embolization to the pulmonary circulation.

The presenting symptoms include dyspnea, chest pain, hemoptysis, cough, and, rarely, syncope or cardiovascular collapse. The examining physician may detect tachycardia, tachypnea, cyanosis, splinting, a loud pulmonic component of the second heart sound, hypotension, or findings of venous thrombophlebitis. Unfortunately, these symptoms and signs are all nonspecific so that the diagnosis of pulmonary embolism is commonly, even usually, missed. Chest radiography is most often abnormal, showing atelectasis, pleural effusion, or infiltrate, but these findings are of little help in making a specific diagnosis. The electrocardiogram may show signs of right heart strain, such as right axis deviation or an $S_1Q_3T_3$ pattern, but these are only present in 15% of patients. The arterial blood gas typically reveals hypoxemia and hypocapnia, but even a normal Po_2 does not exclude the diagnosis. Therefore the utility of these tests is in excluding an alternative diagnosis such as pneumonia, rib fracture, or myocardial infarction, rather than in establishing a diagnosis of pulmonary embolism.

These difficulties in making a diagnosis of a life-threatening, yet treatable, disease have prompted the development of sophisticated diagnostic strategies and procedures. For example, convincing evidence of deep venous thrombosis, while no proof of pulmonary embolization, provides a rationale for anticoagulation. Positive evidence of venous thrombosis, therefore, usually makes the question of embolism unimportant. Leg studies can therefore often aid the physician to avoid risky or invasive tests.

Ventilation-perfusion lung scanning helps the clinician greatly since a normal scan excludes pulmonary embolism. A high-probability lung scan is similarly useful since the likelihood of pulmonary embolism is in excess of 80%. This is high enough to warrant treatment of all such patients, even though a few who do not have pulmonary embolism will be anticoagulated. The utility of low- and intermediate-probability scans is debated, so that when clinical suspicion remains, most experts recommend pulmonary angiography. A pulmonary angiogram is an invasive but safe and accurate means of establishing the presence of clot in the pulmonary artery.

Treatment of the patient with pulmonary embolism consists of anticoagulation to prevent recurrent embolization, thrombolysis to dissolve the embolus and its thrombotic source, or inferior vena caval interruption to prevent reembolization from the legs or pelvis.

Pulmonary embolism and the related disorder of venous thrombosis are particularly challenging problems in pregnancy. In this condition, more than in any other pulmonary disorder, the care of the pregnant woman differs from that of her nonpregnant counterpart (Table 6–5). Because of the many subtly different considerations, management of venous thromboembolism is best carried out in consultation with a specialist.

Effect of Pregnancy on Thromboembolism

Pregnancy, and especially the postpar-

TABLE 6–5.
Management of Thromboembolism: Differences Comparing Pregnant and Nonpregnant Patients

Nonpregnant	Pregnant
Noninvasive leg studies very useful	Noninvasive leg studies may be compromised by compression of vena cava
^{125}I-fibrinogen useful in the diagnosis of calf vein thrombosis	^{125}I-fibrinogen contraindicated
Thrombolytic therapy can be considered	Thrombolytic therapy is risky, and contraindicated near term
Greenfield filter is placed below the renal veins	Greenfield filter is placed suprarenally since the left ovarian vein empties into the left renal vein
Partial thromboplastin time is used to titrate dose of heparin	Heparin levels may be preferred
Warfarin sodium is preferred for long-term anticoagulation	Warfarin crosses the placenta and is avoided due to congenital malformations
Underlying hypercoagulable state is rare	Hypercoagulable states may be relatively more common
Heparin-dihydroergotamine is useful for perioperative prophylaxis against venous thromboembolism	Heparin-dihydroergotamine is contraindicated

tum state, are risk factors for venous thrombosis and pulmonary embolism. The incidence of deep venous thrombosis in pregnancy may be as high as 5 in 1,000 deliveries[139] and is further increased post partum.[140] Postpartum calf vein thrombi were detected by iodine 125–fibrinogen scanning in 3% of deliveries.[141] Women who undergo cesarean section are particularly susceptible to deep venous thrombosis, which is 3 to 16 times more common than in women delivered vaginally.[140] Fortunately, pulmonary embolism is much less common, affecting only 1 in 2,000 pregnancies.[142, 143] Nevertheless, in a study of causes of maternal mortality in the state of Massachusetts, pulmonary embolism ranked second only to trauma.[144] Similar results were reported in a national study of maternal deaths.[145]

Several anatomic, physiologic, and biochemical changes during pregnancy and the postpartum period contribute to the increased tendency to thromboembolism. Compression of the inferior vena cava by the enlarged uterus leads to venous pooling in the legs. Hormonal influences may relax venous smooth muscle in the legs, compounding venous stasis. Probably of greatest importance are the changes in coagulation and fibrinolysis that accompany pregnancy. Both increases in procoagulant substances as well as decreases in naturally occurring anticoagulants are found regularly. Coagulation factors VII, VIII, IX, X, and XII increase in the third trimester. Fibrinogen levels increase dramatically by the third month of gestation and by the end of pregnancy are twice normal. At the same time, levels of antithrombin III (AT-III), an endogenous anticoagulant, decrease. Advances in the study of fibrinolysis, responsible for natural dissolution of clots, have shed more light on the hypercoagulable state of pregnancy. Gore and colleagues[146] have detected a decrease in releasable levels of tissue plasminogen activator, a naturally occurring fibrinolytic substance, as early as the first trimester. They[146] and others[147] have also found increases in plasminogen activator inhibitors, such as fast-acting tissue plasminogen activator inhibitor, which might limit the ability of the pregnant woman to lyse early clots. The clinical relevance of each of these potential contributors to the hypercoagulable state of pregnancy is unknown.

Preexistent, underlying hypercoagulable conditions will occasionally manifest as venous thromboembolism during pregnancy. In particular, AT-III deficiency is probably not rare.[148] Tengborn et al.[149] found AT-III deficiency in 2 of 72 women with recurrent thromboembolism in pregnancy and protein C deficiency in one of six patients in whom the assay was conducted. Discovery of one of these hemostatic abnormalities has serious implications, both for the woman as well as

for family members. If these data are confirmed by subsequent investigators, it will be necessary to screen for the presence of hypercoagulable states in all women with thromboembolism in pregnancy.

Diagnosis of Thromboembolism in Pregnancy

The presenting signs and symptoms of pulmonary embolism in pregnancy are no more helpful to the clinician than the typically nonspecific findings seen in nonpregnant women. Creating even more of a challenge, dyspnea and leg edema are commonly present in normal pregnancy. Since physicians are reluctant to perform many of the tests necessary for the diagnosis of pulmonary embolism in a pregnant woman, it is likely that the diagnosis is often missed. Because the consequences of a missed diagnosis are potentially grave for the mother and fetus, it is important to pursue any reasonable clinical suspicion of pulmonary embolism (Fig 6–3).

Ventilation-Perfusion Lung Scanning

Radiologists and obstetricians are occasionally reluctant to perform ventilation-perfusion lung scanning for fear of radiation exposure to the fetus. Fetal exposure using technetium 99m macroaggregated albumin perfusion lung scanning with technetium 99m pentetic acid (DTPA) aerosol ventilation scanning has been calculated by Marcus et al.[150] to be only 50 mrem. This is a minor exposure, amounting to only 10% of the maximum permissible fetal gestational exposure of 500 mrem for radiation workers. The authors concluded that the risk of not performing the test, and thereby possibly failing to make the diagnosis of pulmonary embolism, far outweighed any risk of radiation exposure. More recently, Ponto[151] has reestimated the fetal exposure based on the proximity of the fetus to the maternal bladder, and concluded that the dose may be severalfold higher than previously thought. Nevertheless, he also concluded that the risk of radiation exposure was far less than that of failure to perform the procedure.

Diagnosis of Deep Venous Thrombosis

When the lung scan is nondiagnostic (i.e., not normal and not high-probability), the most reasonable first approach is to look for deep venous thrombosis in the legs, providing an indication for anticoagulation (see Fig 6–3). Noninvasive venous studies of the legs such as Doppler ultrasound, impedance plethysmography, phleborrheography, and duplex ultrasound examination are without risk. In the nonpregnant patient, noninvasive leg studies are extremely useful for the diagnosis of deep venous thrombosis.

Doppler ultrasound involves scanning the large leg veins for patterns of blood flow. Venous flow normally varies in phase with respiration as well as with maneuvers such as squeezing of the calf muscles. These variations in flow cause a detectable Doppler shift. A decrease in the amplitude or the absence of these signals indicates venous obstruction.

Impedance plethysmography utilizes changes in electrical impedance to detect changes in the volume of a leg. Cuff occlusion in the thigh causes measurable engorgement of the leg. Sudden release of the cuff allows rapid emptying of the leg veins and a consequent decrease in leg volume. These volume changes lead to measurable electrical impedance changes whose time course can be compared to normal values. Outflow obstruction

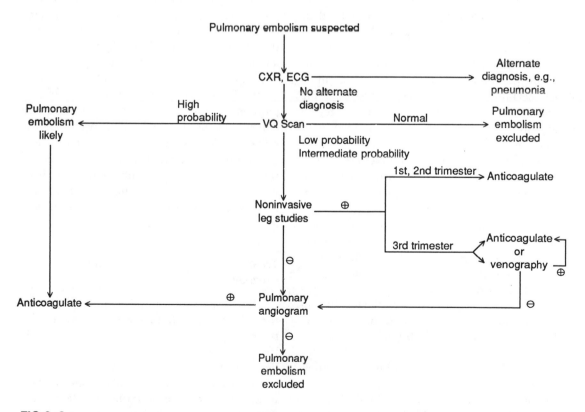

FIG 6–3.
Flow diagram illustrating the steps in evaluation of the pregnant woman when a diagnosis of pulmonary embolism is seriously considered. *CXR* = chest x-ray; *ECG* = electrocardiogram; *VQ* scan = ventilation-perfusion scan.

by clot leads to a detectably slower reduction in leg volume when the thigh cuff is released, compared to normal.

Phleborrheography uses multiple leg cuffs to measure changes in venous waveforms in response to respiration and calf compression. These waveforms are predictably altered by thrombosis.

A newly developed noninvasive method for the diagnosis of venous thrombosis is high-resolution duplex scanning of leg veins. It has been suggested that this new test may be useful in pregnancy but there are no data from which to estimate sensitivity and specificity.[152]

[125]I–fibrinogen scanning is the only noninvasive test that is sensitive for calf vein thrombosis, detecting over 90% of thrombi. Unfortunately, ^{125}I crosses the placenta and enters the fetal circulation. Radioactivity can also be detected in breast milk. Thus, ^{125}I-fibrinogen scanning is contraindicated in pregnancy and while breast-feeding.

Each of these tests is quite sensitive and specific in nonpregnant patients. Their reliability in the last half of pregnancy is much less certain, largely due to compression of the vena cava by the uterus. In one study, 48 asymptomatic patients were assessed with phleborrheography in the second or third trimester, or immediately post partum.[153] The women were carefully placed in a 10-degree reverse Trendelenburg, left lateral position, with knees slightly flexed. Waveforms were normal in all, suggesting that this test, if abnormal, could be taken as an indicator of disease. In a more recent series phleborrheography was performed in several positions in 25 pregnant, healthy women.[154] Venous hemodynamics were greatly affected by position and degree of hip flexion, and waveforms were abnormal in 9 (36%) of the 25.

A reasonable approach, given the conflicting data regarding reliability of noninvasive studies, is to treat on the basis of an abnormal noninvasive test in the first or second trimester. In the third trimester, when a medical center's vascular laboratory has substantial experience in pregnancy, it is also appropriate to anticoagulate for an abnormal result.[155] On the other hand, for the majority of institutions with less experience, since anticoagulation carries substantial risks, abnormal noninvasive studies should generally be confirmed by venography.[140, 142]

Ascending venography is the most accurate test for the detection of deep venous thrombosis. Contrast is injected into the dorsum of the foot and the leg veins are gradually filled. This invasive procedure carries the risks of dye allergy, pain, and the potential for creation of thrombophlebitis. Performance of limited venography, excluding the iliac system, with lead apron shielding of the abdomen, lessens the radiation exposure to the fetus.

Pulmonary Angiography

The gold standard for the diagnosis of pulmonary embolism is pulmonary angiography. This entails greater risk to the fetus than lung scanning, although it is quite safe for the mother. Still, the estimated radiation dose is less than that known to have an effect on the fetus.[140] Deciding when to perform a pulmonary angiogram is probably the most difficult instance of weighing the poorly known risk of an invasive procedure versus the danger of missing the diagnosis. However, unless the clinical suspicion of pulmonary embolism is very low, when leg studies have been unhelpful, an equivocal lung scan should be followed by pulmonary angiography.

Treatment of Thromboembolism in Pregnancy

Treatment of established deep venous thrombosis or pulmonary embolism during pregnancy entails unique risks. Bed rest with leg elevation is indicated for symptomatic relief as well as to minimize the opportunity for reembolization. Oxygen should be given when necessary to ensure maternal and fetal oxygenation. Anticoagulation is the most important aspect of therapy, and should begin with IV heparin. A loading bolus of 7,500 to 10,000 units should be followed by a continuous infusion in a dose sufficient to maintain the activated partial thromboplastin time (PTT) at 1.5 to 2.0 times control. Alternatively, heparin levels can be followed to assess the adequacy of anticoagulation, aiming for 0.3 to 0.4 unit/mL of heparin, using the protamine sulfate neutralization test. It has been suggested that heparin levels may be preferable to the PTT for assessment of heparin therapy in pregnancy.[155, 156] Since pregnancy raises factor VIII and fibrinogen levels, and these factors influence the effect of heparin to prolong the PTT, the adequacy of this test in pregnancy is suspect. Whether there truly is any advantage to the use of heparin levels for the titration of full anticoagulation, however, remains to be shown.

Heparin anticoagulation can typically be achieved with an infusion of 1,000 units/hr, although higher doses are often necessary, especially early in therapy or with massive thrombosis. Heparin acts by combining with AT-III to inhibit the formation of thrombin. It thereby prevents the formation or propagation of clot but does nothing to dissolve clot. Since prevention of reembolization seems to prevent death from pulmonary embolism, heparin is effective therapy. Because of its high molecular weight, heparin does not cross the placenta and is therefore the anticoagulant of choice in pregnancy.

After the acute management with heparin, long-term anticoagulation is required to prevent recurrence of thromboembolism. Oral anticoagulants cross the placenta and enter the fetal circulation. Given between the 6th to 12th weeks of gestation, warfarin results in a typical embryopathy consisting of short stature with stippled epiphyses, nasal hypoplasia, saddle nose, and frontal bossing. Other defects have resulted from administration of oral anticoagulants in the second and third trimesters, probably due to fetal hemorrhage and scarring. These include dorsal midline dysplasia characterized by agenesis of the corpus callosum, Dandy-Walker malformations, and midline cerebellar atrophy, as well as ventral midline dysplasia with optic atrophy.[157] Yet Hall and colleagues[158] concluded that an adverse outcome occurred in one third of pregnancies no matter whether warfarin sodium (Coumadin) or heparin had been given. Subsequently this analysis has been challenged on the basis that the women given heparin had co-morbid conditions and that the adverse outcomes in the heparin patients were overstated. In a reanalysis of the data, heparin was found to be quite safe for the fetus, and thus is the anticoagulant of choice for the continuation of anticoagulation.[157]

Bleeding is the most common complication of heparin anticoagulation, occurring in up to 10% of women.[158] Recent data in general medical patients given adjusted dose (not minidose) subcutaneous heparin suggest a much lower incidence of significant hemorrhage. Heparin may cause thrombocytopenia in approximately 5% of patients, typically occurring 1 week into therapy. Therefore the platelet count should be checked prior to initiation of treatment, then approximately weekly or when clinically indicated. Rarely, this thrombocytopenia is associated with arterial thrombosis, which, of course, necessitates discontinuation of the drug. Heparin has the potential to cause maternal osteoporosis, which is related to dose and duration of therapy. Most reported cases have involved treatment with at least 15,000 units/day, given for at least 6 months,[157] although there is a single case report of severe osteoporosis attributed to heparin after 10,000 units daily for only 36 weeks.[159]

Recommendations

In light of the available evidence, heparin is the anticoagulant of choice in pregnancy. After acute treatment with IV heparin, anticoagulation should be continued with SC heparin given every 12 hours by the patient herself. The dose must be sufficient to prolong the PTT to 1.5 times control at the midpoint of the dosing interval[157] or to achieve heparin levels of 0.3 to 0.4 unit/mL using the protamine sulfate neutralization test. This should be continued at home until delivery.

When anticoagulation is contraindicated, or ineffective in preventing recurrent embolization, or when hemorrhage develops, the mother remains at risk of death from pulmonary embolism. Since most emboli originate as venous thrombi in the legs or pelvis, interruption of the inferior vena cava is effective in preventing reembolization. Transvenous placement of the Greenfield vena caval filter is extremely safe and has replaced open caval ligation. It has been used safely in pregnancy.[160] Since the left ovarian vein empties into the left renal vein, the filter should be placed in the suprarenal vena cava in contrast to the standard infrarenal position.

Streptokinase, urokinase, and tissue plasminogen activator have been advocated in the treatment of pulmonary embolism because of their proved ability to speed clot lysis in the pulmonary circulation as well as in the leg veins. Use in routine management of thromboembolism is controversial, however, because of the risk of hemorrhage. In pregnancy, thrombolytic therapy is relatively contraindicated given the paucity of experience and the substantial risks. Despite this there are several case reports in which lytic therapy has been safely given.[161, 162] Since routine heparin therapy is effective in preventing reembolization and death, thrombolytic therapy should be reserved for the patient who is hemodynamically unstable from massive, proved pulmonary embolism. Thrombolytic therapy is absolutely contraindicated near the time of delivery and shortly post partum due to the risk of hemorrhage.

Emergency pulmonary embolectomy is rarely indicated in pulmonary embolism. The logistics involved in preparing an operating room and assembling a cardiopulmonary pump team makes it rarely practical. By the time the procedure is available, the patient is usually better or has not survived. Despite this, a case in which both mother and infant survived after emergency embolectomy has been reported.[163] Its use can be considered in proven, life-threatening pulmonary embolism when thrombolytic therapy is contraindicated.

Labor, Delivery, and Post Partum Interval

At the time of delivery, a woman who is fully anticoagulated due to recent pulmonary embolism can remain fully anticoagulated if vaginal delivery is anticipated.[140] Except for episiotomy hematomas, full anticoagulation is not associated with increased bleeding during vaginal delivery.[140] Alternatively, the dose of SC heparin can be reduced to 5,000 every 12 hours. In any anticoagulated patient epidural and spinal anesthesia are contraindicated due to the risk of spinal cord hematoma with cord compression. Since heparin does not affect the fetus, there is no increased risk of intracerebral hemorrhage during vaginal delivery. After delivery full anticoagulation should be reinstituted within 12 hours. Then heparin and warfarin should both be given until a therapeutic warfarin effect is achieved. Heparin is then discontinued, while warfarin is maintained for an arbitrary period of from 2[157] to 12[164] weeks.

Nursing is safe during heparin anticoagulation since heparin does not appear in breast milk and is not absorbed from the gastrointestinal tract.[157] Despite the fact that the *Physician's Desk Reference* states that coumarins may pass into the milk of mothers and cause a prothrombinopenic state in the nursing infant, there is convincing evidence from two studies of nursing mothers that oral anticoagulants are also safe.[165, 166]

Oral contraceptives are contraindicated in patients with prior thromboembolic disease due to the risk of recurrence so that an alternative form of contraception should be offered.

Patients With a History of Thromboembolism

Women with a history of prior venous thromboembolism are at substantial risk of a recurrence during pregnancy and the postpartum period. Many questions remain, however, regarding the magnitude of this risk, which women are at highest risk of recurrence, and the optimal management of these patients.

Tengborn et al. surveyed 72 women who became pregnant after a prior pulmonary embolus or deep venous thrombosis.[149] Their 87 pregnancies and deliveries were complicated by 17 episodes of venous thromboembolism (20%), despite the use of heparin prophylaxis in some patients. Others have estimated the risk of recurrent thromboembolism at 4% to 12%.[167, 168]

It may be that women whose thromboembolism was related to an estrogenic stimulus (pregnancy or oral contraceptives) are at higher risk of pregnancy-associated thromboembolism than women whose prior event was related to trauma or nonobstetric surgery. In fact, in the aforementioned survey, all of the recurrences of thromboembolism occurred in women whose first episode was related to a hyperestrogenic influence.[149] One group has suggested venography in women with venous thromboembolism unrelated to pregnancy or oral contraceptives, then recommending prophylaxis only in those with evidence of venous abnormalities.[155] However, until better data become available, it seems most reasonable to consider all women with a prior, well-documented venous thrombosis or pulmonary embolus to be at high risk of recurrence during pregnancy, and therefore deserving of consideration for prophylaxis.

Many prophylactic strategies have been advocated. Unfortunately, it remains unclear whether prophylaxis with heparin is effective or completely safe. Ginsberg and Hirsh[157] suggest an empiric dose of 5,000 units SC every 12 hours until mid–third trimester, then an increase in the dose to prolong the midinterval (6 hours post–injection) PTT to 1.5 times control. Bonnar[139] recommends an empiric increase in dose to 7,500 or 10,000 units each 12 hours in the third trimester.[139] There are insufficient data to evaluate the effectiveness of these regimens, however. In one retrospective analysis, patients with prior thromboembolism given prophylaxis (largely with heparin 5,000 units every 12 hours) were just as likely to have recurrence as those not given prophylaxis.[149] Perhaps the failure to increase dose in the third trimester accounted for the lack

of protection. On the other hand, in one study designed to assess the risks of prophylactic heparin (10,000 units given twice daily throughout pregnancy and labor), 1 of 20 women developed severe, debilitating osteoporosis.[167] In addition, the investigators thought that the withholding of epidural analgesia in the women given heparin might have contributed to maternal and fetal morbidity, although the numbers were too small for certainty.

There is reason to be optimistic that the recent use of heparin assays may lead to safe and effective prophylactic therapies. The activated PTT is an insensitive method to detect the anticoagulant effect of small amounts of heparin. It therefore is an inadequate method on which to base titration of small doses. Recently, sensitive heparin assays have become available, using anti–factor Xa activity. When 26 pregnant women with prior thromboembolism were given prophylactic heparin in a dose to maintain heparin levels between 0.08 to 0.15 unit/mL (measured 3 hours after injection), no thromboembolic complications occurred, bleeding during delivery was not increased, and no spinal fractures were found.[169]

In sum, there is general consensus that women with prior thromboembolism, especially when precipitated by pregnancy or oral contraceptives, should receive some form of heparin prophylaxis during pregnancy, delivery, and post partum. Until new data become available, heparin is best given in an SC dose to achieve heparin levels (using the anti–factor Xa assay) of approximately 0.1 unit/mL throughout pregnancy. Assays should be performed monthly, then increased to weekly in the third trimester. When heparin levels are not available, a dose of 234 units/kg/24 hr, or approximately 7,000 units twice daily, has been suggested.[169]

Other patients at high risk may benefit from prophylaxis as well, including women with preeclampsia, those undergoing cesarean section, or those who have added risk factors such as malignancy, obesity, diabetes, high parity, cardiac disease, or advanced age.[142] Further studies are needed to clarify the role of prophylactic therapy in these risk groups before recommendations can be made. Finally, the fixed drug combination of heparin and dihydroergotamine (Embolex) is contraindicated as a prophylactic strategy in pregnancy as the latter may have potent uterine smooth muscle stimulant and vasoconstrictor actions.

REFERENCES

1. Novy MJ, Edwards MJ: Respiratory problems in pregnancy. *Am J Obstet Gynecol* 1967; 99:1024–1045.

2. Pernoll ML, Metcalfe J, Schlenker TL, et al: Oxygen consumption at rest and during exercise in pregnancy. *Respir Physiol* 1975; 25:285–293.

3. Russell IF, Chambers WA: Closing volume in normal pregnancy. *Br J Anaesth* 1981; 53:1043–1047.

4. Awe RJ, Nicotra MB, Newsom TD, et al: Arterial oxygenation and alveolar-arterial gradients in term pregnancy. *Obstet Gynecol* 1979; 53:182–186.

5. Lucius H, Gahlenbeck H, Kleine HO, et al: Respiratory functions, buffer system, and electrolyte concentrations of blood during human pregnancy. *Respir Physiol* 1970; 9:311–317.

6. Templeton A, Kelman GR: Maternal blood-gases, (PAO_2-PaO_2), physiological shunt and V_D/V_T in normal pregnancy. *Br J Anaesth* 1976; 48:1001–1004.

7. Milne JA: The respiratory response to pregnancy. *Postgrad Med J* 1979; 55:318–324.

8. England SJ, Fahri LE: Fluctuations in alveolar CO_2 and in base excess during the menstrual cycle. *Respir Physiol* 1976; 26:157–161.

9. Weinberger SE, Weiss ST, Cohen WR, et al: State of the art: Pregnancy and the lung. *Am Rev Respir Dis* 1980; 121:559–581.

10. Cugell DW, Frank NR, Gaensler EA, et al: Pulmonary function in pregnancy. I. Serial observations in normal women *Am Rev Tuberc* 1953; 67:568–597.

11. Knuttgen HG, Emerson K Jr: Physiologic response to pregnancy at rest and during exercise. *J Appl Physiol* 1974; 36:549–553.

12. Craig DB, Toole MA: Airway closure in pregnancy. *Can Anaesth Soc J* 1975; 22:665–672.

13. Baldwin GR, Moorthi DS, Whelton JA, et al: New lung functions and pregnancy. *Am J Obstet Gynecol* 1977; 127:235–239.

14. Gilroy RJ, Mangura BT, Lavietes MH: Rib cage and abdominal volume displacements during breathing in pregnancy. *Am Rev Respir Dis* 1988; 137:668–672.

15. Archer GW, Marx GF: Arterial oxygen tension during apnoea in parturient women. *Br J Anaesth* 1974; 46:358–360.

16. Bevan DR, Holdcroft A, Loh L, et al: Closing volume and pregnancy. *Br Med J* 1974; 1:13–15.

17. Garrard GS, Littler WA, Redman CWG: Closing volume during normal pregnancy. *Thorax* 1978; 33:488–492.

18. Milne JA, Mills RJ, Howie AD, et al: Large airways function during normal pregnancy. *Br J Obstet Gynaecol* 1977; 84:448–551.

19. Milne JA, Howie AD, Pack AI: Dyspnoea during normal pregnancy. *Br J Obstet Gynaecol* 1978; 84:448.

20. Gilbert R, Epifano L, Auchincloss JH Jr: Dyspnea of pregnancy: A syndrome of altered respiratory control. *JAMA* 1962; 182:1073–1077.

21. Prowse CM, Gaensler EA: Respiratory and acid-base changes during pregnancy. *Anesthesiology* 1965; 26:381–392.

22. Thomson KJ, Cohen ME: Studies on the circulation in pregnancy. II. Vital capacity observations in normal pregnant women. *Surg Gynecol Obstet* 1938; 66:591–603.

23. Heckler MM: *Public Health Reports*. U.S. Department of Health and Human Services. Public Health Service publication No. 85-50193.

24. Koop CE: Smoking and pregnancy. *Am Pharm* 1986; NS26:34–35.

25. Meyer MB, Tonascia JA: Maternal smoking, pregnancy complications, and perinatal mortality. *Am J Obstet Gynecol* 1977; 128:494–502.

26. Naeye RL, Harkness WL, Utts J: Abruptio placentae and perinatal death: A prospective study. *Am J Obstet Gynecol* 1977; 128:740–746.

27. Chow WH, Daling JR, Weiss NS, et al: Maternal cigarette smoking and tubal pregnancy. *Obstet Gynecol* 1988; 71:167–170.

28. Cnattingius S, Haglund B, Meirik O: Cigarette smoking as risk factor for late fetal and early neonatal death. *Br Med J* 1988; 297:258–261.

29. Shiono PH, Klebanoff MA, Rhoads GG: Smoking and drinking during pregnancy: Their effects on preterm birth. *JAMA* 1986; 82–84.

30. Kleinman JC, Pierre MB, Madans JH, et al: The effects of maternal smoking on fetal and infant mortality. *Am J Epidemiol* 1988; 127:274–282.

31. Werler MM, Pober BR, Holmes LB: Smoking and pregnancy. *Teratology* 1985; 32:473–481.

32. Oster G, Delea TE, Colditz GA: Maternal smoking during pregnancy and expenditures on neonatal health care. *Am J Prev Med* 1988; 4:216–219.

33. Andrews J, McGarry J: A community study of smoking in pregnancy. *J Obstet Gynaecol Br Commw* 1972; 79:1057–1073.

34. Butler NR, Goldstein H, Ross EM: Cigarette smoking in pregnancy: Its influence on birthweight and perinatal mortality. *Br Med J* 1972; 2:127–140.

35. Macarthur C, Knox EG: Smoking in pregnancy: Effects of stopping at different stages. *Br J Obstet Gynaecol* 1988; 95:551–555.

36. Sexton M, Hebel JR: A clinical trial of change in maternal smoking and its effect on birth weight. *JAMA* 1984; 251:911–915.

37. Health and Public Policy Committee, American College of Physicians: Methods for stopping cigarette smoking. *Ann Intern Med* 1986; 105:281–291.

38. Schatz M, Harden K, Forsythe A, et al: The course of asthma during pregnancy, post partum, and with successive pregnancies: A prospective analysis. *J Allergy Clin Immunol* 1988; 81:509–517.

39. Schrier L, Cutler RM, Saigal V: Respiratory failure in asthma during the third trimester: Report of two cases. *Am J Obstet Gynecol* 1989; 160:80–81.

40. Stenius-Aarniala B, Piirila P, Teramo K: Asthma and pregnancy: A prospective study of 198 pregnancies. *Thorax* 1988; 43:12–18.

41. Turner ES, Greenberger PA, Patterson R: Management of the pregnant asthmatic patient. *Ann Intern Med* 1980; 93:905–918.

42. Gluck JC, Gluck PA: The effects of pregnancy on asthma: A prospective study. *Ann Allergy* 1976; 37:164–168.

43. Greenberger PA: Asthma in pregnancy. *Clin Perinatol* 1985; 12:571–584.

44. Smith AP: The effects of intravenous infusion of graded doses of prostaglandins F2a and E2 on lung resistance in patients undergoing termination of pregnancy. *Clin Sci* 1973; 44:17–25.

45. Gordon M, Niswander KR, Berendes H, et al: Fetal morbidity following potentially anoxigenic obstetric conditions. VII. Bronchial asthma. *Am J Obstet Gynecol* 1970; 106:421–429.

46. Bahna SL, Bjerkedal T: The course and outcome of pregnancy in women with bronchial asthma. *Acta Allergol* 1972; 27:397–406.

47. Schatz M, Patterson R, Zeitz S, et al: Corticosteroid therapy for the pregnant asthmatic patient. *JAMA* 1975; 233:804–807.

48. Greenberger PA, Patterson R: Beclomethasone dipropionate for severe asthma during pregnancy. *Ann Intern Med* 1983; 98:478–480.

49. Fitzsimons R, Greenberger PA, Patterson R: Outcome of pregnancy in women requiring corticosteroids for severe asthma. *J Allergy Clin Immunol* 1986; 78:349–353.

50. Greenberger P, Patterson R: Safety of therapy for allergic symptoms during pregnancy. *Ann Intern Med* 1978; 89:234–237.

51. Heinonen OP, Slone D, Shapiro S: *Birth Defects and Drugs in Pregnancy*. Littleton, Mass, Publishing Sciences Group, 1977.

52. Stablein JJ, Lockey RF: Managing asthma during pregnancy. *Compr Ther* 1984; 10:45–52.

53. Carter BL, Driscoll CE, Smith GD: Theophylline clearance during pregnancy. *Obstet Gynecol* 1986; 68:555–559.

54. Gardner MJ, Schatz M, Cousins L, et al: Longitudinal effects of pregnancy on the pharmacokinetics of theophylline. *Eur J Clin Pharmacol* 1987; 31:289–295.

55. Frederiksen MC, Ruo TI, Chow MJ, et al: Theophylline pharmacokinetics in pregnancy. *Clin Pharmacol Ther* 1986; 40:321–328.

56. Yurchek, AM, Jusko WJ: Theophylline secretion into breast milk. *Pediatrics* 1976; 57:518.

57. Altenburger KM: Management of asthma during pregnancy. *N Engl J Med* 1985; 313:517.

58. Schatz M, Zeiger RS, Harden KM, et al: The safety of inhaled β-agonist bronchodilators during pregnancy. *J Allergy Clin Immunol* 1988; 82:686–695.

59. *Physician's Desk Reference,* ed 42. Oradell, NJ, Medical Economics Co, Inc, 1988.

60. Wilson J: Utilisation du cromoglycate de sodium au cours de la grossesse. *Acta Ther* 1982; 8(suppl):45–51.

61. Harris DM: Some properties of beclomethasone dipropionate and related steroids in man. *Postgrad Med J* 1975; 51(suppl):20–25.

62. Morrow-Brown H, Storey G: Beclomethasone dipropionate aerosol in long-term treatment of perennial and seasonal asthma in children and adults: A report of five and half years experience in 600 asthmatic patients. *Br J Clin Pharmacol* 1977; 4(suppl):529S–567S.

63. Snyder RD, Snyder D: Corticosteroids for asthma during pregnancy. *Ann Allergy* 1978; 41:340–341.

64. Munakata M, Abe S, Fujimoto S, et al: Bronchoalveolar lavage during third-trimester pregnancy in patients with status asthmaticus: A case report. *Respiration* 1987; 51:252–255.

65. Gelber M, Sidi Y, Gassner S, et al: Uncontrollable life-threatening status asthmaticus—an indicator for termination of pregnancy by cesarean section. *Respiration* 1984; 46:320–322.

66. Wulf KH, Kunzel W, Lehmann V: Clinical aspects of placental gas exchange, in Longo LD, Bartels H (eds): *Respiratory Gas Exchange and Blood Flow in the Placenta.* Bethesda, Md, Public Health Service, 1972, 505–521.

67. Oppenheimer EH: Lesions in the adrenals of an infant following maternal corticosteroid therapy. *Bull Johns Hopkins Hosp* 1964; 114:146–151.

68. Kepito LE, Kosasky HJ, Shwachman H: Water and electrolytes in cervical mucus from patients with cystic fibrosis. *Fertil Steril* 1973; 24:512.

69. Kredentser JV, Pokrant C, McCoshen JA: Intrauterine insemination for infertility due to cystic fibrosis. *Fertil Steril* 1986; 45:425–426.

70. Polgar G, Denton R: Cystic fibrosis in adults: Studies of pulmonary function and some physical properties of bronchial mucus. *Am Rev Respir Dis* 1972; 85:319–327.

71. Cohen LF, di Sant'Agnese PA, Friedlander J: Cystic fibrosis and pregnancy: A national survey. *Lancet* 1980; 2:842–844.

72. Cystic Fibrosis Foundation: *1974 Report on Survival Studies of Patients With Cystic Fibrosis.* Rockville, Md, Cystic Fibrosis Foundation, 1976.

73. Warwick WJ, Pogue RE, Gerber HU, et al: Survival patterns in cystic fibrosis. *J Chronic Dis* 1975; 28:609–622.

74. Shwachman H, Kulczycki LL: Long-term study of one hundred five patients with cystic fibrosis. *Am J Dis Child* 1958; 96:6–15.

75. Taussig LM, Kattwinkel J, Friedewald WT, et al: A new prognostic score and clinical evaluation system for cystic fibrosis. *J Pediatr* 1973; 82:380–390.

76. Palmer J, Dillon-Baker C, Tecklin JS, et al: Pregnancy in patients with cystic fibrosis. *Ann Intern Med* 1983; 99:596–600.

77. Dooley RR, Braunstein H, Osher AB: Polypoid cervicitis in cystic fibrosis patients receiving oral contraceptives. *Am J Obstet Gynecol* 1974; 118:971–974.

78. Fitzpatrick SB, Stokes DC, Rosenstein BJ, et al: Use of oral contraceptives in women with cystic fibrosis. *Chest* 1984; 86:863–867.

79. Michel BC: Antibacterial therapy in cystic fibrosis. A review of the literature published between 1980 and February 1987. *Chest* 1988; 94(suppl):129S–140S.

80. Valenzuela GJ, Comunale FL, Davidson BH, et al: Clinical management of patients with cystic fibrosis and pulmonary insufficiency. *Am J Obstet Gynecol* 1988; 159:1181–1183.

81. Rayburn W, Wolk R, Mercer N, et al: Parenteral nutrition in obstetrics and gynecology. *Obstet Gynecol Surv* 1986; 41:200–214.

82. Nadler H, Walsh M: Intrauterine detection of cystic fibrosis. *Pediatrics* 1980; 66:690.

83. Alpert SE, Cormier AD: Normal electrolyte and protein content in milk from mothers with cystic fibrosis: An explana-

tion for the initial report of elevated milk sodium concentration. *J Pediatr* 1983; 102:77–80.

84. Maycock RL, Sullivan RD, Greening RR: Sarcoidosis and pregnancy. *JAMA* 1957; 164:158.

85. Reisfeld DR, Yahia L, Laurentia GA: Pregnancy and cardiorespiratory failure in Boeck's sarcoid. *Surg Gynecol Obstet* 1959; 109:412.

86. Scadding JG: Prognosis of intrathoracic sarcoidosis in England. *Br Med J* 1961; 2:1165–1172.

87. O'Leary JA: Ten-year study of sarcoidosis and pregnancy. *Am J Obstet Gynecol* 1962; 84:462–466.

88. Fried KH: Sarcoidosis and pregnancy. *Acta Med Scand* 1964; 176(suppl 425):218–221.

89. Agha FP, Vade A, Amendola MA, et al: Effects of pregnancy on sarcoidosis. *Surg Gynecol Obstet* 1982; 155:817–822.

90. Grossman JH, Littner MR: Severe sarcoidosis in pregnancy. *Obstet Gynecol* 1977; 50(suppl): 81S–84S.

91. Erksine KJ, Taylor KJ, Agnew RAL: Serial estimation of serum angiotensin converting enzyme activity during and after pregnancy in a woman with sarcoidosis. *Br Med J* 1985; 290:269–270.

92. Wilson-Holt N: Post partum presentation of hypercalcemic sarcoidosis. *Postgrad Med J* 1985; 61:627–628.

93. Giesler CF, Buehler JH, Depp R: Alpha-1-antitrypsin deficiency: Severe obstructive lung disease and pregnancy. *Obstet Gynecol* 1977; 49:31–34.

94. Ratto D, Balmes J, Boylen T, et al: Pregnancy in a woman with severe pulmonary fibrosis secondary to hard metal disease. *Chest* 1988; 93:663–665.

95. McKim DA, Dales RE, Lefebvre GG, et al: Nocturnal positive-pressure nasal ventilation for respiratory failure during pregnancy. *Can Med Assoc J* 1988; 139:1069–1071.

96. Jacobs RF, Abernathy RS: Management of tuberculosis in pregnancy and the newborn. *Clin Perinatol* 1988; 15:305–319.

97. Hedvall E: Pregnancy and tuberculosis. *Acta Med Scand* 1953; 147(suppl 286):1–101.

98. Sulavik SB: Pulmonary disease, in Burrow GN, Ferris TF (eds): *Medical Complications in Pregnancy.* Philadelphia, WB Saunders Co, 1975, pp 549–625.

99. Schaefer G, Zervoudakis IA, Fuchs FF, et al: Pregnancy and pulmonary tuberculosis. *Obstet Gynecol* 1975; 46:706–715.

100. Bjerkedal T, Bahna SL, Lehmann EH: Course and outcome of pregnancy in women with pulmonary tuberculosis. *Scand J Respir Dis* 1975; 56:245–250.

101. Good JT, Iseman MD, Davidson PT, et al: Tuberculosis in association with pregnancy. *Am J Obstet Gynecol* 1981; 140:492–498.

102. Kendig EL Jr: The place of BCG vaccine in the management of infants born of tuberculous mothers. *N Engl J Med* 1969; 281:520–523.

103. Present PA, Comstock GW: Tuberculin sensitivity in pregnancy. *Am Rev Respir Dis* 1975; 112:413–416.

104. American Thoracic Society: Treatment of tuberculosis and tuberculous infection in adults and children. *Am Rev Respir Dis* 1986; 134:355–363.

105. Lowe CR: Congenital defects among children born to women under supervision or treatment for pulmonary tuberculosis. *Br J Prev Soc Med* 1964; 18:14–16.

106. Scheinhorn DJ, Angelillo VA: Antituberculous therapy in pregnancy: risks to the fetus. *West J Med* 1977; 127:195–198.

107. Snider DE Jr, Layde PM, Johnson MW, et al: Treatment of tuberculosis during pregnancy. *Am Rev Respir Dis* 1980; 122:65–79.

108. Lewit J, Nebel L, Terracina S, et al: Ethambutol in pregnancy: Observations on embryogenesis. *Chest* 1974; 66:25.

109. Potworowska M, Sianozecka E, Szufladowicz R: Ethionamide treatment and pregnancy. *Polish Med J* 1966; 5:1152–1158.

110. Snider DE, Powell KE: Should women taking antituberculosis drugs breast-feed? *Arch Intern Med* 1984; 144:589.

111. Goodwin RA Jr, Des Prez RM: State of the art: histoplasmosis. *Am Rev Respir Dis* 1978; 117:929–956.

112. Catanzaro A: Pulmonary mycosis in pregnant women. *Chest* 1984; 86(suppl):14S–19S.

113. Hager H, Welt SI, Cardasis JP, et al: Dis-

seminated blastomycosis in a pregnant woman successfully treated with amphotericin-B: A case report. *J Reprod Med* 1988; 33:485–488.

114. Tuthill SW: Disseminated blastomycosis with intrauterine transmission (letter). *South Med J* 1985; 78:1526–1527.

115. Smale LE, Waechter KG: Dissemination of coccidioidomycosis in pregnancy. *Am J Obstet Gynecol* 1970; 107:356–361.

116. Purtilo DT: Opportunistic mycotic infections in pregnant women. *Am J Obstet Gynecol* 1975; 122:607–610.

117. Pappagianis D: Epidemiology of coccidioidomycosis, in Stevens D (ed): *Coccidioidomycosis*. New York, Plenum Press, 1980, pp 63–85.

118. Wack EE, Ampel NM, Galgiani JN, et al: Coccidioidomycosis during pregnancy: An analysis of ten cases among 47,120 pregnancies. *Chest* 1988; 94:376–379.

119. Drutz DJ, Huppert M, Sun SH, et al: Human sex hormones stimulate the growth and maturation of *Coccidioides immitis*. *Infect Immun* 1981; 32:897–907.

120. Powell BL, Drutz DJ, Huppert M, et al: Relationship of progesterone- and estradiol-binding proteins in *Coccidioides immitis* to coccidioidal dissemination in pregnancy. *Infect Immun* 1983; 40:478–485.

121. Ismail MA, Lerner SA: Disseminated blastomycosis in a pregnant woman. *Am Rev Respir Dis* 1982; 126:350–353.

122. Hopwood HG: Pneumonia in pregnancy. *Obstet Gynecol* 1965; 875–879.

123. Benedetti TJ, Valle R, Ledger WJ: Antepartum pneumonia in pregnancy. *Obstet Gynecol* 1982; 144:413–417.

124. Soper DE, Melone PJ, Conover WB: Legionnaire disease complicating pregnancy. *Obstet Gynecol* 1986; 67:10S–12S.

125. Health and Public Policy Committee, American College of Physicians: Pneumococcal vaccine. *Ann Intern Med* 1986; 104:118–120.

126. Advisory Committee on Immunization Practices: Prevention and control of influenza: Part I, vaccines. *MMWR* 1989; 38:297–309.

127. MacKenzie JS, Houghton M: Influenza infections during pregnancy: Association with congenital malformations and with subsequent neoplasms in children, and po-

tential hazards of live virus vaccines. *Bacteriol Rev* 1974; 38:356–370.

128. Kirshon B, Faro S, Zurawin RK, et al: Favorable outcome after treatment with amantadine and ribavirin in a pregnancy complicated by influenza pneumonia: A case report. *J Reprod Med* 1988; 33:179–182.

129. Duong CM, Munns RE: Varicella pneumonia during pregnancy. *J Fam Pract* 1979; 8:277.

130. Brown ZA, Baker DA: Acyclovir therapy during pregnancy. *Obstet Gynecol* 1989; 73:526–531.

131. Straus SE, Ostrove JM, Inchauspe G, et al: NIH conference. Varicella-zoster virus infections. Biology, natural history, treatment, and prevention. *Ann Intern Med* 1988; 108:221–237.

132. Miller E, Cradock-Watson JE, Ridehalgh MKS: Outcome in newborn babies given anti–varicella-zoster immunoglobulin after perinatal maternal infection with varicella-zoster virus. *Lancet* 1989; 2:371–373.

133. Mendelson CL: The aspiration of stomach contents during obstetric anesthesia. *Am J Obstet Gynecol* 1946; 52:191.

134. Thorburn J, Moir DD: Antacid therapy for emergency Caesarean section. *Anaesthesia* 1987; 42:352–355.

135. Hughson WG, Friedman PJ, Feigin DS, et al: Postpartum pleural effusion: A common radiologic finding. *Ann Intern Med* 1982; 97:856–858.

136. Hessen I: Roentgen examination of pleural fluid. *Acta Radiol [Suppl] (Stockh)* 1951; 86:62–64.

137. Parker MA: Prepartum or postpartum pleural effusion (letter). *Ann Intern Med* 1983; 98:413–414.

138. Udeshi UL, McHugo JM, Selwyn Crawford J: Postpartum pleural effusion. *Br J Obstet Gynaecol* 1988; 95:894–897.

139. Bonnar J: Venous thromboembolism and pregnancy. *Clin Obstet Gynaecol* 1981; 8:456.

140. Rutherford SE, Phelan JP: Thromboembolic disease in pregnancy. *Clin Perinatol* 1986; 13:719–739.

141. Friend JR, Kakkar VV: The diagnosis of deep vein thrombosis in the puerperium. *J Obstet Gynaecol Br Commw* 1970; 77:820.

142. Weiner CP: Diagnosis and management of thromboembolic disease during pregnancy.

Clin Obstet Gynecol 1985; 28:107–118.

143. Aaro LA, Juergens JL: Thrombophlebitis associated with pregnancy. *Am J Obstet Gynecol* 1971; 109:1129.

144. Sachs BP, Brown DAJ, Driscoll SG: Maternal mortality in Massachusetts: Trends and prevention. *N Engl J Med* 1987; 316:667–672.

145. Kaunitz AM, Hughes JM, Grimes DA, et al: Causes of maternal mortality in the United States. *Obstet Gynecol* 1985; 65:605–612.

146. Gore M, Eldon S, Trofatter KF, et al: Pregnancy-induced changes in the fibrinolytic balance: Evidence for defective release of tissue plasminogen activator and increased levels of the fast-acting tissue plasminogen activator inhibitor. *Am J Obstet Gynecol* 1987; 156:674–680.

147. Kruithof EKO, Gudinchet A, Bachmann F: Plasminogen activator inhibitor 1 and plasminogen activator inhibitor 2 in various disease states. *Thromb Haemost* 1988; 59:7–12.

148. Johansson L, Hedner U, Nilsson IM: Familial antithrombin III deficiency as pathogenesis of deep venous thrombosis. *Acta Med Scand* 1978; 204:491.

149. Tengborn L, Bergqvist D, Matzsch T, et al: Recurrent thromboembolism in pregnancy and puerperium: Is there a need for thromboprophylaxis? *Am J Obstet Gynecol* 1989; 160:90–94.

150. Marcus CS, Mason GR, Kuperus JH, et al: Pulmonary imaging in pregnancy: Maternal risk and fetal dosimetry. *Clin Nucl Med* 1985; 10:1–4.

151. Ponto JA: Fetal dosimetry from pulmonary imaging in pregnancy: Revised estimates. *Clin Nucl Med* 1986; 11:108–109.

152. Polak JF, O'Leary DH: Deep venous thrombosis in pregnancy: Noninvasive diagnosis. *Radiology* 1988; 166:377–379.

153. Didolkar SM, Koontz C, Schimberg PI: Phleborrheography in pregnancy. *Obstet Gynecol* 1983; 61:363–366.

154. Nicholas GG, Lorenz RP, Botti JJ, et al: The frequent occurrence of false-positive results in phleborrheography during pregnancy. *Gynecol Obstet Surg* 1985; 161:133–135.

155. LeClerc JR, Hirsh J: Venous thromboembolic disorders, in Burrow GN, Ferris TF (eds): *Medical Complications During Pregnancy*. Philadelphia, WB Saunders Co, 1988, pp 202–223.

156. Letsky EA: Thrombo-embolism during pregnancy, in Letsky EA: *Coagulation Problems During Pregnancy*. Edinburgh, Churchill Livingstone, 1985, pp 29–61.

157. Ginsberg JS, Hirsh J: Use of anticoagulants during pregnancy. *Chest* 1989; 95(suppl):156S–160S.

158. Hall JAG, Pauli RM, Wilson KM: Maternal and fetal sequelae of anticoagulation during pregnancy. *Am J Med* 1980; 68:122–140.

159. Griffiths HT, Liu DTY: Severe heparin osteoporosis in pregnancy. *Postgrad Med J* 1984; 60:424–425.

160. Hux CH, Wapner RJ, Chayen B, et al: Use of the Greenfield filter for thromboembolic disease in pregnancy. *Am J Obstet Gynecol* 1986; 155:734–737.

161. Delclos GL, Davila F: Thrombolytic therapy for pulmonary embolism in pregnancy: A case report. *Am J Obstet Gynecol* 1986; 155:375–376.

162. Ludwig H: Results of streptokinase therapy in deep venous thrombosis during pregnancy. *Postgrad Med J* 1973; 20(suppl):65–67.

163. Richards SR, Barrows H, O'Shaughnessy R: Intrapartum pulmonary embolus. *J Reprod Med* 1985; 30:64–66.

164. DeSwiet M: Management of thromboembolism in pregnancy. *Drugs* 1979; 18:478.

165. Orme ML, Lewis PJ, DeSwiet M, et al: May mothers given warfarin breast-feed their infants? *Br Med J* 1977; 1:1564–1565.

166. McKenna R, Cale ER, Vasan U: Is warfarin sodium contraindicated in the lactating mother? *J Pediatr* 1983; 103:325–327.

167. Howell R, Fidler J, Letsky E, et al: The risks of antenatal subcutaneous heparin prophylaxis: A controlled trial. *Br J Obstet Gynaecol* 1983; 90:1124–1128.

168. Lao TT, DeSwiet M, Letsky E, et al: Prophylaxis of thromboembolism in pregnancy: An alternative. *Br J Obstet Gynaecol* 1985; 92:202–206.

169. Dahlman TC, Hellgren SE, Blomback M: Thrombosis prophylaxis in pregnancy with use of subcutaneous heparin adjusted by monitoring heparin concentration in plasma. *Am J Obstet Gynecol* 1989; 161:420–425.

CHAPTER 7

Critical Illness

Jesse B. Hall
Gregory A. Schmidt

Critically ill patients have potential or real multiorgan failure and successful management requires minute-to-minute titration of appropriate supportive therapies while underlying diseases are identified and treated. A discussion organized solely by disease, organ system, or technology of intervention might risk obscuring those principles of understanding that derive from broadly shared pathophysiology. Our approach, based on the general pathophysiology of the critically ill patient, begins with a consideration of the determinants of oxygen delivery and utilization in health and disease followed by discussion of the adequacy of tissue perfusion, focusing on assessment and treatment of hypoperfused states. Next, respiratory failure, the other major cause of diminished oxygen delivery, is highlighted, including the pathophysiology of gas exchange in ventilatory failure and acute hypoxemic respiratory failure during pregnancy. The final part of the chapter stresses therapies used to correct and maintain the internal milieu of the critically ill patient as well as miscellaneous disorders precipitating critical illness.

Pregnancy brings a new consideration to those involved in critical care—the effects of catastrophic illness and its treatment upon the fetoplacental unit. In many cases information on how to approach this problem is far from complete, and clinical decisions are made to optimize maternal well-being, emphasizing that throughout critical illness monitoring and decisions take into account fetal as well as maternal parameters. In essence this requires a team approach consisting not only of the nurse-respiratory therapist-physician unit common to modern intensive care, but an integration of the critical care team with obstetrician and neonatologist as well.

OXYGEN DELIVERY AND UTILIZATION IN CRITICAL ILLNESS

Determinants of Oxygen Delivery

Ongoing supply of key substrates is a prerequisite for normal tissue function and viability. Among such essential substrates are phosphate for synthesis of energy intermediates; glucose, amino acids, and fatty acids for utilization in the Krebs' cycle and other energy-generating pathways; and calcium and magnesium acting as intracellular regulators of contraction and enzyme cofactors. Common to all tissues is a dependence upon oxygen for combustion of organic compounds to fuel cellular metabolism. Continuous delivery of oxygen is achieved by the integrated action of the cardiopulmonary systems which pro-

TABLE 7–1.
Causes of Impaired Oxygen Delivery or Utilization

I. Diminished arterial oxygen content
    A. Anemia
    B. Hypoxemia with desaturation
    C. Carbon monoxide poisoning
II. Hypoperfusion
    A. Low flow shock
        1. Hypovolemia
        2. Cardiac dysfunction
    B. Regional maldistribution in high flow shock
       or adult respiratory distress syndrome?
III. Metabolic block to utilization
    A. Cyanide poisoning
    B. Metabolic inhibition in sepsis?

vide flow of blood with high oxygen content such that oxygen delivery (QO_2) is in excess of oxygen needs or consumption (VO_2). The total amount of oxygen delivered is given by the flow, or cardiac output (Qt), times the arterial oxygen content (CaO_2) or

$$QO_2 = Qt \times CaO_2$$

The arterial oxygen content is determined mainly by the amount of oxygen bound to hemoglobin (1.37 mL O_2/gm Hb × arterial saturation) as limited quantities (0.0031 mL/dL/mm Hg PO_2 [oxygen pressure]) are solubilized in plasma. A number of conditions will impair oxygen delivery or its utilization (Table 7–1). Low flow states (shock) reduce available oxygen despite normal oxygen arterial content. Maldistribution of flow relative to oxygen demand is postulated in sepsis, even though the latter is a "high flow" state in some patients. Arterial oxygen content is decreased in anemia (low hemoglobin) or in the presence of hypoxemia, the latter leading to hemoglobin desaturation. Finally, oxygen delivery may be normal but utilization impaired, as, for example, the metabolic disruption caused by cyanide poisoning. There are also situations where oxygen extraction is defective for unclear reasons, such as in patients with sepsis and/or the adult respiratory distress syndrome (ARDS).[1]

The Relationship of Oxygen Delivery to Consumption

Oxygen delivery under normal conditions (QO_2 = Qt × CaO_2 = 50 dL/min × 21 mL/dL = 1050 mL/min) is in excess of oxygen demand (normal resting VO_2 = 250 mL/min). When oxygen delivery is reduced experimentally or in disease states such as shock, anemia, or hypoxemia, VO_2 is maintained because the tissues extract a greater fraction of the oxygen delivered (extraction fraction = VO_2/QO_2).[1] This is demonstrated in Figure 7–1 *(solid line)*. Note that VO_2 *(ordinate)* remains constant as QO_2 *(abscissa)* falls until a point, termed *critical oxygen delivery*, is reached. Further reduction in delivery causes consumption to fall, and this decrement is associated with the development of anaerobic metabolism, lactic acidosis, and, if persistent, organ failure ensues resulting in death. This critical level of oxygen delivery has been de-

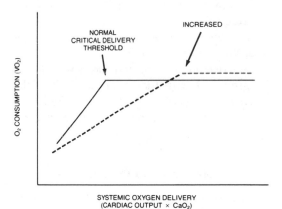

FIG 7–1.
The relationship of oxygen consumption (VO_2) to systemic oxygen delivery: Under normal conditions *(solid line)*, VO_2 remains constant over a wide range of oxygen deliveries until a critical delivery point is reached at which point consumption falls in association with anaerobic metabolism. If not rapidly reversed, tissue dysfunction and death ensue. In certain illnesses (sepsis and adult respiratory distress syndrome) VO_2 is increased and appears dependent on delivery over a wider range of systemic oxygen deliveries *(dashed line)*. (From Schumacker PT, Samsel RW: *Crit Care Clin* 1989; 5:255–269. Used by permission.)

termined in nonpregnant animals and patients and appears to be approximately 7 to 10 mL O_2/min/kg.[1]

This relationship seems to differ in patients with sepsis and/or ARDS.[1, 2] Oxygen consumption is higher on average than in other patient groups, consistent with an increased rate of metabolism, and the slope of the QO_2-VO_2 dependent portion of the curve (ΔVO_2/ΔQO_2, or the extraction fraction) is depressed, suggesting an abnormality in the efficiency of oxygen extraction (*dashed line* in Fig 7–1). This altered relationship has been termed *pathologic supply dependency of oxygen utilization*. Whether such an extraction defect exists on a cellular and metabolic basis or as a result of microcirculatory changes in these disease states remains unclear.[1]

The above formulation provides the background for management of critically ill patients. When anaerobic metabolism has become manifest, resulting in lactic acidosis, the physician must focus on determining and treating underlying causes of inadequate oxygen delivery—typically hypoperfusion, anemia, and hypoxemia—for failure to improve oxygen delivery and reverse the lactic acidosis is associated with high mortality. Since the extraction defect in sepsis and ARDS is less clear, so is the appropriate therapeutic response.

Special Considerations in Pregnancy

Some of the physiologic changes of normal pregnancy might influence oxygen delivery and consumption. There are small increments in arterial PO_2 (to 106–108 mm Hg in the first trimester and 101–104 mm Hg in the third trimester) attributable to hyperventilation,[3] but these have little effect upon oxygen content since hemoglobin saturation is but minimally increased. There is a relative anemia of pregnancy, which reduces oxygen content 20% to 25% to values in the range of 16 vol%,[4] but delivery is maintained at or above prepregnancy levels since there is also an estimated 40% increase in cardiac output.[5] *Of note, therefore, the critically ill pregnant patient relies more upon cardiac output for maintenance of oxygen delivery than do nonpregnant individuals.* Finally, VO_2 increases approximately 20% to 30% in normal pregnancy,[6] although the exact partitioning of this increased consumption between the maternal tissue beds and the fetoplacental unit remains unclear, and during labor there is a further rise in VO_2 to levels 40% to 100% above the nonpregnant baseline.[7]

Data concerning maternal and fetal consequences of conditions that diminish QO_2 come mainly from experiments in animals. Edelstone and colleagues[8] studied regional blood flows and QO_2 in a gravid ewe model of progressive anemia. Hematocrit was lowered from 31% to 8% but QO_2 to the maternal brain and heart was maintained at baseline levels by large increases in flow. Interestingly, there was no flow adjustment in either the uterine or placental beds, resulting in a progressive decline in QO_2. These observations would be consistent with the view that the fetoplacental unit receives near maximal blood flow under normal conditions in late pregnancy, with little ability to adapt to stress by further increases in flow by local vascular adjustment. This would suggest that as one of many parallel maternal tissue beds, the fetoplacental unit is not readily able to compete for diminishing available oxygen by vascular autoregulation.

Nonetheless, in a similar animal model of severe anemia, mother and fetus simultaneously evolved anaerobic metabolism and metabolic acidosis, suggesting that the fetoplacental unit is neither more nor less successful than other tissue beds in maintaining oxygen utilization.[9] That the fetus is able to meet oxygen needs under these conditions is perhaps attributable to the fact that at all levels of PO_2, fetal hemoglobin has a higher affinity for oxygen than maternal hemoglobin. In addition, low arterial PO_2 in the fetus may not constitute tissue hypoxia—as evidenced by the fact that the normal PO_2 in fetal blood is 30 mm Hg, and at least in a primate animal model, brain injury did not occur until PO_2 fell to 9 to 14 mm Hg.[10] It is also likely that significant circulatory and metabolic adjustments can be made by the fetus in response to hypoxic insult. Parer[11] has made the observation that at term the fetus has an estimated 40 mL of available oxygen in blood and tissue stores, with an estimated V_{O_2} of 20 mL/min. This would suggest that conditions causing complete interruption of Q_{O_2} (total placental abruption, complete unbilical cord compression) would result in fetal hypoxia within 2 minutes. The fact that irreversible tissue injury requires much longer periods of hypoxia to occur suggests protective mechanisms are operative at the level of the fetal circulation or peripheral tissues.[11, 12] Parer[11] has suggested these compensations include fetal redistribution of blood flow to vital organs, decreased total V_{O_2} under conditions of hypoxic stress, and prolonged dependence of certain tissue beds on anaerobic metabolism.

Summary

During pregnancy Q_{O_2} is more flow-dependent because hematocrit decreases while cardiac output increases markedly. Oxygen consumption too is increased, rising dramatically in labor. In late pregnancy or near term, the fetoplacental unit appears incapable of augmenting Q_{O_2} significantly by local vascular adjustment. Nonetheless, the fetus may withstand periods of diminished Q_{O_2} because of the avidity of fetal hemoglobin for oxygen relative to maternal hemoglobin, the tolerance of fetal tissues to low P_{O_2}, and fetal circulatory or metabolic adjustments to hypoxic insult. The following management principles derive from the above-described changes:

1. Processes threatening maternal systemic flow are extremely dangerous in pregnancy, and all judgments regarding the adequacy of flow must be made with an understanding that baseline flow is substantially increased.

2. Decrements in placental flow are particularly damaging to fetal viability, especially if superimposed upon other pathology such as anemia and/or hypoxia. Indeed, maternal hypoxemia, via reflex circulatory adjustments causing vasodilation in nonplacental beds and local vasoconstriction of the uterine vasculature, is potentially very injurious to fetal well-being.[13]

3. Distinction between aerobic limits of the mother and fetus are difficult to make clinically. While continuous measurement of transcutaneous P_{O_2} in the fetus is feasible, interpretation of values and prediction of the metabolic state of the fetus is not routine. Secondary phenomena such as fetal heart rate as a measure of well-being are useful but nonspecific for oxygen adequacy and they are late indicators of pathology. In general, the routinely collected parameters of Q_{O_2} and acid-base status in the mother are the best measures of adequacy of Q_{O_2} for both the fetus and the mother.

4. Labor, which represents a tremendous "aerobic load" to the mother, should be avoided or postponed, if possible, when Q_{O_2} is marginal. In this same vein, other aerobic loads, such as respiratory muscle work performed during evolving respiratory failure, can and should be assumed by elective intubation and mechanical ventilation if Q_{O_2} is marginal.

APPROACH TO DISORDERS OF THE CIRCULATION

A bedside approach to the hypoperfused nonpregnant patient begins with distinction between low flow states, caused by inadequate circulating volume and/or "pump" dysfunction, and high flow hypoperfusion typical of septic shock, liver disease, and several other disorders. This approach is readily applied to the critically ill pregnant patient, with the caution that evaluation and management must take into account physiologic alterations associated with gestation and parturition.

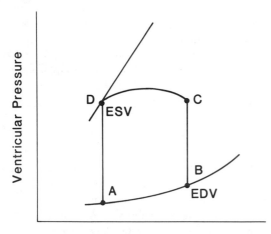

FIG 7–2.
The relationship of ventricular volume to pressure is shown for a complete cardiac cycle. The ventricle fills during diastole from point *A* to point *B* with small pressure changes. Isovolumic contraction occurs from point *B* until point *C,* at which time ventricular pressure exceeds aortic pressure and valve opening occurs. The ventricle then ejects to an end–systolic pressure volume point *(D)* defined by the myocardial contractile state. *ESV* = end–systolic volume; *EDV* = end–diastolic volume.

Left Ventricular Mechanics

As noted, flow is a key determinant of the adequacy of oxygen delivery. When venous return to the heart is adequate, arterial flow is determined by the product of heart rate and stroke volume, and the latter can be analyzed in terms of the pressure-volume characteristics of the ventricle during filling and contraction. Pressure-volume plots are schematized for ventricular function in both diastole and systole in Figure 7–2. As the ventricle begins to fill in early diastole (point *A*), pressure rises minimally but there is a large volume change (from 50 to 120 mL). This is because the normal ventricle is compliant over this range. Diastolic filling is complete at point *B* and ventricular contraction begins. Pressure rises during isovolumic contraction until point *C,* at which time ventricular pressure exceeds aortic pressure and valve opening occurs. Ejection of stroke volume now occurs to a pressure and volume (point *D*) defined by the end-systolic pressure-volume relationship

of the ventricle, determined by the contractile state of the myocardium. Stroke volume is seen to result from the difference between end-diastolic and end-systolic volumes (EDV − ESV).

This analysis permits an explication of both diastolic and systolic dysfunction of the ventricle. Figure 7–3 demonstrates diastolic dysfunction in patients with states such as ischemia or hypertensive cardiomyopathy, which are characterized by chamber stiffness. Note there is an upward and leftward shift of the filling curve, such that ventricular pressure is higher at any given volume. When there is systolic dysfunction, which also occurs in ischemia and cardiomyopathy, there is a downward and rightward displacement of the end-systolic pressure-volume curve, as the ventricle fails to eject to the normal volume. This depressed systolic curve is indicative of impaired contractility of the myocardium.

A number of phenomena and approaches to disease can be outlined with this model. In hypovolemic states, venous return is reduced because of a fall in systemic mean pressure and, as a result, a reduction in the driving

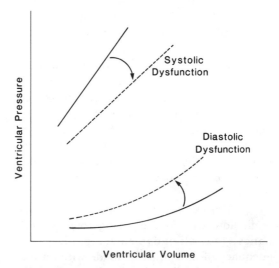

FIG 7–3.
Ventricular dysfunction is represented by a downward and rightward shift of the systolic performance curve (systolic dysfunction) and/or by a shift of the diastolic curve upward and to the left (diastolic dysfunction). See text for discussion.

pressure of flow between the peripheral circulation and the right heart. Because of reduced venous return, diastolic filling is decreased and stroke volume falls. The therapeutic implication is obvious, as volume therapy will restore systemic mean pressure, drive venous return, and allow cardiac output to rise as diastolic filling occurs at a higher end-diastolic volume. The other major cause of low flow and resultant hypoperfusion is ventricular failure, which can be seen to result from either diastolic dysfunction causing a fall in end-diastolic volume at any given filling pressure, or a rise in end-systolic volume due to a depressed systolic function curve (see Fig 7–3). Most commonly, both phenomena are operative in patients with ischemia and/or cardiomyopathy. Therapy here is directed at resolving both diastolic and systolic dysfunction. Resolution of ischemia can improve ventricular "stiffness" and improve diastolic function. Inotropic agents restore contractility and decrease end-systolic volume, represented by a shift of the end-systolic pressure-volume relationship upward and to the left in Figure 7–3. Since inotropes are typically catecholamines with both inotropic action (resulting from β-receptor stimulation) and vasoconstrictor action (due to α-receptor stimulation), it is important that β effects predominate. In cases of ventricular dysfunction, excessive α stimulation may cause elevation of blood pressure at the cost of falling stroke volume. This effect of many of the catecholamines used to support circulatory failure requires that these vasoactive drugs not be titrated solely to the arterial blood pressure but that other measures of flow (cardiac output, urine output, resolution of lactic acidosis) be considered as well. Finally, in patients with low flow shock persisting despite adequate intravascular volume and use of maximal inotropic support, addition of vasodilators within the limits of arterial blood pressure to reduce ventricular afterload will enhance forward flow and improve tissue perfusion.

Physiologic Changes of Pregnancy

When treating pregnant women one should adapt the above principles to the physiologic changes of gestation.[5, 14] Early in pregnancy maternal blood volume increases approximately 40%, associated with increases in stroke volume and cardiac output, although uncertainty exists as to the exact contributions of increased preload and diminished afterload to this increment in flow.[5, 14] This increase in cardiac output seen early in pregnancy is associated with a narrowing of the arterial-venous oxygen content difference (AV O_2 difference), an expected result if QO_2 increases in excess of VO_2. These changes in cardiovascular parameters are summarized in Table 7–2. Potential effects on venous return must also be considered. As early as the 20th to 24th week of pregnancy the gravid uterus causes significant inferior vena caval obstruction, such that an 8% increase in cardiac output can be seen when the pregnant woman is moved from the supine to the lateral recumbent position, thus relieving obstruction.[5] It is important to emphasize that the simple maneuvers of maintaining the ill pregnant patient in a lateral position, or, during emergency procedures, manually elevating or laterally displacing the gravid uterus, can significantly ameliorate this obstruction to flow.[5]

Clinical Assessment and Invasive Monitoring

The initial approach to a critically ill patient is assessment of the state of perfusion, focusing on distinction between high and low flow states. Some requisite information may require invasive hemodynamic measurements. Table 7–3 lists commonly used bedside criteria for hypoperfusion. As each organ system is hypoperfused, a characteristic dysfunction may manifest. Thus, mental status and urine volume are important indicators of adequacy of perfusion. However, during a critical illness there may be other processes

TABLE 7–2.

Alterations in Hemodynamic Variables in Pregnancy

Variable	Typical Change	Time Course
Heart rate (beats/min)	70→85	Rises in 1st trimester
Blood pressure (mm Hg)	125/80→115/70	Falls in 1st trimester returning toward prepregnancy level later
Cardiac output (L/min)	4.5→6.0	40% increase in 1st trimester is maintained throughout pregnancy
Stroke volume (mL)	64→71	Rises in 1st trimester
Systemic vascular resistance (dynes/sec/cm^{-5})	1,250→980	Reaches nadir by midpregnancy
Arteriovenous oxygen content difference (mL/dL)	4.5→3.5	Fall in early pregnancy is followed by a later rise and then variation dependent upon Vo$_2$

which affect these end points. Also, during gestation the physiologic dilation of ureters, which increases the dead space, may make it difficult to assess actual urinary volumes over short periods of time. Tissue hypoxia resulting from hypoperfusion may cause a lactic acidosis, which may manifest by the presence of an increased anion gap. Of importance, all acid-base data from pregnant women should be analyzed in relation to the expected physiologic adjustments during pregnancy: alkalemia and decreased bicarbonate and PCO$_2$ levels (a compensated respiratory alkalosis).

In both high flow and low flow shock states, persistent oliguria and disturbed central nervous system function are observed. In low flow states, broadly divided into either inadequate circulating volume or cardiac dysfunction, compensatory mechanisms usually result in tachycardia and narrowing of the pulse pressure (systolic − diastolic blood pressure) as endogenous catecholamine release occurs. To interpret these heart rate and

blood pressure changes, the baseline of increased heart rate and lowered blood pressure of various stages of pregnancy must be considered. At this point nail bed return is abnormally slow. Hypovolemic shock can be recognized early on by marked orthostatic hypotension. This is difficult to assess in the pregnant patient since the incidence of orthostasis is increased in normal pregnancy, positional changes must take into account the action of the gravid uterus in obstructing flow, and if sudden orthostatic hypotension is elicited, adverse fetal effects may be encountered. In high flow shock or sepsis, pulse pressure is often normal or high despite significant systolic or mean hypotension, since peripheral vascular resistance is low and diastolic runoff in the arterial circulation enhanced. At the bedside this can be appreciated as bounding pulses despite hypotension. Finally, the extremities are often cold and clammy in hypovolemia and cardiogenic shock, but are warm to the touch in high flow states.

Central Hemodynamic Monitoring

Often these bedside criteria are sufficient in and of themselves to assess the state of perfusion of the critically ill patient and to titrate appropriate therapy. Uncomplicated hypovolemia due to massive hemorrhage is such a circumstance, and delay of therapy in order to obtain invasive hemodynamic measurements is not warranted, but there will be many instances in which the patient's volume

TABLE 7–3.

Assessment of Perfusion

Manifestation	Low Flow Shock	High Flow Shock
Mental status	↓	↓
Urine output	↓	↓
Capillary refill	↓	Normal
Extremities	Cold	Warm
Mean blood pressure	↓	↓
Pulse pressure	↓	Normal or ↑
Lactate	↑	↑

TABLE 7–4.
Indications for Pulmonary Artery Catheterization
in Pregnancy

I. Shock
   A. When etiology is unclear
   B. When unresponsive to volume therapy
   C. When accompanied by a high central venous pressure
   D. When vasoactive drug use is contemplated
II. Acute hypoxemic respiratory failure
   A. When accompanied by shock
   B. When mechanical ventilation and positive end-expiratory pressure therapy are instituted
   C. When etiology of pulmonary edema is unclear
III. Hypertensive crises, including preeclampsia/eclampsia
   A. When complicated by pulmonary edema
   B. When complicated by renal or cardiac failure
IV. Routine operative or labor/delivery monitoring
   A. When pulmonary hypertension is present
   B. In severe (class III and IV) congestive heart failure

status is unclear, e.g., in relation to the physiologic changes of pregnancy, the presence of renal disease, the possibility of ventricular dysfunction, etc. Other patients will have suspected or documented ventricular failure requiring vasoactive drug use, or respiratory failure may complicate fluid management. This is when right heart catheterization should be considered, a technology which is routine in the modern intensive care unit, with an acceptable complication rate[15–18] when performed by experienced clinicians. Table 7–4 lists indications for catheterization in the critically ill pregnant patient.[17–19] This list is not exhaustive, nor do all patients with these disorders require this level of monitoring. In our own experience, it is useful for the clinician to pose questions regarding the adequacy of volume resuscitation, the adequacy of ventricular function, and the nature of respiratory failure, if any. If data collected at the bedside, in the aggregate, can answer these questions, further monitoring is not indicated. If the situation remains unclear, invasive characterization of cardiopulmonary function

is warranted to guide management decisions.

During pregnancy right heart catheterization is best performed through the internal jugular vein, because pneumothorax occurs less often with this approach. Subclavian vein catheterization is a second choice, most useful if injury or obesity have obscured neck landmarks or made jugular venipuncture impossible, but the incidence of pneumothorax reported in several series is considerably higher with this approach.[16] Antecubital vein catheterization is often difficult unless surgically placed, and femoral vein catheterization should be avoided during pregnancy because of vena caval obstruction by the uterus when the patient is supine and/or when labor may be in progress or ensue.

Complications of right heart catheterization are listed in Table 7–5. Pneumothorax should occur in less than 0.5% of punctures of the internal jugular vein.[16] Infection can be minimized by careful nursing attention to dressings, limiting manipulation, and changing catheters if monitoring exceeds 72 hours. Pulmonary artery rupture and pulmonary infarction can be avoided by preventing distal migration of the catheter and ensuring that the balloon tip is not overinflated or persistently inflated.[16]

Appropriate catheter positioning can usually be determined without fluoroscopic guidance by monitoring characteristics of each waveform as the catheter is flow-directed through the great veins, right atrium, right ventricle, pulmonary artery, and into a wedge

TABLE 7–5.
Complications of Pulmonary Artery Catheterization

Complication	To Minimize
Pneumothorax	Internal jugular approach
Arrhythmias	Usually self-limited; consider lidocaine for sustained ventricular tachycardia
Pulmonary artery rupture	Avoid overinflation of balloon
Pulmonary infarction	Prevent inadvertent wedging of catheter
Local thrombosis; infection	Do not leave catheter in place for more than 72 hr

A.

B.

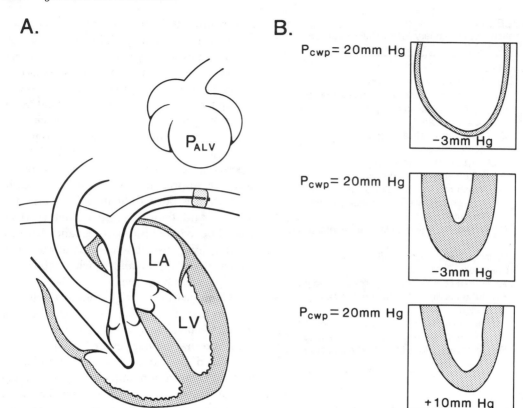

$P_{cwp} = 20mm\ Hg$

−3mm Hg

$P_{cwp} = 20mm\ Hg$

−3mm Hg

$P_{cwp} = 20mm\ Hg$

+10mm Hg

FIG 7–4.
Interpretation of the pulmonary capillary wedge pressure (*PCWP*): In **A,** the PCWP will reflect left ventricular *(LV)* end-diastolic pressure if there is no gradient across the mitral valve or the pulmonary venous circulation. In addition, the catheter *should not reside* in a portion of the lung where alveolar pressure (P_{ALV}) is greater than vascular pressure (zone 1 condition) for reliable assessment of ventricular function. In **B,** the measured PCWP (20 mm Hg) is related to different ventricular volumes. In the uppermost example, ventricular volume is large because the ventricle is normally compliant and transmural pressure is large. In the middle example, ventricular volume is small because the ventricle is thickened and stiff. In the bottom diagram, ventricular volume is small because transmural filling pressure is reduced by positive pressure resulting from mechanical ventilation (see text for explanation).

position (see Fig 7–4), an important consideration in the gravid subject. Extensive reviews of the use of this catheter and the interpretation of data collected are available,[20, 21] but several points will be emphasized. Simultaneous sampling of mixed venous blood from the pulmonary artery and an arterial blood specimen allows determination of the AV O_2 content difference. While cardiac output can be directly measured by thermal dilution with the catheter, substantial error can be present[22] and the interpretation of any given measured flow is difficult, given the physiologic changes that occur with pregnancy. In low flow states, the AV O_2 content difference will widen, typically to greater than

5 vol%, and is a sensitive indicator of inadequate flow. This measurement is easy to obtain and is important. Also, the adequacy of ventricular filling can be difficult to determine since the catheter yields a pressure measurement (pulmonary capillary wedge pressure, or PCWP) and the relationship of this pressure to a given ventricular volume is determined by the compliance of the ventricle and the transmural filling pressure of the ventricle.

The above described concepts are depicted in Figure 7–4. In the left-sided panel (A) of this figure, a pulmonary artery catheter is shown in a wedge position, with occlusion resulting in a static column of blood passing an alveolus and then joining converging pulmonary veins with flow downstream to the left atrium and left ventricle. If no significant pressure drop exists across the mitral valve or the pulmonary venous circuit, and the vascular pressures are not exceeded by alveolar pressure, left ventricular end-diastolic pressure will be closely estimated by PCWP. Thus, mitral stenosis and pulmonary venoocclusive disease, relatively rare diseases, can confound the use of the wedge pressure as an estimate of left ventricular filling. More important is that the catheter may wedge in a portion of the lung where alveolar pressure is greater than pulmonary arterial pressure and measured occlusion pressure will not reflect intravascular pressure at all (termed West zone I conditions). This is more likely to occur in patients who have high alveolar pressures (respiratory failure patients receiving mechanical ventilation and positive end-expiratory pressure, PEEP) and low intravascular pressures (hypovolemia). Indications that this phenomenon is present and confounding interpretation of data include the observation that wedge pressure varies one to one with changes of PEEP, that the catheter appears to be in a nondependent portion of the lung, and that there is failure to obtain a mixed venous specimen.[20]

Even when one has dealt adequately with technical problems of measurement, it may be difficult to relate pressure data to ventricular volume. Of course, the given PCWP is less important to the clinician than the adequacy of diastolic volume to optimize stroke volume and flow. The relationship of pressure to volume in the ventricle, as depicted in Figures 7–2 and 7–3, depends upon the compliance of the ventricle and the extramural pressure. Consider panel B in Figure 7–4. A given PCWP, 20 mm Hg, is shown under three different conditions. At the top of this panel, a ventricle of normal compliance with an extracardiac negative pressure of −3 mm Hg, typical of the negative intrathoracic pressure of a spontaneously breathing healthy adult, is shown. Thus the transmural distending pressure acting upon this normal ventricle will be [20 − (−3)] mm Hg or 23 mm Hg and will be associated with a very large ventricular volume. In the middle diagram, the same wedge pressure is shown in a very stiff (hypertensive, hypertrophied) ventricle. Despite an equal transmural pressure of 23 mm Hg, ventricular volume is small due to the stiffness of the chamber. Finally, another example of a PCWP of 20 mm Hg is shown in the lower diagram, but in this case ventricular compliance characteristics are normal but the patient is receiving mechanical ventilation and PEEP resulting in a positive extramural pressure and a transmural distending pressure of only 10 (20 − 10) mm Hg. Thus ventricular chamber size is near normal and to the clinician might appear to be "stiff" or noncompliant, an artifact of the effect of PEEP.

Such considerations occur frequently in the critically ill patient, making judgments concerning intravascular volume status difficult despite invasive measurements. For these reasons, it would be misleading to list "normal" intravascular pressures or flows for either the pregnant or nonpregnant patient. In essence, data from each individual case must be interpreted in relation to the various physiologic and pathophysiologic circumstances, most of which have been described above. If the state of diastolic filling is unclear, we advocate using the shape of the diastolic filling curve to gauge the effect of a volume challenge. Note from Figure 7–3 that as the ventricle is filled in diastole, the curve eventually rises steeply with large pressure changes associated with small volume changes. In the complex patient with underlying cardiac disease or receiving mechanical ventilation, if the adequacy of ventricular filling is unclear and the patient is hypoperfused, a discrete volume challenge (e.g., 300–500 mL) should be given over a brief period of time. If the PCWP rises precipitously (>3–4 mm Hg), then it is likely that preload reserve has been exhausted. If PCWP remains nearly the same, successive volume challenges can be given until either hypoperfusion has been corrected or evidence of overfilling is present, as suggested by sudden rises in PCWP.

TABLE 7–6.
Causes of Hemorrhagic Shock

First Two Trimesters	Third Trimester
Trauma	Trauma
Disseminated intravascu-	DIC
lar coagulation (DIC)	Placenta previa
Abortion	Marginal sinus rupture
Hydatidiform mole	Placental abruption
Ectopic pregnancy	Uterine rupture
Abdominal pregnancy	

Low Flow States

In the simplest analysis, low flow hypoperfusion exists because of hypovolemia, pump dysfunction, or a combination of both. All critically ill patients require constant attention to the adequacy of diastolic filling, as described above, but in pregnancy there are disorders resulting in sudden and massive hemorrhage and hypovolemic shock, and these will be discussed initially. While postpartum hemorrhage to a level requiring transfusion therapy is not rare,[23] we wish to focus on antepartum causes of bleeding likely to be encountered by the critical care physician assisting in management (see Table 7–6). As noted above, maternal oxygen delivery is more flow-dependent during pregnancy, and uterine blood flow is near maximal at baseline. Maternal hemorrhage sufficient to produce hypotension can thus rapidly produce fetal hypoxia. Accordingly, response to such bleeding must be rapid and definitive.

Hemorrhagic Shock

Trauma has emerged as a frequent cause of maternal and fetal death in the United States[24] and even seemingly minor blunt abdominal trauma can cause significant intraabdominal blood loss. Blood in the pelvis and abdomen can usually be diagnosed by ultrasound, computed tomography, or lavage. Placental abruption occurs with higher incidence in patients with hypertension and high parity, and this complication is more likely to recur in subsequent gestations.[25] When abruption results in fetal death, blood loss averages at least 2 to 3 L but can exceed 5 L and still remain concealed within the uterus.[26]

Disseminated intravascular coagulation can be present in a significant fraction of these patients, which further complicates their hemorrhagic shock.[27]

Placenta previa, which occurs in approximately 1 in 200 pregnancies, does not frequently cause massive hemorrhage in and of itself. However, if inappropriate examination precipitates disruption of the placenta over the cervical os, or if the placenta previa is complicated by invasion of trophoblastic tissue into the myometrium (placenta previa et accreta), then massive hemorrhage may occur.[28] Placenta previa, more common in multiparous, older patients, also has a tendency to recur in subsequent pregnancies. Fetal mortality is 5% to 10%, but can be much higher if maternal shock occurs.[28, 29] Ultrasound has facilitated early diagnosis of many patients.

Uterine rupture may be due to trauma, but can also occur spontaneously, its incidence being 1 in 2,000 or 3,000 pregnancies.[25] The most common setting in which rupture occurs, however, is in the multipara with protracted labor. In overt rupture peritoneal signs may be present due to bleeding at the site of the tear,[4] but substantial blood loss can occur in the absence of such findings.

Management of Hemorrhagic Shock

Management of these patients must be prompt and directed. An overview of management principles is given in Table 7–7.

TABLE 7–7.
Management of Hemorrhagic Shock

Establish IV access with two or three 16-gauge or larger catheters
Massive volume infusion—crystalloid or colloid—while awaiting blood products (pressure bags may assist)
Red cell transfusions; hematocrits during acute bleeding will not reflect ongoing blood loss
Identify associated coagulopathy
Bleeding itself may engender thrombocytopenia or factor deficiency, but do not treat prophylactically
If volume infusion cannot stabilize the patient, consider MAST suit use
Evaluate for surgical/angiographic intervention when stable

MAST = medical antishock trousers.

Identification of patients at risk is of value, in which case venous lines will be in place and blood typing accomplished. In the presence of massive hemorrhage, the following measures are recommended: Two or three large-bore (16-gauge or larger) venous catheters should be in place. Peripheral access is adequate if sufficiently large vessels can be identified and cannulated. Immediate volume replacement is usually not accomplished with blood, since blood bank preparation is not instantaneous. Much discussion is often directed toward crystalloid versus colloid therapy.[30] While it does appear true that treatment with large volumes of crystalloid lowers the colloid oncotic pressure, which may predispose to lung and other tissue edema, a major error in early resuscitation of patients is inadequate volume delivery regardless of fluid chosen. If crystalloids such as lactated Ringer's solution are used, one should be aware that considerably more fluid will be needed (two- to fourfold) than if colloids are utilized to achieve similar degrees of intravascular expansion. Prompt delivery of fluids can be aided by pressure bag applications.

Many forms of shock are associated with rapid development of ventilatory failure.[31] Hypoxemia superimposed on low flow is particularly injurious to fetus and mother. In the setting of any form of respiratory dysfunction and in any patient with persistent shock, elective intubation should be considered, and decision to do so should be made prior to the occurrence of overt hypoxemia or hypercapnea. In the presence of massive hemorrhage and hypotension despite aggressive volume replacement, MAST (*medical antishock trousers*) should be considered, although this is a temporizing measure which limits access to pelvic and abdominal structures.[32, 33] The utility of this intervention is probably based upon local tamponade of bleeding sites and elevation of peripheral vascular resistance, thus preserving critical perfusion pressure to vital organs. It is less likely that this intervention results in an "autotransfusion of blood" from the periphery to the central circulation or enhances venous return.[34] The MAST suit consists of two leg compartments and an abdominal compartment. In the gravid patient the abdominal compartment should not be inflated, and thus in antepartum hemorrhage only the leg compartments should be used. The leg compartments should be inflated separately to 5 mm Hg pressure, and then the abdominal compartment inflated (in postpartum patients). Incremental increases of 5 to 10 mm Hg are made at 5- to 10-minute intervals until bleeding is controlled. The suit should be in place only as long as necessary to initiate definitive therapy (ideally less than several hours) and should be deflated one compartment at a time, in reverse order of inflation, with 5-mm Hg pressure decrements each 15 minutes.

Blood replacement in the form of packed red blood cells should be administered with a goal of achieving a hematocrit of 30% to 35%. This latter determination, however, is difficult to make in acutely bleeding patients because the time required for intravascular volume to equilibrate is variable. Units of packed red cells are typically 250 to 300 mL with hematocrits of 60% to 70%. Massive bleeding in gravidas requires assessment to rule out a coagulopathy. Useful initial tests include peripheral smear, platelet count, prothrombin time (PT), partial thromboplastin time (PTT), and fibrinogen level. Should these tests suggest either excessive factor consumption (disseminated intravascular coagulation, or DIC) or deficient production (liver failure or isolated factor deficiencies), measurement of fibrin degradation products and specific factor levels is useful, although making a distinction between DIC and factor loss may be extremely difficult. The recognition and management of DIC in pregnancy is discussed in Chapter 8. Bleeding itself can lead to DIC,[24] although the most common coagulopathy associated with massive blood loss is thrombocytopenia.[35] Prophylactic platelet transfusion is not recommended, even in cases of massive hemorrhage. If platelet counts fall to 20×10^9/L, or bleeding persists despite platelet counts of 20 to 50×10^9/L, platelet transfusions to a level of 50×10^9/L are indicated.

Another complication, albeit less common, is depletion of circulating clotting factors through blood loss, which requires fresh frozen plasma (FFP). This complication is usually associated with replacement fluids that average two to three times the patient's initial blood volume. Again prophylactic use of this blood component should be avoided because of risks of disease transmission, alloimmunization, and transfusion reactions.[35]

The therapy outlined above, while supportive, is lifesaving and should be continued while prompt surgical evaluation is carried out. As circulatory stability returns, the patient can then be reevaluated in view of a decision to continue conservative management, intervene surgically, or, in selected cases, embolize bleeding sites under angiographic localization.[36-39]

Low Flow Shock Due to Ventricular Dysfunction

A low flow state that persists after adequate volume replacement suggests impairment of "pump" function. At this time, dysrhythmias or ischemia causing inadequate stroke volume must be considered and excluded or identified and corrected.[40] Continuous rhythm monitoring should be routine, and 12-lead electrocardiography, serum enzyme analysis, and echocardiography are helpful in identifying myocardial ischemia.

The most likely cause of pump failure in the peripartum period is congestive heart failure due either to preexisting heart disease or a cardiomyopathy arising de novo or in association with preeclampsia.[41, 42] Metabolic disturbances can worsen ventricular function in underlying cardiomyopathies, and hypocalcemia, hypophosphatemia, acidosis, and hypoxemia should be carefully excluded or corrected.[43, 44]

The supportive management of these patients begins with constant attention to the possibility of preload reserve, as described above. Vasoactive drugs, which may have an adverse effect upon the fetus, are reserved for those circumstances in which hypovolemia has

been resolved and maternal perfusion remains inadequate. At the University of Chicago, patients manifesting cardiogenic shock despite appropriate volume administration receive an infusion of dobutamine[45, 46], an exogenous catecholamine with significant β-receptor activity resulting in positive inotropy. While the α activity of dobutamine in the peripheral circulation is blunted by its β₂-vasodilating effects,[45] this drug may still reduce placental blood flow[47] and therefore it should be reserved for life-threatening conditions. The initial dose of 2 to 3 μg/kg/min can be increased until the desired effect upon flow is achieved. This usually occurs at infusion rates between 5 and 10 μg/kg/min. Of importance, many patients exhibit tachyphylaxis after only 72 hours, and substantial increments in dose schedule may be required to maintain therapeutic effect.[46] Concomitantly, low-dose infusion of dopamine (2–3 μg/kg/min) should be considered in order to preserve splanchnic and renal perfusion.[48] Because dopamine exhibits significant α-stimulatory activity with higher doses, it is not the inotropic drug of first choice. Also, while it is used widely in the critically ill in combination with dobutamine, its use in pregnancy has been limited.[49] Thus it is wise to avoid use of dopamine in patients receiving dobutamine who exhibit acceptable renal function.

When cardiogenic shock persists despite inotropic drug support, cautious attempts at afterload reduction are indicated.[50, 51] Patients with greatly depressed systolic performance demonstrate a significant rise in stroke volume with very small reductions in the pressure at which their ventricles eject. In addition, changes in chamber size achieved with afterload reduction may act to reduce intramural wall stress and myocardial oxygen consumption. In the acute setting, either sodium nitroprusside or nitroglycerin administered intravenously is useful. Sodium nitroprusside has the advantages of rapid onset of action, short duration, and substantial arteriolar and venous vasodilation, but carries the disadvantage of being metabolized to thiocyanate and cyanide, both of which can accumulate

TABLE 7–8.
Vasoactive Drug Use in Pregnancy

Agent	Dose	Purpose	Potential Adverse Effects
Dobutamine	2–15 μg/kg/min (higher doses over time)	Positive inotropy	Arrhythmias Potential ↓ uterine blood flow
Dopamine	1–4 μg/kg/min	Preferential in splanchnic and renal flow	Arrhythmias Potential ↓ uterine blood flow
Nitroprusside*	0–5 μ/kg/min titrated to blood pressure and flow	Afterload and preload reduction	Thiocyanate and cyanide toxicity Hypotension
Nitroglycerin	0–5 μg/kg/min titrated to blood pressure and flow	Afterload and preload reduction	Not as effective as nitroprusside for afterload reduction Hypotension

*Given potential risk to fetus of cyanide toxicity, use should be reserved for cases in which other circulatory manipulations fail to stabilze the mother.

to significant levels in patients receiving high infusion rates for more than 48 to 72 hours. Fetal cyanide poisoning has been described in experimental animal models.[52] Thus, while sodium nitroprusside has been used in pregnancy (most widely in the treatment of hypertensive emergency[53]) we wish to emphasize that *sodium nitroprusside should be used in the management of shock in pregnancy only when all other interventions have failed to establish a stable circulation and when it is essential for maternal well-being. Even under these conditions, the dose and duration of therapy should be minimized.* The initial dose of both nitroglycerin and nitroprusside is 10 to 20 μ/min which can be doubled at 3- to 5-min intervals until stroke volume improves. Patients typically require infusion rates of 30 to 300 μg/min. Hypotension is the limiting factor acutely. Untoward hypotension is more likely in hypovolemic patients since these drugs cause pooling of blood volume in the venous capacitance vessels and is yet one more reason why constant attention to intravascular volume is crucial in managing the hypoperfused patient.[51] If acute afterload reduction is necessary to support cardiac output, the patient should be converted to oral agents for long-term afterload reduction at the earliest possible time to avoid toxicity from long-term nitroprusside infusion. The manifestations of thiocyanate and cyanide toxicity include nausea and anorexia, disorientation, muscle spasm, ventricular ectopy, seizures, and cardiovascular collapse. Toxicity is more

likely to occur at the higher dose levels, especially when infusions have been given for more than 72 hours, or if hepatic or renal dysfunction are present.[52]

There are few data on the prognosis of gravid patients requiring inotropic and afterload reduction for shock, but mortality is high in nonpregnant subjects due to the severity of underlying cardiac injury. Of note, fetal mortality has been estimated to be 10% to 30% with maternal congestive heart failure alone.[41] Delivery should be considered at the point at which the patient can be stabilized. Such patients should, of course, avoid active labor and it is unlikely that the fetus would endure in such circumstances. A summary of vasoactive drug use is given in Table 7–8.

High Flow States (Septic Shock)

The hemodynamic profile of patients with sepsis is quite different from that described above for forms of low flow shock. Septic patients tend to have a hyperdynamic circulation, characterized by high cardiac output and relatively low blood pressure. This statement is equivalent to stating that the systemic vascular resistance is low, since

$$MAP - RAP = CO \times SVR$$

where $MAP - RAP$ is the pressure drop across the peripheral circulation (mean aortic pressure − mean right atrial pressure), CO is the cardiac output, and *SVR* is the systemic vascular resistance. Rearranging,

$$SVR = (MAP - RAP)/CO$$

Thus a low vascular resistance is present when the blood pressure is low for the observed flow.

Although there may be a component of myocardial dysfunction in sepsis,[54] it should be emphasized that flow is high, at least early in the course of the disease. This is also true in the pregnant septic patient.[55] Decreases in stroke volume and depression of stroke work indices are seen, but occur most profoundly late in the course of the disease and are not universally present in frankly hypotensive patients. However, despite high flows, many of the clinical manifestations of low flow hypoperfusion are present, including hypotension, abnormal mental status, oliguria, and lactic acidosis. This has been ascribed to maldistribution of flow, metabolic block to oxygen and other substrate utilization at a cellular level, or combinations of these problems. Convincing data supporting these hypotheses are not available.

While any infection may lead to the circulatory sequelae in septic pregnant patients, pelvic and urinary tract sources predominate.[56] Common antecedents to septic shock are postpartum endometritis after either cesarean section or vaginal delivery, chorioamnionitis, and urinary tract infection including pyelonephritis. Another cause is septic abortion. Thus the peripartum and postabortion periods are when the patients are at greatest risk for sepsis. There are also animal data suggesting that pregnancy increases vulnerability to the systemic effects of bacteremia and endotoxemia.[57, 58] Given the most common infection sites, the bacteriology of sepsis in pregnancy includes a wide variety of aerobic and anaerobic pathogens, often in a polymicrobial setting. Commonly encountered organisms include anaerobic streptococci and bacteroides, *Escherichia coli, Proteus mirabilis, Enterobacter, Klebsiella,* and *Pseudomonas.*[59]

The clinical manifestations of sepsis in-clude the general setting consistent with the underlying site of infection (e.g., premature rupture of membranes as a prelude to chorioamnionitis), followed by temperature perturbation (often with rigor), and then progressive tachycardia and hypotension with a warm periphery and bounding pulse initially, followed by organ system dysfunction as signaled by altered mental status, oliguria, and lactic acidosis. The development of a pulmonary capillary leak is particularly frequent with ARDS and severe hypoxemia, complicating their course.[60] Coagulation abnormalities are also extremely common.

In addition to these bedside and laboratory parameters, invasive characterization of the circulation usually reveals a high cardiac index and heart rate with a low blood pressure.[54, 55] Some patients will have a slightly diminished stroke volume with high flow associated with tachycardia while others may exhibit essentially normal ventricular performance. Seven of 10 pregnant patients reported by Lee et al.[55] had normal or only mildly depressed ventricular function. The systemic vascular resistance index (SVRI) in the eight patients surviving was 885 ±253 dyne-sec/cm^5 m^2 initially and 1672 ±413 dyne-sec/cm^5 m^2 following resolution of their hyperdynamic state. In interpreting systemic vascular resistance in these patients, it is important to note that pregnancy itself results in a 25% decrease from the prepregnancy vascular resistance of 770 to 1500 dyne-sec/cm^5. Thus three useful signs of hemodynamic evolution in sepsis—tachycardia, hypotension, and low systemic vascular resistance—must be interpreted with caution in the gravid patient, particularly in the third trimester. Rapid changes over a brief period of time, however, often signal infection.

Management

Management of the septic gravid patient requires, first and foremost, thorough culturing, including consideration of endometrial sites.[61] Antibiotic therapy is empiric until specific microbiologic data are available, and surgical drainage of appropriate pelvic and abdominal sources may be required. Given the wide range of microbiologic possibilities, broad-spectrum antibiotics should be used initially. Various recommendations have been made,[62] and typical antibiotic choices are shown in Table 7–9.

Fluid administration, which increases preload and flow, may not improve tissue function and does increase the likelihood of development of clinically significant noncardiogenic pulmonary edema (ARDS). In addition, excessive use of vasoactive drugs, especially when titrated to maintain the blood pressure, may cause excessive vasoconstriction which increases afterload resulting in diminished stroke volume and perfusion despite the elevated arterial pressure. Thus, in patients who do not manifest inadequate tissue perfusion and oxygen delivery, tolerance of tachycardia and moderate hypotension may be warranted. Appearance of lactic acidosis or a specific tissue bed dysfunction is an indication for volume loading but the risk of precipitating low-pressure pulmonary edema must be recognized and mechanical ventilatory support instituted if needed. Right heart catheterization is useful at this juncture to titrate volume therapy. If hypoperfusion persists despite volume replacement, further increases in forward flow can be achieved with the use of inotropic agents such as dobuta-

mine, an approach which is of value in a subset of patients who have markedly abnormal ventricular performance.[63] However, there appear to be no clear benefits in the use of inotropic agents in patients with high flow states whose cardiac function is near normal, and one should realize the limitations of their use and be willing to withdraw these drugs if adverse effects are noted.

Several other interventions recommended in the literature have not proved useful in large clinical trials. Recent prospective studies have shown that high-dose corticosteroids do not increase survival or prevent development of acute hypoxemic respiratory failure.[64] Naloxone, a narcotic antagonist, has been anecdotally reported to reverse hypotension in septic shock, but again data are limited with no efficacy being observed in a randomized trial.[65] Neither of these interventions has been studied in any systematic fashion in the gravid patient and therefore routine use is not warranted.

Very promising are trials of immunotherapeutic agents directed against bacterial antigens or exotoxins.[66, 67] Lachman and colleagues[67] investigated the effects of freeze-dried human plasma rich in antilipopolysaccharide (anti-LPS) IgG administered to obstetric and gynecologic patients with sepsis and hypotension. Mortality in anti-LPS–

TABLE 7–9.
Empiric Antibiotic Choices in Sepsis With Pelvic or Urinary Source

Drugs	Intravenous Dose	Comments
1. Ampicillin	150–200 mg/kg/day	Excellent enterococcal coverage
+		
aminoglycoside (gentamicin)	3–5 mg/kg/day after loading	Inadequate *Staphylococcus aureus* coverage Adjust for renal function, follow serum levels of aminoglycoside
2. Above		
+		
clindamycin or	600 mg q8h	Expanded anaerobic coverage
metronidazole	7.5 mg/kg q6h after loading	
3. 2nd-generation cephalosporin (cefoxitin)	1–2 g q 4h	Cephalosporin alone has inadequate enterococcal or *S. aureus* coverage
+		
aminoglycoside		

treated patients was 7.1% as compared to 47.4% in untreated patients, with mean arterial blood pressure rising from 45.1 ± 7.4 mm Hg to 69.1 ± 9.1 mm Hg within 75 minutes of administration of this preparation. Immunotherapeutic agents are not generally available and experience with them remains limited, but genetic engineering should make widely available any effective and safe agents that are identified.

Cardiopulmonary Resuscitation

There are generally accepted guidelines of how to proceed in cardiopulmonary arrest, but appropriate management of the gravid patient is less clear. Clearly, prevention of cardiac arrest would be preferable, and in this regard early support of ventilation prior to respiratory arrest or emergent intubation in the critically ill pregnant woman is crucial.

Several physiologic changes of pregnancy should be taken into account when performing cardiopulmonary resuscitation (CPR). Compression of the inferior vena cava and aorta by the gravid uterus may impede venous return and distal arterial perfusion. The latter may be particularly important for uteroplacental blood flow in the low-pressure perfusion state during CPR. In addition, in late pregnancy the gravid uterus acts as an abdominal binder, resulting in elevation of intrathoracic pressure. Since closed-chest massage appears to create forward flow by alternating intrathoracic pressure,[68] the ability to create flow by this intervention in gravidas may be significantly impaired. DePace and colleagues,[69] for instance, described a patient in whom blood pressure could not be achieved during cardiac massage and cardiac standstill until the uterus was evacuated, after which an immediate pulsatile blood pressure was observed.

These considerations have caused some authors to modify the usual approach to CPR in the pregnant patient. The most thorough review of the subject, by Lee et al,[70] offers an approach outlined in Table 7–10. The key modifications of routine CPR are that the pregnant patient have standard CPR conducted with positioning to decrease aortocaval compression by the uterus. If standard closed-chest massage cannot generate a pulse, particularly in late pregnancy, early consideration of open-chest massage should be made, simultaneous with a decision for emergency cesarean section. In this regard, intensive care units managing critically ill pregnant patients are best organized with a system to call to the bedside all surgical, internal medicine, and anesthesiologic staff necessary to effect such management at the earliest sign of acute deterioration of the circulation of the mother.

RESPIRATORY FAILURE
Pathophysiology of Gas Exchange

Disorders leading to respiratory failure are classified into those causing severe hypoxemia secondary to flooding or collapse of alveoli resulting in a right-to-left shunt as blood traverses nonventilated segments of the lung (type I or acute hypoxemic respiratory failure) and those where there is alveolar hypoventilation with elevation of the arterial carbon dioxide pressure (Pco_2) (type II or ventilatory failure).[71] These two concepts are depicted in Figure 7–5. Hypoxemia due to hypoventilation is readily corrected by small amounts of supplemental oxygen, which causes large increases in alveolar Po_2 and thus corrects arterial desaturation.[71] The underlying hypoventilation remains and requires further diagnosis and treatment. Figure 7–5 further demonstrates that oxygen therapy is relatively ineffective in patients with large intrapulmonary shunts. For example, treatment with 100% oxygen (fractional concentration of inspired oxygen [Fio_2] = 1.0), will result in less than 90% saturation of arterial hemoglobin if shunt fraction (QS/QT) is large (50% in the figure example).

The cause of ventilatory failure may be thought of as an imbalance between the mechanical load on the respiratory system (with resistive and elastic components) and the drive and neuromuscular elements responsible for

TABLE 7–10.
Approach to Cardiopulmonary Resuscitation During Pregnancy*

Time	Resuscitative Action	Diagnostic Action	Pharmacologic Action
0	Chest thump Ventilation (mouth-to-mouth) External cardiac massage	ECG for rhythm Check for pulses and perfusion	IV fluids
	Defibrillate		Ventricular fibrillation— lidocaine

	IV access: central line	Determine gestational age	Supraventricular tachyarrhyth-
			  mia—digitalis/β-blocker as
			  appropriate

1–2 min	Endotracheal intubation +
	  ventilation with oxygen
		Measure arterial blood gases
		Check for pulses and
		  perfusion
		Check fetal heart, sonography
			pH <7.3—NaHCO$_3$
			Asystole/bradyarrhythmia—
			  atropine
			Pulmonary edema—furosemide

2–5 min		ECG for rhythm	Ventricular fibrillation— lidocaine
	Defibrillate as needed	ECG for rhythm	Ventricular fibrillation— bretylium

	Position to move uterus to left	Quick measure of blood pres-
		  sure, pulses, perfusion
			Electromechanical dissocia-
			  tion—calcium chloride,
			  epinephrine (one time only),
			  isoproterenol

		Measure arterial blood gases	pH <7.3—NaHCO$_3$

5–10 min	Continue ventilation + exter-
	  nal massage
	Begin preparation for opera-
	  tive procedure as
	  appropriate
		Check fetal heart, sonography	

	Arterial line	Check for tension pneumo-
		  thorax, cardiac tamponade,
		  hypovolemia	

	Defibrillate as needed	Measure arterial blood gases	pH <7.3—NaHCO$_3$

15 min	Open-chest cardiac massage
	  and/or emergency cesar-
	  ean section as appropriate
		Continue as above	Continue as above

*From Lee RV, Rodgers BD, White LM, et al: Cardiopulmonary resuscitation of pregnant women. *Am J Med* 1986; 81:311–318.
 Used by permission.

performance of the work of breathing.[71, 72] The clinical conditions pertinent to each category are presented in Figure 7–6. Thus, despite normal drive and neuromuscular function, large increases in mechanical load can lead to ventilatory failure. This would be the case, for example, in a young woman with severe asthma. On the other hand, respiratory muscle fatigue and ventilatory failure can evolve in a patient with progressive weakness due to myasthenia gravis, even when lung mechan-ics are normal. In most instances, the cause of ventilatory failure is multifactorial (see Figure 7–6).

Considerations in Pregnancy

A more complete discussion of gestational alterations in pulmonary physiology may be found in Chapter 6 and only the most important changes will be summarized here. In pregnancy, minute ventilation rises in the first trimester to a level at term 40% to 50% greater than values measured post partum. This increase in ventilation exceeds metabolic needs and thus results in hyperventilation with hypocapnea and PCO_2 ranging from 27 to 32 mm Hg. The associated respiratory alkalosis is partially compensated by renal mechanisms such that average plasma pH is only slightly alkalemic, ranging from 7.4 to 7.45, while serum bicarbonate averages 18 to 20 mEq/L. In addition to this increase in minute ventilation, the gravida has an increased elastic load on the respiratory system due to the compressive effects of the uterus on the diaphragm and changes in chest wall compliance in late pregnancy. The latter effect would be expected to be most pronounced in the supine position.

These physiologic changes appear sufficient to reduce pulmonary reserves such that ventilatory failure might be a common complication in gravidas with pulmonary or other problems. However, while dyspnea is an extremely common complaint in pregnancy, ventilatory failure is rare. Gaensler and colleagues[73] observed several women with a 40% to 75% reduction in vital capacity preconception due to lung resection. All carried their pregnancy to term and had few respiratory symptoms. While several authorities suggest that a vital capacity of at least 1 L is necessary for a safe and successful pregnancy, one patient has been reported to have completed pregnancy with a vital capacity of only 0.8 L.[74] Thus, severely reduced lung volume alone, to a level compatible with impairment

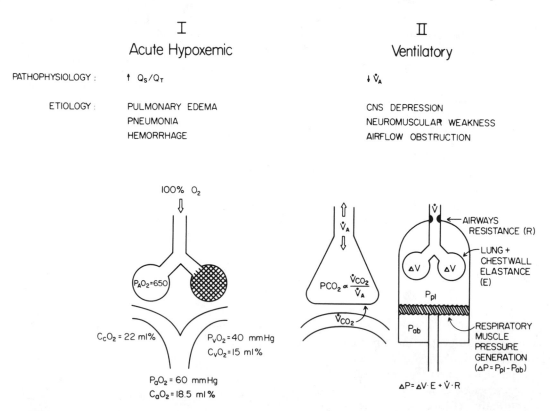

FIG 7–5.
Classification of respiratory failure: In cases in which alveoli are flooded or collapsed (type I respiratory failure) blood will traverse the lung without oxygenation, constituting a right-to-left shunt with the potential for severe hypoxemia with minimal response to oxygen therapy. In ventilatory failure (type II respiratory failure), total alveolar ventilation is reduced due to diminished drive to breathe, neuromuscular dysfunction, or increased loads on the respiratory system. The hallmark of this form of respiratory failure is elevation of the PCO_2 (see text).

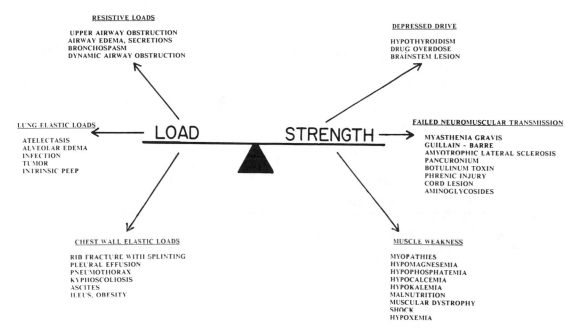

FIG 7–6.
Contributions to ventilatory failure: Conditions which lead to either increased load on the respiratory system (resistive and elastic) or diminished strength (depressed drive, failed neuromuscular transmission, muscle weakness) are given. PEEP = positive end-expiratory pressure. (From Schmidt GA, Hall JB: *JAMA* 1989; 261:3444–3453. Used by permission.)

of ventilatory function in the nonpregnant individual, does not readily predict ability to conceive and carry pregnancy to term.

Ventilatory Failure

Figure 7–6 lists many diseases which contribute to ventilatory failure, none of which predominates among pregnant patients. These include asthma; parenchymal lung diseases such as cystic fibrosis; kyphoscoliosis; neuromuscular diseases such as the Guillain-Barré syndrome and myasthenia gravis; and drug overdose. Patients with a diminished drive to breathe usually exhibit a frankly disturbed sensorium and intubation is often necessary to protect the airway, independent of ventilatory function. Patients with either neuromuscular weakness or increased load or combinations of both tend to exhibit a distinct pattern as they progress to respiratory muscle fatigue and failure—progressively rapid and shallow breathing with increasing use of ac-

cessory muscles of respiration.[71] Thus respiratory rates greater than 35/min, breathlessness precluding speech, accessory muscle use, and patient subjective sense of fatigue all militate for ventilatory support.

There is one report of a patient with severe kyphoscoliosis who required nocturnal ventilatory support with intermittent positive pressure during weeks 30 to 34 of pregnancy until delivery could be accomplished by cesarean section.[75] This patient's forced vital capacity was 640 mL at 14 weeks' gestation and 580 mL at 28 weeks' gestation, with a PCO_2 of 52 mm Hg and PO_2 of 59 mm Hg at 25 weeks' gestation. Positive pressure ventilation was achieved with the use of a tight-fitting mask. In this fashion oxygen administration and ventilation prevented nocturnal desaturation. This novel approach may be applicable to other pregnant patients with chronic ventilatory impairment. In patients with marginal ventilatory function, screening for nocturnal hypoxemia can be accomplished readily with pulse oximetry, a reliable non-invasive means of recording arterial hemoglobin saturation over prolonged periods of time.[76] If significant desaturation occurs during sleep—a period of risk for this complication in patients with chronic obstructive pulmonary disease (COPD) and neuromuscular disease—then various forms of ventilatory support can be contemplated.

Mechanical Support for Ventilatory Failure

If ventilatory failure progresses as judged by the bedside criteria given, then intubation and mechanical ventilation are best accomplished in an elective and controlled fashion. Several difficulties in airway management may be encountered in the critically ill pregnant patient. Delayed gastric emptying due to hormonal factors or mechanical action of the uterus, increased intraabdominal pressure, and diminished competence of the gastroesophageal sphincter may all contribute to an increased risk of aspiration.[77] Upper airway edema (especially in the pharynx) has been described in patients with preeclampsia).[78] It is notable that 40% of maternal deaths associated with general anesthesia in England and Wales from 1976–1978 were related to difficulties in endotracheal intubation.[79] The strong implication of these observations is that airway control should be achieved in an early and elective fashion by skilled personnel.

Stabilization on the ventilator can be achieved with tidal volumes in the range of 10 mL/kg and respiratory rates of 15 to 18, with a goal of eucapnea in the range of 28 to 34 mm Hg for this patient population. While maternal spontaneous hyperventilation does not appear to adversely affect fetal oxygenation,[80] a number of studies in animal models suggest that excessive positive pressure ventilation to a P_{CO_2} causing acute respiratory alkalosis can result in fetal asphyxia, due presumably to metabolic-driven reduction in uteroplacental flow and/or diminished maternal venous return.[81–83] Since positive pressure ventilation may raise intrathoracic pressure and thus impair venous return, it is important that the pregnant patient be managed

in a lateral position whenever possible.

Fetal viability can be maintained throughout pregnancy with mechanical ventilation. Unfortunately, this has too often been accomplished in cases in which maternal death occurs but life support systems are maintained to allow fetal maturation and delivery.[84] When instituted early in the course of progressive ventilatory failure it can stabilize mother and fetus and then permit identification of reversible factors as detailed in Figure 7–6 to allow either safe withdrawal of mechanical support or controlled delivery by cesarean section. These complex decisions are best undertaken by joint discussion among critical care physician, obstetrician, and neonatologist.

Acute Hypoxemic Respiratory Failure

The second major cause of respiratory failure are those disorders causing significant hypoxemia by virtue of intrapulmonary shunting of blood past nonventilated lung units. This occurs when there is diffuse flooding of lung units—the homogeneous lung disease of pulmonary edema—or when nonhomogeneous processes such as acute bacterial pneumonia cause local consolidation of lung units. In this latter cause of acute respiratory failure, hypoxemia can be extreme since blood flow to acutely infected lobes can increase twofold, causing shunt fractions as large as 40% from single-lobe involvement.[85]

Pulmonary edema results when high intravascular pressures, usually in the setting of left ventricular failure, create a hydrostatic pressure gradient driving edemagenesis despite normal lung microcirculatory integrity—so-called cardiogenic or high-pressure edema—or when diffuse injury of the lung results in loss of the oncotic pressure gradient between the vasculature and lung interstitium such that alveoli flood with protein-rich fluid despite normal intravascular pressures—so-called low-pressure edema or ARDS.[86] The distinction between these disorders may often be blurred—any component of volume overload or ventricular diastolic dysfunction can lead to elevation of pulmonary vascular pressures and predispose to edema formation, while any cause of hypooncotic pressure of the circulating blood volume may result in edema formation at a lower hydrostatic pressure.[86]

It has been suggested that pregnancy predisposes to the development of pulmonary edema.[87, 88] One possible reason may be the intravascular volume expansion of 40% to 60% which normally occurs in pregnancy. This would not cause accumulation of lung water unless accompanied by either elevation of lung microvascular pressures or a hypooncotic state. The former does not appear to be the case, as judged by measurements made at the time of cardiac catheterization,[89] although acute fluid shifts from the venous circulation to the central blood compartment may occur in critical illness. Plasma oncotic pressure does fall progressively during gestation, and this fall is greater in women with preeclampsia and is worsened by administration of large volumes of crystalloid during peripartum management.[90, 91] The largest fall in oncotic pressure was noted approximately 18 hours following delivery. This hypooncotic state probably does predispose to lung edema formation. There is no convincing evidence that lung permeability is significantly altered by pregnancy per se. Finally, a number of authors have speculated on the role of catecholamines in producing pulmonary edema in pregnancy,[87] particularly since sympathomimetic agents used for tocolysis can cause lung edema and respiratory failure.

Amniotic Fluid Embolism

Regardless of susceptibility to edema formation, a number of well-recognized causes of acute pulmonary edema have been described. One of the more dramatic presentations is that of amniotic fluid embolism. The incidence of this obstetric catastrophe has been estimated at between 1 in 8,000 and 1 in 80,000[92] and despite its relative rarity amniotic fluid embolism is estimated to account for 1% to 10% of maternal deaths in the United States.[93] Several excellent reviews of

the subject are available,[94, 95] and the remainder of the discussion focuses on amniotic fluid embolism as an example of the clinical dilemma of determining etiology in pregnant patients with pulmonary edema as well as a useful model for treatment approaches to hypoxemic respiratory failure.

Morgan[94] reviewed 272 cases where survival was but 14%, perhaps related to an unwillingness to make the diagnosis except in the most severely ill patients, and thus selecting for those with poor outcome. In addition, this series includes many patients whose management predates modern intensive care. If less advanced disease is recognized and treatment initiated at an earlier point, outcome may improve significantly. The mechanisms of lung and circulatory failure in amniotic fluid embolism are unclear. Amniotic fluid and particulate matter (lanugo hairs, meconium, fat, fetal squamae) may enter the maternal venous circulation via endocervical or uterine veins or at the placental site itself. At least in animals, the amniotic fluid itself may not be sufficient to cause all manifestations of the syndrome—as evidenced by the fact that filtered fluid is relatively innocuous in less than massive amounts.[96] This finding incriminates cellular and other debris present in the fluid embolus as a cause of either mechanical obstruction or a trigger to a maternal systemic reaction. Other possible contributors include prostaglandins present in the fluid or the ability of the embolized fluid to initiate an anaphylactoid reaction. Various risk factors have been reported: (1) tumultuous labor; (2) use of uterine stimulants; (3) meconium in the amniotic fluid; (4) advanced maternal age; (5) multiparity; and (6) intrauterine death, but these risks were identified in retrospective reviews and not all authors agree on the significance of these associations.[94, 95] It is also important to note that while the majority of cases occur as catastrophic complications after difficult labor and delivery, this entity has been reported after normal labor and delivery and has been thought to occur as early as 20 weeks of gestation in the absence of labor.[97]

The clinical manifestations of amniotic fluid embolism are dominated by shock, bleeding secondary to DIC in as many as 40% of patients, and pulmonary edema with respiratory failure.[94, 95] Circulatory failure has been ascribed to various pathophysiologic processes and indeed may vary from patient to patient or over time. Some authors emphasize a component of acute right heart strain, presumed due to embolization of the pulmonary vascular bed and the actions of hypoxia and other mediators to give hypoxic vasoconstriction. Data consistent with this are the acute elevation of pulmonary artery pressure, elevation of the central venous pressures suggesting right heart failure, and the development of hypoperfused state.[95] Certainly in other circumstances, such as thromboembolic disease and right ventricular infarction, acute right ventricular dysfunction appears to be central to the circulatory failure observed. Others have noted elevation of PCWP and a minimal increase in the pulmonary artery diastolic–PCWP (PAD-PCWP) pressure gradient, suggesting that left ventricular dysfunction is more significant than acute right heart failure.[95, 98] While the observation of an elevated PCWP can occur in right heart failure accompanied by a shift of the interventricular septum with compromise of left ventricular volume and diastolic compliance, the latter observation of a small PAD-PCWP pressure difference suggests little change in pulmonary vascular resistance. Albeit made in a limited number of patients undergoing invasive hemodynamic monitoring, these measurements are consistent with some contribution of left ventricular dysfunction. To the extent this is present, the mechanism is unclear.

Management of Amniotic Fluid Embolism.—Initial management of patients with amniotic fluid embolism and cardiovascular collapse is provision of an airway, administration of 100% oxygen and mechanical ventilation to reverse any adverse circulatory effects of hypoxia, as well as treating the frequently present DIC. Again, volume is a suggested first-line therapy until pulmonary artery catheterization can be used to better characterize the circulation. Echocardiography is also useful in determining the degree of pump failure of each ventricle, and informs decisions as to whether or not inotropic support with dobutamine is indicated. The pulmonary artery catheter is also useful from a diagnostic point of view. Pulmonary arterial blood can be sampled and examined cytologically for evidence of abnormal amniotic fluid components—fetal squamous cells, lanugo hairs, etc.[99] This information is very useful to support a diagnosis of amniotic fluid embolism, since pulmonary thromboembolic disease can mimic the cardiovascular presentation. Demonstration of these amniotic fluid elements in the maternal pulmonary circulation is not sufficient to make this diagnosis, however, since they have been observed in patients undergoing pulmonary artery catheterization for other reasons with no manifestations of significant pulmonary arterial embolization.[100] The key elements in diagnosis remain the clinical features of cardiovascular collapse, DIC, and pulmonary edema with acute hypoxemic respiratory failure. Twenty-five percent of these patients, especially those who survive the initial several hours, develop pulmonary edema. The appropriate ventilator and cardiovascular management of these patients will be discussed below.

Tocolytic-Associated and Other Forms of Pulmonary Edema

Other causes of pulmonary edema associated with pregnancy include tocolytic therapy with sympathomimetic amines, eclampsia and other hypertensive disorders, and acid aspiration. In our experience, pulmonary edema associated with tocolytic agents is the most common form of hypoxemic respiratory failure seen during pregnancy. It has been estimated to occur in as many as 4.4% of patients receiving these drugs.[101] Most cases described have resulted from the use of intravenous β-mimetics, particularly ritodrine, terbutaline, isoxuprine, or salbutamol.[101, 102] Some of these patients were receiving concurrent corticosteroids or magnesium sulfate, but these agents are not thought to contribute significantly to the development of lung edema. The incidence of this syndrome is higher in women with twin gestations and most women have intact membranes at presentation. When pulmonary edema develops post partum, the vast majority of cases are encountered within 12 hours of delivery. The development of pulmonary edema more than 24 hours after the discontinuation of these drugs should prompt a search for another cause.[101]

It appears that some alteration related to pregnancy predisposes women to this complication, since it has never been reported during the treatment of asthma with similar high doses of β-agonists. Left ventricular function was normal in those patients assessed echocardiographically and with invasive monitoring.[101] Some authors have speculated that these drugs are capable of producing a pulmonary capillary leak, but data for this are lacking and indeed in animal models β$_2$-sympathomimetic drugs may decrease capillary leakage in the lung and enhance lung liquid clearance.[103, 104] Volume overload may play a very significant role in these patients since (1) large volumes of crystalloid are often given for the reflex tachycardia resulting from sympathomimetic drugs; (2) colloid oncotic pressure is reduced peripartum, increasing susceptibility to hydrostatic edema formation; (3) sodium and water excretion may be impaired in the supine pregnant patient; (4) intravascular volume expansion is an expected alteration of pregnancy; (5) tocolytic agents may increase arginine vasopressin secretion and thus impair water balance; and (6) the response to diuresis is prompt in these patients.[101]

Virtually all patients will manifest tachypnea and tachycardia with crepitations on lung auscultation. Substernal chest pain is noted in approximately 25% of patients.[101] Positive fluid balance is often noted in the hours to days preceding the onset of symptoms. In the largest collected series,[101] the mean arterial PO_2 on room air was 50.4 ±2.9 mm Hg with a PCO_2 of 28.1 ±2.1 mm Hg. This disorder can usually be readily distinguished from acute thromboembolic disease, acid aspiration, and amniotic fluid embolism on the basis of the history and clinical findings.

Clinicians should be aware that the course of this disease is usually benign and that invasive monitoring is not warranted. In the series collected by Pisani and Rosenow,[101] there were only two maternal deaths (3%) and fetal survival was 95%. Patients should be moved to a closely monitored setting such as the intensive care unit. Treatment should consist of discontinuation of tocolytic therapy, oxygen administration to achieve at least 90% saturation of arterial hemoglobin, and diuresis. Response is usually obvious within 12 hours, with resolution of tachypnea and hypoxemia reliable end points for titration of diuretics.

Pulmonary edema can also complicate hypertension.[105, 106] In most cases this appears to be due to excessive volume expansion and elevation of the PCWP, although components of left ventricular failure secondary to increased afterload and even increased lung permeability have been suggested. Regardless of the degree of lung permeability or the component of increased hydrostatic pressure accompanying circulatory abnormalities, it is likely the low oncotic pressure of pregnancy and preeclampsia contributes significantly to edema formation in these patients.[90, 91]

Finally, aspiration is an uncommon but well-described and ominous complication of the peripartum period.[107] The injury due to aspiration of gastric contents is related to the volume of aspirated material, its acidity, the presence of particulate material, the bacterial burden of the aspirated material, and host resistance to subsequent infection.[108] Early injury is a chemical pneumonitis, the extent of which is determined primarily by acidity (pH <6) and volume of aspirate.[109] Some of these patients evolve over several hours to diffuse lung injury with ARDS.[110] A late complication of aspiration 24 to 72 hours after the event is the evolution to bacterial pneumonia, which tends to be focal and polymicrobial.[111]

Management

Pulmonary edema of any cause results in

severe gas exchange abnormalities as well as diminished lung compliance, the latter resulting in increased work of breathing. The patient is severely hypoxemic—her fetus is at risk—and the increased work of breathing places her at risk for progression to respiratory muscle fatigue. Appropriate management should include rapid diagnosis of the etiology of the pulmonary edema, treatment of related disease, and stabilization of the patient with oxygen and mechanical ventilation as necessary. Determination of etiology as either "high"- or "low"-pressure edema is most readily done with pulmonary artery catheterization and measurement of the PCWP. Not all patients will require this intervention—those with evidence of uncomplicated volume overload can undergo an empiric trial of diuresis—but the most severely ill patients can benefit from this information gathering since measurement of vascular pressures helps direct attention to the possibilities of either cardiac dysfunction or direct lung injury, and titration of therapy over time can be enhanced by serial measurement of cardiac output, mixed venous oxygen saturation, and calculation of shunt fraction. In those patients requiring intubation and mechanical ventilation, another useful clue to the cause of pulmonary edema is measurement of the protein content of endotracheal tube suckings—patients with excessive hydrostatic pressure driving edemagenesis will manifest a transudate with low protein content; patients with ARDS typically exhibit a high protein content, close to that of plasma, in the fluid flooding alveoli and the airways.[112]

A patient with pulmonary edema that does not improve rapidly with diuresis should be considered for elective intubation and mechanical ventilation. Clinical information suggesting that this is necessary includes respiratory rates in excess of 30, difficulty achieving arterial saturation with increasing concentrations of oxygen by mask delivery system, and any evidence of respiratory muscle fatigue or circulatory instability complicating acute hypoxemic respiratory failure.

Once intubated, the patient should be placed on 100% oxygen and mechanically ventilated with small tidal volumes (7–8 mL/kg) and high respiratory rates of 24 to 30/min. The low tidal volume approach is preferred because lung stiffness caused by pulmonary edema, as well as the abdominal factors of pregnancy, will cause airway pressures to be high, risking barotrauma. With these guidelines for tidal volume, proximal peak airway pressures can usually be maintained at less than 45 cm H_2O. The pregnant patient should also be placed in a lateral decubitus position to prevent limitation of venous return.

In patients with severe edema and intrapulmonary shunts greater than 30% to 40%, it is difficult to achieve adequate saturation of arterial hemoglobin without resorting to toxic levels of supplemental oxygen.[86] The response of various levels of shunt to supplemental oxygen is shown in Figure 7–7. Note that with shunts approaching 50%, administration of 100% oxygen fails to achieve 90% saturation of arterial blood. Accordingly, positive end-expiratory pressure (PEEP) is added to the ventilator circuit to redistribute lung water out of gas-exchanging regions to reduce shunt and to permit reduction of inspired oxygen to nontoxic levels. There has been considerable debate on the optimal FiO_2 for patients who have substantial lung injury and we recommend titration of PEEP in the early hours of mechanical ventilation aiming at rapidly achieving an FiO_2 of 0.6 or less.

Since PEEP redistributes fluid from the alveoli to the perivascular peribronchiolar interstitial spaces, effectively recruiting alveoli that are collapsed or flooded, improvement in gas exchange is paralleled by improved lung compliance. Therefore, a convenient method of titrating PEEP is to follow lung compliance as measured at the bedside, while incremental PEEP additions are made [respiratory system compliance = tidal volume/(pause airway pressure − PEEP)]. As alveolar recruitment is achieved, compliance will rise. Further additions of PEEP that do not achieve lung water redistribution and instead only increase lung volume will be associated with an unchanged or even reduced compliance. At this point elevated intrathoracic pressures may reduce venous return resulting in tachycardia and hypotension. Use of pulse oximetry during this maneuver will usually confirm improvement in arterial saturation and preclude the need for frequent sampling of arterial blood gases with the associated delay in achieving optimal ventilator settings. Once the shunt has been reduced, FiO_2 can be lowered to achieve 90% to 95% saturation of arterial blood. This approach to adjustment of PEEP and administered oxygen can be applied to optimize the patient in less than 1 hour.[86]

Results from both animal and human

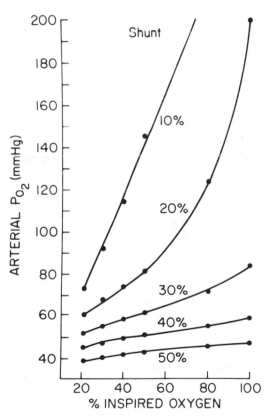

FIG 7–7.
The response of arterial oxygen pressure (PO_2) to changes in the percent of inspired oxygen is shown for varying degrees of intrapulmonary shunt. Note that with large shunts (>30%), there is little change in arterial PO_2 as expired oxygen rises from room air (21%) to 100% oxygen.

studies indicate that PEEP does not reduce total lung water but causes redistribution of water and reduction of shunt.[113] While this is an important intervention, it is but a temporizing measure and, in effect, an escalation of dangerous supportive therapy. Accordingly, once the patient is stabilized, one attempts to reduce lung water. Of course, underlying diseases such as sepsis require therapy. In cases of high-pressure pulmonary edema, most commonly encountered in some preeclamptic patients or the patient with underlying cardiomyopathy, reduction of hydrostatic pressures with diuretics, vasoactive drugs to cause pooling of blood in venous capacitance vessels, and reduction of left ventricular afterload with inotropic support of systolic dysfunction will often rapidly and dramatically improve lung function.[86] Management in low-pressure pulmonary edema is less generally agreed upon. If the mechanisms responsible for the development and continuation of a pulmonary capillary leak were better understood, interventions to break the pathophysiologic sequence of events could be rationalized. Although activation of neutrophils and conceivably lung macrophages play an important role in acute lung injury, prospective trials of agents such as corticosteroids intended to blunt lung injury failed to demonstrate benefit to patients with ARDS.[64, 114] We would argue that the reported trial of corticosteroids in aspiration in nonpregnant patients[114] was hampered by delay of therapy in most patients studied. For the gravid patient, when aspiration is witnessed and therapy can be instituted immediately, we agree with administration of methylprednisolone or an equivalent agent at a dose of 1 g every 6 hours for a total of four doses. Clearly, once pulmonary edema is apparent, this therapy is not indicated.

Our own approach to the circulation in patients with pulmonary edema of any type has been to attempt to reduce PCWP within the limits of an adequate cardiac output.[86, 113] This will reduce the driving pressure to edemagenesis and ideally shorten the duration of potentially dangerous supportive therapy. In making circulatory interventions in patients with low-pressure pulmonary edema, measurements such as cardiac output, mixed venous oxygen tension and saturation, shunt fraction, and PCWP are useful and hence pulmonary artery catheterization is indicated. First one must determine if the patient with low-pressure edema has an adequate cardiac output. A widened AV-O_2 difference (>5 vol%), lactic acidosis, oliguria, and diminished mental status all support the existence of a hypoperfused state, and volume infusion or vasoactive drug administration must be considered. In patients with sepsis and hypotension, if markers of gross tissue hypoperfusion are not present, volume infusion should be used sparingly, if at all, since associated low-pressure edema is likely to worsen.

In those patients with an adequate circulation and pulmonary edema leading to respiratory failure, a cautious reduction of PCWP can be attempted, despite "normal" ventricular filling pressures. Volume reduction can be achieved by various interventions, including phlebotomy and reinfusion of cells to maintain circulating hemoglobin, plasmapheresis, or diuresis. We recommend an approach of seeking the lowest PCWP consistent with an adequate cardiac output, as judged by vital signs, mentation, urine volume, and absence of lactic acidosis. When diuretics are used, interpretation of urine volume and electrolytes is compromised.

In nonpregnant patients, reduction of PCWP to a point of borderline circulatory adequacy can be achieved, and vasoactive drugs such as dobutamine are then used to provide adequate perfusion at a low intravascular volume in an effort to hasten resolution of lung edema, but vasoactive drugs may not be warranted, given our limited knowledge of their effects on uterine and placental blood flow. Nonetheless, many patients can tolerate significant volume reduction with preservation of tissue perfusion.

These general principles of management are enumerated in Table 7–11. With this approach, the patient with acute hypoxemic respiratory failure can be stabilized on the

TABLE 7–11.
Treatment of Low-Pressure Pulmonary Edema (ARDS)

Identify underlying disorders and treat
Early elective intubation
Mechanical ventilation with low tidal volumes and high rates
Least PEEP to achieve 90% saturation of circulating hemoglobin with a nontoxic Fio$_2$
Seek the lowest PCWP consistent with an adequate cardiac output

---

ARDS = adult respiratory distress syndrome; PEEP = positive end-expiratory pressure; Fio$_2$ = fractional concentration of oxygen in inspired gas; PCWP = pulmonary capillary wedge pressure.

ventilator, treated for lung edema, and returned to spontaneous ventilation. Patient resumption of an increased amount of the work of breathing can begin when the intrapulmonary shunt has fallen to 20% or less with less than 5 cm H_2O PEEP. This is a point at which hypoxemia can be prevented with the amount of supplemental oxygen provided by mask systems. Prolonged periods of "weaning" from the ventilator are usually not necessary unless there are intercurrent problems such as diminished drive to breathe, respiratory muscle dysfunction, or persistent abnormalities of lung mechanics. One should also be aware that these severely ill patients do not always require emergent delivery. We have reported a patient with severe hypoxemic respiratory failure requiring mechanical ventilation and PEEP who was stabilized, improved with cautious diuresis, and underwent spontaneous vaginal delivery of a healthy infant while still undergoing mechanical ventilation.[115]

Bacterial Pneumonia

There is one subset of patients with severe hypoxemia requiring a different approach. Patients with acute bacterial lobar pneumonia can experience large intrapulmonary shunts, since the acute inflammation accompanying lung consolidation results in a doubling of blood flow to the involved lung. As a consequence, shunt fractions of 40% and greater are seen.[85] This is an example of nonhomogeneous shunt lung disease, in distinction to the homogeneous lesion of pulmonary edema. In pneumonia, attempts to use PEEP to reduce shunt may have adverse effects. If PEEP results in an increase of lung volume and increase in alveolar pressure in the normally compliant uninvolved lung, alveolar pressures may rise above vascular pressures with a redirection of blood flow to the consolidated lung. This will result in increased shunt and worsened hypoxemia. While the specific bacterial pneumonias are discussed in Chapter 6, the appropriate supportive therapy would be limitation of PEEP therapy, positioning of the patient with noninvolved lung in the dependent position to maximize blood flow to these regions and minimize shunt, and use of high inspired fractions of oxygen for the first 12 to 36 hours, awaiting resolution of the inflammatory phase of the disease. Limited studies in animals have demonstrated actions of prostaglandin inhibitors that may improve gas exchange in lobar pneumonia,[116] but we do not advocate their use in pregnancy because of the possibility of deleterious effects upon the fetus, with ductus arteriosus closure.

MAINTENANCE OF THE INTERNAL ENVIRONMENT

While early death due to hypoxemia is effectively prevented by institution of the therapies outlined above, mortality in disorders such as ARDS remains very high, due to other complications such as malnutrition, nosocomial infection, renal failure, gastrointestinal hemorrhage, airway injury, barotrauma, and thromboembolic disease.[117] Several of these issues will be detailed below with the aim of establishing a physician-directed effort to maintain the appropriate milieu in which recovery from critical illness can occur. The use of prophylactic therapy to prevent thromboembolic complications in the hospitalized gravid patient is described in Chapter 6 text and we will not discuss it here.

Acid-Base Status

As noted, acid-base status in pregnancy is best characterized as that of compensated respiratory alkalosis in which P_{CO_2} and bicarbonate average 30 mm Hg and 18 to 20 mEq/L respectively. While buffering capacity may be preserved, decrements in ventilation with elevation of the P_{CO_2} to prepregnancy levels will result in acidosis. Renal acid excretion in pregnancy appears to be normal.[118] Several descriptive studies have provided information regarding fetal acid-base state during normal labor and delivery.[119] Summarizing these data, in early labor fetal pH averages 7.30 with a P_{CO_2} of 45 mm Hg, with a fall in pH to 7.20 immediately after delivery. This pH drop is largely attributable to a metabolic acidosis, which resolves over the first 60 minutes of neonatal life.

Management

The management of maternal acid-base disturbances should entail several considerations. Exaggeration of the physiologic respiratory alkalosis in the mother carries a theoretical risk of shifting the oxygen-hemoglobin dissociation curve to the left with increased affinity for oxygen and potential interference with off-loading of oxygen to the fetus. While this theoretical possibility has been raised in discussions of a number of critical illnesses, it has never been demonstrated to be clinically relevant. In addition, carbon dioxide diffuses rapidly across the placenta, with a tendency for maintenance of the maternal-fetal gradient. Further leftward shift of the fetal hemoglobin saturation curve may preserve fetal oxygen carrying capacity. Consistent with this compensation is the report by Miller et al.[120] that fetal P_{O_2} decreased only 4 torr when mothers hyperventilated in labor, despite significant increases in maternal and fetal plasma pH. A greater concern regarding alkalosis is that uteroplacental blood flow might be decreased, creating fetal asphyxia on a low flow basis. Experimental data suggesting this occurs was reviewed above in conjunction with the discussion of mechanical ventilation[82, 83] and clearly *hyperventilation causing acute respiratory alkalosis on the ventilator should be avoided.* Additionally, maternal metabolic alkalosis has been shown in animal models to significantly decrease placental blood flow and fetal carotid PO_2.[121, 122] Since most severe metabolic alkalosis in the critically ill is related to treatment phenomena—alkali administration, gastric fluid loss with nasogastric suction, use of diuretics and steroids—careful attention to these therapeutic interventions should prevent most difficulties or permit correction at an early point.

Acidosis may be poorly tolerated by the fetus. Early intervention with mechanical ventilation prior to evolution of hypercapnea and severe acidosis is indicated in gravidas, remembering that a PCO_2 of 40 mm Hg already represents considerable hypercarbia. This is of paramount importance in the patient with an acute load upon the respiratory system, such as status asthmaticus; with diminished drive to breathe, such as drug overdose; or who is manifesting circulatory inadequacy with progressive lactic acidosis. Controlled mechanical ventilation in these circumstances should permit the physician to guarantee an adequate level of ventilation to minimize the extent of acidosis.

Maternal metabolic acidosis occurs in normal labor and delivery, probably as a result of hyperventilation and other muscle activity with associated lactic acid production.[4] These maternal fixed acids pass rapidly to the fetus. The treatment of underlying maternal metabolic acidosis should, of course, be directed at the underlying process, and begin with a distinction between increased and normal anion gap acidoses. The use of bicarbonate to correct pH is controversial for both pregnant and nonpregnant patients.[4, 123, 124] With the administration of bicarbonate, serum carbon dioxide levels will rise and could cause increased acidosis intracellularly or in tissue beds with rapid diffusion of carbon dioxide but slower equilibration of charged species. This is likely to be the case across the placenta, which achieves rapid equilibration of carbon dioxide but a slow rise of fetal bicar-

bonate levels following infusion into the mother. For this reason, if correction of an underlying acidosis or delivery is likely to be achieved within hours, treatment with bicarbonate is not recommended.

Prevention of Gastrointestinal Hemorrhage

There is little to suggest that pregnancy itself results in abnormalities in gastric secretion or vulnerability of the upper gastrointestinal mucosa to ulceration, but critical illness is often complicated by gastric erosion and severe bleeding.[117] In the nonpregnant patient, a number of interventions have been recommended as prophylaxis against this common complication (see Table 7–12). All of them have at least theoretical problems for use in the critically ill pregnant patient.

Holdsworth et al.[125] have shown that the stomach can actually be divided into antral and fundal pouches by the enlarging uterus, making complete mixing of gastric contents unlikely. To the extent this phenomenon is important, agents such as antacids or sucralfate, which act by mixing and neutralizing gastric contents or by direct coating of the gastric mucosa, may fail as prophylaxis against gastric ulceration. On the other hand, histamine receptor blockers such as cimetidine and ranitidine have had limited use in pregnancy but appear to be sufficiently safe for these life-threatening situations. Cimetidine, but not ranitidine, has been shown to have antiandrogen activity and to cause fetal feminization.[126] Finally, a recent study of ulcer prophylaxis in postoperative patients revealed that agents acting to neutralize gastric

TABLE 7–12.
Regimens for Gastrointestinal Hemorrhage Prophylaxis

Agent	FDA Risk Category*	Dose
Sucralfate	B	1 g q4–6h
Antacids	B	q2–3h titrated to pH >4
Ranitidine	B	50 mg q6–8h IV
Cimetidine	B	300 mg q6h IV
*See Preface for description of FDA classification.		

pH (histamine blockers and antacids) resulted in colonization of the upper gastrointestinal tract with nosocomially acquired gram-negative organisms, with a trend toward greater risk for pneumonia with severe sequelae.[127] Should this observation be confirmed in subsequent studies including the pregnant patient, therapy with sucralfate or equivalent drugs might be preferable.

A synthesis of these observations would suggest no agent is ideal. Nonetheless, one safe approach is to start treatment with either sucralfate or antacids. These drugs are usually delivered by nasogastric tube in the critically ill. Periodic sampling of gastric pH should document a pH greater than 6 and no accumulation of gastric residuals. The nasogastric tube should not routinely be hooked to suction and sampling should be kept to a minimum unless evidence of gastric outlet obstruction is present. For patients unable to receive direct instillation of antacids or sucralfate to the stomach, therapy with ranitidine should be considered, particularly if the patient is near term, since this therapy is likely to be given for a relatively brief period of time and the benefits of reduction of risk for gastrointestinal hemorrhage are likely to outweigh fetal risks.

Nutrition

Pregnant patients have been managed with total parenteral nutrition (see Chap. 9) for extended periods of time for disorders such as inflammatory bowel disease, esophageal stricture, and malignancy, but more acute malnutrition such as that associated with critical illness is less well described.[128] Nonetheless, our own impression is that in brief periods of time the pregnant patient without nutritional repletion will become extremely catabolic in the intensive care environment, and our own approach calls for aggressive and early supportive therapy. Accordingly, patients who have not returned to a condition permitting normal oral intake within 3 days of the onset of critical illness should be assessed for nutritional support. Whenever possible, the gut should be used with either bolus gastric feedings by nasogastric tube or duodenal infusions by soft feeding tube. Pregnancy alone will result in calorie requirements close to 40 kcal/kg/day; sepsis, trauma, burns, and recent surgery are likely to increase this requirement. If severe liver disease is not present, 1.5 g/kg/day of protein and approximately 20% of calories administered as lipids are recommended. A variety of enteral feeding supplements will achieve these goals with tolerable infusion rates. Finally, electrolyte disorders are common in patients so managed, and careful attention must be paid to serum calcium, phosphate and magnesium levels with additional supplements given as necessary.

Patients who do not tolerate enteral feeding will require total parenteral nutrition. The same guidelines for total calories and distribution of calories as lipids, carbohydrates, and protein can be used. Some have raised theoretical concerns about the use of intravenous fat emulsions in pregnancy due to possible placental infarction secondary to fat emboli,[129] but such complications have not been reported, and fat emulsions are utilized in our institution.

MISCELLANEOUS DISORDERS

Anaphylaxis

Anaphylaxis is uncommon in the general population and reports in pregnancy are entirely anecdotal.[130] It may occur via an IgE-mediated mechanism, in which a sensitized individual manifests an acute allergic reaction upon antigenic exposure.[131] Various agents, most prominently contrast dyes, are capable of producing a similar clinical picture without antigen-antibody interactions. Under these latter conditions the reaction is often termed "anaphylactoid."

The usual setting in which anaphylaxis is encountered is following insect stings, ingestion of foodstuffs to which the patient is sensitized, and administration of xenogenic sera, contrast media, or various drugs, most especially antibiotics. The clinical manifestations involve the following organ systems: (1) gastrointestinal—with nausea, vomiting, and cramping prominent; (2) skin—with urticaria and pruritus the most common manifestations; (3) respiratory—with laryngedema and airway obstruction as well as bronchospasm seen; and (4) cardiovascular—with vascular collapse and shock. Any combination of these organ system involvements is possible. In pregnancy, the fetus is protected from antibody-mediated phenomena since minimal amounts of IgE cross the placenta. Nonetheless the fetus is at risk if maternal shock or asphyxia occurs.

When recognized, treatment differs little from that in nonpregnant patients and should include (1) intensive care unit monitoring, even in patients with minor skin and gastrointestinal complaints, because of the possibility of progression to more life-threatening manifestations; (2) direct pharmacologic intervention to halt and reverse the allergic reaction; and (3) supportive therapy if airway patency or circulatory adequacy are compromised.[132] For minor manifestations 0.3 to 0.5 mL of epinephrine 1:1000 can be administered subcutaneously concurrently with diphenhydramine, 50 mg intramuscularly. Other histamine blockers, such as ranitidine, have been suggested for use in anaphylaxis but their efficacy is unproven.

In patients with more severe reactions or progression despite the therapy outlined above, epinephrine can be repeated at 10- to 20-minute intervals and 1:10,000 epinephrine can be given intravenously at a dose of 1 to 10 μg/kg as a rapid infusion. Cardiac rhythm must be monitored throughout. Oxygen should be administered and assessment for upper airway obstruction or bronchospasm made. If necessary, the upper airway should be secured by intubation. If present, bronchospasm can be treated with inhaled β-agonists, continued epinephrine administration, aminophylline, and corticosteroids. The last-named would not be expected to be effective for 12 to 24 hours. Finally, if shock develops, aggressive fluid repletion should be carried out with management of the patient in lateral recumbency. If shock persists, agents such as dopamine at high doses (>10 μg/kg/min) or neosynephrine can be given to restore vascular tone. This treatment plan and the appropriate drug doses are outlined in Table 7–13.

TABLE 7–13.
Treatment of Anapyhylaxis

1. Minor manifestations
   A. Epinephrine, 0.3–0.5 mL of 1:1,000 SC, every 30 min
   B. Diphenhydramine, 50 mg IM
2. Major manifestations
   A. Secure an airway
   B. Maximal FIO_2*
   C. Epinephrine, 1:10,000 IV at 1–10 μg/kg
   D. Methylprednisolone, 250 mg
   E. Volume infusion
   F. Consider α agents (dopamine, neosynephrine) for persistent hypotension only *after* volume therapy

*FIO_2 = fractional concentration of oxygen in inspired gas.

Drug Overdose

While drug overdose producing altered mental status, respiratory depression, circulatory or cardiac rhythm instability, or metabolic irregularities is a common cause of admission to the intensive care unit, the magnitude of this problem in the pregnant population is not entirely clear. Thus, while 47% of nearly 200,000 calls to the Poison Control Center of Children's Hospital of Michigan during 1980–1983 were in women, only 111 or 0.07% pertained to drug overdose in pregnancy.[133] Nonetheless, the problem of drug overdose in pregnancy is likely to be encountered in any busy medical center. It is important to note that the general supportive care of these patients is similar for most agents, and indeed maternal outcome is more likely to be determined by the presence or absence and course of respiratory and cardiovascular complications than from the direct drug effects. We will therefore describe general management principles[134] and then discuss a number of agents in greater detail.

Most drug intoxications result from ingestion or intravenous administration, although inhalation of agents, particularly cocaine, is also seen. In cases of oral ingestion, evacuation of the gastrointestinal tract is important, although some would argue against removal of a petroleum product or caustic substance from the stomach.[134, 135] If the patient is fully alert and cooperative, ipecac can be used to induce emesis. If any obtundation is present, particularly early after ingestion and hence likely to progress, evacuation of gastric contents should be conducted after securing an airway. With the airway controlled and protected with an endotracheal tube, a 30–36 F Ewald tube can be used to lavage the stomach clear. Gastric contents can be analyzed for type of pill fragment and toxicologic studies performed for drug identification. It is often the case in the obtunded and uncooperative patient that further sedation is necessary to achieve intubation and manage the patient early on. This is usually sufficient, in addition to the drug ingestion, to suppress ventilatory drive and mandate a period of mechanical ventilation. Ventilatory parameters should be established as described above, targeting eucapnea (in the pregnant patient a PCO_2 of 30 mm Hg is a typical goal) and a PO_2 greater than 60 mm Hg.

Most patients should receive activated charcoal when the stomach is lavaged clear, to bind remaining drug and to absorb the many drug metabolites that are present in the small bowel due to enterohepatic circulation. Charcoal administration can be repeated every 4 to 6 hours followed by an agent such as magnesium citrate to speed gut transit time. Since many drugs can result in significant ileus, the patient must be carefully examined prior to each administration of these agents to prevent undue gastric and bowel distention, with the possible complications of vomiting and aspiration.

Many drug ingestions are polypharmaceutical and self-poisoned patients often give unreliable histories.[136] Thus it is important to seek history from family, police, paramedics,

outside physicians and pharmacists, and observers at the scene as guides to management. Standard references such as the *Poison Index* or regional and national poison control centers accessed by phone are available to identify likely complications and approaches to unusual agents.

Acetaminophen

Acetaminophen should be considered in all drug overdoses since specific antidote therapy is available to blunt the major toxicity of hepatic necrosis.[137–140] If toxicology screens of the blood, urine, or gastric lavage indicate the presence of acetaminophen, maternal serum levels should be determined 12 hours after ingestion. If these levels are above 30 to 40 $\mu g/mL$, treatment with N-acetylcysteine should be started. Nomograms for serum levels at various other times after ingestion are available,[138] although they are based on nonpregnant and even pediatric populations. While experience with acetylcysteine in human pregnancy is largely anecdotal,[137, 139, 140] its use appears warranted if risk of substantial liver injury is present. It is given as a loading dose of 140 mg/kg of a 20% solution, followed by 70 mg/kg every 4 hours for 3 days. If the gastrointestinal tract cannot be used, intravenous administration is possible.[141]

Tricyclic Antidepressants

The growing use of tricyclic antidepressants has resulted in their prominent involvement in drug intoxications. Major toxicities are central nervous system depression, cardiac arrhythmias, cardiovascular collapse, and convulsions.[142] Serum levels are difficult to correlate to risk for major complications but the electrocardiogram at the time of admission to the intensive care unit is useful in this regard. If significant QT interval widening is present, patients are at greater risk for seizures and dysrhythmias.[143] QT widening in and of itself should not be treated with antiarrhythmics but defines a group at risk for development of ventricular ectopy, heart block, and ventricular fibrillation. Management of this overdose would not vary substantially in the pregnant patient. For refractory ventricular arrhythmias phenytoin has been recommended, given as a 10- to 15-mg/kg loading dose over 30 to 40 minutes. Physostigmine has been suggested by some authors for the anticholinergic side effects of these medications (dry mouth, constipation and ileus, urinary retention, tremor, hypertension, hyperthermia, sweating, mydriasis) and even for cardiac toxicity. We do not recommend its routine use. To maintain central nervous system and cardiac function it is extremely important that the patient not become acidotic, since this appears to potentiate toxicity to these organ systems. Thus, ventilatory support should be instituted prior to evolution of hypercapnea, and metabolic acidosis can be treated with slow bicarbonate infusions, if underlying causes cannot be quickly reversed. Arterial blood pH should be maintained at 7.4.

Salicylates

Salicylates are widely available agents that cause a range of clinical abnormalities.[144, 145] The severity of intoxication can be crudely predicted by serum levels taken in the first 6 hours after ingestion. Mild intoxication, usually correlating to serum levels of 30 to 60 mg/dL, is associated with tinnitus, dizziness, headache, and nausea. Hyperventilation is common. As serum levels reach 60 to 90 mg/dL, speech is often slurred, hallucinations can occur, and laboratory irregularities include metabolic acidosis and hypoglycemia. Severe intoxication results from serum levels in excess of 90 mg/dL, with convulsion, coma, pulmonary edema, and worsening metabolic acidosis common findings.

In addition to routine therapy for evacuation of the gastrointestinal tract, several therapeutic interventions are important. Hypoglycemia is present in many patients and blood glucose levels must be closely monitored. Pulmonary edema has been described after massive aspirin ingestion and can result in ARDS. Finally, since salicylates are eliminated by a renal route, excretion can be enhanced by forced diuresis with an alkalinizing solution although, as has been discussed, excessive bicarbonate administration may have adverse consequences on fetal acid-base state and arterial pH should not exceed 7.5.

Cocaine

Given the recent epidemic of cocaine use, it is not surprising to find an ever-growing literature describing acute and chronic toxicities. Chasnoff et al.[146] described a number of pregnant women using cocaine chronically and although not a prospective collection of data there did appear to be an increased risk of abortion among users and possibly an increased incidence of abruptio placentae (also see Chapter 17, Drug Abuse). A number of acute complications of use have been described and include seizures, subarachnoid hemorrhage, myocardial infarction, rhabdomyolysis, cardiac arrhythmias, and renal failure.[147, 148] Increasing observations of poor fetal outcome are likely since the drug not only affects maternal central hemodynamics but has been reported to reduce placental perfusion. Cocaine also crosses the placenta with direct fetal affects. One case report has suggested precipitation of intracranial hemorrhage in a fetus.[149] Critical care physicians should include the possibility of cocaine abuse in their approach to the pregnant patient with central nervous system, circulatory, or renal crises.

Trauma

The incidence of trauma in pregnancy ranges from 6% to 8%[150] with the majority of injuries being minor sprains and lacerations. Nonetheless, death from accidents accounts for 22% of nonobstetric maternal mortality. The causes of major injury include motor vehicle accidents, falls, and penetrating trauma.[151] Certain physiologic changes of pregnancy are important in terms of evaluation and treatment following trauma.[151] Borderline tachycardia may be attributable to pregnancy itself as opposed to indicating loss of blood volume and supine hypotension can result from vena caval obstruction by the normal uterus in late pregnancy. The blood volume expansion by as much as 40% to 50% by the 28th week of gestation must be recognized during evaluation of traumatized pregnant patients, since the usual clinical signs of hypovolemia are insensitive until intravascular volume is reduced 15% to 25%, signaling enormous blood loss in this patient group. The tendency for aspiration to occur during emergent management of the airway has been commented upon.[77-79] Displacement of the urinary bladder into the abdominal cavity beyond 12 weeks of gestation makes it a target for injury, and displacement of abdominal contents cephalad makes visceral injury likely with penetrating trauma of the upper abdomen. Pregnancy may mask findings of peritoneal irritation. Rothenberger et al.[152] reported 12 pregnant patients receiving peritoneal lavage for evaluation of blunt abdominal trauma. Only 2 of these patients exhibited abdominal signs or symptoms, yet 8 had positive lavage and all 8 were positive at laparotomy for intraabdominal bleeding or injury. Finally, there are injuries unique to pregnancy, including placental abruption, uterine rupture, and fetal trauma.

Fetal injuries are uncommon in blunt trauma. Skull fracture has been reported with maternal pelvic fracture, apparently caused by torsion over the gravid uterus.[153] Placental abruption can occur with rapid deceleration injury, and rupture of the amniotic membranes should be sought during pelvic examination. If no vaginal blood or urine is present, phenapthazine (Nitrazine Paper) testing can identify amniotic fluid.[151] In the majority of cases vaginal bleeding will be present as a manifestation of abruption, although Kettel et al. reported several patients with "occult" abruption identified after significant delay following traumatic injury.[154] Abruption can be rapidly complicated by DIC, and evidence for this should be sought in all severely injured pregnant patients. Whether or not trauma involves the uterus, fetal mortality approaches 80% if shock ensues.[155]

Management should be directed first toward the mother, the initial efforts being to determine cardiorespiratory function and extent of injuries, and only then should fetal monitoring be considered. *Again, since maternal shock is the most likely cause of fetal death, the adequacy of the maternal circulation is paramount.* Modalities that are useful in early fetal monitoring include Doppler heart rate and ultrasound evaluation of fetus, placenta, and uterus. If significant hemorrhage is obvious, aggressive fluid replacement as discussed above for hemorrhagic shock is appropriate. Use of the MAST suit is appropriate for shock unresponsive to early fluid resuscitation. Once the patient is cleared for positioning she should be placed in lateral recumbency and uterine lift performed if shock is present. Since needle paracentesis is difficult in the second and third trimester, open peritoneal lavage may be preferable for assessment of blunt abdominal trauma.[156]

If despite all efforts directed at stabilization maternal death occurs with the fetus alive and undelivered, consideration should be made for postmortem cesarean section. Weber[157] reviewed the literature concerning this topic and surveyed over 150 cases. Outcome seemed crucially related to the duration of time between maternal death and delivery. If less than 5 minutes passed, fetal prognosis was excellent; 5 to 10 minutes, good; 10 to 15 minutes, fair; 15 to 20 minutes, poor; and if greater than 20 minutes, fetal survival was unlikely.

REFERENCES

1. Schumacker PT, Cain SM: The concept of a critical oxygen delivery. *Intensive Care Med* 1987; 13:223–229.
2. Kariman K, Burns SR: Regulation of tissue oxygen extraction is disturbed in the adult respiratory distress syndrome. *Am Rev Respir Dis* 1985; 132:109–114.
3. Weinberger SE, Weiss ST, Cohen WR, et al: State of the art: Pregnancy and the lung. *Am Rev Respir Dis* 1980; 121:559–581.
4. Albright GA, Ferguson JE II, Joyce TH III, et al: *Anesthesia in Obstretrics: Maternal, Fetal and Neonatal Aspects.* London, Butterworth Publishers, 1986, pp. 40–63.

5. de Swiet M: The cardiovascular system, in Hytten F, Chamberlain G (eds): *Clinical Phsyiology in Obstetrics.* Oxford, Blackwell Scientific Publications, 1980, pp 3–42.

6. Pernoll ML, Metcalfe J, Schlenker JL, et al: Oxygen consumption at rest and during exercise in pregnancy and postpartum. *Respir Physiol* 1975; 25:285–293.

7. Gemzell CA, Robbe H, Strom G, et al: Observations on circulatory changes and muscular work in normal labour. *Acta Obstet Gynecol Scand* 1957; 36:75–93.

8. Edelstone DI, Paulone ME, Maljovec JJ, et al: Effects of maternal anemia on cardiac output, systemic oxygen consumption, and regional blood flow in pregnant sheep. *Am J Obstet Gynecol* 1987; 156:740–748.

9. Paulone ME, Edelstone DI, Shedd A: Effects of maternal anemia on uteroplacental and fetal oxidative metabolism in sheep. *Am J Obstet Gynecol* 1987; 156:230–236.

10. Adamson K, Myers RE: Perinatal asphyxia—causes, detection, and neurologic sequelae. *Pediatr Clin North Am* 1973; 20:465–472.

11. Parer JT: Uteroplacental circulation and respiratory gas exchange, in Shnider SM, Levison G (eds): *Anesthesia for Obstetrics.* Baltimore, Williams & Wilkins Co, 1987, pp 14–21.

12. Myers RE: Two patterns of perinatal brain damage and their conditions of occurrence. *Am J Obstet Gynecol* 1972; 112:246–276.

13. Greiss FC Jr: Uterine blood flow in pregnancy: An overview, in Moawad AH, Lindheimer MD (eds): *Uterine and Placental Blood Flow.* New York, Masson Publishing, Inc, 1982, pp 19–28.

14. Robson SC, Hunter S, Boys RJ, et al: Serial study of factors influencing changes in cardiac output during human pregnancy. *Am J Physiol* 1989; 256:H1060–H1065.

15. Connors AF Jr, McCaffree R, Gray BA: Evaluation of right-heart catheterization in the critically ill patient without acute myocardial infarction. *N Engl J Med* 1983; 308:263–267.

16. Matthay MA, Chatterjee K: Bedside catheterization of the pulmonary artery: Risks compared with benefits. *Ann Intern Med* 1988; 1091:826–833.

17. Berkowitz RL, Rafferty TD: Invasive hemodynamic monitoring in critically ill pregnant patients: Role of Swan-Ganz catheterization. *Am J Obstet Gynecol* 1980; 137:127–135.

18. Helmkamp BF, Civetta JM, Girtanner R Jr, et al: The Swan-Ganz catheter and its application in the gynecologic patient. *Am J Obstet Gynecol* 1981; 139:628–635.

19. Clark SL, Cotton DB: Clinical indications for pulmonary artery catheterization in the patient with severe preeclampsia. *Am J Obstet Gynecol* 1988; 158:453–458.

20. Clinical Commentary: Pulmonary artery occlusion pressure: Clinical physiology, measurement, and interpretation. *Am Rev Respir Dis* 1983; 128:319–326.

21. Sharkey SW: Beyond the wedge: Clinical physiology and the Swan-Ganz catheter. *Am J Med* 1987; 83:111–120.

22. Elkayam U, Berkley R, Henry WL, et al: Cardiac output by thermodilution. *Chest* 1983; 84:418–421.

23. Watson P: Post-partum hemorrhage and shock. *Clin Obstet Gynecol* 1980; 23:985–1001.

24. Jackson FC: Accidental injury—the problem and the initiatives, in Buchsbaum JH (ed): *Trauma in Pregnancy.* Philadelphia, WB Saunders Co, 1979, p 120.

25. Abdella TN, Sibai BM, Hays JM Jr, et al: Relationship of hypertensive disease to abruptio placentae. *Obstet Gynecol* 1984; 63:365–370.

26. Pritchard JA: Haematological problems associated with delivery, placental abruption, retained dead fetus, and amniotic fluid embolism. *Clin Haematol* 1973; 2:563–586.

27. Hayashi RH: Hemorrhagic shock in obstetrics. *Clin Perinatol* 1986; 13:755–763.

28. Naeye RL: Abruptio placentae and placenta previa: Frequency, perinatal mortality, and cigarette smoking. *Obstet Gynecol* 1980; 55:701–704.

29. Cotton DB, Read JA, Paul RH, et al: The conservative aggressive management of placenta previa. *Am J Obstet Gynecol* 1980; 137:687–695.

30. Rackow EC, Falk JL, Fein LA: Fluid resuscitation in circulatory shock: A comparison of the cardiorespiratory effects of albumin, hetastarch, and saline solutions in patients with hypovolemic and septic

shock. *Crit Care Med* 1983; 11:839–844.

31. Hussain SNA, Roussos C: Distribution of respiratory muscle and organ blood flow during endotoxic shock in dogs. *J Appl Physiol* 1985; 59:1802–1808.

32. Gunning JE: For controlling intractable hemorrhage: The gravity suit. *Contemp Obstet Gynecol* 1983; 22:23–32.

33. Sandberg EC, Pelligra R: The medical antigravity suit for management of surgically uncontrollable bleeding associated with abdominal pregnancy. *Am J Obstet Gynecol* 1983; 146:519–525.

34. Gaffney FA, Thal ER, Taylor WF, et al: Hemodynamic effects of medical antishock trousers (MAST garment). *J Trauma* 1981; 21:931–936.

35. Consensus Conference: Fresh-frozen plasma. *JAMA* 1985; 253:551–554.

36. Angiographic arterial embolization to control hemorrhage in abdominal pregnancy: A case report. *Obstet Gynecol* 1988; 71:456–459.

37. Rosenthal DM, Colapinto R: Angiographic arterial embolization in the management of postoperative vaginal hemorrhage. *Am J Obstet Gynecol* 1985; 151:227–230.

38. Pais O, Glickman M, Schwartz P, et al: Embolization of pelvic arteries for control of postpartum hemorrhage. *Obstet Gynecol* 1980; 55:754–757.

39. Duvauferrier R, Priou G, Tasson D, et al: Emergency uterine embolization in postpartum hemorrhage secondary to coagulopathy. *J Radiol* 1984; 65:285–289.

40. Hankins GDV, Wendel GD, Leveno KJ, et al: Myocardial infarction during pregnancy: A review. *Obstet Gynecol* 1985; 69:139–146.

41. Homans DC: Peripartum cardiomyopathy. *N Engl J Med* 1985; 312:1432–1438.

42. Melvin KR, Richardson PJ, Olsen EGJ, et al: Peripartum cardiomyopathy due to myocarditis. *N Engl J Med* 1982; 307:731–735.

43. Lang RM, Fellner SK, Neumann A, et al: Left ventricular contractility varies directly with blood ionized calcium. *Ann Intern Med* 1988; 108:524–529.

44. Walley KR, Becker CJ, Hogan RA, et al: Progressive hypoxemia limits left ventricular oxygen consumption and contractility. *Circ Res* 1988; 63:849–859.

45. Leier CV, Unverferth V: Diagnosis and drugs five years later: Dobutamine. *Ann Intern Med* 1983; 99:490–496.

46. Leier CV, Heban PT, Huss P, et al: Comparative systemic and regional hemodynamic effects of dopamine and dobutamine in patients with cardiomyopathic heart failure. *Circulation* 1978; 58:466–475.

47. Fishburne JL, Meis PJ, Urban RB, et al: Vascular and uterine responses to dobutamine and dopamine in the gravid ewe. *Am J Obstet Gynecol* 1980; 137:944.

48. Levinson PD, Goldstein DS, Munson PJ, et al: Endocrine, renal and hemodynamic responses to graded dopamine infusions in normal men. *J Clin Endocrinol Metab* 1985; 60:821–826.

49. Kirshon B, Lee W, Mauer MB, et al: Effects of low-dose dopamine therapy in the oliguric patient with preeclampsia. *Am J Obstet Gynecol* 1988; 159:604–607.

50. Widerhorn J, Rubin JN, Frishman WH, et al: Cardiovascular drugs in pregnancy. *Cardiol Clin* 1987; 5:651–674.

51. Miller RR, Fennell WH, Young JB, et al: Differential systemic arterial and venous actions and consequent cardiac effects of vasodilator drugs. *Prog Cardiovasc Dis* 1982; 24:353–373.

52. Palmer RF, Lasseter KC: Drug therapy—Sodium nitroprusside. *N Engl J Med* 1975; 294–297.

53. Rubin PC: Treatment of hypertension in pregnancy. *Clin Obstet Gynaecol* 1986 13:307–317.

54. Parker MM, Shelhamer JH, Bacharach SL: Profound but reversible myocardial depression in patients with septic shock. *Ann Intern Med* 1984; 100:483–490.

55. Lee W, Clark SL, Cotton DB: Septic shock during pregnancy. *Am J Obstet Gynecol* 1988; 159:410–416.

56. Cavanagh D, Knuppel RA, Shepherd JH, et al: Septic shock and the obstetrician/gynecologist. *South Med J* 1982; 75:809–813.

57. Morishima HO, Niemann WH, James LS: Effects of endotoxin on the pregnant baboon and fetus. *Am J Obstet Gynecol* 1978, 131:899–905.

58. O'Brian WF, Golden SM, Davis SE, et al: Endotoxemia in the neonatal lamb. *Am J Obstet Gynecol* 1985; 151:151–671.

59. Blanco JD, Gibbs RS, Castaneda YS: Bac-

teremia in obstetrics: Clinical course. *Obstet Gynecol* 1981; 58:621–626.

60. Fein AM, Lippmann M, Holtzman H, et al: The risk factors, incidence, and prognosis of ARDS following septicemia. *Chest* 1983; 83:40–43.

61. Duff P, Gibbs RS, Blanco JD, et al: Endometrial culture techniques in puerperal patients. *Obstet Gynecol* 1983; 61:217–220.

62. Gonik B: Septic shock in obstetrics. *Clin Perinatol* 1986; 13:741–754.

63. Jardin F, Sportiche M, Bazin M, et al: Dobutamine: A hemodynamic evaluation in human septic shock. *Crit Care Med* 1981; 9:329–332.

64. Luce JM, Montgomery AB, Marks JD, et al: Ineffectiveness of high-dose methylprednisolone in preventing parenchymal lung injury and improving mortality in patients with septic shock. *Am Rev Respir Dis* 1988; 138:62–68.

65. DeMaria A, Heffernan JJ, Grindlinger GA, et al: Naloxone versus placebo in treatment of septic shock. *Lancet* 1985; 1:1363–1365.

66. Natanson C, Parrillo JE: Septic shock. *Anesthesiol Clin North Am* 1988; 6:73–85.

67. Lachman E, Pitsoe SB, Gaffin SL: Antilipopolysaccharide immunotherapy in management of septic shock of obstetric and gynaecological origin. *Lancet* 1984; 981–983.

68. Sanders AB, Meislin HW, Gew GA: The physiology of cardiopulmonary resuscitation. *JAMA* 1984; 252:3283–3286.

69. DePace NL, Betesh JS, Kotler MN: Postmortem cesarean section with recovery of both mother and offspring. *JAMA* 1982; 248:971–973.

70. Lee RV, Rodgers BD, White LM, et al: Cardiopulmonary resuscitation of pregnant women. *Am J Med* 1986; 81:311–318.

71. Hall JB, Wood LDH: Liberation of the patient from mechanical ventilation. *JAMA* 1987; 257:1621–1628.

72. Schmidt GA, Hall JB: Acute on chronic respiratory failure: Assessment and management of patients with COPD in the emergent setting. *JAMA* 1989; 261:3444–3453.

73. Gaensler EA, Patton WE, Verstracten JM, et al: Pulmonary function in pregnancy. III. Serial observations in patients with pulmonary insufficiency. *Am Rev Respir Dis* 1953; 67:779–783.

74. Blood gas measurements in the kyphoscoliotic gravida and her fetus: Report of a case. *Am J Obstet Gynecol* 1975; 121:287–289.

75. McKim DA, Dales RE, Lefebvre GG, et al: Nocturnal positive-pressure nasal ventilation for respiratory failure during pregnancy. *Can Med Assoc J* 1988; 139:1069–1071.

76. Porter KB, Goldhamer R, Mankad A, et al: Evaluation of arterial oxygen saturation in pregnant patients and their newborns. *Obstet Gynecol* 1988; 71:354–357.

77. Baggish MS, Hooper S: Aspiration as a cause of maternal death. *Obstet Gynecol* 1982; 59(suppl):33S.

78. Brock-Utne JG, Downing JW, Seedat F: Laryngeal edema associated with pre-eclamptic toxaemia. *Anaesthesia* 1977, 32:556–558.

79. Tomkinson J, et al: *Report on Confidential Enquiries into Maternal Deaths in England and Wales 1976–1978*. Department of Health and Social Security, Report on Health and Social Subjects No. 26. London, Her Majesty's Stationery Office, 1982.

80. Lumley J, Renou P, Newman W, et al: Hyperventilation in obstetrics. *Am J Obstet Gynecol* 1969; 103:847–855.

81. Levinson G, Shnider SM, deLorimier AA, et al: Effects of maternal hyperventilation on uterine blood flow and fetal oxygenation and acid-base status. *Anesthesiology* 1974; 40:340–347.

82. Parer JT, Eng M, Aoba H, et al: Uterine blood flow and oxygen uptake during maternal hyperventilation in monkeys at cesarean section. Anesthesiology 1976; 32:130–135.

83. Morishima HO, Daniel SS, Adamsons K Jr, et al: Effects of positive pressure ventilation of the mother upon the acid-base state of the fetus. *Am J Obstet Gynecol* 1968; 269–273.

84. Arthur R: Postmortem cesarean section. *Am J Obstet Gynecol* 1978; 132:175–185.

85. Light RB, Mink SN, Wood LDH: Pathophysiology of gas exchange and pulmonary perfusion in pneumoccocal lobar pneumonia in dogs. *J Appl Physiol* 1981; 50:524–530.

86. Hall JB, Wood LDH: *Current Therapy of Respiratory Disease: Pulmonary Edema*. Toronto, BC Decker Inc, 1989; pp 275–280.

87. Feldman JM: Adult respiratory distress syndrome in a pregnant patient with a pheochromocytoma. *J Surg Oncol* 1985; 29:5–7.

88. Cunningham FG, Leveno KJ, Hankins GD, et al: Respiratory insufficiency associated with pyelonephritis during pregnancy. *Obstet Gynecol* 1984; 63:121–125.

89. Groenendijk R, Trimbos JBMJ, Wallenburg HCS: Hemodynamic measurements in preeclampsia: Preliminary observations. *Am J Obstet Gynecol* 1984; 150:232–236.

90. Gonik B, Cotton DB: Peripartum colloid osmotic pressure changes: Influence of intravenous hydration. *Am J Obstet Gynecol* 1984; 150:99–100.

91. Zinaman M, Rubin J, Lindheimer MD: Serial plasma oncotic pressure levels and echoencephalography during and after delivery in severe pre-eclampsia. *Lancet* 1985; 2:1245–1247.

92. Steiner PE, Lushbaugh CC. Maternal pulmonary embolism by amniotic fluid as a cause of obstetric shock and unexpected deaths in obstetrics. *JAMA* 1941; 117:1245.

93. Peterson EP, Taylor HB: Amniotic fluid embolism: An analysis of 40 cases. *Obstet Gynecol* 1970; 35:787–95.

94. Morgan M: Amniotic fluid embolism. *Anaesthesia* 1979; 34:20–30.

95. Clark SL: Amniotic fluid embolism. *Crit Care Obstet* 1986; 13:801–811.

96. Adamsons K, Mueller-Heubach E, Myers RE: The innocuousness of amniotic fluid infusion in the pregnant rhesus monkey. *Am J Obstet Gynecol* 1971; 109:977–83.

97. Meier PR, Bowes WA: Amniotic fluid embolus-like syndrome presenting in the second trimester of pregnancy. *Obstet Gynecol* 1983; 61:31(S).

98. Clark SL, Montz FJ, Phelan JP: Hemodynamic alterations associated with amniotic fluid embolism: A reappraisal. *Am J Obstet Gynecol* 1985; 151:617–623.

99. Dolynuik M, Orfei E, Vania H, et al: Rapid diagnosis of amniotic fluid embolism. *Obstet Gynecol* 1983; 61:28(S).

100. Clark SL, Pavlova Z, Horenstein J, et al: Squamous cells in the maternal pulmonary circulation. *Am J Obstet Gynecol* 1986; 154:104–106.

101. Pisani RJ, Rosenow EC: Pulmonary edema associated with tocoytic therapy. *Ann Intern Med* 1989; 110:714–718.

102. Benedetti TJ: Life-threatening complications of betamimetic therapy for preterm labor inhibition. *Clin Perinatol* 1986; 13:843–852.

103. Berthiaume Y, Staub NC, Matthay MA: Beta-adrenergic agonists increase lung liquid clearance in anesthetized sheep. *J Clin Invest* 1987; 79:335–343.

104. Matthay MA, Wiener-Kronish JP: Resolution of alveolar edema in man: Is active transport an important mechanism? *Am Rev Respir Dis* 1988; 137(suppl):228.

105. Benedetti TJ, Kates R, Williams V, et al: Hemodynamic observations in severe preeclampsia complicated by pulmonary edema. *Am J Obstet Gynecol* 1985; 152:330–334.

106. Mabie AU, William C, Ratts TE, et al: Circulatory congestion in obese hypertensive women: A subset of pulmonary edema in pregnancy. *Obstet Gynecol* 1988; 72:553–558.

107. Hollingsworth HM, Pratter MR, Irwin RS: Acute respiratory failure in pregnancy. *J Intensive Care Med* 1989; 4:11–34.

108. Wynne JW, Modell JH: Respiratory aspiration of stomach contents. *Ann Intern Med* 1977; 466–474.

109. Schwartz DJ, Wynne JW, Gibbs CP, et al: The pulmonary consequences of aspiration of gastric contents at pH values greater than 2.5. *Am Rev Respir Dis* 1980; 121:119–126.

110. Long R, Breen PH, Mayers I, et al: Treatment of canine aspiration pneumonitis: Fluid volume reduction vs. fluid volume expansion. *Am J Physiol* 1988; 65:1736–1744.

111. Gonzales CL, Calia FM: Bacteriologic flora of aspiration-induced pulmonary infections. *Arch Intern Med* 1975; 135:711–714.

112. Fein A, Grossman RF, Jones JG, et al: The value of edema fluid protein measurement in patients with pulmonary edema. *Am J Med* 1979; 67:32–38.

113. Wood LDH, Prewitt RM: Cardiovascular management in acute hypoxemic respiratory failure. *Am J Cardiol* 1981; 47:963–972.

114. Wolfe JE, Bone RC, Ruth WE: Effects of

corticosteroids in the treatment of patients with gastric aspiration. *Am J Med* 1977; 63:719–721.

115. Sosin D, Krasnow J, Moawad A, et al: Successful spontaneous vaginal delivery during mechanical ventilatory support for adult respiratory distress syndrome. *Obstet Gynecol* 1986; 68(3):19S–23S.

116. Mayers I, Breen PH, Gottlieb S, et al: The effects of indomethacin on edema and gas exchange in canine acid aspiration. *J Appl Physiol* 1987; 69:149–160.

117. Pingleton SK: Complications of acute respiratory failure. *Am Rev Respir Dis* 1988; 137:1463–1493.

118. Lim VS, Katz AI, Lindheimer MD: Acid-base regulation in pregnancy. *Am J Physiol* 1976; 231:1764–1770.

119. Eguiluz A, Lopez Bernal A, McPherson K, et al: The use of intrapartum fetal blood lactate measurements for the early diagnosis of fetal distress. *Am J Obstet Gynecol* 1983; 147:949–955.

120. Miller FC, Petrie RH, Arce JJ, et al: Hyperventilation during labor. *Am J Obstet Gynecol* 1974; 120:489–495.

121. Ralston DH, Shnider SM, deLorimier AA: Uterine blood flow and fetal acid-base changes after bicarbonate administration to pregnant ewe. *Anesthesiology* 1974; 40:348–353.

122. Motoyama EK, Rivard G, Acheson F, et al: The effect of changes in maternal pH and PCO2 on the PO2 of fetal lambs. *Anesthesiology* 1967; 28:891–903.

123. Narins RG, Cohen JJ: Bicarbonate therapy for organic acidosis: The case for its continued use. *Ann Intern Med* 1987; 106:615–618.

124. Stacpoole PW: Lactic acidosis: The case against bicarbonate therapy. *Ann Intern Med* 1986; 105:276–278.

125. Holdsworth JD, et al: Mixing of antiacids with stomach contents. *Anaesthesia* 1980; 35:641–650.

126. Parker S, Schade RR, Pohl CR, et al: Prenatal and neonatal exposure of male rats to cimetidine but not rantidine adversely affects subsequent adult sexual functioning. *Gastroenterology* 1984; 86:675–678.

127. Driks MR, Craven DE, Celli BR, et al: Nosocomial pneumonia in intubated patients given sucralfate as compared with antacids or histamine type 2 blockers. *N Engl J Med* 1987; 317:1376–1382.

128. Lee RV, Rogers BD, Young C, et al: Total parenternal nutrition during pregnancy. *Obstet Gynecol* 1986; 68:563–570.

129. Heller L: Parenteral nutrition in obstetrics and gynecology, in Greep, JM, et al: (eds): *Current Concepts in Parenteral Nutrition.* The Hague, Martinus Nijhoff, 1977, p 179.

130. Gallagher JS: Anaphylaxis in pregnancy. *Obstet Gynecol* 1988; 71:491–493.

131. Sheffer AL: Anaphylaxis. *J Allergy Clin Immunol* 1985; 75:227–233.

132. Perkin RM, Anas NG: Mechanisms and management of anaphylactic shock not responding to traditional therapy. *Ann Allergy* 1985; 54:202–208.

133. Rayburn W, Aronow R, DeLancey B, et al: Drug overdose during pregnancy: An overview from a metropolitan poison control center. *Obstet Gynecol* 1984; 64:611–614.

134. Stocker RP, Pratter MR: Poisonings and overdose: General considerations, in Rippe JM, Irwin RS, Alpert JS, et al (eds): *Intensive Care Medicine.* Boston, Little, Brown Co, 1985; pp 901–908.

135. Ng RC: Using syrup of ipecac for ingestion of petroleum distillates. *Pediatr Ann* 1977; 6:43–46.

136. Wright N: An assessment of the unreliability of the history given by self-poisoned patients. *Clin Toxicol* 1980; 16:381–386.

137. Ludmir J, Main DM, Landon MB, et al: Maternal acetaminophen overdose at 15 weeks of gestation. *Obstet Gynecol* 1986; 67:750–751.

138. Rumack BH: Acetaminophen overdose. *Am J Med* 1983; 75:104–108.

139. Byer AJ, Trayler TR, Semner JR: Acetaminophen overdose in the third trimester of pregnancy. *JAMA* 1982; 247:3114–3117.

140. Riggs BS, Bronstein AC, Kulig K, et al: Acute acetaminophen overdose during pregnancy. *Obstet Gynecol* 1989; 74:247–253.

141. Prescott LF, Illingworth RN, Critchley JAJH, et al: Intravenous *N*-acetylcysteine: The treatment of choice for paracetomal poisoning. *Br Med J* 1979; 2:1097–1099.

142. Frommer DA, Kulig KW, Marx JA, et al: Tricyclic antidepressant overdose. *JAMA* 1987; 257:521–526.

143. Boehnert MT, Lovejoy FH Jr: Value of the QRS duration versus the serum drug level in predicting seizures and ventricular arrhythmias after an acute overdose of tricyclic antidepressants. *N Engl J Med* 1985; 313:474–479.

144. Proudfoot AT: Toxicity of salicylates. *Am J Med* 1983; 75:99–103.

145. Hill JB: Salicylate intoxication. *N Engl J Med* 1980; 228:1110–1113.

146. Chasnoff IJ, Burns WJ, Schnoll SH, et al: Cocaine use in pregnancy. *N Engl J Med* 1985; 313:666–669.

147. Pogue VA, Nurse HM: Cocaine-associated acute myoglobinuric renal failure. *Am J Med* 1989; 86:183–186.

148. Cregler LL, Mark H: Medical complications of cocaine abuse. *N Engl J Med* 1986; 315:1495–1500.

149. Chasnoff IJ, Bussey ME, Savich R, et al: Perinatal cerebral infarction and maternal cocaine use. *J Pediatr* 1986; 108:456–459.

150. Buchsbaum HJ: Accidental injury complicating pregnancy. *Am J Obstet Gynecol* 1968; 102:752–769.

151. Bocka J, Courtney J, et al: Trauma in pregnancy. *Ann Emerg Med* 1988; 17:829–834.

152. Rothenberger D, Quattlebaum FW, Zabel J, et al: Diagnostic peritoneal lavage for blunt trauma in pregnant women. *Am J Obstet Gynecol* 1977; 129:479–481.

153. Crosby WM: Trauma during pregnancy: Maternal and fetal injuries. *Obstet Gynecol Surv* 1974; 29:683–699.

154. Kettel LM, Branch DW, Scott JR: Occult placental abruption after maternal trauma. *Obstet Gynecol* 1988; 71:449–453.

155. Rothenberger D, Quattlebaum FW, Perry JF, et al: Blunt maternal trauma: A review of 103 cases. *J Trauma* 1978; 18:173–179.

156. Lavin JP, Polsky SS: Abdominal trauma during pregnancy. *Clin Perinatol* 1983; 14:424–438.

157. Weber CE: Postmortem cesarean section: Review of the literature and case reports. *Am J Obstet Gynecol* 1971; 110:158–168.

CHAPTER 8

Hematologic Disorders

Elizabeth Letsky

Healthy pregnancy is associated with marked changes in the circulating blood which show wide variations. These physiologic adjustments include increases in the blood volume and alterations in the interacting factors involved in hemostasis.

It is not possible to assess accurately the hematologic status of pregnant women by the criteria used for nonpregnant populations and an understanding of hematologic problems in obstetric patients requires familiarity with the dramatic changes in the blood during normal gestation. These changes have special relevance to the most important and potentially hazardous hematologic problems of pregnancy, namely, anemia, thromboembolism, and hemorrhage.

BLOOD VOLUME

Plasma volume and total red cell mass are controlled by different mechanisms, and changes during pregnancy provide a dramatic illustration of this point.

Plasma Volume

Plasma volume rises progressively throughout pregnancy, with a tendency to plateau in the last 8 weeks.[1,2] Most of the rise of about 1,250 mL, from a nonpregnant level of almost 2,600 mL, takes place before 32 to 34 weeks' gestation; thereafter there is relatively little change. The increases seem to correlate with clinical performance and neonatal birth weight. Second and subsequent pregnancies tend to be more successful than the first, with bigger babies and a larger plasma volume increase and women with multiple gestations have proportionately greater increments of plasma volume. Of interest, women with poorly growing fetuses, particularly multigravidas with a history of poor reproductive performance, have correspondingly poor plasma volume responses.

Red Cell Mass

There is a relative paucity of information on gestational increments in red cell mass, a confusing term which expresses the total volume of red cells in the circulation. Furthermore, results of published studies are more variable than those concerning changes in plasma volume. Thus, while all agree that red cell mass increases in pregnancy, there is disagreement as to how much. Also, the extent of the increase is influenced by iron supplementation which causes further increments even in apparently healthy women without clinical evidence of iron deficiency but who on investigation prove to have depleted iron stores (see below).

Accepting 1,400 mL as the average volume of red cells in nonpregnant women will mean that the rise in pregnancy is about 240 mL (18%) for women not receiving iron supplements, and 400 mL (30%) for those who do, with the greatest increments occurring from the end of the first trimester to term. As with plasma volume, the extent of increase is related to conceptus size and is particularly large in association with multiple pregnancy.[3]

Changes in Blood Volume at Parturition and During the Puerperium

When measured meticulously, blood loss at vaginal delivery proves to be slightly more than 500 mL during a singleton birth and almost 1,000 mL after delivery of twins. Cesarean section is associated with an average blood loss of 1,000 mL. Blood volume therefore drops following delivery but remains relatively stable unless the blood loss exceeds 25% of the predelivery volume. There is no compensatory increase in blood volume and there is a gradual fall in plasma volume, due primarily to postpartum diuresis. Increments in red cell mass during pregnancy which are not lost at delivery are slowly reduced as red cells reach the end of their life span. Hematocrit gradually increases and the blood volume returns to nonpregnant levels.

Fluctuations in plasma volume and hematocrit in the first few days following delivery are due to individual responses to dehydration, pregnancy hypervolemia, and the rapidity of blood loss. If blood volume has increased appropriately in pregnancy, losses of 1,000 mL at delivery can be tolerated without causing a significant fall in hemoglobin concentration. Most blood is lost in the first postpartum hour and approximately 80 mL is lost through the vagina during the following 72 hours. Patients with uterine atony, extended episiotomy, or lacerations will, of course, lose much more. If the hematocrit or hemoglobin concentration at 5 to 7 days postdelivery is significantly below predelivery levels, either there was pathologic blood loss at delivery, or blood volume did not increase appropriately in gestation.[4]

Total Hemoglobin

Hemoglobin concentration, hematocrit, and red cell count decrease during pregnancy because expansion of the plasma volume is greater than that of the red cell mass. However, total circulating hemoglobin is greater because of the increase in red cell mass. Published evidence for this rise in total hemoglobin is unsatisfactory and confusing due in part to the varying iron status of the women studied, and it is therefore difficult to cite "physiologic limits" for the expected rise in total hemoglobin.

The lowest normal hemoglobin in the healthy adult *nonpregnant* woman living at sea level is defined as 12.0 g/dL[5], while the mean minimum for pregnancy given in most publications is between 11 and 12 g/dL. In one carefully studied iron-supplemented group the lowest hemoglobin was 10.44 g/dL[6], while the minimum value acceptable to the World Health Organization *(WHO)* is 11.0 g/dL.[5]

IRON METABOLISM IN PREGNANCY

Iron deficiency anemia is the commonest hematologic problem in pregnancy. This topic is dealt with in most obstetric texts and will only be briefly summarized here.

Most body iron is contained in the hemoglobin of circulating and developing red blood cells. Iron exchange is both extremely limited and precisely regulated; a unique feature of balance in the human is that the iron content of the body is controlled largely by a limited variation in absorption and not by excretion. A normal diet supplies about 14 mg of iron each day of which only 1 to 2 mg (5–10%) is absorbed. Absorption, however, is increased when iron stores are depleted, e.g., when there is a low ferritin level and a high concentration of unsaturated transferrin (see below) and also when there is erythroid hyperplasia with a rapid iron turnover. Adult males require 1 mg of iron a day to cover passive losses, while females need another 0.5 to 1.0 mg/day to meet the requirements resulting from menstrual losses.

During pregnancy the average requirement is 4 mg/day, rising from 2.5 mg in early pregnancy to 6.6 mg/day in the last trimester. By far the greatest single demand for iron is that for the expansion of the red cell mass, but iron is also required for the development of fetus and placenta, the total extra requirement being on the order of 700 to 1,400 mg. There is evidence that absorption of dietary iron is enhanced in the latter half of pregnancy, but the maximal daily absorption possible is approximately 3.5 mg/day for a *nonanemic* individual with iron deficiency ingesting an adequate diet, and a reasonable expectation would be an absorption of roughly 2.0 mg/day.[7] It follows that the daily iron requirements of pregnancy can only be met by maximal absorption of dietary iron and mobilization of iron stores.

ABSORPTION OF DIETARY IRON

Heme iron derived from the hemoglobin and myoglobin of animal origin is more effectively absorbed than non-heme iron. Factors interfering with or promoting the absorption of inorganic iron have no effect on the absorption of heme iron. Heme iron also promotes the absorption of inorganic iron. This puts vegetarians at a disadvantage in terms of iron sufficiency. The amount of iron absorbed will also depend very much on the extent of iron stores, the content of the diet, and whether or not iron supplements are given.

It was found, in a carefully controlled study in Sweden,[8] that absorption rates differed markedly between those pregnant women receiving 100 mg ferrous iron supplements daily and those receiving a placebo. Iron absorption increased steadily throughout pregnancy in the placebo group. In the supplemented group there was no increase between the 12th and 24th week of gestation and thereafter the increase was only 60% of the placebo group. After delivery the mean absorption in the placebo group was markedly higher. These differences can be explained by the difference in storage iron between the two groups.[8]

Many women enter pregnancy with already low or depleted iron stores because of demands of previous pregnancies and menstrual losses. They will not be anemic at this stage, a fall in hemoglobin concentration being a late manifestation of iron depletion, but they will be at risk of developing quite severe anemia and other metabolic defects of iron deficiency as pregnancy progresses (see below).

Over the years there have been many studies which have proved without doubt that iron supplements prevent the development of anemia[9–14] and that in women on a good diet who are not apparently anemic at first examination, the mean hemoglobin level can be raised by oral iron therapy throughout pregnancy. The difference in favor of those so treated is most marked at term when the need for adequate hemoglobin is maximal.[6, 12, 15, 16]

IRON DEFICIENCY IN PREGNANCY

Hemoglobin

Reduction in concentration of circulating hemoglobin is a relatively late development in iron deficiency. It is preceded first by depletion of iron stores, then by reduction in serum iron, and finally by detectable decrements in hemoglobin level. Still, this is the simplest non-invasive practical test at our disposal. The normal range of hemoglobin concentration in healthy pregnancy at 30 weeks' gestation in women who have received supplemental iron ranges from 10.0 to 14.5 g/dL, the large variability being related to the changes in blood volume and hemodilution. However, hemoglobin values less than 10.5 g/dL in the second and third trimesters are probably abnormal and require further investigation.

Red Cell Indices

Appearance of red cells on a stained film is a relatively insensitive gauge of iron status

TABLE 8–1.

Red Cell Indices in Iron Deficiency and Thalassemia

Index		Normal Range During Pregnancy	Iron Deficiency	Thalassemia
PCV/RBC	MCV	75–99 fL	Reduced	Very reduced
Hb/RBC	MCH	27–31 pg	Reduced	Very reduced
Hb/PCV	MCHC	32–36 g/dL	Reduced	Normal or slightly reduced

PCV = packed cell volume; RBC = red cell count; Hb = hemoglobin; MCV = mean corpuscular volume; MCH = mean corpuscular hemoglobin; MCHC = mean corpuscular hemoglobin concentration.

in pregnancy. Better information relevant to the diagnosis of iron deficiency in pregnancy is the examination of red cell indices (Table 8–1). The earliest effect of iron deficiency on the erythrocyte is a reduction in cell size (mean corpuscular volume, or MCV) and with the dramatic changes in red cell mass and plasma volume this appears to be the most sensitive indicator of underlying iron deficiency. Hypochromia (low MCH) and a fall in mean corpuscular hemoglobin concentration (MCHC) only appear with more severe degrees of iron depletion.

Of course some women enter pregnancy with already established anemia due to iron deficiency, or with grossly depleted iron stores, and they will quickly develop florid anemia with reduced MCV, MCH, and MCHC. These women do not present any problems in diagnosis. It is those who enter pregnancy in precarious iron balance with a normal hemoglobin who present the most difficult diagnostic problems. Recognition of iron deficiency before a drop in hemoglobin or an effect on indices depends on three noninvasive laboratory tests: ferritin, transferrin saturation, and free erythrocyte protoporphyrin.

Ferritin

This high-molecular-weight glycoprotein circulates at levels ranging from 15 to 300 μg/L in healthy adult females.[17] A level of 12 μg/L or below indicates iron deficiency. Ferritin is stable and not affected by recent ingestion of iron, and appears to reflect the iron stores accurately and quantitatively in the absence of inflammation, particularly in the lower

range associated with iron deficiency which is so important in pregnancy.[18] In the development of iron deficiency a low serum ferritin is the first abnormal laboratory test.

Serum Iron and Total Iron-Binding Capacity (TIBC)

Serum iron, together with the TIBC, is an estimation of transferrin saturation. Reduced transferrin saturation indicates a deficient iron supply to the tissues and this is the second measurement to be affected in the development of iron deficiency.

At this stage erythropoiesis is impaired and there is an adverse effect on iron-dependent tissue enzymes.

In health the serum iron of adult nonpregnant women lies between 13 and 27 μmol/L (70–150 μg/dL), but it demonstrates considerable individual diurnal variation and even fluctuates from hour to hour. The TIBC, which ranges from 45 to 72 μmol/L in the nonpregnant state, rises in association with iron deficiency and decreases in chronic inflammatory states. It is raised in pregnancy because of the increase in plasma volume. In the nonanemic individual the TIBC is approximately one-third saturated with iron.

In pregnancy most report a decrease in both serum iron and percentage saturation of the TIBC, which can be largely prevented by iron supplements. Serum iron, even in combination with TIBC, is not a reliable indication of iron stores because it fluctuates so widely and is affected by recent ingestion of iron and other factors not directly involved with iron metabolism, such as infection. With these reservations a serum iron of less than 12 μmol/L (67 μg/dL) and a TIBC saturation of less than 15% indicate deficiency of iron during pregnancy.

Free Erythrocyte Protoporphyrin (FEP)

Erythroblast protoporphyrin rises when there is defective iron supply to the developing red cell, but there is a misleading increase in patients with chronic inflammatory disease, malignancy, or infection.

In ideal circumstances the above three measurements, combined with the hemoglobin concentration, allow classification of iron-deficient individuals—those with depleted stores (decreased ferritin only), those with severe iron deficiency but as yet no anemia (decreased ferritin and reduced TIBC saturation plus an increased FEP), and those with anemia due to iron deficiency (reduced hemoglobin concentration and iron-deficient indices in addition to decreased ferritin, reduced TIBC saturation, and increased FEP).

Marrow Iron

The most rapid and reliable method of assessing iron stores in pregnancy is by examination of an appropriately stained preparation of a bone marrow sample. In the absence of iron supplementation there is no detectable stainable iron in over 80% of women at term.[6] No stainable iron (hemosiderin) may be visible once the serum ferritin has fallen to below 40 μg/L, but other stigmata of iron deficiency in the developing erythroblasts, particularly the late normoblasts, will confirm that the anemia is indeed due to iron deficiency in the absence of stainable iron. The effects of frequently accompanying folate deficiency will also be apparent (see below).

Management of Iron Deficiency Anemia

Established Iron Deficiency

The management of iron deficiency anemia diagnosed late in pregnancy presents a particular challenge because a satisfactory response has to be obtained in a limited space of time. First, one usually assumes that the woman has failed to take oral supplements. Iron sorbitol citrate can be given as a series of intramuscular injections, but it is associated with toxic reactions such as headache, nausea, and vomiting if given simultaneously with oral iron.[19] Iron dextran (Imferon), an extensively used preparation, can be administered as a series of intramuscular injections or preferably as a total-dose infusion. Rare anaphylactic reactions do occur in the case of intravenous infusions, but usually during the period when the first few milliliters are being administered.[20] For this reason the infusion should initially be administered at a slow rate, carefully observing the patient during the first few minutes. This preparation does not appear to be associated with toxicity if given simultaneously with oral iron.[21]

In the absence of any other abnormality an increase in hemoglobin of 0.8 g/dL/week (1.0 g/dL in the nonpregnant female) can be reasonably expected with adequate treatment. The response is similar whether iron be given orally or parenterally (see below). If there is not enough time to achieve a reasonable hemoglobin for delivery, then transfusion with all its hazards is indicated.

Prophylaxis

Management of iron deficiency in pregnancy focuses primarily on prevention with daily oral supplements. Elemental iron 60 to 80 mg/day starting in early pregnancy maintains hemoglobin in the recognized normal range for gestation, but does not maintain or restore iron stores.[22, 23] The WHO[5] recommends that supplements of 30 to 60 mg/day be given to those pregnant women who have adequate iron stores, and 120 to 240 mg/day to those with none.

Whether all pregnant women need iron is controversial, but if it is accepted that iron is necessary, a bewildering number of preparations of varying expense are available. In those women to whom additional iron cannot be given by the oral route, either because of noncompliance or because of unacceptable side effects, intramuscular injection of iron, 1,000 mg in total, more than ensures iron sufficiency for that pregnancy. This can be administered as a series of daily injections of 100 to 250 mg iron (2–5 mL iron dextran) into alternate buttocks. The injections are painful and may stain the skin, but there is no risk of incurring malignancy at the injection site as once reported.

There is no hematologic benefit in prescribing parenteral as opposed to oral iron, but many women fail to take the prescribed oral preparations and use of the parenteral route ensures that the patient is receiving adequate supplementation.

Side effects of oral iron administration appear related to the quantity administered.[24] Side effects are unusual with any preparation provided the daily dose is reduced to 100 mg and that introduction is delayed until the 16th week of gestation. Some women report gastric symptoms, but the most common complaint is constipation which is usually overcome easily by simple basic measures. Slow-release preparations, which are on the whole more expensive, are said to be relatively free of side effects. This is only because much of the iron is not released at all, is unabsorbed, and excreted unchanged. This means that double doses may have to be given to cover requirements, thereby further increasing expense. Since most women tolerate the cheaper preparations without significant side effects, these should be tried first.

Virtually all preparations used in pregnancy are combined with an appropriate dose of folic acid (see below).

Are Iron Supplements During Pregnancy Necessary?

A review[25] of controlled clinical trials in developed Western countries concluded that there was no beneficial effect of iron administration during pregnancy in terms of birth weight, length of gestation, maternal and infant morbidity, and mortality. Age, economic status, and poor nutrition affected pregnancy outcome, but anemia did not and was simply associated with other risks. Still, from the evidence available it appears that a high proportion of women in reproductive years do lack storage iron[6, 10, 15, 18] and it has been suggested that women at risk for iron deficiency anemia can be identified by estimating the serum ferritin concentration in the first trimester.[26] For instance, Bentley[26] suggests that serum ferritin of less than 50 μg/L in early pregnancy is an indication for daily iron supplements, while women with serum ferritin concentrations of greater than 80 μg/L are unlikely to require iron supplements. Unnecessary supplementation would thus be avoided in women enjoying good nutrition, and any risk to the pregnancy arising from severe maternal anemia would be avoided by prophylaxis and prompt treatment.[26]

A recent investigation at Queen Charlotte's Maternity Hospital, London, is of interest in this respect. Serum ferritin levels were estimated in 669 consecutive women with a hemoglobin concentration of 11.0 g/dL or above who were first seen at 16 weeks' gestation or earlier. These women are drawn from a cosmopolitan, largely well-nourished population. Of this population sample, 552 women (82.5%) had serum ferritin levels of 50 μg/L or below, and would therefore have qualified for routine daily iron supplements by the above criteria, while 80 (12%) had values of less than 12 μg/L and were already iron-deficient at initial examination (despite having a hemoglobin of 11 g/dL or more). Only 51 (7.6%) had ferritins of 80 μg/L or above.[27]

In summary, negative iron balance throughout pregnancy, particularly in the latter half, may lead to iron deficiency anemia in the third trimester. This hazard—together with the increasing evidence of nonhematologic effects of iron deficiency on exercise tolerance, cerebral function, and temperature control—leads to the conclusion that it is safer, more practical, and in the long term less expensive in terms of investigation, hospital admission, and treatment, to give all women iron supplements from 16 weeks' gestation, especially as this would appear to do no harm.[28, 29]

FOLATE DEFICIENCY IN PREGNANCY

Folic acid, together with iron, has assumed a central role in the nutrition of pregnancy.[30] At a cellular level folic acid is reduced first to dihydrofolic acid (DHF) and then to tetrahydrofolic acid (THF), which forms the cornerstone of cellular folate metabolism. It is fundamental, through linkage with L-carbon fragments, both to cell growth and cell division. The more active a tissue is in reproduction and growth, the more dependent it will be on the efficient turnover and supply of folate coenzymes. Bone marrow and epithelial linings are therefore particularly at risk.

Requirements for folate are increased in pregnancy to meet the needs of the fetus, placenta, uterine hypertrophy, and the expanded maternal red cell mass. The placenta transports folate actively to the fetus even in the face of maternal deficiency, but maternal folate metabolism is altered early in pregnancy, like many other maternal functions, before fetal demands act directly.

Laboratory Tests

Plasma Folate

Although few data are available, most agree that plasma folates decrease as pregnancy advances, reaching roughly half nonpregnant values by term.[30] Plasma clearance of folate by the kidneys is more than doubled as early as the eighth week of gestation and while some ascribe importance to urinary losses it is unlikely that increased renal clearance of the vitamin is a major drain on maternal resources, although it can play a marginal role.

Substantial day-to-day variations of plasma folate are possible and postprandial increases have been noted; this will limit its diagnostic value when an occasional sample taken at a casual antenatal clinic visit is considered.

Red Cell Folate

Estimation of red cell folate does not reflect daily or other short-term variations in plasma folate levels, and is thought to give a better indication of overall body tissue levels. However, since red cell turnover is slow, there will be a delay before significant reductions in red blood cell folate concentration are evident. Of interest in this respect is evidence that patients who have a low red cell folate early in pregnancy develop megaloblastic anemia in the third trimester.[30]

Excretion of Formiminoglutamic Acid (FIGLU)

Histidine loading leads to increased FIGLU excretion in the urine when there is folate deficiency. However, because pregnancy is accompanied by altered histamine metabolism and increased urinary excretion of FIGLU, this test is not reliable in the gravid patient.

Red Cell Morphology

There is a physiologic increase in red cell size in healthy iron-replete pregnancy. The MCV rises on average by 4 fL but may be as much as 20 fL.[30] This increase in red cell size is not prevented by folate supplements.

Red blood cell indices may be difficult to interpret as the physiologic macrocytosis may be masked by effects of iron deficiency which results in the production of small red cells (see above). In nongravid patients the hallmark of megaloblastic hematopoiesis is macrocytosis, first identified in routine laboratory investigations by a raised MCV. In pregnancy macrocytosis by nonpregnant standards is the norm and in any event may be masked by iron deficiency. Examination of the blood film may be more helpful. There may be occasional oval macrocytes in a sea of iron-deficient microcytic cells. Hypersegmentation of the neutrophil polymorph nucleus is significant because in normal pregnancy there is a shift to the left, but hypersegmentation is observed in pure iron deficiency, uncomplicated by folate deficiency. Thus, the diagnosis of folate deficiency in pregnancy has to be made ultimately on morphologic grounds and usually involves examination of a suitably prepared marrow aspirate.[30]

Postpartum Events

In the 6 weeks following delivery there is a tendency for all the parameters discussed to return to nonpregnant values. However, should any deficiency of folate have developed and remain untreated in pregnancy, it may present clinically for the first time in the puerperium and its consequences can be detected for many months after delivery. Lactation provides an added folate stress. A folate content of 5 μg/dL of human milk and a yield of 500 mL daily implies a loss of 25 μg folate daily in breast milk. Red cell folate levels in lactating mothers are significantly lower than those of their infant during the first year of life.

Megaloblastic Anemia

The cause of megaloblastic anemia in pregnancy is nearly always folate deficiency (Table 8–2). Vitamin B$_{12}$ is only rarely implicated. A survey of reports from the United Kingdom over the past two decades suggests an incidence ranging from 0.2% to 5.0%, but a considerably greater number of women have megaloblastic changes in their marrow which

TABLE 8–2.
Folic Acid and Pregnancy—Summary

1. Pregnancy is accompanied by a state of negative folate balance even in well-nourished populations.
2. Deficiency in pregnancy can be prevented by oral supplements of 300 μg daily, which should be given with iron.
3. Folate deficiency in the mother has only been shown to cause megaloblastic anemia, which may present for the first time during lactation.
4. Women with multiple pregnancy, chronic hemolytic states, gastrointestinal disease, or on anticonvulsants are at increased risk of deficiency and require special care of folate status.
5. Folate deficiency in the fetus has been shown to be associated with low birth weight in malnourished populations, while association between neural tube defects and other abnormalities and periconceptional folate deficiency awaits confirmation in large multicenter controlled trials.
6. Premature neonates born to folate-deficient mothers are at risk for developing megaloblastic anemia late in infancy.

are not suspected on examination of the peripheral blood only.[30] The incidence of megaloblastic anemia in other parts of the world is considerably greater and is thought to reflect the nutritional standards of the population. While there is much controversy at the moment about the requirement for folate, particularly during pregnancy, WHO recommendations[5] for daily intake are as high as 800 μg in the antepartum period and 600 μg during lactation. Food folates are only partially available and the amount of folate supplied in the diet is difficult to quantify. In Great Britain folate intake in foodstuffs ranges between 129 and 300 μg, while content of 24-hour food collections in various studies in Sweden and Canada averaged 200 μg (range 70–600 μg).[31] Dietary folate deficiency megaloblastic anemia probably occurs in about one third of all pregnant women in the world, despite the fact that folate is found in nearly all natural foods. This is because folate is rapidly destroyed by cooking, especially in finely divided foods such as beans and rice,[32] while green vegetables lose up to 90% of their vitamin content during the first few minutes of boiling.

Effects of dietary inadequacy may be further amplified by frequent childbirth. Several reports have also shown a markedly increased incidence of megaloblastic anemia in multiple pregnancy.[31]

The Fetus and Folate Deficiency

There is an increased risk of megaloblastic anemia occurring in the neonate of a folate-deficient mother, especially if delivery is preterm. There are also data suggesting an association between periconceptional folic acid deficiency and harelip, cleft palate, and, most important of all, neural tube defects.[33–35] The association between folate deficiency and neural tube defects awaits confirmation in a multicenter controlled trial of *pre*pregnancy folate supplementation in susceptible women. This subject has been well reviewed elsewhere.[36]

Prophylaxis

The case for giving prophylactic folate supplements throughout pregnancy is a strong one[30, 37, 38] and the supplement needs to be of the order of 200 to 300 μg pteroylglutamic acid daily. This should be given in combination with iron supplements (see above) and there are several suitable combined preparations available. The risk of adverse effects from folate supplements in a pregnant woman suffering from vitamin B_{12} deficiency is very small, and we are unaware of any reports of subacute combined degeneration of the spinal cord occurring among the thousands of women who have received folate supplements during pregnancy.

Management of Established Folate Deficiency

Once megaloblastic hematopoiesis is established, treatment of folic acid deficiency becomes more difficult, presumably due to megaloblastic changes in the gastrointestinal tract resulting in impaired absorption. Treatment initially, if the diagnosis is made in the antepartum period, should be pteroylglutamic acid 5 mg daily, continued for several weeks after delivery. If there is no response to this therapy parenteral folic acid can be tried.

Pregnancy, Anticonvulsants, and Folic Acid

Folate status is even further compromised in pregnancy if a woman is receiving anticonvulsants, in particular phenytoin and phenobarbital. Although earlier studies suggested that the control of epilepsy became more difficult in pregnant women receiving folate supplements approaching 5 mg daily,[39] more recent studies with supplements between 100 and 1000 μg daily have not substantiated these findings.[40] Also, as anticonvulsant therapy is associated with an increased incidence of congenital abnormality, prematurity, and low birth weight, folate supplements should be given to all epileptic women taking anticonvulsants.

Disorders That May Affect Folate Requirement in Pregnancy

Problems may be caused in pregnancy by disorders which are associated with an increased folate requirement in the nonpregnant state. Women with hemolytic anemia, particularly hereditary hemolytic conditions such as hemoglobinopathies and hereditary spherocytosis, require extra supplements from early pregnancy if development of megaloblastic anemia is to be avoided. The recommended supplement in this situation is 5 to 10 mg orally daily. The anemia associated with thalassemia trait is not strictly due to hemolysis but to ineffective erythropoiesis (see below). However, the increased, though abortive, marrow turnover still results in folate depletion and such women would probably benefit from the routine administration of oral folic acid 5.0 mg daily from early pregnancy.

Folate supplements are of particular importance in the management of sickle cell syndromes during pregnancy if aplastic crises and megaloblastic anemia are to be avoided.

Table 8–2 summarizes a number of important issues concerning folic acid in pregnancy.

VITAMIN B_{12} IN PREGNANCY

Muscle, red cell, and serum vitamin B_{12} concentrations fall during pregnancy.[30] Nonpregnant serum levels of 205 to 1,025 μg/L decrease to 20 to 510 μg/L at term, with low levels in multiple pregnancy. Women who smoke tend to have lower serum vitamin B_{12} levels, which may account for the positive correlation between birth weight and serum levels in nondeficient mothers.

Vitamin B_{12} absorption is unaltered in pregnancy[31] but tissue uptake may be increased by the action of estrogens, as oral contraceptives cause a fall in serum vitamin B_{12}. Cord blood serum vitamin B_{12} is higher than that of maternal blood. The fall in serum vitamin B_{12} in the mother is related to preferential transfer of absorbed vitamin B_{12} to the fetus at the expense of maintaining the maternal serum concentration, but the placenta does not transfer vitamin B_{12} with the same efficiency as it does folate. Low serum vitamin B_{12} levels in early pregnancy in vegetarian Hindus do not fall further, while their infants often have subnormal concentrations. The vitamin B_{12}–binding capacity of plasma increases in pregnancy analogous to the rise in transferrin. The rise is confined to the liver-derived transcobalamin II concerned with transport rather than the leukocyte-derived transcobalamin I, which is raised in myeloproliferative conditions.

Pregnancy does not make a vast impact on maternal vitamin B_{12} stores. Adult stores are of the order of 3,000 μg or more, and vitamin B_{12} stores in the newborn infant are about 50 μg.

Addisonian pernicious anemia is very unusual during the reproductive years. Also, vitamin B_{12} deficiency is associated with infertility, and pregnancy is likely only if the deficiency is remedied. However, severe vitamin B_{12} deficiency may be present without morphologic changes in hematopoietic and other tissues. Pregnancy in such patients may be followed by fetal demise.[31]

Chronic tropical sprue is another cause of vitamin B_{12} deficiency in pregnancy. The megaloblastic anemia in this case is due to a longstanding vitamin B_{12} deficiency to which folate deficiency is added. Cord vitamin B_{12} levels remain above the maternal levels in these cases, but the concentration in the breast milk follows the maternal serum levels.[31]

The recommended intake of vitamin B_{12}, 2 μg/day in the nonpregnant and 3 μg/day during pregnancy,[5] will be met by almost any diet which contains animal products. However, processed foods, including milk products, may lose their vitamin B_{12} content in preparation.[32] Strict vegetarians (vegans) may have a deficient intake of vitamin B_{12} and their diet should be supplemented during pregnancy.

HEMOGLOBINOPATHIES AND PREGNANCY

This group of diseases, characterized by anemia due to genetic defects of hemoglobin, are important to recognize early in pregnancy, or before conception, because (1) other clinical effects may complicate obstetric management and appropriate precautions can be taken; and (2) it is now possible to offer prenatal diagnosis to those women carrying a fetus at risk of a serious defect of hemoglobin synthesis or structure at a time when termination of pregnancy is feasible.[41, 42]

The hemoglobinopathies are inherited defects of hemoglobin, resulting from impaired globin synthesis (thalassemia syndromes) or from structural abnormality of globin (hemoglobin variants), and appreciation of these defects requires some understanding of the structure of normal hemoglobin. The hemoglobin molecule consists of four globin chains each of which is associated with a heme complex. There are three normal hemoglobins in man, Hb A, Hb A_2, and Hb F, each of which contains two pairs of polypeptide globin chains. Synthesis and structure of the four globin chains, α, β, γ, and δ, are under separate control and it is obvious that only conditions affecting the synthesis of Hb A ($\alpha_2\beta_2$), which constitutes over 95% of the total circulating hemoglobin in normal adults, will be of significance for the mother during pregnancy. α-Chain production is under the control of four genes, two inherited from each parent, and the α-chains are common to all three hemoglobins. β-Chain production, on the other hand, is under the control of only two genes, one inherited from each parent.

The Thalassemia Syndromes

The thalassemia syndromes, the commonest of the genetic blood disorders, constitute a vast public health problem in many parts of the world. The basic defect, a reduced rate of globin chain synthesis, results in red cells being formed with an inadequate hemoglobin content. These syndromes are divided into two main groups, the α- and β-thalassemias, depending on whether the α- or β-globin chain synthesis of adult hemoglobin (Hb A $[\alpha_2\beta_2]$) is depressed.

β-Thalassemia

Thalassemia major, homozygous β-thalassemia, was the first identified form of the thalassemia syndromes. Since the first cases were described in children of Greek and Italian immigrants, the disease was named thalassemia from the Greek *thalassa* meaning the sea, or in the classical sense, the Mediterranean. We know now that the distribution is virtually worldwide, although the defect is concentrated in a broad band which does include the Mediterranean and the Middle East. If both parents are carriers of β-thalassemia the newborn has a 1 in 4 chance of acquiring thalassemia major. The carrier rate in Great Britain is around 1 in 10,000 compared with 1 in 7 in Cyprus, and there are 300 to 400 patients with thalassemia major in Britain today, while over 100,000 babies are born worldwide with the condition each year.

At one time a child born with homozygous β-thalassemia would die in the first few years of life from anemia, congestive cardiac failure, and intercurrent infection, but since the advent of transfusion therapy survival has been prolonged into the teens and early twenties. The concomitant management problem has become one of iron overload derived mainly from the transfused red cells. This results in hepatic and endocrine dysfunction, but most important of all, myocardial damage, the cause of death being cardiac failure in the vast majority of cases. Puberty is delayed or incomplete and there has only been a very rare case report of successful pregnancy in a truly transfusion-dependent thalassemic girl.[43] It remains to be seen how effective recently instituted intensive iron chelation programs or future plans to use molecular biology will be.

The Diagnosis and Management of Thalassaemia in Pregnancy.—There are occasions when survival is possible without regular transfusion in thalassemia major, but these patients usually manifest severe bone deformities due to massive expansion of marrow tissue. Although iron loading still occurs from excessive gastrointestinal absorption, stimulated by the accelerated but ineffective marrow turnover, it is much slower than in those who are transfused, and such patients may conceive. Extra daily folate supplements should be given but iron in any form is contraindicated. The anemia should be treated by transfusion during the antenatal period.

Perhaps the commonest problem associated with hemoglobinopathies and pregnancy is the anemia developing in the antenatal period in women who have thalassemia minor, heterozygous β-thalassemia. They can be identified by the presence (as in α-thalassemia) of small poorly hemoglobinized red blood cells (low MCV and MCH) (see Table 8–1). The level of hemoglobin may be normal or slightly below the normal range. The diagnosis will be confirmed by finding a raised concentration of Hb A_2 ($\alpha_2\delta_2$) with or without a raised Hb F ($\alpha_2\gamma_2$), excess α-chains combining with δ- and γ-chains because of the relative lack of β-chains.

Women with β-thalassemia minor require the usual *oral* iron and folate supplements in the antenatal period. Oral iron for a limited period will not result in significant iron loading, even in the presence of replete iron stores, but parenteral iron should *never* be given. A serum ferritin estimation would be advisable early in pregnancy, and if iron stores are found to be high, iron supplements can be withheld. Many women with thalassemia minor enter pregnancy with depleted iron stores (as do many women with normal hemoglobin synthesis). To cover the requirements of ineffective erythropoiesis, folic acid 5 mg daily is recommended (see above). If

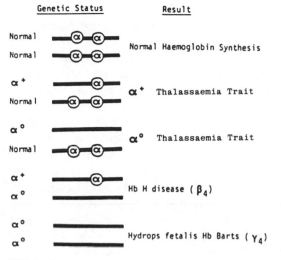

Genetic Status		Result

FIG 8–1.
Normal alpha gene status and the various forms of α-thalassemia resulting from gene deletion.

the anemia does not respond to oral iron and folate, and intramuscular folic acid has been tried, transfusion is indicated to achieve an adequate hemoglobin for delivery at term

α-Thalassemia

α-Thalassemia, unlike β-thalassemia, often, but not always, a gene deletion defect (Fig 8–1), is found most often in individuals of Chinese descent. There are two forms of α-thalassemia trait, the result of inheriting two or three normal alpha genes instead of the usual four. They are called α^0- and α^+-thalassemia. Hb H disease is an intermediate form of α-thalassemia in which there is only one functional alpha gene. Hb H is the name given to the unstable hemoglobin formed by tetramers of the beta chain (β_4), when there is a relative lack of α-chains. α-Thalassemia major, in which there are no functional alpha genes (both parents having transmitted α^0-thalassemia), is incompatible with life, and fetuses inheriting this defect usually develop hydrops and only survive a matter of hours if born alive, often prematurely. The condition is common in Southeast Asia. The name Hb Barts was given to tetramers of the γ-chain of fetal hemoglobin (γ_4) which forms in utero when no α-chains are made.

The Diagnosis and Management of α-Thalassemia in Pregnancy.—During pregnancy, with its stress on the hemopoietic system, carriers of α-thalassemia, particularly those with α^0-thalassemia (two defective genes), may become anemic. They can be identified by the finding of abnormal red cell indices (see Table 8–1). They have reductions MCV and MCH, although the MCHC is usually within the normal range (see Table 8–1). These changes are often minimal in α^+-thalassemia (see Fig 8–1) but this condition is not so important as α^0-thalassemia in terms of maternal anemia, genetic counseling, and prenatal diagnosis. The diagnosis can only be confirmed by globin chain synthesis studies or by DNA analysis of nucleated cells. There is no abnormal hemoglobin made, or excess or lack of one or other of the normal hemoglobins (cf. β-thalassemia). These women need iron and folate supplements throughout the antepartum period. Sometimes intramuscular folic acid is helpful but parenteral iron should *never* be given. If the hemoglobin is not thought to be adequate for delivery at term, transfusion is indicated.

Patients with Hb H disease have a chronic hemolytic anemia and have 5% to 30% Hb H in their peripheral blood. This can be identified on hemoglobin electrophoresis. They have a normal life expectancy but do require daily oral folate supplements to cover the demands of increased marrow turnover. During pregnancy it is recommended to give women with Hb H disease 5 mg folate daily. They will transmit either α^0- or α^+-thalassemia to their offspring.

Pregnancy with an α-thalassemia hydrops is associated with severe, sometimes life-threatening, preeclampsia (cf. severe rhesus hemolytic disease). Vaginal deliveries are associated with obstetric complication, due to the large fetus and very bulky placenta. If routine screening of the parents (see below) indicates that the mother is at risk of carrying such a child, both parents having α^0-thalassemia, she should be referred, as early as possible in pregnancy, for prenatal diagnosis so that termination of an affected pregnancy can be carried out before these severe obstetric complications with a nonviable fetus develop.

Hemoglobin Variants

Over 250 structural variants of the globin chains of normal human hemoglobin have been described, but the most important by far, both numerically and clinically, is sickle cell hemoglobin (Hb S). This is a variant of the β-globin chain where there is one amino acid substitution at the sixth position, a glutamine replacing a valine residue. Hb S has the unique physical property that, despite being a soluble protein in its oxygenated form, in its reduced state the molecules become stacked on one another, forming tactoids, which distort the red cells to the characteristic shape that gives the hemoglobin its name. Because of their rigid structure these sickled cells tend to block small blood vessels. The sickling phenomenon occurs particularly in conditions of lowered oxygen tension but may also be favored by acidosis or dehydration and cooling, which cause stasis in small blood vessels.

Sickle Cell Syndromes

The sickling disorders include the heterozygous state for sickle cell hemoglobin, sickle cell trait (Hb AS); homozygous sickle cell disease (Hb SS); compound heterozygotes of Hb variants, the most important of which is sickle cell–Hb C disease (Hb SC); and sickle cell thalassemia. Although these disorders are more commonly seen in black people of African origin, they can be seen in Saudi Arabians, Indians, and peoples of the Mediterranean.

The characteristic feature of homozygous sickle cell anemia (Hb SS) is occurrence of periods of health punctuated by periods of crisis. Between 3 and 6 months of age, when normal Hb A production usually becomes predominant, a chronic hemolytic anemia develops—the hemoglobin level being between 6 g/dL and 9 g/dL. Even if the hemoglobin is in the lower part of the range, symptoms due to anemia are surprisingly few because of

the low affinity of Hb S for oxygen, which facilitates oxygen delivery to the tissues. The acute episodes due to intravascular sickling are of far greater practical importance since they cause vascular occlusion resulting in tissue infarction. The affected part is painful and the clinical manifestations are extremely variable, depending on the site at which sickling takes places. Sickling crises are often precipitated by infection and may be exacerbated by any accompanying dehydration. Most deaths are due to massive sickling following an acute infection. Prognosis depends greatly on environment: in Africa, a large proportion of children with this disorder die within the first 5 years and probably less than 10% reach adulthood. In the West Indies, however, where prompt treatment and prophylaxis of infection are more easily available, many women with sickle cell disease need management during pregnancy.[44] Thomas et al.,[45] reviewing 241 mortalities from homozygous sickle cell disease in the West Indies, found that 10 were associated with pregnancy and often due to pulmonary embolus which has even been reported with heterozygotes.[46] This may of course be a chance association. Renal complications are a constant finding; there is a progressive inability to concentrate urine, and subtle protein and potassium-secreting defects and hematuria are common. These deficits result from sickling in the renal medullary circulation. Inability to concentrate the urine adequately makes pregnant women with the sickling disorders unduly prone to dehydration during labor. Also, perhaps due to the antialdosterone actions of progesterone, hyperkalemia has been reported in pregnant women with sickle cell disease at levels of renal dysfunction below those observed in nongravid individuals with Hb SS disease.[47]

Sickle cell–hemoglobin C disease (Hb SC) is a milder variant of Hb SS with normal or near-normal levels of hemoglobin. One of the dangers of this condition is that, owing to its mildness, neither the woman nor her obstetrician may be aware of its presence. These women are at risk of massive, sometimes fatal, sickling crises during pregnancy and particularly in the puerperium. It is therefore vital that the abnormality be detected, preferably before pregnancy, so that the appropriate precautions can be taken. Clinical manifestations of the doubly heterozygous condition, sickle cell thalassemia, are usually indistinguishable from Hb SS; those who make detectable amounts of Hb A are usually less severely affected but still at risk from sickling crises during pregnancy.

Sickle cell trait (Hb AS) results in no detectable abnormality under normal circumstances although it is easily diagnosed by specific investigations including hemoglobin electrophoresis (see below). Affected subjects are not anemic, even under the additional stress of pregnancy, unless there are additional complications, and sickling crises occur only in situations of extreme anoxia, dehydration, and acidosis.

Management of Sickle Cell Syndromes

At present there is no effective long-term method of reducing the liability of red cells to sickle in vivo. Once a crisis is established, there is no evidence that alkali, hyperbaric oxygen, vasodilators, plasma expanders, urea, or anticoagulants are of any value. Where beneficial effects have been reported they can usually be attributed to the meticulous care and supportive therapy received by the patient, rather than to the specific measures themselves. Adequate fluid administration alone probably accounts for the benefit.

Contraception and Sickle Cell Syndromes.—Methods of contraception vary,[48] but problems arise from the assumption that patients with sickle cell syndromes are at increased risk of thromboembolism if they use oral contraception. The patient's risk is less than that of pregnancy and there are almost no data to suggest that these patients run a greater risk than any other patients using low-estrogen preparations.[49] The usual contraindications hold true, of course, and patients should be monitored meticulously for alterations in blood pressure and liver function.

Sickle Cell Disease and Pregnancy.— Women with sickle cell disease present special problems in pregnancy.[50, 51] Fetal loss is high, and thought to be due to both impaired oxygen supply and sickling infarcts in the placental circulation.[49] Abortion, preterm labor, and other complications are more common than in women with normal hemoglobin. Although many women with sickle cell disease have no complications, the outcome in any individual case is always in doubt. The only consistently successful way of reducing the incidence of complications due to sickling is by regular blood transfusions at approximately 6-week intervals, to maintain the proportion of Hb A at 60% to 70% of the total.[52] Between 3 and 4 units of blood are given at each transfusion. This regimen has two effects: (1) it dilutes the circulating sickle hemoglobin and (2) by raising the hemoglobin, reduces the stimulus to the bone marrow and therefore the amount of sickle hemoglobin produced. However, the trade-off of such a regimen includes alloimmunization and of course all the other problems of transfusion including hepatitis and human immunodeficiency virus (HIV) transmission.

Sickle cells have a shorter life span than normal red cells and so the effect of each successive transfusion is more beneficial. If this regimen has been instituted, a general anesthetic may be given with safety and sickling crises in the course of normal labor are much less likely. The management of sickle cell syndromes in pregnancy in the United Kingdom is a relatively recent problem and longitudinal data are lacking here. It is clear on review of the extensive American literature that although risks remain higher for pregnancy complicated by sickle cell disease, modern obstetric care alone, without transfusion, has reduced the maternal morbidity and mortality dramatically and also improved fetal outcome.[50] Increasing numbers of obstetric centers have adopted prophylactic transfusion regimens but the real benefit of such regimens remains to be proved by a large trial with contemporary controls.[53] At the time of writing one such trial is in progress in Great Britain, while a smaller multicenter trial in the United States suggests that outcome is similar in women transfused prophylactically compared to those transfused only when indications arise.[54]

One of the most worrying complications of transfusion of Hb SS patients has been the development of atypical red cell antibodies, resulting from the fact that the donor populations differ in ethnic origin from the recipients and carry different minor red cell antigens. This has resulted in extreme difficulties in finding compatible blood,[55, 56] even in hemolytic disease of the newborn.[51] The general consensus from the United States in 1990, based on the results of one multicenter randomly controlled trial,[54] is that it is wiser to give close obstetric supervision and deliver women where there are special care baby units available. Transfusion should only be given in preparation for general anesthesia or where there is evidence of maternal distress.[49, 51] If the disorder presents late in pregnancy and there is more urgency because, for instance, the woman is profoundly anemic or is suffering a crisis, exchange transfusion can be used. Standard exchange transfusion regimens for sickle cell disease have been used with success in a large number of pregnant patients, as described in most hematology tests.

The worry concerning aspiration pneumonitis, hypoxia, and other perioperative pulmonary problems may be avoided by using regional anesthesia, but substitutes the risk of hypotension and venous pooling in the vessels of the lower extremities. Wrapping the legs in elastic bandages and elevating them will reduce venous pooling and subsequent hypotension. Although a number of patients with sickle cell disease have been reported to have suffered pulmonary emboli,[45, 49] there is no good evidence to incriminate regional anesthesia as a significant additional risk factor.

No special preparation with blood transfusion is required in pregnancy for women with sickle cell trait (Hb AS). However, as in patients with Hb SS, it is essential that hypoxia and dehydration are avoided during anesthesia and labor, particularly in the immediate postdelivery period. In fact, the majority of unexpected deaths associated with Hb S have occurred in patients with sickle cell trait in the immediate postoperative or postpartum period.[57]

Screening for Hemoglobinopathies

The single most important pregnancy precaution is for the woman's partner to be screened, so that the couple can be advised of the risk of a serious hemoglobin defect in their offspring. Screening procedures vary from location to location and often only involve high-risk populations. Figure 8–2 is a schema used at Queen Charlotte's Maternity Hospital, London, which serves a cosmopolitan population. This involves examination of red cell indices (see Table 8–1) hemoglobin electrophoresis, and, where indicated, quantitation of Hb A_2 and Hb F on every sample of blood taken at initial examination.

If a hemoglobin variant or thalassemia is found, the partner is requested to attend so that his blood can also be examined. By this means the chances of a serious hemoglobin defect in the fetus may be assessed early in pregnancy and the parents advised of the potential hazard and offered prenatal diagnosis by fetal blood sampling.[58]

MISCELLANEOUS ANEMIC DISORDERS

Bone Marrow Aplasia

There have been sporadic case reports of refractory hypoplastic anemia, sometimes recurrent, developing in gravid women and appearing to be related in some way to the pregnancy.[59] Occasionally gestation occurs when chronic acquired aplastic anemia is present as an underlying disease. It has been generally considered that in both these situations pregnancy exacerbates the marrow depression, causing rapid deterioration, and the gestation should be terminated. It is true that many cases do remit spontaneously after termination,[60] but there is no record of excessive hemorrhage at delivery despite profound thrombocytopenia. Supportive measures in this situation are improving and pregnancy should be maintained as long as the health of the mother is not seriously impaired.[61]

There are a few cases in the literature of reversible pure red cell aplasia associated with pregnancy. One report describes the course of relapsing pure red cell aplasia during three pregnancies.[62] Anemia can be profound and supportive red cell transfusions are necessary, but the outcome is generally good if there are no other interacting complications.

Autoimmune Hemolytic Anemia

The rare combination of autoimmune hemolytic anemia (AIHA) and pregnancy carries great risks to both the woman and the fetus. Very careful antenatal supervision and adjustment of steroid therapy is required.[63] There have been a number of reports in which women have been treated with steroids and other immunosuppressives (e.g., azathioprine) throughout pregnancy for a variety of conditions including immune thrombocytopenic purpura (ITP), systemic lupus, erythematosus, AIHA, and some forms of malignancy. The problems with their use are essentially those encountered in nonpregnant patients, but more frequent monitoring and adjustment are required due to the rapidly changing blood volume and changes in the circulating hormones during the antenatal and postnatal periods. There is also concern about the possible effects of azathioprine on the reproductive performance of female offspring.

POLYCYTHEMIA RUBRA VERA AND PREGNANCY

Polycythemia rubra vera (PRV), a myeloproliforative disease involving a pluripotent hematopoietic stem cell, is an uncommon disorder with an estimated incidence of 1 in 50,000. It affects women less often than men,

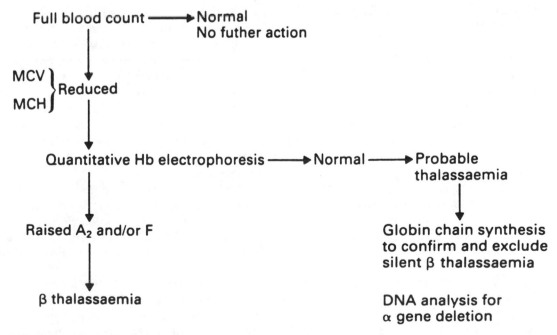

FIG 8–2.
Schema for identifying thalassemia carriers. MCV = mean corpuscular volume; MCH = mean corpuscular hemoglobin; Hb = hemoglobin.

usually appearing in the seventh decade of life, and is therefore only rarely encountered in pregnant women.

Reports in the literature are very sparse; only 15 pregnancies in nine women were recorded in a review published in 1983.[64] The maternal outcome in the few reports available is usually good, but there is an increased incidence of pregnancy-induced hypertension and perinatal mortality is high due to the frequent occurrence of abortion, stillbirth, and preterm delivery. Control of hematologic parameters is best achieved by repeated phlebotomy designed to maintain the hematocrit at a value of less than 45% in order to reduce the associated hazards of abnormal bleeding, thrombosis, and tissue hypoxia. Prophylactic antithrombotic measures during the intrapartum and postpartum period have been recommended because of the associated hypercoaguloability in uncomplicated pregnancy.[64] Low-dose heparin would appear to be the treatment of choice.

THROMBOCYTHEMIA (THROMBOCYTOSIS) AND PREGNANCY

Essential and primary thrombocythemia (thrombocytosis), a myeloproliferative disorder which usually affects subjects beyond the childbearing age, is characterized by an isolated high platelet count and is associated with both hemorrhagic and thromboembolic phenomena. We are aware of but a single report in the literature[66] of isolated thrombocytosis in pregnancy, but have observed two pregnant patients at our hospital and believe the condition may occur more frequently. If it is not accompanied by polycythemia, then the treatment of choice should be low-dose aspirin (75 mg/day) to inhibit platelet aggregation and thrombosis; this should be instituted when the platelet count exceeds $800 \times 10^9/L.$[65] Cytoxic agents have been used in this disease but such therapy ought to be avoided in gestation. There have also been reports of recurrent late abortions associated with thrombocythemia which were successfully managed with aspirin.[66] The two asymptomatic women with platelet counts around $1,000 \times 10^9/L$ at our hospital were managed throughout pregnancy with aspirin and no complications occurred in either mother or fetus.

PAROXYSMAL NOCTURNAL HEMOGLOBINURIA

This rare condition of unknown etiology, which occurs primarily in young adults, is believed to be due to an acquired change in the bone marrow stem cell, giving rise to populations of defective red cells, granulocytes, and platelets. The intrinsic defect in the red cell makes it particularly sensitive to lysis by complement. Paroxysmal nocturnal hemoglobinuria (PNH) varies widely in severity; it usually begins insidiously, and hemoglobinuria as a presenting symptom is found in only 25% of all patients. The laboratory diagnosis is made with a series of special tests which demonstrate the sensitivity of the patient's red cells to lysis by complement.

More important complications arise from the defective platelets and granulocytes produced by the abnormal clone of stem cells, leading to thrombosis, infection, and ultimately, marrow aplasia.[67, 68] The fertility rate in PNH is thought to be low, and experience with pregnancies in patients with PNH is limited to fewer than 50 cases reported in the English-language literature. Although more recently there have been reports of successful maternal and fetal outcome of pregnancies associated with PNH,[69–71] safe, effective contraception needs to be considered. There has been one report of cerebral vein thrombosis in a woman with PNH associated with use of an oral contraceptive.[72] An intrauterine device is contraindicated in the presence of thrombocytopenia and granulocytopenia. If pregnancy is embarked upon, the main hazards appear to be spontaneous abortion and serious thrombotic events, mainly in the puerperium. Hepatic vein thrombosis is the most common thrombotic complication, having a maximum incidence post partum; antepartum pulmonary embolism has also been reported. Prophylactic transfusions with washed red cells, which are not a source of extrinsic complement, and maintaining the hematocrit between 25% and 30% to suppress the production of abnormal cells have been recommended in the first trimester.[73]

Low-dose heparin has been shown to be ineffective prophylaxis against thrombosis in at least one case in the antepartum period.[65] It has been suggested therefore that full anticoagulation should be used to treat any thrombotic episode in the antepartum period and that full anticoagulation be used prophylactically in the puerperium.[73]

HEMATOLOGIC MALIGNANCIES

See Chapter 12 for a discussion of leukemia and lymphoma in pregnancy.

COAGULATION DEFECTS

Hemostasis and Pregnancy

Healthy hemostasis depends on normal vasculature, platelets, coagulation factors, and fibrinolysis. These act together to confine the circulating blood to the vascular bed and arrest bleeding after trauma. Normal pregnancy is accompanied by dramatic changes in the coagulation and fibrinolytic systems where there is a marked increase in some of the coagulation factors, particularly fibrinogen. Fibrin is laid down in the uteroplacental vessel walls and fibrinolysis is suppressed. These changes, together with the increased blood volume, help to combat the hazard of hemorrhage at placental separation, but play only a secondary role to the unique process of myometrial contraction which reduces blood flow to the placental site. They also produce a vulnerable state for intravascular clotting, which is expressed as a whole spectrum of disorders

in pregnancy ranging from thromboembolism to bleeding due to disseminated intravascular coagulation.[74] To make more understandable the pathophysiology and management of these disorders, a short account follows of hemostasis during pregnancy and how it differs from that in the nonpregnant state.

It is not known how vascular integrity is normally maintained but it is clear that platelets have a key role to play since conditions in which their number is depleted or their function is abnormal are characterized by widespread spontaneous capillary hemorrhages. It is thought that the platelets in health are constantly sealing microdefects in the vasculature, by forming minifibrin clots, the unwanted fibrin being removed by a process of fibrinolysis. Generation of prostacyclin appears to be the physiologic mechanism which protects the vessel wall from excess deposition of platelet aggregates, and explains the fact that contact of platelets with healthy vascular endothelium is not a stimulus for thrombus formation.[75]

Prostacyclin (prostaglandin I_2, or PGI_2) is the principal prostanoid synthesized by blood vessels, a powerful vasodilator and a potent inhibitor of platelet aggregation. Moncada and Vane[75] have proposed that there is a balance between the production of prostacyclin by the vessel wall and the production of the vasoconstrictor and powerful aggregating agent thromboxane by the platelet.

When injury is minor, small platelet thrombi form and are washed away by the circulation, as described above, but the extent of the injury is an important determinant of the size of the thrombus and whether or not platelet aggregation is stimulated (see below). Prostacyclin synthetase is abundant in the intima and progressively decreases in concentration from the intima to the adventitia, whereas the proaggregating elements increase in concentration from the subendothelium to the adventitia. It follows that severe vessel damage or physical detachment of the endothelium will lead to the development of a large thrombus as opposed to simple platelet adherence.

There are several conditions in which production of prostacyclin could be impaired, thereby upsetting the normal balance. Deficiency of prostacyclin production has been suggested in platelet consumption syndromes such as hemolytic-uremic syndrome and thrombotic thrombocytopenic purpura.[76] Prostacyclin production has also been shown to be reduced in fetal and placental tissue from preeclamptic pregnancies, and the current role of prostacyclin in the pathogenesis of preeclampsia is undergoing active investigation (see Chap. 1, Hypertension).

Platelets in Pregnancy

Observations concerning the platelet count during normal pregnancy conflict, but the majority consensus is that there is a small decrement in the platelet count near term.[77] Unfortunately, few studies obtained data on a longitudinal basis and in none of them was a within-patient analysis performed. The most recent studies, many surveying larger populations with the use of automated counting equipment, suggest that if mean values for platelet concentration are analyzed throughout pregnancy, there is a downward trend,[78] even though all values may be within the accepted nonpregnant range.[77, 79, 80]

There is conflicting evidence[81, 82] of increased platelet turnover and low-grade platelet activation as pregnancy advances, resulting in a larger proportion of younger platelets with a greater mean platelet volume.[78, 79] Most investigators agree that low-grade chronic intravascular coagulation within the uteroplacental circulation is a part of the physiologic response of all women to pregnancy. This is partially compensated and it is not surprising that the platelets should be involved showing evidence either of increased turnover or in some cases a reduction in number.

One study[83] demonstrated significantly more aggregated platelets in a small number of women during late pregnancy and the puerperium compared to nonpregnant controls. In another study, patients with a normal pregnancy were compared to nonpregnant controls, and were shown to have a significantly lower platelet count and an increase in circulating platelet aggregates.[84] In vitro the platelets were shown to be hypoaggregable. This was interpreted as suggesting platelet activation during pregnancy causing platelet aggregation and followed by exhaustion of platelets.[84]

Earlier publications suggesting that there was no evidence of changes in platelet function[85] or differences in platelet life span[81] between healthy nonpregnant and pregnant women have to be reevaluated in the face of more recent investigations, but it is clear that normal pregnancy has little significant effect on the screening parameter that is usually measured, namely the platelet count.

The problem remains in defining "completely normal pregnancy." Certain disease states specific to pregnancy have profound effects on platelet consumption, life span, and function. For example, a decrease in platelet count has been observed in pregnancies with fetal growth retardation[86] and the life span of platelets is shortened significantly, even in mild preeclampsia.

Arrest of Bleeding After Trauma

An essential function of the hemostatic system is a rapid reaction to injury that remains confined to the area of damage. This requires a control mechanism which will stimulate coagulation after trauma, and also limit the extent of the responses. The substances involved in the formation of the hemostatic plug normally circulate in an inert form, until activated at the site of injury. The role of platelets is of less importance in injury involving large vessels, because platelet aggregates are of insufficient size and strength to breach the defect. The coagulation mechanism is of major importance here, together with vascular contraction.

Coagulation System

The end result of blood coagulation, the formation of an insoluble fibrin clot from the soluble precursor fibrinogen in the plasma, involves a complex interaction of clotting fac-

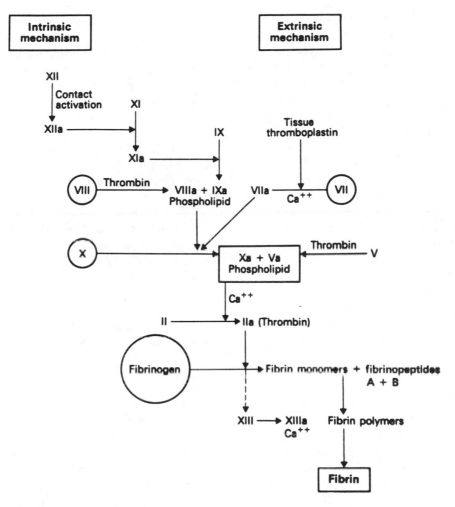

FIG 8–3.
The factors involved in blood coagulation and their interactions. The circled factors show significant increases in pregnancy.

tors, and a sequential activation of a series of proenzymes—the coagulation cascade (Fig 8–3). When a blood vessel is injured, blood coagulation is initiated by activation of factor XII by collagen (intrinsic mechanism) and activation of factor VII by thromboplastin release (extrinsic mechanism) from the damaged tissues. Both the intrinsic and extrinsic mechanisms are activated by components of the vessel wall and both are required for normal hemostasis. Strict divisions between the two pathways do not exist and interactions between activated factors in both pathways have been shown. They share a common pathway following the activation of factor X.

The intrinsic pathway (or contact system) proceeds spontaneously but is relatively slow, requiring 5 to 20 minutes for visible fibrin formation. All tissues contain a specific lipoprotein, thromboplastin (particularly concentrated in lung and brain), which markedly increases the rate at which blood clots. The placenta is also very rich in tissue factor (thromboplastin), which will produce fibrin formation within 12 seconds; the acceleration of coagulation is brought about by bypassing the reactions involving the contact (intrinsic) system (see Fig 8–3). Since blood coagulation is strictly confined to the site of tissue injury in normal circumstances, powerful control mechanisms must be at work to prevent dissemination of coagulation.

Normal pregnancy is accompanied by major changes in the coagulation system, with increases in levels of factors VII, VIII, and X and a particularly marked increase in the level of plasma fibrinogen[87] (see Fig 8–3), which is probably the chief cause of the accelerated erythrocyte sedimentation rate observed during pregnancy. The effect of pregnancy on the coagulation factors can be detected from about the third month of gestation, and the amount of fibrinogen in late pregnancy is at least double that of the nonpregnant state.[87]

The Naturally Occurring Anticoagulants.—Mechanisms that limit and localize the clotting process at sites of trauma are critically important for protection against generalized thrombosis and also to prevent spontaneous activation of those powerful procoagulant factors which circulate in normal plasma.

The recent investigation of healthy hemostasis switched emphasis from the factors that promote clotting to those that prevent generalized and spontaneous activation of these factors. Space requirements limit an account of the complex interactions and biochemistry of all of these factors and only those of major importance in hemostasis and their relevance to pregnancy will be mentioned here. The balance of procoagulant and inhibitory factors is discussed well in a review article.[88]

Antithrombin III.—Antithrombin III (AT-III) is considered to be the main physiologic inhibitor of thrombin and factor Xa. Heparin greatly enhances the reaction rate of enzyme AT-III interaction and this is the rationale for the use of low-dose heparin as prophylaxis in patients at risk for thromboembolism postoperatively, in pregnancy, and in the puerperium. An inherited deficiency of AT-III is one of the few conditions in which a familial tendency to thrombosis has been described.

AT-III is synthesized in the liver. Its ac-

tivity is low in cirrhosis and other chronic diseases of the liver, as well as in protein-losing renal disease, disseminated intravascular coagulation, and hypercoagulable states. The commonest cause of a small reduction in AT-III is the use of oral contraceptives; this effect is related to the estrogen content of the pill.

During pregnancy there is little change in AT-III level but there is some decrease at parturition and an increase in the puerperium.[89]

Protein C-thrombomodulin-protein S.— *Protein C* inactivates factors V and VIII in conjunction with its cofactors thrombomodulin and protein S. To exert its effect protein C, a vitamin K–dependent anticoagulant synthesized in the liver, must be activated by an endothelial cell cofactor termed *thrombomodulin*. The importance of the protein C-thrombomodulin-protein S system is exemplified by the absence of thrombomodulin in the brain where the priority for hemostasis is higher than for anticoagulation.

Many kindreds with a deficiency or a functional deficit of protein C with associated recurrent thromboembolism have been described.[90] Purpura fulminans neonatalis is the homozygous expression of protein C deficiency with severe thrombosis and neonatal death.[91]

Protein S, also a vitamin K-dependent glycoprotein, acts as a cofactor for activated protein C by promoting its binding to lipid and platelet surface, thus localizing the reaction. Several families have been described with protein S deficiency and thromboembolic disease.

Data on protein C and protein S levels in healthy pregnancy are sparse. One study showed a significant reduction in functional protein S levels during pregnancy and the puerperium.[92] More recently, 14 patients followed longitudinally throughout gestation and post partum showed a rise of protein C within the normal nonpregnant range during the second trimester. In contrast, free protein S fell from the second trimester onward but remained within the confines of the normal range.[93]

As Salem[94] has noted:

> Although the era of natural anticoagulants has only just begun, the system has grown in complexity in a very short time. There is little doubt that more components will be recognised in the near future which will allow a better and more thorough understanding of the mechanisms underlying venous and arterial thromboembolism.[94]

Fibrinolysis

Fibrinolytic activity, an essential part of the dynamic, interacting hemostatic mechanism, is dependent on plasminogen activator in the blood (Fig 8–4). Fibrin and fibrinogen are digested by plasmin, an enzyme derived from an inactive plasma precursor, plasminogen.

Increased amounts of activator are found in the plasma after strenuous exercise, emotional stress, surgical operations, and other trauma. Tissue activator can be extracted from most human organs with the exception of the placenta. Tissues especially rich in activator include the uterus, ovaries, prostate, heart, lungs, thyroid, adrenals, and lymph nodes. Activity in tissues is concentrated mainly around blood vessels, veins showing greater activity than arteries.

The inhibitors of fibrinolytic activity are of two types: antiactivators (antiplasminogens) and the antiplasmins. Inhibitors of plasminogen include ϵ-aminocaproic acid (EACA)

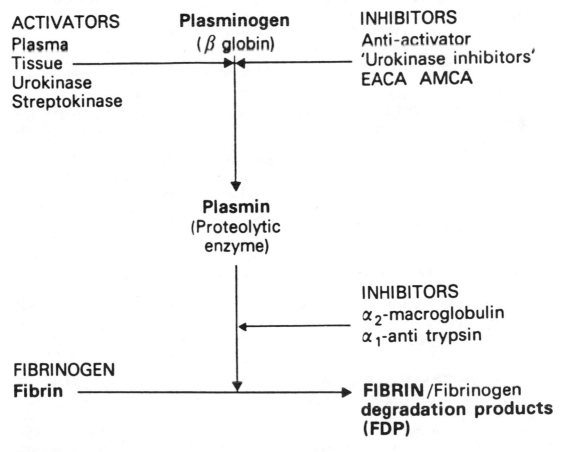

FIG 8–4.
Components of the fibrinolytic system. EACA = ϵ-aminocaproic acid; AMCA = tranexamic acid.

and tranexamic acid (AMCA). Aprotinin (Trasylol) is another antiplasminogen which is commercially prepared from bovine lung.

Platelets, plasma, and serum exert a strong inhibitor action on plasmin. Normally, plasma antiplasmin levels exceed levels of plasminogen and hence the levels of potential plasmin; otherwise we would dissolve away our connecting cement! When fibrinogen or fibrin is broken down by plasmin, fibrin degradation products are formed; these comprise the high-molecular-weight split products X and Y, and smaller fragments, A, B, C, D, and E. When a fibrin clot is formed, 70% of fragment X is retained in the clot, Y, D, and E being retained to a somewhat lesser extent. Blood should be taken for estimation of fibrin degradation products by clean venipuncture. The tourniquet should not be left on too long since venous stasis also stimulates fibrinolytic activity. The blood should be allowed to clot in the presence of an antifibrinolytic agent such as EACA to stop the process of fibrinolysis which would otherwise continue in vitro.

Plasma fibrinolytic activity is decreased during pregnancy, remains low during labor and delivery, and returns to normal within 1 hour of delivery of the placenta.[95] The rapid return to normal fibrinolytic activity following delivery of the placenta and the fact that the placenta has been shown to contain inhibitors which block fibrinolysis suggest that inhibition of fibrinolysis during pregnancy is mediated by the placenta.

Summary of Changes in Hemostasis in Pregnancy and Delivery

Changes in the coagulation system during normal pregnancy are consistent with a continuing low-grade process of coagulant activity. Using electron microscopy, fibrin deposition can be demonstrated in the intervillous space of the placenta and in the walls of the spiral arteries supplying the placenta.[96] As pregnancy advances, the elastic lamina and smooth muscle of these spiral arteries are replaced by a matrix containing fibrin. This allows expansion of the lumen to accommodate an increasing blood flow and reduces the vascular resistance of the placenta. At placental separation during normal childbirth, a blood flow of 500 to 800 mL/min has to be reduced within seconds, or serious hemorrhage will occur. Myometrial contraction plays a vital role in securing hemostasis by decreasing blood flow to the placental site. Rapid closure of the terminal part of the spiral artery will be further facilitated by removal of the elastic lamina. The placental site is rapidly covered by a fibrin mesh following delivery. The increased levels of fibrinogen and other coagulation factors will be advantageous to meet the sudden demand for hemostatic components.

The changes also produce a vulnerable state for intravascular clotting and a whole spectrum of disorders involving coagulation which occur in pregnancy.[74] (For a discussion of venous thromboembolism in pregnancy, see Chapter 6, p. 218.)

Disseminated Intravascular Coagulation

The changes in the hemostatic system and the local activation of the clotting system during parturition carry with them a risk not only of thromboembolism but also of disseminated intravascular coagulation (DIC). This results in consumption of clotting factors and platelets, leading in some cases to severe, particularly uterine and sometimes generalized, bleeding.[97]

The first problem with DIC is in its definition. It is never primary but always secondary to some general stimulation of coagulation activity by release of procoagulant substances into the blood (Fig 8–5). Hypothetical triggers of this process in pregnancy include the leaking of placental tissue fragments, amniotic fluid, incompatible red cells, or bacterial products into the maternal circulation. There is a great spectrum of manifestations of the process of DIC (Table 8–3), ranging from a compensated state with no clinical manifestations but evidence of increased production and breakdown of coagulation factors, to the condition of massive uncontrollable

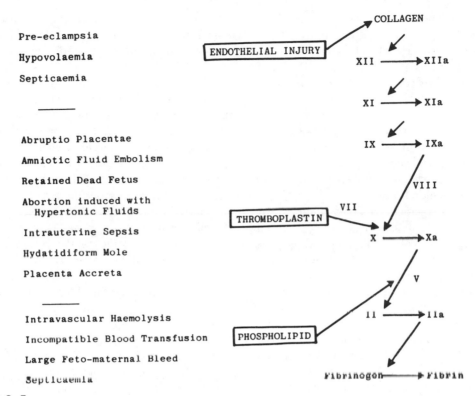

FIG 8–5.
Trigger mechanisms of disseminated intravascular coagulation during pregnancy. Interactions occur in many of these obstetric complications.

hemorrhage with very low concentrations of plasma fibrinogen, pathologically raised levels of fibrin degradation products, and variable degrees of thrombocytopenia. Further cause for confusion is that there appears to be a transitory state of intravascular coagulation during the whole of normal labor, maximal at the time of birth.[98-100]

Fibrinolysis is stimulated by DIC, and the fibrin degradation products resulting from the process interfere with the formation of a firm fibrin clot, causing a vicious circle which results in further disastrous bleeding. These degradation products also interfere with myometrial function and possibly cardiac function and therefore in themselves aggravate both hemorrhage and shock. Obstetric conditions associated with DIC include abruptio placentae, amniotic fluid embolism, septic abortion and intrauterine infection, retained dead fetus, hydatidiform mole, placenta accreta, preeclampsia and eclampsia, and prolonged shock from any cause (see Fig 8–5).

Despite the advances in obstetric care and highly developed blood transfusion services, hemorrhage still constitutes a major factor in maternal mortality and morbidity. There have been many reports concerning small series of patients or individual patients with coagulation failure during pregnancy. However, no significant controlled trials of the value of the many possible therapeutic measures seems to have been carried out, due probably to the paucity of patients with these problems in any one center. Also, the complex and variable nature of the conditions associated with DIC, which are often self-correcting and treated with a variety of measures, makes it difficult to draw helpful conclusions from anecdotal published reports.

Hematologic Management of the Bleeding Obstetric Patient With a Coagulation Defect

(See also Chapter 7, p. 242, for a discussion of hemorrhagic shock.) Because of the urgency of the situation there should be a routine planned practice agreed to by a hematologist, physician, anesthesiologist, obstetrician, and nursing staff in all maternity units, to deal with this situation whenever it arises.

It is imperative that the source of bleeding, often an unsuspected uterine or genital laceration, be located and dealt with. Prolonged hypovolemic shock, or indeed shock from any cause, may also trigger DIC and this may lead to hemostatic failure and further prolonged hemorrhage.

The management of hemorrhage is virtually the same whether the bleeding is caused or augmented by coagulation failure. The clinical condition usually demands urgent treatment and there is no time to wait for results of coagulation factor assays or sophisticated tests of fibrinolytic system activity for precise definition of the extent of hemostatic failure. Blood may be taken for this purpose and analyzed at leisure once the emergency is over.

The simple rapid tests recommended below will establish the competence or otherwise of the hemostatic system. In the vast majority of obstetric patients, coagulation failure results from a sudden transitory episode of DIC triggered by a variety of conditions (see Fig 8–5).

As soon as there is any concern about a patient bleeding from any cause, venous blood should be taken by a quick, efficient, nontraumatic technique and delivered into a set of tubes kept in an emergency pack with a set of laboratory request forms previously made out which require only that the patient's name and identification number be added to them.

Heparin characteristically prolongs the partial thromboplastin time and thrombin time out of proportion to the prothrombin time. As little as 0.05 unit/mL of heparin will prolong the coagulation test times. It is customary, though not desirable, to take blood for coagulation tests from lines which have been washed through with fluids containing heparin to keep them patent. It is almost impossible to overcome the effect of such fluids on the blood passing through such a line, however much blood is taken and discarded before obtaining a sample for investigation. Useful rapid screening tests for hemostatic

TABLE 8–3.
Spectrum of Severity of Disseminated Intravascular Coagulation (DIC): Its Relationship to Specific Complications in Obstetrics

Stage*	Severity of DIC	In Vitro Findings	Obstetric Condition Commonly Associated
1	Low-grade compensated	FDPs ↑ Increased soluble fibrin complexes Increased VIIIRAg:VIIIC ratio Coagulation screen normal	Preeclampsia/eclampsia Retained dead fetus
2	Uncompensated but no hemostatic failure	FDPs ↑ Fibrinogen ↓ Platelets ↓ Factors V and VIII ↓ Clotting times prolonged	Small abruption Preeclampsia/eclampsia
3	Rampant with hemostatic failure	Platelets ↓ ↓ Gross depletion of coagulation factors, particularly fibrinogen FDPs ↑ ↑	Abruptio placentae Amniotic fluid embolism Preeclampsia/eclampsia

FDPs = fibrin degradation products; ↑ = increased; ↑ ↑ = markedly increased; ↓ = decreased; ↓ ↓ = markedly decreased.
*Rapid progression from stage 1 to stage 3 is possible unless appropriate action is taken.

failure include the platelet count, partial thromboplastin time (which tests intrinsic coagulation), prothrombin time (which tests extrinsic coagulation), thrombin time, and estimation of fibrinogen.

The measurement of fibrin degradation products provides an indirect test for fibrinolysis. In obstetric practice the measurement of fibrin degradation products is usually part of the investigation of suspected acute or chronic DIC. In the acute situation raised fibrin degradation products only confirm the presence of DIC, but are not diagnostic, and once the specimen is taken the laboratory measurement should be delayed until the emergency is over. Of the tests of coagulation the thrombin clottable fibrinogen in a citrated sample of plasma is the most valuable overall rapid screen of hemostatic competence of coagulation factors. The thrombin time of normal plasma is adjusted in the laboratory to 10 to 15 seconds, and the fibrin clot that is formed is firm and stable. In the most severe forms of DIC there is no clottable fibrinogen in the sample, and no fibrin clot appears even after 2 to 3 minutes. Indication of severe DIC is obtained usually by a prolonged thrombin time with a friable clot, which may dissolve on standing owing to fibrinolytic substances present in the plasma. Prolongation of the thrombin time is observed not only with depleted fibrinogen but in conditions where fibrin degradation products are increased.

There is no point whatsoever in the physician or nursing staff wasting time trying to perform bedside whole-blood clotting tests. Such estimation of whole-blood clotting time furnishes little information of practical value and only creates more panic. The valuable hands at the bedside are of more use doing the things they are trained to do in this emergency situation rather than wasting time performing a test which is time-consuming, of little value or significance unless performed under strictly controlled conditions, and which will not contribute much, if anything, to management. The alerted laboratory worker will be able to provide helpful results on which the physician can act within half an hour of receiving the specimen in the laboratory.

Treatment.—Treatment of severe hemorrhage includes prompt and adequate volume replacement to avoid renal shutdown. If effective circulation is restored without too much delay, fibrin degradation products will be cleared from the blood mainly by the liver, which will further aid restoration of normal hemostasis. This is an aspect of management which is often not appropriately emphasized.[101] Since various treatment regimens are outlined in Chapter 7 on critical care, remarks here will relate only to the controversies and complications of the various therapies.

There is much controversy around which plasma substitute to give a bleeding patient. The choice lies between simple crystalloids and artificial colloids, or the very expensive preparations of human albumin (albuminoids). If crystalloids are used, two or three times the volume of estimated blood loss should be administered because the crystalloid remains in the vascular compartment for a shorter time than do colloids.

Infusion of plasma substitutes, i.e., plasma protein, dextran, gelatin, and starch solutions, may result in adverse reactions. Although the incidence of severe reactions is rare, they are diverse in nature, varying from allergic urticarial manifestations and mild fever to life-threatening anaphylactic reactions due to spasm of smooth muscle, with cardiac and respiratory arrest.[102]

Dextrans adversely affect platelet function, may cause pseudoagglutination, and interfere with interpretation of subsequent blood grouping and crossmatching tests. They are therefore contraindicated in the pregnant woman who is bleeding since there is such a high chance of there being a serious hemostatic defect. Dextrans are also associated with allergic anaphylactoid reactions. The anaphylactoid reactions accompanying infusion of dextrans are probably related to IgG and IgM antidextran antibodies which have subsequently been found in high concentrations in all patients with severe reactions.[103]

Whole blood may be the treatment of choice in coagulation failure associated with obstetric disorders,[104] but whole fresh blood is no longer generally available because there is insufficient time to complete hepatitis surface antigen, HIV (human immunodeficiency virus) antibody, and blood grouping tests before it is released from the transfusion center. Cytomegalovirus and Epstein-Barr virus are examples of other infections not screened for which may be transmitted in fresh blood rather than stored blood. Their viability diminishes rapidly on storage at 4°C. The use of fresh frozen plasma followed by bank red cells provides all the components, apart from platelets, present in whole blood and allows the plasma from the freshly donated unit to be used to make the much needed blood components.[105]

Plasma Component Therapy.—Fresh frozen plasma contains all the coagulation factors present in plasma obtained from whole blood within 6 hours of donation. Frozen rapidly and stored at −30°C, the factors are well preserved for at least 1 year. Plasma stored at −20°C does degenerate and should be used within 6 months of preparation. Freeze-dried plasma is deficient in factors V and VIII and carries a risk of transmitting hepatitis and acquired immunodeficiency syndrome (AIDS). It can be of value in providing colloid in the management of hemorrhage. Concentrated fibrinogen, which also carries considerable risk of hepatitis and/or AIDS, should not be used in obstetric hemorrhage. Administration may result in a sharp fall in levels of AT-III, suggesting that the concentrate may aggravate intravascular coagulation[87] by adding fuel to the fire. Fresh frozen plasma provides abundant fibrinogen together with factors V and VIII, which are also depleted, and the coagulation inhibitor AT-III.

Platelets are not present in fresh frozen plasma and their functional activity rapidly deteriorates in stored blood. A patient with persistent bleeding and a very low platelet count (<20 × 10⁹/L) may be given concentrated platelets, although they are very seldom required in addition to fresh frozen plasma to achieve hemostasis. Indeed, it has been suggested that platelet transfusions are more likely to do harm than good in this situation since most concentrates contain some damaged platelets which might in themselves provide a fresh trigger or mediator of DIC in the existing stage.[106] A spontaneous recovery from the coagulation defect is to be expected once the uterus is empty and well contracted, provided that blood volume is maintained by adequate replacement monitored by central filling pressures and urinary output.

Stored whole blood, even under optimal conditions, undergoes deleterious changes. The oxygen affinity of red cells increases, inhibiting unloading of oxygen from hemoglobin in hypoxic tissues. Plasma ionic concentrations of potassium and hydrogen increase but these changes are not significant until after 4 weeks of shelf life. Platelets deteriorate rapidly within the first 24 hours and after 72 hours they have lost all hemostatic function.

If the blood loss is replaced only by stored bank blood, which is deficient in the labile clotting factors V and VIII and platelets, then the circulation will rapidly become depleted in these essential components of hemostasis even if there is no DIC initially as the cause of hemorrhage. It is advisable to transfuse 1 unit of fresh frozen plasma for every 6 to 8 units of bank red cells administered.

The single most important component of hemostasis at delivery is contraction of the myometrium stemming the flow from the placental site. Massive transfusion of all clotting factors and platelets will not stop hemorrhage if the uterus is atonic. Vaginal delivery will make less severe demands on the hemostatic mechanism than delivery by cesarean section, which requires the same hemostatic competence as any other major surgical procedure.

DIC in Selected Clinical Conditions

In Vitro Detection of Low-Grade DIC.—Rampant uncompensated DIC results in severe hemorrhage, with the characteristic laboratory findings described above. Low-grade DIC, however, does not usually give rise to any clinical manifestations although the condition is a potentially hazardous one for both mother and fetus. Many in vitro tests have been claimed to detect low-grade compensated DIC and space does not allow an account of all of these. Evaluation should include review of the blood film for telltale signs such as red blood cell fragmentation.

Fibrin Degradation Products.—Estimation of these will give some indication of low-grade DIC if they are significantly raised when fibrinogen, platelets, and screening tests of hemostatic function appear to be within the normal range (see Table 8–3).

Soluble Fibrin Complexes.—The action of thrombin on fibrinogen is crucial in DIC. Thrombin splits two molecules of fibrinopeptide A and two molecules of fibrinopeptide B from fibrinogen. The remaining molecule is called a fibrin monomer and polymerizes rapidly to fibrin (see Fig 8–3).

Free fibrinopeptides in the blood are a specific measure of thrombin activity and high levels of fibrinopeptide A have been shown to be associated with compensated DIC in pregnancy.[100]

Soluble fibrin complexes made up of fibrin-fibrinogen dimers are increased in conditions of low-grade DIC. These complexes are generated during the process of thrombin generation and the conversion of soluble fibrinogen to insoluble fibrin. Levels of soluble fibrin complexes are increased in patients with severe preeclampsia and with a retained dead fetus.[107]

Factor VIII.—During normal pregnancy the levels of both factor VIII–related antigen (VIIIR:Ag) and factor VIII coagulation activity (VIII:C) rise in parallel.[108, 109] An increase in the ratio of factor VIIIR:Ag to factor VIII:C has been observed in conditions accompanied by low-grade DIC whether associated with pregnancy or not. An increase in the ratio has been observed in pregnancy with a retained dead fetus and with preeclampsia[110] without any alteration in the simple screening tests of hemostatic function previously described.

The stages in the spectrum of severity of

DIC (see Table 8–3) are not strictly delineated and there may be rapid progression from low-grade compensated DIC, as diagnosed by the paracoagulation tests described above, to the rampant form with hemostatic failure.

Abruptio Placentae.—Premature separation of the placenta, or abruptio placentae, is the most frequent obstetric cause of coagulation failure. This problem is dealt with in detail in most obstetric texts. However, many of the problems in this situation are common to other conditions associated with DIC in pregnancy, (e.g., amniotic fluid embolism, retained dead fetus) and management controversies exist such that further discussion here is warranted.

Clinical Presentation.—Abruptio placentae can occur in apparently healthy women with no clinical warning or in the context of established preeclampsia. It is possible that clinically silent placental infarcts may predispose to placental separation by causing low-grade abnormalities of the hemostatic system such as increased factor VIII consumption and raised fibrin degradation products.[111]

There is a wide spectrum in the severity of hemostatic failure in this condition which appears to be related to the degree of placental separation. Only 10% of patients with abruptio placentae show significant coagulation abnormalities. In some small abruptions there is a minor degree of failure of hemostatic processes and the fetus does not succumb (see Table 8–3). When the uterus is tense and tender and no fetal heart can be heard, the separation and retroplacental bleeding are extensive. No guide to the severity of the hemorrhage or coagulation failure will be given by the amount of vaginal bleeding. For example, there may be no external vaginal blood loss, even when the placenta is completely separated, the fetus is dead, the circulating blood is incoagulable, and there is up to 5 L of concealed blood loss resulting in hypovolemic shock.

Diagnosis and Treatment.—Hemostatic

failure may be suspected if there is persistent oozing at the site of venipuncture or bleeding from the mucous membranes of the mouth or nose. Simple rapid screening tests will confirm the presence of DIC. There will be a low platelet count, greatly prolonged thrombin time, low fibrinogen, together with raised fibrin degradation products (see Table 8–3), due to secondary fibrinolysis stimulated by the intravascular formation of fibrin.[112] The mainstay of treatment is to restore and maintain the circulating blood volume. This not only prevents renal shutdown and further hemostatic failure caused by hypovolemic shock, but helps clearance of fibrin degradation products which in themselves act as potent anticoagulants. It has also been suggested that they inhibit myometrial activity, and serious postpartum hemorrhage in women with abruptio placentae has been found to be associated with high levels of fibrin degradation products.[113] High levels of fibrin degradation products may also have a cardiotoxic effect resulting in low cardiac output and reduced blood pressure despite a normal circulating blood volume.

If the fetus is dead the aim should be prompt vaginal delivery avoiding soft tissue damage, once correction of hypovolemia is underway. There is no evidence that the use of oxytocic agents aggravates thromboplastin release from the uterus.[114] Following the emptying of the uterus, myometrial contraction will greatly reduce bleeding from the placental site and spontaneous correction of the hemostatic defect usually occurs shortly after delivery, if the measures recommended above have been taken. However, postpartum hemorrhage is a not infrequent complication and is the commonest cause of death in abruptio placentae.[115]

In cases where the abruption is small and the fetus is still alive, prompt cesarean section may save the baby, if vaginal delivery is not imminent. Fresh frozen plasma, bank red cells, and platelet concentrates should be available to correct the potentially severe maternal coagulation defect. In rare situations where vaginal delivery cannot be stimulated and hemorrhage continues, cesarean section is indicated even in the presence of a dead fetus. In these circumstances normal hemostasis should be restored as far as possible by the administration of fresh frozen plasma and platelet concentrates, if necessary, as well as by transfusing red cells before surgery is undertaken.

Despite extravasation of blood throughout the uterine muscle, its function is not impaired and good contraction will follow removal of the fetus, placenta, and retroperitoneal clot. Regional anesthesia or analgesia is contraindicated. Expansion of the lower limb vascular bed resulting from regional block can add to the problem of uncorrected hypovolemia; in the presence of hemostatic failure there is the additional hazard of bleeding into the epidural space.[87]

In recent years, heparin has been used to treat many cases of DIC, whatever the cause. There is, however, no objective evidence to demonstrate that its use in abruptio placentae decreases morbidity and mortality although anecdotal reports continue to suggest this.[116] Very good results have been achieved without the use of heparin.[101] Its use, with an intact circulation, would be sensible to break the vicious circle of DIC, but in the presence of already defective hemostasis with a large bleeding placental site, it may prolong massive local and generalized hemorrhage.[117]

Treatment with antifibrinolytic agents such as EACA or aprotinin can result in blockage of small vessels of vital organs, such as the kidney or brain, with fibrin. Such agents are therefore contraindicated, although Bonnar[87] suggests that delayed severe and prolonged hemorrhage from the placental site several hours postdelivery may respond to their use if all other measures fail.

It has been suggested[113, 118] that aprotinin may be helpful in the management of abruptio placentae, particularly in those cases with uterine inertia associated with high levels of fibrin degradation products. There is a high incidence (1.5%) of abruptio placentae in the obstetric admissions (18,000 per annum) at the Groote Schuur Obstetric Unit, Cape

Town, where the first study was carried out. Intravenous administration of aprotinin in eight patients with abruptio placentae and uterine inertia together with other prompt supportive measures resulted in a rapid re-coordination of uterine activity as well as a steady fall in serum fibrin degradation product levels and a progressive rise in platelet count. The selection of aprotinin as opposed to EACA depended on its alleged anticoagulant activity in addition to its well-known antifibrinolytic properties. An anticoagulant effect would make it a less hazardous agent in view of intravascular deposition of fibrin in vital organs and particularly useful in the management of hemorrhage due to DIC. However, in vitro studies indicate that very high concentrations are required to have any anticoagulant effect.[119] Another study[120] showed that high concentrations of aprotinin appeared to inhibit the contact phase of co-agulation only and the authors concluded that the drug would be a relatively weak anticoagulant in doses liable to be achieved in vivo. It would of course have no direct effect on the extrinsic coagulation pathway, which is activated in the course of DIC due to abruptio placentae. However, Nordstrom and colleagues[121] showed that DIC in dogs, induced by injection of thromboplastin, was partially inhibited if they were treated prophylactically with aprotinin.

In recent years, obstetricians appear unconvinced of the benefits of aprotinin in the treatment of DIC and abruptio placentae. Prompt supportive measures alone, maintaining central blood volume and replacing blood loss together with essential coagulation factors, will of course result in reduction in fibrin degradation products. This will improve myometrial function and contribute to the return of healthy hemostasis.

One patient with recurrent abruptio placentae successfully treated with the fibrinolytic inhibitor tranexamic acid has been reported[122]; the compound is related to EACA. Investigations in this woman suggested abnormally increased fibrinolytic activity in the 26th week of her third pregnancy. The previous two pregnancies had been complicated by abruptio placentae associated with a neonatal death and a stillbirth, respectively. The intravenous administration of tranexamic acid following a small vaginal bleed resulted in restoration of normal coagulation status and the bleeding stopped; oral administration was continued. Another small bleed occurred at 33 weeks' gestation, and was treated again with intravenous tranexamic acid. The eventual successful outcome of this pregnancy was attributed by the authors to the use of this agent, but there may have been many other variables involved.

Amniotic Fluid Embolism.—(See Chap. 7, p. 253).

Induced Abortion.—Changes in hemostatic components consistent with DIC have been demonstrated in patients undergoing abortion induced with hypertonic solutions of saline and urea.[123–127] This combination appears to be particularly hazardous in comparison to the use of urea and prostaglandin or oxytocin.[128] The stimulus appears to be the release of tissue factor into the maternal circulation from the placenta which is damaged by the hypertonic solutions. In later pregnancy DIC has been described with both dilation and evacuation[129] and also with prostaglandin and oxytocin termination.[130] The hemorrhage resulting may be massive and has resulted in maternal deaths. Prompt restoration of the blood volume and transfusion with red cells and fresh frozen plasma, as described above, should resolve the situation which, once the uterus is empty, is self-limiting.

Intrauterine Infection.—Endotoxic shock associated with septic abortion and antepartum or postpartum intrauterine infection can trigger DIC.[131, 132] Infection is usually with gram-negative organisms. Fibrin is deposited in the microvasculature owing to endothelial damage by the endotoxin, and secondary red cell intravascular hemolysis with characteristic fragmentation, so-called microangiopathic hemolysis, is characteristic of the condition. Septic shock and abortion are detailed further in Chapters 7, p. 245, and 13.

Purpura Fulminans.—This rare complication of infection sometimes occurs in the puerperium, precipitated by gram-negative septicemia. Extensive hemorrhage occurs into the skin in association with DIC. The underlying mechanism is unknown but there appears to be an acute activation of the clotting system resulting in the deposition of fibrin thrombi within blood vessels of the skin and other organs.[133] The extremities and face are usually involved first, the purpuric patches having a jagged and erythematous border, which can be shown histologically to be the site of a leukocytoclastic vasculitis. Rapid enlargement of the lesions, which become necrotic and gangrenous, is associated with shock, tachycardia, and fever. Without treatment the mortality rate is high and among those who survive, digit or limb amputation may be necessary. The laboratory findings are those of DIC with leukocytosis. In this situation treatment with heparin should be started as soon as the diagnosis is apparent. It will prevent further consumption of platelets and coagulation factors. It should always be remembered, however, that bleeding from any site in the presence of defective coagulation factors will be aggravated by the use of heparin. Survival in purpura fulminans is currently much improved because of better supportive treatment for the shocked patient and effective control of the triggering infection, together with heparin therapy.

Acute Fatty Liver of Pregnancy.—Acute fatty liver of pregnancy (AFLP) is an unusual complication of pregnancy discussed in Chapter 10, but included in this section because it is often associated with variable degrees of DIC which contribute significantly to its morbidity and mortality.[117, 134] Only the hematologic aspects will be discussed here.

Early diagnosis and subsequent delivery are believed essential for improving survival of both mother and child. Most patients have prodromal symptoms for at least 1 week before jaundice develops. One reported series[135] draws attention to a characteristic blood picture of neutrophilia, thrombocytopenia, and normoblasts. Some of the blood films available for review also showed basophilic stippling and giant platelets and the authors suggest that these appearances might help toward an early diagnosis of AFLP. However, these features are not specific to AFLP and may be seen in any condition of additional stress on a bone marrow already working to capacity in the last trimester or pregnancy.

DIC complicating severe liver failure is an extremely complex topic. In AFLP the hemostatic defect is frequently resistant, probably owing to prolonged activation of coagulation combined with very low to undetectable AT-III levels.[117, 136, 137] The replacement of AT-III with plasma or concentrate to shorten the period of DIC and thereby decrease morbidity and mortality in AFLP has been suggested[117] and an AT-III concentrate has been used in the successful management of a patient with AFLP.[138] Heparin therapy can be very dangerous.[139]

Conclusions

Disseminated intravascular coagulation is always a secondary phenomenon and the mainstay of management is therefore to remove the initiating stimulus if possible.

With rampant DIC and hemorrhage, recovery will usually follow delivery of the patient provided that the blood volume is maintained and shock due to hypovolemia is prevented. An efficiently acting myometrium postdelivery will stem hemorrhage from the placental site. Measures taken to achieve a firm contracted uterus will obviously contribute one of the most important factors in preventing continuing massive blood loss from the placental site.

It is of interest that the maternal mortality of DIC associated with placental abruption is less than 1%,[140] whereas that associated with infection and shock may be as high as

50% to 80%, depending on the underlying disorder.[141] There is no doubt that the major determinant of survival is the identification of the underlying trigger and our ability to manage this successfully.

Acquired Primary Defects of Hemostasis

Thrombocytopenia

The commonest platelet abnormality encountered in clinical practice is thrombocytopenia, and pregnancy is no exception. Progress through the years has effected dramatic reductions in maternal and fetal mortality and morbidity, but maternal thrombocytopenia remains a difficult management problem during pregnancy and can also have profound effects on fetal and neonatal well-being. The causes and management of maternal and fetal thrombocytopenia have been reviewed.[142] Emphasis here will be on those conditions which cause particular diagnostic and management problems in obstetric practice.

A recent prospective study of 2,263 healthy women delivering during 1 year at a Canadian obstetric center[143] showed that 112 (8.3%) had mild thrombocytopenia at term (platelet counts 97–150 $\times$ 10^9/L). The frequency of thrombocytopenia in their offspring was no greater than that of babies born to women with platelet counts in the normal range and none of these infants had a platelet count of less than 100 $\times$ 10^9/L. This supports an earlier study[84] (see above) showing decreased platelet counts and an increase in circulating aggregates in women with normal pregnancies compared to nonpregnant controls.

A low platelet count is seen most frequently in association with DIC (as already described). Sometimes severe megaloblastic anemia of pregnancy is accompanied by thrombocytopenia, but the platelet count rapidly returns to normal after therapy with folic acid.[87] Toxic depression of bone marrow megakaryocytes in pregnancy can occur in association with infection, certain drugs, and alcoholism. Neoplastic infiltration may also result in thrombocytopenia. Probably the single most important cause of isolated thrombocytopenia is autoimmune thrombocytopenic purpura (AITP), which is a disease primarily of young women in the reproductive years.[144]

Autoimmune Thrombocytopenia

The diagnosis of autoimmune thrombocytopenia was formerly made when extremely low platelet counts were found to be associated with normal or increased numbers of megakaryocytes in the bone marrow. There are now more reliable tests for demonstrating the responsible IgG antibody.[145, 146] The antibody is directed against and coats the platelet, which is rapidly removed from the circulation by the reticuloendothelial system. It is possible with these new tests to distinguish between IgG antibodies, which can cross the placenta, and IgM antibodies, which do not,[146] and also to identify platelet-bound antibody and the more dangerous free IgG antibody in the maternal plasma.[147, 148] Much of the published literature[149–151] consists of retrospective analyses of women suffering from idiopathic thrombocytopenic purpura (ITP), managed throughout pregnancy without the advantage of these tests which identify specific platelet autoantibodies. However, there are still centers where these laboratory investigations are not freely available, and cases apparently occur when antibodies are undetectable, so that diagnosis and management may have to be planned without their aid. The direct antiglobulin test (Coombs test) and tests to exclude systemic lupus erythematosus (SLE), such as anti-DNA antibodies and antinuclear factor, must be done in all patients that present with immune thrombocytopenia, as this may be the first manifestation of a more generalized autoimmune disease.

The IgG platelet autoantibody may cross the placenta and cause immune destruction of fetal platelets. Hedge[152] has analyzed the reported cases in the literature from 1950–1983 suggesting an overall prevalence of neonatal thrombocytopenia of 52%, with significant morbidity in 12%. The incidence increases to 70% of deliveries if maternal platelet counts are less than 100×10^9/L at term, and the probability of fetal thrombocytopenia increases with the severity of maternal thrombocytopenia.

However, even in the asymptomatic mother with relatively high platelet counts ($>100 \times 10^9$/L), the incidence of neonatal thrombocytopenia is about 20%. These risk factors are modified further by previous maternal splenectomy. In this situation the incidence of neonatal thrombocytopenia and morbidity is increased even if the mother has a normal platelet count.[149] One study of 41 pregnancies in 38 patients with AITP from Canada[153] showed that the maternal platelet count was not related to the platelet count in the fetus, but that maternal platelet–associated antibody was predictive of infant platelet count.

The maternal platelet count should be checked regularly during pregnancy and if it falls below 20×10^9/L, steroid therapy is indicated. This should be tapered to the lowest dose that provides safe platelet counts.[144, 149] It has been suggested[152] that high doses of steroids to elevate platelet counts at or near term should be avoided since they may increase the transplacental passage of IgG antibody and thus expose the fetus to greater risk of severe thrombocytopenia.[147] In my experience this is a theoretical hazard never seen in practice.

Although reviews of management have associated splenectomy during pregnancy with high fetal loss rates[149] and even an approximate 10% maternal mortality rate in the past,[154] modern supportive measures and improved surgical practices have reduced the fetal loss rate considerably and the risk of a maternal mortality is now negligible.[155] Nonetheless, splenectomy is almost never indicated in the pregnant patient with ITP given the success of medical management; however, removal of the spleen remains an option if all other attempts to increase the platelet count fail.

Because the IgG antibody will cross the placenta and may lead to increased fetal platelet destruction and thrombocytopenia, the major risk to the fetus is intracranial bleeding during delivery. If there is any question that a vaginal delivery will be difficult because of cephalopelvic disproportion, premature labor, etc., elective cesarean section should be carried out. It has also been recommended by several authors[149] that if the maternal platelet count is less than 100×10^9/L, indicating active ITP, cesarean section should be performed. McMillan[144] states that this is indicated if the spleen is absent regardless of platelet count. If, however, one has access to reliable reproducible platelet antibody tests, and no appreciable IgG platelet-bound or free maternal autoantibody can be demonstrated, this rule need not apply. If an easy vaginal delivery is expected in a term baby, this should present no more risk of intracranial bleeding than does a cesarean section. It should be remembered that a cesarean section in the presence of maternal thrombocytopenia carries considerable risk of hemorrhage from incisions (not from the placental site, which is protected by normal myometrial contraction). Although transfused platelets will have a short life in the maternal circulation due to the antibody, they will help to achieve hemostasis of the wound, and should be standing by for the mother at delivery, but only given if she bleeds excessively. This has never occurred in my experience, however low the platelet count. The unnecessary transfusion of platelet concentrates in the absence of hemostatic failure may stimulate more autoantibody and increase the severity of maternal thrombocytopenia. Whatever the mode of delivery, maternal soft tissue damage should be avoided as far as possible.

A method for direct measurement of the fetal platelet count in scalp blood, obtained transcervically prior to or early in labor, has been described.[156] The authors recommend that cesarean section be performed in all cases where the fetal platelet count is less than 50×10^9/L. This approach is more logical than a decision about the mode of delivery based on the maternal platelet count and splenectomy status, but it is not without risk, gives false-positive results, and demands urgent action on the results obtained. If reliable platelet antibody tests are available and have been performed throughout the antenatal period, the decision concerning the need for cesarean section and its timing can be taken at leisure; this can be based on a rational assessment of disease activity and the risk to the mother and fetus. In the future, decisions about the route of delivery may well be made on the basis of fetal platelet count determined by ultrasound-guided transuterine fetal blood sampling,[155] as early reports with this method have already occurred.[157, 158]

The recent introduction of intravenous infusion of immunoglobulin in the management of AITP has made the difficult decision regarding delivery much easier. It is known that intravenous administration of monomeric polyvalent human IgG in doses greater than those produced endogenously prolongs the clearance time of immune complexes by the reticuloendothelial system (RES). It is thought that in AITP such a prolongation of clearance of IgG-coated platelets by the RES results in an increase in the number of circulating platelets, but the mechanism is as yet unknown.

The successful use of high-dose intravenous IgG in the treatment of childhood AITP in the early 1980s led to its adoption in the management of severe cases of maternal AITP in pregnancy. Used in the recommended doses of 0.4 mg/kg for 5 days by intravenous transfusion, it results in a consistent and predictable response in platelet count in over 80% of reported cases. Platelets begin to rise on about the fourth day of infusion and peak about 5 days later; remission lasts for about 3 weeks. Most patients achieve a platelet count within the normal range, some rise to safe but still thrombocytopenic levels, and a very few fail to respond or have an extremely sluggish response, but it will be clear within 5 or 6 days if the patient is the rare nonresponder.

IgG given intravenously can cross the placenta and should provoke an identical response in the fetus "at risk," but this has never been proved (see below). Anecdotal reports of the value of intravenous IgG in the management of AITP in pregnancy have appeared in the literature but so far no large series have been published.[158–160] Morgenstern et al.[161] suggest that if infusion is started 10 to 14 days before the expected date of delivery, benefits should be threefold: (1) Vaginal delivery will be safe. (2) The neonatal platelet count should be normal. (3) An instrumented delivery or even cesarean section, if necessary, may be undertaken without the hazard of maternal bleeding.

Hegde[152, 162] recommends the use of IgG, as described above, in all patients with platelet counts of less than 75 to 100 × 10^9/L. However, this therapy is very expensive (e.g., in Great Britain the cost is £2,500 (approx. $4,175) or more for one 5-day course) and in my limited experience asymptomatic women with platelet counts of 50 to 70 × 10^9/L will often deliver babies with normal platelet counts and need no supportive therapy, even to cover cesarean section. Also, at Queen Charlotte's Maternity Hospital we have had a severely thrombocytopenic infant born to a woman who was a partial responder to intravenous IgG and who had received several 5-day courses before delivery. More recent reports suggest that the transplacental effect of intravenous IgG is not reliable and even exogenous IgG does not cross the placenta.[159] There is no doubt about the value of IgG in selected cases of severe and particularly non–steroid-responsive pregnant women with AITP, but its indiscriminate use in moderately severe cases would have to be shown to dramatically improve both maternal and fetal outcome to justify the high cost.

No active measures need be taken in the infant with nonsymptomatic thrombocytopenia once delivery is negotiated successfully, unless surgery is necessary or other trauma is inflicted. The platelet count in the newborn may fall further in the first few days of life despite static or falling maternally derived antibody concentration, perhaps because of the development of the neonatal splenic circulation and more efficient removal of IgG-coated platelets.

The platelet count usually rises to normal

levels within the first month of life, but occasionally thrombocytopenia persists for up to 12 or even 16 weeks. Intravenous hydrocortisone and platelet transfusion can be used in more severely thrombocytopenic infants with evidence of skin and mucosal bleeding.

Even without the introduction of more recent aids to diagnosis of activity of disease and before the discovery of the effects of intravenous IgG, the maternal death rate had fallen from 8% to 9% in 1950 to virtually zero. The outlook for the fetus, which previously had a death rate of up to 26%, is also much more promising.[150, 163]

Thrombocytopenia and SLE.—SLE is frequently complicated by thrombocytopenia, but this is seldom severe, less than 5% of cases having platelet counts below $30 \times 10^9/L$ during the course of the disease.[164] Thrombocytopenia is often the first presenting feature and may antedate any other manifestations by months or even years. Such patients are often labeled as suffering from AITP, unless appropriate additional tests are carried out. Platelet-associated IgG is often found on testing but it is not clear whether this is due to antiplatelet antibody, immune complexes, or both. The management of isolated thrombocytopenia associated with SLE in pregnancy does not differ substantially from that of AITP, but immunosuppressive therapy should not be reduced or discontinued during pregnancy.[165] However, the main management problem of SLE and pregnancy is the complication of the variably present in vitro lupus anticoagulant and its paradoxical association with in vivo thromboembolism and recurrent fetal loss (see Chap. 11, Rheumatic Disease).

Preeclampsia and Platelets.—Thrombocytopenia can occur in association with preeclampsia and its severity seems to be related directly to disease activity. The mechanism appears to be multifactorial and may result from a selective intravascular consumption of platelets without significant fibrinogen consumption as postulated in thrombotic thrombocytopenic purpura (see below) or it may be part of the picture of DIC. Now that most centers have electronic automated platelet counting facilities, thrombocytopenia is becoming an important simple differentiating variable in the categorization and management of the high-risk pregnant patient. (See also Chap. 1, Hypertension.)

Thrombotic Thrombocytopenic Purpura (TTP) and Hemolytic-Uremic Syndrome (HUS)

These conditions share so many features that they should probably be considered as one disease with pathologic effects confined largely to the kidney in HUS and being more generalized in TTP.

These conditions are extremely rare and fewer than 70 cases have been reported in pregnancy.[166] HUS usually presents in the postpartum period with renal failure.

Diagnosis of TTP is based on the classic clinical pentad of fever, microangiopathic hemolytic anemia, thrombocytopenia, neurologic symptoms, and renal abnormalities.[166] Symptoms can be quite variable but fluctuating neurologic abnormalities and hemorrhagic manifestations of thrombocytopenia predominate. The disease is often rapidly progressive and fatal. The role of DIC in TTP has been the subject of speculation by many authors, as evidence of a true consumptive coagulopathy is absent in most patients. The levels of fibrinogen and the labile coagulation factors V and VIII are usually within the normal range. The most consistent abnormalities appear to be the presence of fibrin degradation products and a prolonged thrombin time. Laboratory evidence of DIC is minimal and when present is probably secondary to severe intravascular hemolysis.[167, 168]

An essential requisite of the pathogenesis is damage to the wall of small vessels. There is no doubt that local intravascular coagulation contributes to the vascular damage. In HUS the hyaline material laid down on basement membranes and occluding glomerular arterioles is rich in fibrin, and in TTP the occluding material in arterioles and capillaries is also rich in fibrin, but as noted, laboratory and clinical evidence of DIC has only rarely been documented in association with TTP.[169, 170] Plasminogen activator is absent from the wall of occluded vessels in TTP, but whether this is a primary or secondary effect is not clear. Plasma of patients with TTP causes heightened aggregability of platelets from normal donors which has led to the suggestion that the plasma lacks an inhibitor, allowing intravascular platelet aggregation and leading to widespread microvascular damage. Remission was induced and the defect corrected by administration of fresh frozen plasma.[171] Some suggest that the missing inhibitor of platelet aggregation is a stimulator of prostacyclin production,[172] but whether this deficiency is cause or effect is still not clear.[168] Circulating prostacyclin levels were low in four cases reported by Machin and colleagues,[173] while prostacyclin synthesis–stimulating factors were noted to be low in two cases noted by Stratta et al.[174] Some patients fail to remit on simple plasma infusions but respond to plasmapheresis or exchange transfusion, reinforcing the suggestion that soluble immune complexes are responsible for vascular damage leading to organ dysfunction. It has also been suggested that the capacity of the reticuloendothelial system to clear potentially damaging substances such as immune complexes, soluble fibrin monomer complexes, and platelet microaggregates is greatly reduced in TTP and HUS, a factor that may relate to the genesis of these diseases.[170]

A crucial problem when dealing with TTP is to establish a correct diagnosis,[166, 169] because this condition can be confused with severe preeclampsia[175] (see Table 1–3) and placental abruption, especially if DIC is triggered (although DIC is uncommon in TTP).

Unlike fatty liver of pregnancy there is no evidence that prompt delivery affects the course of HUS or TTP favorably. Most clinicians would recommend delivery if these conditions are present in late pregnancy so that the mother can be treated vigorously without fear of harming the fetus.[168]

Once the correct diagnosis has been made, the management of TTP is the same in principle whether the patient is pregnant or not. The fetus is involved only insofar as it may suffer from placental insufficiency, but it is not directly involved in the disease process. Prompt and repeated plasmapheresis or intensive plasma exchange using fresh frozen plasma seem to be the only measures in modern practice which have altered the outcome of this condition which had previously an extremely high fatality rate.[166, 169, 176] In the interim or if plasmapheresis is unavailable, fresh frozen plasma, as a source of the missing inhibitory factor, and antiplatelet agents, such as dipyridamole or low-dose aspirin (which will not interfere with prostacyclin production), should be considered.[170, 174] If these measures fail, then infusions of prostacyclin, steroids, immunosuppressants, and splenectomy may be tried, but their value is not clear from the few reports in the literature.[166, 169, 170] There are only isolated recent reports of the efficacy of modern treatment of TTP during pregnancy. The similarity between TTP and HUS might be of great importance in the light of the successful management of HUS in pregnancy using prostacyclin infusions,[177] although more recent reports of its use have been disappointing.[178]

Inherited Platelet Defects, Qualitative Platelet Abnormalities

Serious bleeding disorders due to genetic abnormalities of platelet function are rare, the inheritance being autosomal recessive. Clinically, the signs and symptoms are similar to those of von Willebrand's disease, with skin and mucosal hemorrhages. Spontaneous bruises are common but hemarthroses are not. Although these disorders can lead to life-threatening hemorrhage, particularly after surgery or trauma, the bleeding tendency is usually mild. The essential defect is intrinsic to the platelet. Bleeding time is prolonged and platelet function tests are abnormal, showing reduced aggregation and/or adhesion. In thrombasthenia (Glanzmann's disease), the platelets appear morphologically normal but they fail to aggregate with collagen adenosine diphosphate (ADP) or ristocetin. In the very rare Bernard-Soulier syndrome, the aggregation defect is similar but the platelets have a characteristically abnormal giant appearance. Serious bleeding episodes in pregnancy have been treated with plasmapheresis and fresh platelet concentrate infusions.[179]

Thrombocytopenia.—Genetically determined thrombocytopenia may be associated with aplastic anemia or isolated megakaryocytic aplasia. The thrombocytopenia-absent radius (TAR) syndrome is thought to be an autosomal recessive defect and has been successfully diagnosed prenatally by examination of fetal blood sample.[180, 181] Patients with May-Heggelin anomaly, an autosomal dominant condition with variable thrombocytopenia and giant platelets, may receive platelet concentrates to achieve hemostasis at delivery and should be offered prenatal diagnosis.[142]

Factor VIII Antibody

An inhibitor of antihemophilic factor is a rare cause of hemorrhage in previously healthy postpartum women, less than 50 cases having been described.[182–186] These inhibitors are immunoglobulins, as are the factor VIII antibodies found in treated hemophiliacs.[186] Nearly all postpartum coagulation defects of this type have been noted by in vitro testing to be directed against factor VIII and only two have been reported to be anti–factor IX antibodies.

Etiology

The etiology of antibodies to factor VIII:C is complex; its appearance in nonhemophilic individuals is usually attributed to an autoimmune process, or, in postpartum women, to alloimmunization. There are no differences, however, between maternal and fetal factor VIII and neutralization of both maternal and fetal factors by the antibody is similar. In fact, presently there is no definite evidence that factor VIII antigen allotypes exist. If the antibody and bleeding tendency resulted from stimulation of the maternal immune system by fetal factor VIII, one would expect such antibody to reappear after some of the subsequent pregnancies (by analogy with rhesus sensitization), but relapses have not been reported. The variable nature of the disorder argues in favor of a more complex pathogenesis. Indeed, there is an association between factor VIII antibodies and autoimmune disorders such as rheumatoid arthritis and SLE, and there is the well-known alteration of immune reactivity in normal pregnancy. These two observations suggest that a likely explanation of postpartum factor VIII antibodies is that of a temporary breakdown in the mother's tolerance to her own factor VIII (or factor IX).

Clinical Manifestations

The patient usually presents within 3 months (reported range 3 days–17 months) of delivery with severe and sometimes life-threatening bleeding, extensive painful bruising, bleeding from the gastrointestinal and genitourinary tracts, and occasional hemarthroses. The diagnosis is established on the basis of characteristic laboratory findings. Prothrombin time and thrombin time are normal but the partial thromboplastin time is greatly prolonged and is not corrected by the addition of normal plasma or factor VIII. While the IgG antibodies cross the placenta and are detectable in plasma of newborns that have decreased factor VIII, there have been no reports of hemorrhagic problems in offspring.

Management

These gravidas should be managed through an expert coagulation unit. Treatment of the acute bleeding episode is difficult because conventional amounts of factor VIII may just enhance antibody formation and fail to control the bleeding. Immunosuppressive agents in combination with corticosteroids have been suggested to reduce the antibody production.[182]

In one reported case[185] after failure of therapy with factor VIII concentrate and fresh plasma, improvement in the clinical status was achieved by administration of an anti-inhibitor coagulation complex (Autoplex), a preparation of pooled fresh plasma containing precursors and activated clotting factors. The mechanism of action of Autoplex is unknown. It does not suppress or destroy the inhibitor but seems to control the acute hemorrhagic diathesis.[185]

The natural history is for the antibody to disappear gradually, usually within 2 years. Women should be advised to avoid further pregnancy until coagulation returns to normal, although in the one documented case where conception occurred in the presence of clinically active antibody, it disappeared during the course of the pregnancy.[186]

Inherited Primary Defects of Hemostasis

It is important to recognize these uncommon conditions not only because the morbidity and mortality they cause in the sufferer is almost completely preventable by correct diagnosis and treatment, but also because carriers of the most devastating of these conditions, particularly the X-linked hemophilias, can be identified and prenatal diagnosis offered.

However, because of the profound changes in hemostasis during normal pregnancy, it is desirable to establish a correct diagnosis with appropriate family studies before conception so that appropriate management and chorion villus sampling, in conditions where DNA prenatal diagnosis is feasible, can be planned in advance.

Severe congenital disorders of hemostasis are nearly always apparent early in life while milder forms may go unrecognized until adult life and are more of a diagnostic challenge. Patients with thrombocytopenia or platelet function abnormalities suffer primarily from mucosal bleeding, with epistaxis, gingival and gastrointestinal bleeding, and menorrhagia. Bleeding occurs immediately after surgery or trauma and may not occur at all if primary hemostasis can be achieved with suturing. In contrast, patients with coagulation disorders typically suffer deep muscle hematomas and hemarthroses. Bleeding after trauma or surgery may be immediate or delayed.

A history of previous vaginal deliveries without undue bleeding does not exclude a significant coagulopathy because of the increase in coagulation factors, particularly factor VIII, during normal pregnancy, and the fact that a healthy myometrium is the most important hemostatic factor at parturition. In contrast, it is not uncommon for adult patients to have significant bleeding after surgery because of previously undiagnosed inherited hemostatic disorders, due to the fact that surgery imposes a challenge on the hemostatic mechanisms which far exceeds anything encountered in everyday life.

Complete laboratory evaluation of a patient giving a history of "easy bleeding" or "bruising" is time-consuming and expensive and a history of significant previous hemostatic challenges should be obtained. For example, a patient who has undergone tonsillectomy without transfusion or special treatment and lived to tell the tale cannot possibly have an inherited hemostatic disorder! Of more relevance perhaps is a history of dental extractions where hemorrhage can occur with both platelet disorders and coagulopathies. If prolonged bleeding has occurred and particularly if blood transfusion has been required, then a high index of suspicion of a congenital hemorrhagic disorder is justified. In such cases, even if initial laboratory screening tests—partial thromboplastin time, prothrombin time, platelet count, and bleeding time—are normal, the diagnosis should be vigorously pursued in consultation with an expert hematologist.

The most common congenital coagulation disorders are von Willebrand's disease, factor VIII deficiency (hemophilia A), and factor IX deficiency (hemophilia B). Less common diseases include factor XI deficiency, abnormal or deficient fibrinogen, and deficiency of factor XIII (fibrin stabilizing factor). All other coagulation factor disorders are extremely rare. The most frequent disorder of platelet function is von Willebrand's disease.

von Willebrand's Disease

von Willebrand's disease[187] is the commonest of all inherited hemostatic disorders. The incidence of overt disease is about 1 in 10,000, similar to that of hemophilia A, but because subclinical forms of the disorder are common the total incidence of von Willebrand's disease is greater than that of hemophilia. In contrast to hemophilia (an X-linked condition) von Willebrand's disease has an autosomal inheritance and equal incidence in males and females, and therefore is the most frequent genetic hemostatic disorder encountered in obstetric practice.

Nature of the Defect.—Von Willebrand's disease is a disorder of the von Willebrand factor portion of the human factor VIII complex. Factor VIII circulates as a complex of two proteins of unequal size. There is a low-molecular-weight portion of factor VIII:C (290,000) which promotes coagulation linked to a large multimer known as von Willebrand factor (factor VIII:vWF) or factor VIIIR:Ag (factor VIII-related antigen). Factor VIII circulates as polymers ranging in size from 800,000 to more than 10,000,000 daltons. The biosynthesis of factor VIII:C coded for by the X chromosome is reduced or abnormal in hemophilia A. The larger factor VIII:vWF serves as a "carrier" for factor VIII:C, is under separate autosomal control, and is unaffected in hemophilia. Von Willebrand's factor appears to stabilize the small coagulant protein or perhaps protect it from proteolytic digestion. Reduction in factor VIII:vWF usually leads to comparable decrease in factor VIII:C activity.

Von Willebrand's factor is the major protein in plasma that promotes platelet adhesion, forming a bridge between the subendothelial collagen and a specific receptor on the platelet membrane. The large multimeric forms of factor VIII:vWF appear to have the greatest physiologic effect in promoting this adhesion, which is the first step in coagulation in vivo, followed by platelet aggregation. However, in vitro tests of platelet aggregation will be entirely normal in von Willebrand's disease because the initial step is bypassed and different platelet receptors are activated when they are exposed to collagen, ADP, or thrombin in standard laboratory conditions. The platelet abnormality in von Willebrand's disease can be studied in vitro using the antibiotic ristocetin, which takes advantage of the fact that it will agglutinate platelets by a mechanism involving factor VIII:vWF. The most sensitive test for detection of von Willebrand's disease is the ristocetin cofactor assay, which is normal in less than 10% of patients with the disorder. This functional assay for von Willebrand's factor shows the best correlation with clinical manifestations of the disease. If the patient's own platelet-rich plasma is used in this test system, the ristocetin aggregation is normal in more than one third. However, the direct ristocetin platelet aggregation test may be useful in the diagnosis of one of the variants of von Willebrand's disease, type IIb (see below).

Clinical Manifestations.—Presenting symptoms and signs are primarily those of a platelet defect, namely spontaneous mucous membrane and skin bleeding, with prolonged bleeding following trauma or surgery. In addition, there is a variable secondary defect of factor VIII coagulant activity and if this is severely depressed there may be clinical manifestations of a coagulation disorder. The most frequent problem encountered in the nonpregnant female is menorrhagia, which may be quite severe at times. Patients with mild abnormalities may be asymptomatic and picked up only after excessive hemorrhage following trauma or related to surgery. The severity of the disorder does not run true within families and fluctuates from time to time in the same individual.

Subtypes of von Willebrand's Disease.—Type I von Willebrand's disease, which accounts for 80% of all cases, is inherited as an autosomal dominant trait. The protein is qualitatively normal but there is a reduction in factor VIII activity, both coagulation activity and platelet function being affected in roughly equal proportions. The condition is usually mild.

Type II von Willebrand's disease is characterized by the absence of the large multimers of von Willebrand's factor which seem to be essential for normal platelet function. In type IIa the large and intermediate-size multimers are absent from both plasma and platelets. This disease accounts for less than 10% of all cases. Another 5% of cases belong to the subtype IIb in which the large multimers are absent in the plasma but present in the platelets. Types IIc and IId and pseudo–von Willebrand's disease have also been described on the basis of multimeric pattern and distribution of factor VIII:vWF and inheritance. Type III is a rare, apparently autosomal recessive form of the disorder. There is absence of in vitro factor VIII:C, factor VIII:vWF, and ristocetin cofactor activity, as well as a severe bleeding disorder. It is in these cases that couples at risk may seek prenatal diagnosis. It must be obvious from the discussion so far that any woman with von Willebrand's disease or a history suggestive of this complex disorder who is contemplating pregnancy or already pregnant must be managed by a unit which has access to expert hemostatic advice. The subtype must be identified correctly because this has serious implications in terms of optimum management (see below).

Treatment.—There are several forms of treatment for von Willebrand's disease, the choice of management depending on the severity and type of the disease. The aim is to correct the platelet and coagulation disorder by achieving normal levels of factor VIII coagulant activity and a bleeding time within the normal range, and the key feature in treatment is replacement of von Willebrand's factor and factor VIII:C by administering plasma concentrates. In less severe cases the vasopressin analogue L-desamino-8-arginine vasopressin (desmopressin acetate, DDAVP) has been used with success. Contraceptive hormones have been used with success in the treatment of menorrhagia in von Wille-

brand's disease.[185] Also, and of importance, aspirin and related anti-inflammatory drugs should not be prescribed to patients with von Willebrand's disease, as these drugs compromise platelet function and prolong the bleeding time markedly in patients with platelet/coagulation disorders.

While replacement therapy using cryoprecipitate or fresh frozen plasma is the mainstay of therapy, large volumes may be required to secure hemostasis. However, this does not usually cause any problems, especially during delivery. Cryoprecipitate is also the product of choice to cover nonurgent surgery. In the past, factor VIII concentrates were not recommended in the management of von Willebrand's disease because in commercial preparation the factor promoting platelet adhesion was lost and although factor VIII coagulant activity was enhanced, ristocetin cofactor activity was unaffected and the bleeding time remained prolonged. Recently produced concentrates are said to retain some von Willebrand activity and have the advantage, being heat-treated, of reducing the risk of infection.

In modern practice the replacement therapy used has to be a local decision, based on the relative disadvantages of pooled sterilized products versus the superior efficacy and hazard of transmitting infection using cryoprecipitate.

Desmopressin.—This vasopressin analogue has been shown to cause release of von Willebrand's factor from endothelial cells where it is synthesized and stored, resulting in raised plasma levels of both ristocetin cofactor and of factor VIII:C. It is therefore of benefit to patients with von Willebrand's disease and hemophilia A. It is particularly effective in mildly affected patients and may in some cases replace the use or need for blood products in patients undergoing surgery. Toxicity associated with the use of this product has been trivial. Occasional patients experience flushing and dizziness.[187] The theoretical risk of water intoxication and hyponatremia due to the antidiuretic hormone effect has not been observed using the current dosage schedules. The recommended dose is an intravenous infusion of 0.3 μg/kg given over 30 minutes with a total dose of 15 to 25 μg. This may be repeated every 12 to 24 hours.[188] Patients with mild type I von Willebrand's disease would be expected to derive maximal benefit from this mode of treatment. Factor VIII:C levels are dramatically increased provided that the baseline level is more than 10%. The effect of the use of desmopressin on the bleeding time is controversial but a review of the literature[188] shows that in vitro ristocetin cofactor levels increase and there is an overall reduction in clinical bleeding.

In patients with severe type III von Willebrand's disease, the drug will have no effect and replacement therapy must be used. In type IIb von Willebrand's disease the use of desmopressin is contraindicated. In vivo platelet aggregation and severe thrombocytopenia will follow the infusion although it does transiently improve the plasma multimeric pattern.

von Willebrand's Disease and Pregnancy.—A rise in both factor VIII:C and von Willebrand's factor is observed in normal pregnancy. Patients with all but the severest forms of von Willebrand's disease show a similar but variable rise in both these factors, although there may not be a reduction in the bleeding time.[189–191]

After delivery, normal women maintain an elevated factor VIII:C level for at least 5 days. This is followed by a slow fall to baseline levels over 4 to 6 weeks. The duration of factor VIII activity post partum in women with von Willebrand's disease seems to be related to the severity of the disorder. Those women with severer forms of the condition may have a rapid fall in factor VIII procoagulant and platelet hemostatic activity. They are then at risk of quite severe secondary postpartum hemorrhage.

What is the hemorrhagic risk during pregnancy and delivery for women with von Willebrand's disease? An analysis of published reports of 33 pregnancies in 22 women showed abnormal bleeding in 9 (27%) pregnancies at the time of abortion, delivery, or post partum.[191]

Because of this high reported incidence of bleeding, some workers in the field recommend aggressive treatment with prophylactic replacement therapy in the form of cryoprecipitate given at delivery and in the puerperium. Although this may be necessary in severer forms of the disease[188] there is no evidence that this is so in the most frequent type I and milder type II forms of the disorder.[191] However, type IIb patients may develop thrombocytopenia and require cryoprecipitate at delivery.[192]

The consensus is that the most important determinant for abnormal hemorrhage at delivery is a low factor VIII:C plasma level. The vast majority of women will have increased their factor VIII:C production to within the normal range (50%–150%) by late gestation and although cryoprecipitate should be standing by at delivery it probably will not be needed to achieve hemostasis.

There is virtually no place for desmopressin in the antepartum period because if a rise in factor VIII is possible under the influence of the drug (milder cases), then it will have been achieved during the stimulus of pregnancy itself. However, desmopressin has an obvious valuable place in the management of women with von Willebrand's disease in the puerperium when factor VIII levels fall once the uterus is empty, and secondary hemorrhage could occur.

The Hemophilias

The hemophilias are inherited disorders associated with reduced or absent coagulation factors VIII or IX with an incidence of approximately 1 in 10,000.[193] *Hemophilia A,* which is associated with deficiency of factor VIII, is more common, while about one sixth of the 3,000 to 4,000 cases in Great Britain today have a condition known as *Christmas disease* which is due to a lack of coagulation factor IX (hemophilia B). Clinical manifestations of the two conditions are indistinguishable, the symptoms and signs being variable and depending on the degree of the lack of the coagulation factors concerned. Severe disease with frequent spontaneous bleeding (particularly hemarthroses) is associated with clotting factor levels of 0% to 1%. Less severe disease is found in subjects with clotting factors of 1% to 4%. Spontaneous bleeding and severe bleeding after minor trauma are rare in cases with coagulation factor levels between 5% and 30%; the danger is that the condition may be clinically silent but during the course of major surgery or following trauma, such subjects will behave as though afflicted with the very severest form of hemophilia. Unless the defect is recognized and the lacking coagulation factor replaced, such patients will continue to bleed. Inheritance of both hemophilias is X-linked recessive, being expressed in the male and carried by the female.

The risks in pregnancy for a female carrier of hemophilia are twofold:

1. She may, due to lyonization (random deletion of the X chromosome in every cell), have very low factor VIII or IX levels and be at risk of excessive bleeding, particularly following a traumatic or surgical delivery.
2. Fifty percent of her male offspring will inherit hemophilia while 50% of her daughters will be carriers like herself. This has important implications now that prenatal diagnosis of these conditions is possible.

Management of Hemophilia in Pregnancy

On average, female carriers of hemophilia do not have clinical manifestations but in rare individuals in whom the factor VIII:C or IX levels are unusually low (10%–30% of normal), abnormal bleeding may occur after trauma or surgery.[194] It is important to identify carriers prior to pregnancy, not only to provide genetic counseling but so that appropriate provision can be made for those cases

with pathologically low coagulation factor activities. Fortunately, the level of the deficient factor tends to increase during the course of pregnancy, as in normal women. In fact, there are anecdotal reports of female homozygotes for hemophilia A with uneventful and successful pregnancies.[195] Hemorrhage post partum does not appear to be a consistent feature, particularly if delivery is by the vaginal route at term with little or no soft tissue damage. The effect of pregnancy on factor VIII:C levels in these rare cases has not been studied.

If the factor VIII level remains low in carriers of hemophilia A, replacement therapy should be given in order that factor VIII levels are maintained above 50% to cover delivery and treatment continued for 3 to 4 days post partum in the event of a normal vaginal delivery. Replacement levels will have to be maintained for a longer period after cesarean deliveries or if there has been extensive soft tissue damage. Before factor VIII concentrates were sterilized by heat treatment they were avoided because they exposed the woman unnecessarily to the hazards of multiple donations.

Desmopressin has been shown to be of benefit in patients with mild hemophilia, as with Von Willebrand's disease (see above). However, the storage pools of factor VIII released during treatment may become exhausted and tachyphylaxis does occur.[188] There are no controlled studies concerning the use of desmopressin during pregnancy although this drug has been used safely in pregnant women with diabetes insipidus. Still, and as noted previously, if the stimulus of pregnancy has not raised the level of factor VIII as an expected physiologic response in mild hemophilia, it is unlikely that desmopressin will do so.

Clinical problems occur more often in carriers of factor IX deficiency (Christmas disease) than in those women who carry factor VIII deficiency.[194] In the exceptionally rare situations where the factor IX level is very low and remains low during pregnancy, the patient should be managed with fresh frozen plasma to cover delivery and for 3 to 4 days post partum. This is preferable to factor IX concentrates, which are prepared from multiple donors and contain factors II, VII, and X, as well as factor IX and therefore carry a much greater thrombogenic hazard adding to the innate risk of thromboembolism in pregnancy. However, fresh frozen plasma will carry the remote hazard (in the United Kingdom) of transmitting HIV infection.[195] These patients should be managed in a unit with access to expert advice, 24-hour laboratory coagulation service, and immediate access to the appropriate plasma components required for replacement therapy.

Factor XI Deficiency (Plasma Thromboplastin Antecedent [PTA] Deficiency)

This rare coagulation disorder, less common than the hemophilias, occurs more frequently than the very rare inherited deficiencies of the remaining coagulation factors. It is inherited as an autosomal recessive trait, and occurs predominantly in Ashkenazi Jews. Usually only the homozygotes have clinical evidence of a coagulation disorder though occasionally carriers may have a bleeding tendency. The disease is mild and spontaneous hemorrhages and hemarthroses are rare, but the danger is that profuse bleeding may follow major trauma or surgery if no prophylactic plasma is given.[189] Diagnosis is made by finding a prolonged partial thromboplastin time, and a low factor XI level in a coagulation assay system in which all other tests are normal. Management consists of replacement with fresh frozen plasma as prophylaxis for surgery or to treat bleeding. Fresh frozen plasma is also indicated at labor.

The effective hemostatic level of factor XI has a half-life of around 2 days. To cover surgery or delivery women can be treated with fresh frozen plasma in an initial dose of 20 mL/kg followed by a maintenance dose of 5 mL/kg daily until primary healing is established.

Genetic Disorders of Fibrinogen (Factor I)

Fibrinogen is synthesized in the liver, has a molecular weight of 340,000, and circulates in plasma at a concentration of 300 mg/dL. Both quantitative and qualitative genetic abnormalities are described.

Afibrinogenemia or Hypofibrinogenemia

These are rare autosomal recessive disorders resulting from reduced fibrinogen synthesis. Most patients with hypofibrinogenemia are heterozygous.

Afibrinogenemia is characterized by a lifelong bleeding tendency of variable severity. Prolonged bleeding after minor injury, and easy bruising are frequent symptoms. Menorrhagia can be very severe. Spontaneous deep tissue bleeding and hemarthroses are rare, but severe bleeding can occur after trauma or surgery and several patients have suffered intracerebral hemorrhages.

In afibrinogenemia all screening tests of coagulation are prolonged but corrected by addition of normal plasma or fibrinogen. A prolonged bleeding time may be present. The final diagnosis is made by quantitating the concentration of circulating fibrinogen.

Plasma or cryoprecipitate may be used as replacement therapy to treat bleeding and cover surgery or delivery. The in vivo half-life of fibrinogen is between 3 and 5 days. Initial replacement should be achieved with 25 mL plasma per kilogram and daily maintenance with 5 to 10 mL/kg for 7 days.

Congenital hypofibrinogenemia has been associated with recurrent early miscarriages and with recurrent placental abruption.[196]

Dysfibrinogenemia

Congenital dysfibrinogenemia is an autosomal dominant disorder. In contrast to patients with afibrinogenemia, patients with this disorder are often symptom-free. Some have a bleeding tendency; others have been shown to have thromboembolic disease. The diagnosis is made by demonstrating a prolonged thrombin time with a normal immunologic fibrinogen level.

Affected women, like those with hypofibrinogenemia, may have recurrent spontaneous abortion or repeated placental abruption.[196]

Factor XIII Deficiency (Fibrin Stabilizing Factor Deficiency)

This is an autosomal recessive disorder classically characterized by bleeding from the umbilical cord during the first few days of life and later by ecchymoses, prolonged posttraumatic hemorrhage, and poor wound healing. Bleeding is usually delayed and characteristically of a slow oozing nature. Intracranial hemorrhage has been described in a significant proportion of reported cases. Spontaneous recurrent abortion with excessive bleeding occurs in association with factor XIII deficiency.[197] All standard coagulation tests are normal. Diagnosis of severe deficiency is made by the clot solubility test, as normal fibrin clots will not dissolve when incubated overnight in 5M urea solutions, whereas the unstable clots formed in the absence of factor XIII will.

Factor XIII has a half-life of 6 days to 2 weeks and only 5% of normal factor XIII levels are needed for effective hemostasis; therefore patients can be treated with fresh frozen plasma in doses of 5 mL/kg, which can be repeated every 3 weeks. Using this therapy pregnancy has progressed safely to term in a woman who had previously suffered repeated fetal losses. Because of the high incidence of intracranial hemorrhage, replacement therapy should be recommended for all patients who are known to have factor XIII deficiency.[197]

Other Plasma Factor Disorders

Congenital deficiencies of factors II, V, VII, and X are extremely rare and the reader is referred to a review of hereditary coagulopathies in pregnancy for an account of their diagnosis and special management problems.[189]

REFERENCES

1. Hytten F: Blood volume changes in normal pregnancy, in Letsky EA (ed): Haematological disorders in pregnancy. *Clin Haematol* 1985; 14:601–612.
2. Pirani BBK, Campbell DM, McGillivray I: Plasma volume in normal pregnancy. *Obstet Gynacol Br Common* 1973; 80:884–887.
3. Letsky EA: The haematological system, in Hytten FE, Chamberlain GVP (eds): *Clinical Physiology in Obstetrics*, ed 2. Oxford, England, Blackwell Scientific Publications, 1990, pp 43–78.
4. Peck TM, Arias F: Hematologic changes associated with pregnancy. *Clin Obstet Gynecol* 1979; 22:785–798.
5. World Health Organization: *Nutritional Anaemias*, Technical Report Series No. 503, 1972, Geneva, World Health Organization.
6. de Leeuw NKM, Lowenstein L, Hsieh YS: Iron deficiency and hydremia in normal pregnancy. *Medicine (Baltimore)* 1966; 45:291–315.
7. Finch CA, Cook JD: Iron deficiency. *Am J Clin Nutr* 1984; 39:471–477.
8. Svanberg B: Absorption of iron in pregnancy. *Acta Obstet Gynecol Scand [Suppl]* 1975; 48:7–108.
9. Lund CJ: Studies on the iron deficiency anemia of pregnancy including plasma volume, total hemoglobin, erythrocyte protoporphyrin in treated and untreated normal and anemic patients. *Am J Obstet Gynecol* 1951; 62:947–961.
10. Magee HE, Milligan EHM: Haemoglobin levels before and after labour. *Br Med J* 1951; 2:1307–1310.
11. Gatenby PBB: The anaemias of pregnancy in Dublin. *Pro Nutr Soc* 1956; 15:115–119.
12. Morgan EH: Plasma iron and haemoglobin levels in pregnancy. The effect of oral iron. *Lancet* 1961; 1:9–12.
13. Chanarin I, Rothman D, Berry V: Iron deficiency and its relation to folic acid status in pregnancy. Results of a clinical trial. *Br Med J* 1965; 1:480–485.
14. Chisholm J: A controlled clinical trial of prophylactic folic acid and iron in pregnancy. *J Obstet Gynaecol Br Comm* 1966; 73:191–196.

15. Fenton V, Cavill I, Fisher J: Iron stores in pregnancy. *Br J Haematol* 1977; 37:145–149.

16. Taylor DJ, Mallen C, McDougall N, et al: Effect of iron supplements on serum ferritin levels during and after pregnancy. *Br J Obstet Gynaecol* 1982; 89:1011–1017.

17. Jacobs A, Miller F, Worwood M, et al: Ferritin in serum of normal subjects and patients with iron deficiency and iron overload. *Br Med J* 1972; 4:206–208.

18. Thompson WG: Comparison of tests for diagnosis of iron depletion in pregnancy. *Am J Obstet Gynecol* 1988; 159:1132–1134.

19. Scott JM: Iron sorbitol citrate in pregnancy anaemia. *Br Med J* 1963; 2:354–357.

20. Clay B, Rosenburg B, Sampson N, et al: Reactions to total dose intravenous infusion of iron dextran (Imferon). *Br Med J* 1965; 1:29–31.

21. Scott JM: Toxicity of iron sorbitol citrate. *Br Med J* 1962: 2:480–481.

22. Fleming AF, Martin JD, Hahnell R, et al: Effects of iron and folic acid antenatal supplements on maternal haematology and fetal well-being. *Med J Aust* 1974; 2:429–436.

23. de Leeuw NKM, Lowenstein L, Tucker EC, et al: Correlation of red cell loss at delivery with changes in red cell mass. *Am J Obstet Gynecol* 1968; 100:1092–1101.

24. Hallberg I, Ryttinger L, Solvell L: Side effects of oral iron therapy. *Acta Med Scand [Suppl]* 1966; 459:3–10.

25. Hemminki E, Starfield B: Routine administration of iron and vitamins during pregnancy: Review of controlled clinical trials. *Br J Obset Gynaecol* 1978; 85:404–410.

26. Bentley DP: Iron metabolism and anaemia in pregnancy, in Letsky EA (ed): Haematological disorders in pregnancy. *Clin Haematol* 1985; 14:613–628.

27. Letsky EA: Anaemia in obstetrics, in Studd J (ed): *Progress in Obstetrics and Gynaecology*, Vol 6. Edinburgh, Churchill Livingstone, 1987, pp 23–58.

28. Kullander S, Kallen B: A prospective study of drugs and pregnancy. *Acta Obstet Gynecol Scand* 1976; 55:287–295.

29. Sheldon WL, Aspillaga MO, Smith PA, et al: The effects of oral iron supplementation on zinc and magnesium levels during pregnancy. *Br J Obset Gynaecol* 1985; 92:892–898.

30. Chanarin I: Folate and cobalamin, in Letsky EA (ed): Haematological disorders in pregnancy. *Clin Haematol* 1985; 14:629–641.

31. Chanarin I: Megaloblastic anaemia in pregnancy, in *The Megaloblastic Anaemias*, ed 2. Oxford, England, Blackwell Scientific Publications, 1979, pp 466–490.

32. Herbert V: Biology of disease—megaloblastic anaemias. *Lab Invest* 1985; 52:3–19.

33. Smithells RW, Sheppard S, Schorah CJ, et al: Possible prevention of neural-tube defects by periconceptional vitamin supplementation. *Lancet* 1980; 1:339–340.

34. Laurence KM, James N, Miller MH, et al: Double-blind randomised controlled trial of folate treatment before conception to prevent recurrence of neural tube defects. *Br Med J* 1981; 282:1509–1511.

35. Smithells RW, Newin NC, Seller MJ, et al: Further experience of vitamin supplementation for prevention of neural tube defect recurrences. *Lancet* 1983; 1:1027–1031.

36. Elwood JM: Can vitamins prevent neural tube defects? *Can Med Assoc J* 1983; 129:1088–1092.

37. Baumslag N, Edelstein T, Metz J: Reduction of incidence of prematurity of folic acid supplementation in pregnancy. *Br Med J* 1970; 1:16–17.

38. Iyengar L: Folic acid requirements of Indian pregnant women. *Am J Obstet Gynecol* 1971; 111:13–16.

39. Reynolds EH: Anticonvulsants, folic acid and epilepsy. *Lancet* 1973; 1:1376–1378.

40. Hiilesmaa VK, Teramo K, Granstrom M-L, et al: Serum folate concentrations during pregnancy in women with epilepsy: Relation to anti-epileptic drug concentrations, number of seizures and fetal outcome. *Br Med J* 1983; 287:577–579.

41. Weatherall DJ: Prenatal diagnosis of inherited blood diseases, in Letsky EA (ed): Haematological disorders in pregnancy. *Clin Haematol* 1985; 14:747–774.

42. Nicolaides KH, Rodeck CH, Mibashan R: Obstetric management and diagnosis of haematological disease in the fetus. *Clin Haematol* 1985; 14:775–805.

43. Goldfarb AW, Hochner-Celnikier D, Beller U, et al: A successful pregnancy in transfusion dependent homozygous β-thalassaemia: A case report. *Int J Gynaecol Obstet* 1982; 20:319–322.

44. Serjeant GR: Sickle haemoglobin and pregnancy. *Br Med J* 1983; 287:628–630.

45. Thomas AN, Pattison C, Serjeant GR: Causes of death in sickle-cell disease in Jamaica. *Br Med J* 1982; 285:633–655.

46. Van Dinh T, Boor PJ, Garza JR: Massive pulmonary embolism following delivery of a patient with sickle cell trait. *Am J Obstet Gynecol* 1982; 143:722–724.

47. Lindheimer MD, Richardson DA, Ehrlich EN, et al: Potassium homeostasis in pregnancy. *J Reprod Med* 1987; 32:517–526.

48. Samuels-Reid JH, Scott RB, Brown WE: Contraceptive practices and reproductive patterns in sickle cell disease. *J Natl Med Assoc* 1984; 76:879–883.

49. Charache S, Neibyl JR: Pregnancy in sickle cell disease, in Letsky EA (ed): Haematological disorders in pregnancy. *Clin Haematol* 1985; 14:720–746.

50. Charache S, Scott J, Niebyl J, et al: Management of sickle cell disease in pregnant patients. *Obstet Gynecol* 1980; 55:407–410.

51. Tuck SM, Studd JWW, White JM: Pregnancy in sickle cell disease in the United Kingdom. *Br J Obstet Gynaecol* 1983; 90:112–117.

52. Huehns ER: The structure and function of haemoglobin: Clinical disorders due to abnormal haemoglobin structure, in Hardisty RM, Weatherall DJ (eds): *Blood and Its Disorders,* ed 2. Oxford, England, Blackwell Scientific Publications, 1982, p 365.

53. Tuck SM, James CE, Brewster EM, et al: Prophylactic blood transfusion in maternal sickle cell syndromes. *Br J Obstet Gynaecol* 1987; 94:121–125.

54. Koshy M, Burd L, Wallace D, et al: Prophylactic red cell transfusions in pregnant patients with sickle cell disease. *N Engl J Med* 1988; 319:1447–1452.

55. Miller JM, Horger EO, Key TC, et al: Management of sickle haemoglobinopathies in pregnant patients. *Am J Obstet Gynecol* 1981; 141:237–241.

56. Tuck SM, James CE, Brewster EM, et al: Prophylactic blood transfusion in maternal sickle cell syndromes. *Br J Obstet Gynaecol* 1987; 94:121–125.

57. Pastorek JG II, Saseiler B: Maternal death associated with sickle cell trait. *Am J Obstet Gynecol* 1985; 151:295–297.

58. Weatherall DJ, Letsky EA: Genetic haematological disorders, in Wald NJ (ed): *Antenatal and Neonatal Screening.* Oxford, England, Oxford University Press, 1984, pp 155–191.

59. Taylor JJ, Studd JWW, Green ID: Primary refractory anaemia and pregnancy. *J Obstet Gynaecol Br Comm* 1968; 75:963–968.

60. Evans IL: Aplastic anaemia in pregnancy remitting after abortion. *Br Med J* 1968; 3:166–167.

61. Lewis SM, Gordon Smith EC: Aplastic and dysplastic anaemias, in Hardisty RM, Weatherall DJ (eds): *Blood and Its Disorders,* ed 2. Oxford, England, Blackwell Scientific, 1982, pp 1229–1268.

62. Picot C, Triadou P, Lacombe C, et al: Relapsing pure red-cell aplasia during pregnancy. *N Engl J Med* 1984; 311:196.

63. Chaplin H, Cohen R, Bloomberg G, et al: Pregnancy and idiopathic auto-immune haemolytic anaemia. A prospective study during 6 months gestation and 3 months post-partum. *Br J Haematol* 1973; 24:219–229.

64. Ferguson JE, Ueland K, Aronson WJ: Polycythemia rubra vera and pregnancy. *Obstet Gynecol* 1983; 62:16S–20S.

65. Snethlage W, Tengate JW: Thrombocythaemia and recurrent late abortions. Normal outcome of pregnancies after anti-aggregatory treatment. *Br J Obstet Gynaecol* 1986; 93:386–388.

66. Spencer JAD: Paroxysmal nocturnal haemoglobinuria in pregnancy. *Br J Obstet Gynaecol* 1980; 87:246–248.

67. Vermylen J, Blockmans D, Spitz B, et al: Thrombosis and immune disorders, in Chesterman N (ed): Thrombosis and the vessel wall. *Clin Haematol* 1986; 15:395.

68. Dacie JV, Lewis SM: Paroxysmal nocturnal haemoglobinuria: Clinical manifestations, haematology and nature of the disease. *Ser Haematol* 1972; 5:3–23.

69. Beresford CJ, Gudex DJ, Symmans WA: Paroxysmal nocturnal haemoglobinuria and pregnancy. *Lancet* 1986; 2:1396–1397.

70. De Gramont A, Krulik M, Debray J: Paroxysmal nocturnal haemoglobinuria and pregnancy. *Lancet* 1987; 1:868.

71. Jacobs P, Wood L: Paroxysmal nocturnal haemoglobinuria and pregnancy. *Lancet* 1986; 2:1099.

72. Fitzpatrick C: Birth control and paroxys-

mal nocturnal haemoglobinuria. *Lancet* 1987; 1:1260.

73. Hurd WH, Miodovnik M, Stys SJ: Pregnancy associated with paroxysmal noctural haemoglobinuria. *Obstet Gynecol* 1982; 60:742–746.

74. Letsky EA: Coagulation problems during pregnancy, in Lind T (ed): *Current Reviews in Obstetrics and Gynaecology,* vol 10. Edinburgh, Churchill Livingstone, 1985, pp 1–133.

75. Moncada MD, Vane JR: Arachidonic acid metabolites and the interactions between platelets and blood-vessel walls. *N Engl J Med* 1979; 300:1142–1147.

76. Lewis PJ: The role of prostacyclin in pre-eclampsia. *Br J Hosp Med* 1982; 62:1048–1052.

77. Sill PR, Lind T, Walker W: Platelet values during normal pregnancy. *Br J Obstet Gynaecol* 1985; 92:480–483.

78. Fay RA, Hughes AO, Farron NT: Platelets in pregnancy: Hyperdestruction in pregnancy. *Obstet Gynecol* 1983; 61:238–240.

79. Beal DW, de Masi AD: Role of the platelet count in the management of the high-risk obstetric patient. *J Am Osteopath Assoc* 1985; 85:252–255.

80. Fenton V, Saunders K, Caville I: The platelet count in pregnancy. *J Clin Pathol* 1977; 30:68–69.

81. Rakoczi I, Tallian F, Bagdan YS, et al: Platelet lifespan in normal pregnancy and pre-eclampsia as determined by a non-radio-isotope technique. *Thromb Res* 1979; 15:553–556.

82. Wallenberg HCS, Van Kessel PH: Platelet lifespan in normal pregnancy as determined by a non-radioisotopic technique. *Br J Obstet Gynaecol* 1978; 85:33–36.

83. Lewis PJ, Boylan P, Friedman LA, et al: Prostacyclin in pregnancy. *Br Med J* 1980; 280:1581–1582.

84. O'Brien WF, Saba HI, Knuppel RA, et al: Alterations in platelet concentration and aggregation in normal pregnancy and pre-eclampsia. *Am J Obstet Gynecol* 1986; 155:486–490.

85. Romero R, Duffy TP: Platelet disorders in pregnancy. *Clin Perinatol* 1980; 7:327–348.

86. Redman CWG, Bonnar J, Bellin C: Early platelet consumption in pre-eclampsia. *Br Med J* 1978; 1:467–469.

87. Bonnar J: Haemostasis and coagulation disorders in pregnancy, in Bloom AL, Thomas DP (eds): *Haemostasis and Thrombosis,* ed 2. Edinburgh, Churchill Livingstone, 1987, pp 570–584.

88. Lammle B, Griffin JH: Formation of the fibrin clot: The balance of procoagulant and inhibitory factors, in Ruggeri ZM (ed): Coagulation disorders. *Clin Haematol* 1985; 14:281–342.

89. Hellgren M, Blomback M: Blood coagulation and fibrinolysis in pregnancy, during delivery and in the puerperium. *Gynecol Obstet Invest* 1981; 12:141–154.

90. Bertina RM, Briet E, Engesser L, et al: Protein C deficiency and the risk of venous thrombosis. *N Engl J Med* 1988; 318:930–931.

91. Seligsohn U, Berger A, Abend M, et al: Homozygous protein C deficiency manifested by massive venous thrombosis in the newborn. *N Engl J Med* 1984; 310:559–562.

92. Comp PC, Thurnau GR, Welsh J, et al: Functional and immunologic protein S levels are decreased during pregnancy. *Blood* 1986; 68:881–885.

93. Warwick R, Hutton RA, Goff L, et al: Changes in protein C and free protein S during pregnancy and following hysterectomy. *J R Soc Med* 1989; 82:591–594.

94. Salem HH: The natural anticoagulants, in Chesterman CN (ed): Thrombosis and the vessel wall. *Clin Haematol* 1986; 15:371–391.

95. Bonnar J, Prentice CRM, McNicol GP, et al: Haemostatic mechanism in uterine circulation during placental separation. *Br Med J* 1971; 2:564–567.

96. Sheppard BL, Bonnar J: The ultrastructure of the arterial supply of the human placenta in early and late pregnancy. *J Obstet Gynaecol Br Comm* 1974; 81:497–511.

97. Talbert IM, Blatt PM: Disseminated intravascular coagulation in obstetrics. *Clin Obstet Gynecol* 1979; 22:889–900.

98. Gilabert J, Aznar J, Parilla J, et al: Alterations in the coagulation and fibrinolysis system in pregnancy, labour and puerperium, with special reference to a possible transitory state of intravascular coagulation during labour. *Thromb Haemost* 1978; 40:387–396.

99. Stirling Y, Woolf L, North WRS, et al: Haemostasis and normal pregnancy.

Thromb Haemost 1984; 52:176.

100. Wallmo L, Karlsonn K, Teger-Nilsson A-C: Fibrinopeptide and intravascular coagulation in normotensive and hypertensive pregnancy and parturition. *Acta Obstet Gynecol Scand* 1984; 63:637–640.

101. Pritchard JA: Haematological problems associated with delivery, placental abruption, retained dead fetus and amniotic fluid embolism. *Clin Haematol* 1973; 2:563–580.

102. Doenicke A, Grote B, Lorezn W: Blood and blood substitutes in management of the injured patient. *Br J Anaesth* 1977; 49:681–688.

103. Richter AW, Hedin HI: Dextran hypersensitivity. *Immunol Today* 1982; 3:132–138.

104. Phillips LP: Transfusion support in acquired coagulation disorders. *Clin Haematol* 1984; 13:137–150.

105. Boulton FE, Letsky E: Obstetric haemorrhage: Causes and management. *Clin Haematol* 1985; 14:683–728.

106. Sharp AA: Diagnosis and management of disseminated intravascular coagulation. *Br Med Bull* 1977; 33:265–272.

107. Hafter R, Graeff H: Molecular aspects of defibrination in a reptilase treated case of "dead fetus syndrome." *Thromb Res* 1975; 7:391–399.

108. Fournie A, Monrozies M, Pontonnier G, et al: Factor VIII complex in normal pregnancy, pre-eclampsia and fetal growth retardation. *Br J Obstet Gynaecol* 1981; 88:250–254.

109. Whigham KAE, Howie PW, Shaf MM, et al: Factor VIII related antigen and coagulant activity in intrauterine growth retardation. *Thromb Res* 1979; 16:629–638.

110. Caires D, Arocha-Pinango CL, Rodriguez S, et al: Factor VIIIR:Ag/Factor VIII:C and their ratios in obstetrical cases. *Acta Obstet Gynecol Scand* 1984; 63:411–416.

111. Redman CWG: Coagulation problems in human pregnancy. *Postgrad Med J* 1979; 55:367–371.

112. Estelles A, Aznar J, Gilabert J: A quantitative study of soluble fibrin monomer complexes in normal labour and abruptio placentae. *Thromb Res* 1980; 18:513–519.

113. Sher G: Pathogenesis and management of uterine inertia complicating abruptio placentae with consumption coagulopathy. *Am J Obstet Gynecol* 1977; 129:164–170.

114. Bonnar J: Haemorrhagic disorders during pregnancy, in Hathway WE, Bonnar J (eds): *Hemostatic Disorders of the Pregnant Woman and Newborn Infant*. New York, John Wiley & Sons, 1987, pp 76–103.

115. Department of Health and Social Security: *Report on Health and Social Subjects 26: Report on Confidential Enquiries into Maternal Deaths in England and Wales 1982–1984*. 1989, London, Her Majesty's Stationery Office.

116. Thragarajah S, Wheby MS, Jarn R, et al: Disseminated intravascular coagulation in pregnancy. The role of heparin therapy. *J Reprod Med* 1981; 26:17–24.

117. Feinstein DI: Diagnosis and management of disseminated intravascular coagulation: The role of heparin therapy. *Blood* 1982; 60:284–287.

118. Sher GI, Statland BE: Abruptio placentae with coagulopathy: A rational basis for management. *Clin Obstet Gynecol* 1985; 28:15–23.

119. Amris CJ, Hilden M: Anticoagulant effects of Trasylol: In vitro and in vivo studies. *Ann NY Acad Sci* 1968; 116:612–691.

120. Prentice CRM, McNicol GP, Douglas A: Studies on the anticoagulant action of aprotinin ('Trasylol'). *Thromb Diath Haemorrh* 1970; 24:1265–1272.

121. Nordstrom S, Blomback B, Blomback M, et al: Experimental investigations on the antithromboplastic and antifibrinolytic activity of Trasylol. *Ann NY Acad Sci* 1968; 146:701–714.

122. Astedt B, Nilsson IM: Recurrent abruptio placentae treated with the fibrinolytic inhibitor tranexamic acid. *Br Med J* 1978; 1:756–757.

123. Grundy MFB, Craven ER: Consumption coagulopathy after intra-amniotic urea. *Br Med J* 1976; 2:677–678.

124. MacKenzie IZ, Sayers L, Bonnar J, et al: Coagulation changes during second trimester abortion induced by intra-amniotic prostaglandin E_{2+} and hypertonic solutions. *Lancet* 1975; 2:1066–1069.

125. Spivak JL, Sprangler DB, Bell WR: Defibrination after intraamniotic injection of hypertonic saline. *N Engl J Med* 1972; 287:321–323.

126. Stander RW, Flessa HC, Gluck HC, et al: Changes in maternal coagulation factors after intra-amniotic injection of hypertonic saline. *Obstet Gynecol* 1971; 37:321–323.

127. Van Royen EA: *Haemostasis in Human Pregnancy and Delivery.* (thesis). University of Amsterdam, 1974.

128. Burkman RT, Bell WR, Atizenza MF, et al: Coagulopathy with midtrimester induced abortion. Association with hyperosmolar urea administration. *Am J Obstet Gynecol* 1977; 127:533–536.

129. Davis G: Midtrimester abortion. Late dilation and evacuation and DIC. *Lancet* 1972; 2:1026.

130. Savage W: Abortion: Methods and sequelae. *Br J Hosp Med* 1982; 27:364–384.

131. Graeff H, Ernst E, Bocaz JA: Evaluation of hypercoagulability in septic abortion. *Haemostasis* 1976; 5:285–294.

132. Steichele DF, Herschlein HJ: Intravascular coagulation in bacterial shock. Consumption coagulopathy and fibrinolysis after febrile abortion. *Med Welt* 1968; 1:24–30.

133. McGibbon DH: Dermatological purpura, in Ingram GIC, Brozovic M, Slater NCP (eds): *Bleeding Disorders—Investigation and Management.* Oxford, England, Blackwell Scientific Publications, 1982, pp 220–242.

134. Laursen B, Frost L, Mortensen JZ, et al: Acute fatty liver of pregnancy with complicating disseminated intravascular coagulation. *Acta Obstet Gynecol Scand* 1983; 62:403–407.

135. Burroughs AK, Seong NG, Dojcinoov DM, et al: Idiopathic acute fatty liver of pregnancy in 12 patients. *Q J Med* 1982; 51:481–497.

136. Hellgren M, Hagnevik K, Robbe H, et al: Severe acquired antithrombin III deficiency in relation to hepatic and renal insufficiency and intra-uterine death in late pregnancy. *Gynecol Obstet Invest* 1983; 16:107–108.

137. Liebman HA, McGehee WG, Patch MJ, et al: Severe depression of antithrombin III associated with disseminated intravascular coagulation in women with fatty liver of pregnancy. *Ann Intern Med* 1983; 98:330–333.

138. Laursen B, Mortensen JZ, Frost L, et al: Disseminated intravascular coagulation in hepatic failure treated with antithrombin III. *Thromb Res* 1981; 22:701–704.

139. Goodlin RC: Acute fatty liver of pregnancy. *Acta Obstet Gynecol Scand* 1984; 63:379–380.

140. Pritchard JA, Brekken AL: Clinical and laboratory studies on severe abruptio placentae. *Am J Obstet Gynecol* 1967; 57:681–695.

141. Mant MJ, King EG: Severe acute disseminated intravascular coagulation. A reappraisal of its pathophysiology, clinical significance and therapy, based on 47 patients. *Am J Med* 1979; 67:557–563.

142. Colvin BT: Thrombocytopenia, in Letsky EA (ed): Haematological disorders in pregnancy. *Clin Haematol* 1985; 14:661–681.

143. Burrows RF, Kelton JG: Incidentally detected thrombocytopenia in healthy mothers and their infants. *N Engl J Med* 1988; 319:142–145.

144. McMillan R: Chronic idiopathic thrombocytopenic purpura. *N Engl J Med* 1981; 304:1135–1147.

145. Hegde UM, Gordon-Smith EC, Worrledge SM: Platelet antibodies in thrombocytopenic patients. *Br J Haematol* 1977; 56:191–197.

146. Van Leeuwen EF, Helmerhorst FM, Engelfriet CP, et al: Maternal autoimmune thrombocytopenia and the newborn. *Br Med J* 1981; 283:104.

147. Cines DB, Dusak B, Tomaski A, et al: Immune thrombocytopenic purpura and pregnancy. *N Engl J Med* 1982; 306:826–831.

148. Hegde UM, Bowes A, Powell DK, et al: Detection of platelet bound and serum antibodies in thrombocytopenia by emzyme linked assay. *Vox Sang* 1981; 41:306–312.

149. Carloss HW, McMillan R, Crosby WH: Management of pregnancy in women with immune thrombocytopenic purpura. *JAMA* 1980; 144:2756–2758.

150. Terao T, Oike J, Kobayashi T, et al: Pregnancy complicated by idiopathic thrombocytopenic purpura. *J Obstet Gynecol* 1981; 2:1–10.

151. Territo M, Finkelstein J, Oh O: Management of autoimmune thrombocytopenia in pregnancy and the neonate. *Obstet Gynecol* 1973; 41:579–582.

152. Hegde UM: Immune thrombocytopenia in pregnancy and the newborn. *Br J Obstet Gynaecol* 1985; 92:657–659.

153. Kelton JG, Inwood MJ, Barr RM, et al: The prenatal prediction of thrombocytopenia in mothers with clinically diagnosed

immune thrombocytopenia. *Am J Obstet Gynecol* 1982; 144:449–454.

154. Bell WR: Hematologic abnormalities in pregnancy. *Med Clin North Am* 1977; 61:165–203.

155. Martin JN, Morrison JC, Files JC: Autoimmune thrombocytopenia purpura: Current concepts and recommended practices. *Am J Obstet Gynecol* 1984; 150:86–96.

156. Scott JR, Cruickshank DP, Kochenou RMD, et al: Fetal platelet counts in the obstetric management of immunologic thrombocytopenia purpura. *Am J Obstet Gynecol* 1980; 136:495–499.

157. Moise KJ, Carpenter RJ, Cotton DB, et al: Percutaneous umbilical cord sampling in the evaluation of fetal platelet counts in pregnant patients with autoimmune thrombocytopenia purpura. *Obstet Gynecol* 1988; 72:346–350.

158. Scioscia AL, Grannum PAT, Copel JA, et al: The use of percutaneous umbilical blood sampling in immune thrombocytopenia purpura. *Am J Obstet Gynecol* 1988; 159:1066–1068.

159. Davies SV, Murray JA, Gee H, et al: Transplacental effect of high-dose immunoglobulin in idiopathic thrombocytopenia (ITP). *Lancet* 1986; 1:1098–1099.

160. Tchernia G, Dreyfus M, Laurian Y, et al: Management of immune thrombocytopenia in pregnancy: Response of infusions of immunoglobulins. *Am J Obstet Gynecol* 1984; 148:225–226.

161. Morgenstern GR, Measday B, Hegde UM: Auto-immune thrombocytopenia in pregnancy. New approach to management. *Br Med J* 1983; 287:584.

162. Hegde U: Immune thrombocytopenia in pregnancy and the newborn: A review. *J Infect* 1987; 15(supple 1):55–58.

163. Epstein RD, Longer EL, Conbey JT: Congenital thrombocytopenic purpura. Purpura haemorrhage in pregnancy and the newborn. *Am J Med* 1950; 9:44–56.

164. Hughes GRV: Systemic lupus erythematosus, in Hughes GRV (ed): *Connective Tissue Diseases*, ed 3. Oxford, England, Blackwell Scientific Publications, 1987, pp 3–71.

165. Varner MW, Meehan RT, Syrop CH, et al: Pregnancy in patients with systemic lupus erythematosus. *Am J Obstet Gynecol* 1983; 145:1025–1037.

166. Pinette MG, Vintzileos AM, Ingardia CJ: Thrombotic thrombocytopenia purpura as a cause of thrombocytopenia in pregnancy: Literature review. *Am J Perinatol* 1989; 6:55–57.

167. Bukowski RM: Thrombotic thrombocytopenic purpura. *Prog Hemost Thromb* 1982; 287–337.

168. de Swiet M: Some rare medical complications of pregnancy. *Br Med J* 1985; 290:2–4.

169. Atlas M, Barkai G, Menszer J, et al: Thrombotic thrombocytopenic purpura in pregnancy. *Br J Obstet Gynaecol* 1982; 89:476–479.

170. Ingram GIL, Brozovic M, Slater NGP: Thrombotic thrombocytopenic purpura, in Ingram GIC, Brozovic M, Slater NCP (eds): *Bleeding Disorders—Investigation and Management*. Oxford, England, Blackwell Scientific Publications, 1982, pp 131–135.

171. Lian EC, Harkness DR, Byrnes JJ, et al: Presence of a platelet aggregating factor in the plasma of patients with thrombotic thrombocytopenic purpura (TTP) and its inhibition by normal plasma. *Blood* 1979; 53:333–336.

172. Remuzzi G, Misiani R, Marchesi D, et al: Haemolytic-uraemic syndrome. Deficiency of plasma factor(s) regulating prostacyclin activity? *Lancet* 1978; 2:871–872.

173. Machin SJ, Defrey NG, Vermylen J, et al: Prostacyclin deficiency in thrombotic thrombocytopenic purpura (TTP) and the haemolytic uraemic syndrome (HUS). *Br J Haematol* 1981; 49:141–142.

174. Stratta P, Cavavese CK, Bussolino P, et al: Haemolytic anaemia syndrome. *Lancet* 1988; 2:424–425.

175. Weiner CP: Thrombotic microangiopathy in pregnancy and the post-partum period. *Semin Hematol* 1987; 24:119–129.

176. Ambrose A, Welham RT, Lefalo RC, et al: Thrombotic thrombocytopenia purpura in early pregnancy. *Obstet Gynecol* 1985; 66:267–272.

177. Webster J, Rees AJ, Lewis PJ, et al: Prostacyclin deficiency in haemolytic uraemic syndrome. *Br Med J* 1980; 281:271.

178. Machin SJ: Thrombotic thrombocytopenic purpura. *Br J Haematol* 1984; 56:191–197.

179. Peaceman AM, Katz AR, Laville M: Bernard-Soulier syndrome complicating preg-

nancy: A case report. *Obstet Gynecol* 1989; 73:457–459.

180. Daffos F, Forestier F, Kaplan C, et al: Prenatal diagnosis and management of bleeding disorders with fetal blood sampling. *Am J Obstet Gynecol* 1988; 158:939–946.

181. Nicolaides KH, Rodeck CH, Mibasham RS: Obstetric management and diagnosis of haematological disease in the fetus, in Letsky EA (ed): Haematological disorders in pregnancy. *Clin Haematol* 1985; 14:775–804.

182. Coller BS, Hultin MB, Homer LW, et al: Normal pregnancy in a patient with a prior post partum factor VIII inhibitor: With observations on pathogenesis and prognosis. *Blood* 1981; 58:619–624.

183. Marengo-Rowe AJ, Murff G, Leveson JE, et al: Haemophilia-like disease associated with pregnancy. *Obstet Gynecol* 1972; 40:56–64.

184. O'Brien JR: An acquired coagulation defect in a woman. *J Clin Pathol* 1954; 7:22–25.

185. Reece EA, Fox HE, Rapoport F: Factor VIII inhibitor: A cause of severe postpartum haemorrhage. *Am J Obstet Gynecol* 1982; 144:985–987.

186. Voke J, Letsky E: Pregnancy and antibody to factor VIII. *J Clin Pathol* 1977; 30:928–932.

187. Holmberg L, Nilsson IM: Von Willebrand disease, in Ruggeri AM (ed): Coagulation disorders. *Clin Haematol* 1985; 14:461–488.

188. Linkler CA: Congenital disorders of haemostasis, in Laros RK (ed): *Blood Disorders in Pregnancy*. Philadelphia, Lea & Febiger, 1986, p 160.

189. Caldwell DC, Williamson RA, Goldsmith JC: Hereditary coagulopathies in pregnancy. *Clin Obstet Gynecol* 1985; 28:53–72.

190. Chediak JR, Alban CM, Maxey B: Von Willebrand's disease and pregnancy: Management during delivery and outcome of offspring. *Am J Obstet Gynecol* 1986; 155:618–624.

191. Conti M, Mari D, Conti E, et al: Pregnancy in women with different types of von Willebrand disease. *Obstet Gynecol* 1986; 68:282–285.

192. Rich ME, Williams SB, Sacher RA, et al: Thrombocytopenia associated with pregnancy in a patient with type IIb von Willebrand's disease. *Blood* 1987; 69:786–789.

193. Jones P: Developments and problems in the management of hemophilia. *Semin Hematol* 1977; 14:375–390.

194. Luscher JM, McMillan CW: Severe factor VIII and IX deficiency in females. *Am J Med* 1978; 65:637.

195. Acheson D: Department of Health and Social Security press release, 1987.

196. Ness PM, Budzynski AZ, Olexa SA, et al: Congenital hypofibrinogenemia and recurrent placental abruption. *Obstet Gynecol* 1983; 61:519–523.

197. Kitchens CS, Newcomb TF: Factor XIII. *Medicine* 1979; 658:413–429.

CHAPTER 9

Gastrointestinal and Pancreatic Disease

Robert Modigliani

Pierre Bernades

Pregnancy may cause a number of physiologic changes of the digestive tract but the only well-demonstrated effects are the modifications of esophageal function and intestinal motility. Nausea and vomiting (including hyperemesis gravidarum) and gastroesophageal reflux are very frequent during pregnancy but the most interesting problems are the management of generally preexisting diseases such as peptic ulcer or inflammatory bowel disease.

EFFECT OF PREGNANCY ON THE PHYSIOLOGY OF THE DIGESTIVE TRACT AND PANCREAS

The pressure of the lower esophageal sphincter is decreased during pregnancy,[1, 2] probably starting during the second trimester, becoming maximal by the end of gestation, and normalizing within a few days after delivery.[2] Peristaltic wave velocity in the distal esophagus also decreases significantly in pregnant women.[3] In contrast, studies to determine if pregnancy affects the gastric emptying have produced conflicting results,[4, 5] while the influence of gestation on gastric acid secretion is poorly understood. Experiments performed on pregnant rats demonstrate gastric acid hypersecretion that is partly attributable to increased vagal tonus[6]; however, no changes in gastric secretion were observed in a small number of third-trimester pregnant women.[7] The alterations in esophageal function are probably related to pregnancy-induced hormonal changes,[8] especially to increased estrogen[9] and chorionic gonadotropic hormone levels.[10] There is no proof that gastroesophageal motor function is modified by increased abdominal pressure secondary to uterine enlargement.[8]

Gastrointestinal transit time, measured by the lactulose breath test,[11] is significantly prolonged in the second and third trimesters of pregnancy when compared to the first trimester or postpartum period. This prolonged transit time has been tentatively attributed to the effects of hormones, especially progesterone. There are no available data on pancreatic function in pregnancy.

ENDOSCOPY AND RADIOLOGY IN PREGNANCY

Upper gastrointestinal tract endoscopy and colonoscopy[12] may be performed throughout pregnancy without increased risk.

TABLE 9–1.
Presentation and Management of Hypermesis
Gravidarum

Clinical presentation	Onset during the first month of gestation
	Intractable vomiting
	Fluid and electrolyte disturbances
	Nutritional deficiency
	Liver function abnormalities
Management	Fluid and electrolyte replacement
	Vitamin B supplementation
	Metoclopramide IV
	Supportive psychotherapy (may be useful in selected cases)
	Total parenteral nutrition (in most severe cases)

Abdominal ultrasound is without risk during gestation in the investigation of liver, biliary tract, and pancreatic abnormalities. Occasionally computed tomography is required, especially in the diagnosis of pancreatic diseases; in such instances sections should be localized to the pancreatic area in order to minimize fetal radiation exposure (see Chap. 18 regarding the risks of diagnostic radiation).

Fluoroscopy should be avoided during early pregnancy because of the doses of radiation required and the accompanying risk to the fetus. Also, other techniques such as small bowel series, endoscopic retrograde cholangiopancreatography, percutaneous transhepatic cholangiography, and angiography should be postponed until after delivery unless essential for maternal evaluation and therapy.

UPPER DIGESTIVE TRACT DISORDERS

Nausea and Vomiting

Nausea and vomiting are very common symptoms in early pregnancy. In a prospective study vomiting was reported in 56% of 9,098 gravidas in the first trimester.[13] Symptoms usually begin shortly after the first missed menstrual period and disappear by the fourth month of pregnancy. Generally, nausea and vomiting occur in the morning and rarely persist throughout the day. These symptoms are mild and the patient does not develop fluid and electrolyte disturbances. No demonstrable gastrointestinal lesion is present and the cause of these symptoms remains obscure. Paradoxically, women who vomit have a decreased risk for fetal loss and preterm delivery. They are more likely to vomit in subsequent pregnancies than women who do not experience emesis.[13] Also, such patients should be advised to eat small carbohydrate-rich meals and avoid high-fluid intake, especially in the morning.[14] When vomiting is severe, treatment with antiemetic drugs may be necessary; recommended medications are promethazine (FDA category C) or metoclopramide (FDA category B), which are believed to have no adverse fetal effects, but adequate studies are still lacking.[15] Side effects of metoclopramide include somnolence and galactorrhea (due to stimulation of prolactin secretion).

Hyperemesis Gravidarum

Hyperemesis gravidarum (Table 9–1), or pernicious vomiting of pregnancy, is a condition defined by intractable vomiting leading to fluid and electrolyte disturbances and nutritional deficiency. The onset of symptoms occurs mainly during the first month of gestation and remits by the end of the first trimester. Some patients may also experience increased salivation. This condition may be accompanied by liver dysfunction characterized by elevation in transaminases and bilirubin levels.[9] (See also Chap. 10, p. 347.)

The pathogenesis of hyperemesis gravidarum is poorly understood, though a recent case-control study of 419 affected patients demonstrated that younger age, multiparity, and obesity were significantly associated with an increased risk of hyperemesis.[9] Possible pathogenic factors include the elevated estrogen level of pregnancy and increased circulating chorionic gonadotropin.[10] Some believe psychologic factors underlie this disorder; however, epidemiologic evidence does not support this contention.[9]

Treatment of this condition requires hospitalization for fluid, electrolyte, and vitamin replacement.[10, 14] Supportive psychotherapy may be useful in selected cases. In cases of intractable vomiting, metoclopramide can be administered intravenously. Generally, vomiting resolves promptly under treatment. However, there are instances of severe disease in which total parenteral nutrition is necessary.[16]

Gastroesophageal Reflux

Pyrosis (heartburn), regurgitation, or both, occur in nearly half of pregnant women, mainly during the last trimester of pregnancy.[8] Symptoms are mild and resolve spontaneously after delivery. Upper digestive endoscopy is usually not performed and symptomatic treatment is prescribed. However, in very severe cases, endoscopy is indicated and may demonstrate esophagitis. Gastroesophageal reflux is related to alterations of the lower esophageal sphincter and esophageal motility during the last 6 months of gestation. The mechanism of these changes in unclear, but may be related to pregnancy-induced hormonal changes.[8]

Treatment of pyrosis should be limited to (1) raising the head of the bed when pyrosis occurs at night; (2) avoiding factors which decrease lower esophageal sphincter tone (smoking, alcohol, fatty meals); and (3) prescription of drugs without risk to the fetus, such as antacids (aluminum and magnesium hydroxides) and alginate, all of which are poorly absorbed, if at all.[14] Prescription of metoclopramide should be reserved for severe cases. Drugs which inhibit gastric secretion, such as histamine H_2-receptor antagonists (cimetidine and ranitidine; both FDA category B), should generally be prescribed only when severe esophagitis is demonstrated by endoscopy. These drugs appear to have minimal risk when used during the last 3 gestational months.[15]

Peptic Ulcer

The relationship between pregnancy and peptic ulcer disease is poorly understood, but it appears that neither the incidence nor the risk of recurrence of peptic ulcer are increased during gestation. For example, in one study of life events related to stress, pregnancy was not listed as a factor associated with gastric ulcer.[17] Furthermore, the incidence of peptic ulcer is low in young adult women; in Copenhagen County during 1963–1968, the mean annual incidence in 20- to 40-year-old women was about 0.1 per 1,000 for gastric ulcer and 0.2 to 0.5 per 1,000 for duodenal ulcer.[18] This may be one reason why complications of peptic ulcer, such as hemorrhage and perforation, are extremely unusual during pregnancy.

When peptic ulcer is associated with pregnancy, the primary problem concerns the appropriate choice of antiulcer medications (Table 9–2). Among the available agents,

TABLE 9–2.
Use of Antiulcer Drugs During Pregnancy

Drug	FDA Risk Category*	1st Trimester	2nd, 3rd Trimesters	Comment
Sucralfate	B	Yes	Yes	Not absorbed
Antacids	B	Yes	Yes	Poorly absorbed
Cimetidine	B	No	Yes	No adverse fetal effect known
Ranitidine	B	No	Yes	No adverse fetal effect known
Nizatidine	C	No	?	Insufficient data
Famotidine	B	No	?	Insufficient data
Omeprazole	C	No	No	Insufficient data
Misoprostol	X	No	No	May provoke uterine contraction and abortion or premature delivery

*See Preface for description of FDA risk categories.

prostaglandins (misoprostol) are clearly contraindicated both in gravidas and women who may conceivably be pregnant as these eicosanoids provoke uterine contractions and may lead to abortion.[19] Sucralfate, which acts locally on the gastrointestinal mucosa, is not absorbed to any significant degree and is a reasonable first drug, especially in the first trimester.[15] Antacids may also be prescribed because they too are poorly absorbed, but if aluminum hydroxide is used, dosage reduction will be necessary to avoid worsening the physiologic constipation of pregnancy. If sucralfate and/or antacids are ineffective, an H_2-receptor antagonist can be prescribed during the second and third trimesters of pregnancy.[15] Cimetidine or ranitidine are preferable to more recently available H_2-receptor antagonists (e.g., nizatidine, famotidine) because the former two have been subjected to many years of postmarketing surveillance. While evaluation of their safety in gestation is still incomplete, available data in pregnant women are encouraging and these agents appear to have no serious adverse fetal effects.[15] Cimetidine and ranitidine cross the placenta and are excreted in breast milk. Ranitidine is preferable to cimetidine because the former has no obvious antiandrogenic effects. Omeprazole, an inhibitor of H^+, K^+-adenosinetriphosphatase (H^+, K^+-ATPase), is the most potent antisecretory drug currently available. However, because of insufficient data on its use in pregnant women, we do not recommend its use during gestation. Treatment of an active gastric or duodenal ulcer should be continued for 4 to 6 weeks. It is not necessary to document healing with endoscopy if the patient is asymptomatic, and in most instances maintenance therapy is not required.

INFLAMMATORY BOWEL DISEASE

Fertility

Most studies of fertility in women with inflammatory bowel disease (IBD) are flawed because of problems such as short follow-up and because little attention is given to prior medical advice regarding contraception, intent to conceive, or fertility of the male partner.

Although earlier reports suggested that women with ulcerative colitis had decreased fertility, recent data indicate that this is not true.[20, 21] In one carefully conducted study,[22] 81% (119/147) of women with ulcerative colitis has conceived either shortly before their colitis began or during the subsequent follow-up. If voluntary avoidance of pregnancy was taken into account (12.2%), then the incidence of true infertility decreased to 6.8%, a figure that was similar to that of the general population (which was 10%). Whether impaired fertility is more common in patients with chronically active ulcerative colitis is unknown.

Variable, but at times high rates of infertility have been reported for women with Crohn's disease.[23–27] These discrepancies are probably due, at least in part, to differences in methodology. In one case-control study,[27] however, the number of children born to patients with Crohn's disease was decreased to 57% of those in paired controls. This difference was present after (but not before) onset of the disease. Whether the anatomic location of the disease process has an effect on fertility is controversial.[23, 25] The European epidemiologic study concluded that disease location had no influence on fertility.[27]

Reasons for reduced fertility in Crohn's disease have not been investigated, but are probably multiple. These include reduced sexual activity due to active disease, perineal disease, and fear that the disease might become worse or the fetus might be damaged. Involvement of ovaries or fallopian tubes in the inflammatory process is also possible, although not documented. It should also be borne in mind that sulfasalazine causes reversible infertility in the male,[28] due probably to the sulfapyridine component. This problem may not be present with use of the newer 5-aminosalicylate (5-ASA) preparation.[29]

In summary, fertility appears to be normal in ulcerative colitis and reduced in Crohn's disease. The cause for the latter decrement is unclear.

Effect of Inflammatory Bowel Diseases on Pregnancy

Ulcerative Colitis

Table 9–3 summarizes the outcome of 978 pregnancies in women with ulcerative colitis reported in seven major series published since 1965.[21, 22, 30–35] The overall figures are similar to the general population, and the average patient has a very good chance of a normal full-term delivery. The probability of having a spontaneous abortion is significantly higher in women with active disease at conception than in women with inactive ulcerative colitis (7/19 vs. 9/133, $P < .005$, according to a Danish series[33]). The proportion of babies with low birth weight, however, was similar to that in the general population.[33] Also, in one case-controlled study, ulcerative colitis had no effect on duration of pregnancy, mode of delivery, or the frequency of gestational complications.[34]

Crohn's Disease

Table 9–4 summarizes seven major series published since 1970 describing outcome in 688 pregnancies in women with Crohn's disease.[23–26, 31, 35, 36] The pattern is similar to that seen in ulcerative colitis, but spontaneous abortions seem to be slightly more frequent in Crohn's disease. This appears to be the case primarily when the disease is active at the time of conception[26, 36] or in women who had undergone bowel resection before pregnancy.[36] One group also noted an increase in the prematurity rate of these two subgroups.[36] In the case-control study cited above,[27] the risk of prematurity (defined as delivery more than 3 weeks before the expected date of confinement) was 16% in a large group of women with a variety of forms of Crohn's disease compared to 7% in controls ($P < .03$), the risk

being independent of the anatomic site of the disease process.

Effect of Pregnancy on Inflammatory Bowel Disease

Ulcerative Colitis

When ulcerative colitis is inactive at conception, approximately 30% of the patients experience exacerbation of their disease during the 9 months of pregnancy and the first 3 postpartum months,[21, 22, 33] a figure which does not differ from the rate at which ulcerative colitis recurs among nonpregnant women of comparable age.[33] Relapses are more likely to occur in the first trimester.[22, 33] Sixty to eighty percent of women in whom ulcerative colitis is active at the start of pregnancy are likely to experience either no change or a worsening of their symptoms during pregnancy[22, 33] despite medical treatment.

In the past, ulcerative colitis presenting during pregnancy was associated with a 15% maternal mortality rate and was considered quite dangerous. More recently, the initial presentation during pregnancy appears to have been adequately controlled by medical treatment, and maternal mortality no longer seems to occur.[22] Recent studies have also failed to support another traditional view,[21] that presentation of disease in the puerperium is associated with a poor clinical course.[22, 33] The effect of successive pregnancies on ulcerative colitis is variable and one cannot use the outcome of one pregnancy to predict the course in a second.[30]

Crohn's Disease

When Crohn's disease is inactive at conception, risk of reactivation is about 25% and does not appear to be greater than in nonpregnant women of comparable age.[36] Relapses seem to occur more frequently in the first trimester[26, 36] and in the puerperium,[36] and those occurring during pregnancy do not seem to be especially severe. If the patient has clinically active disease at the time of con-

TABLE 9–3.
Effect of Ulcerative Colitis on Pregnancy

Series (yr)	Pregnancy (n)	Spontaneous Abortion (%)	Induced Abortion (%)	Normal Full-Term Baby (%)	Premature (%)	Malformation (%)	Stillbirth (%)
De Dombal et al.[21] (1965)	107	6.0	5	84	—	3.0	2.0
McEwan[30] (1972)	50	8.0	2	88	0	0	2.0
Willoughby & Truelove[22] (1980)	209	11.0	4	81.5	—	2.5	1.0
Mogadam et al[31] (1981)	309	0.5	0	97	1.0	1.0	0.5
Levy et al[32] (1981)	60	12.0	3	83.5	1.5	0	0
Nielsen et al[33] (1983)	173	9.0	13	71	5.0	2.0	0
Baioco & Korelitz[35] (1984)	70	13.0	3	74	7.0	3.0	0
Total	978	Mean 7.0	4	85	2.0	1.5	0.5

TABLE 9–4.
Effect of Crohn's Disease on Pregnancy

Series (yr)	Pregnancy (n)	Spontaneous Abortion (%)	Induced Abortion (%)	Normal Full-Term Baby (%)	Premature (%)	Malformation (%)	Stillbirth (%)
Fielding & Cooke[23] (1970)	98	13.0	1.0	80.0	4.0	—	2.0
De Dombal et al.[24] (1972)	60	5.0	1.5	87.0	0	2.0	5.0
Homan & Thorbjarnarson[25] (1976)	42	16.5	7.0	69.0	2.5	2.5	2.5
Mogadam et al[31] (1981)	222	3.0	—	94.5	1.0	1.0	0.5
Khosla et al[26] (1984)	80	28.0	0	70.0	0	1.0	1.0
Baioco & Korelitz[35] (1984)	77	11.5	6.5	73.0	4.0	2.5	2.5
Nielsen et al[36] (1984)	109	9.0	17.5	56.0	14.0	0	3.5
Total	688	Mean 10	4.5	79.0	3.5	1.0	2.0

ception she is likely to have continuing problems throughout that gestation, as only 35% of such patients improve during pregnancy.[26] Also, Crohn's disease occurring for the first time in the puerperium is not necessarily associated with a more severe course, and active disease does not seem to be associated with increments in maternal mortality.[23, 26]

Although therapeutic abortion has been previously advised in pregnant patients with inflammatory bowel disease,[37] it is now generally agreed upon that inflammatory bowel disease per se is not an indication for terminating pregnancy.[22, 33, 34]

Pregnancy and Surgery for Inflammatory Bowel Disease

Pregnancy in Women With Previous Surgery

After Proctocolectomy for Ulcerative Colitis.—Pregnancy has been reported in a small series of women who had previously undergone proctocolectomy and ileostomy. Normal vaginal delivery was the most frequent outcome and cesarean section, essentially for severe perineal scarring following the previous abdominoperineal resection,[38] was necessary in 20% to 40% of cases.[21, 30, 38] The major complications of ileostomy during pregnancy were stomal dysfunction, bowel obstruction, ileostomy prolapse, and nipple valve retraction.[39] Pregnancy has also been observed after ileal pouch–anal anastomosis; a transient deterioration of anorectal function during the last trimester of pregnancy manifested by an increased stool frequency and a need for greater voluntary effort for defecation has been reported.[40] Continence was maintained in four of these patients who underwent vaginal delivery. Routine cesarean section does not appear to be indicated when an ileal pouch–anal anastomosis is present.[40]

After Bowel Resection for Crohn's disease.—Prior bowel resection has been reported to be associated with a decrease in the rate of full-term delivery (62% vs. 83%), and with increases in rates of prematurity (20% vs. 5%) and spontaneous abortion (13% vs. 4%) in Crohn's disease. These differences were, however, not statistically significant and their clinical importance is uncertain.[36]

Surgery for Inflammatory Bowel Disease During Pregnancy

Operative procedures in pregnant women with inflammatory bowel disease are rarely needed, but seem to carry a considerable risk. Of 16 women with ulcerative colitis operated on during pregnancy,[21, 30, 33] 4 maternal deaths occurred and only 9 healthy babies were delivered; the relative contributions of maternal disease and surgery per se to these outcomes are unclear. Nevertheless, if its indication is clear, surgery should not be delayed in the pregnant patient since procrastination may lead to deterioration of both maternal and fetal health.

Influence of Medical Therapy for Inflammatory Bowel Disease on Pregnancy Course and Outcome

Sulfasalazine and Its New Derivatives

Sulfasalazine and one of its metabolites, sulfapyridine, cross the placenta and the concentrations are similar in cord and maternal serum.[41] Concentrations of 5-ASA, the other metabolite of sulfasalazine, are very low because of its poor absorption.

There are a few anecdotal reports[42, 43] of congenital abnormalities associated with the use of sulfasalazine during pregnancy; however, the incidence of fetal complications has not been reported to be increased in large series of women treated with this drug for inflammatory bowel disease. In another report,[31] however, there was an increased risk of fetal complications in women receiving sulfasalazine but this seems to have been due to inflammatory bowel disease activity rather than to drug toxicity.[22, 26, 33, 36] A national survey in the United States concluded that the frequency of fetal complications was even lower than in the general population.[31]

Sulfonamides displace bilirubin from albumin and thus have the potential to provoke neonatal kernicterus. However, at the concentrations of sulfasalazine and sulfapyridine measured in cord blood, displacement of bilirubin is negligible and in fact has not been a problem in the series quoted here. This drug does interfere with folic acid absorption by the small bowel and since folates are important for fetal development, 1 mg of folic acid twice daily should be prescribed to pregnant women who take sulfasalazine. There are no data on the use of the new salicylates (5-ASA and olsalazine) during pregnancy, but they are likely to be safe. It is generally agreed that sulfasalazine may be safely given during nursing.[41–45]

Corticosteroids

Corticosteroids cross the placenta, but cortisol is rapidly converted to the less active cortisone.[46] Prednisone and prednisolone levels in the fetal circulation are only 10% of those in the maternal circulation.[47] A variety of corticosteroid compounds are teratogens in animals,[15] but there is little evidence that steroids are harmful to the human fetus. While anecdotal instances of fetal abnormalities have been reported, there is no evidence of an increased incidence of congenital defects based on observations in several large prospective studies,[15] as well as in hundreds of patients with inflammatory bowel disease.[22, 26, 30, 33, 35, 36] In the national survey quoted above,[31] pregnant patients with ulcerative colitis who were receiving steroids (with or without sulfasalazine) displayed similar outcomes (in terms of spontaneous abortion, developmental defects, prematurity, small-for-gestational-age infants, and stillbirths) compared to untreated patients. On the contrary, patients with Crohn's disease receiving steroids had more complications than the untreated group, this difference being attributed by the authors to disease activity rather than to the drugs themselves.[31]

There is a theoretical risk that steroids may suppress the fetal hypothalamus-pituitary-adrenal axis. This risk, however, appears to be extremely low, even for women receiving long-term maintenance high-dose schedules.

Suppression was not noted in one study of 185 pregnant patients with inflammatory bowel disease receiving steroids.[31] Finally, only minimal quantities of prednisolone (0.07%– 0.25% of a single test dose) enter breast milk[48] and nursing should not be proscribed.

Azathioprine and 6-Mercaptopurine

Azathioprine and 6-mercaptopurine ought not to be used in pregnancy because of a high incidence of fetal abnormality reported in animals,[49, 50] as well as several problems reported in humans, including thymic hypoplasia, lymphopenia, reduced serum immunoglobulin concentration, and chromosome breaks.[51, 52] Some even suggest that exposure to these drugs is sufficient reason for pregnancy termination.[53] However, deliveries of normal infants following maternal prenatal use of azathioprine have been reported, mainly in the renal transplantation literature[54, 55] (see Chap. 2). Also, women with inflammatory bowel disease receiving 6-mercaptopurine who became pregnant against advice and chose not to have a therapeutic abortion usually delivered normal offspring.[56] There is also concern about fertility and mutagenic effects in future offspring. Thus, despite absence of convincing data on their toxicity, azathioprine or 6-mercaptopurine ought to be avoided for 3 months prior to conception and through pregnancy. The decision to discontinue the drug, however, may be difficult, especially in some azathioprine- or 6-mercaptopurine-responsive patients in whom the risk of reactivation of the disease is as high as 40% during the year following interruption of drug therapy.[57] In these patients the risk to pregnancy is great if medication is stopped.

Metronidazole

Metronidazole (FDA category B) is prescribed in Crohn's disease, especially when perianal and perineal lesions are present. This drug is mildly fetotoxic when administered intraperitoneally to pregnant mice, but its effect in humans is unclear. In one survey of a large number of pregnant women treated with metronidazole, no increase in the incidence of congenital abnormalities was observed.[15]

TABLE 9–5.
Use of Drugs for Inflammatory Bowel Disease During Gestation

Drug	FDA Risk Category*	Use in Pregnancy	Comment
Corticosteroids	B	Yes	As in nonpregnant women
Sulfasalazine	B	Yes	Supplement with folic acid
Newer salicylates (mesalazine, olsalazine)	?	?	Insufficient data
Azathioprine	D	No	Avoid except in severe chronic active Crohn's disease
Metronidazole	B	No	Insufficient data

*See Preface for description of FDA risk categories.

Antidiarrheals

First-trimester use of diphenoxylate hydrochloride–atropine sulfate (FDA category C) (Lomotil) has been associated with malformations in a small number of infants.[15] Both agents are excreted in breast milk and atropine may inhibit lactation. Therefore, the routine use of this antidiarrheal is not recommended in pregnancy and should be avoided in nursing mothers. Loperamide (FDA category B) safety has not been established in pregnancy and paregoric should not be used in gravid patients. Kaolin and pectin are not absorbed and they are probably safe during pregnancy.

A summary of the use of drugs for inflammatory bowel disease during gestation is given in Table 9–5.

Prepregnancy Counseling and Contraception

Young women with inflammatory bowel disease should be reassured about their ability to become pregnant and to have a normal baby. They should be advised to start a pregnancy while the disease is in remission or under good medical control. However, they cannot be told that there is no risk of transmitting inflammatory bowel disease to their offspring since 10% to 20% of patients have at least one relative with inflammatory bowel disease.

Oral contraception has been associated with an increased risk for Crohn's disease, remission of symptoms having been noted following discontinuance of the drug.[58] In fact, a recent community-based case-control study convincingly shows that there is no association between oral contraceptive use and Crohn's disease and concludes that oral contraceptives are not contraindicated in this disease.[59a]

Summary

1. Inflammatory bowel diseases do not influence pregnancy outcome except for a moderate increase in the spontaneous abortion rate, and only if the disease is active.

2. Pregnancy does not increase the risk of disease exacerbation; if the disease is active at conception, the patient is likely to have continuing symptoms during pregnancy.

3. Steroids and sulfasalazine should be used in pregnancy in the same way as they are in nonpregnant women (since they do not appear to be harmful to the fetus), the most important therapeutic aim being the rapid control of the disease; the major threat to the pregnancy comes from the disease activity itself and not from the medication.

4. Azathioprine (or 6-mercaptopurine) should be avoided during pregnancy except in the small group of severe chronic active and azathioprine-dependent Crohn's disease patients.

PANCREATITIS IN PREGNANCY

Acute Pancreatitis

Until recently, pregnancy has been considered among the causes of acute pancreatitis.[59] However, the prevalence of acute pancreatitis is no more frequent in pregnant than in nonpregnant women[60] and most instances of disease in gravid patients are a result of other associated pathology. In one study involving 282 women presenting with acute pancreatitis, 7 patients developed disease during pregnancy and 13 did so within 5 months after delivery.[61] Acute pancreatitis was associated with gallstones in 18 of the 20 women (pregnancy is a recognized risk factor for biliary lithiasis[62]), with type I hyperlipoproteinemia in one instance, and with alcohol abuse in another.[61] These data confirm that pregnancy itself should no longer be considered as a cause of acute pancreatitis.[63]

Diagnosis of acute pancreatitis currently rests on demonstrating elevated serum levels of pancreatic enzyme levels and abnormalities on abdominal ultrasound, although the latter may not visualize the pancreas in 30% of cases of acute pancreatitis. Computed tomography is rarely necessary, but if felt to be indicated tomographic images should be limited to the pancreatic region to reduce fetal x-ray exposure. Diagnosis of acute pancreatitis can be difficult in pregnant women and gestational complications such as ectopic pregnancy have to be excluded. However, diagnosis of complications such as acute fatty liver or hyperemesis gravidarum are generally easy to distinguish from acute pancreatitis. Clinical severity in most cases of acute pancreatitis during pregnancy is mild.[61] The best treatment is intravenous fluids while restricting oral intake. Nasogastric suction is not necessary except when nausea and vomiting are present. When acute pancreatitis is severe, the patient should be hospitalized in an intensive care unit. Total parenteral nutrition can be performed if necessary[16, 64] (see below).

Except in very severe forms maternal mortality is low.[61] However, there is an increased risk of abortion when pancreatitis occurs in early pregnancy and an increased risk of premature labor when it occurs in late pregnancy.[59] When acute pancreatitis is secondary to biliary lithiasis, surgery is recommended,[61] and the gravid state should not be a deterrent for such action (see Chap. 10, p. 353, for discussion of biliary lithiasis).

Chronic Pancreatitis

Pregnancy in women with chronic pancreatitis is infrequent, as this is a disease where (1) male predominance is high (90% of cases) and (2) mean age at the onset of the disease is about 40 years.[65] When present, chronic pancreatitis does not seem to influence the course of pregnancy. If steatorrhea is present, pancreatic enzymes can be prescribed because they are not systemically absorbed.[15]

MISCELLANEOUS

Constipation

The incidence of constipation is as high as 38% at some time during pregnancy, and this condition affects 20% of third-trimester gravidas.[66] Also, rare examples of megacolon have been reported during pregnancy.[67] The safest way to treat constipation is to prescribe bulk-forming preparations containing psyllium hydrophilic mucilloid, or bran[66] if classic dietary measures (such as increasing vegetables and fruits in the diet) are not sufficient. Certain laxatives which should not be prescribed during pregnancy include anthraquinone derivatives (possible increased risk of fetal malformations), castor oil (which may initiate uterine contractions), mineral oil (which may induce malabsorption of fat-soluble vitamins), and hyperosmotic saline laxatives (sodium retention in the mother). For other laxatives such as phenolphthalein, bisacodyl, senna, and lactulose, the risk-benefit ratio is unknown and they too are best avoided, especially during the first trimester.

TABLE 9–6.
Recommended Daily Allowances for Pregnant Patients*

Mineral or trace element	Nutrition	
	Enteral	Parenteral
Calcium	1,200 mg	250 mg
Phosphorus	1,200 mg (38mM)	30–45mM
Magnesium	450 mg (37.5 mEq)	10–15 mEq
Zinc	20 mg	2.55–3.0 mg
Copper	2–3 mg[†]	0.5–1.5 mg
Manganese	2.5–5.0 mg[†]	0.15–0.8 mg
Iodine	175 μg	
Iron	10 + 30–60 mg supplemental iron	3–6 mg
Chromium	0.05–0.2 mg[†]	10–15 μg
Selenium	0.05–0.2 mg	20–40 μg[‡]
Vitamins		
A	1,000 μg RE	3,000 IU (retinol)[§]
D	400 IU	200 IU[¶]
E	10 mg α-TE[‖]	10 IU
K**	—	0.03–1.5 μg/kg
Ascorbic acid	60 mg	100 mg
Thiamine (B_1)	1.5 mg	3 mg
Riboflavin (B_2)	1.7 mg	3.6 mg
Niacin (B_3)	15 mg	40 mg
Pantothenic Acid (B_5)	7 mg	15 mg
Pyridoxine (B_6)	2.2 mg	4 mg
B_{12}	4 μg	5 μg
Folic acid	800 μg	400 μg
Biotin	200 μg	60 μg
Energy	300 kcal above basal requirements	
Protein	30 g above basal requirements	

RE = retinol equivalents; α-TE = α-tocopherol equivalents.
*From Kirkby DF, Fiorenza V, Craig RM: *JPEN* 1988; 12:72–80. Used by permission.
[†]Estimated safe and adequate daily dietary intakes for nonpregnant patients.
[‡]Recommended intravenous dose for stable patients.
[§]One RE = 0.3 μg of retinol.
[¶]One IU = 0.025 μg of vitamin D (cholecalciferol).
[‖]α-Tocopherol equivalents: 1 mg *d*-α-tocopherol = 1 α-TE.
**No specific recommendation for normal persons due to synthesis by intestinal bacteria. Parenteral administration is suggested for patients on prolonged intravenous nutrition.

Celiac Disease

Celiac disease may present in the postpartum period, sometimes as an acute diarrheal illness with evidence of severe malabsorption[68]; increased nutritional demands due to pregnancy may unmask preexisting latent celiac disease. This is probably true for any malabsorption syndrome.

Parenteral Feeding

Total parenteral nutrition (TPN) use has been reported in approximately 60 pregnant women[16] for a variety of illnesses, including hyperemesis gravidarum,[69] pancreatitis, and inflammatory bowel disease (Table 9–7). There are no specific guidelines for TPN in pregnancy, although recommended daily al-

TABLE 9–7.
Diseases for Which Intravenous Nutrition Has Been
Used in Pregnancy

Digestive diseases
  Hyperemesis gravidarum
  Pancreatitis
  Pancreatic carcinoma
  Ulcerative colitis
  Crohn's disease
  Short-bowel syndrome
  Jejunoileal bypass
  Bowel obstruction
  Diabetic gastroparesis
  Esophageal injury
  Esophagocolonogastrostomy with aspiration
  Partial hepatectomy
  Cholecystitis
  Chronic abdominal pain
Other disorders
  Anorexia nervosa
  Congenital myotonic dystrophy
  Paroxysmal nocturnal hemoglobinuria
  Burn
  Leukemia

lowances for pregnant women have been proposed (Table 9–6). At present, each of the major components (amino acids), hypertonic glucose, and fat emulsion) contains a product warning stating that its safety to mother and fetus is not known. Data on the use of hypertonic glucose are conflicting but the few published cases suggest that its judicious use is not contraindicated. The use of fat emulsion in pregnancy remains controversial because of theoretical risks of maternal ketonemia, premature labor, fat accumulation in the placenta, and pulmonary complications in neonates.[16] However, the few available reports of its use to date have not revealed serious maternal and fetal adverse effects. Pregnancy in patients on home parenteral nutrition has been reported.[70]

REFERENCES

1. Fisher RS, Roberts GS, Grabowski CJ, et al: Altered lower esophageal sphincter function during early pregnancy. *Gastroenterology* 1978; 74:1233–1237.

2. Van Thiel DH, Gavaler JS, Joshi SN, et al: Heartburn of pregnancy. *Gastroenterology* 1977; 72:666–668.

3. Ulmsten U, Lindstrom G: Esophageal manometry in pregnant and nonpregnant women. *Am J Obstet Gynecol* 1978; 132:260–264.

4. O'Sullivan GM, Sutton AJ, Thompson SA, et al: Noninvasive measurement of gastric emptying in obstetric patients. *Anesth Analg* 1987; 66:505–511.

5. Simpson KH, Stakes AF, Miller M: Pregnancy delays paracetamol absorption and gastric emptying in patients undergoing surgery. *Br J Anaesth* 1988; 60:24–27.

6. Takeuchi K, Okabe S: Factors related to gastric hypersecretion during pregnancy and lactation in rats. *Dig Dis Sci* 1984; 29:248–255.

7. O'Sullivan GM, Bullingham RES: The assessment of gastric acidity and antacid effect in pregnant women by a non-invasive radiotelemetry technique. *Br J Obstet Gynaecol* 1984; 91:973–978.

8. Galmiche JP, Denis P: Reflux gastro-oesophagien et grossesse: une énigme physiopathologique non resolue! *Gastroenterol Clin Biol* 1982; 6:421–423.

9. Depue RH, Berstein L, Ross RK, Judd HL, Henderson BE: Hyperemesis gravidarum in relation to estradiol levels, pregnancy outcome, and other maternal factors: A seroepidemiologic study. *Am J Obstet Gynecol* 1987; 156:1137–1141.

10. Riely CA: Case studies in jaundice of pregnancy. *Semin Liver Dis* 1988; 8:191–199.

11. Lawson M, Kern F Jr, Everson GT: Gastrointestinal transit time in human pregnancy: prolongation in the second and third trimesters followed by postpartum normalization. *Gastroenterology* 1985; 89:996–999.

12. Donaldson RM: Management of medical problems in pregnancy—inflammatory bowel disease. *N Engl J Med* 1985; 312:1616–1619.

13. Klebanoff MA, Koslowe PA, Kaslow R, et al: Epidemiology of vomiting in early pregnancy. *Obstet Gynecol* 1985; 66:612–616.

14. Atlay RD, Weekes ARL: The treatment of gastrointestinal disease in pregnancy. *Clin Obstet Gynaecol* 1986; 13:335–347.

15. Lewis JH, Weingold AB: The use of gastrointestinal drugs during pregnancy and lactation. *Am J Gastroenterol* 1985; 80:912–923.

16. Kirkby DF, Fiorenza V, Craig RM: Intravenous nutritional support during pregnancy. *JPEN* 1988; 12:72–80.

17. Thomas J, Greig M, Pipper DW: Chronic gastric ulcer and life events. *Gastroenterology* 1980; 78:905–911.

18. Bonnevie O: Changing demographics of peptic ulcer disease. *Dig Dis Sci* 1985; 30(suppl):8S–14S.

19. Lauritsen K, Rask-Madsen J: Prostaglandin analogues. *Clin Gastroenterol* 1988; 2:621–628.

20. Miller JP: Inflammatory bowel disease in pregnancy: A review. *J R Soc Med* 1986; 79:221–225.

21. De Dombal FT, Watts JM, Watkinson G, et al: Ulcerative colitis in pregnancy. *Lancet* 1965; 2:599–602.

22. Willoughby CP, Truelove SC: Ulcerative colitis in pregnancy. *Gut* 1980; 21:469–474.

23. Fielding JF, Cooke WT: Pregnancy and Crohn's disease. *Br Med J* 1970; 2:76–77.

24. De Dombal FT, Burton IL, Goligher JC: Crohn's disease and pregnancy. *Br Med J* 1972; 3:550–553.

25. Homan WP, Thorbjarnarson B: Crohn's disease and pregnancy. *Arch Surg* 1976; 111:545–547.

26. Khosla R, Willoughby CP, Jewell DP: Crohn's disease and pregnancy. *Gut* 1984; 25:52–56.

27. Mayberry JF, Weterman IT: European survey of fertility and pregnancy in women with Crohn's disease: A case control study by European collaborative group. *Gut* 1986; 27:821–825.

28. O'Morain C, Smethurst P, Dore CJ, et al: Reversible male infertility due to sulphasalazine. Studies in man and rats. *Gut* 1984; 25:1078–1084.

29. Mulder CJJ, Tytgat GNJ, Dekker W, Terpstra: Pentasa in 70 patients with severe side effects or allergy to sulphasalazine. *Gastroenterology* 1988; 94:A313.

30. McEwan HP: Ulcerative colitis in pregnancy. *Proc R Soc Med* 1972; 65:279–281.

31. Mogadam M, Dobbins WO, Korelitz BI, et al: Pregnancy in inflammatory bowel disease: Effect of sulfasalazine and corticosteroids on fetal outcome. *Gastroenterology* 1981; 80:72–70.

32. Levy N, Roisman I, Teodor I: Ulcerative colitis in pregnancy in Israel. *Dis Colon Rectum* 1981; 24:351–354.

33. Nielsen OH, Andreasson B, Bondesen S, et al: Pregnancy in ulcerative colitis. *Scand J Gastroenterol* 1983; 18:735–742.

34. Porter RJ, Stirrat GM: The effects on inflammatory bowel disease on pregnancy: A case-controlled reprospective analysis. *Br J Obstet Gynaecol* 1986; 93:1124–1131.

35. Baioco PJ, Korelitz BI: The influence of inflammatory bowel disease and its treatment on pregnancy and fetal outcome. *J Clin Gastroenterol* 1984; 6:211–216.

36. Nielsen OH, Andreasson B, Bondesen S, et al: Pregnancy in Crohn's disease. *Scand J Gastroenterol* 1984; 19:724–732.

37. Crohn BB, Yarnis H, Crohn EB, et al: Ulcerative colitis and pregnancy. *Gastroenterology* 1956; 30:391–403.

38. Barwin BN, Harley JMG, Wilson W: Ileostomy and pregnancy. *Br J Clin Pract* 1974; 26:256–258.

39. Gopal KA, Amshel AL, Shonberg IL, et al: Ostomy and pregnancy. *Dis Colon Rectum* 1985; 28:912–916.

40. Metcalf A, Dozois RR, Beart RW, et al: Pregnancy following ileal pouch-anal anastomosis. *Dis Colon Rectum* 1985; 28:859–861.

41. Jarnerot G, Into-Malmberg MB, Esbjorner E: Placental transfer of sulphasalazine and sulphapyridine and some of its metabolites. *Scand J Gastroenterol* 1981; 16:693–697.

42. Craxi A, Pagliarello F: Possible embryotoxicity of sulphasalazine. *Arch Intern Med* 1980; 140:1674.

43. Newman NM, Correy JF: Possible teratogenicity of sulphasalazine. *Med J Aust* 1983; 1:528–529.

44. Jarnerot G, Andresen S, Esbjorner E, et al: Albumin reserve for binding bilirubin in maternal and cord serum under treat-

ment with sulphasalazine. *Scand J Gastroenterol* 1981; 16:1049–1055.

45. Jarnerot, Into-Malmberg MB: Sulphasalazine treatment during breast feeding. *Scand J Gastroenterol* 1979; 14:869–871.

46. Murphy BEP, Clark SJ, Donald IR, et al: Conversion of maternal cortisol to cortisone during placental transfer to the human fetus. *Am J Obstet Gynecol* 1974; 118:538–541.

47. Beitins IZ, Bayard F, Ances IG, et al: The transplacental passage of prednisone and prednisolone in pregnancy near term. *J Pediatr* 1972; 81:936–945.

48. McKenzie SA, Selley JA, Agnew JE: Secretion of prednisolone into breast milk. *Arch Dis Child* 1975; 50:894–896.

49. Reimers TJ, Sluss PM: 6-Mercaptopurine treatment of pregnant mice: Effect on second and third generation. *Science* 1978; 205:65.

50. Scott JR: Fetal growth retardation associated with maternal administration of immunosuppressive drugs. *Am J Obstet Gynecol* 1976; 128:668–676.

51. Cote CJ, Meuwissen HJ, Pickering RJ: Effect on the neonate of prednisone and azathioprine administered to the mother during pregnancy. *J Pediatr* 1974; 85:324–328.

52. Price HV, Salaman JR, Laurence KM, et al: Immunosuppressive drugs and the foetus. *Transplantation* 1976; 21:294–298.

53. Sorokin JJ, Levine SM: Pregnancy and inflammatory bowel disease: A review of the literature. *Obstet Gynecol* 1983; 62:247–252.

54. Erkman J, Blythe JG: Azathioprine therapy complicated by pregnancy. *Obstet Gynecol* 1972; 40:708–710.

55. Registration Committee of the European Dialysis and Transplant Association: Successful pregnancies in women treated by dialysis and kidney transplantation. *Br J Obstet Gynaecol* 1980; 87:839–845.

56. Korelitz BI: Fertility and pregnancy in inflammatory bowel disease, in Kirsner JB, Shorter RG (eds): *Inflammatory bowel disease,* ed 3. Philadelphia, Lea & Febiger, 1988, pp 319–326.

57. O'Donoghue DP, Dawson AM, Powell-Tuck J, et al: Double blind withdrawal trial of azathioprine as maintenance treatment for Crohn's disease. *Lancet* 1978; 2:955–957.

58. Mendeloff AP, Calkins BM: The epidemiology of idiopathic inflammatory bowel disease, in Kirsner JB, Shorter RG (eds): *Inflammatory bowel disease,* ed 3. Philadelphia, Lea & Febiger, 1988, pp 3–34.

58a. Lashner BA, Kane SV, Hanover SB: Lack of association between oral contraceptive use and Crohn's disease: A community-based matched case-control study. *Gastroenterology* 1989; 97:1442–1449.

59. Young KR: Acute pancreatitis in pregnancy: Two case reports. *Obstet Gynecol* 1982; 60:653–657.

60. Durr GH: Acute pancreatitis, in HT Howatt, H. Sarles, (eds): *The Exocrine Pancreas.* London, WB Saunders, 1979, pp 352–401.

61. McKay AJ, O'Neill J, Imrie CW: Pancreatitis, pregnancy and gallstones. *Br J Obstet Gynaecol* 1980; 87:47–50.

62. Scragg RKR, McMichael AJ, Seamark RK: Oral contraceptives, pregnancy, and endogenous oestrogen in gallstone disease. A case control study. *Br Med J* 1984; 288:1795–1799.

63. Steer ML: Etiology and pathophysiology of acute pancreatitis, in Go VLW, Gardner JD, Brooks FP, et al (eds): *The Exocrine Pancreas: Biology, Pathobiology, and Diseases.* New York, Raven Press, 1986, pp 465–474.

64. Weinberg RB, Sitrin MD, Adkins GM, et al: Treatment of hyperlipidemic pancreatitis in pregnancy with total parenteral nutrition. *Gastroenterology* 1982; 83:1300–1305.

65. Worning H: Chronic pancreatitis: Pathogenesis, natural history and conservative treatment. *Clin Gastroenterol* 1984; 13:871–894.

66. Anderson AS, Whichlow MJ: Constipation during pregnancy: Dietary fibre intake and the effect of fibre supplementation. *Hum Nutr Appl Nutr* 1985; 39A:202–207.

67. Sheld HH: Megacolon complicating pregnancy. A case report. *J Reprod Med* 1987; 32:239–42.

68. Stewart K, Willoughby JMT: Postnatal presentation of coeliac disease. *Br Med J* 1988; 297:1245.

69. Levine MG, Esser D: Total parenteral nutrition for the treatment of severe hyperemesis gravidarum: Maternal nutritional effects and fetal outcome. *Obstet Gynecol* 1988; 72:102–107.

70. Mughal MM, Shaffer JL, Turner M, et al: Nutritional management of pregnancy in patients on home parenteral nutrition. *Br J Obstet Gynaecol* 1987; 94:44–49.

CHAPTER 10

Liver and Biliary Tract Diseases

Alfred L. Baker

Liver disease, although uncommon in pregnancy, poses a significant challenge to the clinician because of the large number of diagnostic possibilities (Table 10–1). Some liver diseases that occur during pregnancy carry a substantial risk for the mother and fetus. A prompt, accurate diagnosis is necessary for appropriate management and optimal results.

THE LIVER IN NORMAL PREGNANCY

Morphology

Although interstitial and intravascular volumes increase markedly, especially in the third trimester of pregnancy, there is no corresponding increase in the size of the liver.[1, 2] The gross morphology of the organ remains normal. Therefore, hepatomegaly in pregnant women suggests liver disease. Many pregnant women develop spider angiomas and palmar erythema, probably due to increased circulating estrogen levels, findings which ordinarily regress following delivery. In women who have had several pregnancies, however, spider angiomas and palmar erythema may persist. These findings during pregnancy do not necessarily indicate the presence of underlying liver disease.

During normal pregnancy, histologic liver abnormalities are frequent but nonspecific. Percutaneous needle liver biopsy specimens demonstrate that the size of the liver cells is often more variable than in normal subjects who are not pregnant.[3] Nuclear size may also be increased. Mild fatty infiltration and portal triad inflammatory infiltrates are occasionally present.[3]

TESTS OF HEPATIC AND BILIARY FUNCTION

Serum Bilirubin and Tests for Cholestasis

The normal range of values in several liver chemistry tests is altered in pregnancy whereas others remain unchanged (Table 10–2). For instance, total serum bilirubin rises slightly in a few pregnant women.[4] The serum alkaline phosphatase concentration also increases during pregnancy. Levels rise gradually during the first two trimesters and accelerate more sharply in the last trimester when they may be four times the upper limit of normal nonpregnant values. This increase is due mainly to an isoenzyme of alkaline phosphatase that is placental in origin.[5, 6] In addition, small increases in the bone isoenzyme of alkaline phosphatase have also been reported. In any event, the source of a raised serum alkaline phosphatase can be determined by techniques such as serum electrophoresis or heat denaturation.[5–7] The increased values usually return to nonpregnant levels within 2 or 3 months of delivery. A fall in serum alkaline

TABLE 10–1.
Liver Diseases in Pregnancy

Liver diseases specifically related to pregnancy
  Preeclampsia and eclampsia
  Hepatic rupture and infarction
  Acute fatty liver of pregnancy
  Tetracycline-induced fatty liver
  Intrahepatic cholestasis of pregnancy
  Hyperemesis gravidarum
  Budd-Chiari syndrome
Liver diseases coincidental to pregnancy
  Acute viral hepatitis
  Drug-induced hepatitis
  Fulminant hepatic failure
  Acute cholecystitis and biliary tract calculus
    disease
  Pyelonephritis and other bacterial infections
Pregnancy superimposed on chronic liver diseases
  Chronic hepatitis
  Cirrhosis and portal hypertension
  Wilson's disease
  Liver tumors
  Pregnancy following liver transplantation

phosphatase before delivery has been associated with fetal death, perhaps due to placental dysfunction.[8] Estrogen administration may also raise the serum alkaline phosphatase in nonpregnant subjects.[9] Thus, since total serum bilirubin and alkaline phosphatase both increase in gestation, only markedly elevated levels can be taken as clear evidence of liver disease in pregnancy.

Raised levels of 5'-nucleotidase and γ-glutamyl transpeptidase usually suggest cholestasis in nonpregnant patients, and can be used to establish that a raised serum alkaline phosphatase is of hepatic origin. Both of these enzymes are increased in normal pregnancy,[10–12] and γ-glutamyl transpeptidase can also be raised by chronic alcohol consumption. Thus, a test to determine the major isoenzyme contributing to an elevated serum alkaline phosphatase is probably best for detecting cholestasis in pregnancy.

Aminotransferases and Serum Proteins

In contrast to the tests described above, the aspartate (AST) and alanine (ALT) aminotransferases remain normal throughout pregnancy, as does the serum lactic dehydro-

genase. These enzymes are most useful in detecting the presence of necroinflammatory diseases such as hepatitis. The levels may increase during labor and delivery, but the rise is rarely more than twice the usual normal values.[10] The levels usually fall to normal within a day or two of delivery.

Total plasma albumin content is usually unaltered during pregnancy, but the serum albumin concentration decreases, reaching levels as low as 60% of normal nonpregnant values. Part of the decrease may be due to hemodilution, owing to the large increase in plasma volume during pregnancy. A decrease in the serum albumin concentration is often a feature of chronic liver disease in nonpregnant patients. A fall in the serum albumin alone cannot be taken as evidence of chronic liver disease in pregnancy. Total globulin levels are usually unchanged, although the alpha and beta fractions are mildly increased, perhaps due to increased stimulation or responsiveness of the immune system in pregnancy.

Lipids and Other Proteins

Blood lipids are also altered during pregnancy. Serum trygliceride levels rise as pregnancy progresses and reach a maximum at the end of the first trimester; the rate of very-low-density lipoprotein (VLDL) secretion by

TABLE 10–2.
Liver Chemistry Tests in Normal Pregnancy

Test	Values
Total serum bilirubin	Unchanged; slightly raised in a few patients
Alkaline phosphatase	Up to 3-fold increased
5'-nucleotidase	Slightly raised
γ-Glutamyl trans-peptidase	Slightly raised
Aspartate/alanine aminotransferase	Unchanged
Albumin	Decreased 20%
Globulin	Unchanged or slightly raised
α-globulin	Slightly raised
β-globulin	Slightly raised
Probthrombin time	Unchanged
Ceruloplasmin	Raised
Cholesterol	Raised up to 2-fold

the liver also increases. Serum cholesterol levels often rise to twice the usual upper limit of normal. For this reason raised serum cholesterol levels, often present in nonpregnant patients with cholestasis, do not provide specific evidence of liver dysfunction during pregnancy.

The concentrations of a number of other clinically important proteins are also altered in normal pregnancy. Ceruloplasmin levels rise as term approaches, and in patients with Wilson's disease may increase to normal values.[13] Therefore, this test may not be reliable in the diagnosis of Wilson's disease during pregnancy. The increase appears to be due to the effects of estrogens. Fibrinogen and factors VII, VIII, and X are also increased during pregnancy, probably due to the rising serum estrogen concentration. The prothrombin time remains normal.

Some plasma hormone binding proteins synthesized by the liver are also increased during pregnancy and in a manner similar to that following ingestion of estrogens by nonpregnant subjects. These changes result in alterations in circulating hormone levels, including thyroxin, cortisol, estrogens, testosterone, and vitamin D.

LIVER DISEASES SPECIFICALLY RELATED TO PREGNANCY

Preeclampsia and Eclampsia (see also Chap. 1)

Clinical Features.—Liver involvement in preeclampsia is the most common cause of abnormal liver chemistry tests in pregnant patients. Some liver dysfunction may be detected in up to 50% of patients with preeclampsia, but its true frequency is unknown.[14]

Preeclampsia is primarily a disease of the third trimester and when the disease affects the liver the patients usually present with right upper quadrant and/or epigastric pain, but do not often manifest clinical jaundice. Nevertheless, hospitalization and aggressive management of the preeclampsia are indicated. In very severe cases jaundice, usually due to intravascular hemolysis, may occur and there is risk of maternal and fetal mortality.[15] Such patients have the so-called HELLP syndrome with *h*emolytic anemia, *e*levated *l*iver enzyme values, and *l*ow *p*latelet counts. Hepatic encephalopathy, however, is not a feature of this illness. Resolution of liver injury along with the features of preeclampsia usually occurs within the first 2 days following delivery, but recovery may take up to 1 week.

The diagnosis may be delayed in patients with minimal evidence of other preeclamptic signs such as raised blood pressure and proteinuria.[16, 17] On occasion a patient who has failed to seek prenatal care early in gestation presents late in pregnancy with features that predominantly involve the liver. Hepatitis and fulminant hepatic failure as well as acute fatty liver of pregnancy should of course be considered, but the physician should also maintain a high index of suspicion that preeclampsia may be the sole culprit (see Table 1–3). In such cases the prognosis is better once the fetus is delivered.

Liver Chemistry Tests.—Liver chemistry tests are ordinarily only mildly abnormal in patients with liver disease associated with preeclampsia. Aminotransferases are elevated but modestly, and total serum bilirubin generally does not exceed 2–3 mg/dL (34–50 μmol/L). With severe disease, as when patients manifest the HELLP syndrome, jaundice may be more marked and the aminotransferases as high as 2,000 IU/L (33.3 μkat/L). Alkaline phosphatase may also become markedly raised. In such cases laboratory evidence of disseminated intravascular coagulation is often present, with schistocytes and burr cells present on a blood smear along with thrombocytopenia, and occasionally prolongation of the prothrombin time. The serum ammonia level is generally normal or only mildly increased.

Histologic Changes.—The main histologic feature in the liver in patients with preeclampsia is the presence of fibrin thrombi in the sinusoids, most frequently in periportal regions.[16, 17] Some patients have microscopic areas of periportal hemorrhage. Periportal hemorrhages are more frequent in patients with severe disease and may predispose to the development of intrahepatic hemorrhage or subcapsular hematoma.[16] Lobular disarray and occasional foci of hepatocellular necrosis may be present, but in uncomplicated cases there is little evidence of an inflammatory infiltrate. In fatal cases, hemorrhage may be marked, and the findings of centrilobular ischemia may be superimposed on the other features of the disease.

Pathogenesis.—The liver injury associated with preeclampsia and eclampsia appears to be part of the systemic vasculopathy underlying the illness.[19] Segmental vascular spasm has been suggested as an underlying cause of preeclampsia and eclampsia, and in the liver this could result in localized vascular injury, thromboplastin activation, platelet aggregation, and fibrin deposition. Regional liver perfusion might vary considerably, and could produce endothelial tears and localized hemorrhages. These changes could result in hepatocellular necrosis and predispose patients to liver hemorrhage and infarction.

Diagnosis.—When evidence of preeclampsia is unequivocal and the clinical and laboratory features of liver injury are typical, the diagnosis should be established rapidly and without difficulty (See Table 1–3, Chap. 1). When the signs of preeclampsia such as hypertension and proteinuria are absent or minimal, there may be confusion with hepatitis, either viral or drug-induced, or acute fatty liver of pregnancy. Patients with acute fatty liver of pregnancy often appear to have preeclampsia, but nausea and vomiting are more marked than in preeclamptic patients with liver disease. Patients with viral hepatitis usually do not have preeclampsia, and the aminotransferases are usually more elevated. Discontinuation of medications, or prescribing chemically unrelated drugs for important medical conditions, may help to exclude drug hepatitis. Serologic tests for hepatitis A and hepatitis B may help to establish a diagnosis, and shortly a test for hepatitis C will be available.

Maternal and Fetal Effects and Management.—The effects on the mother and fetus are mainly those of preeclampsia or eclampsia rather than the mild liver disease. Hospitalization and aggressive management of preeclampsia is indicated even for patients with mild disease. (see Chap. 1). If liver disease is present and progressing, especially where there is evidence of disseminated intravascular coagulation, most authorities recommend induction of labor and prompt delivery.[14, 15, 20] When right upper quadrant or epigastric pain is present, along with liver disease, an ultrasound examination should be considered to search for evidence of intrahepatic hemorrhage or subcapsular hematoma.[21, 22] Once delivery is accomplished, the clinical features of the liver disease and the liver chemistry test abnormalities resolve, usually within a day or two. There is no evidence of permanent liver damage following recovery from this disorder.

Hepatic Rupture and Infarction

Hepatic hemorrhage is a complication of severe preeclampsia and eclampsia. This diagnosis should be considered in any patient with preeclampsia or eclampsia who has severe right upper quadrant abdominal pain.[21, 22] Evidence of disseminated intravascular coagulation is usually present. Hepatomegaly with a mass in the area of the liver has also been reported.[22] The liver chemistry tests are generally only mildly elevated and resemble those of other patients with preeclampsia. Early reports emphasized the difficulty in establishing the diagnosis, but the availability of ultrasound and computed tomography examination have probably increased the recognition of hepatic hemorrhage.

The livers of patients with severe preeclampsia or eclampsia may have periportal hemorrhages that become confluent and result in the development of hematomas. These are almost always located in the right lobe of the liver; dissection may result in a subcapsular hematoma, and this often presents on the anterior surface of the liver. Rarely, these hematomas may become infected and become hepatic abscesses. Minor trauma from nausea and vomiting or labor may be sufficient to cause intraperitoneal rupture. Abdominal pain often worsens suddenly in such patients. Abdominal distention may be progressive, and evidence of peritonitis may develop. Shock and a fall in hematocrit are usually present.[23–26] A diagnostic paracentesis is helpful and may reveal the presence of blood in the peritoneal cavity. Some patients with a similar clinical picture may develop areas of hepatic infarction, particularly if the course has been marked by episodes of hypotension.[27]

There is a risk of fetal and maternal death with these conditions. For intrahepatic hemorrhage or subcapsular hematoma without rupture, most authorities recommend immediate repair of the patient's coagulation deficits and delivery by cesarean section.[26, 27] If hepatic rupture is present, immediate cesarean section along with exploration of the liver bed is indicated. A variety of approaches have been described, including ligation of the hepatic artery, repair of the site of hepatic rupture, or hepatic lobectomy, depending on the extent of the liver damage.[28–31] Despite prompt management, sepsis, renal failure, and continued disseminated intravascular coagulation may complicate the course, resulting in death in 50% of patients.

Acute Fatty Liver of Pregnancy

Clinical Features.—Acute fatty liver of pregnancy was once considered to be a rare disease with high mortality. Early recognition is one reason for the recently described improvements in outcome.[32] The onset of this disease is usually after the 34th week of pregnancy, although cases have been observed as early as the 32nd week. In most patients the onset is insidious, although it may occasionally be abrupt; initial features include anorexia, nausea, headache, and fatigue followed by jaundice. The symptoms invariably progress if delivery does not occur, and vomiting and abdominal pain usually develop. Abdominal pain is often localized to the right upper quadrant, but it may be diffuse. Radiation to the back suggests concomitant pancreatitis, which has been reported in a number of patients with acute fatty liver of pregnancy.[33] Mental confusion and evidence of diffuse bleeding caused by disseminated intravascular coagulation are grave manifestations in patients with progressive disease. Renal failure with marked azotemia, acidosis, and hypoglycemia may develop as the disease progresses (see Chap. 2). Fetal death may occur, followed by spontaneous delivery of a stillborn infant. The symptoms rapidly abate with parturition in most patients, but death sometimes occurs despite prompt delivery, probably owing to the presence of marked complications.

Most patients are young and primiparous, although the disease has been reported at any reproductive age and even after several normal pregnancies. Acute fatty liver of pregnancy is more frequent in patients that are pregnant with twins. The features of preeclampsia are present in some patients, leading some authors to suggest a common etiology for acute fatty liver of pregnancy and the liver disease of preeclampsia.[32]

Liver Chemistry Tests.—Jaundice typically develops a few days after the onset, but the serum bilirubin is rarely above 10 mg/dL (171 μmol/L), unless hemolysis or renal failure are present. The aminotransferases are moderately elevated, but usually do not exceed 300 IU/L (5.0 μkat/L), unless the disease is complicated by hypotension or sepsis. The serum alkaline phosphatase is markedly raised, and the prothrombin time and partial thromboplastin time are prolonged in most patients. The serum ammonia is usually moderately elevated, even in early disease, and values may reach tenfold normal in patients who develop coma.

The white blood cell count sometimes reaches levels of 30,000/mm³. An increased

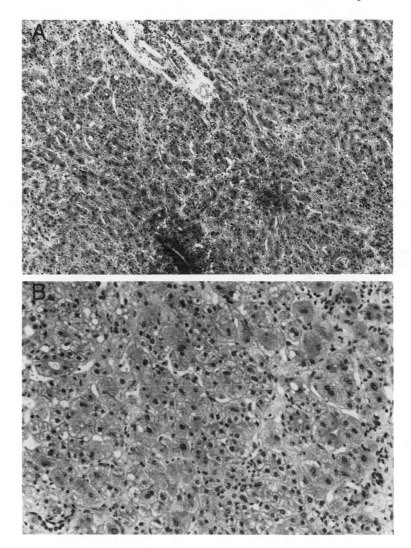

FIG 10–1.
Photomicrographs of a liver biopsy from a 27-year-old primagravida with acute fatty liver of pregnancy. She was admitted in the 37th week with abdominal pain, nausea, confusion, and jaundice. Liver chemistry tests revealed total serum bilirubin 5.4 mg/dL (92 μmol/L), alkaline phosphatase 587 units/L (9.8 μkat/L), AST 268 units/L (4.48 μkat/L), ALT 183 units/L (3.05 μkat/L), and prothrombin time 6 seconds prolonged. She delivered a stillborn fetus 12 hours later. The biopsy was performed 4 days after delivery because of persistently abnormal liver chemistry tests. **A,** low-power views showing intact hepatic architecture with little increased fibrosis (Masson trichrome, original magnification ×20). **B,** high-power view showing typical features of microvesicular fatty infiltration. Note the pale, vacuolated cytoplasm and central placement of the nuclei (HE, original magnification, ×60).

serum uric acid level is commonly present, but the cause is unclear. In patients with severe illness, laboratory evidence of intravascular hemolysis is often present, including schistocytes, burr cells, and normoblasts on a blood smear, depressed fibrinogen and antithrombin III levels, and raised fibrin degradation products.[34, 35]

Histologic Features.—The liver biopsy findings in patients with acute fatty liver of pregnancy are characterized by microvesicular fatty infiltration[36] (Fig 10–1). This feature is more marked in the centrilobular areas of the liver, but may be overlooked in some patients. A special fat stain, such as oil red O, of unfixed tissue may aid in making the diagnosis. The hepatocyte nuclei remain in a central position in the cell, rather than eccentric as in fatty infiltration of the liver due to other causes. Inflammation and necrosis are not ordinarily a part of the histologic findings in acute fatty liver of pregnancy, but these features may be present in patients with sepsis or hypotension.

These features appear to be entirely reversible, based on reports of repeat biopsy findings in a few patients after disease resolution.[37] In addition, no permanent structural liver damage results from this disease.

Pathogenesis.—The pathogenesis of acute fatty liver of pregnancy is still uncertain. The presence of microvesicular fatty infiltration and hyperammonemia has raised the possibility of an underlying metabolic disorder resembling Reye's syndrome, a disease that has a similar picture.[38] Electron microscopy reveals mitochondrial enlargement in both disorders. However, the mitochondria in acute fatty liver of pregnancy display dense bodies and these are generally absent in Reye's syndrome. Marked cytoplasmic vacuolization is present in Reye's syndrome but is not a feature of acute fatty liver of pregnancy.[38, 39]

Tetracycline is no longer utilized in pregnancy, but it also produces a similar picture. Patients with acute fatty liver of pregnancy rarely have a history of exposure to this drug. In addition, tetracycline can produce fatty liver in nonpregnant patients.

Effects on Mother and Fetus.—Acute fatty liver of pregnancy was first recognized as a disease distinct from fulminant hepatic failure in 1940.[40] Early reports suggested that this complication of pregnancy was rare, but examples have been more frequent in recent years, probably because of better recognition. Maternal and fetal mortality were reported to be as high as 90% in some earlier studies,[40–45] but reports in the last 10 years have shown a maternal mortality below 25%, perhaps due to earlier recognition and prompt delivery.[32, 39, 46–53] Perinatal mortality, although improved, is still significant because of the number of stillbirths.

Diagnosis.—Acute fatty liver of pregnancy is most often confused with liver injury from preeclampsia or eclampsia early in the course of the disease (see Table 1–3). Although preeclampsia is present in many patients with acute fatty liver of pregnancy, abdominal pain and nausea and vomiting are more characteristic of patients with acute fatty liver of pregnancy. Intravascular hemolysis, present to some degree in patients with HELLP, usually does not appear until late in the course of acute fatty liver of pregnancy, when other features of the disorder help to establish the diagnosis. Ultrasonography and computed tomography have been suggested as noninvasive approaches to establish the diagnosis, but their sensitivity and specificity have yet to be determined.[54–56]

Fulminant hepatic failure may also resemble acute fatty liver in pregnancy in some instances. Abdominal pain is usually absent in patients with fulminant hepatic failure. Patients with fulminant hepatic failure usually do not have the marked increase in serum alkaline phosphatase and uric acid typical of acute fatty liver of pregnancy, but the aminotransferases are more elevated.

Management.—Early recognition and prompt delivery have improved the prognosis of acute fatty liver of pregnancy for both mother and infant in recent years. Thus a prompt diagnosis is a key to obtaining improved outcome in such patients. Once the diagnosis is established, the patient should be treated aggressively, particularly for the coagulopathy. Fresh frozen plasma should be administered to correct the prothrombin time and partial thromboplastin time. Patients should receive adequate intravenous dextrose to manage hypoglycemia, and acidosis, if present, should be repaired. Platelet transfusions and red blood cell transfusions may also be needed, depending on the clinical situation. Lactulose can be administered for treatment of hepatic encephalopathy.

Once the patient has been resuscitated, prompt delivery should be accomplished. Some authors have suggested that this be performed by cesarean section, but the outcome is good with vaginal delivery as well when this can be carried out. Despite these measures, liver disease may progress. Liver transplantation should be considered for such patients if there is no contradiction.[57] The disease ordinarily does not recur with subsequent pregnancies.[58]

Tetracycline-Induced Fatty Liver

Previous reports document that intravenous administration of tetracycline is occasionally associated with the development of fatty liver which has histologic and clinical features similar to acute fatty liver of pregnancy.[59] There are a few reports of this complication following oral tetracycline administration. It has also been reported after intravenous administration in nonpregnant patients, but the risk seems greatly increased with pregnancy.[60, 61] Fatalities have been frequent and have occurred as early as 6 days after beginning the drug. Although the pathogenesis of this lesion is uncertain, it is thought to be related to inhibition of protein synthesis in the liver. Tetracycline is no longer prescribed to pregnant women because of the availability of safer alternative drugs. When the diagnosis of acute fatty liver of pregnancy is considered, a history of tetracycline administration should nonetheless be sought.

Intrahepatic Cholestasis of Pregnancy

Clinical Features.—Intrahepatic cholestasis of pregnancy (obstetric cholestasis, benign cholestasis of pregnancy, obstetric hepatosis, recurrent jaundice of pregnancy) is a common cause of liver disease in pregnancy and may be more frequent than is presently recognized. A recent prospective study of 297 pregnancies showed that 10% had elevated postprandial serum bile acid levels. Most women in this group complained of pruritus and may have had a mild form of intrahepatic cholestasis of pregnancy.[62]

Approximately two thirds of patients present in the third trimester, although the disease has been diagnosed as early as the second gestational month. Pruritis is usually the initial symptom and may be generalized. It frequently involves the palms and soles as in other types of cholestatic liver disease. This symptom is followed in a few days by dark urine, but only a minority of patients develop jaundice. Insomnia and irritability are frequent complaints attributed to the itching, but otherwise the patient's sense of well-being is preserved. Excoriations may be present. The illness resolves within a day or two of delivery. There is no abdominal pain, anorexia, nausea, or vomiting and the liver is not enlarged or tender.

Liver Chemistry Tests and Histologic Features.—The serum alkaline phosphatase is generally raised above the level ordinarily seen in pregnancy, and serum bile acid concentrations may increase ten- to 100-fold.[63, 64] Most patients have raised total and conjugated serum bilirubin levels, but the values rarely exceed 5 mg/dL (85 μmol/L). The aminotransferases are generally mildly elevated, but may be normal in some patients. The prothrombin time is usually normal but may become prolonged when there is marked cholestasis or when cholestyramine is administered.

The clinical features, along with the liver chemistry tests, generally begin to improve shortly after delivery. The serum alkaline phosphatase may remain somewhat elevated for several months.

Liver biopsies demonstrate preserved hepatic architecture with no increase in fibrosis (Fig. 10–2). Bile plugs are present, mainly in pericentral canaliculi, but there is little evidence of cell injury. A mild portal triaditis may be present in some patients. The disorder is not associated with permanent liver damage.

Pathogenesis.—This disease is most frequent in Scandinavians, Bolivians, and Chileans, and the incidence is as high as 25% in certain native Indian kindreds in the last-named country.[65–69] In addition, familial studies from northern Europe and the United States show an increased prevalence with a mendelian dominant pattern with variable penetrance, perhaps due to polygenic or environmental influences. A sex-limited mendelian dominant pattern has also been proposed.[70]

Estrogens appear to be the main injurious factor in susceptible women. Patients previously exposed to oral contraceptives or other estrogen-containing medications usually have a history suggestive of cholestasis in response to these medications, and repeated pregnancies are almost always associated with recurrent intrahepatic cholestasis of pregnancy.[71, 72] Estrogens decrease the canalicular transport

maximum for bile acids and other constituents of bile, suggesting a generalized effect on canalicular bile secretion.[73, 74] Back-diffusion of bile acids through the cannaliculus, decreased membrane fluidity, or decreased Na^+, K^+ adenosine triphosphatase (ATPase) activity may be involved.[75–76] The precise mechanism of the toxic effect on hepatocytes is uncertain, however.

Effects on Mother and Fetus.—Early studies suggested that the prognosis of this condition was benign, but more recent reports indicate that intrahepatic cholestasis of preg-

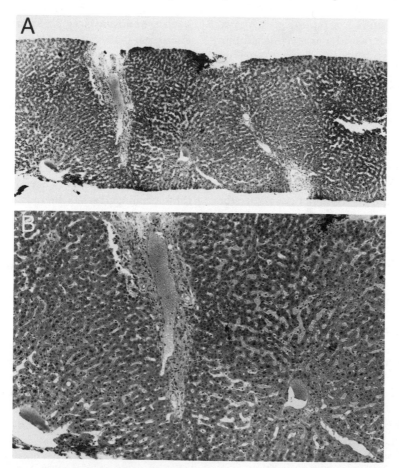

FIG 10–2.
Photomicrographs of a liver biopsy from a 20-year-old primagravida with intrahepatic cholestasis in the 35th week. She had marked pruritus, but the physical examination was normal. Liver chemistry tests showed total serum bilirubin 2.3 mg/dL (39 μmol/L), alkaline phosphatase 468 units/L (7.80 μkat/L), AST 44 units/L (0.73 μkat/L), ALT 36 units/L (0.60 μkat/L), and prothrombin time normal. **A,** low-power view showing intact hepatic architecture. Note that there is a mild portal triad inflammation infiltrate (Masson trichrome, original magnification, ×20) **B,** high-power view showing several bile plugs typical of this lesion (HE, original magnification, ×60).

nancy carries a significant risk for both mother and fetus.[77-79] Postpartum maternal hemorrhage is an occasional complication, perhaps related to prolongation of the prothrombin time caused by malabsorption of vitamin K resulting from cholestasis.[80] Up to 60% of infants may be premature, and low birth weights and fetal distress occur in up to one third of cases. Perinatal mortality may be as high as 3.5%.[79] Increased levels of sulfated and unsulfated bile acids have been found in the blood of fetuses from mothers with intrahepatic cholestasis of pregnancy, suggesting that they may be involved in fetal injury.[81] Women with a history of intrahepatic cholestasis of pregnancy also have an increased risk for developing cholesterol gallstones, probably a result of the effects of increased estrogen levels on bile secretion.[82]

Diagnosis.—The characteristic clinical features, especially severe pruritus in an otherwise healthy patient with a markedly elevated serum alkaline phosphatase, usually permit differentiation from other liver diseases associated with pregnancy. Patients with viral hepatitis and acute fatty liver of pregnancy usually have anorexia and manifest greater elevations in aminotransferase levels. If hypertension and proteinuria are present, acute fatty liver of pregnancy or preeclampsia should also be considered in the differential diagnosis. Liver chemistry results in patients with extrahepatic cholestasis due to gallstones may resemble those in intrahepatic cholestasis of pregnancy. The absence of abdominal pain, however, suggests the latter disease. Also, ultrasound examination of the extrahepatic bile ducts, gallbladder, and liver help to exclude gallstones and provide evidence of bile duct obstruction.

Management.—The treatment of intrahepatic cholestasis of pregnancy consists of symptomatic management of the pruritus, repair of the coagulopathy, and close observation for fetal distress and premature delivery. Cholestyramine (FDA category C), probably the drug of choice for management of itching,

is effective in a majority of cases. Doses of 4 g should be administered in juice or water before breakfast, after breakfast, and before lunch, dinner, and at bedtime. Side effects include anorexia, constipation, and prolongation of the prothrombin time due to vitamin K binding by the drug. Thus patients ingesting this drug should receive oral vitamin K 10 mg daily, and the prothrombin time should be monitored during therapy. Also, several oral medications can be bound by cholestyramine and should not be administered at the same time. In instances where the prothrombin time has been prolonged, treatment with oral vitamin K was usually successful. Recent reports suggest that administration of *S*-adenosylmethionine, an important methyl donor in hepatic transmethylation reactions, improves the symptoms and liver chemistry test abnormalities of intrahepatic cholestasis of pregnancy.[83] However, these observations await confirmation and proof of safety before this drug can be recommended for treatment of intrahepatic cholestasis of pregnancy.

Hyperemesis Gravidarum

Hyperemesis gravidarum, which occasionally involves the liver, is also discussed in Chapter 9. Liver chemistry tests are abnormal only in occasional patients.[27, 84-86] The total serum bilirubin rarely exceeds 5 mg/dL (85 μmol/L), the aminotransferases are generally only mildly raised (less than fivefold), while the serum alkaline phosphatase and prothrombin time are usually normal. Transient abnormalities of thyroid function tests may occur in up to 40% of patients, but their significance is unknown as clinical hyperthyroidism is rarely present.[87] Resolution generally occurs after a few days of in-hospital management, and the pregnancy proceeds without further problems.

Histologic features are poorly defined in this disease. Some authors have found evidence of cholestasis, while others have reported fatty infiltration or mild nonspecific changes.

TABLE 10–3.
Characteristics of the Three Major Types of Viral Hepatitis

	Hepatitis A	Hepatitis B	Non-A, Non-B Hepatitis
Virus type	RNA	DNA	?
Size	27 nm	42 nm	?
Major route of transmission	Fecal/oral	Parenteral	Parenteral
Incubation period	14–50 Days	14–180 Days	14–180 Days
Maternal/fetal transmission	Rare	Frequent	Probably occurs
Acute hepatitis	Yes	Yes	Yes
Fulminant hepatic failure	Yes	Yes	Yes
Chronic hepatitis/cirrhosis	No	Yes	Yes
Carrier state	No	Yes	Yes

Budd-Chiari Syndrome

Budd-Chiari syndrome, a disorder characterized by thrombotic occlusion of the hepatic veins, is a rare complication of pregnancy.[88, 89] Most reported cases presented within a few weeks of delivery, but in several onset occurred during pregnancy. The increased synthesis of factors II, VII, and X, as well as of fibrinogen, observed in normal pregnancy may be a predisposing factor. Budd-Chiari syndrome has also been reported in association with oral contraceptives, where a similar hypercoagulable state could have been involved in the pathogenesis.

The onset may be acute, with the rapid development of abdominal pain and distention and sometimes jaundice. Hepatomegaly is usual, and ascites of high protein content is almost always present. The aminotransferases are often markedly raised when the onset is rapid, but jaundice is present in only half the cases. In some patients the onset is insidious, occurring over many months. Liver chemistry tests are usually moderately raised, while the symptoms may be mild.

Liver biopsy demonstrating centrilobular congestion combined with hepatic venography provide the most definitive diagnostic approach, while Doppler flow ultrasonography and computed tomography may also be helpful.[90] Treatment is often unsatisfactory, and the prognosis guarded.[88, 89, 91] Anticoagulation with heparin or clot lysis by streptokinase seem to be helpful in some cases.[92] On occasion, side-to-side portacaval shunt has decompressed the liver and led to a positive outcome.[93] Liver transplantation has been performed successfully in a few of these patients.[94]

LIVER DISEASES COINCIDENTAL TO PREGNANCY

Acute Viral Hepatitis

Clinical Features.—Several viruses have been identified as causing acute hepatitis and commercially available tests permit the physician to establish a specific diagnosis in many instances (Table 10–3). The clinical features are generally similar, regardless of the type, and all are characterized by an initial prodromal illness with a variety of nonhepatic symptoms. The onset is often abrupt with hepatitis A and is typically more insidious with hepatitis B and non-A, non-B hepatitis. There may be an influenza-like illness, and accompanying low-grade temperature elevations. Arthralgias, skin rash, and other multisystem features may also be present, particularly with hepatitis B. Jaundice usually follows in a few days focusing attention on the liver and bringing the patient to medical attention. However, anicteric disease accounts for over half the cases in adults. Anorexia and nausea along with altered bowel habits are frequent during the prodromal and early period of clinical jaundice. Improvement usually begins after a week or two, and in patients with hepatitis A and hepatitis B this is usually progressive. Recovery is complete within several weeks in over 90% of patients.

Although patients with hepatitis A and

hepatitis B usually recover within 3 to 4 months of onset, the illness is prolonged in occasional individuals, lasting 6 to 12 months or more, and yet the outcome is benign. The clinical features and liver chemistry tests are variable in such patients, but features suggestive of ongoing acute hepatitis generally persist.[95] Liver biopsies are often performed to exclude serious complications of hepatitis, such as chronic hepatitis, and the results generally show features typical of biopsies from patients with classic acute hepatitis. The explanation for the continued activity of hepatitis A is unknown.

Occasional individuals with hepatitis B may have prolonged infection which evolves to chronic active hepatitis and ultimately to cirrhosis, or they may enter into a chronic hepatitis B carrier state which may persist for years.[96] Non-A, non-B hepatitis has a more variable course, as initial periods of improvement are often punctuated by exacerbations in clinical symptoms and liver chemistry tests. Half of the infected patients develop chronic hepatitis, and up to 20% of these ultimately develop cirrhosis.

Patients with the hepatitis B carrier state may develop disease reactivation.[97] This has been observed most commonly in hemodialysis patients and individuals with malignant tumors who require chemotherapy, but has also been observed as a spontaneous occurrence in some hepatitis B carriers. Patients with a reactivation of hepatitis B typically develop clinical features suggestive of the acute disease, along with positive tests for HBe-Ag, indicating increased viral replication.[98]

Delta hepatitis is a unique illness in that it infects only individuals who already have hepatitis B.[99] Patients may be coinfected with hepatitis B and delta hepatitis, or delta hepatitis may superinfect hepatitis B carriers. Delta hepatitis usually manifests as a more severe illness than that produced by hepatitis B virus alone, and the risk of developing fulminant hepatic failure is increased in such patients. Delta hepatitis has been observed most often in patients from the Mediterranean though in the United States it is mainly diagnosed in drug addicts.

Liver Chemistry Tests.—Patients with acute hepatitis, regardless of the etiology, usually have markedly raised aminotransferases, generally exceeding 500 IU/L (8.33 μkat/L), when jaundice is present. If the illness is anicteric, the increase in aminotransferases is often attenuated. In patients with uncomplicated disease the serum albumin does not fall below the level usually seen in pregnancy, and the globulin levels remain normal, as does the prothrombin time. The blood count usually remains normal, except for development of a mild lymphocytosis during the acute phase of the illness.

Histologic Features.—Liver biopsy findings in patients with uncomplicated viral hepatitis generally include spotty necrosis throughout the hepatic lobule. Hydropic change and eosinophilic bodies are present, along with reticuloendothelial cell activation and a mild portal triaditis. The inflammatory cell infiltrate is comprised mainly of lymphocytes. Necrosis is rarely confluent in uncomplicated disease.

Serologic Tests for the Cause of Acute Viral Hepatitis.—Once the clinical features and liver chemistry tests point to a diagnosis of hepatitis, appropriate serologic tests can establish a specific cause in most patients (Table 10–4). In acute hepatitis A, antibodies of the IgM class develop shortly after the onset of the clinical illness and persist for a few months; antibodies of the IgG class develop more slowly but persist throughout life and serve as a marker of previous infection with this virus. The hepatitis B surface antigen is positive in 95% of patients with acute hepatitis B, even late in the prodromal period of the illness. Hepatitis B "e" antigen also becomes positive at this time and indicates viral replication; it usually persists for only a few days. Antibodies to the hepatitis B core antigen (anti-HBc IgM) typically develop after the onset of jaundice in acute hepatitis B and persist for a few years but are replaced by antibodies of the IgG class which remain as markers of previous infection for several years. Antibodies to the hepatitis B surface antigen (anti-HBs) usually appear only after the clinical illness has resolved. During the "window period," after HBsAg disappears but before anti-HBs appears, anti-HBc may be the only marker indicative of recent acute hepatitis B. Shortly, a test for hepatitis C antibody will become commercially available. Hepatitis C virus is the main cause of posttransfusion non-A, non-B hepatitis. Preliminary reports suggest that it will be useful for identifying patients with chronic illness, but that conversion in acute, self-limited disease may not always occur or may be detected only after disease resolution.[100]

Effects on Mother and Infant.—Acute hepatitis has little adverse maternal effect during pregnancy in patients in the United States and Western Europe except for rare fulminant hepatic failure, a life-threatening complication.[101] The risk however seems greater in underdeveloped countries. The precise explanation for the difference is uncertain but may be related to malnutrition. Acute hepatitis, particularly late in pregnancy, may induce premature labor, but this seems to have little adverse fetal effect.[102] Maternal-fetal transmission of hepatitis A may occur, particularly when the disease occurs late in pregnancy.[103]

Maternal-fetal transmission is the major risk to the infant born to a mother with acute hepatitis B.[103–105] Previous investigations have shown that up to 90% of infants born to mothers positive for HBsAg and HBeAg develop neonatal hepatitis. In these patients estimates for the development of cirrhosis and hepatocellular carcinoma in adolescence and adulthood range as high as 25%.[106–109] Although the risk of infection is less when tests for HBeAg are negative, the chance of maternal-fetal transmission may still be as high as 25%.

Most mothers with hepatitis B infection have the hepatitis B carrier state rather than acute hepatitis B, so the symptoms may be mild or inapparent. Hepatitis B infections are more common in the Orient and Africa, as well as in countries around the Mediterranean where maternal-fetal transmission is thought to be a major route of infection.

Management.—Management of acute hepatitis in pregnancy usually includes monitoring the patient's fluid and dietary intake to see that weight and hydration are maintained and encouraging activity as tolerated by the patient's symptoms. If marked anorexia or vomiting are present, hospitalization may be required for intravenous fluid administration.

Maternal Prophylaxis.—On occasion, the physician may be asked to recommend prophylactic measures for a pregnant woman exposed to hepatitis. If there has been sexual or needle-stick exposure to hepatitis B, hepatitis B immune globulin should be adminis-

TABLE 10–4.
Serologic Tests in Three Major Forms of Viral Hepatitis

	Hepatitis A (HA)	Hepatitis B (HB)	Non-A, Non-B Hepatitis*
Acute hepatitis	Anti-HA IgM	HBsAg, anti-HBc IgM	Anti-HC
Fulminant hepatic failure	Anti-HA IgM	HBsAg, anti-HBc IgM	Anti-HC
Chronic hepatitis/cirrhosis	—	HBsAg, anti-HBc IgM, anti-HBc IgG	Anti-HC
Carrier state	—	HBsAg, anti-HBc IgM, anti-HBc IgG	Anti-HC
Past infection	Anti-HA IgG	Anti-HBs	?

Anti-HA = antibody to HA Ag; Anti-HC = antibody to hepatitis C (HC) antigen; anti-HBc = antibody to HB core antigen (HBcAg); Anti-HBs = antibody to HB surface antigen (HBsAg).
*Preliminary data only for anti-HC test. Conversion following acute infection may take up to several months, whereas patients with chronic illnesses are usually positive.

TABLE 10–5.
Prophylaxis for Infants Born to Mothers With Hepatitis

Type	Trimester		
	First	Second	Third
Hepatitis A (HA)			
Acute infection	None	None	ISG 0.5 mL at birth optional
Hepatitis B (HB)			
Acute infection	None	None	HBIG 0.5 mL at birth; HB vaccine at birth or within 1 mo; repeat 1 and 6 mo later
Carrier state, chronic hepatitis, cirrhosis	HBIG 0.5 mL at birth; HB vaccine at birth or within 1 mo; repeat 1 and 6 mo later	HBIG 0.5 mL at birth; HB vaccine at birth or within 1 mo; repeat 1 and 6 mo later	HBIG 0.5 mL at birth; HB vaccine at birth or within 1 mo; repeat 1 and 6 mo later
Hepatitis non-A, non-B			
Acute infection	None	None	ISG 0.5 mL at birth optional
High-risk mother but no prenatal care	—	—	HBIG 0.5 mL at birth; await HBsAg test results for further prophylaxis

ISG = immune serum globulin; HBIG = HB immune serum globulin; HBsAg = HB surface antigen.

tered as soon as possible in a dose of 0.1 mL/ kg body weight. If there is likely to be continued sexual exposure to a partner with hepatitis B, the hepatitis B vaccine should be administered as for any adult exposed repeatedly to hepatitis B. Prophylactic measures for a pregnant woman with sexual exposure to a partner who may have non-A, non-B hepatitis are not well established, but the physician may wish to prescribe immune serum globulin 0.1 mL/kg. Similar prophylaxis might also be considered if there is a familial occurrence or exposure to a "point-source" epidemic of hepatitis A.

Infant Prophylaxis.—For infants born to mothers with acute hepatitis A infection, the physician may wish to administer immune serum globulin 0.5 mL at the time of birth, even though the risk of maternal-fetal transmission is small (Table 10–5).

Because of the high risk of maternal-fetal transmission of hepatitis B, screening for the presence of HBsAg early in the third trimester of pregnancy is recommended (see Table 10–5).[110] As many as 16,500 births may occur yearly in the United States in HBsAg-positive patients, and a third of these may have HBeAg as well. Up to 3,500 of these infants may be-

come chronic HBsAg carriers, some of whom develop chronic active hepatitis with cirrhosis and hepatocellular carcinoma in adolescence or adulthood. Occasionally, infants also develop fulminant hepatic failure shortly after birth.

Several studies on the practicality of universal screening programs support the cost-effectiveness of determining HBsAg in all pregnant patients.[110–114] Prophylactic measures are effective in preventing neonatal transmission in up to 90% of infants. The small proportion of infants that are not protected by prophylaxis, approximately 10%, appears to be due to transplacental transmission of the infection.[105]

Prophylactic measures should include hepatitis B immune serum globulin 0.5 mL given by intramuscular injection at birth, along with an initial injection of the hepatitis B vaccine, either 5 μL of the recombinant yeast vaccine or 10 μL of the human serum-derived vaccine.[115–118] The initial vaccination can be administered when the infant is physiologically stable but within 1 month of birth; the vaccination should be repeated 1 month and 6 months later to achieve maximal benefit. Infants born to mothers without prenatal testing in high-risk groups should receive hepatitis B immune serum globulin, and additional prophylactic measures should await the results of HBcAg tests.

Infants born to HBsAg-positive mothers receiving vaccination should be tested for HBsAG and anti-HBs at 12 to 18 months after birth. If anti-HBs alone is present, the infant has had a complete immunologic response to vaccination and is protected from infection for up to 5 years. Infants who have HBsAg at the time of screening probably acquired it in utero.

As noted, delta hepatitis virus can only infect individuals who have hepatitis B. Coinfection with the two agents in the perinatal period might be expected, but to date there is little evidence of neonatal delta hepatitis infection.[119] Prophylactic measures for hepatitis B should help to prevent this infection.

Guidelines for prophylaxis of non-A, non-B hepatitis are not yet well established (see Table 10–5). The availability of new tests for hepatitis C in the next several years will doubtless clarify this issue, at least for this main bloodborne non-A, non-B virus. Physicians may wish to administer immune serum globulin in a dose similar to that used for prophylaxis of hepatitis A to infants born to mothers that have acute hepatitis which appears to be due to non-A, non-B hepatitis.

Drug-Induced Hepatitis

Drug-induced liver injury is uncommon during pregnancy. Physicians are understandably concerned about the adverse effects of medications on fetal development, so the use of medications in pregnant women is limited. There is no drug that has an unequivocally increased risk of producing hepatic injury in pregnant women except for tetracycline. As noted, the risk of tetracycline-induced fatty infiltration of the liver is greatest when given intravenously, although cases have been reported after oral administration. A recent Public Health Service study suggested that the risk of development of isoniazid-induced hepatitis might be increased in pregnancy.[120] However, most physicians withhold isoniazid prophylaxis during pregnancy. Fetal death has been reported after maternal overdose with acetaminophen.[121]

Some drugs prescribed to gravidas are occasionally associated with hepatic injury. These include antiemetics, antibiotics, sedative-hypnotics, analgesics, and antihypertensives. Most produce a picture that resembles hepatitis, although some drugs characteristically produce cholestasis. Reactions that resemble hepatitis are generally regarded as potentially more serious, although cholestatic drug reactions may persist for weeks or months before complete resolution occurs. Drugs of the chlorpromazine class, particularly prochlorperazine (Compazine), are sometimes used to control nausea during pregnancy, but occasionally produce cholestasis. The patient generally improves promptly when the drug is discontinued. Most physicians who treat pregnant patients prescribe needed antibiotics for a clearly established diagnosis. The risk of liver injury is small.

Heartburn is a common problem in pregnancy, and H_2 blockers may be prescribed on occasion. Cimetidine and ranitidine sometimes produce mild hepatocellular injury or cholestasis. Improvement is prompt when the drug is stopped. Alpha-methyldopa is still a widely used antihypertensive agent, but has occasionally been associated with life-threatening hepatic injury.

It may be difficult to determine whether a patient's liver injury is caused by a drug. The simplest approach may be to discontinue the medication and substitute a chemically unrelated drug if continued therapy is necessary. Finally, transplant patients receiving azathioprine (Imuran) sometimes experience elevations in their enzymes, which decrease when the dose is lowered.

Fulminant Hepatic Failure

A rare complication of acute hepatitis of whatever etiology is the development of fulminant hepatic failure. This occurs in less than 1 in 100 cases. This illness begins with typical features of acute hepatitis with progressive jaundice leading to the development of hepatic encephalopathy within 8 weeks of onset.[122] Progressive liver failure may develop, including evolution to hepatic coma, the development of ascites, and peripheral edema. The course may be complicated by infections, including pneumonia, sepsis, and urinary tract infections, as well as gastrointestinal hemorrhage and renal failure. Cerebral edema is frequent and often contributes to death.

At the onset liver chemistry tests show markedly raised aminotransferases, along with prolongation of the prothrombin time, which is refractory to parenteral vitamin K_1 administration. The bilirubin may rise to levels of 20 to 30 mg/dL (340 to 510 μmol/L), and in patients whose disease progresses, the aminotransferases may fall markedly.

Death rates may be as high as 80% to 90% in patients who develop grade 4 hepatic encephalopathy, and some investigators have proposed treatment with liver transplantation for this group.[123] Treatments such as corticosteroids, plasma exchange, and charcoal hemoperfusion are ineffective.[124, 125]

Fulminant hepatic failure may be confused with acute fatty liver of pregnancy and liver injury from preeclampsia and eclampsia, particularly when the illness occurs in late pregnancy. During the initial period of the illness, the aminotransferases are generally highest in fulminant hepatic failure, while the serum alkaline phosphatase rises less markedly than in preeclampsia and acute fatty liver of pregnancy. In all of these diseases, including fulminant hepatic failure, delivery is usually the best treatment. Parturition usually results in resolution of acute fatty liver of pregnancy and preeclampsia or eclampsia, and there is little evidence that delivery increases maternal mortality in fulminant hepatic failure. In fact, it may improve the infant's chance of survival.

Acute Cholecystitis and Biliary Tract Calculus Disease

Clinical Features.—Acute cholecystitis presents with the abrupt onset of right upper quadrant or epigastric pain, usually with anorexia and nausea. Vomiting is usually not prominent unless there is associated pancreatitis or choledocholithiasis (common bile duct

stone). The pain is generally steady in nature but may fluctuate in intensity over periods of 30 minutes to an hour. Attacks usually last for several hours up to a day or so and may be accompanied by fever as high as 38.5°C. Localized tenderness over the area of the gallbladder (Murphy's sign) is frequent in nonpregnant patients but is difficult to detect if the episode occurs toward term when the uterus is considerably enlarged. There is no evidence of an increased occurrence of acute cholecystitis during pregnancy.

Pancreatitis may also occur, particularly if a stone is impacted even transiently at the distal end of the common bile duct. Choledocholithiasis is a serious complication of gallstone disease that is usually associated with jaundice and temperature elevation. Patients with these conditions usually have more vomiting and abdominal pain. Although temperature elevation is more common in uncomplicated cholecystitis, abdominal pain and tenderness are also more marked with these conditions.

Aside from acute cholecystitis, some patients have brief episodes of biliary tract pain that last only a few hours and often resolve spontaneously. They also have nonspecific symptoms, such as brief episodes of right upper quadrant abdominal pain lasting only a few minutes, persistent right upper quadrant abdominal fullness, fatty food intolerance, or increased flatus and eructation. Investigation of these complaints may reveal the presence of gallstones, but this finding does not account for the symptoms.[126] On further investigation, such individuals may have irritable bowel syndrome, peptic ulcer disease, gastroesophageal reflux, or other gastrointestinal problems. Cholecystectomy usually does not relieve the symptoms.

Laboratory Tests.—Patients with acute cholecystitis often have an increased white blood cell count, due to a raised neutrophil count. Liver chemistry tests are ordinarily within normal limits unless there is a choledocholithiasis. However, with marked inflammation of the gallbladder, there may be a mild increase in the aminotransferases, suggestive of mild injury to the liver surrounding the gallbladder bed. When there is biliary tract involvement, the serum alkaline phosphatase is ordinarily elevated above the levels expected in normal pregnancy, and jaundice is usually evident. The aminotransferases are usually only mildly raised, and the serum albumin does not fall below the usual levels observed in pregnancy. If biliary tract involvement is prolonged, particularly when antibiotics of the cephalosporin class are used, the prothrombin time may be prolonged, suggestive of serious hepatic involvement. This abnormality usually improves with administration of parenteral vitamin K_1 10 mg daily for several days, indicating that hepatic synthetic function is present. Patients with prolonged biliary tract pain or nonspecific symptoms generally do not have abnormalities of the liver chemistry test or hemogram. Raised serum amylase results have been observed frequently by some investigators, suggesting that subclinical pancreatitis probably related to passage of a common duct stone may be more frequent in this condition than is presently recognized.[127]

Pathogenesis.—Cholelithiasis and acute cholecystitis are clearly more prevalent in women than men.[128, 129] However, the prevalence of gallstones is similar in the two sexes until puberty. Early menarche, multiple pregnancies, and/or ingestion of other estrogen-containing drugs are some of the factors that account for the increased prevalence in women.[129] Increasing age, obesity, and American Indian heritage, particularly of the Pima and Chippewa tribes, are other important risk factors. Individuals who have a history of periods of rapid weight gain and loss due to dieting also have an increased risk of gallstone formation.

Approximately 90% of gallstones in Western countries are comprised of cholesterol, which is insoluble in a water solution. The main factor which determines its solubility in bile is the relative percent molar concentrations of cholesterol, bile salts, and phospholipids. Factors that increase cholesterol secretion into bile or decrease bile salt secretion into bile increase the risk of gallstone formation. δ-Aminolevulinic acid synthetase, the rate-limiting enzyme in hepatic cholesterol synthesis, is probably under genetic control. Bile acid secretion into bile is mainly controlled by the hepatic 7α-cholesterol hydroxylase. This rate-limiting enzyme for bile salt synthesis declines with age, perhaps providing a partial explanation for the increased risk of gallstones with aging. Pregnant women have increased cholesterol saturation of bile, probably because estrogen inhibits bile salt secretion.[129–130]

It is clear that subjects without cholesterol gallstones have a limited capacity to solubilize additional cholesterol in bile, and most subjects, whether or not gallstones are present, usually have bile that is supersaturated with cholesterol after periods of fasting. These observations suggest that additional factors are important in the development of cholesterol gallstones, particularly nucleating factors in bile.[131, 132] Cholesterol precipitation is more rapid in the filtered gallbladder bile from patients with gallstones than in those without despite similar relative percent molar cholesterol content. In addition, a small aliquot of filtered bile from a patient with gallstones induces rapid nucleation of cholesterol in bile from a patient with no stones. Thus, while cholesterol saturation of bile seems to be necessary for cholesterol gallstone formation, additional factors, particularly nucleating factors, seem to be essential to stone formation.

Gallbladder dysfunction may also play a role, particularly in women.[130, 133, 134] Using quantitative ultrasound, pregnant women have an increased gallbladder volume after fasting and empty the gallbladder more slowly and less completely than do nonpregnant controls. Gallbladder emptying is also less complete in women taking medications containing estrogen. Gallbladder function returns to normal after such medications are stopped and following delivery in pregnant patients.

Effects on Mother and Fetus.—There

is no clear increase in the incidence of acute cholecystitis during pregnancy, and the course of the disease seems to be similar to that in nonpregnant patients. However; risk of the development of gallstone is increased in patients who have had previous pregnancies. There is no clear increase in fetal risk consequent to maternal cholelithiasis unless infection supervenes.

Management.—Emergency laparotomy is considered by many surgeons to be the standard treatment for acute cholecystitis. In the first trimester, surgery carries an increased risk of abortion. While operations late in gestation may provoke premature delivery, the risk is less than in early gestation. However, since acute attacks usually subside in a day or two with conservative therapy, this may be the preferred approach.[135] Still, some authorities report greater success with a surgical approach, but this difference probably reflects differences in patient selection.[136] In any event, maternal safety is predominant, and pregnancy itself should not preclude surgery. Hospitalization, bowel rest perhaps with nasogastric suction, and antibiotics, if there is evidence of infection, should be the initial approach to treatment. Surgery should be considered when patients fail to improve in 24 to 72 hours or who have recurrent attacks, as well as those who have symptomatic common bile duct stones. Patients with prolonged biliary tract pain or nonspecific abdominal symptoms in whom gallstones are detected for the first time during pregnancy should be observed. Cholecystectomy is not indicated for this group. Episodes of pain may recur during pregnancy, but recent studies of the natural history in nonpregnant patients with mild symptoms suggest that only a few will develop acute cholecystitis requiring surgery in a follow-up period of 2 years.

Although unnecessary medications should be avoided during gestation, patients requiring surgery can probably receive analgesics such as meperidine (FDA category B) or morphine (FDA category B) safely; in addition, if the clinical evidence suggests the presence of bacterial infection, antibiotics should be administered as to nonpregnant patients, since adverse effects of these drugs have not been clearly documented.

Pyelonephritis and Other Bacterial Infections

Pyelonephritis is discussed in greater detail in Chapters 2 and 13. Of note is that symptomatic infection of the kidney may be associated with liver chemistry abnormalities.[137, 138] Increased alkaline phosphatase above levels normal for pregnancy and raised aminotransferases are frequently present, and total serum bilirubin may be slightly elevated. Jaundice, however, is uncommon unless a β-hemolytic organism is involved. The abnormality subsides when the infection is controlled.

The cause of the liver abnormalities is uncertain but may be related to the effect of circulating toxic products of bacterial metabolism on the liver. Similar abnormalities have been described in nonpregnant patients with serious bacterial infection involving different organ systems.[139] Specific antibodies have not been implicated.

PREGNANCY SUPERIMPOSED ON CHRONIC LIVER DISEASE

Chronic Hepatitis

Chronic hepatitis encompasses a group of necroinflammatory diseases, varying widely in severity and persisting for 6 months or more. Causes include hepatitis B as well as non-A, non-B hepatitis (hepatitis C). Some patients, particularly those in their teens and twenties, may have "autoimmune" chronic hepatitis characterized by evidence of multisystem involvement and positive seroimmunologic tests such as antinuclear antibodies. There may be no history of blood transfusions or evidence of multisystem involvement, in which case the disease is termed *idiopathic chronic hepatitis*.[140, 141]

Prognosis is related not only to etiology but also to histologic severity.[141] In addition, patients with more severe liver damage are more likely to have complications with pregnancy. Liver biopsies from patients with *chronic persistent hepatitis* show portal triad inflammatory infiltrates comprised mainly of lymphocytes which are confined mainly to the portal triads. The limiting plate, the row of hepatocytes which abut the portal triad, is intact, but there may be occasional foci of inflammation in the parenchyma. Most patients are asymptomatic or have only mild fatigue. The aminotransferases are ordinarily no more than fivefold elevated. The serum albumin does not fall below the level expected in pregnancy, and the prothrombin time is normal. The total serum bilirubin is only slightly elevated. Such patients require no therapy and have a good prognosis. Patients with *chronic active hepatitis* have liver biopsies which show portal triad inflammatory infiltrates extending into the parenchyma; piecemeal necrosis, entrapment of hepatocytes in the periportal inflammatory reaction, is present, but there is no confluent necrosis. Patients are generally more symptomatic than those with chronic persistent hepatitis and may be markedly jaundiced, particularly those with autoimmune chronic hepatitis. The aminotransferases sometimes approach the levels in patients with acute hepatitis, but serum albumin and the prothrombin time are generally within normal limits. As with chronic persistent hepatitis, the prognosis is generally good, and the development of cirrhosis is uncommon. Treatment with corticosteroids is indicated only for patients with severe clinical illness.

Chronic active hepatitis with bridging is clearly more severe and has a guarded prognosis. Biopsies from these patients show extensive necrosis which extends (bridges) from portal triad to central vein and sometimes involves the necrosis of multiple hepatic lobules. Although some patients are severely ill with jaundice, ascites, and hepatic encephalopathy, others have only mild fatigue. Liver chemistry tests likewise vary widely, although patients with the most severe disease often have marked elevations of the total serum bil-

irubin along with prolongation of the prothrombin time and depression of the serum albumin below that ordinarily seen in pregnancy. Some patients have the histologic features of cirrhosis in addition to chronic active hepatitis and are classified as *chronic active hepatitis with cirrhosis*. Patients in this category usually have evidence of ongoing chronic active hepatitis, as well as the features of cirrhosis.

Patients with histologic evidence of bridging or cirrhosis in addition to chronic hepatitis should receive treatment with corticosteroids, particularly if serologic tests are negative for hepatitis B and there is no history of blood transfusions. Patients with autoimmune and idiopathic chronic hepatitis generally show marked clinical improvement with such therapy. In addition, histologic disease severity often subsides, and survival is clearly improved.

Although patients with hepatitis B and non-A, non-B hepatitis respond poorly to corticosteroids, preliminary data suggest that interferon-α may be beneficial. However, relapse is frequent when this medication is stopped, and with present dosage schedules there is no clear evidence of prolonged benefit.

Maternal and Fetal Effects and Management.—Chronic persistent hepatitis and chronic active hepatitis carry no clear increased risk during pregnancy, unless hepatitis B is the cause, in which case transmission to the infant is likely. Pregnancies have been reported in at least 28 of these patients without any harmful maternal effects; in addition, the delivery of healthy term infants has been the rule.[142]

In contrast, when pregnancy is superimposed on severe chronic hepatitis, the risk of maternal and fetal death is increased. Occasionally, chronic hepatitis may first be suspected early in pregnancy. Because histologic severity is a key prognostic marker and important in determining therapy, a liver biopsy should be performed. Patients with severe forms of chronic hepatitis should be treated with corticosteroids if there is no history of blood transfusion or evidence of hepatitis B infection. The patient's liver condition usually improves as the pregnancy progresses, and the risk to the mother and fetus declines. We are unaware of reports describing the use of interferon-α during pregnancy.

Cirrhosis and Portal Hypertension

Clinical Features.—Although most types of cirrhosis have been reported in women of childbearing age, cirrhotic patients who become pregnant ordinarily have a history of some form of chronic hepatitis. Occasional patients have primary biliary cirrhosis or alcoholic cirrhosis, but other causes are unusual during pregnancy. Fertility is decreased in cirrhotic women, probably due to amenorrhea and nonovulatory cycles. In addition, fetal loss is increased. Malnutrition and altered hepatic sex steroid metabolism probably contribute to these problems.

Ordinarily, the physician will be aware that a pregnant patient has cirrhosis because of previous investigations, which often include liver biopsy. In addition, a history of some form of hepatitis or the presence of positive serologic tests for hepatitis B or antinuclear antibodies may be present. Physical findings suggestive of the presence of cirrhosis may also be helpful. These include a firm liver and an enlarged spleen, spider angiomas, palmar erythema, or ascites. Liver chemistry tests may show abnormalities typical of the causative disease; in addition, a serum albumin below the usual level seen in pregnancy and prolongation of the prothrombin time may be present with more severe disease.

Maternal and Fetal Effects.—Pregnancy has a variable course in cirrhotic patients, but the risk is mainly related to the degree of portal hypertension and the likelihood of esophageal variceal hemorrhage.[143–146] The presence of hepatocellular failure, indicated by decreased hepatic synthetic function with or without jaundice, may also be important. In a study of 95 patients with cirrhosis due mainly to chronic hepatitis, 23 had esophageal varices and 18 bled during the course of the pregnancy. Of the patients without varices, most developed no substantial change in liver function. However, liver chemistry tests worsened in a few, along with the development of jaundice. There were 7 abortions and 10 stillbirths.[147]

Management.—Despite the risks, many women can be managed successfully through pregnancy despite the presence of cirrhosis. If esophageal varices are present before pregnancy, some form of portacaval shunting may be recommended.[146, 147] The course of pregnancy for women with previous portacaval shunts has generally been smooth, and the likelihood of successful vaginal delivery appears to be high. However, stillbirths have occurred in some patients.[147]

If the patient is already pregnant but the stage of pregnancy is early, the risk for the mother must be balanced against her wish to carry the pregnancy to term. An upper gastrointestinal tract endoscopy should probably be performed to search for esophageal varices in any pregnant patient with chronic liver disease. Successful portacaval decompressive surgery can usually be accomplished, but there is some risk of spontaneous abortion.[147, 148] If deranged synthetic function is present, particularly prolongation of the prothrombin time refractory to the administration of vitamin K_1, termination of the pregnancy should be considered.

Even if large esophageal varices are present, which carry an increased risk of hemorrhage, some patients can be managed through pregnancy to successful vaginal delivery.[149, 150] Once labor begins, prompt delivery should be accomplished, either vaginally or by cesarean section as dictated by obstetric considerations. Because of increased abdominal pressure, prolonged labor may increase the likelihood of bleeding. Careful attention should be given to the management of the coagulopathy that accompanies cirrhosis in some patients. This may require the administration of fresh frozen plasma to correct the prothrombin time and of platelet packs to repair thrombocytopenia. Since the risk of post-partum hemorrhage is increased in these patients, the coagulopathy should be treated aggressively for 24 to 48 hours after surgery, or until the risk of hemorrhage has subsided.

Wilson's Disease

Wilson's disease is a rare disorder of copper metabolism which has an autosomal recessive pattern of inheritance. Decreased biliary copper excretion appears to be the main defect in this disease, leading to an increase in total body copper with markedly raised levels in the liver, brain, and other tissues. The disease often mimics one of the stages of chronic hepatitis. Some patients present with fulminant hepatic failure or cirrhosis. Neurologic manifestations sometimes predominate, but liver disease is present in these as well.

The diagnosis should be considered in any patient with features of hepatitis where the etiology is not clear. The diagnosis can be suspected when features of neurologic Wilson's disease are present in a patient with liver disease that resembles chronic hepatitis. These include loss of fine hand movement and decreased coordination in early disease. The Kayser-Fleischer ring may be present on slit-lamp examination.

The serum ceruloplasmin level is usually markedly decreased and helps to establish the diagnosis, but the level is often raised in pregnancy. Measurement of 24-hour urine copper content is often more helpful in pregnant patients. A liver biopsy performed for direct measurement of copper content is the most sensitive diagnostic test.

Treatment with penicillamine is recommended for most patients, and even advanced neurologic disease may respond to therapy.

Maternal and Fetal Effects and Management.—Because of the improved outcome of Wilson's disease patients treated with penicillamine, more women with this illness are becoming pregnant. While some reports suggest that penicillamine (FDA class D) has toxic effects on the fetus, the largest single study recorded 29 healthy births in 18 mothers.[151] There was no evident fetal toxicity from penicillamine, and the deliveries were uncomplicated. Indeed, the risk of pregnancy in patients with untreated Wilson's disease, or in patients with documented disease whose penicillamine therapy is stopped, seems to be greater. Hepatic decompensation has been reported in at least four patients as the pregnancy progressed, resulting in maternal death in two and stillbirths in two. These observations suggest that patients with Wilson's disease who become pregnant should continue their treatment throughout the pregnancy.

Liver Tumors

Liver adenomas were uncommon before the introduction of oral contraceptives, suggesting that these drugs may be involved in the pathogenesis.[152] Cases have been discovered during pregnancy and the puerperium, and hepatic rupture with maternal and fetal death has sometimes resulted.[153–155] Regression of hepatic tumors after cessation of oral contraceptives can occur, and the tumors do not always regrow with pregnancy and the concomitant increased circulating estrogen concentrations.

Focal nodular hyperplasia, a highly vascular benign tumor, has also been reported in pregnancy.[156] Increased circulating estrogen concentrations are thought to contribute to bleeding but not necessarily to tumor development. Rupture during pregnancy has also been reported with these tumors, posing a risk to both mother and fetus.[157]

Hepatocellular carcinomas and cholangiocarcinomas are sometimes diagnosed in pregnancy and carry a risk for the mother and fetus because of accompanying cirrhosis with hemorrhage, tumor rupture, and metastases.[158, 159] Circulating estrogen levels may contribute to growth and bleeding of these tumors, as with benign liver tumors.

Because of the limited clinical data, guidelines for management must be tentative. If a woman with a previously diagnosed hepatic tumor becomes pregnant, conservative management and monitoring with serial ultrasonography seems prudent. If the lesion is near the surface of the liver, rupture may be more likely and surgery may be warranted after the first trimester. If a mass in the liver is first discovered during pregnancy, Doppler flow ultrasonography may help to determine the vascularity of the lesion and the diagnosis. A conservative approach is probably best, but surgery may be considered for lesions that appear to carry a risk of hemorrhage, particularly after the first trimester.

Pregnancy Following Liver Transplantation

Liver transplantation is performed increasingly for the management of end-stage liver disease, when conventional therapy has ceased to be effective. The liver diseases for which transplantation is often recommended include chronic hepatitis, cryptogenic cirrhosis, and fulminant hepatic failure, diseases which may affect young women. Thus it is not surprising that successful pregnancies have been reported following liver transplantation. With immunosuppression consisting of azathioprine and prednisone, one mother had an uncomplicated vaginal delivery of a term infant; another mother had vaginal delivery of two term pregnancies.[160, 161] A third mother had abruptio placentae, and spontaneous delivery occurred at 28 weeks; however, both the mother and the infant survived and subsequently did well.[162] Four additional successful pregnancies that resulted in vaginal deliveries at term have been reported which used cyclosporine and prednisone as immunosuppressive agents; one mother also received a small dose of azathioprine.[163–166]

The precise risk of pregnancy following liver transplantation is uncertain because of the limited clinical experience. However, results in women with renal transplantation taking azathioprine and prednisone seem to have been quite successful when organ function had been good. Most physicians who manage patients that have had liver transplants recommend avoidance of pregnancy,

at least in the first year following the procedure, when immunosuppressive medications are being adjusted and the risk of complications such as acute rejection is still significant. A therapeutic abortion should probably be considered for patients during this period. After the first year, patients who are functioning well and have stable liver function on minimal immunosuppression may find the uncertain risk of pregnancy acceptable. A therapeutic abortion might be considered for those who do not wish to accept this risk.

The risk to the fetus is mainly related to the injurious potential of the medications used to maintain immunosuppression. Ample clinical experience suggests that prednisone has little, if any, untoward effects on the fetus. However, azathioprine in the doses used to maintain immunosuppression following liver transplantation probably does carry a small but significant risk of teratogenicity. Cyclosporine may be associated with growth retardation and the drug has been identified in the placenta, amniotic fluid, and fetal blood. (See Chap. 2 for further discussion of these immunosuppressive agents.)

REFERENCES

1. Haemmerli UP: Jaundice during pregnancy with special emphasis of recurrent jaundice during pregnancy and its differential diagnosis. *Acta Med Scand [Suppl]* 1967; 44:1–9.
2. Combes B, Shibata H, Adams R, et al: Alterations in sulfobromophthalein sodium removal mechanisms from blood during normal pregnancy. *J Clin Invest* 1963; 42:1431–1442.
3. Ingerslev M, Teilum G: Biopsy studies on the liver in pregnancy. II. Liver biopsy in normal pregnant women. *Acta Obstet Gynecol Scand* 1945; 25:352–360.
4. Kessler WB, Andros JG: Hepatic function during pregnancy and puerperium. *Obstet Gynecol* 1964; 23:372–379.
5. Kaplan MM: Alkaline phosphatase. *N Engl J Med* 1972; 286:200–202.
6. Kaplan MM: Serum alkaline phosphatase—Another piece is added to the puzzle. *Hepatology* 1986; 6:526–528.

7. Mestery D, Leroux ML, Perry WF: Effect of dialysis on tissue and serum alkaline phosphatase heat stability. *Clin Biochem* 1975; 8:18–22.

8. Sussman H, Bowman M, Lewis JL: Placental alkaline phosphatase in maternal serum during normal and abnormal pregnancy. *Nature* 1968; 218:359.

9. Mueller MN, Kappas A: Estrogen pharmacology. I. The influence of estradiol and estriol on hepatic disposal of sulfobromophthalein (BSP) in man. *J Clin Invest* 1964; 43:1905–1914.

10. Cerutti R, Ferrari S, Grella P, et al: Behavior of serum enzymes in pregnancy. *Clin Exp Obstet Gynecol* 1976; 3:22.

11. Kreek MJ, Sleisenger MH, Jeffries GH: Recurrent cholestatic jaundice of pregnancy with demonstrated estrogen sensitivity. *Am J Med* 1967; 43:795–803.

12. Kreek MJ, Weser E, Sleisenger MH, et al: Idiopathic cholestasis of pregnancy. The response to challenge with the synthetic estrogen, ethinyl estradiol. *N Engl J Med* 1967; 277:1391–1395.

13. Spechler SJ, Koff RS: Wilson's disease in diagnostic difficulties in the patient with chronic hepatitis and hypoceruloplasminemia. *Gastroenterology* 1980; 78:803–806.

14. Weiner CP: The clinical spectrum of preeclampsia. *Am J Kidney Dis* 1987; 9:312–316.

15. Sibai BM, Taslimi MM, El-Nazer A, et al: Maternal-perinatal outcome associated with the syndrome of hemolysis, elevated liver enzymes, and low platelets in severe preeclampsia-eclampsia. *Am J Obstet Gynecol* 1986; 155:501–509.

16. Rolfes DB, Ishak KG: Liver disease in toxemia of pregnancy. *Am J Gastroenterol* 1986; 81:1138–1144.

17. Minakami H, Oka N, Sato J, et al: Preeclampsia: A microvesicular fat disease of the liver? *Am J Obstet Gynecol* 1988; 159:1043–1047.

18. Aarnoudse JG, Houthoff HJ, Weits J, et al: A syndrome of liver damage and intravascular coagulation in the last trimester of normotensive pregnancy. A clinical and histopathological study. *Br J Obstet Gynaecol* 1986; 93:145–155.

19. Roberts JM, Taylor RN, Musci TJ, et al: Preeclampsia: An endothelial cell disorder. *Am J Obstet Gynecol* 1989; 161:1200–1204.

20. Erkkola R, Ekblad U, Kero P, et al: HELLP syndrome. *Ann Chir Gynaecol* 1987; 202:26–28.

21. Stalter KD, Sterling WA: Hepatic subcapsular hemorrhage associated with pregnancy. *Surgery* 1985; 98:112–114.

22. Manas KJ, Welsh JD, Rankin RA, et al: Hepatic hemorrhage without rupture in preeclampsia. *N Engl J Med* 1985; 312:424–426.

23. Westergaar L: Spontaneous rupture of the liver in pregnancy. *Acta Obstet Gynecol Scand* 1980; 59:559–561.

24. Aziz S, Merrell RC, Collins JA: Spontaneous hepatic hemorrhage during pregnancy. *Am J Surg* 1983; 146:680–682.

25. Ibrahim N, Payne E, Owen A: Spontaneous rupture of the liver in association with pregnancy. Case report and review of the literature. *Br J Obstet Gynaecol* 1985; 92:539–540.

26. Heller TD, Goldfarb JP: Spontaneous rupture of the liver during pregnancy. *NY State J Med* 1986; 86:314–316.

27. Riely CA: Case studies in jaundice of pregnancy. *Sem Liver Dis* 1988; 8:191–199.

28. Ekberg H, Leyon J, Jeppsson B, et al: Hepatic rupture secondary to pre-eclampsia—Report of a case treated conservatively. *Ann Chir Gynaecol* 1984; 73:350–353.

29. Gonzalez GD, Rubel HR, Giep NN, et al: Spontaneous hepatic rupture in pregnancy: Management with hepatic artery ligation. *South Med J* 1984; 77:242–245.

30. Goodlin RC, Anderson JC, Hodgson PE: Conservative treatment of liver hematoma in the postpartum period. *J Reprod Med* 1985; 30:368–370.

31. Loevinger EH, Vujic I, Lee WM, et al: Hepatic rupture associated with pregnancy: Treatment with transcatheter embolotherapy. *Obstet Gynecol* 1985; 65:281–284.

32. Reily CA, Latham PS, Romero R, et al: Acute fatty liver of pregnancy. A reassessment based on observations in nine patients. *Ann Intern Med* 1987; 106:703–706.

33. Hatfield AK, Stein JH, Greenberger NJ, et al: Idiopathic acute fatty liver of pregnancy. Death from extrahepatic manifestations. *Dig Dis Sci* 1972; 17:167–178.

34. Bernuau J, Degott C, Nouel O, et al: Non-fatal acute fatty liver of pregnancy. *Gut* 1983; 24:340–344.

35. Liebman HA, McGehee WG, Patch MJ, et al: Severe depression of antithrombin III associated with disseminated intravascular coagulation in women with fatty liver of pregnancy. *Ann Intern Med* 1983; 98:330–333.

36. Rolfes DB, Ishak KG: Acute fatty liver of pregnancy: A clinicopathologic study of 35 cases. *Hepatology* 1985; 5:1149–1158.

37. Duma RJ, Dowling DA, Alexander HC, et al: Acute fatty liver of pregnancy. Report of a case studied with serial liver biopsies. *Ann Intern Med* 1965; 63:051–058.

38. Weber FL, Snodgrass PJ, Powell DE, et al: Abnormalities of hepatic mitochondrial urea-cycle enzyme activities and hepatic ultrasound in acute fatty liver of pregnancy. *J Lab Clin Med* 1979; 94:27–41.

39. Kaplan MM: Acute fatty liver of pregnancy. *N Engl J Med* 1985; 313:367–370.

40. Sheehan HL: The pathology of acute cellular atrophy and delayed chloroform poisoning. *J Obstet Gynaecol Br Emp* 1940; 47:43–61.

41. Ober WB, Le Compte PM: Acute fatty metamorphosis of the liver associated with pregnancy. *Am J Med* 1955; 19:743–758.

42. Kahil ME, Fred HL, Brown H, et al: Acute fatty liver of pregnancy. A report of two cases. *Arch Intern Med* 1964; 113:63–69.

43. Fast BB, Roulston TM: Idiopathic jaundice of pregnancy. *Am J Obstet* 1964; 88:314–320.

44. Breen KJ, Perkins KW, Mistilis SP, et al: Idiopathic acute fatty liver of pregnancy. *Gut* 1970; 11:822–825.

45. Cano RI, Delman MR, Pitchumoni CS, et al: Acute fatty liver of pregnancy. Complication by disseminated intravascular coagulation. *JAMA* 1975; 231:159–161.

46. Scully RE, Galdabini JJ, McNeely BU: Case Records of the Massachusetts General Hospital. *N Engl J Med* 1981; 304:216–224.

47. Sherlock S: Acute fatty liver of pregnancy and the microvesicular fat diseases. *Gut* 1983; 24:265–269.

48. Hou SH, Levin S, Ahola S, et al: Acute fatty liver of pregnancy. Survival with early cesarean section. *Dig Dis Sci* 1984; 29:449–452.

49. Ebert EC, Sun EA, Wright SH, et al: Does early diagnosis and delivery in acute fatty liver of pregnancy lead to improvement in maternal and infant survival? *Dig Dis Sci* 1984; 29:453–455.

50. Pockros PJ, Peters RL, Reynolds TB: Idiopathic fatty liver of pregnancy: Findings in ten cases. *Medicine* 1984; 63:1–11.

51. Reily CA: Acute fatty liver of pregnancy. *Dig Dis Sci* 1984; 29:456–457.

52. Cammu H, Velkeniers B, Charels K, et al: Idiopathic acute fatty liver of pregnancy associated with transient diabetes insipidus. Case report. *Br J Obstet Gynaecol* 1987; 94:173–178.

53. Brown MS, Reddy KR, Hensley GT, et al: The initial presentation of fatty liver of pregnancy mimicking acute viral hepatitis. *Am J Gastroenterol* 1987; 82:554–557.

54. Foster KJ, Dewbury KC, Griffith AH, et al: The accuracy of ultrasound in the detection of fatty infiltration of the liver. *Br J Radiol* 1980; 53:440–442.

55. Campillo B, Bernuau J, Witz MO, et al: Ultrasonography in acute fatty liver of pregnancy. *Ann Intern Med* 1986; 105:383–384.

56. McKee CM, Weir PE, Foster JH, et al: Acute fatty liver of pregnancy and diagnosis by computed tomography. *Br Med J* 1986; 292:291–292.

57. Ockner SA, Brunt EM, Cohn SM, et al: Fulminant hepatic failure caused by acute fatty liver of pregnancy treated by orthotopic liver transplantation. *Hepatology* 1990; 11:59–64.

58. Breen KJ, Perkins KW, Schenker S, et al: Uncomplicated subsequent pregnancy after idiopathic fatty liver of pregnancy. *Obstet Gynecol* 1972; 40:813–815.

59. Kunelis CT, Peters JL, Edmondson HA: Fatty liver of pregnancy and its relationship to tetracycline therapy. *Am J Med* 1965; 38:359–377.

60. Peters RL, Edmondson HA, Mikkelson WP, et al: Tetracycline-induced fatty liver in nonpregnant patients: A report of six cases. *Am J Surg* 1967; 113:622–632.

61. Schultz JC, Adamson JS, Workman WN, et al: Fatal liver disease after intravenous administration of tetracycline in high dosage. *N Engl J Med* 1963; 269:999–1004.

62. Lunzer M, Barnes P, Byth K, et al: Serum bile acid concentrations during pregnancy

and their relationship to obstetric cholestasis. *Gastroenterology* 1986; 91:825–829.

63. Heikkinen J, Maentausta O, Ylostalo P, et al: Changes in serum bile acid concentrations during normal pregnancy, in patients with intrahepatic cholestasis of pregnancy and in pregnant women with itching. *Br J Obstet Gynaecol* 1981; 88:240–245.

64. Kirkinen P, Ylostalo P, Heikkinen J, et al: Gallbladder function and maternal bile acids in intrahepatic cholestasis of pregnancy. *Eur J Obstet Gynecol Reprod Biol* 1984; 18:29–34.

65. Shaw D, Frohlich J, Wittmann BA, et al: A prospective study of 18 patients with cholestasis of pregnancy. *Am J Obstet Gynecol* 1982; 142:621–625.

66. Laatikainen T, Ikonen E: Serum bile acids in cholestasis of pregnancy. *Obstet Gynecol* 1977; 50:313–318.

67. Reyes H, Gonzales MC, Ribalta J, et al: Prevalence of intrahepatic cholestasis of pregnancy in Chile. *Ann Intern Med* 1978; 88:487–393.

68. Reyes H, Taboada G, Ribalta J: Prevalence of intrahepatic cholestasis of pregnancy in La Paz, Bolivia. *J Chronic Dis* 1979; 32:499–504.

69. Svanborg A, Ohlsson S: Recurrent jaundice of pregnancy. *Am J Med* 1959; 27:40–49.

70. Holzbach RT, Sivak DA, Braun WE: Familial recurrent intrahepatic cholestasis of pregnancy: A genetic study providing evidence for transmission of a sex-limited, dominant trait. *Gastroenterology* 1983; 85:175–179.

71. Eisale A, Jarvinen PA, Luukkainen T: Hepatic impairment during the intake of contraceptive pills: Clinical trial with postmenopausal women. *Br Med J* 1964; 2:426–427.

72. Adlercreutz H, Ikonen E: Oral contraceptives and liver damage. *Br Med J* 1964; 2:1133–1134.

73. Heikel TAJ, Lathe GH: The effect of oral contraceptive steroids on bile secretion and bilirubin Tm in rats. *Br J Pharmacol* 1970; 38:593–601.

74. Frezza M, Chiesa L, Pozzato G, et al: Alteration in sulfobromphthalein hepatic storage capacity(s) in non-pregnant women previously affected with intrahepatic cholestasis of pregnancy (ICP). *Acta Obstet Gynecol Scand* 1986; 65:577–580.

75. Vore M: Estrogen cholestasis: Membranes, metabolites, or receptors? *Gastroenterology* 1987; 93:643–647.

76. Jaeschke H, Trummer E, Krell H: Increase in biliary permeability subsequent to intrahepatic cholestasis by estradiol valerate in rats. *Gastroenterology* 1987; 93:533–538.

77. Fisk NM, Storey GNB: Fetal outcome in obstetric cholestasis. *Br J Obstet Gynaecol* 1988; 95:1137–1143.

78. Roszkowski I, Miedzinska DP: Jaundice in pregnancy II. Clinical course of pregnancy and delivery and condition of the neonate. *Am J Obstet Gynecol* 1968; 101:500–503.

79. Wilson BR, Haverkamp AD: Cholestatic jaundice of pregnancy: New perspectives. *Obstet Gynecol* 1979; 54:128–134.

80. Reyes H, Radrigan ME, Gonzalez MC, et al: Steatorrhea in patients with intrahepatic cholestasis of pregnancy. *Gastroenterology* 1987; 93:584–590.

81. Laatikainen TJ, Lehtonen PJ, Hesso AE: Fetal sulfated and nonsulfated bile acids in intrahepatic cholestasis of pregnancy. *J Lab Clin Med* 1978; 92:185–193.

82. Svanborg A, Ohlsson S: Recurrent jaundice of pregnancy. *Am J Med* 1959; 27:40–49.

83. Frezza M, Pozzato G, Chiesa L, et al: Reversal of intrahepatic cholestasis of pregnancy in women after high dose S-adenosyl-L-methionine administration. *Hepatology* 1984; 4:274–278.

84. Adams RH, Gordon J, Combes B: Hyperemesis gravidarum. I. Evidence of hepatic dysfunction. *Obstet Gynecol* 1968; 31:659–664.

85. Larrey D, Rueff B, Feldman G, et al: Recurrent jaundice caused by recurrent hyperemesis gravidarum. *Gut* 1984; 25:1414–1415.

86. Jamfelt-Samsioe A, Eriksson B, Waldenstrom J, et al: Serum bile acids, gamma glutamyl transferases, and routine liver function tests in emetic and non-emetic pregnancies. *Gynecol Obstet Invest* 1986; 21:169–176.

87. Swaminathan R, Chin RK, Lao CTH, et al: Thyroid function in hyperemesis gravidarum. *Acta Endocrinol [Suppl] (Copenh)*

1989; 120:155–160.

88. Parker RGF: Occlusion of the hepatic veins in man. *Medicine* 1959; 38:369–412.

89. Mitchell MC, Boitnott JK, Kaufman S, et al: Budd-Chiari syndrome: Etiology, diagnosis and management. *Medicine* 1982; 61:199–218.

90. Baert AL, Fevery J, Marchal G, et al: Early diagnosis of Budd-Chiari syndrome by computed tomography and ultrasonography: Report of five cases. *Gastroenterology* 1983; 84:587–595.

91. Sparano J, Chang J, Trasi S, et al: Treatment of the Budd-Chiari syndrome with percutaneous transluminal angioplasty: Case report and review of the literature. *Am J Med* 1987; 82:821–828.

92. Cassel GA, Morley JE: Hepatic vein thrombosis treated with streptokinase. *S Afr Med J* 1974; 48:2319–2320.

93. Malt RA, Dalton JC, Johnson RG, et al: Side-to-side portacaval shunt versus nonsurgical treatment of Budd-Chiari syndrome. *Am J Surg* 1978; 136:387–390.

94. Putnam CW, Porter KA, Weil R III, et al: Liver transplantation for Budd-Chiari syndrome. *JAMA* 1976; 236:1142–1143.

95. Lysy Y, Medina A, Shouval D, et al: Fatal relapsing viral hepatitis A infection during pregnancy. *Isr J Med Sci* 1988; 24:681–683.

96. Shah N, Ostrow D, Altman N, et al: Evolution of acute hepatitis B in homosexual men to chronic hepatitis B. *Arch Intern Med* 1985; 145:881–882.

97. Mohite BJ, Rath S, Bal V, et al: Mechanisms of liver cell damage in acute hepatitis B. *J Med Virol* 1987; 22:199–210.

98. Davis GL, Hoofnagle JH: Reactivation of chronic type B hepatitis presenting as acute viral hepatitis. *Ann Intern Med* 1985; 102:762–765.

99. Colombo M, Cambieri R, Rumi MG, et al: Long-term delta superinfection in hepatitis B surface antigen carriers and its relationship to the course of chronic hepatitis. *Gastroenterology* 1983; 85:235–239.

100. Alter HJ, Purcell RH, Shih JW, et al: Detection of antibody to hepatitis C virus in prospectively followed transfusion recipients with acute and chronic non-A, non-B hepatitis. *N Engl J Med* 1989; 321:1494–1500.

101. Baker VV, Cefalo RC: Fulminant hepatic failure in the third trimester of pregnancy: A case report. *J Reprod Med* 1985; 30:229–231.

102. Adams RH, Combes B: Viral hepatitis during pregnancy. *JAMA* 1965; 192:195–198.

103. Tong MJ, Thursby M, Rakela J, et al: Studies on the maternal-infant transmission of the viruses which cause acute hepatitis. *Gastroenterology* 1981; 80:999–1004.

104. Franks AL, Berg CJ, Kane MA, et al: Hepatitis B virus infection among children born in the United States to Southeast Asian refugees. *N Engl J Med* 1989; 321:1301–1305.

105. Mitsuda T, Mori T, Ookawa N, et al: Demonstration of mother-to-infant transmission of hepatitis B virus by means of polymerase chain reaction. *Lancet* 1989; 1:886–888.

106. Arevalo JA: Hepatitis B in pregnancy. *West J Med* 1989; 150:668–674.

107. Chang MH, Hwang LY, Hsu HC, et al: Prospective study of asymptomatic HBsAg carrier children infected in the perinatal period: Clinical and liver histologic studies. *Hepatology* 1988; 8:374–377.

108. De Potter CH, Robberecht E, Laureys G, et al: Hepatitis B related childhood hepatocellular carcinoma: Childhood hepatic malignancies. *Cancer* 1987; 60:414–418.

109. Tong MJ, Govindarajan S: Primary hepatocellular carcinoma following perinatal transmission of hepatitis B. *West J Med* 1988; 148:205–208.

110. Prevention of perinatal transmission of hepatitis B virus: Prenatal screening of all pregnant women for hepatitis B surface antigen. *MMWR* 1988; 37:341–346.

111. Chen DS, Hsu NHM, Sung JL, et al: A mass vaccination program in Taiwan against hepatitis B virus infection in infants of hepatitis B surface antigen-carrier mothers. *JAMA* 1987; 257:2597–2603.

112. Arevalo JA, Washington E: Cost-effectiveness of prenatal screening and immunization for hepatitis B virus. *JAMA* 1988; 259:365–369.

113. Cruz AC, Frentzen BH, Behnke M: Hepatitis B: A case for prenatal screening of all patients. *Am J Obstet Gynecol* 1987; 156:1180–1183.

114. Kumar ML, Dawson NV, McCullough AJ, et al: Should all pregnant women be screened for hepatitis B? *Ann Intern Med*

1987; 107:273–277.

115. Beasley RP, Chin-Yun Lee G, Roan CH, et al: Prevention of perinatally transmitted hepatitis B virus infections with hepatitis B immune globulin and hepatitis B vaccine. *Lancet* 1983; 2:1099–1102.

116. Wong VCW, Reesink HW, Reerink-Brongers EE, et al: Prevention of the HBsAg carrier state in newborn infants of mothers who are chronic carriers of HBsAg and HBeAg by administration of hepatitis B vaccine and hepatitis B immunoglobulin. *Lancet* 1984; 2:921–926.

117. Stevens CE, Toy PT, Tong MJ, et al: Perinatal hepatitis B virus transmission in the United States. Prevention by passive-active immunization. *JAMA* 1985; 253:1740–1745.

118. Stevens CE, Taylor PE, Tong MJ, et al: Yeast-recombinant hepatitis B vaccine: Efficacy with hepatitis B immune globulin in prevention of perinatal hepatitis B virus transmission. *JAMA* 1987; 257:2612–2616.

119. Ramia S, Bahakim H: Perinatal transmission of hepatitis B virus-associated hepatitis D virus. *Ann Inst Pasteur Virol* 1988; 139:285–290.

120. Franks AL, Binkin NJ, Snider DE, et al: Isoniazid hepatitis among pregnant and postpartum hispanic patients. *Public Health Rep* 1989; 104:151–155.

121. Haibach H, Akhter JE, Muscato MS, et al: Acetaminophen overdose with fetal demise. *Am J Clin Pathol* 1984; 82:240–242.

122. Davidson TC: The management of fulminant hepatic failure, in: Schaffer F, Popper H (eds): *Progress in Liver Diseases,* vol 3. New York, Grune & Stratton, Inc, 1970, pp 282–398.

123. Emond JC, Aran PP, Whitington PF, et al: Liver transplantation in the management of fulminant hepatic failure. *Gastroenterology* 1989; 96:1583–1588.

124. Report of the European Association for Study of the Liver: Randomized trial of steroid therapy in acute liver failure. *Gut* 1979; 20:620—623.

125. O'Grady JG, Gimson AES, O'Brien CJ, et al: Controlled trials of charcoal hemoperfusion and prognostic factors in fulminant hepatic failure. *Gastroenterology* 1988; 94:1186–1192.

126. Chesson RR, Gallup DG, Gibbs RL, et al:

Ultrasonographic diagnosis of asymptomatic cholelithiasis in pregnancy. *J Reprod Med* 1985; 30:920–922.

127. Block P, Kelly TR: Management of gallstone pancreatitis during pregnancy and the postpartum period. *Surg Gynecol Obstet* 1989; 168:426–428.

128. Jorgensen T: Gall stones in a Danish population: Fertility period, pregnancies, and exogenous female sex hormones. *Gut* 1988; 29:433–439.

129. Thistle JL: Gallstones in women. *Med Clin North Am* 1974; 58:811–816.

130. Kern F, Everson GT, DeMark B, et al: Biliary lipids, bile acids, and gallbladder function in the human female. *J Clin Invest* 1981; 68:1229–1242.

131. Van Erpecum KJ, Van Berge Henegouwen GP, Stoelwinder B, et al: Bile concentration is also a factor for nucleation of cholesterol crystals and cholesterol saturation index in gallbladder bile of gallstone patients. *Hepatology* 1990; 11:1–6.

132. Hoover EL, Jaffe BM, Webb H, et al: Effects of female sex hormones and pregnancy on gallbladder prostaglandin synthesis. *Arch Surg* 1988; 123:705–708.

133. Braverman DZ, Johnson ML, Kern F Jr: Effects of pregnancy and contraceptive steroids on gallbladder function. *N Engl J Med* 1980; 302:362–364.

134. Radberg G, Asztely M, Cantor P, et al: Gastric and gallbladder emptying in relation to the secretion of cholecystokinin after a meal in late pregnancy. *Digestion* 1989; 42:174–180.

135. Hiatt JR, Hiatt JCG, Williams RA, et al: Biliary disease in pregnancy: Strategy for surgical management. *Am J Surg* 1986; 151:263–265.

136. Dixon NP, Faddis DM, Silberman H: Aggressive management of cholecystitis during pregnancy. *Am J Surg* 1987; 154:292–294.

137. Sworn MJ, Innew WM: Perpartum hepatic dysfunction and xanthogranulomatous pyelonephritis. *Br J Urol* 1973; 45:327–328.

138. Vermillion SE, Morlock CG, Bartholomew LG, et al: Nephrogenic hepatic dysfunction secondary to tumefactive xanthogranulomatous pyelonephritis. *Ann Surg* 1971; 171:171–176.

139. LaMont JT, Isselbacher KJ: Postoperative jaundice. *N Engl J Med* 1978; 288:305–308.

140. Czaja AJ: Strategies in the management of chronic active hepatitis. *Surv Dig Dis* 1984; 2:233–243.

141. Lashner BA, Jonas RB, Tang HS, et al: Chronic hepatitis: Disease factors at diagnosis predictive of mortality. *Am J Med* 1988; 85:609–614.

142. Infeld DS, Borkowf HI, Varma RR: Chronic-persistent hepatitis and pregnancy. *Gastroenterology* 1979; 77:524–527.

143. Whelton MJ, Sherlock S: Pregnancy in patients with hepatic cirrhosis. Management and outcome. *Lancet* 1968; 2:995–997.

144. Cheng YS: Pregnancy in liver cirrhosis and/or portal hypertension. *Am J Obstet Gynecol* 1977; 128:812–822.

145. Borhanmanesh F, Haghighi P: Pregnancy in patients with cirrhosis of the liver. *Obstet Gynecol* 1970; 36:315–324.

146. Wilbanks GD, Klinges KG: Pregnancy after portacaval shunt. Report of 2 cases and review of the literature. *Obstet Gynecol* 1967; 29:44–49.

147. Schreyer P, Caspi E: Cirrhosis—pregnancy and delivery: A review. *Obstet Gynecol Surv* 1982; 37:304–314.

148. Reisman TM, O'Leary JA: Portacaval shunt performed during pregnancy in a case report. *Obstet Gynecol* 1971; 37:253–254.

149. Hermann RE, Esselstyn CG: The potential hazard of pregnancy in extrahepatic portal hypertension. *Arch Surg* 1967; 95:956.

150. Yip DM, Baker AL: Liver diseases in pregnancy. *Clin Perinatol* 1985; 12:683–694.

151. Scheinberg IH, Sternlieb I: Pregnancy in penicillamine-treated patients with Wilson's disease. *N Engl J Med* 1975; 293:1300–1302.

152. Klatsin G: Hepatic tumors: Possible relationship to the use of oral contraceptives. *Gastroenterology* 1977; 73:386–394.

153. Stenwig AE, Solgaard T: Ruptured benign hepatoma associated with an oral contraceptive. A case report. *Virchows Arch [Pathol Anat]* 1975; 367:337–343.

154. Berg JW, Ketelaar RJ, Rose ER, et al: Hepatomas and oral contraceptives. *Lancet* 1974; 2:349–350.

155. Motsay GJ, Gamble WG: Clinical experience with hepatic adenomas. *Surg Gynecol Obstet* 1972; 134:415–418.

156. Whelan TJ, Baugh GH, Chandor S: Focal nodular hyperplasia of the liver. *Ann Surg* 1973; 177:150–158.

157. Schenken JR: Hepatocellular adenomas: Relationship of contraceptives? *JAMA* 1976; 236:559–561.

158. Purtilo DT, Clark JV, Williams R: Primary hepatic malignancy in pregnant women. *Am J Obstet Gynecol* 1975; 121:41–44.

159. Roddie TW: Haemorrhage from primary carcinoma of the liver complicating pregnancy. *Br Med J* 1957; 1:31–39.

160. Walcott WO, Derick DE, Jolley JJ, et al: Successful pregnancy in a liver transplant patient. *Am J Obstet Gynecol* 1978; 132:340–341.

161. Meyers RL, Schmid R, Newton JJ: Childbirth after liver transplantation. *Transplantation* 1980; 29:432–434.

162. Newton ER, Turksay N, Kaplan M, et al: Pregnancy and liver transplantation. *Obstet Gynecol* 1988; 71:499–500.

163. Penn I, Makowski EL: Parenthood in kidney and liver transplant recipients. *Transplant Proc* 1981; 13:36–39.

164. Venkataramanan R, Koneru B, Wang CC, et al: Cyclosporine and its metabolites in mother and baby. *Transplantation* 1988; 46:468–469.

165. Haagsma EB, Visser GHA, Klompmaker IJ, et al: Successful pregnancy after orthotopic liver transplantation. *Obstet Gynecol* 1989; 74:442–443.

166. Sims CJ, Porter KB, Knuppel RA: Successful pregnancy after a liver transplant. *Am J Obstet Gynecol* 1989; 161:532–533.

CHAPTER 11

Rheumatic Disease

Michael D. Lockshin

Maurice L. Druzin

Rheumatic disease comprises those illnesses characterized by sterile inflammation, the joints, skin, and kidney being the most frequently involved organs. Other shared pathology in the collagen diseases is blood vessel inflammation. Infections and local (traumatic) anatomic disease of individual joints are not considered to be primary rheumatic illnesses.

The most frequent rheumatic illnesses encountered in pregnant women are systemic lupus erythematosus (SLE), rheumatoid arthritis, juvenile (rheumatoid) arthritis, and scleroderma. Other forms of collagen disease are occasionally seen: dermatomyositis, Takayasu arteritis, polyarteritis nodosa, and Wegener's granulomatosis. Diseases categorically different from the collagen diseases, but most conveniently described here, include inborn errors of collagen metabolism (Ehlers-Danlos, Marfan's syndromes) and miscellaneous musculoskeletal complaints (hip replacement, tendonitis, disc disease, and low back pain).

In collagen disease, pregnancy management issues center on a few specific questions. Is there any organ system impairment or disability that will compromise pregnancy, delivery, or child care? Are the kidneys involved? Does the patient have hypertension? Does the patient have antiphospholipid antibody? Does the patient have anti-Ro/La antibody? Be-

cause SLE is the commonest collagen disease in which pregnancy is encountered, and because most known pregnancy complications occur in SLE patients, SLE is used as an example; lesser discussions accompany the other diseases.

PHYSIOLOGIC ADAPTATIONS IN PREGNANCY WHICH MAY INFLUENCE THE COURSE OF RHEUMATOLOGIC DISORDERS

Gestational events relevant to the collagen diseases fall into four major groups: (1) volume and blood pressure changes (cardiac, renal/hypertensive complications), (2) coagulation control mechanisms (thrombocytopenias and circulating anticoagulants), (3) immunologic (complement kinetics, immune complexes, humoral and cellular immunity), and (4) hormonal changes.[1]

Patients with collagen diseases can have renal, vascular, and cardiac compromise and may not be able to tolerate the increments in intravascular volume which occur during pregnancy.[2, 3] Rheumatic renal disease may be renovascular, glomerular, or tubulointerstitial. The extrarenal vascular bed may lack sufficient compliance to accommodate the increased fluid volume. Subclinical forms of myocarditis or valvulitis are also common. Pericarditis is frequent in patients with collagen diseases. Thus, when fluid volumes increase during pregnancy, congestive cardiomyopathy, valvular insufficiency, "stiff ventricle" syndrome, and constrictive pericarditis due to subclinical disease may become apparent.

Coagulation systems change during pregnancy[4–8] (see Chap. 8). Platelet survival decreases. To compensate, in normal women platelet production increases, resulting in no net change in the peripheral platelet count. Pregnant patients with collagen diseases may manifest thrombocytopenia, but this event also occurs commonly in several complications of pregnancy such as preeclampsia, abruption, amniotic fluid embolism, and intrauterine fetal demise. Therefore, when decreases in platelet count are present, the cause may be difficult to define.

Immunologic alterations characterize both pregnancy and all the connective tissue diseases. In pregnancy, cell-mediated immunity is generally depressed, as reflected by altered lymphocyte tests, decreased T/B lymphocyte ratios, increased suppressor-helper T cell ratios, and decreased lymphocyte-monocyte ratios.[9–14] Cutaneous and antibody responses, including responses to specific microbial antigens, are selectively depressed,[15] as are cellular measures of inflammation.[16] In SLE, which is characterized by decreased T cell suppressor function, pregnancy paradoxically normalizes this function.[17] Some of these suppressive and immunoregulatory phenomena have been attributed to direct effects of pregnancy-associated plasma protein A,[18–20] alpha fetoprotein,[21] and increases in endogenous corticosteroids.[22] In pregnancy, immunoglobulin-secreting cells increase,[20, 23] inflammatory responses decrease, plasma proteins change,[24] and circulating immune complexes may be present.[25–31] In addition, patients with rheumatoid arthritis treated with gamma globulin eluted from human placenta improve.[32] The immunology of pregnancy is reviewed in detail elsewhere.[33, 34]

Hypergammaglobulinemia occurs universally in patients with collagen diseases as a diffuse immunologic B cell hyperreactivity occurs. T suppressor function in most reports is diminished while T helper function is increased. A variety of cytokine abnormalities involving both decreased interferon and variably altered interleukins are reported, as are reductions of leukocyte and erythrocyte membrane receptors for complement and immune complexes. Each of the collagen diseases is associated with a specific HLA-DR or -B type; some of the immunologic abnormalities common to the collagen diseases themselves may be HLA-linked.[35] Relevance of some of the same immunologic abnormalities to primary infertility or to fetal loss has been suggested but there are few direct and no definitive studies of cellular or cytokine abnormalities in pregnant patients with collagen diseases.

Clinically measured complement reflects the balance between synthesis and consumption of rate-limiting complement components.[30–45] In an uncomplicated pregnancy, total C3, C4, and CH50 are normal or raised relative to normal nonpregnant levels. For example, C3, normally 80 to 120 mg/dL; C4 normally 15 to 50 mg/dL; and CH50, normally 150 to 300 units/mL, often rise to 200 mg, 75 mg, and greater than 300 units/mL, respectively, in late pregnancy. Measures of some classic pathway activation products (C3a, C4a, C5a), but of not others (C1s-C1 inhibitor complex), suggest that low-grade classic pathway activation normally occurs in pregnancy.[46–48] The normal clinical levels of C3, C4, and CH50 in pregnancy imply increased synthesis of complement components. In nonpregnant patients with collagen diseases, activation of both the classic and the alternative complement pathways and decreased synthesis of complement components occur. Pregnant patients with collagen disease are often hypocomplementemic and this issue is discussed in detail in the section on SLE. However, hypocomplementemia has been described in preeclampsia.[38, 39, 43]

Hyperestrogenemia and other complex hormonal changes characterize normal pregnancy. These alterations are potentially detrimental to patients with SLE, since hyperestrogenic states may characterize, and therefore be partly responsible for the occurrence of, SLE. Similarly, pregnancy-associated protein and hypercortisolism have been proposed as explanations for improvement of rheumatoid arthritis during pregnancy.[49-53.]

IMPORTANT QUESTIONS FOR ALL RHEUMATIC DISEASES

Does Pregnancy Influence the Course of Disease?

The question of whether pregnancy influences the course of disease depends on a clear understanding of the natural history of the disorder in question and upon clear definitions of exacerbation or improvement. For rarer diseases, neither the natural history nor the measurement of exacerbation is exact. Because physiologic gestational events may cause a variety of symptoms, the patient's health may worsen, although, in a technical sense, her disease has not. The importance of this distinction is that, in the symptomatically worsening patient, treatment directed against the primary illness (on the assumption that it has become "active") may be misguided. Changes which may mimic the primary disease are blood volume–induced cardiovascular, renal, hematologic, and pulmonary compromise and pregnancy-induced thrombocytopenia.

Does the Disease Influence Pregnancy?

Whether preclinical rheumatic disease influences fertility is unclear.[54-57] Recent retrospective studies suggest that patients destined to develop rheumatoid arthritis or scleroderma have subnormal fertility prior to clinical recognition of their illnesses,[55] but other studies reject this hypothesis.[54-58] The necessarily retrospective nature of the studies and the use of ethnically different populations prevent clear resolution of the contradictions.

End-organ dysfunction due to collagen disease may, when superimposed on the physiologic changes of pregnancy, produce a variety of clinical problems. Obviously, women with no cardiopulmonary, hematologic, or renal impairment endure pregnancy without incident. Neurologic and musculoskeletal impairment, which may influence delivery, may have little impact on the antecedent pregnancy. However, medications that must be continued during pregnancy, such as anti-inflammatory agents, corticosteroids, antihypertensives, and anticonvulsants, may adversely affect the fetus. Finally, maternal antibodies may cross the placenta and affect the infant.

SYSTEMIC LUPUS ERYTHEMATOSUS

Definition and Clinical Course

Lupus erythematosus (LE) occurs in two clinical forms. *Discoid LE* is a dermatologic illness characterized by a scarring rash, no visceral illness, and negative laboratory investigations. *Systemic lupus erythematosus* (SLE) is defined by abnormalities of multiple organ systems and by serologic abnormalities.[59] (Table 11–1). Since rash, including the discoid type, may be present in patients with SLE, differentiation from the discoid variety of the disease cannot be made on the characteristics of the rash alone, and both forms have to be viewed with caution in pregnancy. For instance, the newborn of the pregnant patient with discoid disease is at risk to develop neonatal lupus.

The cause of SLE is unknown. It is commoner in blacks, hispanics, and orientals than in whites.[60] HLA-DR3 and the C4 null allele are excessively represented among SLE patients.[61] The reason for female predominance is unknown. Both men and women with SLE share a variant of estrogen metabolism that renders them feminized by biochemical, but not by clinical, criteria. Hyperestrogenism in women with SLE may approach that of normal pregnancy.[49-53, 62, 63] Although hyperestrogenism has been proposed to explain the female predominance of SLE, such hormonal

TABLE 11–1.

American Rheumatism Association Criteria for the Classification of Systemic Lupus Erythematosus (SLE)*

1. Malar rash (flat erythema, sparing nasolabial folds)
2. Discoid rash (raised patches with follicular plugging and scarring)
3. Photosensitivity (skin rash after sun exposure)
4. Oral ulcers (painless oral or nasopharyngeal, observed by a physician)
5. Arthritis (nonerosive, involving two or more joints, observed by a physician)
6. Serositis (pleurisy or pericarditis, confirmed by a physician)
7. Renal disorder (>0.5 g/day proteinuria or cellular casts)
8. Neurologic disorder (seizures or psychosis)
9. Hematologic disorder (hemolytic anemia or leukopenia [<4000 WBC/mm³ on two or more occasions] or thrombocytopenia [<100 × 10⁹/L] or lymphopenia [<1,500/mm³ on two or more occasions])
10. Immunologic disorder (positive LE cell preparation or anti-DNA (double-stranded) antibody or anti-Sm antibody or biologic false-positive test for syphilis for at least 6 mo)
11. Antinuclear antibody in the absence of drugs known to induce SLE

*Criteria are designed for classification of patient populations for purposes of making published reports uniform. The criteria are not used for the diagnosis of an individual patient. Persons fulfilling four or more criteria serially or simultaneously may be classified as having SLE in such studies.

changes are not thought relevant to gestational outcome.

The commonest findings of SLE are arthritis, rash, pleuropericarditis, fever, photosensitivity, lymphadenopathy, alopecia, and Raynaud's phenomenon. Renal and neurologic diseases occur in half or fewer of patients. Mucosal ulcers and necrotizing vasculitis occur in a minority. A given patient may exhibit any combination or all of these manifestations in any degree of severity. Typically an SLE patient has periods of disease exacerbation ("flare") and periods of remission. These occur at unpredictable intervals.

The arthritis of SLE affects the distal extremities symmetrically, most frequently the hands, wrists, elbows, knees, and ankles. It is rare for the spine or hips to be involved. The arthritis resembles that of rheumatoid arthritis but is more variable from day to day and is much less likely to cause bone erosions or permanent deformity. SLE patients, especially when treated with high-dose corticosteroid, frequently develop osteonecrosis of the hip or other joints. This painful complication is distinct from lupus arthritis. It restricts hip range of motion and frequently leads to joint replacement surgery.

Lupus rashes are usually slightly raised and erythematous; they may flake or ulcerate and resolve with hyper- or hypopigmentation. Characteristically such rashes occur on the cheeks and over the bridge of the nose (the "butterfly") but are also common on the chin, hair line, upper chest, upper back, and lateral surface of the upper arms. A telangiectatic erythema of the palms and about the nail beds is also common. Alopecia begins frontally in lupus. Broken hairs on the forehead are characteristic and diffusely thinned hair is also quite common.

Pleuropericarditis is often painful, transient, and with small or no recordable effusion. Lymphadenopathy is prominent in the neck and axillae; it can occasionally be quantitatively important enough to suggest lymphoma. Fever may be of any type; hectic, spiking is usual, but low-grade persistent fever also occurs. Photosensitivity is the development of increased rash or the worsening of any SLE symptom after (usually rather intense) sun exposure. Renal disease is extremely variable. There are several forms of lupus nephropathy which may produce variable degrees of hematuria, proteinuria, hypertension, and renal insufficiency. The course may range from stable minimal proteinuria with normal renal function over decades to severe nephrotic syndrome, as well as anuric renal failure, within days of onset. Neurologic disease is also extremely variable. Psychosis, delirium, coma, stroke, seizures, movement disorders, myelopathy, and peripheral neuropathies occur. Mucosal ulcers are shallow, painless ulcers on the hard palate or nasal septum; nasal septal perforation may occur. These ulcers are uncommon and are not noted by the patient, but they have diagnostic importance. Necrotizing vasculitis of a polyarteritis nodosa type, with major vascular occlusion and extremity and visceral gangrene, is rare but catastrophic.

In SLE the (nonspecific) antinuclear antibody test is nearly always positive in high titer[64] (Table 11–2). Many normal persons, patients with other illnesses, and apparently normal pregnant women may also have positive tests for antinuclear antibodies in low titer. Over 80% of patients with SLE have antinative (double-stranded [ds]) DNA antibodies. Anti-Sm antibody is positive in approximately one third of SLE patients. Anti-dsDNA and anti-Sm antibodies are the only antibodies specific for SLE. Nonspecific antibodies, commonly present in SLE and patients with other collagen disorders, include antibodies to denatured (single-stranded) DNA, Ro (SSA), La (SSB), and RNP. Approximately 10% of patients have a lupus anticoagulant; approximately 40% have anticardiolipin antibody.[65–68] Serum complement is frequently reduced in patients with active glomerulonephritis but is typically normal in patients with active nonrenal SLE.[64] SLE patients have increased B cell function and diminutions in suppressor T cell function, macrophage function, cell surface complement receptors, and interferon. About 25% of SLE patients have a positive test for rheumatoid factor. Skin biopsy may show inflammatory change or immunoglobulin and complement deposition at the dermo-epidermal junction. Renal biopsy aids in categorizing different forms of nephropathy for prognostic and/or treatment purposes. Immunoglobulin, complement, and immune complexes are demonstrable at sites of inflammation in biopsy specimens.

Routine laboratory tests demonstrate variable degrees of anemia, which is commonly that of chronic illness but may be associated with Coombs' antibody and severe hemolysis, leukopenia, usually in the range of 3,000 WBCs/mm³ (3.0 × 10⁹ L), and thrombocytopenia.[69–74] The last occurs in two forms in nonpregnant patients: (1) chronic, low-grade, with platelet counts averaging 50 to 70

× 10⁹/L, and (2) recurrent, severe, idiopathic thrombocytopenic purpura (ITP)–like, with counts reaching life-threatening levels. Urinalysis may demonstrate hematuria, pyuria, cylinduria, and proteinuria; renal function may be impaired. Erythrocyte sedimentation rate is almost always elevated. Both aspartate and alanine aminotransferases may be abnormal in patients taking nonsteroidal anti-inflammatory drugs, but are seldom abnormal in otherwise uncomplicated SLE. Alkaline phosphatase is often abnormal with or without the ingestion of nonsteroidal anti-inflammatory drugs.

Patients with SLE are treated with non-steroidal anti-inflammatory drugs (usually for arthritis or fever), corticosteroid preparations (for many indications), antimalarial drugs (usually for rash or for steroid-sparing effect), and immunosuppressive agents such as cyclophosphamide or azathioprine (for severe disease, especially glomerulonephritis). The disease can be rapidly fatal, but more than 90% of patients are alive more than 10 years from first diagnosis. Most SLE patients spend more time in remission than in exacerbation. Despite this list of problems encountered by the SLE patient, most SLE patients capable of becoming pregnant are not desperately ill.

TABLE 11–2.
Laboratory Abnormalities Commonly Found in Patients With Systemic Lupus Erythematosus (SLE)

Autoantibodies	Frequency
Antinuclear	>90%
Anti-DNA (double-stranded)	>80%
Anti-DNA (single-stranded)	50%
Anti-Sm	30%
Anti-Ro/SSA	25%
Anti-La/SSB	20%
Anti-RNP	25%
Rheumatoid factor	25%
Anticardiolipin	40%
Lupus anticoagulant	20%
Other findings	
Anemia, leukopenia, thrombocytopenia	
Coombs' antibody	
Increased erythrocyte sedimentation rate	
Proteinuria, cylindruria, hematuria, pyuria	
Abnormal blood urea nitrogen, creatinine	
Decreased complements (C3, C4, CH50)	

Does Pregnancy Influence the Course of SLE?

An accurate assessment of the effect of gestation on disease activity of SLE depends upon a precise and accurate definition of disease exacerbation (flare). Unfortunately there is no consensus regarding the definition of *flare* of SLE.[75] Most flare scoring systems identify and quantify rash, arthritis, fever, nephritis, and cytopenias. Further complicating the issue is the fact that thrombocytopenia and proteinuria can occur in pregnant patients in the absence of SLE, and attribution of proteinuria or thrombocytopenia in the pregnant patient to either active SLE or to pregnancy complications is often difficult. Correct attribution depends on the time of onset during the pregnancy and on the coexistence or absence of pregnancy-independent phenomena, such as lymphadenopathy or inflammatory arthritis.

By global criteria (e.g., statement by physician or patient that disease is worse or better) flare is uncommon in SLE pregnancy. The supposition that pregnancy induces flare, or that pregnancy brings out new disease in women who would be well were they not pregnant, is unproved.[76–78] Early case reports identified individual patients who had pregnancy-related exacerbation; studies in which patients served as their own controls have suggested that manifestations of the disease were more likely to occur during a given month of pregnancy than during one when the woman was not pregnant (reviewed in references 76 and 78). However, when pregnant patients are matched with demographically and clinically similar controls there does not appear to be a difference between pregnant patients and those who are not pregnant, either during pregnancy or for the first postpartum year.[76] In the authors' experience, exacerbation occurs in under 15% of all pregnancies, a rate consistent with that of a nonpregnant population. It is also the authors' experience, but not that of others,[77] that exacerbations are not related to disease activity prior to pregnancy.

Thrombocytopenia.—Thrombocytopenia is common in SLE pregnancy, especially in those patients with antiphospholipid antibody.[47] Thrombocytopenia during gestation in patients with SLE occurs in four patterns: Firstly, thrombocytopenia occurring early, usually prior to gestational week 15, a nadir of greater than 50×10^9/L, remaining constant, and not responding to corticosteroid therapy, occurs in association with antiphospholipid antibody. This type of thrombocytopenia usually remits after delivery, whether or not treatment is administered, and usually recurs with subsequent pregnancies. The antiphospholipid-thrombocytopenic form of the disease is usually not accompanied by signs of SLE activity in other organ systems; and erythrocyte destruction with increased serum lactic dehydrogenase (LDH) is uncommon. Aspirin may reverse the thrombocytopenia.[77a]

A second type of thrombocytopenia occurring late, usually after 25 weeks, is most often associated with impending or present preeclampsia. This form of thrombocytopenia tends to worsen as pregnancy progresses, is associated with signs of fetal jeopardy, and remits after delivery. It too is not associated with signs or symptoms of active SLE, but biochemical and clinical manifestations of preeclampsia or the HELLP (hypertension, elevated liver enzymes, low platelets) syndrome may be present.

There is a third, abrupt, and severe (often $<10 \times 10^9$/L) form of the ITP type which also occurs most often with no other signs of active SLE. Thrombocytopenia, due to other causes, such as drugs and hematologic malignancy, must be excluded by bone marrow examination. It is our experience that this type of thrombocytopenia generally responds to high-dose corticosteroid. Intravenous gamma globulin has been successfully used as a therapeutic (temporizing) measure to accomplish delivery. In a minority of patients splenectomy is necessary. The fourth type is a variable, moderate ($50–120 \times 10^9$/L) thrombocytopenia that is persistent over long periods of time and which responds to prednisone. This type is diagnosed by the simultaneous presence of other manifestations of active SLE: vascular disease, as manifest by renal or neurologic worsening and by "vas-

TABLE 11–3.
Relative Frequency of Causes of
Thrombocytopenia in Systemic Lupus
Erythematosus (SLE) Pregnancies*

No thrombocytopenia	76%
Thrombocytopenia	24%
Anticardiolipin syndrome	8%
Active SLE	7%
Preeclampsia	9%
Idiopathic thrombocytopenic purpura–type	<1%

*Authors' unpublished observations, 1990.

culitic" skin rashes. Erythrocyte fragmentation is common; serum LDH levels are often elevated.

Unfortunately, there is no specific test that clearly differentiates one type of thrombocytopenia from another in gravid patients with SLE. Nonpregnant patients with SLE commonly have immunoglobulin, complement, and immunoglobulin-containing immune complexes on their platelets. Tests seeking platelet-associated immunoglobulin or anti-platelet antibodies are potentially useful if the diagnosis of SLE has not been made, but if the diagnosis of SLE is known, platelet-associated immunoglobulin tests seldom help in the differential diagnosis. In our experience (Table 11–3), approximately one fourth of all SLE patients experienced thrombocytopenia ($<150 \times 10^9$/L) during pregnancy. The frequencies of antiphospholipid antibody syndrome, active SLE, and pregnancy-induced hypertension were equally distributed.

Renal Disease.—In patients with renal disease proteinuria may increase during gestation because glomerular filtration has (normally) increased, because of preeclampsia, or because of active SLE[79–85] (see also Chap. 2, Renal Disorders). Clinical signs of active SLE, rising anti-DNA antibody titer and the appearance of erythrocyte casts in the urine, are evidence favoring the diagnosis of lupus glomerulonephritis. Normal serum complement argues against the diagnosis of active lupus glomerulonephritis. Rapid worsening over days is more common in preeclampsia than in active SLE. Hypertension, thrombocyto-

penia, hypocomplementemia, and hyperuricemia may occur in both lupus nephritis and preeclampsia. Although renal biopsy might distinguish the two, biopsy is not generally feasible. In women with preexisting renal disease who develop preeclampsia, renal function usually returns to its prepregnancy baseline, but exceptions exist, especially in patients with moderately or severely impaired renal function before conception[86] (see Chap. 2).

Total hemolytic complement and levels of C3 and C4, often low in active lupus nephritis, may also be abnormal in the pregnant SLE patient who does not have apparent active disease. Very sensitive measures of classic pathway activation, such as C4a, abnormal in active lupus nephritis, are also abnormal in normal pregnancies. Less sensitive measures (C1s-C1 inhibitor complex) are most often normal in lupus pregnancy with proteinuria.[46–48] Measures of alternative pathway complement activation (Ba and Bb) are abnormal in active lupus nephritis but normal in lupus pregnancies with proteinuria that is not due to active SLE. A consensus is developing that measurement of alternative pathway complement activation products or of C1s-C1 inhibitor complex may be the clearest way to determine whether new proteinuria in the pregnant patient is due to active SLE or to a pregnancy complication. However, these tests are not yet widely available, and therefore distinctions between lupus nephritis and preeclampsia must be made by clinical criteria (Table 11–4).

Skin, Joint, and Neurologic Involvement.—It is common for pregnancy erythemas, particularly of the face and hands, to suggest active SLE skin rashes. Areas where there has been prior rash frequently become more erythematous as cutaneous blood flow increases. With experience, distinguishing between active SLE rash and pregnancy-induced change is not difficult. Patients who suddenly discontinue hydroxychloroquine often have exacerbation of rash.[87]

Arthritis is common in SLE. Pregnant patients with the disease often complain of joint "achiness" (authors' experience). As ligaments loosen in late pregnancy joint effusions occur. The decision that a given patient's joint complaints are due to active SLE rather than to normal physiologic changes of pregnancy depends on the demonstration that the joint effusion is new or inflammatory, e.g., has increased warmth or heat, or has over 10,000 WBCs/mm³ (10 × 10⁹/L) synovial fluid or that extraarticular manifestations of SLE are present.

Neuropsychiatric events of SLE include strokes, seizures, psychoses, and demyelination or transverse myelitis.[88–90] In our experience, neurologic events during the course of pregnancy are rare. There is no indication that any specific neurologic event, including chorea,[89] is induced by pregnancy. In a patient with seizures, hypertension, and renal failure, the distinction between eclampsia and fulminant renal and neurologic SLE may be difficult. The circumstances in which the events occur, the presence of other clinical and serologic (rising anti-DNA antibody) evidence of active SLE, and response to therapy may all be required to make the distinction.

Does SLE Influence the Course of Pregnancy?

Global flare in its worst manifestations will seriously complicate pregnancy. However, malignant forms of SLE are rarely seen in pregnant patients, and there is no general experience described. More common are exacerbations involving single organ systems.

Renal disease predisposes pregnant patients to develop hypertension.[3, 91, 92] With regard to its effect on gestation, lupus nephropathy differs little from glomerulonephritis complicated by hypertension of other etiologies (see Chap. 2, p. 59). In our experience with 125 completed SLE pregnancies, only 15% entered pregnancy with preexisting renal involvement. Of the women with preexisting kidney disease, 63% developed preeclampsia, (or aggravation of their hypertension and proteinuria), while preeclampsia developed in 14% of women without preexisting renal disease. Because so few women entered pregnancy with kidney disease, the majority of patients developing preeclampsia did not have preexisting kidney disease.

Most patients with severe lupus glomerulonephritis develop hypertension, proteinuria, and accelerated loss of renal function and have poor pregnancy outcomes. However, there are rare exceptions in which patients with severe renal disease have successful gestations. There are even reported instances of women with lupus nephritis severe enough to necessitate hemodialysis who were able to discontinue dialysis and carry a gestation to term; others have delivered while maintained on dialysis therapy (authors' experience).[78] Patients with extreme degrees of nephrosis have also completed successful pregnancies and others with severe glomerulonephritis

TABLE 11–4.
Comparison Between Preeclampsia and Lupus Nephritis

Clinical Measures	Preeclampsia	Lupus Nephritis
C3, C4, CH50	May be low	Commonly low
Urinalysis	Red blood cell (RBC) casts rare	RBC casts frequent
Onset of proteinuria	Commonly abrupt	Gradual or abrupt
Hepatic aminotransferases	May be increased	Rarely abnormal
Quantity of proteinuria	Will not differentiate	
Thrombocytopenia	Will not differentiate	
Hyperuricemia	Will not differentiate	
Hypertension	Will not differentiate	

have been treated with high-dose corticosteroids and improved during gestation.

Anemia can be severe enough to threaten fetal well-being. It is common for SLE patients who are not pregnant to have hematocrits in the low 30s. In pregnant SLE patients, hematocrits in the low 20s may occur. Except for the occasional gravida with important IgG Coombs' hemolytic antibody (which may be transmitted to the fetus), there is nothing specific about the severe anemia that occurs in SLE patients. One probable consequence of the anemia, however, is an increased incidence of fetal growth retardation.

IgG-associated thrombocytopenia may be transmitted to the fetus, but most infants born of mothers with SLE-associated thrombocytopenia have normal platelet counts. In our studies, thrombocytopenia itself was not an independent predictor of fetal death. In patients with antiphospholipid antibody, thrombocytopenia did not add an independent risk factor for fetal death.[93–95]

Neuropsychiatric disease has little direct influence on pregnancy outcome. Fetal injury from hypoxia during seizures or self-abuse during psychosis are possible. If phenobarbital is used as an anticonvulsant, neonatal sedation or drug withdrawal may occur. Other manifestations of SLE do not appear to influence the course of pregnancy.

Does SLE Affect Infant Outcome?

SLE has an important general effect on the fetus: fetal death, intrauterine growth retardation, and prematurity are common. The frequency of these complications will vary according to the frequencies of preexisting hypertension, renal disease, and antiphospholipid antibodies in the study population. Published figures for these abnormalities vary from less than 10% to more than 50% of reported SLE pregnancies.[56, 77, 79, 80, 93, 94, 96, 97] Other than the frequency of their occurrence, these events in SLE patients do not differ from similar events occurring in non-SLE patients. Thrombocytopenia and hemolytic anemia are

rare events occurring in infants of mothers with IgG antiplatelet and Coombs' antibodies. Anti-DNA antibody, also transmitted to the infant, has no apparent pathologic effect.[98, 99] Antiphospholipid antibody for the most part is not transmitted to the fetus.

Mothers with anti-Ro (SSA), anti-La (SSB), and rarely anti-U1RNP antibody, whether or not they have a clinical diagnosis of SLE, may deliver a child with neonatal lupus.[100–102] Approximately one third of all SLE patients have one or more of these antibodies. Neonatal lupus consists of any or all of the following: a (usually transient) photosensitive rash, thrombocytopenia, hemolytic anemia, and congenital complete heart block.[103–105] It is probable that maternal HLA-DR3 increases the risk that the infant will develop this syndrome.[106] Among all SLE patients with anti-Ro antibody, the risk that a liveborn child will have any manifestation of neonatal lupus is about 25%,[107] and that it will have definite neonatal lupus, about 13%. The risk for congenital complete heart block is less than 3%. The risk of recurrence of neonatal lupus rash is also about 25%.[108] The risk for heart block may be increased if the mother has high-titer anti-Ro. Heart block may possibly be predicted by maternal antibody to both anti-48 kD Ro and anti-52 kD La bands identified by immunoblot.[109, 110] Neither these bands nor anti-Ro titer predict noncardiac manifestations of neonatal lupus. There are clinical suspicions that infants of mothers with anti-Ro antibody and discoid LE or Sjögren's syndrome are more likely to develop neonatal lupus than are infants of SLE mothers who have anti-Ro. Several published studies of dizygotic twin pregnancies have been discordant for congenital complete heart block and neonatal lupus rash, suggesting that transmission of maternal antibody alone is not sufficient to produce the syndrome.[107, 111, 112] Neonatal lupus also occurs in infants of mothers who are clinically normal. Some of these latter develop SLE many years after the birth of an infant with neonatal lupus.[113]

There are few data regarding pregnancies

in which the father had SLE. It appears there are no known effects of paternal SLE on the infant, regardless of the clinical condition or serologic status of the father. However, there may be an increased risk of subsequent SLE in those instances where SLE is familial.

Management of the Pregnant Woman With SLE (Table 11–5)

Thrombocytopenia.—Treatment of thrombocytopenia in a pregnant patient with lupus depends on clear definition of the cause of the thrombocytopenia. Thrombocytopenia associated with antiphospholipid antibody may respond to 80 mg/day aspirin (authors' experience).[77a] Aspirin interferes with platelet aggregation and may worsen antiplatelet antibody-type thrombocytopenia. Corticosteroid therapy is not contraindicated. Prednisone, 30 to 60 mg/day, should therefore be prescribed if the diagnosis is uncertain. Response to prednisone takes several days to 2 to 3 weeks to occur.

Fluorinated corticosteroids (dexamethasone and betamethasone) should not be used during pregnancy unless there is intent to treat the fetus, since these drugs easily cross the placenta.[114–118] In experimental mice, dexamethasone induced longstanding immunologic and endocrinologic impairment in the offspring of females treated during gestation; a potential for harm is therefore present, but, similar problems have not been reported in humans.[116] Pulse intravenous methylprednisolone also reaches the infant (as do dexamethasone or betamethasone) and could potentially cause long-term damage.[114–116]

When thrombocytopenia is life-threatening ($<30 \times 10^9$/L), or if delivery is imminent, temporary remission of thrombocytopenia may be obtained by infusing platelets (response within minutes, duration hours to 2 days) or intravenous aggregate-free IgG (response within days, duration 2–3 weeks).[119–122] This latter treatment, however, cannot be used on a long-term basis. It adds to the volume load of patients already at risk for hypertension or congestive cardiomyopathy. The infused antibody is also transmitted to the fetus and theoretically adds a volume load to the fetus, increases fetal blood viscosity, and inhibits fetal immunoglobulin synthesis. However, normal children have been delivered of mothers receiving immunoglobulin therapy.[119–123] Splenectomy is a last-resort measure in the treatment of thrombocytopenia. It is rarely used in nonpregnant patients and is unlikely ever to be recommended in pregnant patients.

Anemia.—Corticosteroid therapy is the treatment of choice for anemia (hemolytic or anemia of chronic disease), if treatment is necessary, and if anemia is not due to vitamin or iron deficiency, or to sickle cell disease, glucose-6-phosphate dehydrogenase (G6PD) deficiency, or other Coombs-negative hemolysis. In most cases the indication for treatment is fetal rather than maternal. Potential problems with corticosteroid therapy include glucose intolerance and hypertension, which of course must be carefully watched for. Transfusions are occasionally also necessary.

Renal Disease (see also Chap. 2).—Treatment of SLE nephritis in the pregnant patient is identical to treatment in the nonpregnant patient, with the following exceptions: The risk of hypertension as a side effect of corticosteroid therapy may be greater in the pregnant patient. Also, there is no accumulated experience with pulse bolus corticosteroid in pregnancy. Azathioprine, commonly used in nonpregnant patients, may be used in pregnant patients, but there are also reports about its toxicity.[124–127] The largest experience is with renal transplant patients who conceive, where for the most part few problems arise (see Chap. 2, p. 63). However cytopenias and malformations have occurred,[126, 127] especially with doses above 2.2 mg/kg. Cyclophosphamide, also commonly used in nonpregnant patients, is contraindicated in pregnancy, unless felt to be critical for maternal health and/or survival.

Low-dose aspirin may prevent preeclampsia in non-SLE women identified as being at high risk for developing preeclamp-

TABLE 11–5.
Nonobstetric Monitoring of the Pregnant Systemic
Lupus Erythematosus (SLE) Patient

1. Database for initial visit: complete blood count including platelet count, urinalysis, creatinine clearance, anticardiolipin antibody, lupus anticoagulant, anti-Ro antibody, complement screen (C3, C4, C50, or assay available) and anti-DNA antibody titer
2. Monthly: platelet count*
3. Each trimester: creatinine clearance,* 24-hr urine protein (if screening urinalysis abnormal),* anticardiolipin antibody, complement screen, anti-DNA antibody

(Erythrocyte sedimentation rate is often elevated in uncomplicated pregnancy and is not useful to follow)
*More frequently if abnormal.

sia; however, this treatment is considered experimental at the time of this writing[128–130] (see Chap. 1, p. 13). There is no systematic study of the use of aspirin for this purpose in women with SLE nephritis. In the authors' experience aspirin may be of benefit and is not apparently harmful. There are reports of closure of the ductus arteriosus when indomethacin is used close to term,[131] and further reports of prolonged labor and increased peripartum bleeding when aspirin is used close to term.[132, 133] While intracerebral bleeding and premature ductus closure are serious complications, such life-threatening events are in fact rare in aspirin-treated patients.

Skin, Joint, and Neurologic Involvement.—Rashes may be treated with topical or systemic corticosteroid, but the latter treatment can often be deferred to the postpartum period. There are insufficient data concerning the use of antimalarial drugs during pregnancy, and these drugs should therefore be avoided.[87] Although nonsteroidal drugs, commonly used for lupus arthritis, may be safe in pregnancy, here too experience with full antiarthritis doses is limited and it is potentially safer to treat pregnant patients with lupus arthritis with small doses of prednisone. Neurologic events are treated identically in pregnant and nonpregnant patients.

Monitoring and Treatment of the Fetus

Fetal growth and development in SLE patients may be threatened by four problems: (1) disease activity, (2) decreased renal function, (3) antiphospholipid antibody, and (4) anti-Ro antibody. Factors concerning active disease that affect the fetus include maternal fever or anemia; with renal disease the degree of azotemia, presence of hypertension, or superimposed preeclampsia may also jeopardize fetal well-being. Antiphospholipid antibodies may also cause fetal growth retardation as well as a high frequency of in utero death. In patients with anti-Ro or anti-La antibody, congenital complete heart block is an in utero risk. Evaluation for noncardiac manifestations of neonatal lupus is indicated in the neonatal period in the offspring of these patients.

Gestation complicated by SLE obviously necessitates implementation of all obstetric surveillance and management used in the high-risk setting. In addition, it is necessary to check platelet counts, creatinine clearance, and urinary protein. In women with anti-Ro or anti-La antibody, fetal echocardiography, seeking evidence of heart block or other cardiac dysfunction, is appropriate in the second trimester. Fetal growth rate and placental volume and appearance may also be monitored by sonography, and late fetal well-being by fetal heart rate testing.[134–137] During gestational weeks 25 to 30, nonreactive tests are relatively common. Occurrence of bradycardia is predictive of potential fetal compromise. Later in gestation any nonreactive test is abnormal; bradycardia may indicate a need to deliver, even at early gestational ages. The potential role of umbilical artery waveform determinations is not yet known.

In utero treatment of the fetus affected by heart block would be ideal; however, there is no known effective therapy. Dexamethasone or betamethasone, which reach the fetus, and plasmapheresis have been attempted.[123] After delivery the cardiac lesion does not appear to progress; early delivery may therefore be indicated for the fetus with diminishing cardiac function, as measured by fetal echocardiography or by the appearance of signs of congestive heart failure.

Labor, Delivery, and the Puerperium

The timing and route of delivery may be influenced by SLE-related phenomena such as severe maternal systemic illness, thrombocytopenia, and total hip replacement in addition to the presence of fetal heart block as discussed above. Most often, however, delivery decisions are guided solely by standard obstetric criteria. Thirty-eight percent of our patients underwent operative delivery (Table 11–6). In 28% the indications were fetal distress, prior cesarean, and other reasons not specific for SLE. In the remaining 10% fetal distress associated with antiphospholipid antibody, thrombocytopenia, and maternal illness were the indications. Osteonecrosis of the hip, with or without joint replacement, should lead one to consider an operative rather than vaginal delivery.

There is little information about the use of tocolytics or stimulators of labor in SLE pregnancy. We have used ritodrine, magnesium sulfate, and prostaglandin suppositories without incident.

At delivery, "stress" corticosteroid doses (usually 100 mg of hydrocortisone every 8 hours from onset of labor until 24 hours postdelivery) are administered to patients currently or recently taking corticosteroids. Prophylactic antibiotic coverage (usually a cephalosporin plus gentamicin or vancomycin plus gentamicin) is indicated in women with artificial joint replacements undergoing vaginal or cesarean delivery.

At one time clinicians increased the dose of or started steroid therapy in the puerperium, anticipating that pregnancy had an adverse influence on SLE in the first 2 postpartum months. This flare during the puerperium has not been borne out in a case-controlled, prospective trial,[76] and we do not recommend prophylactic alterations of steroid therapy following delivery.

Breast-Feeding and Counseling

There are no specific studies favoring or countermanding breast-feeding by SLE patients. There is often insufficient milk production in these patients, although the reasons for this are unclear (e.g., disease activity, steroid therapy, or perhaps the fact that premature infants nurse poorly). Also lupus rashes frequently occur on the breasts, making breast-feeding painful. Finally, some potential hazardous drugs or their products (e.g., azathioprine) may be secreted in breast milk and thus it may be prudent to advise against breast-feeding in gravidas receiving such agents. The American Academy of Pediatrics considers prednisone treatment compatible with breast-feeding.

Data from uncontrolled studies have revealed a higher frequency of SLE complications in women taking oral contraceptives,[138, 139] and therefore barrier methods or intrauterine devices are preferred. However, the risks associated with oral contraceptives are not high, and thus if a patient declines use of mechanical methods, it is the practice of the authors to permit oral contraceptives, especially the current low-estrogen formulations.

SLE is a strongly familial disease, the probability of a second first-degree relative being afflicted being approximately 1%. Inheritance of SLE is linked to the HLA type DR3.[35] In twin studies, concordance of illness in identical twins surpasses 70%, whereas in

TABLE 11–6.
Frequency of and Indications for Cesarean Section in 125 Systemic Lupus Erythematosus (SLE) Pregnancies*

No cesarean section	62%
Cesarean section	38%
Non-aPL*† fetal distress or ineffective labor	16%
aPL fetal distress	7%
Prior cesarean	5%
Preeclampsia	5%
Maternal thrombocytopenia	3%
Maternal miscellaneous	2%

*Unpublished observations of the authors.
†aPL = antiphospholipid antibody.

fraternal twins concordance is that of other first-degree relatives.[140] The risk of neonatal lupus may also be HLA-DR3-related. Women with anti-Ro antibody have an approximately 25% risk of delivering a child with any manifestation of neonatal lupus.[106, 107, 108] Finally, when counseling prospective parents, one must consider and discuss the possibility of maternal disability or death. Willingness to accept the responsibilities of child rearing under these potential circumstances is important.

ANTIPHOSPHOLIPID ANTIBODY SYNDROME

Definition and Clinical Course

Antiphospholipid antibody is a general term describing antibodies of any immunoglobulin class which react with cardiolipin (or other negatively charged phospholipids) in enzyme-linked immunosorbent assays (ELISAs) or radioimmunoassays, which have lupus anticoagulant activity, or which react in a serologic test for syphilis.[141–144] Lupus anticoagulant is measured by screening for inhibitors of any of several measures of phospholipid-dependent coagulation and then confirming a positive result with a mixing experiment (in which normal plasma does not correct the abnormality). There is marked variability among assays for lupus anticoagulant.[145, 146] The most sensitive assays are the kaolin clotting time, Russell's viper venom time, and activated partial thromboplastin time using dilute thromboplastin. International standards exist for the ELISA assay for anticardiolipin antibody. Concordance of anticardiolipin antibody and lupus anticoagulant (when lupus anticoagulant is measured by very sensitive tests) is high but not complete; patients with either antibody alone occur.[96] Discordance between serologic tests for syphilis and the lupus anticoagulant on ELISA assays is fairly common, possibly because the former emphasizes low-titer IgM antibody while the latter tests more typically identify IgG antibodies.[141]

Approximately one half of patients with antiphospholipid antibody do not have SLE ("primary antiphospholipid antibody syndrome"). Of these, a minority have relatives with SLE or other collagen disease. Clinical characteristics of this syndrome include vascular occlusive events, other neurologic syndromes (e.g., multi-infarct dementia, white matter disease, and demyelinating myelopathies), thrombocytopenia, livedo reticularis, valvular heart disease, and recurrent fetal death.[142–144]

IgG anticardiolipin antibody is more commonly present than is IgM or IgA; IgM and IgA anticardiolipin antibody are usually found only in persons with IgG as well. Spontaneous anticardiolipin antibody is usually of IgG2 and IgG4 subclass, and has λ light chain predominance rather than κ. Because IgG2, IgG4, and IgM do not readily cross the placenta, anticardiolipin antibody is seldom found in cord blood. Persons with low-titer VDRL reactivity most often have IgM anticardiolipin antibody, which has IgG1 and IgG3 and κ predominance. When maternal IgG1 antiphospholipid antibody is present it is transmitted to the fetus. Anticardiolipin antibody, usually of low titer and of IgM isotype, occurs in patients treated with chlorpromazine and in patients with a variety of infections, including enteric infections and *Pneumocystis carinii*. When it is present in these circumstances, the clinical complications associated with spontaneous antibody do not occur.[93, 96, 97, 148–152]

Whether or not SLE is present, persons with IgG anticardiolipin antibody have a high frequency of midpregnancy fetal death.[65–68] In most, but not all, laboratories the simultaneous or isolated presence of IgA or IgM anticardiolipin antibody isotypes does not change the probability of fetal death, nor does the simultaneous presence of lupus anticoagulant or thrombocytopenia. Antibody directed against other phospholipids, for instance phosphatidylserine, in most investigators' hands, does not improve prognosis.[94] Those few women with lupus anticoagulant, but not anticardiolipin antibody, suffer a fetal risk similar to that of women with anticardiolipin

TABLE 11–7.
Probability of Current Fetal Death, According to Antiphospholipid
Antibody Level and History of Prior Fetal Death*

GPL Units[†]	No. Fetal Deaths/Total (%)			
		Multipara		
	Primipara	No Prior Fetal Death	Prior Fetal Death	All
0–16	2/15(13)	1/16(6)	6/22(27)	9/53(17)
17–39	1/6(17)	1/7(14)	1/3(33)	3/16(19)
41–80	1/5(20)	—	5/8(63)	6/13(46)
>80	3/7(43)	1/1(100)	11/15(73)	15/23(65)
Total	7/33(21)	3/24(13)	23/48(48)	33/105(31)

*From Lockshin MD, Druzin ML, Qamar T: *Am J Obstet Gynecol* 1989; 160:439–443. Used by permission.
[†]International standard unit for IgG antiphospholipid concentration.

antibody. Identification of IgG subclass and anticardiolipin antibody affinity do not increase the predictive power of anticardiolipin antibody for fetal death.[95, 153]

Does Pregnancy Influence the Course of Antiphospholipid Antibody Syndrome?

Primary antiphospholipid antibody syndrome consists of episodic symptoms such as thrombotic events and arterial occlusive diseases. There is no evidence that the frequency of these events is increased during pregnancy, but treatment of patients with prior thrombotic events with aspirin or heparin may have reduced the rate of thrombosis relative to that described in the literature. Thrombocytopenia is common in antiphospholipid antibody pregnancies, and often remits at the conclusion of a pregnancy. Livedo reticularis does not change during pregnancy.

Does the Antiphospholipid Antibody Syndrome Influence the Course of Pregnancy and/or Fetal Outcome?

The most striking effect of antiphospholipid antibody is its association (as either anticardiolipin antibody or lupus anticoagulant) with midpregnancy fetal death (Table 11–7). The usual course is as follows: Early pregnancy is uneventful except for the possible occurrence of thrombocytopenia. Fetal growth rate then slows, usually after 15, most often at 25, gestational weeks. Prospective monitoring reveals, in succession, nonreactive fetal heart rate testing, diminished fetal motion, diminished amniotic fluid, diminished placental size, spontaneous bradycardia, and if delivery does not take place, fetal death. During the course of these events, the mother, whether or not she has SLE, demonstrates no evidence of illness other than thrombocytopenia.

The likelihood that fetal death will occur is directly related to the titer of IgG anticardiolipin antibody and to maternal history of prior fetal death.[94] Women with SLE, anticardiolipin antibody greater than 80 GPL units, and a prior fetal death have an 73% probability of having current fetal death (see Table 11–7). Lupus anticoagulant is usually not titered, but there is a correlation between strength of anticoagulant measured by seconds in the chosen clotting test and probability of fetal death. Prognosis does not necessarily improve if the anticoagulant activity is corrected since, with treatment, lupus anticoagulant often returns to normal but anticardiolipin antibody does not.

In addition to fetal death, prematurity and/or intrauterine growth retardation occur in this syndrome. While there appear to be no formal follow-up studies of infant survivors of antiphospholipid antibody syndrome, informal surveys suggest that except for the known sequelae of growth-retarded and premature infants of any cause, these children develop normally.

The pathogenesis of this syndrome is

not known. Occlusive, vasculopathy, due to placental intraluminal thrombosis or to endothelial cell proliferation, has been suggested.[154–158] Placental infarcts have been recorded but do not invariably occur. Placentas are usually very small for fetal size. Other placental lesions have been described in patients with SLE[159, 160] because in earlier studies SLE and antiphospholipid antibody syndrome were not distinguished. Whether these lesions also are characteristic of antiphospholipid antibody syndrome is unknown.

Management of the Antiphospholipid Antibody Syndrome

Maternal Management.—Maternal monitoring consists of measuring platelet count, lupus anticoagulant, and anticardiolipin antibody in early pregnancy. In women with strongly positive tests, repetition of the last two is unnecessary, since decrease in titer does not permit relaxation of vigilance. In women with low titer or negative tests, repetition at least once each trimester is useful, since an occasional patient demonstrates an increasingly abnormal test as pregnancy progresses, and the overall prognosis is that of the highest titer seen during the pregnancy.[93–96, 147–151] Even when initially normal, the platelet count should be repeated monthly, since thrombocytopenia may occur at any time.

The best treatment of the mother with high-titer antiphospholipid antibody has not been firmly established. Since IgM and low-titer IgG anticardiolipin antibody are not as a rule associated with poor fetal outcome, there is a strong argument for closely monitoring and against arbitrarily treating women with antibodies with these characteristics. A biologic false-positive test for syphilis, in the absence of IgG anticardiolipin antibody and in the absence of lupus anticoagulant is not associated with increased fetal risk, and need not be treated. Since primiparas and women with prior liveborn children even with high-titer antiphospholipid antibody have an approximately 50% probability of having a live-born child, there is also a strong argument for close monitoring without treatment of these women. Since first-trimester miscarriages have many causes, and second-trimester fetal deaths are more characteristic of antiphospholipid antibody syndrome than are first-trimester losses, the argument for treating women who have lost only first-trimester pregnancies is not compelling. However, a consensus panel convened to design and interpret therapeutic trials has recently suggested that treatment be offered to those with high titer antiphospholipid antibody (>35 GPL units/mL) or lupus anticoagulant and a history of second- or third-trimester fetal death not attributable to other causes.

Three forms of treatment have been proposed (Table 11–8), and are reviewed in reference 94. In reports describing limited numbers of patients, prednisone, 40 to 60 mg/day, was credited with achieving liveborn results in women with lupus anticoagulant and prior fetal deaths. These studies were uncontrolled, have included growth-retarded and premature infants as "successes," and permitted concomitant aspirin therapy. Aspirin, 80 to 300 mg/day, or aspirin plus prednisone (varying doses) also has its strong advocates. In one large but uncontrolled experience comparing aspirin and prednisone in women with high-titer IgG anticardiolipin antibody and prior fetal loss, aspirin improved fetal prognosis only slightly, whereas high-dose prednisone seemed to worsen it.[94] The explanation for the latter was the high frequency of preeclampsia in prednisone-treated patients. Aspirin therapy may prevent both preeclampsia and recurrent intrauterine growth retardation (see Chap. 1). Many physicians recommend that aspirin be continued for 1 month post partum, as prophylaxis for the potential complication of thrombosis, although this is unproven. Some physicians also prescribe dipyridamole (FDA category C), 25 mg four times daily, with aspirin, but there are no good data on the risks and benefits of this therapy and therefore we advise against routine use of this drug. Subcutaneous heparin, approximately 10,000 units twice daily, has

TABLE 11–8.
Treatment Recommendations for Pregnant Women With APL Antibody*†

Patient	Recommendation
High-titer APL antibody (IgG >40 GPL units)	
Primipara	No therapy initially; if thrombocytopenia occurs, aspirin, 80 mg/day
Multipara, most recent prior pregnancy liveborn	No therapy initially; if thrombocytopenia occurs, aspirin, 80 mg/day
Multipara, most recent prior pregnancy failure <15 wk	No therapy initially; if thrombocytopenia occurs, aspirin, 80 mg/day
Multipara, most recent prior pregnancy failure ≥15 wk without other explanation	Aspirin, 80 mg/day, starting after pregnancy confirmed
	or
	Aspirin, 80 mg/day, starting after pregnancy confirmed, plus prednisone, 15 mg b.i.d. to be tapered after 4 wk or as clinical condition indicates
	or
	Aspirin, 80 mg/day, for weeks 1–16, then subcutaneous heparin, 10,000 units b.i.d. for weeks 17–36, then aspirin, 80 mg/day
Low-titer APL antibody (IgG 16–40 GPL units)	
Primipara	No therapy
Multipara, no prior fetal loss	No therapy
Multipara, prior fetal loss, pre-eclampsia, or intra-uterine growth retardation	Aspirin, 80 mg/day, starting after pregnancy confirmed
Normal APL antibody (IgG <16 GPL units)	
Primipara	No therapy
Multipara, prior pre-eclampsia	Aspirin, 80 mg/day, starting after pregnancy confirmed
Multipara, all others	No therapy indicated by APL antibody

*From Lockshin MD, Qamar T, Levy R: Anticardiolipin and related antibodies, thrombosis and fetal death, in Scott JS, Bird HA (eds): *Pregnancy, Auto-immunity and Connective Tissue Disorders.* Oxford, England, Oxford University Press, 1990, pp 204–205. Used with permission.
†These suggestions have been made by different investigators in experimental protocols. No single therapy has been proven successful.

also been used, but again there are no defin-itive data regarding the effectiveness of this therapy, although several controlled treat-ment trials of its use were in progress in 1989. In the United States warfarin sodium (FDA category D) (Coumadin) is considered to be teratogenic and should not be used in preg-nancy, though it may be used post partum.

Fetal Management.—Monitoring of fe-tal growth and development, as outlined for patients with SLE, is essential. Identification of slowing fetal growth or other abnormalities is indication for pharmacologic intervention, and, for viable infants, to deliver when fetal distress is clearly identified. There are no spe-cial fetal risks other than those of prematurity and growth retardation. Premature closure of the ductus arteriosus is a theoretical concern in infants of aspirin-treated women but it has not been reported. Choice of route of delivery is determined by standard obstetric criteria, including maternal and fetal platelet count.

Breast-Feeding and Counseling

There are no published reports regarding breast-feeding in women with antiphospho-lipid antibody syndrome. Since many of live-born infants are premature or growth-re-tarded, breast-feeding is often impossible. Those that have been able to breast-feed have done so uneventfully.

Since both oral contraceptives and anti-phospholipid antibody syndrome are associ-ated with a high frequency of vascular oc-clusive events, it is unwise to prescribe oral contraceptives to patients with antiphospho-lipid antibody. Those electing an early preg-nancy termination should receive prophylactic aspirin, 80 to 300 mg/day for 1 month post partum.

Antiphospholipid antibody is a familial phenomenon;[161] the frequency of a rheumatic illness, such as SLE, in family members is high. Women with antiphospholipid antibody may have an unusual frequency of HLA-DR7 or the C4 null allele. There are no known

genetic fetal abnormalities associated with antiphospholipid antibody.

Most studies indicating that antiphos-pholipid antibody has high risk for throm-bosis or fetal death have begun with the event (thrombosis or prior fetal death) or diagnosis (SLE) and measured the antibody; cross-sec-tional studies of populations suggest much lower risks.[65–68] Prospective studies indicate that the occurrence of a vascular event cannot be predicted by changes in antibody titer.[162] Discussion of these uncertainties is appropri-ate, since both parents may have strong feel-ings about suggested therapies. They should be told that there are as yet no prospective studies which provide firm estimates of risks except perhaps for that of fetal death, nor are there good estimates of the likelihood that the patient will eventually develop SLE. There are no known risks to the surviving infant beyond those of prematurity and/or intra-uterine growth retardation.

MIXED CONNECTIVE TISSUE DISEASE, UNDIFFERENTIATED CONNECTIVE TISSUE DISEASE, AND FORME FRUSTE SLE

An important proportion of patients sus-pected of having SLE do not fulfill clinical (at least four American Rheumatism Association criteria)[59] or serologic criteria (anti-native DNA or anti-Sm antibody) for SLE.[163–166] Most of these patients have some of the non-specific SLE symptoms of arthritis, serositis, fever, lymphadenopathy, or Raynaud's phe-nomenon, but usually do not have the specific SLE symptoms of butterfly rash or glomer-ulonephritis. They often have cytopenias and positive antinuclear antibody tests. Although by definition they do not have anti-DNA or anti-Sm antibodies, they may have anti-sin-gle-stranded DNA, anti-Ro, anti-La, anti-RNP, or antibodies directed against other cy-toplasmic or nuclear antigens. Patients with sclerodactyly, Raynaud's phenomenon, pleu-risy, and myositis who have extremely high-titer antibody to RNP and who do not have anti-DNA or anti-Sm have mixed connective tissue disease (MCTD). Patients with similar overlapping features of SLE, scleroderma, and dermatomyositis who do not have anti-RNP, or who have insufficient other features to allow a definitive diagnosis, have undifferentiated connective tissue disease (UCTD). Persons with miscellaneous nonspecific symptoms and livedo reticularis, recurrent thromboses, recurrent fetal death, and thrombocytopenia, who have lupus anticoagulant and/or anticardiolipin antibody have the antiphospholipid antibody syndrome (see above). None of these syndromes is static; over time each may evolve into classic SLE or into another connective tissue disease.

Pregnancy

Although there are case reports or small series regarding pregnancy and MCTD or UCTD, there is no organized body of literature on this topic. Patients with any of these syndromes may carry anti-Ro/La antibodies or antiphospholipid antibodies. For these reasons patients with MCTD or UCTD must be monitored through pregnancy in a manner similar to that appropriate for a patient with classic SLE. Treatment is directed to the organ systems involved, not to the specific diagnosis, and is similar to that used for SLE. Similarly, counseling is that relevant to SLE.

SJÖGREN'S SYNDROME

The Sjögren's syndrome symptom complex consists of parotid hypertrophy, lacrimal hypertrophy, keratoconjunctivitis sicca, and xerostomia. Sjögren's syndrome may exist without a complicating connective tissue disease (primary) or with any of the defined connective tissue diseases (secondary). Diagnosis is established by biopsy of a lacrimal or salivary gland, or by demonstration of keratitis sicca by standard ophthalmologic techniques. Typically, patients with Sjögren's syndrome have many immunologic abnormalities, including antinuclear antibody and rheumatoid

factor. Approximately 70% of patients with Sjögren's syndrome have anti-Ro (SSA [Sjögren's syndrome-A]) and anti-La (SSB [Sjögren's syndrome-B]) antibodies. Treatment for the symptoms of Sjögren's syndrome itself, independent of pregnancy, includes nonsteroidal anti-inflammatory drugs, corticosteroids, and topical artificial tears and artificial saliva. Patients with primary Sjögren's syndrome are prone to develop malignant lymphoma.

Pregnancy

Management of gestation in patients with secondary Sjögren's syndrome is not different from that of the accompanying connective tissue disease. For patients with primary Sjögren's syndrome treatment is not altered by the presence of pregnancy. It is important to determine anti-Ro/La antibodies in any pregnant patient with Sjögren's syndrome, and to anticipate neonatal lupus in those found to be positive. As for all patients with collagen-vascular disease, since the risk for congenital heart block in patients negative for anti-Ro/La or anti-RNP antibodies is very small, it is not necessary to fetal echocardiography on patients with negative tests. Nevertheless, there is a clinical suspicion, but no definitive data, that indicates that Sjögren's patients are more likely than are other anti-Ro antibody-positive patients to deliver children with neonatal lupus.[167] Counseling should reflect these objectives.

RHEUMATOID ARTHRITIS

Rheumatoid arthritis is defined by its major characteristic: chronic, inflammatory, destructive, symmetric arthritis. Sustained joint inflammation for at least 3 months is required to make the diagnosis. The disease occurs at any age, but has its most common onset in the twenties to forties. Women predominate among patients by approximately 2:1. All races are affected equally. The disease is familial; HLA-DR4 is commonly present.[35]

The clinical pattern of rheumatoid arthritis is less variable than that of SLE. Most commonly, onset is insidious. The disease has periods of remission and periods of exacerbation. The joints show proliferative synovitis; erosions of cartilage and subchondral bone occur, leading to permanent deformity. Chronic arthritis of the hips or knees is most likely to affect obstetric care.

Rheumatoid arthritis is a systemic disease. Weight loss, fatigue, and lymphadenopathy are frequent. A minority of patients develop subcutaneous nodules. Serious visceral disease is rare and occurs late. It includes pulmonary fibrosis, pleuropericarditis, neuropathy, and vasculitis. A minority of patients with rheumatoid arthritis develop severe crippling illness.

The laboratory abnormalities include a modest anemia, moderate leukocytosis, and almost invariably an elevated erythrocyte sedimentation rate. Approximately 80% of patients have a moderate to strongly positive test for rheumatoid factor, but this test is frequently also positive in other collagen diseases and in infectious illnesses. The diagnosis of rheumatoid arthritis is a clinical diagnosis which may be supported by the laboratory; the diagnosis is never made by the laboratory alone. The cause of rheumatoid arthritis is unknown. Treatment of rheumatoid arthritis includes nonsteroidal anti-inflammatory drugs in full doses, remission-inducing agents such as the gold compounds, penicillamine, hydroxychloroquine, and methotrexate; low-dose corticosteroid; and immunosuppressive agents such as azathioprine or cyclophosphamide. Joint replacement and other orthopedic procedures are frequently performed.

Pregnancy

Patients with rheumatoid arthritis frequently experience amelioration of their illness during pregnancy. Explanations for this phenomenon include the increased production of endogenous corticosteroid, pregnancy-associated plasma protein A (PAPP-A), and other products. Improvement of illness during pregnancy occurs in approximately two thirds of all rheumatoid patients and about half of the patients suffer exacerbations post partum.[55, 168–174]

There are no special risks to the fetus other than those related to maternal therapy. It is controversial whether patients with rheumatoid arthritis have excessive fetal wastage.[54, 55, 167, 168] Some but not all retrospective studies suggest a higher-than-normal frequency of pregnancy loss even before the clinical appearance of the illness.[168–170] Low-titer antiphospholipid antibody occurs in patients with rheumatoid arthritis but there has been no excess fetal wastage attributed to it. Anti-Ro antibody also occurs, but much less frequently than in SLE patients. Detailed information about risk of neonatal lupus in children of patients with rheumatoid arthritis is not available; since rheumatoid arthritis is primarily associated with HLA-DR4, and the risk of neonatal lupus is increased in children of women with HLA-DR3, the risk is likely very low. Management of the pregnancy, and counseling of the parents, can therefore be optimistic, cautious, and expectant.

Management During Pregnancy.—The articular disease of rheumatoid arthritis is best managed by the patient's rheumatologist. Since cervical spine disease, especially C1–2 subluxation, is common, a particular concern is the potential for worsening of preexisting atlantoaxial subluxation during the period of late pregnancy when ligaments loosen. Joint infection during bacteremia related to labor is another concern.

Management of arthritis during pregnancy is compromised by the potential fetal toxicity of gold, penicillamine, hydroxychloroquine, methotrexate, azathioprine, and cyclophosphamide. Of these, gold (FDA category C), hydroxychloroquine, and azathioprine have been used during pregnancy without apparent ill effect, but published experience is small. Cyclophosphamide and methotrexate (FDA category D) are highly teratogenic and contraindicated during pregnancy unless the mother's life is in jeopardy.

Aspirin and low-dose corticosteroid may be used with little fear of fetal injury. There are no specific hazards known regarding other nonsteroidal anti-inflammatory drugs, but little experience has accumulated regarding their use in pregnancy (see Table 11–9).

Before delivery the team managing the patient must take special care to identify the patient's disabilities joint by joint. It is important that the patient's rheumatologist or orthopedist review with the obstetrician and nurses the range of motion and permissible activities of the rheumatoid patient during labor. Points for special emphasis are hip and knee range of motion and the potential risks of forcible flexion and extension of the neck. Temporomandibular arthritis may prevent wide opening of the mouth. If motion of the neck, hips, or knees is markedly restricted, elective cesarean section may be necessary. If intubation is planned, an anesthesiologist familiar with managing a patient with neck and temporomandibular arthritis must be available.

Breast-feeding is usually possible, but arthritis of the shoulders, elbows, hands, and wrists may cause considerable discomfort for the mother. Normal handling of a young child may be severely compromised by maternal arthritis.

ANKYLOSING SPONDYLITIS AND OTHER HLA-B27 SPONDYLOARTHRITIS

Ankylosing spondylitis, Reiter's syndrome, and other illnesses associated with HLA-B27 have extreme (>90%) male predominance. Very little information is available regarding pregnancies in women with these diseases.[173] Their predominant manifestations are lower extremity, sacroiliac, hip, and spinal inflammatory arthritis. Many patients have concomitant inflammatory eye disease, most typically anterior uveitis. Inflammatory aortitis occurs in severe cases. Pain and restricted motion of the hips and lower back are typical.

Patients with ankylosing spondylitis have normal fertility. Other than the specific anatomic problems that might restrict delivery, they have no known unusual problems with pregnancy.[173]

PROGRESSIVE SYSTEMIC SCLEROSIS (SCLERODERMA)

Progressive systemic sclerosis (PSS) is rarer than the preceding illnesses. It also has female predominance (3:1) and is familial. Its onset is often between the ages of 20 and 40 years. Its first symptom is usually severe Raynaud's phenomenon (90% of patients). Later, edema of the hands, feet, or face occurs, then tightening of the skin of the affected areas. Usually the changes are gradual; occasionally they are abrupt. Some groups have suggested that fertility is reduced before the onset of PSS, but other studies deny that this occurs.[55, 50, 170, 175]

Although the skin is the most obvious organ involved, visceral disease may be prominent. Most common is pulmonary fibrosis. Esophageal dysmotility, duodenal and jejunal dilatation, cardiac arrhythmia, pulmonary hypertension (with or without pulmonary fibrosis), myositis, and, uncommonly, an abrupt hyperreninemic, hypertensive, oliguric renal failure, also occur. Prognosis of PSS is dictated by the visceral disease. Occurrence of cardiac or renal involvement frequently predicts death within a few months to years. Pulmonary hypertension is rare but devastating when it occurs. Patients with a variant of PSS, called CREST syndrome (for *c*alcinosis, *R*aynaud's, *e*sophageal dysmotility, *s*clerodactyly [scleroderma limited to the fingers as opposed to proximal or central scleroderma], and *t*elangiectasia), develop pulmonary hypertension late in the course of the illness, but have little other visceral disease, and thus have a generally good prognosis. Mixed connective tissue disease frequently evolves into PSS.

The primary lesion in PSS is not clearly known, but intimal proliferation of vascular beds of affected areas is prominent. Most patients have vasospasm and in vasospastic states they tolerate fluid loads poorly. Their inability to handle fluid loads poses the greatest threat to pregnancy management. Intense Raynaud's phenomenon, hypertension, or any degree of renal insufficiency, is an important clue to this problem.

The diagnosis is clinical, supported by the laboratory. Skin biopsy shows perivascular inflammatory infiltrate and collagen deposition. Most patients have a positive test for antinuclear antibody, usually occurring in a speckled or nucleolar pattern. A majority of patients have antibody to Scl-70 (topoisomerase I). Patients with the CREST variant often have anticentromere antibody. An important proportion of patients with Raynaud's phenomenon have mild PSS, not easily recognizable on casual examination. These patients usually lead normal lives and do not develop important visceral disease.

There is no effective treatment for PSS. Vasodilators, d-penicillamine, and immunosuppressive drugs are sometimes used. Except for patients with inflammatory myositis or hemolytic anemia, corticosteroids are seldom useful. Angiotensin converting enzyme inhibitors are lifesaving in patients with renal crisis. By reducing intravascular fluid volume, diuretics increase renin secretion and may precipitate renal crisis in patients with PSS. They can also cause a lethal decrease in cardiac output in patients with pulmonary hypertension.

Pregnancy

A small literature suggests that patients with recognized PSS do not tolerate pregnancy well.[58, 175, 176] The problems they encounter are related to their nondistensible vascular beds and to renal, cardiac, and pulmonary insufficiency. Severe preeclampsia, congestive heart failure, pulmonary hypertension, pulmonary insufficiency, and renal insufficiency may occur in the mother and prematurity in the newborn. One must note that renal crisis, pericarditis, pulmonary hy-

pertension, and cardiac arrhythmias are prognostically poor signs in patients with PSS.[177, 178] Although unusual, these may occur in pregnant patients and may be lethal.

Management focuses on individual organ system capacities. Intolerance of PSS patients to large fluid volumes must be anticipated. Wound healing is normal despite cutaneous fibrosis, so cesarean section can be performed without incident. Intubation may be complicated by the small opening of the mouth characteristic of PSS patients. Esophageal dysmotility and reflux esophagitis are very common in gravidas with PSS. The latter is treated in the standard ways: small meals, elevating the head of the bed, and antacids. H_2-blocking agent may also be necessary.[179] If esophageal stricture occurs, dilatation may be warranted.

Counseling.—There are no special caveats other than the above risks to pregnancy in patients with PSS if they are not taking D-penicillamine, chlorambucil (both FDA category D), or other drugs that may have adverse fetal effects. These women, however, must be told that due to an anecdotal literature of sudden and unanticipated lethal problems (see above), some authorities proscribe pregnancy. No matter how mild their current symptoms, they must be followed closely in a high risk center if they conceive. There is a low risk of PSS or other collagen diseases in family members, but no special problems identified in neonates of women with PSS. Furthermore, the progressive nature of PSS and the likelihood of progressive disability should be considered in giving advice to the family.

DERMATOMYOSITIS

This is a rare affliction characterized by inflammatory myositis with (dermato-) or without (poly-) a specific skin rash involving the eyes, forehead, shoulders, upper arms, and periungual areas. Female predominance is the rule. There is a bimodal distribution of age of onset: childhood to 25 years of age, and 50 years and greater. In older but not in younger patients malignancies are frequently associated with dermatomyositis/polymyositis. The disease is chronic, with remissions and relapses. Progressive proximal muscle weakness is the rule. Pulmonary fibrosis is the commonest visceral manifestation; weakness of the muscles of the upper airway sometimes leads to aspiration or respiratory failure, a particular danger in late pregnancy.

In active disease, the laboratory shows elevated muscle enzymes; creatine kinase and aspartate aminotransferase abnormalities are most prominent. Muscle enzymes do not reflect muscle strength: there may be profound weakness with trivially abnormal or normal chemical tests. To monitor a patient, direct testing of the strength of relevant muscle groups must be done serially. Electromyography may show muscle irritability in a myositic pattern. Skin and muscle biopsy may show characteristic inflammatory changes and muscle necrosis. Antinuclear antibody may be positive, and there may be demonstrable autoantibodies to a specific antigen known as Jo-1. Corticosteroids, usually in high doses, and immunosuppressive agents, especially methotrexate, are the basic forms of treatment. Withdrawal of therapy frequently leads to relapse.

Pregnancy

Gravid women with dermatomyositis experience problems related to their specific organ system disabilities, and often have nonspecifically complicated pregnancies. The literature related to pregnancy in this illness consists of case reports cited in a referenced review.[180] Muscle fatigue and respiratory impairment are the greatest dangers for the pregnant patient. Unlike patients with myasthenia gravis, patients with dermatomyositis have no pathogenic autoantibody that crosses the placenta and causes muscle weakness in the fetus. Pulmonary fibrosis may compromise respiratory reserve, especially in late pregnancy. There are few definitive data, but uterine muscle may theoretically be weak,

though anecdotally this has not proved to be the case. Muscle strength and pulmonary function must be repeatedly monitored during pregnancy and delivery. Maternal fatigue or respiratory embarrassment should be anticipated. Monitoring of serum levels of muscle enzymes is of lesser importance.

The risk to the fetus is that of the mother's therapy and of the complications she suffers during pregnancy. Because the disease is rare and variable in severity, specific management, counseling, and breast-feeding decisions must be ad hoc in most instances.

VASCULITIS

Clinical vasculitis syndromes constitute rare forms of inflammatory connective tissue diseases. Little literature or experience has accumulated regarding pregnancy in women with these illnesses. Of the many forms of vasculitis, because of the demography of the illnesses, five types are most likely to be encountered.

Leukocytoclastic Vasculitis

Leukocytoclastic vasculitis (cutaneous vasculitis, palpable purpura) occurs in young women and is often associated with another systemic rheumatic disease (most characteristically Sjögren's syndrome or cryoglobulinemia). Leukocytoclastic vasculitis also occurs in several chronic infectious diseases, most notably chronic gonococcemia and bacterial endocarditis. These diagnoses must be considered in patients with leukocytoclastic vasculitis, but they are uncommon causes. Leukocytoclastic vasculitis not associated with infection generally runs an indolent course, and causes recurrent outbreaks of purpuric lesions or cutaneous ulcers on the lower legs. Patients frequently have myalgias and fatigue. Visceral manifestations include peripheral neuropathy and slowly progressive glomerulonephritis. The latter manifestation is characterized by hematuria, proteinuria, and, over years, gradual diminution of creatinine clearance. Hypocomplementemia is frequent. Although corticosteroids, antimalarial drugs, colchicine, and occasionally plasmapheresis are prescribed, the course of the illness is not markedly altered by treatment. There is no published experience concerning pregnancy and leukocytoclastic vasculitis. In our personal experience the indolent nature of the illness has resulted in uneventful pregnancies. Hypocomplementemia with mild glomerulonephritis occurred in some cases.

Takayasu Arteritis

Takayasu arteritis is a rare disease of inflammatory arteritis of the aorta and great vessels; the brachiocephalic arteries are more commonly involved than are the lower extremity vessels. Renal artery involvement and ensuing renovascular hypertension is also common. The rare pulmonary and coronary artery involvement is potentially life-threatening. Symptoms and physical findings reflect alternating constriction and aneurysmal dilatation of affected vessels. Pulselessness is common, as is hypertension and aortic insufficiency (due to valve root dilatation). Patients often present with signs or symptoms of vascular occlusion: transient ischemic cerebral symptoms, arm or leg claudication, or incidental discovery of an absent pulse. A small proportion have symptoms of an inflammatory collagen disease at onset: severe myalgias, fever, and elevated erythrocyte sedimentation rate. Tuberculosis is frequently associated with Takayasu arteritis. Measurement of blood pressure is particularly difficult since hypertension measured in the right arm may be normotension in the cerebral vessels and hypotension in the left arm or pelvic circulation, depending on the specific anatomy of the patient's disease. Thus the diagnosis of preeclampsia based on conventional blood pressure measurement may be inordinately difficult.

Diagnosis is most often made by imaging the great vessels. Angiography is the gold standard for diagnosis, but magnetic resonance imaging can suffice for both diagnosis and staging. Occasionally a surgical biopsy first indicates the diagnosis. In patients with inflammatory signs of active disease, prednisone is the primary therapy. An occasional nonresponding patient may enter remission with cyclophosphamide. Many patients are able to discontinue therapy after a few months to years. In the absence of inflammation the presence of vascular deformities does not justify treatment; return of absent pulses is rare.

There is a small experience with pregnancy in women with Takayasu arteritis.[181–185] They do reasonably well, but renovascular occlusive disease, pulmonary hypertension, and cardiac insufficiency remain as important problems. Strict attention to monitoring the patient's cerebral and uterine circulation is important. Babies do not appear to suffer any special problems.

Polyarteritis Nodosa

Polyarteritis nodosa is a rare, frequently fatal, disease, most commonly found in older men, but occasionally seen in young women. Its onset is usually abrupt, with severe myalgias, fever, visceral or digital infarction, and mononeuritis multiplex. A minority of patients have evidence of recent hepatitis B infection and persistent hepatitis B surface antigenemia. Diagnosis is made by muscle biopsy, which demonstrates necrotizing arteritis, or by angiography, which demonstrates small aneurysms. With treatment with corticosteroid and (on occasion) cyclophosphamide, approximately half the patients undergo remission. Most of the remaining patients die within the first year of illness. The end-organ damage suffered during active disease remains when patients enter remission. Renal insufficiency and hypertension are the most frequently encountered late residua.

Pregnancy.—Other than rare case reports of polyarteritis nodosa in pregnancy,[186, 187] there is little information about gestation in women with this disease. Still, because of an anecdotal literature documenting maternal demise, especially when renal involvement and hypertension are present, many counsel women with this disease against conceiving. In any event close scrutiny at a high-risk center is warranted for gravidas with polyarteritis nodosa.

Wegener's Granulomatosis

Wegener's granulomatosis is a rare illness that occurs in limited (upper and lower airway disease) and in generalized form (upper and lower airway disease, glomerulonephritis, and systemic necrotizing vasculitis). Its histopathology, which is required for diagnosis, is granulomatous necrotizing vasculitis. Tuberculosis, fungal infections, lymphomatoid granulomatosis, and sarcoidosis present similar pathologic findings and must be excluded. Wegener's granulomatosis occurs most frequently after the age of 50 and has a slight male predominance. Like other collagen diseases, Wegener's granulomatosis has remissions and exacerbations. Potentially rapidly lethal, Wegener's granulomatosis may be controlled, but not cured, with the combination of prednisone and cyclophosphamide. Infectious complications of the lungs and upper airways are common in patients with chronic illness. Marked deformity of the nasal bridge, and tracheal and bronchial stenosis, are late sequelae.

Pregnancy.—There is very little experience with pregnancy in this illness. Because of the frequent use of cyclophosphamide and the potential for rapidly progressive renal failure, pregnancy should be discouraged. Although a mild exacerbation may be controlled with prednisone, if the patient rapidly deteriorates during pregnancy, cyclophosphamide should be administered despite the pregnancy because the potential for maternal death is very high. There is no substantial literature on the effect of this illness on the fetus.

Erythema Nodosum

Erythema nodosum is a common, benign form of inflammatory illness that resembles but is not a true vasculitis. It has abrupt onset, with striking swelling about the feet and ankles and characteristic painful, raised nodules on the lower leg that evolve and subside as bruises without scarring over several days to a few weeks. Erythema nodosum may be triggered by infections, drugs, certain diseases, and possibly pregnancy (erythema nodosum gravidarum). In developed countries the most common infectious organisms that trigger erythema nodosum are the streptococcus, tubercle bacillus, and *Histoplasma* and *Coccidioides* organisms. Oral contraceptives are prominent among the drugs that induce erythema nodosum.

Noninfectious diseases that induce erythema nodosum are sarcoidosis, ulcerative colitis, and regional enteritis involving the colon. Nonsteroidal anti-inflammatory medications are effective therapy in most cases; severe cases may respond to low-dose corticosteroid therapy. Treatment of an inciting infection or removal of an identified trigger agent is mandatory. Recovery is complete. There is no known harm to the fetus in pregnancies of women with erythema nodosum. Management and counseling focus on the search for a treatable cause.

MISCELLANEOUS RHEUMATIC OR CONNECTIVE TISSUE DISEASES

Inborn Errors of Collagen Metabolism

Marfan's syndrome is an autosomal dominant illness characterized by elongated extremities, lenticular dislocation, scoliosis, mitral valve prolapse, and tendency to sudden death due to cardiac arrhythmia or aortic aneurysm dissection, or rupture. The physical defects associated with Marfan's syndrome resemble those of homocystinuria. Management consists of extremely tight control of blood pressure and avoidance of strenuous Valsalva maneuvers to protect against aortic dissection. Antibiotic prophylaxis for cardiac valvular disease is appropriate[188, 189] (see Chap. 5, p. 159). Elective cesarean section may be appropriate.

The Ehlers-Danlos syndromes consist of any of several inborn abnormalities of collagen synthesis. Depending on the specific abnormality, patients have recurrent joint dislocations or thin, easily tearing skin. Risks in pregnancy are those of joint dislocation and, very rarely, uterine rupture. In both illnesses there is likelihood that the fetus will be affected.[190] Since Marfan's syndrome is autosomal dominant, half of the infants will be affected, but Ehlers-Danlos consists of several different syndromes, which are autosomal dominant, autosomal recessive, or X-linked, variable penetrance being the rule. Specific predictions about the fetus cannot be made unless the biochemical lesion in the mother has been defined.[190]

Congenital and Other Hip Disease

Hip disease of any kind may interfere with normal delivery. In a woman with abnormal hips, abduction or external rotation may be extremely painful or impossible. Forcing these motions may cause dislocation or fracture. Antibiotic prophylaxis during delivery is necessary for patients with total joint replacements. The regimen used in 1989 at the Hospital for Special Surgery (New York) was gentamicin 1.5 mg/kg (maximum 80 mg), every 8 hours in two doses, plus ampicillin, 2 g every 8 hours in two doses, both commencing 30 to 60 minutes prior to delivery.

Back Pain, Sciatica, and Other Nerve Compression Syndromes

The common causes of back pain in young women include soft tissue "sprains," intervertebral disc ruptures, and spondylolisthesis. The altered body mechanics of pregnancy frequently cause exacerbation of a previously present abnormality. In collagen disease patients taking corticosteroids, osteoporotic vertebral collapse is another possible cause. Inflammatory spondylitis (Reiter's disease and ankylosing spondylitis) is rare in women. Labor and delivery may be complicated post partum by infectious sacroiliitis. Rarely seen by obstetricians, infectious sacroiliitis or osteitis pubis most commonly occurs after genitourinary manipulation and recent parturition is one of many associated preceding events.[191]

Uncomplicated low back pain consists of sharp pain in the lumbar area, clearly related to movement, often absent at rest. Unlike inflammatory spondylitis, mechanical forms of back pain worsen with activity. First episodes in young people usually subside spontaneously within days to weeks. Subsequent episodes are more prolonged. With lateral disc ruptures or severe spondylolisthesis, nerve root compression causing pain, paresthesias, or motor weakness in a sciatic or more localized distribution may occur. Examination demonstrates lumbar paravertebral muscle spasm. Sensory and motor examination may demonstrate localized nerve injury. Radiographic studies of the spine (anteroposterior, lateral and oblique lumbar spine films, myelography, computed tomography), helpful in assessing the problem, should not under most circumstances be done in the pregnant patient. Magnetic resonance imaging easily outlines disc herniation. Its safety in pregnancy is not yet certain (see Chap. 18).

If there is no motor impairment, appropriate treatment is analgesics, heating pads to the back, and bed rest. Back exercises, routinely prescribed for nonpregnant patients, are awkward and uncomfortable to perform in late pregnancy. If motor nerve impairment is present, surgical intervention is usually necessary. In preparation for surgery, for protection of the fetus, magnetic resonance imaging is preferable to computed tomography. Because of the risks, detailed consultation with appropriate specialists, and with the patient and her spouse, is required.

Occasional patients may suffer pain along the lateral thigh, radiating to the knee, markedly worsened by walking or by abduction of the leg against gravity. They have marked tenderness over the greater femoral trochanter. Such patients most commonly suffer trochanteric bursitis. In most acute cases this is easily handled with intrabursal injection of a corticosteroid preparation. In patients with chronic pain, or who refuse injection, analgesic medication may suffice. Dysesthetic pain in the medial thigh and occasionally lower abdomen may be due to meralgia paresthetica, another form of nerve root compression.[192] This frequently subsides after delivery. Analgesic medication is appropriate. Carpal tunnel syndrome is also common in pregnancy.[193] Mild cases can be treated with resting splints; injection of a corticosteroid preparation into the wrist and/or carpal tunnel is an alternative or subsequent treatment. Since the syndrome frequently subsides after delivery, carpal tunnel release is a last-resort form of therapy for the pregnant patient. Sur-

gical release is always indicated, however, if there is thenar atrophy or weakness of thumb adduction.

DRUG THERAPY OF RHEUMATIC DISEASE DURING PREGNANCY

Many patients with rheumatic disease must continue their regular medications during pregnancy. Table 11–9 provides guidelines to the commonly used drugs.[169, 194] (See also the Preface for the FDA pregnancy risk classification and a discussion of pharmacologic therapy during gestation.)

TABLE 11–9.
Drug Therapy of Rheumatic Disease During Pregnancy

Drug	Safety	FDA Risk Category*	Comments
Aspirin[†]	C/D[‡]	Variable; depends on dose and time of use	May be protective against fetal death in antiphospholipid antibody syndrome; may cause maternal and fetal bleeding if administered near term; high dose (sufficient for treatment of arthritis) probably safe; low dose may be protective against preeclampsia
Naproxen[†] and ibuprofen[†]	B/D[‡]	Variable; depends on dose and time of use	Experience largely accumulated through treatment of headache; no major teratogenicity noted
Indomethacin[†]	B/D[‡]	Variable; depends on dose and time of use	Rare cases of fetal pulmonary hypertension
Prednisone	B	Appears safe	Trivial passage across placenta; safe in lactation but may suppress milk production
Methylprednisolone	B	Probably safe	Similar to prednisone, but fewer data available
Dexamethasone	C	Probably safe	Important transfer across placenta; used to induce fetal lung maturation
Betamethasone	C	Probably safe	Similar to dexamethasone
Hydroxychloroquine	?	Questionable safety	Small published experience indicating safety but theoretical risk of fetal eye damage
Azathioprine	D	Safety uncertain	Large experience with renal transplant patients indicates no immediate danger to offspring if maternal dose is <2 mg/kg/day; rare reports of multiple abnormalities including immunodeficiencies
Cyclophosphamide	D	Dangerous	Abortifacient; highly teratogenic; use only when felt to be lifesaving
Chlorambucil	D	Dangerous	Similar to cyclophosphamide
Heparin	B[§]	Appears to be safe	Anticoagulant of choice; usually given SC twice daily; dose control essential for safety; unclear risk of maternal osteoporosis
Warfarin	D	Teratogenic and possibly fetotoxic	Fetal warfarin syndrome when given in 1st trimester; may cause CNS defects when used in 2nd/3rd trimesters; risk of severe neonatal hemorrhage when given near term

*See the Preface for a discussion of the FDA pregnancy risk classification.
[†]All inhibitors of prostaglandin synthetase activity may inhibit labor and prolong gestation. There is also a risk of in utero closure of the ductus arteriosus, particularly when used after the 34th gestational week.
[‡]Risk category D when used in the third trimester.
[§]Assigned by editors.

REFERENCES

1. Clapp JF, Seaward BL, Sleamaker RH, et al: Maternal physiologic adaptations to early human pregnancy. *Am J Obstet Gynecol* 1988; 159:1456–1460.

2. Artherton JC, Green R: Renal function in pregnancy (editorial). *Clin Sci* 1983; 65:449–455.

3. Lindheimer MD, Katz AI: The kidney and hypertension in pregnancy, in Brenner BM, Rector FC Jr (eds): *The Kidney* ed 4. Philadelphia, WB Saunders Co, 1990, in press.

4. Vaziri ND, Toohey K, Powers D, et al: Activation of intrinsic coagulation pathway in pre-eclampsia. *Am J Med* 1986; 80:103–107.

5. Sill PR, Lind T, Walker W: Platelet values during normal pregnancy. *Br J Obstet Gynaecol* 1985; 92:480–483.

6. Stirling Y, Woolf L, North WRS, et al: Hemostasis in normal pregnancy. *Thromb Haemost* 1984; 52:176–182.

7. Burrows RF, Kelton JG: Incidentally detected thrombocytopenia in healthy mothers and their infants. *N Engl J Med* 1988; 319:142–145.

8. Pekonen F, Rasi V, Ammala M, et al: Platelet function and coagulation in normal and preeclamptic pregnancy. *Thromb Res* 1986; 43:553–560.

9. Coulam CB, Silverfeld JC, Kazmar RE, et al: T-lymphocyte subsets during pregnancy and the menstrual cycle. *Am J Reprod Immunol* 1983; 4:88–90.

10. Fizet D, Bousquet J, Piquet Y, et al: Identification of a factor blocking a cellular cytotoxicity reaction in pregnant serum. *Clin Exp Immunol* 1983; 52:648–654.

11. Gregory CD, Lee H, Rees GB, et al: Natural killer cells in normal pregnancy: Analysis using monoclonal antibodies and single-cell cytotoxicity assays. *Clin Exp Immunol* 1985; 62:121–127.

12. Gusdon JP Jr, Heise E, Quinn DK, et al: Lymphocyte subpopulations in normal and preeclampsia pregnancy. *Am J Reprod Immunol* 1984; 5:28–31.

13. Okudaira K, Diaz-Jouanen E, Lockshin MD, et al: Changes in anti-lymphocyte and anti-Ia antibodies during pregnancy in systemic lupus erythematosus. *Clin Immunol Immunpathol* 1986; 40:259–264.

14. Valdimarsson H, Mulholland C, Fridriksdottir V, et al: A longitudinal study of leucocyte blood counts and lymphocytic responses in pregnancy: A marked early increase of monocyte-lymphocyte ratio. *Clin Exp Immunol* 1983; 53:437–443.

15. Kumar A, Madden DL, Nankervis GA: Humoral and cell-mediated immune responses to herpesvirus antigens during pregnancy. *J Clin Immunol* 1984; 4:12–18.

16. Normann SJ, Schardt M, Sorkin E: Effect of pregnancy on cellular inflammation. *Br J Exp Pathol* 1982; 63:432–437.

17. Frajman M, Diaz-Jouanen E, Alcocer-Varela J, et al: Effect of pregnancy on functions of circulating T cells from patients with systemic lupus erythematosus: Correction of T-cell suppression and autolog. *Clin Immunol Immunopathol* 1983; 29:94–102.

18. Bischof P, Duberg S, Sizonenko MT, et al: In vitro production of pregnancy-associated plasma protein A by human decidua and trophoblast. *Am J Obstet Gynecol* 1984; 148:13–18.

19. Bishof P, Lauber K, Girard JP, et al: Circulating levels of pregnancy proteins and depression of lymphoblastogenesis during pregnancy. *J Clin Lab Immunol* 1983; 12:93–96.

20. Bischof P, Lauber K, de Wurstemberger B, et al: Inhibition of lymphocyte transformation by pregnancy-associated plasma protein-a (PAPP-A). *J Clin Lab Immunol* 1982; 7:61–65.

21. Toder V, Blank M, Gleicher N, et al: Immunoregulatory mechanisms in pregnancy. II. Further characterization of suppressor lymphocytes induced by alpha-fetoprotein in lymphoid cell culture. *J Clin Lab Immunol* 1983; 11:149–154.

22. Stites DP, Siiteri PK: Steroids as immunosuppressants in pregnancy. *Immunol Rev* 1983; 75:117–137.

23. Carter J, Dresser DW: Pregnancy induces an increase in the number of immunoglobulin-secreting cells. *Immunology* 1983; 49:481–490.

24. Laurell CB, Rannevik A: Comparison of plasma protein changes induced by danazol, pregnancy, and estrogens. *J Clin*

Endocrinol Metab 1979; 49:719–725.

25. d'Amelio R, Bilotta P, Pachi A, et al: Circulating immune complexes in normal pregnant women and in some conditions complicating pregnancy. *Clin Exp Immunol* 1979; 37:33–37.

26. Theofilopoulos AN, Gleicher N, Pereira AB, et al: The biology of immune complexes and their possible role in pregnancy. *Reprod Immunol* 1981; 93–114.

27. Gleicher N, Adelsberg BR, Liu TL, et al: Immune complexes in pregnancy. (III) Immune complexes in immune complex–associated conditions. *Am J Obstet Gynecol* 1982; 142:1011–1015.

28. Masson PL, Delire M, Cambiaso C: Circulating immune complexes in normal human pregnancy. *Nature* 1977; 266:542–543.

29. Pope RM, Yoshinoya S, Rutstein J, et al: Effect of pregnancy on immune complexes and rheumatoid factors in patients with rheumatoid arthritis. *Am J Med* 1983; 74:973–979.

30. Schena FP, Manno C, Selvaggi L, et al: Behaviour of immune complexes and the complement system in normal pregnancy and pre-eclampsia. *J Clin Lab Immunol* 1982; 7:21–36.

31. Rote NS, Caudle MR: Circulating immune complexes in pregnancy, pre-eclampsia, and autoimmune diseases: Evaluation of Raji cell enzyme-linked immunosorbent assay and polyethylene glycol precipitation methods. *Am J Obstet Gynecol* 1983; 14:267–273.

32. Combe B, Cosso B, Clot J, et al: Human placenta-eluted gammaglobulins in immunomodulating treatment of rheumatoid arthritis. *Am J Med* 1985; 78:920–928.

33. Weinberg ED: Pregnancy-associated depression of cell-mediated immunity. *Rev Infect Dis* 1984; 814–831.

34. Persellin RH: Inhibitors of inflammatory and immune responses in pregnancy serum. *Clin Rheum Dis* 1981; 7:769–780.

35. McDermott M, McDevitt H: The immunogenetics of rheumatic diseases. *Bull Rheum Dis* 1988; 38:1–10.

36. Adelsberg BR: The complement system in pregnancy. *Am J Repro Immunol* 1983; 38–44.

37. Devoe LD, Taylor RL: Systemic lupus erythematosus in pregnancy. *Am J Obstet Gynecol* 1979; 135:473–479.

38. Kitzmiller JL, Stoneburner L, Yelenosky PF, et al: Serum complement in normal pregnancy and pre-eclampsia. *Am J Obstet Gynecol* 1973; 117:312–315.

39. Koslowski JP, Guiget M, Taquoi G, et al: Complément (C3 et CH50) et immuno-globulines sériques au cours de la toxémie gravidique. *J Gynecol Obstet Biol Reprod (Paris)* 1978; 7:923–931.

40. Levy DL, Cox A, Leffell MS, et al: Serum complement activity in pre-term pregnancies: Relationship to duration of ruptured membranes and clinical infection. *AJRI* 1982; 2:142–147.

41. Hopkins P, Belmont HM, Buyon J, et al: Increased levels of anaphylatoxins in systemic lupus erythematosus predict flares of the disease and may elicit vascular injury in lupus cerebritis. *Arthritis Rheum* 1988; 31:632–641.

42. Ogston D, Walker J, Campbell DM: C1 inactivator level in pregnancy. *Thromb Res* 1981; 23:453–455.

43. Prall RH, Kantor FS: Serum complement in eclamptogenic toxemia. *Am J Obstet Gynecol* 1966; 95:530–533.

44. Tedder RS, Nelson M, Eisen V: Effects of serum complement of normal and pre-eclamptic pregnancy and of oral contraceptives. *Br J Exp Pathol* 1975; 56:389–395.

45. Teisner B, Hau J, Tucker M, et al: Circulating C3, C4, and C3 split products (C3c and C3d) during normal pregnancy. *Am J Reprod Immunol* 1982; 2:309–311.

46. Buyon JP, Cronstein BN, Morris M, et al: Serum complement values (C3 and C4) to differentiate between systemic lupus activity and pre-eclampsia. *Am J Med* 1986; 81:194–200.

47. Lockshin MD, Harpel PC, Druzin ML, et al: Lupus pregnancy. II. Unusual pattern of hypocomplementemia and thrombocytopenia in the pregnant patient. *Arthritis Rheum* 1985; 28:58–66.

48. Lockshin MD, Qamar T, Redecha P, et al: Hypocomplementemia with low C1s-C1 inhibitor complex in systemic lupus erythematosus. *Arthritis Rheum* 1986;

29:1467–1472.

49. Lahita RG, Bradlow HL, Fishman J, et al: Estrogen metabolism in systemic lupus erythematosus. *Arthritis Rheum* 1982; 25:843–846.

50. Lahita RG, Bradlow HL, Kunkel HG, et al: Alterations of estrogen metabolism in systemic lupus erythematosus. *Arthritis Rheum* 1979; 22:1195–1198.

51. Lahita RG, Bucala R, Bradlow HL, et al: Determination of 16 alpha-hydroxyestrone by radioimmunoassay in systemic lupus erythematosus. *Arthritis Rheum* 1985; 28:1122–1127.

52. Bucala R, Lahita RG, Fishman J, et al: Increased levels of 16 alpha hydroxyesterone-modified proteins in pregnancy and in systemic lupus erythematosus. *J Clin Endocrinol Metab* 1985; 60:841–847.

53. Cousins L, Rigg L, Hollingsworth D, et al: Qualitative and quantitative assessment of the circadian rhythm of cortisol in pregnancy. *Am J Obstet Gynecol* 1983; 145:411–416.

54. McHugh NJ, Reilly PA, McHugh LA: Pregnancy outcome and autoantibodies in connective tissue disease. *J Rheumatol* 1989; 16:42–46.

55. Siamopoulou-Mavridou A, Manoussakis MN, Mavridis AK, et al: Outcome of pregnancy in patients with autoimmune rheumatic disease before the disease onset. *Ann Rheum Dis* 1988; 47:982–987.

56. Fraga A, Mintz G, Orozco J, et al: Sterility and fertility rates, fetal wastage and maternal morbidity in systemic lupus erythematosus. *J Rheumatol* 1974; 1:293–298.

57. Grimes DA, Lebolt SA, Grimes KR, et al: Systemic lupus erythematosus and reproductive function: A case-control study. *Am J Obstet Gynecol* 1985; 153:179–186.

58. Steen VD, Conte C, Day N, et al: Pregnancy in women with systemic sclerosis. *Arthritis Rheum* 1989; 32:151–157.

59. Tan EN, Cohen AS, Fries JF, et al: The 1982 revised criteria for the classification of systemic lupus erythematosus. *Arthritis Rheum* 1982; 25:1271–1277.

60. Fessel WJ: Systemic lupus erythematosus in the community. *Arch Intern Med* 1974; 134:1027–1035.

61. Wilson WA, Perez MC, Michalski JP, et al: Cardiolipin antibodies and null alleles of C4 in black Americans with systemic lupus erythematosus. *J Rheumatol* 1988; 15:1768–1772.

62. Jungers P, Nahoul K, Pelissier C, et al: Étude des androgenes plasmatiques chez les femmes atteinte du lupus érythèmateux disséminé. *Presse Med* 1983; 12:685–688.

63. Lavalle C, Gonzalez-Barcena D, Graef A, et al: Gonadotropins pituitary secretion in systemic lupus erythematosus. *Clin Exp Rheumatol* 1984; 2:163–165.

64. Lloyd W, Schur PH: Immune complexes, complement, and anti-DNA in exacerbations of systemic lupus erythematosus (SLE). *Medicine (Baltimore)* 1981; 60:208–217.

65. Harris EN, Chan JKH, Asherson RA, et al: Thrombosis, recurrent fetal loss and thrombocytopenia. Predictive value of the anticardiolipin antibody test. *Arch Intern Med* 1986; 146:2153–2156.

66. Kalunian KC, Peter JB, Middlekauff HR, et al: Clinical significance of a single test for anti-cardiolipin antibodies in patients with systemic lupus erythematosus. *Am J Med* 1988; 85:602–608.

67. Petri M, Rheinschmidt M, Whiting-O'Keefe Q, et al: The frequency of lupus anticoagulant in systemic lupus erythematosus. *Ann Intern Med* 1987; 106:524–531.

68. Cronin ME, Biswas RM, Van der Straeton C, et al: IgG and IgM anticardiolipin antibodies in patients with lupus with anticardiolipin antibody associated clinical syndromes. *J Rheumatol* 1988; 15:795–798.

69. Lee SL, Miotti AB: Disorders of hemostatic function in patients with systemic lupus erythematosus. *Semin Arthritis Rheum* 1975; 4:241–252.

70. Godeau P, Herreman G, Raby C, et al: Coagulation et lupus érythèmateux aigu disséminé. *Sem Hop Paris* 1977; 53:609–612.

71. Gladman DD, Urowitz MB, Tozman EC, et al: Haemostatic abnormalities in systemic lupus erythematosus. *Q J Med* 1983; 52:424–433.

72. Stratta P, Canavese C, Valmaggia P, et

al: Coagulation and fibrinolysis study in systemic lupus erythematosus: Haematological, urinary and tissue parameters. *Thromb Haemos* 1981; 46:575–580.

73. Sergent JS, Sherman RL, Al-Mondihiry H: Fibrinogen catabolism in systemic lupus erythematosus. *Arthritis Rheum* 1976; 19:195–198.

74. Miller MH, Urowitz MB, Gladman DD: The significance of thrombocytopenia in systemic lupus erythematosus. *Arthritis Rheum* 1983; 26:1181–1186.

75. Liang MH, Socher SA, Roberts WN, et al: Measurement of systemic lupus erythematosus activity in clinical research. *Arthritis Rheum* 1988; 31:817–825.

76. Lockshin MD, Reinitz E, Druzin ML, et al: Lupus pregnancy. Case-control prospective study demonstrating absence of lupus exacerbation during or after pregnancy. *Am J Med* 1984; 77:893–898.

77. Mintz G, Niz J, Gutierrez G, et al: Prospective study of pregnancy in systemic lupus erythematosus. Results of a multidisciplinary approach. *J Rheumatol* 1986; 13:732–739.

77a. Alarcon-Segovia D, Sanchez-Guerrero J: Correction of thrombocytopenia with small dose aspirin in the primary antiphospholipid antibody syndrome. *J Rheumatol* 1989; 16:1359–1361.

78. Lockshin MD: Pregnancy does not cause systemic lupus erythematosus to worsen. *Arthritis Rheum* 1989; 32:665–670.

79. Hayslett JP: Effect of pregnancy on patients with SLE. *Adv SLE* 1983; 2:127–132.

80. Hayslett JP, Lynn RI: Effect of pregnancy in patients with lupus nephropathy. *Kidney Int* 1982; 18:207–220.

81. Imbasciati E, Surian M, Bottino S, et al: Lupus nephropathy and pregnancy. *Nephron* 1984; 36:46–51.

82. Surian M, Imbasciati E, Cosci P, et al: Glomerular disease and pregnancy. *Nephron* 1985; 36:101–105.

83. Jungers PM, Dougados M, Pelissier C, et al: Lupus nephropathy and pregnancy. *Arch Intern Med* 1982; 142:771–776.

84. Devoe LD, Loy GL, Spargo BH: Renal histology and pregnancy performance in systemic lupus erythematosus. *Clin Exp Hypertens [B]* 1983; 2:325–240.

85. Leppert P, Tisher CC, Sheng SCS, et al: Antecedent renal disease and the outcome of pregnancy. *Ann Intern Med* 1979; 90:747–751.

86. Hou S: Pregnancy in women with chronic renal disease. *N Engl J Med* 1985; 312:836–839.

87. Parke AL: Antimalarial drugs, systemic lupus erythematosus and pregnancy. *J Rheumatol* 1988; 15:607–610.

88. Kaell AT, Shetty M, Lee BCP, et al: The diversity of neurologic events in systemic lupus erythematosus. *Arch Neurol* 1986; 43:273–276.

89. Wolf RE, McBeath JG: Chorea gravidarum in systemic lupus erythematosus. *J Rheumatol* 1985; 12:992–993.

90. Marabani M, Zoma A, Hadley D, et al: Transverse myelitis occurring during pregnancy in a patient with systemic lupus erythematosus. *Am Rheum Dis* 1989; 48:160–162.

91. Plouin PF, Milliez J, Breart G, et al: Rein, hypertension et grossesse. *Nouv Presse Med* 1982; 11:1625–1630.

92. Druzin ML: Pregnancy induced hypertension and pre-eclampsia: The fetus and the neonate, in Rubin PC (ed): *Handbook of Hypertension*. Vol 10: *Hypertension in Pregnancy*, Amsterdam, Elsevier, 1988, pp 267–289.

93. Lockshin MD, Qamar T, Druzin ML, et al: Antibody to cardiolipin, lupus anticoagulant and fetal death. *J Rheumatol* 1987; 14:259–262.

94. Lockshin MD, Druzin ML, Qamar T: Prednisone does not prevent recurrent fetal death in women with antiphospholipid antibody. *Am J Obstet Gynecol* 1989; 160:439–443.

95. Gharavi AE, Harris EN, Lockshin MD, et al: IgG subclass and light chain distribution of anticardiolipin and anti-DNA antibodies in systemic lupus erythematosus. *Ann Rheum Dis* 1988; 47:286–290.

96. Petri M, Golbus M, Anderson R, et al: Antinuclear antibody, lupus anticoagulant, and anticardiolipin antibody in women with idiopathic habitual abortion. *Arthritis Rheum* 1987; 30:601–606.

97. Unander AM, Norberg R, Hahn L, et al: Anticardiolipin antibodies and complement in 99 women with habitual abor-

tion. *Am J Obstet Gynecol* 1987; 156:114–119.

98. Beck JS, Oakley CL, Rowell NR: Transplacental passage of antinuclear antibody (studies in infants of mothers with SLE) *Arch Dermatol* 1966; 93:656–663.

99. Cruveiller J, Harpey JP, Veron P, et al: Lupus érythèmateux systémique/transmission de manifestations clinques et de facteurs biologiques de la mère au nouveau-né. *Arch Fr Pediatr* 1970; 27:195–209.

100. Miyagawa S, Kitamura W, Yuoshioka J, et al: Placental transfer of anticytoplasmic antibodies in annular erythema of newborns. *Arch Dermatol* 1981; 117:569–572.

101. Provost TT, Watson RM, Gammon WR, et al: The neonatal lupus syndrome associated with U1RNP (nRNP) antibodies. *N Engl J Med* 1987; 316:1135–1138.

102. Ramsey-Goldman R, Hom D, Deng J-S, et al: Anti-SSA antibodies and fetal outcome in maternal systemic lupus erythematosus. *Arthritis Rheum* 1986; 29:1269–1273.

103. Watson RM, Lane AT, Barnett NK, et al: Neonatal lupus erythematosus. *Medicine (Baltimore)* 1984; 63:362–378.

104. Watson R, Kang JE, May M, et al: Thrombocytopenia in the neonatal lupus syndrome. *Arch Dermatol* 1988; 124:560–563.

105. Weston WL, Harmon C, Peebles C, et al: A serologic marker for neonatal lupus. *Br J Dermatol* 1982; 107:377–382.

106. Lee LA, Bias WB, Arnett FC, et al: Immunogenetics of the neonatal lupus syndrome. *Ann Intern Med* 1983; 99:592–596.

107. Lockshin MD, Bonfa E, Elkon K, et al: Neonatal lupus risk to newborns of mothers with systemic lupus erythematosus. *Arthritis Rheum* 1988; 31:697–701.

108. McCune AB, Weston WL, Lee LA: Maternal and fetal outcome in neonatal systemic lupus erythematosus. *Ann Intern Med* 1987; 106:518–523.

109. Buyon JP, Ben-Chetrit E, Karp S, et al: Acquired congenital heart block: Pattern of maternal antibody response to biochemically defined antigens of the SSA/Ro-SSB/La system in neonatal lupus. *J Clin Invest* 1989; 84:627–634.

110. Buyon JP, Pompeo L, Elkon K, et al: Characterization by immunoblot of the immune response to SSA/Ro associated with congenital heart block. *Arthritis Rheum* 1989; 34:S104.

111. Callen JP, Fowler JF, Kulick KB, et al: Neonatal lupus erythematosus occurring in one fraternal twin. *Arthritis Rheum* 1985; 28:271–275.

112. Harley JB, Kaine JL, Fox OF, et al: Ro (SS-A) antibody and antigen in a patient with congenital complete heart block. *Arthritis Rheum* 1985; 28:1321–1325.

113. Kasinath BS, Katz AL: Delayed maternal lupus after delivery of offspring with congenital heart block. *Arch Intern Med* 1982; 142:2317.

114. Anderson GG, Rotchell Y, Kaiser DG: Placental transfer of methylprednisolone following maternal intravenous administration. *Am J Obstet Gynecol* 1981; 140:699–701.

115. Semchyshyn S, Zuspan RP, Cordero L: Cardiovascular response and complications of glucocorticoid therapy in hypertensive pregnancies. *Am J Obstet Gynecol* 1983; 145:530–533.

116. Eishi Y, Hirokawa K, Hatakeyama S: Long-lasting impairment of immune and endocrine systems of offspring induced by injection of dexamethasone into pregnant mice. *Clin Immunol Immunopathol* 1983; 26:335–349.

117. Smith BT, Torday JS: Steroid administration in pregnant women with autoimmune thrombocytopenia. *N Engl J Med* 1982; 306:744–745.

118. Hensleigh PA, Herzenberg LA, Lipman SH, et al: Transient immunologic effects of betamethasone in human pregnancy after suppression of pre-term labor. *Am J Reprod Immunol* 1983; 4:83–87.

119. Besa EC, MacNab MW, Solan AJ, et al: High-dose intravenous IgG in the management of pregnancy in women with idiopathic thrombocytopenic purpura. *Am J Hematol* 1985; 18:373–379.

120. Fehr J, Hofmann V, Kappeler U: Transient reversal of thrombocytopenia in idiopathic thrombocytopenic purpura by high-dose intravenous gamma globulin. *N Engl J Med* 1982; 306:1254–1258.

121. Newland AC, Boots MA, Patterson KG:

Intravenous IgG for autoimmune thrombocytopenia in pregnancy. *N Engl J Med* 1984; 310:261–262.

122. Scott JR, Branch DW, Kochenour NK, et al: Intravenous immunoglobulin treatment of pregnant patients with recurrent pregnancy loss caused by antiphospholipid antibodies and Rh immunization. *Am J Obstet Gynecol* 1988; 159:1055–1056.

123. Buyon JP Swersky SH, Fox HE, et al: Intrauterine therapy for presumptive fetal myocarditis with acquired heart block due to systemic lupus erythematosus. *Arthritis Rheum* 1987; 30:44–49.

124. Meehan RT, Dorsey KT: Pregnancy among patients with systemic lupus erythematosus receiving immunosuppressive therapy. *J Rheumatol* 1987; 14:252–258.

125. Sharon E, Jones J, Diamond H, et al: Pregnancy and azathioprine in systemic lupus erythematosus. *Am J Obstet Gynecol* 1974; 118:25–28.

126. Dewitte DB, Buick MK, Cyran SE, et al: Neonatal pancytopenia and severe combined immunodeficiency associated with antenatal administration of azathioprine and prednisone. *J Pediatr* 1984; 105:625–628.

127. Fein A, Gross A, Serr DM, et al: Effect of Imuran on placental and fetal development in rats. *Isr J Med Sci* 1983; 19:73–75.

128. Schiff E, Peleg E, Goldenberg M, et al: The use of aspirin to prevent pregnancy-induced hypertension and lower the ratio of thromboxane A_2 to prostacyclin in relatively high risk pregnancies. *N Engl J Med* 1989; 321:351–356.

129. Benigni A, Gregorini G, Frusca T, et al: Effect of low dose aspirin on fetal and maternal generation of thromboxane by platelets in women at risk for pregnancy-induced hypertension. *N Engl J Med* 1989; 321:357–362.

130. Wallenburg HCS, Makovitz JW, Dekker GA, et al: Low-dose aspirin prevents pregnancy-induced hypertension and pre-eclampsia in angiotensin-sensitive primigravidae. *Lancet* 1986; 1:1–3.

131. Moise KJ, Huhta JC, Sharif DS, et al: Indomethacin in the treatment of premature labor. Effects on the fetal ductus arteriosus. *N Engl J Med* 1988; 319:327–331.

132. Himmelstein DU: Aspirin and maternal or neonatal hemostasis (letter). *N Engl J Med* 1983; 308:281.

133. Stuart MJ, Gross SJ, Elrad H, et al: Effects of acetylsalicylic-acid ingestion on maternal and neonatal hemostasis. *N Engl J Med* 1982; 307:909–912.

134. Druzin ML, Fox A, Kogut E, et al: The relationship of the nonstress test to gestational age. *Am J Obstet Gynecol* 1985; 153:386–389.

135. Druzin ML, Gratacos J, Keegan KA, et al: Antepartum fetal heart rate testing. VII. The significance of fetal bradycardia. *Am J Obstet Gynecol* 1981; 139:194–198.

135. Druzin ML, Gratacos J, Paul RH, et al: Antepartum fetal heart rate testing. XII. The effect of manual manipulation of the fetus on the nonstress test. *Am J Obstet Gynecol* 1985; 151:61–64.

136. Druzin ML, Lockshin M, Edersheim TG, et al: Second-trimester fetal monitoring and preterm delivery in pregnancies with systemic lupus erythematosus and/or circulting anticoagulant. *Am J Obstet Gynecol* 1987; 157:1503–1510.

137. Buyon JP, Swersky SH, Fox HE, et al: Intrauterine therapy for presumptive fetal myocarditis with acquired heart block due to systemic lupus erythematosus. *Arthritis Rheum* 1987; 30:44–49.

138. Chapel TA, Burns RE: Oral contraceptives and exacerbation of lupus erythematosus. *Am J Obstet Gynecol* 1971; 110:366–369.

139. Garovich M, Agudelo C, Pisko E: Oral contraceptives and systemic lupus erythematosus. *Arthritis Rheum* 1980; 23:1396–1398.

140. Block SR, Winfield JB, Lockshin MD, et al: Studies of twins with systemic lupus erythematosus. A review of the literature and presentation of 12 additional sets. *Am J Med* 1975; 59:533–552.

141. Koskela P, Vaarala O, Makitalo R, et al: Significance of false positive syphilis reactions and anticardiolipin antibodies in a nationwide series of pregnant women. *J Rheumatol* 1988; 15:70–73.

142. Alarcon-Segovia D, Sanchez-Guerrero J: Primary antiphospholipid antibody syndrome. *J Rheumatol* 1989; 16:1014.

143. Asherson RA: A "primary" antiphospho-

lipid syndrome? (editorial). *J Rheumatol* 1988; 15:1742–1746.

144. Harris EN, Gharavi AE, Hughes GRV: Anti-phospholipid antibodies. *Clin Rheum Dis* 1985; 11:591–609.

145. Lesperance B, David M, Rauch J, et al: Relative sensitivity of different tests in the detection of low titer lupus anticoagulants. *Thromb Haemost* 1988; 60:217–219.

146. Triplett DA, Brandt JT, Musgrave KA, et al: The relationship between lupus anticoagulants and antibodies to phospholipid. *JAMA* 1988; 259:550–554.

147. Cowchock S, Smith JB, Gocial B: Antibodies to phospholipids and nuclear antigens in patients with repeated abortions. *Am J Obstet Gynecol* 1986; 155:1002–1010.

148. Howard MA, Firkin BG, Healy DL, et al: Lupus anticoagulant in women with multiple spontaneous miscarriage. *Am J Hematol* 1987; 26:175–178.

149. Lockshin MD, Druzin ML, Goei S, et al: Antibody to cardiolipin as a predictor of fetal distress or death in pregnant patients with systemic lupus erythematosus. *N Engl J Med* 1986; 313:152–156.

150. Branch DW, Scott JR, Kochenour NK, et al: Obstetric complications associated with the lupus anticoagulant. *N Engl J Med* 1985; 313:1322–1326.

151. Derue GJ, Englert HJ, Harris EN, et al: Fetal loss in systemic lupus: Association with anticardiolipin antibodies. *J Obstet Gynaecol* 1985; 5:207–209.

152. Lubbe WF, Palmer SJ, Butler WS, et al: Fetal survival after prednisone suppression of maternal lupus-anticoagulant. *Lancet* 1983; 1:1361–1363.

153. Tsutsumi A, Koike T, Ichikawa K, et al: IgG subclass distribution of anticardiolipin antibody in patients with systemic lupus erythematosus. *J Rheumatol* 1988; 15:1764–1767.

154. Abramowsky CR: Lupus erythematosus, the placenta, and pregnancy: A natural experiment in immunologically mediated reproductive failure. *Prog Clin Biol Res* 1981; 70:309–320.

155. Abramowsky CT, Vegas ME, Swinehart G, et al: Decidual vasculopathy of the placenta in lupus erythematosus. *N Engl J Med* 1980; 303:668–672.

156. de Wolf F, Carreras LO, Moerman P, et al: Decidual vasculopathy and extensive placental infarction in a patient with repeated thromboembolic accidents, recurrent fetal loss and a lupus anticoagulant. *Am J Obstet Gynecol* 1982; 142:829–834.

157. Hanley JG, Gladman DD, Rose TH, et al: Lupus pregnancy. A prospective study of placental changes. *Arthritis Rheum* 1988; 31:358–366.

158. Labarrere CA, Catoggio LJ, Mullen EG, et al: Placental lesion in maternal autoimmune disease. *Am J Reprod Immunol* 1986; 12:78–87.

159. Bresnihan B, Oliver M, Grigor RR, et al: Immunological mechanism for spontaneous abortion in systemic lupus erythematosus. *Lancet* 1977; 2:1205–1207.

160. Grennan DM, McCormick JN, Wojtacha D, et al: Immunological studies of the placenta in systemic lupus erythematosus. *Ann Rheum Dis* 1978; 37:129–134.

161. Matthay F, Walshe K, Mackie IJ, et al: Familial occurrence of the antiphospholipid antibody syndrome. *J Clin Pathol* 1989; 42:495–497.

162. Sturfelt G, Nived O, Norberg R, et al: Anticardiolipin antibodies in patients with systemic lupus erythematosus. *Arthritis Rheum* 1987; 30:382–388.

163. Lazaro MA, Maldonado-Cocco JA, Catoggio LJ, et al: Clinical and serologic characteristics of patients with overlap syndrome: Is mixed connective tissue disease a distinct clinical entity? *Medicine (Baltimore)* 1989; 68:58–65.

164. Lockshin MD: What is SLE? *J Rheumatol* 1989; 16:419–420.

165. LeRoy EC, Maricq HR, Kahaleh MB: Undifferentiated connective tissue syndrome. *Arthritis Rheum* 1980; 23:341–343.

166. Kaufman RL, Kitridou RC: Pregnancy in mixed connective tissue disease: Comparison with systemic lupus erythematosus. *J Rheumatol* 1982; 9:549–555.

167. Herreman G, Betous F, Batisse PH, et al: Blocs aurico-ventriculaires détectés in utero chez 2 enfants dont la mère a un syndrome de Sjögren. *Nouv Presse Med* 1982; 11:657–660.

168. Kaplan D: Fetal wastage in patients with rheumatoid arthritis. *J Rheumatol* 1986; 13:875–877.

169. Ostensen M, Husby G: Ensuring a

healthy pregnancy for the woman with severe RA. *J Musculoskeletal Med* 1988; 5:13–25.

170. Cecere FA, Persellin RH: The interaction of pregnancy and the rheumatic diseases. *Clin Rheum Dis* 1981; 7:747–768.

171. Benhamou CL, Brandely M: Influence de la grossesse et de l'état hormonal sur la polyarthrite rhumatoïde. *Presse Med* 1983; 12:2223–2224.

172. Ostensen M, Aune B, Husby G: Effect of pregnancy and hormonal changes on the activity of rheumatoid arthritis. *Scand J Rheumatol* 1983; 12:69–72.

173. Ostensen M, Husby G: A prospective clinical study of the effect of pregnancy on rheumatoid arthritis and ankylosing spondylitis. *Arthritis Rheum* 1983; 26:1155–1159.

174. Ostensen M, Lundgren R, Husby G, et al: Studies on humoral immunity in pregnancy: Immunoglobulins, alloantibodies and autoantibodies in healthy pregnant women and in pregnant women with rheumatoid arthritis. *J Clin Lab Immunol* 1983; 11:143–147.

175. Ballou SP, Morley JJ, Kushner I: Pregnancy and systemic sclerosis. *Arthritis Rheum* 1984; 27:295–298.

176. Malia RG, Greaves M, Rowlands LM, et al: Anticardiolipin antibodies in systemic sclerosis: Immunological and clinical associations. *Clin Exp Immunol* 1988; 73:456–460.

177. McWhorter JE IV, Leroy EC: Pericardial disease in scleroderma (systemic sclerosis) *Am J Med* 1974; 57:566.

178. Cannon PJ, Hasser M, Case DB, et al: The relationship of hypertension and renal failure in scleroderma (progressive systemic sclerosis) to structural and functional abnormalities of the renal cortical circulation. *Medicine (Baltimore)* 1974; 53:1–46.

179. Anad S, Van Thiel DH: Prenatal and neonatal exposure to cimetidine results in gonadal and sexual dysfunction in adult males. *Science* 1982; 218:493–494.

180. Gutierrez G, Dagnino R, Mintz G: Polymyositis/dermatomyositis and pregnancy. *Arthritis Rheum* 1984; 27:291–294.

181. Ayers MA: Takayasu syndrome and pregnancy: A ten-year-follow up. *Am J Obstet Gynecol* 1974; 120:562–563.

182. Nagey DA, Fortier KJ, Hayes BA, et al: Takayasu's arteritis in pregnancy: A case presentation demonstrating absence of placental pathology. *Am J Obstet Gynecol* 1983; 147:463–465.

183. Winn HN, Setaro JF, Mazor M, et al: Severe Takayasu's arteritis in pregnancy: The role of central hemodynamic monitoring. *Am J Obstet Gynecol* 1988; 159:1135–1136.

184. Wong VCW, Wang RYC, Tse TF: Pregnancy and Takayasu's arteritis. *Am J Med* 1983; 75:597–601.

185. Ishikawa K, Matsuura S: Occlusive thromboaortopathy (Takayasu's disease) and pregnancy. *Am J Cardiol* 1982; 50:1293–1300.

186. De Beukelaer MM, Travis LB, Roberts DK: Polyarteritis nodosa and pregnancy. *South Med J* 1973; 66:613–615.

187. Owen J, Hauth C: Polyarteritis nodosa in pregnancy: A case report and brief literature review. *Am J Obstet Gynecol* 1989; 160:606–607.

188. Pyeritz RE: Maternal and fetal complications of pregnancy in the Marfan syndrome. *Am J Med* 1981; 71:784–789.

189. Snir E, Levinsky L, Salomon J, et al: Dissecting aortic aneurysm in pregnant women without Marfan disease. *Surg Gynecol Obstet* 1988; 167:461–465.

190. Rowe DW, Shapiro JR: Diseases associated with abnormalities of structural proteins, in Kelly WN, Harris ED, Ruddy S, et al (eds): *Textbook of Rheumatology,* ed 2. Philadelphia, WB Saunders Co, 1985, pp 1621–1644.

191. Lockshin MD, Brause BD: Infectious arthritis. *DM* 1982; 28:9.

192. Nakano KK: Entrapment neuropathies , in Kelley WM, Harris ED Sr, Ruddy S (eds): *Textbook of Rheumatology,* ed 2. Philadelphia, WB Saunders Co, 1985, pp 1766–1777.

193. Nakano KK: Entrapment neuropathies, in Kelley WN, Harris ED Sr, Ruddy S (eds): *Textbook of Rheumatology,* ed 2. Philadelphia, WB Saunders Co, 1985, pp 1621–1644.

194. Hill LM, Kleinberg F. Effects of drugs and chemicals on the fetus and newborn. *Mayo Clin Proc* 1984; 59:755–765.

CHAPTER 12

Neoplastic Disorders

Stephanie F. Williams
Richard L. Schilsky

Cancer is the second leading cause of death in women during the reproductive years. Malignancy is estimated to complicate the course of approximately 1 in 1,000 pregnancies. When cancer occurs in a pregnant woman it is devastating and anxiety-provoking. Both the patient and physician will have to contemplate difficult therapeutic options.

This chapter describes the effects pregnancy has upon the natural history of cancer, as well as the effects of therapy upon the pregnancy, the progeny, and upon gonadal function. We describe specific neoplastic disorders during pregnancy and discuss the impact that pregnancy has on staging and treatment planning.

THE EFFECTS OF PREGNANCY ON THE NATURAL HISTORY OF CANCER

Cancer and pregnancy may have some common features in that foreign antigens, in one case tumor-associated antigens and in the other fetal antigens, are tolerated by the patient. Recent observations suggest similar immunologic alterations in both states: depressed cellular immunity, the presence of a blocking antibody (an IgG immunoglobulin) that permits tolerance to antigenic tissue, the presence of immunosuppressive substances such

as human chorionic gonadotropin, and increased suppressor T lymphocytes.[1, 2] Despite these factors, which can potentially facilitate tumor growth, the incidence of cancer in pregnant women is no greater than in nonparous women of the same age. Indeed, in most cases it is probable that pregnancy itself does not alter the course of a coexistent cancer.[3] The diagnostic workup and therapeutic choices, however, may be influenced by the pregnancy and by the concern for fetal outcome.

Hormonal Effects

Pregnancy produces various changes in the hormonal milieu of a woman that could potentially influence the course of a coexistent malignancy. Anecdotal reports suggest that certain tumors such as melanoma are increased in frequency in pregnant patients. Evidence for a hormonal influence in melanoma includes pigmentation of nevi during puberty, hyperpigmentation associated with pregnancy, increased melanocyte-stimulating hormone in pregnancy, the presence of estrogen receptors in 46% of melanomas, and reports of regression of disease during hormonal manipulation.[4] However, other data indicate that the incidence of melanoma in pregnant and nonparous women is the same.[5] Two studies have suggested that pregnant patients

TABLE 12–1.
Physiologic Changes During Pregnancy That May Alter Drug Metabolism

Increased plasma volume
Decreased serum albumin concentration
Enhanced hepatic detoxification of drugs
Decreased gastric emptying
Increased glomerular filtration rate
Pharmacologic third space—?amniotic fluid

with melanoma may have a worse prognosis than nonparous patients.[6, 7] Both studies found a worse survival in pregnant patients; however, these patients had advanced-stage disease at diagnosis and truncal lesions, which carry a poor prognosis. When matched with nonpregnant patients with the same prognostic factors, survivals were similar. It is therefore not possible to say with certainty that pregnancy adversely affects the course of patients with malignant melanoma.

Breast cancer is a tumor that is often responsive to hormonal manipulation, yet there is little convincing evidence that breast cancer is accelerated by the hormonal changes in pregnancy. In fact, estriol, an estrogen produced during pregnancy, may exert a protective effect against carcinogenesis.[8] As in nonparous women of the same age group, it is the spread of the cancer to axillary lymph nodes at diagnosis that is prognostically significant, not the pregnancy itself. However, it is often difficult to detect an early breast carcinoma in a pregnant patient because of the associated changes in breast tissue during this time. Thus, a delay in diagnosis during pregnancy may be more detrimental than the hormonal influence of pregnancy.

Drug Metabolism During Pregnancy

The pregnant state can potentially alter the therapeutic effectiveness of cancer chemotherapy by effects on drug metabolism (Table 12–1). Plasma volume increases, which may lead to drug dilution and changes in volume of distribution.[9] Albumin concentration decreases, which may lead to increased concentrations of nonprotein-bound drug in the circulation.[10] Hepatic function and renal excretion are enhanced, which may alter drug clearance and pharmacodynamics.[11, 12] Gastric emptying is decreased, especially late in pregnancy, which may alter absorption and bioavailability of oral agents.[13] A major concern, especially for methotrexate administration, is the possibility that amniotic fluid could act as a pharmacologic third space, resulting in delayed drug clearance and increased toxicity. Amniotic fluid has not as yet been reported to act in this way but concern is still appropriate. Little information is available on the clinical pharmacology of cytotoxic drugs administered during pregnancy. Clearly, the physiologic changes that accompany pregnancy could have a significant influence on the already narrow therapeutic index of these agents.

Whether the placenta can act as a barrier to chemotherapeutic drug entry from the maternal circulation to the fetus is unknown but probably depends to some extent on the characteristics of the drug in question. Agents that are of low molecular weight, high lipid solubility, nonionized, and loosely bound to plasma protein may readily cross the placenta.[10, 11] A number of chemotherapeutic agents have these characteristics. In addition, if chemotherapeutic agents cross the placenta into the fetal circulation, the metabolism and excretion of these agents are likely to be abnormal because the fetal liver and kidneys are functionally immature. Thus, the fetus could be exposed to high concentrations of antineoplastic agents that cannot be efficiently metabolized or excreted, thus placing the fetus at risk for drug toxicity. Potential teratogenic effects of cancer chemotherapy are discussed below.

Effects of Delayed Diagnostic and Therapeutic Interventions

There is no clear evidence that the state of pregnancy alters the course of a cancer by influencing tumor growth and metastatic potential. Poor results of treatment of cancer during pregnancy are more likely due to delay in diagnosis with subsequent delay in initiating appropriate therapy. Because of concern for the developing fetus, many procedures that might lead to definitive diagnosis or accurate staging may be avoided. Therapeutic strategies have to be carefully considered depending upon the type of cancer and may require some modification. A decision to continue or terminate a pregnancy can only be made after careful, frank, and deliberate discussions about the risks and benefits to the patient and developing fetus, and based on a full knowledge of the extent of disease and the prognosis.

THE EFFECTS OF CANCER THERAPY ON PREGNANCY

Embryology

In order to appreciate the potential effects of antineoplastic therapy upon the fetus, a brief review of fetal development is necessary (Table 12–2). The first phase of gestation is implantation, which occurs in the first 2 weeks following conception. Therapeutic interventions during this phase can result in a high number of spontaneous abortions. The second to eighth weeks of gestation represent the period of major organogenesis. All major organs and organ systems are formed during this period (first trimester). During this period, the developing embryo is most susceptible to teratogenic effects of drugs and radiation. Most congenital malformations found at birth begin during this critical period. Many organ systems have self-limited

development; however, others, such as the nervous system, eye, respiratory, and hematopoietic systems, continue to develop and remain sensitive throughout intrauterine development. The final phase of fetal development beginning with the third month of gestation is a period characterized by maturation of tissues and growth (second and third trimesters). Insults during this period can result in growth retardation. These insults consist not only of therapy-related causes but also disease-related effects.

Congenital malformations are defined as gross structural defects present at birth.[14] The possible deleterious effects of cancer therapy must be compared with fetal loss and congenital malformation in "normal" pregnancies. Approximately 10% to 15% of pregnancies result in miscarriage or spontaneous abortion. Liveborn infants have a 2% to 3% risk of a significant congenital malformation. The fetal consequences of cancer therapy may be related to drug dosage, fetal gestational age, and type and combination of chemotherapy and radiotherapy as well as duration of therapy. Other factors related to the patient's treatment and disease process can also affect fetal development: immunosuppression from chemotherapy can lead to opportunistic infections that can infect the developing fetus, and nutritional deficiencies secondary to anorexia from cancer and its therapy can be detrimental to the developing fetus. The interplay of all these factors is complex and makes it difficult to implicate a single cause of fetal abnormalities that may result from treatment during pregnancy.

TABLE 12–2.
Summary of Effects of Antineoplastic Therapy on the Developing Fetus Related to Gestational Age

Gestational Period	Time	Effects of Therapy	Comments
Implantation	Fertilization–week 2	Spontaneous abortion	
Organogenesis	Weeks 2–8	Congenital malformations	Nervous system, eye, respiratory, and hematopoietic systems continue to develop throughout gestation
Growth and development	Week 9–term	Growth retardation	More subtle effects may not be apparent until some time after birth

Chemotherapeutic Agents

Currently available antineoplastic drugs can prolong the lives of many patients with cancers such as lymphomas, leukemia, trophoblastic tumors, sarcomas, and breast cancer. Chemotherapeutic agents are nonspecific in selecting target cells and usually affect rapidly dividing cells. The harmful effects of these agents on the embryo or fetus are not well described (Table 12–3). Though the teratogenic potential of chemotherapeutic agents is clearly demonstrable in animals, extrapolation from animal data to humans may not be reliable.[15–17] Chemotherapeutic agents affect both normal and neoplastic cells by a variety of different mechanisms. The fetal consequences of exposure to cytotoxic drugs may be related to drug dose, fetal gestational age at the time of exposure, possible synergism of combinations of drugs, and combination chemotherapy and radiotherapy.[18] In addition, the placenta may create a biologic barrier to some antineoplastic agents.[19]

The exact nature and incidence of fetal effects after chemotherapy administration to pregnant women are not known. Many case reports have been published that describe both normal and abnormal outcomes following chemotherapy exposure during pregnancy. Several reviews allow some conclusions to be drawn. In general, antimetabolites carry a significant risk to the fetus. Aminopterin, a folate antagonist, is a known abortifacient when administered during the first trimester.[20] Other antimetabolites may be less potent. Maloney[21] studied 21 pregnant women with acute leukemia treated with 6-mercaptopurine and found no teratogenic effects in surviving children. Nicholson's review[22] of 185 pregnancies suggested that less than 8% of infants were congenitally malformed if the drugs were administered during the first trimester. He also noted that exposure in the later trimesters was not associated with increased risk of congenital malformation, but 40% of the exposed infants were of low birth weight. Sweet and Kinzie[23] commented that the risk of fetal malformation was 5% after

exposure to nonaminopterin antimetabolites was excluded.

Mauer et al.[24] reported a case of a trisomy C in an aborted fetus of a patient treated with cytosine arabinoside and thioguanine, two antimetabolites, during her second trimester. Another report discussed an infant with multiple anomalies after third-trimester exposure to busulfan.[25] Thus, there appears to be no safe drug or timing of exposure. In addition, long-term sequelae not apparent at birth can develop. Although an infant exposed to antineoplastic therapy in utero may appear normal, one must observe the child for any delayed effects on the cardiac, pulmonary, and central nervous (CNS) systems. In addition, the child's fertility may ultimately be affected. Finally, exposure to teratogenic drugs in utero may predispose to the development of later malignancies in the child. This has been demonstrated by the relationship between exposure to diethylstilbestrol (DES) in utero and the development of clear cell vaginal carcinoma in young women.[26]

There are some generalizations that one can state. First, there is no entirely safe cytotoxic drug or timing of exposure to the developing fetus; however, not all pregnancies so affected will produce a bad outcome. Second, antimetabolites, particularly antifolates, appear to produce an increased risk of spontaneous abortion and congenital malformations, especially after first-trimester exposure.[20–24] Third, lactating women on chemotherapy should avoid nursing; the secretion of these drugs into milk is as yet not well established. The patient and her family should be advised of all potential risks before embarking on cytotoxic chemotherapy of any type.

Radiation Therapy (see also Chap. 18)

Ionizing radiation is an important treatment modality for malignant lymphomas such as Hodgkin's disease and for many solid tumors, particularly breast carcinoma. The fetal effects of radiation exposure include growth

TABLE 12–3.
Commonly Used Antineoplastic Agents

Agent	Most Common Neoplasm	FDA Classification*	Comments
Anti-metabolites			
Methotrexate	Lymphomas Lymphoid leukemias Breast cancer Trophoblastic malignancies	D	Has caused fetal death and/or congenital anomalies; defective oogenesis has been reported
5-Fluorouracil (5-FU)	Breast cancer Gastrointestinal tumors	D	Adverse effect on fetal development in humans is not well established but is teratogenic in laboratory animals
6-Thioguanine	Acute leukemias	D	Potential teratogen; has been shown to be teratogenic in rats; there are no adequate and well-controlled studies in pregnant women
6-Mercaptopurine (6-MP)	Acute leukemias	D	Women receiving 6-MP in the 1st trimester have an increased incidence of abortion; the risk of malformation in offspring surviving 1st-trimester exposure is not accurately known
Cytosine arabinoside	Acute leukemias Lymphomas	C	Two cases of congenital malformation have been reported after 1st-trimester exposure; there have been multiple reports of normal offspring after in utero exposure
Antitumor antibiotics			
Doxorubicin	Acute lymphoblastic leukemia Breast cancer Sarcoma Ovarian carcinoma	D	Safe use during pregnancy has not been established; concern about long-term cardiac effects after in utero exposure
Daunorubicin	Acute nonlymphocytic leukemia	D	Safe use during pregnancy has not been established; concern about long-term cardiac effects after in utero exposure
Dactinomycin	Sarcomas Uterine cancer	C	Adverse effect on fetal development in humans is not well established; malformations occur in laboratory animals
Bleomycin	Lymphomas Squamous cell carcinomas	D	Adverse effect on fetal development in humans is not well established; malformations occur in laboratory animals; may have long-term pulmonary sequelae
Alkylating agents			
Cyclophosphamide	Breast carcinoma Lymphomas Ovarian carcinoma Chronic leukemias	D	Safe use in early pregnancy has not been established; can cause amenorrhea and infertility; excreted in breast milk
Melphalan	Ovarian carcinoma Chronic leukemias Multiple myeloma	D	No adequate and well-established studies in pregnant women

(Continued)

TABLE 12–3 (cont.).
Commonly Used Antineoplastic Agents

Agent	Most Common Neoplasm	FDA Classification*	Comments
Busulfan	Chronic leukemias	D	One case of malformed infant after in utero exposure and radiotherapy and 6-MP; several cases of normal offspring; can cause infertility; there are no adequate or well-controlled studies in pregnant women
Steroids			
Prednisone	Lymphomas Leukemias Breast carcinoma	B	Minimal risk to fetus; however, infants born of women on steroids need to be watched for hypocortisolism
Antiestrogens			
Tamoxifen	Breast cancer Uterine cancer	D	No well-controlled studies have been performed in pregnancy
Others			
Cisplatin	Ovarian cancer Sarcoma Bladder cancer	D	Safe use in pregnancy has not been established
Vincristine	Leukemia Lymphomas	D	Adverse effect on fetal development is not well documented
Vinblastine	Choriocarcinoma Breast cancer Lymphomas	D	No adequate well-controlled studies performed in pregnancy
Etoposide	Lymphomas Leukemias	D	Induces chromosomal aberrations

*See Preface for description of FDA drug classification.

retardation, microcephaly, and eye abnormalities. These effects are related to dose, dose rate, and gestational age. Even prior to implantation, the embryo is susceptible to the lethal effects of in utero radiation exposure. During the period of major organogenesis, radiation exposure can lead to congenital malformations. Later in pregnancy, radiation exposure can lead to growth retardation, though the still developing eye, nervous system, and hematopoietic system remain susceptible to the damaging effects of ionizing radiation.[18] There is no safe dose of radiation during pregnancy, but radiation damage follows a dose-response curve. Studies of atomic bomb survivors of Nagasaki and Hiroshima[27, 28] have provided important information about the relationship of gestational age and radiation dose in producing fetal abnormalities. The highest risk of fetal damage after such intense exposure ([>0.5 Gy] [100 rad = 1 Gy]) occurred when radiation exposure was during the first 20 weeks of gestation. In clinical practice, radiation exposure generally occurs with diagnostic radiographic procedures[29] and this topic is discussed in detail in Chapter 18.

Therapeutic radiation to supradiaphragmatic areas can be accomplished with abdominal shielding. Nonetheless, significant scatter can occur to the enlarging uterus in the third trimester.[30] Subdiaphragmatic, in particular pelvic, irradiation is hazardous. This is true of diagnostic as well as therapeutic radiology. Procedures such as lymphangiograms and computed tomographic (CT) scans of the abdomen and pelvis expose the fetus to fairly high doses of radiation (up to 0.05–0.1 Gy) and should be avoided unless essential for diagnostic or therapeutic purposes. Diagnostic ultrasound and magnetic resonance imaging may be relatively safe to perform during pregnancy, although the exact role of magnetic resonance imaging in staging most malignancies is not well established.[31, 32]

The long-term effects of fetal irradiation are not entirely known. Sweet and Kinzie reported an increased risk of leukemia and other cancers after low-dose radiation exposure. Other studies have not substantiated this claim.[33] However, children exposed to radiation in utero should be observed carefully as secondary malignancies can have a long latency period. Similarly, the exact incidence of sterility in these children is unknown, as is the potential for transmission of genetic diseases through chromosomal damage.

Ionizing radiation, like chemotherapeutic agents, can have a spectrum of effects upon the developing fetus depending upon dose and gestational age. As one attempts to stage the pregnant patient with cancer, one must determine the appropriate and safest diagnostic radiologic procedures. Alternatives such as ultrasound may be more advisable. Therapeutic radiation also requires careful consideration and one must advise the patient of all the potential risks.

EFFECTS OF ANTINEOPLASTIC THERAPY UPON GONADAL FUNCTION

Oogenesis

As more patients are treated and survive longer after antineoplastic therapy, many toxic effects have been recognized. Among these are acute and chronic effects upon gonadal function. Since antineoplastic therapy affects proliferating and rapidly self-renewing cell populations, the germ cell lines are particularly susceptible. Younger women undergoing antineoplastic therapy who are successfully treated may wish to resume a normal life style and questions of fertility and sexual function may be particularly problematic.

In order to understand the effects of antineoplastic therapy, such as chemotherapy and radiotherapy, a brief review of gonadal development in women will be presented. The mature female germ cells are direct descendants of the primordial germ cells which appear in the wall of the yolk sac and migrate toward the primitive sex glands by the beginning of the fifth gestational week. Once the primordial germ cells have arrived in the female gonad they differentiate into oogonia. These cells then undergo multiple mitotic divisions and some differentiate into the larger primary oocytes. By the seventh gestational month, the surviving primary oocytes have entered the first meiotic division which will eventually reduce the diploid chromosome number to half prior to fertilization. The primary oocyte, together with its surrounding epithelial cells, is known as the primordial follicle. Thus, women are born with a fixed number of germ cells which are not self-perpetuating after birth.[14]

At birth, the primary oocytes have completed prophase of the first meiotic division and have entered a resting stage between prophase and metaphase. The primary oocytes do not complete their first meiotic division until puberty is reached. The total number of primary oocytes at birth is estimated at between 700,000 to 2 million, the majority of which will become atretic. At puberty, the primordial follicles develop into mature graafian follicles and the first meiotic division is completed. Following puberty, follicular growth is a continuous process and ovulation occurs in a cyclic fashion. With each ovarian cycle, a number of follicles begin to develop, although usually only one reaches maturity. The others degenerate and become atretic.[14] An important point to realize is that some oocytes, reaching maturity late in reproductive life, have been dormant after prophase in the first meiotic division for 40 years or more. Since the incidence of children with congenital chromosomal abnormalities increases with maternal age, extended meiotic division may make the primary oocyte vulnerable to damage. This may be important when potentially teratogenic chemotherapy is administered to women at this time.

Effects of Therapy

Antineoplastic therapy is most likely to affect the process of follicular growth and maturation. There are no reliable animal models to study the effects of chemotherapeutic agents on ovarian function. Most information comes from clinical studies that rely upon menstrual and reproductive histories and serum hormone levels. Effects of antineoplastic therapy on the ovary are primarily follicle destruction and fibrosis with resultant hormonal changes and amenorrhea. An autopsy study of leukemia patients who received chemotherapy did not reveal a decrease in the primary follicles but a marked reduction in secondary follicles.[34] As a result of follicle destruction, amenorrhea ensues accompanied by sustained elevation of serum follicle-stimulating hormone (FSH) and luteinizing hormone (LH) and a fall in serum estradiol. Clinical signs and symptoms are similar to those of natural menopause and include vaginal atrophy, endometrial glandular hypoplasia, "hot flashes," and vaginal dryness with dyspareunia. The onset and duration of amenorrhea appear to be both chemotherapy dose- and age-related with younger patients able to tolerate large cumulative doses before becoming amenorrheic and having a greater likelihood of resumption of menstruation after completing therapy.[35]

Among antineoplastic drugs, alkylating agents are most commonly used and are the most frequent cause of ovarian dysfunction. Early clinical trials of single alkylating agents revealed amenorrhea as a common side effect. The early clinical trials of busulfan therapy for chronic myeloproliferative disorders demonstrated the onset of permanent amenorrhea in patients receiving doses varying from 0.5 to 14 mg/day for at least 3 months.[36, 37] Cyclophosphamide has been noted to cause amenorrhea in at least half of premenopausal women receiving 40 to 120 mg/day for an average of 18 months.[38, 39] Ovarian biopsy demonstrated arrest of follicular maturation and absence of ova in some patients.

Two studies in early breast cancer patients treated with adjuvant chemotherapy have suggested that the onset of amenorrhea and resumption of menses is related to patient age and total dose administered.[40, 41] These patients received cyclophosphamide in combination with other chemotherapeutic agents. Amenorrhea occurred in the majority of patients, with permanent amenorrhea in all patients over 40 years of age following a mean cumulative cyclophosphamide dose of 5.2 g. Amenorrhea occurred in patients under 40 years of age but only after a higher mean total dose of cyclophosphamide (9.3 g). Menses returned to all but two of these patients within 6 months of discontinuing chemotherapy. A study examined ovarian function in women receiving melphalan alone or in combination with the antimetabolite 5-fluorouracil (5-FU), and demonstrated amenorrhea in 22% of patients younger than 39 but in 73% of patients older than 40 years.[42] Among other classes of chemotherapeutic agents, high-dose methotrexate, an antimetabolite, does not appear to have immediate ovarian toxicity,[43] but etoposide, a topoisomerase II inhibitor, produces age- and dose-related amenorrhea following a mean total dose of 5 g.[44]

Combination chemotherapy used to treat advanced Hodgkin's disease frequently leads to ovarian failure. At least half of the women treated with MOPP (nitrogen mustard, vincristine, procarbazine, prednisone) will become amenorrheic. The risk is clearly related to the age of the patient at the time of treatment.[45–52] In the amenorrheic patients, serum FSH and LH are elevated consistent with primary ovarian failure. In one study, almost 90% of women over the age of 25 at the time of treatment developed permanent amenorrhea.[48] In addition, the onset of amenorrhea occurred within 1 year of stopping therapy in patients over 39 years of age, while younger patients had a gradual decrease in frequency of menses over several years.

The effects of radiation therapy on ovarian function are not as well defined. However, ovarian toxicity also appears to be related to age and total dose administered. Of patients treated with abdominopelvic radiotherapy for Hodgkin's disease, women younger than 20 years of age have a greater than 70% chance of retaining normal menses, whereas by age 30, the chance decreases to 20% and all older

TABLE 12–4.
Summary of Effects of Antineoplastic Therapy on the Ovary

1. Chemotherapy and radiotherapy can lead to follicle destruction with resultant amenorrhea
2. The onset and duration of ovarian failure is age- and total dose–related
3. In single-agent chemotherapy trials and adjuvant chemotherapy studies, women under 40 years of age can have return of normal menses
4. Combination chemotherapy is more likely to cause permanent ovarian failure in women over 25 years of age

women become sterile.[53] An operative procedure, oophoropexy, has been devised to shield the ovaries from megavoltage irradiation by moving the ovaries to the midline of the pelvis behind the uterus.[54] This has been shown to protect ovarian function in about half of the women receiving pelvic radiotherapy.

Can the ovary also be protected from the adverse effects of chemotherapy administration? An early report suggested that the ovarian follicles could be protected by inducing ovarian suppression with oral contraceptives.[55] However, more recent studies with a larger patient population and longer follow-up have not confirmed this benefit.[51, 52]

It appears that the majority of women treated with antineoplastic therapy will have premature ovarian failure (Table 12–4). This appears to be age- and total dose-related. Women who maintain normal menstrual function may have diminished fertility and premature menopause. Continued, long-term prospective follow-up is necessary to determine the risks of ovarian failure and early menopause in these patients.

SPECIFIC NEOPLASTIC DISEASES

Breast Cancer

The most frequent cancer in women is breast carcinoma, which accounts for approximately 45,000 deaths per year.[56] About 15% of all breast cancers occur in women under 40 years of age and about 3% occur during pregnancy. More than 90% of breast abnormalities and more than 75% of breast cancers are detected by patients themselves. Early diagnosis greatly improves the results of breast cancer treatment. Thus, breast self-examination is an essential component of programs to facilitate early detection.

Treatment of early-stage (I, II) breast cancer is primarily surgical with adjuvant chemotherapy or hormonal therapy used to improve survival in certain subsets of patients, i.e., premenopausal patients with axillary lymph nodes involved with tumor[57, 58] (Table 12–5). More advanced-stage breast cancer (III, IV) carries a much poorer prognosis and in premenopausal patients often requires aggressive combination chemotherapy. Breast cancer that expresses steroid hormone receptors (estrogen, progesterone) is not common in young premenopausal patients but if present can be treated with hormonal manipulation that might also interfere with ovarian function.

Diagnosis.—When a suspicious lesion is found in the breast of a pregnant or lactating woman, the physician must make every effort to expedite evaluation. Diagnosis is more difficult during pregnancy and lactation because of hypervascularity, increased size, and engorgement of glandular tissue. Careful serial examinations can be valuable but must not delay definitive diagnosis and risk disease dissemination. Typically, a delay in diagnosis averages 2 to 7 months for pregnant patients.[59] Thus, a disproportionately high number of patients present with axillary node involvement, which may reflect this delay in diagnosis. The histologic types of breast cancer in pregnant women are similar and not

TABLE 12–5.
Prognostic Factors in Primary Breast Cancer

Patient age
Size of primary tumor
Number of positive axillary lymph nodes
Hormone receptor status
Nuclear grade of malignant cells
Elevated *neu* oncogene expression

more aggressive than those in nonpregnant patients.

Mammography is a good noninvasive test that should precede biopsy of any suspicious lesion. Mammography may delineate other areas of subclinical involvement. It can be performed safely at low radiation dose, usually less than 1 rad per breast, with abdominal shielding. However, because of dense breast tissue present in pregnant or lactating patients, mammography is not a sensitive screening procedure during pregnancy. Suspicious lesions, either on palpation or imaging, should be biopsied. Needle biopsies can be safely performed with local anesthesia if the expertise is available. If not, an excisional biopsy is necessary. Tissue can then be sent for both estrogen receptor (ER) and progesterone receptor (PR) assays, realizing that most premenopausal breast cancer patients have low levels of ER and PR. Nevertheless, these assays may provide important information necessary to determine optimal therapy.

Treatment.—The treatment approach in pregnant or lactating women is the same as that for nonpregnant women. The therapeutic approach can be separated into the treatment of localized or locoregional disease and systemic therapy.[60, 61]

Local therapy consists of surgery, a modified radical mastectomy (MRM), or lumpectomy followed by radiation therapy. Recently, a large prospective randomized clinical trial has shown the efficacy of these two approaches to be equivalent.[62] Surgery and radiation therapy do pose a risk to the fetus.[63] The risk of spontaneous abortion during mastectomy is about 1%. Local radiotherapy to the chest can produce significant local scatter to the enlarging uterus even with proper shielding although this is not absolutely prohibitive and should not delay timely therapeutic intervention. There is now a growing body of evidence that women with stage I (i.e., node-negative) breast cancer may benefit in disease-free survival with adjuvant chemo- or hormonal therapy.[64]

Once tumor involves the axillary lymph nodes in premenopausal patients, adjuvant chemotherapy is indicated. The presence of axillary lymph node involvement correlates with the presence of occult disseminated metastases[57, 58] and adjuvant therapy attempts eradication of occult metastases. As previously discussed, most antineoplastic drugs are potentially teratogenic; thus, in early pregnancy, a decision regarding therapeutic abortion may be necessary. During the third trimester, therapy may be delayed a week or two until the fetus is viable ex utero. There have been reports of normal children born following systemic chemotherapy as discussed above; however, the numbers of reported cases are too few and adequate follow-up is not available to allow for definitive statements about long-term adverse effects.

In locally advanced or disseminated breast cancer (stages III and IV), systemic chemotherapy poses substantial risk to the fetus. Commonly used chemotherapy programs include cyclophosphamide, methotrexate, 5-FU (CMF) and cyclophosphamide, Adriamycin, 5-FU (CAF). Hormonal manipulation can be utilized in patients with ER- and/or PR-positive tumors.

Although the breast cancers occurring during pregnancy and lactation tend to present at later stages with more frequent nodal and disseminated disease (which may be due to delay in diagnosis), the prognosis is only slightly less favorable than in nonpregnant women on a stage-by-stage comparison.[65] The 5-year survival rates for each clinical stage are as follows: stage I, 90%; stage II, 37%; stage III, 15%; stage IV, 0%. The results are similar for therapy in each trimester of pregnancy or post partum for similar stages.

If breast cancer occurs during pregnancy, surgery is the treatment of choice for local disease (see Table 12–6). If adjuvant chemotherapy is necessary because of tumor involving the axillary lymph nodes, CMF should be avoided in the first trimester because of the antimetabolite methotrexate. Since one could potentially lose the therapeutic efficacy of adjuvant chemotherapy by waiting 6 months for

TABLE 12–6.
Guidelines for Evaluation and Treatment of Breast Cancer During Pregnancy

1. Definitive diagnosis of a breast mass should *NOT* be delayed.
2. Early-stage disease, i.e., stages I and II, requires multimodality therapy which should *NOT* be delayed because appropriate therapy has a significant positive influence upon survival:
   a. For first-trimester patients, consider therapeutic abortion before definitive surgery with or without radiotherapy *and* adjuvant chemotherapy.
   b. For second- or third-trimester patients, the pregnancy can be continued with some fetal risk, as discussed previously, during therapy which includes surgery with or without radiotherapy *and* adjuvant chemotherapy.
3. For advanced local breast cancer, i.e., stage III, the same above considerations apply. These patients will require chemotherapy.
4. For metastatic stage IV, breast cancer therapy is palliative and if necessary can be delayed.

delivery, CAF could be an alternative regimen in the first trimester. Treatment of metastatic breast cancer is truly palliative and treatment during pregnancy should only be undertaken for life-threatening indications such as hepatic metastases, CNS involvement, and compromised blood counts due to bone marrow involvement.

Hematologic Malignancies

Leukemia.—Acute leukemias are of two basic types: myeloid (AML) or lymphocytic (ALL). Both present with evidence of bone marrow failure due to suppression of normal blood stem cells by the leukemic clones. Bone marrow failure is manifested by suppression of normal blood counts resulting in neutropenia, anemia, and thrombocytopenia which can lead to life-threatening complications. If left untreated, patients with acute leukemia will die of infections or bleeding complications within 3 months of diagnosis.[66] With the use of aggressive combination chemotherapy and blood product transfusion support, a subset of patients with acute leukemia can obtain long-term survival and potential cure.

The incidence of acute leukemia in preg-

nancy is less than 1 in 75,000.[67] Approximately 300 pregnancies associated with leukemias, both acute and chronic, have been reported in the literature.[67–72] Acute leukemia constitutes 50% of these cases, with AML being more common than ALL, as is also true in nonpregnant women with acute leukemia. The main objectives in obstetric and medical management are to obtain remission, to maintain that remission long enough for the fetus to become viable, and to achieve delivery. Acute leukemia offers a great challenge as maternal mortality is high, with perinatal mortality estimated at 36% to 39%.[67] Chronic myelogenous leukemia (CML) represents most of the remaining cases of leukemia during pregnancy. This disorder frequently has an indolent clinical course initially and can be conservatively managed with careful observation and leukapheresis to reduce excessive leukocyte counts. Transformation of CML into blast phase presents problems similar to those that occur in AML. Chronic lymphocytic leukemia is an indolent disease of older patients and rarely occurs in patients of childbearing age.

There is no well-defined treatment approach for acute leukemia during pregnancy. Intensive combination chemotherapy is necessary and can prolong the life of the patient. Cytotoxic chemotherapy is potentially dangerous to the fetus, although the risk to any particular individual cannot be determined. Along with direct toxic effects of cytotoxic drugs, pregnancy is jeopardized by the prolonged period of anemia, thrombocytopenia, and infection that frequently accompany treatment of acute leukemia. The cornerstone of therapy for AML is cytosine arabinoside (ara-C) and anthracycline antibiotics such as daunorubicin. Combination chemotherapy for ALL consists of vincristine, prednisone, asparaginase, and methotrexate. CML in its chronic phase can be controlled with allkylating agents such as busulfan but will require intensive therapy during blastic transformation.

Patients diagnosed with acute leukemia during pregnancy also require aggressive

TABLE 12–7.
Classification of Non-Hodgkin's
Lymphoma—Working Formulation

Low grade
    A. Small lymphocytic plasmacytoid
    B. Follicular small cleaved cell
    C. Follicular mixed, small cleaved
       and large cell
Intermediate grade
    D. Follicular large cell
    E. Diffuse small cleaved cell
    F. Diffuse mixed, small and large
       cell
    G. Diffuse large cell
High grade
    H. Large cell, immunoblastic
    I. Lymphoblastic lymphoma
    J. Small noncleaved cell (Burkitt's)

chemotherapy to obtain remission, since without therapy acute leukemia is rapidly fatal. Thus, therapy cannot be delayed and its institution is considered a medical emergency. If therapy is initiated during the first trimester, there is an increased risk of fetal abnormalities and one may need to consider therapeutic abortion; however, therapy during the second or third trimester has not been clearly shown to increase fetal risk.[73–75] Leukemia therapy does not preclude a successful pregnancy. Hopefully, with improved chemotherapeutic regimens and suportive care, the life expectancy of mothers with leukemia can be improved.

Lymphoma

Malignant lymphomas can be divided into two main histopathologic groups: Hodgkin's disease (HD) and non-Hodgkin's lymphomas (NHLs). The NHLs can be further divided into three groups, low-grade, intermediate-grade, and aggressive lymphomas[76] (Table 12–7), that reflect the clinical behavior and prognoses of these disorders. Lymphomas are staged according to extent of nodal disease above and below the diaphragm (stages I, II, III) and presence of extranodal disease (stage IV) according to the Ann Arbor staging system (Table 12–8). Advanced-stage disease, in particular extranodal disease, generally has a worse prognosis. In addition, the presence of constitutional symptoms such as fever, night sweats, and weight loss greater than 10% of usual body weight over 6 months (B symptoms) portends more disseminated disease and a poorer prognosis. HD is readily treatable and curable 70% of the time with radiotherapy, combination chemotherapy, or a combination of the two depending upon stage of disease.[77] Indolent (low-grade) NHLs frequently present as advanced-stage but have a long natural history. Therapy is palliative for most patients. Aggressive NHL is rapidly fatal if left untreated but potentially can be cured with aggressive combination chemotherapy in over 50% of patients with advanced-stage disease (stages II, III, IV).[78–80]

It is estimated that 1 in 1,000 to 1 in 6,000 pregnancies are complicated by lymphomas.[81] HD is the most common lymphoma occurring in younger women during their reproductive years. NHL generally occurs in older individuals. There are fewer than 20 reports of NHL complicating pregnancy.[81–83] Pregnancy and lactation may complicate the management of patients with Burkitt's lymphoma, a particularly aggressive lymphoma which is rapidly fatal if untreated. In the gravid or lactating woman, Burkitt's lymphoma has a predilection for the breast.[83, 84] Because the breasts swell dramatically, this may be mistaken for mastitis and treated as such, thereby delaying diagnosis and therapy. Otherwise, pregnancy appears not to influence the course of lymphomas.

The approach to staging and therapy in

TABLE 12–8.
Ann Arbor Staging Criteria

Stage	Disease Extent
I	Involvement of a single lymph node group or a single extralymphatic site
II	Involvement of two or more lymph node groups on the same side of the diaphragm
III	Involvement on both sides of the diaphragm
IV	Diffuse or disseminated disease
A	Asymptomatic
B	Fever, sweats, weight loss >10% of body weight (not pruritus)

TABLE 12–9.
Management Guidelines for Pregnant Patients With
Lymphoma

1. Diagnostic and staging evaluation should be performed expeditiously.
2. For Hodgkin's disease, if unable to completely evaluate the abdomen because of a large, gravid uterus, combination chemotherapy will be necessary with or without radiotherapy.
3. For non-Hodgkin's lymphoma, therapy can be tailored to histologic subtype:
   a. Low-grade lymphomas may not require therapy if there is no major visceral compromise, i.e., liver, kidney, bone marrow, CNS.
   b. Intermediate- and high-grade lymphomas will require therapy no matter what gestational age is involved. If patient is in the first trimester, therapeutic abortion should be considered before the institution of definitive therapy. Therapy during later trimesters carries all the risks to the fetus as previously mentioned.

pregnant patients must be individualized. Many patients with low-grade indolent lymphomas or early-stage HD late in the third trimester can be allowed to deliver prior to staging and therapy. The approach to staging is more complicated in gravid patients with extensive disease and/or in early pregnancy. The purpose of staging is to detect disease in nodal or extranodal sites such as the bone marrow, liver, and CNS. In the nonpregnant patient, minimal evaluation includes a physical examination, chest radiographs, bone marrow biopsy, and imaging of the abdomen with CT or nuclear scans.[85] Lymphangiography can be extremely useful in evaluating abdominal lymph nodes in HD. It can be accomplished in pregnant patients if a *single* abdominal film is taken 24 hours after injection of contrast to minimize radiation risks.[86] For pregnant patients, the minimum number of radiographic studies should be performed that will allow therapy decisions to be made; however, the diagnostic evaluation should not be delayed. Only a small number of patients with HD require staging laparotomy if radiotherapy is to be their only therapeutic option. If combined-modality therapy or chemotherapy alone is to be utilized, staging laparotomy is not necessary; thus, in most cases, it can be avoided.

Once staging is accomplished, treatment should be started as soon as possible (see Table 12–9). Localized disease above the diaphragm can be treated with radiotherapy and abdominal shielding. Extensive disease on both sides of the diaphragm or involving extralymphatic sites is more complicated. Extensive low-grade or indolent NHL may not require immediate therapy if there is no serious compromise of major organ systems such as ureteral obstruction. Advanced-stage, intermediate-grade, and aggressive NHL will require combination chemotherapy to halt progression of tumor growth and offer the possibility of cure. For advanced-stage HD that would require chemotherapy (stages IIIB, IVA, IVB), therapy could be delayed until after organogenesis when fetal risks may be less. The potential risks to the developing fetus depend upon drugs, drug dose, and timing during development as discussed previously.

Following therapy for HD, amenorrhea may occur, particularly in older patients. Younger patients, who may not have permanent amenorrhea, should not conceive until they have been in continuous remission for 2 years.[81] Recurrences are most likely to occur within this period. The risk of fetal abnormalities following successful treatment for HD has not been carefully defined although one study suggests that there may be an increased risk of future pregnancies resulting in spontaneous abortion and in fetal abnormalities if there has been prior therapy with radiation and chemotherapy.[87] Most studies, however, demonstrate no increased risk of spontaneous abortion or fetal abnormalities following treatment for HD greater than the risks prevailing in the general population.

Malignant Melanoma

Melanoma accounts for 1% of all cancers diagnosed in the United States. The peak incidence is in the third and fourth decades of life. The exact incidence during pregnancy is unknown. The effect of pregnancy on the course of melanoma is controversial and has been discussed above. Melanoma can be a very unpredictable disease. There are reports of spontaneous regression, although once it has metastasized it is usually rapidly fatal.

Diagnosis is made by biopsy. Any suspicious skin change in a pregnant patient should prompt immediate biopsy and therapeutic intervention. Staging systems have been devised by Clark[88] and Breslow[89] and are based upon depth of local invasion. The development of regional or distant metastatic disease correlates with the thickness of the cancerous lesion. Patients with lesions of intermediate thickness, 0.76 to 3.99 mm, have a 50% to 60% risk of metastases to regional nodes and a 20% risk of distant metastases. Treatment consists of wide local excision and regional lymphadenectomy.[90] Patients with melanomas greater than 4 mm in thickness have more than an 80% risk of distant metastatic disease. Other poor prognostic features include ulceration of the lesion, truncal location, and presence of nodal metastases.

Distant metastatic disease may be treatable with systemic chemotherapy. Metastases in skin, soft tissue, or lymph nodes have response rates of 30% to 50%. However, metastases to liver, bone, and/or brain have response rates of less than 20%. Dacarbazine (DTIC-Dome) is the agent of choice with response rates of 20%.[91] Combination chemotherapy has been attempted without clear evidence of superior results.[92] Immunotherapy with bacille Calmette-Guérin (BCG) vaccine is helpful in localized skin lesions and interleukin-2, a lymphokine, may have a limited role.[93] Early diagnosis and therapy is essential to obtaining long-term survival. Even if metastatic disease is present during pregnancy, the low probability of response to chemotherapy may not justify exposing the fetus to such treatment unless the tumor is rapidly progressive and symptomatic.

Gynecologic Malignancies

Cervical Carcinoma.—As a group, gynecologic malignancies, and in particular cervical carcinoma, are as common in pregnant women as is breast carcinoma. It is es-

timated that there is one gynecologic cancer for every 407 pregnancies.[97] Almost 80% of these are cervical carcinoma. Indeed, it has been estimated that 2.7% to 3.5% of all cervical cancers occur in pregnant patients.[95]

The diagnostic approach is the same as in nonpregnant women. Vaginal examinations and Papanicolaou smears are part of routine prenatal evaluation and are important in screening for premalignant and malignant cervical lesions. There are no pathophysiologic changes in the cervix that occur during pregnancy that mimic premalignant or malignant lesions. Pregnant patients with cytologic evidence of dysplasia but without clinically apparent lesions can be followed closely with colposcopy. If no severe changes occur, patients can be allowed to deliver and then undergo postpartum evaluation.[96, 97] Conization should be avoided during pregnancy unless frank anaplasia is found on the smear. Under these circumstances, a cone biopsy is invaluable in determining depth of invasion.

Cervical cancer in the nonpregnant patient is a treatable malignancy with 10-year survival rates of 45% to 50% overall. It can be cured by radiotherapy, by surgery, or by the combination of the two if discovered before metastatic disease is present. The approach to metastatic disease is palliative, not curative. There is no difference in the manner in which cervical cancer behaves in the pregnant versus nonpregnant patient. The cure rate is similar in the two groups.[97, 98]

Cervical cancer tends to be a slow-growing malignancy and rarely progresses rapidly from in situ to invasive cancer. Thus, the disease can be closely followed during the course of pregnancy. In cases where the carcinoma has invaded more than 3 mm into the stroma when discovered, therapy must be instituted. FIGO (International Federation of Obstetrics and Gynecology) stage IA, microinvasive disease, can be treated conservatively in pregnant patients.[96–98] FIGO stage IB, more invasive disease, should be treated with a third-trimester cesarean hysterectomy.[95] FIGO stages II, III, and IV, frankly invasive, malignant, and advanced disease, are treated with radiotherapy, both external beam and brachytherapy, and chemotherapy. It may be feasible to allow the fetus to mature to viability if this occurs in the third trimester, especially for FIGO stage IV where therapy is only palliative, not curative. It is not advisable to allow a woman to deliver vaginally through a cancerous cervix, which may bleed excessively. To institute effective curative therapy, lesions must be discovered and treated early.

Ovarian Cancer.—The incidence of ovarian malignancies is from 1 in 9,000 to 1 in 25,000 pregnancies. Nulliparous women have a higher incidence[99] of this disease suggesting that pregnancy may protect against the development of ovarian tumors. About 5% of ovarian masses found during pregnancy are malignant; in contrast, up to 20% of ovarian masses have been reported to be malignant in nonpregnant patients.[99–101] Ovarian masses are easily found during pregnancy because of the routine use of ultrasound. Patients with masses greater than 5 cm persisting into the second trimester may require laparotomy or laparoscopy for diagnosis.[99–102]

The key prognostic variables in ovarian cancer are histology, grade, and stage. Early-stage (FIGO I, II) ovarian cancer can be cured with surgery. More advanced stages (FIGO III, IV) will require combination chemotherapy with only a very small fraction of these patients potentially cured. A large proportion of ovarian tumors occurring during pregnancy are of unusual histologic types and have a low-grade histology.[103] Thus, unilateral oophorectomy may be appropriate in some cases. More poorly differentiated but localized neoplasms may require adjuvant chemotherapy such as oral melphalan following surgery. For the advanced stages (FIGO III, IV), combination chemotherapy with cisplatin-based regimens can lead to complete responses but few cures. Pregnancy itself does not appear to adversely affect survival.[99, 102, 103] Once again the institution of chemotherapy for advanced stages of disease

carries risk to the fetus but may be beneficial to the mother and improve her survival. Thus, for advanced-stage disease, postoperative chemotherapy should be administered as indicated.

Choriocarcinoma.—Choriocarcinomas occur rarely during normal pregnancy. Thirty cases have been reported.[104–106] Pregnant patients with choriocarcinoma are considered to have a poorer prognosis than nonpregnant patients.[106] Methotrexate, an antimetabolite, has been an extremely active agent against this tumor but also poses great risk to the developing fetus. It has been used in combination with other chemotherapeutic agents such as actinomycin D and cyclophosphamide. Patients with metastases to the brain or liver should receive radiotherapy to those areas. Human chorionic gonadotropin levels can be followed as tumor markers and used to judge duration of therapy. The Duke Trophoblastic Disease Center demonstrated survival figures of 60% for patients with choriocarcinoma following term gestation compared with 95% in nonpregnant patients with trophoblastic malignancy.[105, 107] Chemotherapy is the treatment of choice for choriocarcinoma and should be instituted without delay. If this occurs during the first trimester, one may need to consider therapeutic abortion since the degree of fetal risk may be unacceptable. Patients treated for choriocarcinoma with methotrexate have been reported to undergo subsequent successful pregnancies following therapy.[106] The risks of fetal malformations in subsequent pregnancies are no greater than for the general population.

Vulvar and Vaginal Cancer.—Since the majority of patients with vulvar carcinoma are in an older age group, its association with pregnancy is rare.[94, 103, 108] There have been fewer than 50 cases reported. Vaginal carcinoma is even rarer with 11 reported cases of squamous cell carcinoma and 3 reported cases of adenocarcinoma in women with a history of exposure to DES. Diagnosis is made by physical examination, Papanicolaou smear, and biopsy.

There is no evidence that pregnancy adversely affects vulvar or vaginal cancers. Therapy of vulvar tumors is surgical. For invasive lesions, a radical vulvectomy and groin dissection may be necessary. This can be deferred in third-trimester patients until after delivery.[108] The experience with vaginal malignancies is more limited and therapy consists of surgery, radiation, or both.[103] There is not enough experience with these malignancies during pregnancy to draw meaningful conclusions.

Endometrial Cancer.—Only 8% of cases of endometrial cancer occur in women under the age of 40. Eight cases associated with pregnancy have been reported. Most patients had well-differentiated tumors and were found to have limited-stage disease. Only one patient had deep invasion of the myometrium and was reported to have died of her disease.[94, 103] Thus, no definite conclusions about this tumor's behavior during gestation can be made.

Other Tumors

Thyroid Cancer.—Thyroid cancer occurs with an estimated frequency of 2.2 per 100,000 cases each year. Less than half are in women in the reproductive age group. Patients with a history of thyroid irradiation for benign conditions are at increased risk.[109] Ultrasound-guided fine-needle aspiration of thyroid nodules for cytology is a useful diagnostic procedure. Most of these tumors are well-differentiated papillary carcinomas. Treatment for well-differentiated tumors such as papillary and follicular carcinomas as well as medullary carcinomas should be surgical with total thyroidectomy and lymph node dissection if indicated[110] (see Table 12–10). Patients with well-differentiated thyroid cancers should take thyroid hormone postoperatively to reduce recurrence.[111] Radioactive iodine for diagnostic purposes, ablation, or treatment for metastatic disease should not be used during pregnancy, as this poses risk to the fetus since the fetal thyroid gland will also take up the isotope.[112] Pregnancy does not appear to have an adverse effect on the biology of this tumor.[109, 113] (See also Chapter 4, p. 124.)

Gastrointestinal Cancer

These neoplasms are relatively rare in women of childbearing age and not often associated with pregnancy. The incidence of colorectal cancer during pregnancy is estimated to be between 0.02% and 0.002%. There are probably fewer than 200 cases of rectal cancer reported in pregnancy and 19 cases of colon cancer.[59, 114, 115] There are 3 cases of gastric cancer reported in the English literature and

TABLE 12–10.
Management Guidelines for Thyroid Carcinoma

Histology	Stage	Therapy of Choice
Well-differentiated		
Papillary + Follicular	Localized	Surgery and thyroid suppression with hormone or [131]I*
	Metastatic	Radioactive iodine (^{131}I)*
Medullary	Localized	Surgery/radiotherapy ([131]I* or megavoltage)
	Metastatic	Chemotherapy†
Anaplastic	Localized	Surgery/radiotherapy
	Metastatic	Combination chemotherapy†

*Should not be used during pregnancy.
†Decisions regarding chemotherapy during pregnancy must be individualized, decisions being influenced by gestational age and extent and site of tumor.

TABLE 12–11.
Summary of Management Recommendations

1. Diagnostic and therapeutic strategies have to be individualized depending upon the tumor, its prognosis, and the gestational stage. However, evaluation and therapy of treatable lesions needs to proceed rapidly.
2. The potential for fetal risk from antineoplastic therapy is greatest in the first trimester.
3. During the first trimester, folate antagonists should be avoided.
4. During the first trimester, radiation exposure to the pelvis should be limited to essential diagnostic and therapeutic interventions necessary to preserve the life of the mother and fetus.

44 in the Japanese literature. Hepatocellular carcinomas are rare in the United States. Women who use contraceptive pills have an increased incidence of benign hepatocellular adenomas which have a propensity to rupture and cause intraabdominal hemorrhage.[116]

There are several conditions that can occur in young women that predispose to gastrointestinal cancer: ulcerative colitis, familial polyposis, Gardner's syndrome, and villous tumors. These patients require frequent surveillance with annual colonoscopy and biopsies of any suspicious lesions. Delay in diagnosis is, unfortunately, common, as many of the symptoms can be attributable to the pregnancy itself. Any persistent rectal bleeding, changing bowel habits, weight loss, or nausea and vomiting in late pregnancy should be investigated. Digital rectal examination can detect many rectal cancers. Colonoscopy can be performed with care during pregnancy. Diagnostic barium radiographs pose some radiation risk to the fetus and should be performed only if benefits of early diagnosis clearly outweigh fetal risks (see Chap. 18).

The chance for cure of these tumors depends upon whether the tumor is resectable. Chemotherapy has produced disappointing results and thus can be avoided in pregnancy. Although numbers in reported series are too small to make meaningful statements concerning survival, no pregnant patient with colon cancer has survived 5 years.[117] Only a few patients with rectal cancer have been long-term survivors.[118] In many of these cases, di-

agnosis and adequate therapy was delayed.

Other Tumors

Sarcomas are rare tumors but can occur in women in their childbearing years. They can be primary osseous tumors or soft tissue tumors. Over 50 cases have been reported to date; all required therapy and were not affected by the hormonal state of pregnancy.[119–121] Other tumors reported during pregnancy include parathyroid carcinoma, primary brain tumors, and multiple myeloma.

Summary

Malignancies occurring in women of childbearing age include breast cancer, cervical carcinoma, hematologic malignancies, and malignant melanoma. Pregnancy does not appear to affect adversely the outcome of most tumors. However, delay in diagnosis has contributed to an increase in mortality. Thus, rapid diagnosis is essential to increasing the probability of successful therapy. The approach to malignancy during pregnancy needs to be individualized and involves input from the mother, obstetrician, oncologist, and pediatrician (Table 12–11). Therapy, whether by radiation or with antineoplastic drugs, has the greatest potential for fetal risk during the first trimester but more acceptable risk in the second and third trimesters. If chemotherapy is to be given, folate antagonists should be avoided early in pregnancy as they pose a great risk to the fetus. Similarly, high-dose radiotherapy to the pelvis should be avoided in early pregnancy. One must weigh the risk to the mother's life posed by her malignancy versus the harmful effects of antineoplastic therapy upon the fetus. There are as yet many unanswered questions concerning long-term effects of the cancer and its therapy upon the surviving child. Many difficult issues arise when cancer complicates pregnancy and the solutions are not always obvious, but acceptable alternatives can often be devised based upon a thorough knowledge of the prognosis and natural history of the tumor, the effects of treatment on the fetus, and a strong and compassionate doctor-patient relationship.

REFERENCES

1. Gleicher N, Deppe G, Cohen CJ: Common aspects of immunologic tolerance in pregnancy and malignancy. *Obstet Gynecol* 1979; 54:335–342.

2. Gleicher N, Seigel I: Common denominators of pregnancy and malignancy. *Prog Clin Biol Res* 1981; 70:339–353.

3. Mitchell MS, Capizzi RL: Neoplastic diseases, in Burrow GN, Ferris TF (eds): *Medical Complications of Pregnancy.* Philadelphia, WB Saunders Co, 1988, pp 540–569.

4. Riberti C, Marola G, Bertani A: Malignant melanoma: The adverse effect of pregnancy. *Br J Plast Surg* 1981; 34:338–339.

5. Nieminen N, Remes N: Malignancy during pregnancy. *Acta Obstet Gynecol Scand* 1970; 49:315.

6. Shiu MH, Schottenfeld D, Maclean B, et al: Adverse effect of pregnancy on melanoma: A reappraisal. *Cancer* 1976; 37:181–187.

7. Houghton AN, Flannery J, Viola MV: Malignant melanoma of skin occurring during pregnancy. *Cancer* 1980; 45:1540–1548.

8. Donegan WL: Breast cancer and pregnancy. *Obstet Gynecol* 1977; 50:244.

9. Pirani BBK, Campbell DM, MacGillivray I: Plasma volume in normal first pregnancy. *Br J Obstet Gynaecol* 1973; 80:884–887.

10. Mucklow JC: The fate of drugs in pregnancy. *Clin Obstet Gynaecol* 1986; 13:161–175.

11. Redmond GP: Physiologic changes during pregnancy and their implications for pharmacologic treatment. *Clin Invest Med* 1985; 8:317–322.

12. Powis G: Anticancer drug pharmacodynamics. *Cancer Chemother Pharmacol* 1985; 14:177–183.

13. Davison JS, Davison MC, Hay DM: Gastric emptying time in late pregnancy and labour. *Br J Obstet Gynaecol* 1970; 77:37–41.

14. Langman J: *Medical Embryology,* ed 3. Baltimore, Williams & Wilkins Co, 1975.

15. Chaube S, Murphy ML: The teratogenic effects of the recent drugs active in cancer chemotherapy. *Adv Teratol* 1968; 3:181–237.

16. Sieber SM, Adamson RH: Toxicity of anti-neoplastic agents in man: Chromosomal aberrations, antifertility effects, congenital malformations and carcinogenic potential. *Adv Cancer Res* 1975; 22:57–155.

17. Brent RL: Evaluating the alleged teratogenicity of environmental agents. *Clin Perinatol* 1986; 13:609–613.

18. Orr JW Jr, Shingleton HM: Cancer in pregnancy. *Curr Probl Cancer* 1983; 8:1–50.

19. Roboz J, Gleicher N, Wu K, et al: Does doxorubicin cross the placenta? *Lancet* 1979; 2:1382–1383.

20. Shaw EB, Steinbach HL: Aminopterin-induced fetal malformation. *Am J Dis Child* 1968; 115:477–482.

21. Maloney WC: Management of leukemia in pregnancy. *Ann NY Acad Sci* 1964; 114:857–867.

22. Nicholson HO: Cytotoxic drugs in pregnancy. *J Obstet Gynecol Br Commw* 1968; 75:307–312.

23. Sweet DL Jr, Kinzie J: Consequences of radiotherapy and anti-neoplastic therapy for the fetus. *J Reprod Med* 1976, 17:241–246.

24. Mauer LH, Forcier RJ, McIntyre OR: Fetal group C trisomy after cytosine arabinoside and thioguanine. *Ann Intern Med* 1971; 75:809–810.

25. Boros SJ, Reynolds JW: Intrauterine growth retardation following third trimester exposure to busulfan. *Am J Obstet Gynecol* 1977; 129:111–112.

26. Herbst AL, Ulfelderlt H, Poskanzer DC, et al: Adenocarcinoma of the vagina: Association of material stilbestrol therapy with tumor appearance in young women. *N Engl J Med* 1971; 284:878–881.

27. Blot WJ, Miller RW: Mental retardation following *in utero* exposure to the atomic bombs of Hiroshima and Nagasaki. *Radiology* 1973; 106:617–619.

28. Plummer G: Anomalies occurring in children exposed *in utero* to the atomic bomb in Hiroshima. *Pediatrics* 1952; 10:687–692.

29. Brent RL: Irradiation in pregnancy, in Gerbie AB, Sciarra JJ (eds): *Gynecology and Obstetrics,* New York, Harper & Row Publishers, 1981, pp 1–22.

30. Doll DC, Ringenberg S, Yarbro JW: Management of cancer during pregnancy. *Arch Intern Med* 1988; 148:2058–2064.

31. Stark DD, McCarthy SM, Filly RA, et al: Intrauterine growth retardation: Evaluation by magnetic resonance. *Radiology* 1985; 155:425–427.

32. Cohen JM, Weinreb JC, Low TW, et al: MR imaging of a viable full-term abdominal pregnancy. *AJR* 1985; 145:407–408.

33. Court-Brown WM, Soll R, Hill RB: Incidence of leukemia after exposure to diagnostic radiation *in utero*. *Br Med J* 1960; 2:1539–1545.

34. Kuhajdu FP, Haupt HM, Moore GW, et al: Gonadal morphology in patients receiving chemotherapy for leukemia: Evidence for reproductive potential and against a testicular tumor sanctuary. *Am J Med* 1982; 72:759–767.

35. Gradishar WJ, Schilsky RL: Effects of cancer treatment on the reproductive system *CRC Crit Rev Oncol Hematol* 1988; 8:153–171.

36. Louis J, Umargi LR, Best WR: Treatment of chronic granulocytic leukemia with Myeleran. *Arch Intern Med* 1956; 97:299–308.

37. Galton DAG, Till M, Wiltshaw E: Busulfan: Summary of clinical results. *Ann NY Acad Sci* 1958; 68:967–973.

38. Uldall PR, Kerr DNS, Tacchi D: Sterility and cyclophosphamide. *Lancet* 1972; 1:693–694.

39. Warne GL, Fairley KF, Hobbs JB, et al: Cyclophosphamide-induced ovarian failure. *N Engl J Med* 1973; 289:1159–1162.

40. Samaan NA, DeAsis DM, Buydar AU, et al: Pituitary-ovarian function in breast cancer patients on adjuvant chemo-immunotherapy. *Cancer* 1978; 41:2084–2087.

41. Dnistrian AM, Schwartz MK, Fracchia AA, et al: Endocrine consequences of CMF adjuvant therapy in pre-menopausal and post-menopausal breast cancer patients. *Cancer* 1983; 51:803–807.

42. Fisher B, Sherman B, Rockette H, et al: L-phenylalanine mustard in the management of pre-menopausal patients with primary breast cancer. *Cancer* 1979; 44:847–857.

43. Shamberger RC, Rosenberg SA, Seipp CA, et al: Effects of high dose methotrexate and vincristine on ovarian and testicular functions in patients undergoing postoperative adjuvant treatment of osteosarcoma. *Cancer Treat Rep* 1981; 65:739–746.

44. Choo YC, Chan SYW, Wong LC, et al: Ovarian dysfunction in patients with gestational trophoblastic neoplasia treated with short intensive courses of etoposide. *Cancer* 1985; 55:2348–2352.

45. Morgenfeld MC, Goldberg V, Parisier H, et al: Ovarian lesions due to cytostatic agents during the treatment of Hodgkin's disease. *Surg Gynecol Obstet* 1972; 134:826–828.

46. Sherins R, Winokur S, De Vita VT Jr, et al: Surprisingly high risk of functional castration in women receiving chemotherapy for lymphoma (abstract). *Clin Res* 1975; 23:343A.

47. Chapman RM, Sutcliffe SB, Malpas JS: Cytotoxic-induced ovarian failure in women with Hodgkin's disease I. Hormone function. *JAMA* 1979; 242:1877–1881.

48. Schilsky RL, Sherins RJ, Hubbard SM, et al: Long-term followup of ovarian function in women treated with MOPP chemotherapy for Hodgkin's disease. *Am J Med* 1981; 71:552–556.

49. Horning SJ, Hoppe RT, Kaplan HS, et al: Female reproductive potential after treatment of Hodgkin's disease. *N Engl J Med* 1981; 304:1377–1382.

50. Andrieu JM, Ochoa-Molina ME: Menstrual cycle, pregnancies, and offspring before and after MOPP therapy for Hodgkin's disease. *Cancer* 1983; 52:435–438.

51. Whitehead E, Shalet SM, Blackledge G, et al: The effect of combination chemotherapy on ovarian function in women treated for Hodgkin's disease. *Cancer* 1983; 52:988–993.

52. Specht L, Hansen MM, Geisler C: Ovarian function in young women in long-term remission after treatment for Hodgkin's disease stage I or II. *Scand J Haematol* 1984; 32:265–270.

53. Hornig SJ, Hoppe RT, Kaplan HS, et al: Female reproductive potential after treatment for Hodgkin's disease. *N Engl J Med* 1981; 304:1377–1382.

54. Ray GB, Trueblood HW, Enright LP, et al: Oophoropexy: A means of preserving ovarian function following pelvic megavoltage radiotherapy for Hodgkin's disease. *Radiology* 1970; 96:175–180.

55. Chapman RM, Sutcliffe SB: Protection of

ovarian function by oral contraceptives in women receiving chemotherapy for Hodgkin's disease. *Blood* 1981; 58:849–851.

56. Cancer Statistics, 1989. *CA* 1989; 39:3–20.

57. Bonadonna G, Brussamolina M, Valagusa P, et al: Combination chemotherapy as an adjuvant treatment in operable breast cancer. *N Engl J Med* 1976; 294:405–410.

58. Fisher B, Redmond C, Fisher ER, et al: The contribution of recent NSABP clinical trials of primary breast cancer therapy to an understanding of tumor biology. *Cancer* 1980; 46:1009–1025.

59. Donegan WL: Cancer and pregnancy. *CA* 1983; 33:194–214.

60. King RM, Welch JS, Martin JK, et al: Carcinoma of the breast associated with pregnancy. *Surg Gynecol Obstet* 1985; 160:228–232.

61. Parente JT, Amsel M, Lerner R, et al: Breast cancer associated with pregnancy. *Obstet Gynecol* 1988; 71:861–864.

62. Fisher B, Bauer M, Margolese R: Five-year results of a randomized clinical trial comparing total mastectomy and segmented with or without radiation in the treatment of breast cancer. *N Engl J Med* 1985; 312:665–673.

63. Byrd BF Jr, Bayer DS, Robertson JC, et al: Treatment of breast tumors associated with pregnancy and lactation. *Ann Surg* 1962; 155:904–947.

64. Fisher B, Redmond C, Dimitrov NV, et al: A randomized clinical trial evaluating sequential methotrexate and fluorouracil in the treatment of patients with node-negative breast cancer who have estrogen-receptor-negative tumors. *N Engl J Med* 1989; 320:473–478.

65. Riberio GG, Palmer MK: Breast carcinoma associated with pregnancy: A clinician's dilemma. *Br Med J* 1977; 2:1524–1527.

66. Wiernick PH: Acute leukemias of adults, in DeVita VT Jr, Hellman S, Rosenberg SA (eds): *Cancer—Principles and Practices of Oncology*, ed 2. Philadelphia, JB Lippincott Co, 1985, pp 1711–1737.

67. McClain CR: Leukemia in pregnancy. *Clin Obstet Gynecol* 1974; 17:185–194.

68. Raich PC, Curet LB: Treatment of acute leukemia during pregnancy. *Cancer* 1975; 36:861–862.

69. Bitran JD, Roth DG: Acute leukemia during reproductive life: Its course, complications and sequelae for fertility. *J Reprod Med* 1976; 17:225–231.

70. Miller JB: Chronic myelogenous leukemia and the myeloproliferative diseases during the child-bearing years. *J Reprod Med* 1976; 17:217–224.

71. Lilleyman JS, Hill AS, Anderson KJ: Consequences of acute myelogenous leukemia in early pregnancy. *Cancer* 1977; 40:1300–1303.

72. Doney KC, Kraemer KG, Shepard TH: Combination chemotherapy for acute myelocytic leukemia during pregnancy: Three case reports. *Cancer Treat Rep* 1979; 63:369–371.

73. Gokal R, Durant J, Baum JD, et al: Successful pregnancy in acute monocytic leukemia. *Br J Cancer* 1976; 34:299–302.

74. Okun DB, Groncy PK, Siegler L, et al: Acute leukemia in pregnancy: Transient neonatal myelosuppression after combination chemotherapy in the mother. *Med Pediatr Oncol* 1979; 7:315–319.

75. Dora P, Slater IM, Armentrout SA: Successful pregnancy during chemotherapy for acute leukemia. *Cancer* 1981; 47:845–846.

76. National Cancer Institute Sponsored Study of Classifications of Non-Hodgkin's Lymphomas: Summary and description of a working formulation for clinical usage. *Cancer* 1982; 49:2112–2135.

77. Longo DL, Young RC, Wesley M, et al: Twenty years of MOPP therapy for Hodgkin's disease. *J Clin Oncol* 1986; 4:1295–1306.

78. Armitage JO, Dick FR, Corder MP, et al: Predicting therapeutic outcome in patients with diffuse histiocytic lymphoma treated with cyclophosphamide, adriamycin, vincristine, and prednisone (CHOP). *Cancer* 1982; 1695–1702.

79. Fisher RI, DeVita VT Jr, Hubbard SM, et al: Diffuse aggressive lymphomas: Increased survival after alternating flexible sequences of ProMACE and MOPP chemotherapy. *Ann Intern Med* 1983; 98:304–309.

80. Klimo P, Connors JM: MACOP-B chemotherapy for the treatment of diffuse large cell lymphoma. *Ann Intern Med* 1985; 102:596–602.

81. Sweet DL Jr: Malignant lymphoma: Im-

plications during the reproductive years and pregnancy. *J Reprod Med* 1976; 17:198–208.

82. O'Dell RF: Leukemia and lymphoma complicating pregnancy. *Clin Obstet Gynecol* 1979; 22:859–870.

83. Jones DED, d'Avignon MB, Lawrence, et al: Burkitt's lymphoma: Obstetric and gynecologic aspects. *Obstet Gynecol* 1980; 56:533–536.

84. Durodola JT: Burkitt's lymphoma presenting during lactation. *Int J Gynaecol Obstet* 1976; 14:225–231.

85. Williams SF, Golomb HG: Perspective on staging approaches in the malignant lymphomas. *Surg Gynecol Obstet* 1986; 163:193–201.

86. Thomas PRM, Biochem D, Peckham MJ: The investigation and management of Hodgkin's disease in the pregnant patient. *Cancer* 1976; 38:1443–1451.

87. Holmes GE, Holmes FF: Pregnancy outcome of patients treated for Hodgkin's disease: A controlled study. *Cancer* 1978; 41:1317–1322.

88. Clark WH, Jr: The histogenesis and biologic behavior of primary human malignant melanoma of the skin. *Cancer Res* 1960; 29:705–727.

89. Breslow A: Thickness, cross-sectional areas and depth of invasion in the prognosis of cutaneous melanoma. *Ann Surg* 1970; 172:902–908.

90. Balch CM, Murad TM, Soong SJ, et al: Tumor thickness as a guide to surgical management of clinical stage I melanoma patients. *Cancer* 1979; 43:883–888.

91. Comis RL: DTIC (NSC-45388) in malignant melanoma: A perspective. *Cancer Treat Rep* 1976; 165–175.

92. Mastrangelo MJ, Baker AR, Katy HR: Cutaneous melanoma, in DeVita VT Jr, Hellman S, Rosenberg SA (eds): *Cancer—Principles and Practices of Oncology*, ed 2. Philadelphia, JB Lippincott Co, 1985, pp 1371–1422.

93. Rosenberg SA: Adoptive immunotherapy of cancer using lymphokine activated killer cells and recombinant interleukin-2, in DeVita VT Jr, Hellman S, Rosenberg SA (eds): *Important Advances in Oncology*. Philadelphia, JB Lippincott Co, 1986, pp 55–91.

94. Lutz MH, Underwood PB Jr, Rozier JC, et al: Genital malignancy in pregnancy. *Am J Obstet Gynecol* 1977; 129:536–542.

95. Sablinska R, Tarlowska L, Stelmachow J: Invasive carcinoma of the cervix associated with pregnancy: Correlation between patient age, advancement of cancer and gestation, and results of treatment. *Gynecol Oncol* 1977; 5:363–373.

96. Gilotra PM, Lee FY, Krupp RJ, et al: Carcinoma in situ of the cervix uteri in pregnancy. *Surg Gynecol Obstet* 1976; 142:396–398.

97. Hoskins WJ, Perez C, Young RL: Gynecologic tumors, in DeVita VT, Hellman S, Rosenberg SA (eds): *Cancer: Principles and Practice of Oncology*, ed 3. Philadelphia, JB Lippincott Co, 1989, pp 1099–1161.

98. Hacker NF, Bereck JS, Lagasse LD, et al: Carcinoma of the cervix associated with pregnancy. *Obstet Gynecol* 1982; 59:735–746.

99. Chung A, Birnbaum SJ: Ovarian cancer associated with pregnancy. *Obstet Gynecol* 1973; 41:211–214.

100. Munnell EW: Primary ovarian cancer associated with pregnancy. *Clin Obstet Gynecol* 1963; 6:983–993.

101. Hess LW, Peaceman A, O'Brien WF, et al: Adrenal mass occurring with intrauterine pregnancy: Report of fifty-four patients requiring laparotomy for definitive management. *Am J Obstet Gynecol* 1988; 158:1029–1034.

102. Young RC, Fuks Zvi, Hoskins WJ: Cancer of the ovary, in DeVita VT, Hellman S, Rosenberg SA (eds): *Cancer: Principles and Practice of Oncology*, ed 3. Philadelphia, JB Lippincott Co, 1989, pp 1162–1196.

103. DeSaia RJ, Creasman WT: *Clinical Gynecologic Oncology*, ed 2. St Louis, CV Mosby Co, 1984.

104. Miller JM Jr, Surwitt EA, Hammond CB: Choriocarcinoma following term pregnancy. *Obstet Gynecol* 1979; 53:207–213.

105. Cunanan RG Jr, Lipper J, Tancinco PA: Choriocarcinoma of the ovary with coexisting normal pregnancy. *Obstet Gynecol* 1980; 55:669–672.

106. Brewer JI, Mayur MT: Gestational choriocarcinoma. *Am J Surg Pathol* 1981; 5:267–277.

107. DuBeshter B, Berkowitz RS, Goldstein

DP, et al: Metastatic gestational tropho-blastic disease: Experience at the New England Trophoblastic Disease Center, 1965 to 1985. *Obstet Gynecol* 1987; 69:390–395.

108. Collins CG, Barclay DL: Cancer of the vulva and cancer of the vagina in pregnancy. *Clin Obstet Gynecol* 1973; 6:927–942.

109. Asteris GT, DeGroot LJ: Thyroid cancer: Relationship to radiation exposure and pregnancy. *J Reprod Med* 1976; 17:209–216.

110. Cunningham MP, Slaughter DP: Surgical treatment of disease of the thyroid gland in pregnancy. *Surg Gynecol Obstet* 1970; 131:486–488.

111. Norton JA, Doppman JL, Jensent RT: Cancer of the Endocrine System, in DeVita VT, Hellman S, Rosenberg SA (eds): *Cancer: Principles and Practice of Oncology*, ed 3. Philadelphia, JB Lippincott Co, 1989, pp 1269–1344.

112. Brill AB, Forgotson EH: Radiation and congenital malformations. *Am J Obstet Gynecol* 1964; 90:1149–1168.

113. Burrow GN: The thyroid in pregnancy. *Med Clin North Am* 1975; 59:1089–1098.

114. Girard RM, Lamarche J, Ballot R: Carci-noma of the colon associated with pregnancy. *Dis Colon Rectum* 1981; 24:473–475.

115. Nesbitt JC, Moise KJ, Sawyers JL: Colo-rectal carcinoma in pregnancy. *Arch Surg* 1985; 120:636–640.

116. Kent DR, Nissen ED, Nissen SE, et al: Effect of pregnancy on liver tumor associated with oral contraceptives. *Obstet Gynecol* 1978; 51:148–151.

117. Green LK, Harris RE, Massey RM: Cancer of the colon during pregnancy. *Obstet Gynecol* 1975; 46:480–483.

118. O'Leary JA, Pratt JH, Simmonds RE: Rectal carcinoma and pregnancy: A review of 17 cases. *Obstet Gynecol* 1967; 30:862–868.

119. Lysyj A, Bergquist JR: Pregnancy complicated by sarcoma. Report of two cases. *Obstet Gynecol* 1963; 21:506–509.

120. Cantin J, McNeer GP: The effect of pregnancy on the clinical course of sarcoma of the soft somatic tissues. *Surg Gynecol Obstet* 1967; 125:28–32.

121. Pratt CB, Rivera G, Shank E: Osteosar-coma during pregnancy. *Obstet Gynecol* 1977; 50:245–265.

CHAPTER 13

Bacterial, Fungal, and Parasitic Infections

Stephen J. Pedler

Katherine E. Orr

THE EFFECTS OF PREGNANCY ON THE IMMUNE SYSTEM

Changes in the Immune System

Many studies of the effect of pregnancy on the immune system have been performed, many of which have attempted to explain nonrejection of the fetus by the mother. If changes in the maternal immune status do occur, we might also expect to see alteration in the immune response to infection and immunization.

Humoral immunity to infectious disease can be assessed by measurement of total immunoglobulin levels and by the antibody response to immunization. Levels of IgA and IgM do not change significantly in pregnancy[1] and although there is a decrease in serum IgG this appears to be a result of hemodilution or redistribution. In addition, the antibody response to a variety of immunizing agents such as influenza vaccine or tetanus toxoid are normal,[1] and it appears that pregnancy does not affect the humoral immune response to infection.

However, the effect of pregnancy on cell-mediated immunity (CMI) is less clear. There is considerable evidence[2] from clinical observations that those infections in which CMI is an important means of defense are more common or more severe in pregnancy. These include infections such as listeriosis,[3] malaria,[4] and coccidioidomycosis.[5] Unfortunately, it has not been possible to correlate these findings with laboratory evidence of depressed CMI. Skin testing with a variety of antigens appears to be normal, as are T4/T8 cell numbers.[1] Some studies have shown a reduction in lymphocyte responsiveness to phytohemagglutinin, but this may simply reflect increased monocyte activity during pregnancy. Nevertheless, depression of CMI undoubtedly occurs in pregnancy and may be of such a degree as to increase susceptibility to infection.

Immunization in Pregnancy

As discussed above, there is no evidence of a reduced response to a variety of vaccines in pregnancy. Immunization may be performed, therefore, provided that the benefits outweigh the potential risk. Live attenuated viral or bacterial vaccines should not, as a general rule, be given as these vaccines cause a (usually) subclinical infection in the mother and may cause fetal infection as well.[6, 7] One exception to this rule is bacille Calmette-Guérin (BCG) vaccine when an unimmunized mother has been exposed to tuberculosis, as this vaccine has been given to pregnant women without adverse effect to the fetus.[8] Inactivated bacterial vaccines and toxoids may be given during pregnancy, but for most of these agents the potential for harm to the fetus is not known.[8]

BACTERIAL INFECTIONS

Urinary Tract Infection

Urinary tract infection is a common disorder in both pregnant and nonpregnant women and is in fact the most common medical complication of pregnancy.[9] (See also Chap. 2, p. 50.) Bacteriuria of pregnancy comprises three distinct but interlinked clinical entities: asymptomatic (or covert) bacteriuria, acute cystitis, and acute pyelonephritis.

Bacteriuria is detected in 2% to 10% of pregnant women.[10] This is not significantly different from the incidence in nonpregnant women, and there is no evidence to suggest that pregnancy increases the prevalence of this infection. In nonpregnant women of childbearing age, bacteriuria is not usually persistent, it has a high spontaneous cure rate, and if repeated episodes do occur, these are often self-limiting. Finally, in the absence of renal tract abnormality, nonpregnant women with bacteriuria rarely develop acute pyelonephritis. Bacteriuria of pregnancy, however, tends to be persistent, has a low spontaneous cure rate, and if untreated approximately 20% to 30% of pregnant women with covert bacteriuria will go on to develop acute pyelonephritis.[11] It is because of this risk that all pregnant women are routinely screened for the presence of asymptomatic bacteriuria at their first prenatal assessment.

Significant Bacteriuria

Bacteriuria is defined as the presence of bacteria in the urine, and it can occur as a result of infection or colonization by, or contamination with, organisms normally found in the anterior urethra and periurethral area. Colonization is the transient occurrence of bacteria in the urine causing no host injury, while infection implies the presence of actively multiplying organisms within the urinary tract which are causing some degree of injury to the host.

As the presence of bacteriuria alone does not establish the diagnosis of urinary tract infection, the concept of significant bacteriuria was developed to distinguish between contamination and true infection.[12] Most urine specimens which have become contaminated during collection contain less than 100 organisms per milliliter and the term *significant bacteriuria* describes the presence of organisms in freshly voided urine in numbers greater than 100,000/mL. Pyuria often accompanies significant bacteriuria, and its measurement may be a useful indication of host injury and no help to differentiate between colonization and infection.

Generally, the isolation of a single pure species of organism in significant numbers from two consecutive, freshly voided midstream specimens of urine, with or without the presence of pyuria, is considered diagnostic of a urinary tract infection. There may be exceptions, however, as recent workers have isolated organisms in counts as low as 100/mL from young women with acute dysuria and urinary tract infections,[13] and mixed infections can occasionally occur.

Pathogenesis of Urinary Tract Infection

The urinary tract is usually sterile, apart from the anterior urethra which may harbor small numbers of normal skin flora and anaerobes. Bacteria enter the urine most commonly via the ascending route from the perineum through the urethra, but hematogenous and lymphatic spread of organisms to the urine may occur. In general terms, urinary tract infections become established when the body's natural host defenses are overcome by intrinsic or extrinsic host risk factors, bacterial virulence factors, the size of the original inoculum, or any combination of the above.

Natural host defenses which normally prevent the development of infection include the flushing effect of micturition which physically removes many potential pathogens. The chemical composition of the urine itself may be an important factor; for example, urines of high or low osmolality, high urea content, low pH, and those with high concentrations of organic acids may all inhibit bacterial growth.[14] Intact mucosal surfaces throughout the urinary tract and their mucopolysaccharide covering, which the uroepithelial cells secrete, help to prevent bacterial invasion and may be the site of local immunity. Uromucoid,[15] a mannose-rich compound secreted into the urine by renal tubular cells, may act as a defense mechanism by binding certain mannose-sensitive *Escherichia coli*, and therefore preventing their adherence to the urinary tract mucosa. Finally, the length of the urethra is important, especially in the male, in reducing the risk of acquiring an ascending infection from the periurethral area.

Intrinsic host risk factors which result in urinary obstruction, stasis, or reflux increase the risk of developing infection. Examples include congenital valves or stenosis occurring in the urethra or ureter, urinary calculi, polycystic kidneys, neurologic disturbance of normal bladder function, and bladder neck obstruction caused, for example, by prostatic hypertrophy. Abnormalities of the urine itself may predispose to infection; for example, glycosuria in patients with diabetes mellitus may encourage bacterial multiplication, and the urine from pregnant women has been found to have a more suitable pH for the growth of common urinary pathogens than that of non-pregnant women.[14] Women are at greater risk of developing urinary tract infections than men at all ages except in the neonate. This is in part due to the shorter female urethra. In women, sexual intercourse may be an important predisposing risk factor, facilitating entry of periurethral organisms into the bladder.[16–18] Urinary tract infections become increasingly common with age, and they also occur more frequently in patients with blood

groups A and AB.[19] Other blood groups may be involved in the pathogenesis of urinary tract infections, as women with blood group P have been found to be at greater risk of developing recurrent episodes of pyelonephritis than P-negative women.[20]

Extrinsic risk factors in the establishment of urinary infections include trauma, surgery, and instrumentation of the urinary tract.[21] The most important of these is probably urinary catheterization. After a single urinary catheterization procedure, less than 1% of healthy, ambulatory patients will develop a urinary infection.[22] In the presence of an indwelling urinary catheter, however, the prevalence of urinary tract colonization and infection increase with time so that after 3 days, 10% will become infected and this figure rises to 50% after 10 to 14 days.[23]

Many bacteria are able to multiply in urine, but certain bacteria possess virulence factors which help them to overcome the natural host defenses and establish infection. Uropathogenic *E. coli*, for example, possess specialized surface structures, known as pili or fimbriae, which mediate the adherence of the bacterium to specific carbohydrate or glycolipid receptors found on uroepithelial cells. Other postulated virulence factors include endotoxin and hemolysin production, and the possession of capsular material.

Aerobic gram-negative bacilli, selected from the fecal reservoir, predominate as the cause of urinary tract infections. Of community acquired urinary infections, 80% to 90% are caused by *E. coli*, and this also applies to bacteriuria of pregnancy. Other coliforms such as *Klebsiella, Proteus,* and *Enterobacter* spp. may be found. *Staphylococcus saprophyticus* and fecal streptococci may be isolated, while group B streptococci may account for 5% of urinary tract infections in pregnant women. More rarely, organisms such as *Salmonella* spp., anaerobic bacteria, *Gardnerella vaginalis, Mycobacterium* spp., *Chlamydia trachomatis, Mycoplasma hominis,* and *Ureaplasma urealyticum* have been associated with urinary tract infections, and *Candida albicans* may occasionally infect the urinary tract, especially in diabetics, patients who have had repeated courses of antibiotics, or in the immunocompromised.

Asymptomatic Bacteriuria of Pregnancy

Asymptomatic bacteriura refers to the presence of significant bacteriuria ($>10^5$ colony-forming units/mL) in the absence of any symptoms. It is found in 2% to 10% of the population,[9] and although it can occur in all ages, it may pose a serious threat in pregnant women.

Asymptomatic bacteriuria is generally an early feature of pregnancy. It is usually detected at the first prenatal assessment during the first trimester, rarely appears for the first time after 12 weeks, and it is possible that in most patients the asymptomatic bacteriuria actually antedates the pregnancy. Asymptomatic bacteriuria of pregnancy is important because, if untreated, 20% to 30% of patients will subsequently develop acute pyelonephritis, usually in the third trimester.[11] This is in contrast to the 1% of women without asymptomatic bacteriuria at the first prenatal assessment who go on to develop acute pyelonephritis later in pregnancy. If asymptomatic bacteriuria is treated, then the attack rate of acute pyelonephritis later in pregnancy is lowered to approximately 3%.[11] It is for this main reason that asymptomatic bacteriuria is actively sought and treated in early pregnancy and then followed by microbiologic surveillance until delivery.

Although a common condition, the management of asymptomatic bacteriuria of pregnancy is usually undertaken by the obstetrician, and will not be considered in further detail here.

Acute Cystitis in Pregnancy

Acute cystitis is characterized by significant bacteriuria ($>10^5$ colony-forming units/mL) associated with lower urinary tract symptoms such as frequency, urgency, dysuria, and suprapubic discomfort, but in the absence of systemic symptoms.

The incidence of acute cystitis of pregnancy is approximately 1.3%.[24] It is believed to be a distinct clinical entity, being quite different from asymptomatic bacteriuria of pregnancy in several ways.[24] Acute cystitis most often occurs in the second trimester of pregnancy, whereas new-onset asymptomatic bacteriuria is rare after 12 weeks. Sixty-four percent of women with acute cystitis of pregnancy have had a negative initial prenatal screening culture, compared with only 20% of cases of asymptomatic bacteriuria. There is evidence that the infection is localized to the bladder in up to 94% of cases of acute cystitis of pregnancy, while in up to 50% of cases of asymptomatic bacteriuria there may be occult renal involvement.[25, 26] Acute cystitis usually responds rapidly to appropriate therapy, has a relatively low recurrence rate of 17% (compared to about 35% for asymptomatic bacteriuria[24]), and is not associated with the same increased risk of developing acute pyelonephritis as asymptomatic bacteriuria of pregnancy.

Acute cystitis presents clinically as the symptom complex of frequency and urgency of micturition, dysuria, suprapubic discomfort, and sometimes frank hematuria. Constitutional symptoms such as fever and loin tenderness are absent. The diagnosis is confirmed by quantitative urine culture performed on two consecutive, carefully collected midstream specimens of urine. The isolation of more than 100,000 colony-forming units/mL of urine is still generally felt to indicate significant bacteriuria, although some workers feel that the criterion should be lowered to more than 100 colony-forming units/mL for acute cystitis caused by coliforms in young women.[13]

The antimicrobial agent used to treat gravidas with lower urinary tract infection should be safe to use in pregnancy, well absorbed orally, excreted by the kidney, and concentrated in the urine. Three drugs which fulfill these criteria, and with which the majority of cases of bacteriuria of pregnancy may be treated, are nitrofurantoin, an oral cephalosporin, or amoxicillin (all FDA category B). The most appropriate length of treatment is still unclear. Most workers advocate a 7-

TABLE 13–1.
The Treatment of Asymptomatic Bacteriuria
and Cystitis in Pregnancy

1. Standard courses of treatment: 7–10 days	
Ampicillin	500 mg qid
Amoxicillin	250 mg tid
Nitrofurantoin*	50 mg qid
Cephalexin	250 mg bid
2. Long-term prophylaxis	
Nitrofurantoin*	50 mg at night
Cephalexin	250 mg at night

*The use of nitrofurantoin macrocrystals may reduce the incidence of gastrointestinal side effects.

to 10-day course which will cure 75% to 80% of cases,[27] but shorter courses, including single-dose therapy, are being evaluated.[28, 29] (See Table 13–1 for recommended therapy of bacteriuria of pregnancy.)

Following treatment, the patient should be carefully monitored. This may be most convenient at a clinic specially held for such case follow-up.[30] Urine specimens should be checked 1 to 2 weeks after the initial therapy has been finished, and then at 4- to 6-week intervals until delivery, so that treatment failures and recurrent infections can be discovered.

Recurrent infection may either be a relapse or a reinfection. A relapsing infection may be diagnosed when the same strain of the same species of organism is reisolated after appropriate therapy. It may be considered as a treatment failure and most occur less than 5 days and usually within 2 weeks of finishing a course of treatment. A relapsing infection may suggest the presence of a urinary tract abnormality, or may signify renal involvement in the initial infection. Relapsing infections should be treated with a prolonged (2–3-week) course of an appropriate antimicrobial agent. Reinfections, however, are caused by a different strain of organism following successful initial therapy. These infections usually occur more than 3 weeks after treatment and are normally limited to the bladder. Reinfections identify women who, despite initial successful therapy, are at increased risk of developing repeated episodes of bacteriuria of

pregnancy. These may be treated with repeated courses of appropriate antibiotics each time they occur, or long-term, low-dose suppressive antimicrobial chemotherapy may be considered until delivery. Suitable prophylactic regimens are given in Table 13–1.

Women who have suffered from recurrent urinary tract infections during pregnancy should also be followed up in the postpartum period for further infections, and, if necessary, investigated for the presence of an underlying abnormality of the urinary tract.

Acute Pyelonephritis

Acute pyelonephritis is characterized by the presence of bacteriuria associated with symptoms and signs indicating upper urinary tract involvement. It complicates 1% to 2% of pregnancies and is probably one of the commonest reasons for hospital admission in a pregnant woman.[9]

Pregnancy does not increase the risk of a patient developing bacteriuria, but it dramatically increases the risk of developing acute pyelonephritis. Most cases of acute pyelonephritis (60%–70%) follow untreated or inadequately treated cases of asymptomatic bacteriuria in early pregnancy.[11] Studies have shown that 20% to 30% of pregnant women with untreated asymptomatic bacteriuria will go on to develop acute pyelonephritis, while with appropriate treatment this figure falls to 3%.[11] In women with asymptomatic bacteriuria of pregnancy, a past medical history of symptomatic urinary tract infections further increases the risk of developing acute pyelonephritis by a factor of four.[31]

Certain physiologic changes which occur during normal pregnancy may predispose to the development of acute pyelonephritis in women with asymptomatic bacteriura.[32] These include the so-called hydronephrosis of pregnancy, or progressive dilatation of the renal pelves and ureters which starts in the first trimester and is more frequently seen and more marked on the right, a reduction in bladder tone, and an increased tendency for pooling of residual urine in the bladder after micturition (see Chap. 2, p. 42). These alterations are thought to occur in response to changing hormonal influences and mechanical obstruction caused by the expanding uterus and may promote ascending urinary infection by impairing normal urinary flow.

There is evidence of asymptomatic renal involvement, or subclinical pyelonephritis, in up to 50% of patients with asymptomatic bacteriuria of pregnancy,[25, 26] which underlines the close association between these two clinical entities. It is, however, sometimes difficult to localize the level of infection in the urinary tract without performing invasive procedures such as bladder washouts or ureteric catheterization. It is thought that the presence in the urine of bacteria coated with antibody (IgA), which can be demonstrated by a fluorescent antibody test (FAT), is suggestive of tissue infection in the kidney. Positive FAT results have been found in only 6% of patients with acute cystitis during pregnancy, but were present in 50% of patients with asymptomatic bacteriuria of pregnancy and 75% of pregnant women with acute pyelonephritis.[26] The normal morphologic changes thought to predispose to ascending urinary tract infections during pregnancy regress dramatically after the pregnancy is terminated, mostly reaching prepregnancy status by the third postpartum month.[32]

Acute pyelonephritis of pregnancy is a serious systemic illness which may adversely affect the health of both mother and fetus. It is associated with an increased incidence of premature rupture of membranes and premature labor, with the delivery of low-birth-weight infants, and with an increased perinatal mortality. It is also associated with maternal complications. Bacteremia occurs in 15% to 20%, and endotoxic shock in up to 3% of gravidas with acute pyelonephritis.[33, 34] Recurrence is seen in approximately 19% of cases.[35]

The diagnosis of acute pyelonephritis is primarily clinical. It usually presents with sudden onset of a high spiking fever and loin pain in 85% of cases, lower urinary tract symptoms of frequency, urgency, and dysuria in 40%, nausea and vomiting in 25%, and sometimes with headache and general malaise.[10] The diagnosis should be confirmed by quantitative culture of a carefully taken urine specimen, and bacterial counts of less than 100,000/mL of urine may sometimes be significant in clinically diagnosed cases of acute pyelonephritis.[10] Blood cultures should also be taken as approximately 15% to 20% of patients with acute pyelonephritis will have an associated bacteremia, and up to 3% will develop endotoxic shock with its attendant morbidity and mortality.[33, 34]

A patient with suspected acute pyelonephritis should be admitted to hospital, given supportive treatment, and after the appropriate cultures have been taken, started on empiric intravenous antibiotic therapy which may be reviewed when the responsible organism and its sensitivities are known. Coliforms, including *E. coli*, are the commonest cause of acute pyelonephritis and a second- or third-generation cephalosporin provides suitable empiric therapy which is relatively safe to use in pregnancy. Aminoglycosides are not contraindicated in pregnancy if they are required to treat serious infections such as acute pyelonephritis, although there may be a small risk of causing auditory or vestibular nerve damage in the fetus. In recent years, many gram-negative bacilli have acquired resistance to ampicillin, and this agent can no longer be recommended as first-line empiric therapy for acute pyelonephritis. The use of "extended-spectrum" penicillins, such as piperacillin, may be considered instead.[35] Most patients will start to respond after 48 to 72 hours of appropriate therapy, and if after this time there is continued fever and evidence of sepsis, then an obstructive lesion of the urinary tract should be sought and treated. Urinary calculi are the commonest cause of obstruction, and as nearly 90% are radio-opaque, a plain abdominal x-ray is justified, if necessary for diagnostic purposes. If the plain abdominal film is negative, but an obstructive lesion is still suspected, then an intravenous pyelogram (IVP) may be indicated. In this case, the number of radiographs taken after contrast injection should be reduced.[35] Ultrasound scan of the abdomen may also be a useful diagnostic procedure. There is no consensus regarding the duration of treatment of uncomplicated pyelonephritis. We recommend approximately 2 weeks while others have suggested courses as long as 3 to 5 weeks.

After treatment, women should receive regular follow-up with repeated urine cultures in order to detect recurrent infections. Some workers recommend instituting continuous, low-dose suppressive antibiotic therapy until term in women who have had an episode of acute pyelonephritis, and this has been shown to reduce the overall recurrence rate from approximately 19% to 3%.[36] Urinary surveillance, and appropriate therapy when indicated has been found to be as effective as long-term suppressive therapy with nitrofurantoin[37] (see Table 13–1).

As with acute cystitis, microbiologic surveillance should continue in the postpartum period, to detect recurrent urinary tract infections, and at this stage investigations for an underlying abnormality of the renal tract may be considered.

Bacteremia and Septic Shock

General Aspects

Bacteremia, with or without the classic picture of septic shock, is not a common condition in the pregnant woman. It has been estimated that even in the presence of localized infection, the incidence of bacteremia is no more than 10%,[38] and true septic shock is even less frequent. The mortality is generally lower in pregnant women than in other patients, presumably because many of the risk factors associated with poor prognosis are absent.[39, 40] These include particularly advanced age and the presence of underlying disease. Nevertheless, sepsis is associated with significant morbidity and mortality and deserves mention here. (See also Chap. 7, p. 245).

Pathophysiology of Septic Shock.— Septic shock has been studied extensively, especially with regard to shock originating from infection with gram-negative bacteria ("gram-

negative shock"). It is important to remember that shock may also result from infection with gram-positive bacteria, and indeed it is not possible to distinguish clinically between shock due to these different groups of organisms. The most important virulence factor of gram-negative bacteria is endotoxin, a lipoidal agent contained within the bacterial cell wall. This material has a number of profound biologic effects, which are further discussed below. Gram-positive bacteria do not possess endotoxin, yet may still produce septic shock, so the possession of endotoxin is clearly not the whole explanation. There is evidence that pregnancy may increase susceptibility to the effects of endotoxin[41, 42] and it has been suggested that the pregnant patient should, at least in this respect, be considered a compromised host.[38]

Fever is a common finding in patients with bacteremia or shock. In infected patients fever is the result of the action on the hypothalamus of endogenous pyrogen, itself released from circulating monocytes and tissue macrophages by the action of endotoxin, phagocytosis of bacteria, or the presence of antigen-antibody complexes. The rigors which often accompany fever are presumably an attempt to generate more heat in response to the elevated set-point in the hypothalamic "thermostat."

In addition to causing fever, endotoxin has a variety of additional properties.[43] It activates the complement system by both the classic and alternative pathways with the release of vasoactive substances. Endotoxin activates the clotting cascade with eventual consumption of platelets and clotting factors, in turn leading to hemorrhage due to insufficiency of these factors (disseminated intravascular coagulation, DIC). Finally, it also stimulates the release of a number of vasoactive compounds which increase vascular permeability and vasodilation. The final result may be reduced cardiac output leading to lowered organ perfusion, tissue hypoxia, acidosis, and cell death.

The Clinical Syndrome of Septic Shock.—The clinical features of septic shock

TABLE 13–2.
The Clinical Features of Septic Shock

Initial Presentation	Later Features and Complications
Fever	Skin rashes
Rigors	Renal failure
Hypotension	Adult respiratory distress
Initial vasodilation,	syndrome
then vasoconstriction	Disseminated intravascular
Mental confusion	coagulation

are summarized in Table 13–2. The presentation may initially be of a febrile patient (with warm rather than cold extremities due to the initial vasodilation), possibly with rigors, tachycardia, and mental confusion. This may rapidly progress to the full syndrome of shock with cold extremities, hypotension, DIC, multiple organ failure, and adult respiratory distress syndrome.

Bacteremia and septic shock in the pregnant woman may be due to a number of causes, which are summarized in Table 13–3.[44] Acute pyelonephritis is dealt with in an earlier section of this chapter while the other causes are discussed in detail below.

Management of Bacteremia and Septic Shock.—Management consists of supportive measures needed to maintain cardiac, pulmonary, and renal function plus appropriate antimicrobial agents.[44] For a discussion of the therapeutic measures other than antimicrobials, the reader is referred to Chapter 7, p. 245. Antibiotic treatment will be discussed under the individual conditions.

One additional therapy which has excited considerable attention recently deserves to be further discussed. This is the therapeutic use of antilipopolysaccharide antibodies aimed at neutralizing circulating endotoxin.[45–48] In one study[45] antibodies were obtained by immunizing volunteers with a strain of *E. coli* and there was a statistically significant difference in mortality between patients treated with the specific antiserum compared to those given a control serum. Investigators in South Africa[46] obtained antilipopolysaccharide antibodies by fractionating plasma donations to a blood

bank. The serum was given to patients suffering from septic shock, which in the majority of cases was due to septic abortion. Again, a statistically significant difference in mortality was observed between the treated and control groups. Results from subsequent studies have been rather variable[49] and further investigation is needed, as is an assured supply of antiserum.

Septic Abortion

Before the ready availability of contraception and before the termination of pregnancy was permitted by law, patients with severe endometritis resulting from illegal termination of pregnancy were seen frequently.[50] Fortunately, this condition is now unusual in both the United States and the United Kingdom, although it may still occasionally be seen and may occur following spontaneous abortion and termination of pregnancy in hospitals.

The clinical features of septic abortion include fever, lower abdominal pain, and a vaginal discharge which may be foul-smelling due to the presence of anaerobic bacteria. These features may be accompanied by the symptoms and signs of septic shock. A wide range of bacteria may be found in such patients, including aerobic gram-negative bacilli such as *E. coli*, *Klebsiella*, and *Proteus*, staphylococci, streptococci, and anaerobic organisms. *Clostridium perfringens* may be found and may be associated with a high mortality rate.[51]

The management of septic abortion consists of two approaches: firstly, the removal of retained products of conception, and secondly, appropriate antibiotic therapy. Supportive management of shock, if present, will

TABLE 13–3.
The Etiology of Bacteremia in Pregnancy*

Ante Partum	Post Partum
Urinary tract infection	Postpartum endometritis
Acute pyelonephritis	Urinary tract infection
Chorioamnionitis	Surgical wound infection
Septic abortion	
Listeriosis	

*For the causative organisms, see the relevant sections.

also be required. Due to the wide range of possible infecting organisms, the initial empiric therapy will be broad-spectrum in nature. It is the authors' practice (in the United Kingdom) to recommend an initial combination of ampicillin, gentamicin, and metronidazole, with suitable changes being made when the results of the cultures of blood and products of conception are available. A cephalosporin such as cefuroxime or cefoxitin may be used in place of the aminoglycoside in patients with renal dysfunction. In the United States clindamycin plus gentamicin (or another aminoglycoside) would be a suitable alternative. If clostridial sepsis is suspected, penicillin G in high doses should be given; 3 million units every 4 hours would be suitable in patients with normal renal function. (Clostridial sepsis, especially in relation to acute renal failure, is discussed in Chap. 2, p. 50.)

Puerperal Fever (Postpartum Endometritis)

Before the advent of a better understanding of asepsis, puerperal fever was a much-feared complication of pregnancy; group A β-hemolytic streptococcus was a common cause and was associated with a high mortality rate. Infection due to this organism is now most unusual, and endogenous vaginal flora are responsible in most cases, but postpartum endometritis is still a significant cause of morbidity in obstetric patients.[52]

The most important risk factor in the development of this condition is cesarean section,[38, 52, 53] and this procedure is also associated with a greater severity of infection. Prolonged rupture of membranes is also associated with increased risk of infection,[53] but fetal monitoring probably does not increase the risk.[54, 55] Clinically, most patients present with fever plus offensive lochia, although progression to septicemia and shock may occur. Indeed, postpartum endometritis is the commonest cause of septic shock in the obstetric patient.[38]

The infection is often polymicrobial[56, 57] and is usually due to those organisms found in the vagina. These include gram-negative bacilli such as *E. coli*, *Klebsiella*, and *Proteus*, group B streptococci, fecal streptococci, *G. vaginalis*, and anaerobes such as anaerobic cocci and various species of *Bacteroides*. Anaerobes form a significant component of the postpartum vaginal flora possibly due to the presence of blood. *Chlamydia trachomatis* and genital mycoplasmas may also be found in this infection.

Specimens for bacteriology should be collected before commencing treatment. In addition to blood cultures, it may be possible to collect specimens from the uterine cavity by passing a swab through the cervix. Contamination of the swab with vaginal material may lead to misleading results, and the use of double- or triple-lumen devices will avoid this.[56, 58] A Gram's stain of a carefully collected swab may yield useful information on which to base treatment. A urine sample and a cesarean section wound swab should also be collected.

Treatment of Endometritis.—The antibiotic treatment of this infection will usually need to be empiric in nature until the results of cultures are known. Whatever agent or agents are chosen, they must possess activity against anaerobes, gram-negative aerobes, and streptococci. In the United Kingdom the combination of ampicillin and gentamicin, or perhaps a second-generation cephalosporin such as cefuroxime, plus metronidazole would be frequently employed. In the United States a combination of clindamycin and gentamicin or single-agent therapy with an agent such as cefoxitin is generally used.[59]

Because of the risk of endometritis associated with cesarean section, many obstetricians now routinely given antibiotics as prophylaxis to patients undergoing this procedure and this has been shown to be of proven efficacy in a number of studies.[52, 60, 61] When true prophylaxis is given (as opposed to the treatment of an already established infection) it should be of short duration to cover the time of surgery; single-dose prophylaxis is commonly used. The antimicrobials used are the same as those used for treatment.

TABLE 13–4.
Clinical Features of Syphilis

Stage of Infection	Clinical Features
Primary	Primary chancre (firm, painless ulcer at the site of inoculation); may be multiple; regional lymphadenopathy is also present
Secondary	Skin rashes—may be macular, papular, or pustular in type; the whole body may be involved, but involvement of the palms of the hands and soles of the feet is suggestive of syphilis
	Systemic symptoms—pyrexia, general malaise, weight loss, arthralgia
	Generalized lymphadenopathy
	Skin plaques (condylomata lata), particularly in the perineal region and in skin folds
	Mucous patches and erosions on mucous membranes
	Central nervous system involvement may be asymptomatic or produce an aseptic meningitis
	Other organs—hepatitis, glomerulonephritis, arthritis, etc.
Latent	Positive serologic tests without clinical symptoms
Late (tertiary)	Gummas of skin, bone, and other organs
	Cardiovascular syphilis
	Neurosyphilis

Sexually Transmitted Diseases

Syphilis

Although the incidence of syphilis declined in both the United Kingdom and the United States following World War II, it has recently begun to increase again in the United States.[62, 63] The main concern which stems from the occurrence of syphilis in the pregnant woman is for the fetus, since in the mother clinical presentation and treatment are similar to that in the nonpregnant patient. It should be possible to completely prevent congenital syphilis by diligent prenatal care, but this has not been achieved.[64, 65] It follows that all those who take part in the health care of

the pregnant woman must remain aware of the possibility of this infection. Most cases of syphilis in pregnancy will be detected by prenatal serologic screening but cases may also be detected by contact tracing or by clinical presentation to a physician or obstetrician.[66]

Syphilis is caused by the spirochete *Treponema pallidum*. The classic pathologic feature of syphilis is an obliterative endarteritis and this can be seen in biopsies of lesions at all the stages of syphilis, from the primary chancre to the gummas of tertiary disease.

The clinical symptoms and signs[67] of syphilis are numerous and to cover them in detail is beyond the scope of this chapter. Table 13–4 lists the main features of the various stages of syphilis. Primary syphilis usually presents as a hard, painless single genital ulcer (chancre), although multiple ulcers may occur. The absence of pain serves to distinguish the chancre of syphilis from herpes simplex, but if the chancres become infected with other bacteria diagnostic confusion may result. Secondary syphilis may cause a wide variety of clinical manifestations and it should be remembered that the primary chancre and the lesions of secondary syphilis are potentially infective to physicians, nurses, and other health care personnel.

Not every fetus of an infected mother will acquire the disease but if fetal infection does occur the consequences are potentially serious. Infection of the fetus occurs most frequently during the second and third trimesters and during the early stages of maternal infection when there is the highest degree of spirochetemia.[68] The effects on the pregnancy may be to cause late abortion, stillbirth, or a congenitally infected neonate.[68]

There are a wide variety of clinical signs in the neonate with congenital syphilis[67] and these are listed in Table 13–5. Latent infection may be present without overt clinical manifestations.[68] A recent study[65] found that of 50 neonates with congenital infection, 31 (62%) were symptomatic at birth and that there was a high incidence of preterm delivery (39%) and/or low birth weight (38%).

TABLE 13–5.
Clinical Features of Congenital Syphilis

Early signs
Skin rash—including bullae, papular, or maculo-
  papular forms
Mucous membrane lesions—mucous patches, and in
  the nose a rhinitis giving "snuffles"
Osteochondritis and perichondritis
Hepatosplenomegaly and hepatitis
Failure to thrive
Later signs
Interstitial keratitis
Eighth nerve deafness
Clutton's joints—bilateral painless joint effusions,
  usually in the knees
Maldeveloped teeth, such as peg-shaped, notched
  central incisors (Hutchinson's teeth) and mulberry
  molars
Saddle nose and prominent mandible
Frontal bone bossing
Saber shins (anterior bowing of the tibia)
Neurosyphilis

Management of Syphilis in Pregnancy.—Serologic screening for syphilis should be performed in all pregnant women. Failure to do this may lead to some cases of active infection being missed, but serologic screening cannot be relied upon to detect all cases of syphilis in pregnancy since some women may be in the early stages of the disease when serology is negative or may acquire the infection later.[66] The different tests available for syphilis serology are potentially confusing and it may be useful to briefly review these tests, which fall into two groups, the nonspecific and the specific tests.

The original "nonspecific" test for syphilis was the Wasserman reaction, now superseded in most laboratories by the Venereal Disease Research Laboratory (VDRL) test. These tests detect so-called reaginic antibodies (not to be confused with IgE) which may appear as a result of treponemal infection and as a result of a variety of other conditions, including pregnancy itself ("biologic false-positives"). A list of causes of false-positive reaginic tests is given in Table 13–6. Interestingly, it has been suggested that false-positive tests for syphilis may be an early indicator of an immunologic disorder and that such pa-

tients should be assessed with this in mind (see Chap. 11 for a discussion of anti-phospholipid antibody syndrome).[69] These tests continue to be widely used because they are inexpensive, easy to perform, and can be automated. Their role is mainly as a screening test but the antibody titer declines with successful treatment and can be used to follow the efficacy of therapy.

A positive nonspecific test must be confirmed by a specific test such as the *T. pallidum* hemagglutination assay (TPHA) or the fluorescent treponemal antibody test (FTA). Once positive, these tests remain so for life and cannot therefore be used to follow the efficacy of therapy. It should be noted that previously treated syphilis will continue to give positive results in specific tests and that although they are specific for treponemal infection, other infections such as yaws or pinta will cause both the specific and the nonspecific tests to become positive. This should be remembered when assessing patients from countries where these infections are endemic.

Although syphilis in pregnancy will most often be diagnosed by prenatal serologic

TABLE 13–6.
Causes of False-Positive Results of Serologic Tests for Syphilis

Test	Cause
Nonspecific (WR, VDRL, rapid plasma reagin, etc.)	Pregnancy
	Elderly patients
	Drug addiction
	Connective tissue and auto-immune diseases
	Other treponemal infections—yaws, pinta, bejel
	Other infectious diseases including, e.g., mycobacterial infections; other spirochetal infections such as leptospirosis, borreliosis, and Lyme disease; infectious mononucleosis; malaria
Specific tests	Treated syphilis in the past—these tests may remain positive for life
	Other treponemal infections, even if successfully treated

WR = Wasserman reaction; VDRL = Venereal Disease Research Laboratory.

TABLE 13–7.
Treatment Regimens for Syphilis in Pregnancy*

Primary syphilis or secondary or latent syphilis of less than 1 year's duration	Benzathine penicillin 2.4 million units IM as a single dose *or* aqueous procaine penicillin 600,000 units IM once daily for 10 days *or* (for penicillin-hypersensitive patients) oral erythromycin 500 mg qid for 15 days[†]
Syphilis of more than 1 year's duration (except neurosyphilis)	Benzathine penicillin 2.4 million units IM once weekly for 3 wks *or* aqueous procaine penicillin 600,000 units IM once daily for 15 days *or* (for penicillin-hypersensitive patients) oral erythromycin 500 mg qid for 30 days[†]
Congenital syphilis	Penicillin G 50,000 units/kg body weight daily IV in 2 divided doses for 10 days *or* (if CSF findings normal) benzathine penicillin 50,000 units/kg body weight IM in single dose

*Data from references 66, 71, 72.
†Compliance may be a problem with the extended courses of erythromycin, and serologic follow-up is essential.

screening, a patient with syphilis may present to a physician with symptoms suggestive of the infection. In the very early stages of the disease serology may be negative, but the diagnosis may be made by examining a serous exudate from a chancre or other lesion by dark-ground microscopy for the motile spiral organism.[70]

The treatment of choice for syphilis is penicillin G. A variety of therapeutic regimens have been suggested,[66, 68, 71, 72] which are similar in dose and duration of treatment. In penicillin-allergic patients erythromycin may be used but it does not cross the placenta reliably[73, 74] and an infant born to a mother treated with erythromycin should be re-treated with penicillin.[66] Alternatively, an attempt may be made to desensitize the mother before treating with penicillin.[75] Table 13–7 gives

details of treatment regimens. A possible complication of treatment is the Jarisch-Herxheimer reaction, which is due to the release of endotoxin from the killed spirochetes. This effect usually lasts for less than 24 hours and is manifested by fever, rigors, general malaise, and possibly shock with hypotension and tachycardia. For this reason, and to ensure compliance with treatment, it has been advocated that patients be hospitalized at least for the first day or two of therapy.[67]

After delivery, the infant should be followed up with serologic tests using a nonspecific test to give a result which can be quantified. Antibodies of maternal origin may be detected in the infant but the titer should decrease within 2 to 3 months. Failure of the titer to fall, or a rise in the titer, is an indication to treat the child even if the mother received effective treatment. In such infants a specimen of cerebrospinal fluid (CSF) should also be examined for abnormalities such as a raised white cell count, raised protein, or lowered glucose, or a positive VDRL test. Penicillin is again the treatment of choice (see Table 13–7) but benzathine penicillin produces very low CSF levels of penicillin[76] and should not be used if CSF abnormalities are found. Infants should be followed up for at least 2 years (3 if CSF abnormalities were detected). All mothers should also be followed up with repeat VDRL or another quantitative nonspecific test for 2 years.

Gonorrhea

Gonorrhea caused by the gram-negative coccus *Neisseria gonorrhoeae*,[77] is one of the commonest sexually transmitted diseases in the world.[62, 63] Pathologically, gonorrhea is characterized by direct invasion of the tissues by the organism with resultant tissue destruction and an acute inflammatory reaction.[78] In order to initiate infection the organism must first attach to the mucosa, which may be facilitated by the pili which freshly isolated, virulent gonococci produce.[79, 80] As with other gram-negative organisms *N. gonorrhoeae* possesses a lipopolysaccharide endotoxin within its cell wall which is cytotoxic and may therefore be implicated in the tissue damage that occurs. Other than this the organism produces no other toxins that have been identified so far.

Gonorrhea is usually spread by sexual contact, or from an infected mother to a newborn infant. Although the organisms is highly susceptible to drying, under favorable conditions it can survive outside the body for several hours. A recent outbreak in a household was attributed to the use of a communal washcloth.[81] However, the occurrence of gonorrhea in a child should normally lead the clinician to suspect possible child abuse.

The clinical features of gonorrhea are summarized in Table 13–8. In women, gonorrhea produces a cervicitis; the organism may also spread to the urethra and rectum. Vaginitis does not occur because the organism does not infect stratified squamous epithelium. Symptoms compatible with pelvic inflammatory disease may occur in up to 10% to 20% of infected women while disseminated gonococcal infection is thought to occur in about 1% of patients. It is of interest that strains which cause disseminated infection are rather different from those causing localized disease; they may produce few local symptoms, often belong to the arginine-uracil-hydroxuridine (AHU) auxotype and to particular outer membrane protein I serotypes, are resistant to the bactericidal action of serum, and are often highly sensitive to penicillin.[82, 83]

Because gonorrhea is such a common infection it is inevitable that it will be regularly seen in the pregnant woman. The incidence in pregnancy is reportedly lower in the United Kingdom (less than 1%)[84] than in the United States (2%–5%).[85] This is unlikely to be related to diagnostic laboratory methods since similar methods are in use in both countries. There is no evidence that the pregnant patient is more susceptible to gonorrhea but it has been suggested that disseminated gonococcal infection may be more common in pregnant than in nonpregnant women. Recent studies do not confirm this.[80] There seems little doubt, however, that gonorrhea in pregnancy

is associated with an increased incidence of chorioamnionitis, preterm delivery, and premature rupture of the membranes.[80, 85–87] In addition, the delivery of a baby by an infected mother may lead to orogastric infection and ophthalmia neonatorum.

Management of Gonorrhea in Pregnancy.—In the United States it is standard practice to take routine specimens from the cervix for culture from all pregnant women at the first prenatal consultation and to collect

TABLE 13–8.
The Clinical Features of Gonorrhea in Women

Site of Infection	Clinical Features
Genital	Often asymptomatic; may present as vaginal discharge, dysuria, or abdominal pain; physical examination may yield few findings, but a mucopurulent discharge may be apparent at the cervix
Anorectal	Usually asymptomatic, but may cause proctitis with a mucopurulent discharge and tenesmus
Pharyngeal	Usually asymptomatic but a sore throat may occur
Pelvic infection	Ascending infection from the cervix may lead to salpingitis and endometritis (pelvic inflammatory disease) and other organisms may also be present, such as streptococci, gram-negative bacilli, and anaerobes; clinical features include lower abdominal pain, fever, cervical discharge, and menstrual abnormalities
Perihepatitis	Usually due to chlamydial infection, but can result from the direct spread of gonococci from the fallopian tube or from bacteremia; typical presentation is with acute right upper abdominal pain and tenderness
Disseminated infection	Typically presents as arthralgia with swollen joints, together with fever, tenosynovitis, and a skin rash which is often purpuric or pustular; frank septic arthritis may occur; rare complications include meningitis and endocarditis

TABLE 13–9.
Diagnostic Methods for Gonorrhea

Specimens	Appropriate specimens include urethral, rectal, and cervical swabs; other specimens may be collected as appropriate, such as throat swabs, joint fluid, or blood cultures
Microscopy	Specimen is stained by Gram's stain and examined for the typical gram-negative kidney bean–shaped diplococci which are often seen inside polymorphs; note that microscopy of throat swabs is unlikely to be helpful as there are large numbers of commensal neisseriae in the pharyngeal flora
Culture	Culture is performed on media containing antibiotics to suppress the normal flora which may overgrow the gonococcus; typical media include modified Thayer-Martin medium and New York City medium; specialized blood culture media are not required for the isolation of this organism from blood and conventional media may be used
Rapid methods	An enzyme immunoassay kit (Gonozyme, Abbott Laboratories) is available which detects the presence of gonococcal antigen in clinical specimens; this provides a rapid result (in about 2 hr)

repeat specimens during pregnancy in women at high risk of gonococcal infection. This is generally not done in the United Kingdom due to the lower incidence of gonorrhea in pregnancy.[84] However, this practice makes the provision of a satisfactory contact-tracing service mandatory; otherwise, asymptomatic contacts of patients with gonorrhea will go untreated.

Diagnostic methods are given in Table 13–9. The mainstay of the diagnosis of gonorrhea is the isolation of the organism from clinical specimens. In experienced hands there is a very high correlation (greater than 95%) between gram-stained smears of urethral exudates from symptomatic males and culture, but this is much reduced (50%–70%) in en-

docervical smears from women.[88] Optimum culture results are obtained when the culture plate is inoculated in the clinic immediately the specimen has been collected. If this is not possible the swab should be placed in suitable transport medium such as Stuart's or Amies medium, both of which will maintain the viability of the organism for 6 to 12 hours.[88]

Dry swabs must never be sent as the organism dies rapidly when dried. If delays in transport of more than 12 hours are anticipated, a nutritive transport system may be used.[88] Rapid diagnostic methods for gonorrhea are becoming available, such as enzyme-linked immunoassay (ELISA),[89] direct immunofluorescence,[90] and DNA hybridization,[91] but although they approach the sensitivity and specificity of Gram's stain in male urethral specimens, they are not as satisfactory in female cervical specimens or specimens from other sites. They also suffer from the disadvantage that unless culture is also performed, antibiotic susceptibility testing is not possible.

The treatment of uncomplicated genital gonorrhea[72, 92–94] is relatively straightforward. A large number of different regimens have been tried[92] but much of this work has been done in uncomplicated gonorrhea in men. The treatment of gonorrhea in pregnancy is complicated by the need to consider fetal as well as maternal toxicity; for this reason certain effective antimicrobial agents, such as the tetracyclines (which are contraindicated in pregnancy) and ciprofloxacin, the safety of which has not been proved, cannot be used. Appropriate regimens for use in pregnancy are given in Table 13–10. Once delivery has occurred, treatment with tetracycline, 500 mg four times daily, or doxycycline, 100 mg twice daily, both for 7 days, or ciprofloxacin, 250 mg in a single dose, may be given if desired. It must be remembered that some of these drugs, notably the tetracyclines, are excreted in breast milk and may lead to toxic effects in the infant.

An additional problem is the increasing incidence of antibiotic-resistant gonococci. The most commonly encountered strains are those which produce a β-lactamase (penicillinase-producing *N. gonorrhoeae*, or PPNG) which is genetically encoded by a plasmid, an extra-chromosomal circular strand of DNA. First reported in the United Kingdom and United States in 1976, PPNG has considerably increased in incidence in the United States; in 1986, 16,648 cases of infection were recorded.[93] These strains are, however, much less common in the United Kingdom.

Penicillin resistance may also be chro-mosomally mediated, rather than by a plasmid. Such strains (chromosomally mediated resistant *N. gonorrhoeae*, or CMRNG) may also show resistance to other agents including cephalosporins, spectinomycin, and tetracycline. Chromosomally mediated resistance does not always lead to treatment failures[93] but outbreaks have been described due to organisms exhibiting resistance of clinical sig-

---

TABLE 13–10.
Treatment Regimens for Gonorrhea in the Pregnant Woman*†

1. Uncomplicated genital or anorectal infection
   1st choice: Ceftriaxone 250 mg IM
   Alternative regimens: Spectinomycin 2 g IM (FDA category B)
   or
   Amoxicillin 3.0 g plus (FDA category B)
   Probenecid 1 g orally†
   or
   Procaine penicillin 4.8 million units IM plus probenecid 1.0 g orally†

2. Pharyngeal infection
   As for anogenital infection, except that spectinomycin and amoxicillin are less effective and should not be used

3. Disseminated gonococcal infection
   Initial inpatient therapy—1st choice:
   Ceftriaxone 1 g IM or IV q24h (FDA category B)
   or
   Ceftizoxime 1 g IV q8h (FDA category B)
   or
   Cefotaxime 1 g IV q8h (FDA category B)
   Initial inpatient therapy—2nd choice:
   Spectinomycin 2 g IM q12h (β-lactam-allergic patients)
   or
   Penicillin G 3 million units IV q6h†
   or
   Ampicillin 1 g q6h†

   Posthospitalization treatment:
   Reliable patients with uncomplicated disease may be discharged 24–48 hr after symptoms resolve and complete a total of 1 wk of antibiotic therapy with one of the following oral regimens:
   Cefuroxime axetil 500 mg bid
   or
   Amoxicillin 500 mg with clavulanic acid tid†
   or
   Amoxicillin 500 mg qid†

*Patients should also be treated presumptively for *Chlamydia* with erythromycin base or stearate 500 mg qid for 7 days because of the high incidence of concomitant infection in patients with gonorrhea.
†Regimens of choice are based on 1989 recommendations of the Centers for Disease Control[72] and reflect the spread of penicillinase-resistant *Neisseria gonorrhoeae* in the United States. In areas where such strains are rare, penicillin and its derivatives remain agents of choice.

nificance. Finally, sporadic cases and clusters of infection due to tetracycline-resistant *N. gonorrhoeae* have been described, in which resistance is plasmid-mediated and has resulted in treatment failures in patients treated with tetracycline alone.

The treatment of choice for PPNG is ceftriaxone or a similar cephalosporin such as cefotaxime or cefuroxime. In the United States, PPNG is now so common that ceftriaxone is standard therapy unless the strain is known to be β-lactamase-negative, or in nonendemic areas (PPNG accounts for less than 1% of all gonococci) (see Table 13–10). Spectinomycin is an alternative, but its safety in pregnancy is not established nor is it suitable for the treatment of pharyngeal gonorrhea.[94]

Disseminated gonococcal infection should initially be treated in hospital with a parenteral cephalosporin such as ceftriaxone in the United States and other areas with a significant incidence of penicillinase-producing strains, or with intravenous penicillin in other geographic locations (see Table 13–10). Provided a satisfactory clinical response has occurred, treatment may be changed to oral therapy after 3 days of parenteral treatment. In all cases of gonorrhea, treatment failure does occasionally occur, and repeat specimens should be taken 7 days after the end of treatment to check for bacteriologic cure. Concomitant infection with *N. gonorrhoeae* and *C. trachomatis* is common[80]; chlamydial infection in pregnancy should be treated with erythromycin (see below).

Chlamydial Infection

Infection with *Chlamydia trachomatis* is the commonest sexually transmitted disease in Europe and the United States.[62, 63, 95] The organism itself is an obligate intracellular parasite with a complex life cycle. The infective state (the elementary body) exists outside the cell but is incapable of dividing. To reproduce, the elementary body is first attached to the cell and then is taken up into it. There it develops into the reticulate body, which undergoes binary fission forming the large intracytoplasmic inclusion bodies visible on light microscopy. The reticulate bodies develop into elementary bodies and the cell then ruptures to release them.

This organism can cause a variety of clinical manifestations.[96] In developing countries, immunotypes A through C cause endemic trachoma. In developed countries genital infections (due to immunotypes D–K) are extremely common and conjunctivitis may be seen in neonates or in adults.

Genital infection in males appears most frequently as urethritis, but also as epididymitis or proctitis. Infection may be asymptomatic. In women the majority of infections are asymptomatic; the organism may cause a cervicitis and is associated with pelvic inflammatory disease and perihepatitis.

Lymphogranuloma venereum is a genital infection due to the L1, L2, and L3 immunotypes of *C. trachomatis*, which may also involve other organs. The disease is most frequently seen in Third World countries but is occasionally encountered in the United States and Europe. It presents as a painless genital ulcer which heals within a few days. Local lymphadenopathy occurs some weeks later; the enlarged nodes are painful, become fixed and matted, and eventually ulcerate through the overlying skin (bubo formation). Systemic involvement may occur with symptoms of fever, rigors, malaise, and arthralgia.

Chlamydial Infection in Pregnancy.—It has been estimated that the prevalence of chlamydial infection in pregnant women ranges from 2% to 30%.[96] The effects of chlamydial infection on pregnancy have not been fully defined.[85, 87, 96] It has been associated with preterm delivery, premature rupture of membranes, and low-birth-weight babies, but these associations have not been proved. An infected mother may transmit the infection in a high proportion (perhaps up to 70%) of cases to the child during delivery[96] resulting in neonatal conjunctivitis and/or pneumonia.

At present, routine screening for chlamydial infection in pregnancy is not performed. The diagnosis of infection is not

TABLE 13–11.
Treatment Regimens for Chlamydial Infection

1. During pregnancy	Oral erythromycin base or stearate* 500 mg qid for 7 days
2. After delivery if the mother is *NOT* breast-feeding	Oral tetracycline 500 mg qid daily for 7 days *or* Oral doxycycline 100 bid for 7 days
3. Neonatal infection	Erythromycin base or stearate* 50 mg/kg body weight/day in 4 divided doses for 14–21 days

*Erythromycin estolate is contraindicated in pregnancy as it may produce severe hepatotoxicity

straightforward, as it requires tissue culture, ELISA, or immunofluorescent microscopy. In many women who are sexual contacts of infected persons, laboratory diagnosis is often not attempted and treatment is given empirically. If it is decided to attempt to confirm a clinical diagnosis, either isolation of the organism or demonstration of its presence in clinical material may be performed. It should be noted that the organism is found associated with epithelial cells and not with pus.[97] Purulent or mucopurulent exudate should be removed from the site of infection before taking the specimen, which should be collected by scraping the affected surface to ensure sufficient numbers of epithelial cells. Swabs or other material for culture must be placed into chlamydial transport medium, which contains antibiotics to inhibit the growth of other bacteria that may be present. Ordinary bacterial transport medium is quite unsuitable and must not be used.

The diagnosis of lymphogranuloma venereum may be made by isolating the organism from material aspirated from a bubo, but serologic diagnosis may also be useful, as it may in the diagnosis of neonatal pneumonia.[97] Serology is unlikely to be of use in localized genital infection due to the D–K immunotypes of *C. trachomatis*.

The treatment of chlamydial infection is straightforward. In the nonpregnant woman, or after delivery if the mother is not breast-feeding, a tetracycline is the treatment of choice.[96] Erythromycin (FDA category B) should be used in pregnancy and in the neonate. Treatment regimens are given in Table 13–11.

Chancroid

The causative organism of chancroid is *Haemophilus ducreyi*, a small gram-negative bacillus. The disease is unusual in developed countries, although its incidence may be increasing[98] and it is considerably more common in men than in women.

Clinically, chancroid presents as a painful papule which breaks down to form an ulcer. The ulcers are painful with an irregular outline and undermined edges. Although most commonly located on the genitalia and perineal area, they may be found in extragenital sites. There is an accompanying regional lymphadenopathy which usually results in bubo formation, with matted, fixed lymph nodes which drain through the overlying skin through fistulas. This appearance often leads to diagnostic confusion with lymphogranuloma venereum (see above).

The diagnosis is made by culturing the causative organism from the ulcer or from the buboes.[99] Superficial swabs of the ulcer surface are usually contaminated with other bacteria and the ulcer should be cleaned with sterile saline before sampling. *Haemophilus ducreyi* will not grow on conventional media and if this condition is suspected the laboratory should be informed before collecting the specimen.

Treatment for the nonpregnant patient is either erythromycin or trimethoprim-sulphamethoxazole (TMP-SMZ, co-trimoxazole).[71, 72, 99] Since the use of TMP-SMZ may not be desirable in pregnancy, erythromycin in a dose of 500 mg four times daily for at least 10 days is recommended.

Granuloma Inguinale

The causative organism of this condition is *Calymmatobacterium granulomatis*, a gram-negative bacillus. The organism is very difficult to culture in vitro and the diagnosis is made by microscopy of suitable specimens. As with chancroid, this infection is much more common in developing countries and is rarely seen in developed nations.[99]

The initial lesion of granuloma inguinale is a painless papule which breaks down into an ulcer, which then enlarges by local spread. The ulcer is painless unless secondarily infected and regional lymphadenopathy and bubo formation do not occur. Multiple lesions may be present due to autoinoculation from the original lesion onto other sites, and extragenital lesions may be present. Scar formation occurs as the lesion heals and this may lead to urethral stricture or genital lymphedema. Rarely, disseminated infection may occur.

The diagnosis is made by histologic examination of biopsies of the lesion. The characteristic *Donovan bodies* are groups of bipolar staining bacteria within histiocytes.

A variety of therapeutic regimens have been described[99] and tetracycline, TMP-SMZ, chloramphenicol, and gentamicin have been shown to be effective in the nonpregnant population. In the gravida erythromycin (500 mg four times daily) has been used but is probably less effective[100]; TMP-SMZ may also be used but the problems of this agent in pregnancy should be remembered (see below).

Other Bacterial Infections

Infective Endocarditis

Several studies have shown that the risk of infective endocarditis in the pregnant woman is very low, even in patients with heart disease.[101, 102] Nevertheless, there seems little doubt that bacteremia may occur during delivery and there is therefore at least a potential risk of endocarditis. It is a vexed question whether or not antibiotic prophylaxis should be given to pregnant patients at risk. There is evidence to suggest that this is unnecessary,[103] yet, as Durack[104] has pointed out, this does not help the physician caught in the malpractice dilemma! At the present time the case for antibiotic prophylaxis in pregnancy remains unproven and each patient must be assessed individually. The exceptions are patients with prosthetic heart valves and those who have had one or more previous episodes of infective endocarditis, since these groups of patients are at particular risk and should be given prophylaxis.

Prophylaxis, if given, should be directed principally against the fecal streptococci. The recommendations in Table 13–12 are those of the authors and are based on those of the British Society for Antimicrobial Chemotherapy.[105] (See also Chap. 5.)

Listeriosis

Listeria monocytogenes is a small gram-positive bacillus widely distributed in the environment. It has been isolated from many sources, including sewage, water, and soil, plus many different animals and the feces of asymptomatic humans.

There is little doubt that pregnancy predisposes the individual to listeriosis for reasons that are unknown. Cell-mediated immunity is an important defense against listeriosis, and the disease is found in patients with such conditions as lymphomas and in those receiving immunosuppressive therapy.[3] Alterations in cell-mediated immunity do occur in pregnancy (see above) and pregnant women exhibit increased susceptibility to certain other infections associated with depressed cell-mediated immunity. In the United Kingdom, attack rates have been calculated as 14 per 100,000 known conceptions,

TABLE 13–12.
Prophylaxis of Infective Endocarditis in Pregnancy

At onset or induction of labor	Ampicillin 1 g IM or IV plus gentamicin 120 mg IM or IV
Every 8 hr until delivery	Ampicillin 500 mg IM or IV plus gentamicin 80 mg IM or IV
In penicillin-allergic patients	Vancomycin 1 g12h until delivery, plus gentamicin in the above dosages

Note: All doses assume normal renal function.

0.3 per 100,000 adults under the age of 75, and 1.4 per 100,000 adults over 75 years.[106] Figures for the United States are similar.

Statistics from the United States and the United Kingdom show that about one third of confirmed cases of listeriosis occur in pregnant women. For example, in 1988 in the United Kingdom there were 291 confirmed cases of which 115 (39%) were pregnancy-associated.[106] The majority of the remaining cases occurred in immunocompromised patients, although the disease also occurs in otherwise healthy persons. The infection may be acquired from animal contact, contaminated milk,[107] and other foods such as coleslaw[108] or soft cheeses.[109] The organism has also been found in precooked meals designed for rapid reheating,[110] and concern has been expressed that inadequate heating could lead to infection. However, although well-documented foodborne outbreaks of listeriosis have occurred, the role of food in the occurrence of sporadic cases is much less certain.[111]

In the immunocompromised patient listeriosis usually presents as septicemia or meningitis.[112] In pregnant women the presentation is of a febrile illness with rigors and myalgia or arthralgia, which is usually self-resolving. There are several possible consequences of maternal infection, which is most commonly seen in the third trimester. The fetus may be entirely unaffected[113] or stillbirth or premature delivery may occur. Infection in utero may lead to granulomatosis infantiseptica, a specific condition ascribed to the organism comprising disseminated infection and multiple abscess formation. Late neonatal infection may also occur when the organism is acquired either during birth or as a result of cross-infection in the nursery.[112] In such neonates the presentation is usually as septicemia with or without meningitis.

Management.—Recent concern in the United Kingdom has stemmed from the presence of *L. monocytogenes* in soft cheeses and precooked meals. As a result advice has been given[106] that pregnant women should not eat ripened soft cheeses (e.g., of the Brie or Camembert type), but hard cheeses, cottage cheese, and processed cheeses have not been implicated in this problem. It has also been advised that precooked meals be thoroughly reheated before consumption.[106]

Listeriosis should be borne in mind when a pregnant woman presents with a febrile illness of unknown origin. The diagnostic method of choice is blood culture; the organism may also be isolated from vaginal swabs and urine. A serologic test for circulating antibodies is available, but gives a retrospective diagnosis and is therefore more useful for epidemiologic purposes.

The treatment of choice for listeriosis is ampicillin[112] in a dose of 500 mg four times daily, which is usually combined with gentamicin in neonates or immunocompromised patients. In the pregnant woman the efficacy of treatment in preventing fetal infection is unknown. Erythromycin (1 g four times daily intravenously) may be used in penicillin-sensitive patients.

Use of Antimicrobial Agents in Pregnancy

General Aspects

In addition to the usual criteria applied in selecting an antimicrobial agent (see Table 13–13), there are two further points which must be considered in the pregnant patient. These are the problem of potential fetal and/or maternal toxicity and the physiologic changes in pregnancy which may affect the dose, frequency, and route of administration.

Pregnancy is associated with a significant increase in the volume of distribution of a drug, and this in turn may lead to reduced maternal serum concentrations. In addition, renal blood flow and the glomerular filtration rate are elevated, leading to an increase in clearance of drugs excreted by this route. Absorption of an orally administered agent is variable and may be reduced in the pregnant woman as a result of reduced gastrointestinal motility. These factors might theoretically require an increase in dose or more frequent administration, but in practice the significance of these changes is unclear. Most antimicrobial agents have a high therapeutic ratio and the usual full adult doses should be used.[114] An exception is the aminoglycoside group, and measurement of serum levels of these drugs should be performed and doses adjusted accordingly.

Transfer of Antimicrobials Across the Placenta and Into Breast Milk

Transfer of a drug across the placenta depends on a number of factors. Since most drug transfer occurs by diffusion, agents with low molecular weight, high lipid solubility, and a low degree of protein binding are more readily transferred than others. The degree of drug transfer increases with gestation due to reduced thickness of the placental barrier.

The excretion of antimicrobial agents into breast milk has not been studied in detail and for many agents little is known. The same factors affecting cross-placental transfer also affect the penetration of antimicrobials into breast milk. It should be noted that even for agents that reach high concentrations in milk, the actual amount of drug taken in by the infant is very small, and in most cases would not be therapeutically sufficient. Nor would it be likely to lead to dose-related side effects. However, it may be sufficient to cause hypersensitivity reactions, idiosyncratic side effects, and reactions in infants with enzyme deficiencies, such as glucose-6-phosphate dehydrogenase deficiency. The pharmacokinetics and safety of antimicrobial agents in pregnancy have been reviewed in detail by Chow and Jewesson.[73]

In Table 13–13, which summarizes the use of antibacterial agents in pregnancy, an attempt has been made to assess the safety of the agent to the fetus and any additional hazards to the mother resulting from pregnancy. Toxic effects which occur independently of pregnancy have not been listed. The United States Food and Drugs Administration (FDA) rating has also been given; for readers unfamiliar with this system, details can be found in the references[115, 116] and in the Preface.

FUNGAL INFECTIONS

Superficial fungal infections of the skin and mucous membranes are common and in many people are irritating and uncomfortable rather than a cause of serious illness. For that reason, the use of many antifungal agents available for the treatment of superficial infections, especially those administered systemically, is generally not justified in pregnancy because the benefit does not outweigh the potential risk. On the other hand, systemic mycoses, which are very uncommon in pregnant women, are associated with a high degree of morbidity and mortality, and it may be necessary to consider the use of antifungals which are known to be potentially toxic to the fetus.

Superficial Fungal Infections

Dermatophyte Infections

The dermatophytes are filamentous fungi (i.e., molds) which infect keratinized tissue, so that infection of skin, nail, and hair are seen. The causative fungi comprise three genera, *Microsporum, Epidermophyton,* and *Trichophyton.* It should be noted that while *Epidermophyton* is usually restricted to skin infections, *Microsporum* may cause skin or hair infections, and *Trichophyton* may be found in all three tissues. A large variety of different species are present within these genera and may be classified according to their source, which may be human, soil, or animal. This is of some clinical importance as the inflammatory reaction resulting from the infection (and hence the severity of symptoms produced) is less with human strains than with those from soil or animals.

Clinical Manifestations.—Dermatophytosis of the skin may be found in a wide variety of sites and may present in the classic appearance of "ringworm"—a gradually enlarging circular lesion with an erythematous edge and central healed area. The lesion is often scaly and itchy and vesicles may occa-

TABLE 13–13.
Antibacterial Agents in Pregnancy

Agent	Placental Passage	Excretion in Breast Milk	Comments	FDA Rating*	References
Penicillins					
Penicillin G	Readily crosses placenta to produce fetal serum levels of up to 100% maternal levels	Trace levels only	Safe for use in pregnancy	B	146, 147
Ampicillin, amoxicillin	As for penicillin G	Low or trace levels only	Safe for use in pregnancy	B	148
Amoxicillin/ clavulanate	As for penicillin G	Low or trace levels only	Limited experience but no evidence of fetal toxicity	—	27
Carbenicillin	Not known	Not known	Limited experience suggests no evidence of fetal toxicity	B	
Flucloxacillin	Low, probably due to high degree of protein binding	Trace levels only	No evidence of fetal toxicity	Not used in the United States	
Nafcillin	As for flucloxacillin	Trace levels only	No evidence of fetal toxicity	B	
Cephalosporins					
Cephalothin	Low degree of transfer only	Low or trace levels only	No evidence of fetal toxicity	B	149, 150
Cephalexin	Moderately, especially in late pregnancy	Trace levels only	Safe for use in pregnancy	B	151, 152
Cefuroxime	Moderate, fetal serum levels 20%–30% of maternal levels	Trace levels only	No evidence of fetal toxicity	B	153, 154
Ceftazidime	Not known	Trace levels only	No evidence of fetal toxicity, but experience is limited	—	
Imipenem	Not known	Not known	No experience of its use in pregnancy; there is evidence of fetal toxicity in animal studies using high doses	—	
Aminoglycosides					
Gentamicin	Moderately; fetal serum levels of up to 40% of maternal levels are achieved	Not known	Fetal ototoxicity may potentially occur but degree of risk to fetus is unknown	C	76, 155, 156
Tobramycin	As for gentamicin	Not known	As for gentamicin	D	157
Netilmicin	Not known	Not known	As for gentamicin	—	

	Placental transfer	Breast milk	Comment	Category	References
Amikacin	As for gentamicin	Not known	As for gentamicin	C	158, 159
Other antibacterials					
Chloramphenicol	Readily; fetal serum levels up to 100% of maternal levels	High levels achieved, up to 50% of serum levels	Circulatory collapse ("gray baby syndrome") may occur if given in late pregnancy or labor; the drug should be avoided except for life-threatening infections	C	160
Ciprofloxacin	Not known	Not known	Arthropathy has been demonstrated in young animals and use of this agent is not recommended in pregnancy	—	161
Clindamycin	Moderately	Low to moderate levels (10%–20% of serum levels)	No evidence of fetal toxicity	B	73, 74
Erythromycin	Crosses placenta to a low and variable extent	High, up to 100% of serum levels	Erythromycin estolate is contraindicated due to potential for reversible hepatotoxicity in mother; erythromycin does not cause fetal toxicity	B	73, 74, 162
Fusidic acid	Not known	Not known	Limited clinical experience in pregnancy has not shown evidence of fetal toxicity		
Metronidazole	See Table 13–17				
Nalidixic acid	Yes, but only to a small extent	Low levels are achieved	Although there is no evidence of fetal toxicity, use of nalidixic acid is not recommended in pregnancy	B	73, 163
Nitrofurantoin	Readily; fetal serum levels up to 100% of maternal levels	Low levels are achieved	Many years of clinical experience has shown nitrofurantoin to be safe for use in pregnancy	B	164
Spectinomycin	Not known	Not known	There is no evidence of fetal toxicity due to this agent	B	73
Tetracycline	Readily; fetal serum levels up to 100% of maternal levels	Moderate to high levels are found in breast milk, but bioavailability is low due to chelation with calcium	All tetracyclines are contraindicated in pregnancy due to fetal toxicity (teeth discoloration and inhibition of bone growth) and maternal toxicity (acute fatty liver and renal failure) In nursing mothers absorption from breast milk is minimal but use of these agents is not recommended	D	165–169

(Continued)

TABLE 13–13 (cont.).
Antibacterial Agents in Pregnancy

Agent	Placental Passage	Excretion in Breast Milk	Comments	FDA Rating*	References
Trimethoprim	Readily; fetal serum levels up to 100% of maternal levels	High, levels up to 100% of serum levels	Teratogenic in animals due to mode of action (folate antagonism); not recommended in pregnancy, especially in first trimester Trimethoprim may precipitate megaloblastic anemia in pregnant women, which may be prevented by administration of folinic acid	C	73, 170
Sulfamethoxazole	Readily crosses the placenta	Low levels oly	May potentially cause kernicterus if given to mother in late pregnancy; not recommended in pregnancy	B (rated D at term)	73, 170
Vancomycin	Not known	Not known	Experience is very limited; drug should be used only when there is an absolute indication for it	C	

*For description of the FDA pregnancy risk classification see the Preface.

sionally be present. In the hair, alopecia is common and may be accompanied by scales and vesicle or pustule formation. Dermatophytosis of the nail usually presents as discoloration and thickening of the nail with subsequent distortion.

Diagnosis.—Dermatophyte infections may resemble a large number of other conditions, including other fungal infections, and laboratory diagnosis should be performed. Appropriate specimens include skin scrapings, infected hair or nail scrapings, and clippings. Culture should be performed in all cases as microscopy may give false-negative results, particularly in nail infections.

Treatment.—Dermatophytosis may be treated with either topical or systemic antifungal agents. The treatment of choice for dermatophytosis of the skin is a topical imidazole agent such as clotrimazole or miconazole. Both of these agents have been used in pregnancy for many years without evidence of adverse effects and absorption from the skin is minimal.[117] In extensive disease a systemic agent given by mouth such as griseofulvin or ketoconazole (both FDA category C) could be considered in the nonpregnant patient, but these agents are relatively contraindicated in pregnancy (Table 13–16). Infections of the hair and nails do not respond to topical therapy. Since both griseofulvin and ketoconazole are relatively contraindicated in the pregnant woman, treatment of these conditions should be postponed until after delivery.

Superficial Candidiasis

Clinical Presentation.—*Candida albicans*, a yeastlike fungus, is a common organism which forms part of the normal flora of the gastrointestinal and female genital tracts, and infection is therefore usually endogenous. There are three common clinical syndromes. Oral candidiasis presents as numerous white patches on the tongue and other areas of the mouth, which can be scraped off to leave a

painful, bleeding surface. This condition is particularly associated with the use of broad-spectrum antibiotics, diabetes mellitus, prosthetic teeth, and human immunodeficiency virus (HIV) infection. Cutaneous candidiasis most frequently occurs in intertriginous areas where the skin is moist and macerated, such as the perineal or perianal areas or under the breasts. It appears as a superficial erythematous lesion often with vesicle formation. Vaginal candidiasis is also seen in patients with diabetes mellitus or in those taking antibiotics, but it is also more frequent in pregnant women. This condition presents as a thick white vaginal discharge accompanied by itching, which may be severe.

Treatment.—The treatment for superficial candidiasis is a topical antifungal agent. Various agents are available, including the polyenes (amphotericin B, nystatin) or imidazoles such as clotrimazole or miconazole. Topical nystatin and imidazoles have been used for many years in pregnant women without evidence of harm,[118] although care should clearly be taken when inserting the agent into the vagina. Oral and cutaneous candidiasis will usually respond to repeated applications of one of these agents but vaginal candidiasis may be less easy to treat and recurrence is common. Excellent results have been described in nonpregnant women with the use of orally absorbed agents such as fluconazole and itraconazole,[119] but the safety of these agents in pregnancy has not been established and they should not be used at the present time.

Deep or Systemic Fungal Infections

Fungal infections, other than superficial infection of the skin or mucous membranes, are rare in pregnancy. It is convenient to consider such infections as either being opportunistic infections, occurring in a host whose defenses are in some way compromised, or as due to one of the so-called pathogenic fungi, which may cause infection in an otherwise healthy host.

TABLE 13–14.
Predisposing Causes of Systemic Fungal Infection

Immunosuppression
  Congential immunodeficiency states
  Hematologic malignancy
  Neutropenia from any cause
  Renal, liver, cardiac, and bone marrow
    transplantation
  Aquired Immunodeficiency syndrome (AIDS)
  Corticosteroid and cytotoxic therapy
Other predisposing causes
  Broad-spectrum antibiotic therapy
  Indwelling intravenous cannulas
  Indwelling prosthetic devices (e.g., artificial heart
    valves)
  Diabetes mellitus (associated with mucormycosis)

Opportunistic Infections

These infections are a potential result of a wide variety of disorders which in some way interfere with the normal host defenses. Table 13–14 gives a list of such disorders. In pregnancy, these disorders are no more common than in the nonpregnant woman of childbearing age although there is evidence of a reduction in cell-mediated immunity in pregnancy and of an increased risk of coccidioidomycosis.[5] It is likely that as HIV infection becomes more widespread in females, pregnant women with the acquired immunodeficiency syndrome (AIDS) may be seen more frequently with a concomitant increase in systemic fungal infection. The commonest fungi seen in such disorders are *Candida albicans* and related species; Table 13–15 gives a list of the more common fungi found to cause systemic infections. It should be noted that the so-called pathogenic fungi may also occur as opportunistic infections.

It is beyond the scope of this chapter to discuss these infections in detail. Clinically, they exhibit a variety of clinical manifestations, including fungemia, fungal pneumonia, meningitis, endocarditis, and infection of a wide range of other organs. The diagnosis is often made on clinical grounds and may not be confirmed microbiologically. Isolation of the organism may be attempted from relevant specimens such as blood, cerebrospinal fluid (CSF), or biopsy tissue, or the organism may be demonstrated in biopsies by histology.

Antibody detection is generally unhelpful and detection of fungal antigens in body fluids is not yet widely available, with the exception of cryptococcal antigen in serum and CSF.

A number of antifungal agents are now available for the treatment of these infections, but many have the disadvantage of significant maternal or fetal toxicity (see Table 13–16). Since these infections are likely to be life-threatening the use of such agents may be justified. For all fungi amphotericin B remains an effective treatment, and may be combined with 5-flucytosine in infections due to yeasts. 5-Flucytosine should not be used alone as the organism may rapidly become resistant to it. Miconazole or ketoconazole are possible alternatives in patients unable to tolerate amphotericin, and recently newer imidazoles such as fluconazole and itraconazole have shown promise.[119]

The Pathogenic Fungi

These are fungi which are capable of causing disease in the otherwise healthy individual and include infections such as histoplasmosis, coccidioidomycosis, cryptococcosis, and blastomycosis. These infections generally present as chest infections and are therefore discussed in Chapter 6. Cryptococcal infection, however, may also present as a meningitis, often of slow onset over several weeks, with headache, personality changes, and neurologic disorder. Cryptococcal meningitis may be diagnosed by isolation of the organism from CSF or by the detection of cryptococcal antigen in CSF or serum. Standard treatment consists of the combination of

TABLE 13–15.
Fungi Found in Opportunistic Fungal Infection

Yeast and yeastlike fungi
  Candida albicans
  Other *Candida* spp., e.g., *C. tropicalis*
  Torulopsis glabrata
  Cryptococcus neoformans
Filamentous fungi
  Aspergillus spp.
  Agents of mucormycosis—*Mucor, Absidia,
    Rhizopus,* etc.

TABLE 13–16.
Antifungal Agents in Pregnancy

Agent	Placental Passage	Excretion in Breast Milk	Comments	FDA Category*	References
Amphotericin B	Moderately; about 33%–50% of maternal serum level	Not known	No evidence of fetal toxicity, but experience is limited	B	171
5-Flucytosine	Not known	Not known	Teratogenic in animal (rat) studies; has been used safely in pregnancy but is not recommended; benefit vs. risk must be assessed carefully	C	172, 173
Fluconazole	Not known	Not known	Safety in pregnancy not established	—	
Griseofulvin	Moderately well, but variable	Not known	Teratogenic and fetotoxic in animal studies; contraindicated in pregnancy	C	174, 175
Ketoconazole	Not known	Not known	Teratogenic in high doses in rats; safety in pregnancy not established	—	
Miconazole	Not known	Not known	Fetotoxic at high doses in animals; safety in pregnancy not established but there are no reports of fetal or maternal toxicity from topical use; absorption from skin or vagina is minimal	B	117, 145, 176

*For description of FDA pregnancy risk classification, see Preface.

amphotericin B plus 5-flucytosine,[120, 121] but recently excellent results have been achieved with the new imidazole fluconazole.[121–123] Unfortunately, relapse of infection is frequent and survivors may be left with permanent neurologic damage.

PROTOZOAL AND HELMINTH INFECTIONS

Although there is reasonably wide experience of many antibacterial agents in pregnancy, much less is known about the use of antiprotozoal or antihelminthic agents. For this reason, the question of the benefit of treatment versus the risk must be judged even more carefully then normally. Some infections, particularly those due to helminths, may not pose a threat to the mother or fetus and can safely be left untreated until after delivery. Others, such as malaria, are medical emergencies and urgent treatment, even with potentially hazardous agents, is justified. The use of antiparasitic agents in pregnancy is presented in Table 13–17. Since safe, effective treatment may not be available, prevention of these infections is of great importance and therefore at least a basic knowledge of the life cycle of the parasite is necessary.

Protozoal Infections

Giardiasis

Giardiasis is caused by a flagellate protozoan, *Giardia lamblia*. It is an endemic infection throughout the world although for reasons discussed below it is much more commonly seen in developing nations.

The life cycle of this organism is simple. The infection is acquired by ingesting the infectious cyst form of the parasite. The organism excysts in the small bowel to release the active, motile trophozoite which lives and multiplies in the duodenum and upper jejunum. As the organism passes down the gut it encysts so that the encysted form rather than the trophozoite is seen in feces, although in severely affected patients the trophozoite

may also be found. The cysts may be ingested by another individual, either by direct contact with a sufferer or by ingesting contaminated food or water. Prevention of this infection therefore hinges on the provision of safe water supplies and effective sewage disposal.

Clinically, giardiasis produces a syndrome of diarrhea, often with evidence of steatorrhea, abdominal pain, nausea, and flatulence.[124] Symptoms usually persist for at least 1 week and often for several weeks. Most cases resolve spontaneously if untreated, but a small proportion will enter a chronic course with persistent diarrhea and malabsorption. In pregnancy, giardiasis may cause a patient on the borderline of adequate nutrition to become malnourished.

The diagnosis is made by the examination of feces for cysts or trophozoites. If fecal examination is negative, duodenal aspirates may be examined for the trophozoite. The treatment of choice is metronidazole, but the safety of this agent has not yet been established in pregnancy, and it should therefore be used only when considered essential. An appropriate dose would be 400 mg three times daily for 7 days. Short-duration, high-dose regimens (such as 2 g daily for 3 days[124]) should not be used in pregnancy,[125] and quinacrine, often used outside of pregnancy in the United States, should also be avoided.[73]

Amebiasis

Entamoeba histolytica is a ubiquitous pathogen although infection with this protozoan is much more frequently seen in developing countries. The patient is infected by ingesting the infective cyst form which then excysts in the gut, the trophozoite inhabiting the large bowel. Infection is acquired, as with giardiasis, by direct contact with another person, or by ingesting contaminated water or food.

Most individuals infected with this organism are asymptomatic cyst passers. Symptomatic patients experience abdominal pain, frequent small stools containing blood and mucus, fever, and malaise. Potential complications include bowel perforation with resultant fecal peritonitis and extraintestinal

TABLE 13–17.
Antiparasitic Agents in Pregnancy

Agent	Placental Passage	Excretion in Breast Milk	Comments	FDA Category*	References
Cloroquine	Readily crosses placenta	Very low levels only	No evidence of fetal toxicity in doses used for treatment and prophylaxis of malaria	C	73, 135, 140, 145
Primaquine	Not known	Not known	Increased risk of intravascular hemolysis and methemoglobinemia in fetus; contraindicated in pregnancy	C	73
Pyrimethamine	Yes	Levels of 20%–40% of serum levels achieved	Teratogenic in animal studies; not recommended in pregnancy except in life-threatening infection (see text)	C	132, 139
Quinine	Yes	Low levels, about 15% of serum levels	Potential abortifacient, but not in doses used for treatment of malaria; may induce severe hypoglycemia (see text)	D	4, 138, 145
Spiramycin	Readily crosses placenta	High levels achieved	No evidence of fetal toxicity	—	4, 131, 145
Metronidazole	Readily crosses placenta	High levels achieved, approaching serum levels	No evidence of fetal toxicity, but is mutagenic and carcinogenic in animals in high doses; short-course, high-dosage regimens should not be used	B	177–180
Mebendazole	Not known	Not known	Teratogenic and fetotoxic in rats; contraindicated in pregnancy	—	142–144
Niclosamide	Not known	Not known	Experience is limited, but no evidence of animal or human fetal toxicity	—	145
Piperazine	Not known	Not known	Not recommended in first trimester but may be safe for use in late pregnancy	B	143, 144
Pyrantel	Not known	Not known	Experience is very limited and drug is not recommended in pregnancy	C	143–145

*For description of FDA pregnancy risk classification, see Preface.

TABLE 13–18.
Clinical Presentation of
Congenital Toxoplasmosis

Central nervous system
  Microcephaly
  Intracranial calcification
  Mental retardation
  Encephalitis
  Hydrocephalus
Choroidoretinitis and blindness
Jaundice
Anemia and thrombocytopenia
Pneumonitis

disease, most frequently in the liver. In pregnancy a syndrome of fulminating amebiasis may be seen with a rapid onset of severe colitis, abdominal distention, bowel perforation, and peritonitis.[126, 127] This condition may be seen at all stages of pregnancy and is associated with a high mortality rate.[127]

The diagnosis is made by the detection of cysts in stool specimens. In patients with acute, symptomatic infection, trophozoites may be detected by microscopy of a fresh stool specimen or material obtained at endoscopy. Invasive disease stimulates antibody formation and serologic diagnosis is available.

The treatment of choice for extraintestinal or symptomatic intestinal amebiasis is metronidazole,[128] in a dose of 800 mg three times daily for 5 days. In nonpregnant patients asymptomatic cyst passers should be treated, if only to avoid the transmission of infection to another person. Concern about the safety of antiamebic agents in the pregnant woman means that in the authors' opinion it is justifiable to refrain from treating asymptomatic infection until after delivery. Metronidazole is less effective in treating asymptomatic infection and diloxanide furoate, 500 mg three times daily for 10 days, should be used in nonpregnant patients. The safety of this agent during gestation has not been established.

Toxoplasmosis

Toxoplasma gondii, a sporozoan parasite, is found worldwide and has both a sexual reproductive cycle (in felines) and an asexual cycle in other mammals and in birds. Cats, the definitive host for the parasite, acquire infection either by ingesting infective oocysts or by eating meat containing tissue cysts. In the cat intestine the parasite undergoes sexual reproduction and oocysts are excreted in the cat's feces. Other animals become infected by ingesting the oocysts or tissue cysts; sporozoites are liberated in the intestine and enter the blood. The organism may proceed to infect any organ but has a predilection for the brain and skeletal muscle. Infection stimulates an effective immune response and the organism eventually becomes localized in tissue cysts, although the parasite within the cyst remains viable and may become reactivated if the immune status of the patient is compromised.

Humans are infected either by ingesting oocysts or by ingesting tissue cysts as a result of eating the undercooked meat of an infected animal. The incidence of infection varies among different countries and regions. In the United States and United Kingdom, up to 70% of women of childbearing age may be susceptible[129] and the incidence of maternal toxoplasmosis has been estimated at 1 to 10 per 1,000 pregnancies.[130]

Clinically, toxoplasmosis is often asymptomatic in immunocompetent individuals. Possible symptoms include fever, malaise, myalgia, and a skin rash, accompanied by generalized lymph node enlargement and splenomegaly. Atypical lymphocytes are present in peripheral blood. The clinical presentation of toxoplasmosis is not altered during pregnancy and the danger from this infection is to the fetus rather than the mother. Toxoplasmosis may lead to spontaneous abortion, stillbirth, or congenital infection of the fetus. It has been shown that fetal infection only occurs if the mother acquires infection during pregnancy and will not occur if the mother is infected before conception.[4] The risk of fetal infection increases with gestation but the severity of the infection is correspondingly reduced.[4, 131] It has been estimated that acute toxoplasmosis in pregnancy gives rise to an overall risk of fetal infection of approximately 60%, and an 11% risk of severe fetal damage or death.[4] Congenital infection may lead to a wide range of clinical results, which are summarized in Table 13–18.

The diagnosis of toxoplasmosis is confirmed by serologic tests for IgG and IgM. Interpretation of the results obtained is given in Table 13–19.

If acute toxoplasmosis is detected early in pregnancy, termination of the pregnancy may be offered to the mother. If this is not possible, chemotherapy may be offered. The most effective treatment is a combination of a sulfonamide plus pyrimethamine but the latter is a folate antagonist, has been shown to be potentially teratogenic (at least in laboratory animals),[132] and is not recommended for use in the first trimester. The alternative is spiramycin, a macrolide antibiotic similar to erythromycin, which is widely used in France but not in the United States or United Kingdom. This should be given in a dosage regimen of 3 g daily until after delivery.[133] In studies in France,[131, 133] spiramycin has been shown to reduce but not abolish the risk of congenital infection.[131]

As treatment is not completely reliable it is essential to advise the pregnant woman to avoid contact with cat feces (for example, in cat litter) and not to eat undercooked meat during pregnancy.[129] There is, however, some doubt about the efficacy of such preventive measures.[134] It has been recommended[4] that all pregnant women be screened for immunity to *Toxoplasma* at their first prenatal clinic visit. This is part of standard obstetric practice in France, where it has been shown to be effective when coupled with treatment for acute disease if detected,[133] but this is not done in the United Kingdom or United States.

Malaria

Malaria is caused by four species of sporozoan parasites belonging to the genus *Plasmodium* (*P. falciparum*, *P. vivax*, *P. ovale*, and *P. malariae*). Infection is acquired when the individual is bitten by a female anopheline mosquito seeking a blood meal. The infective sporozoite form of the parasite is present in the salivary glands of the mosquito and is injected into the circulation at the time of feeding. The sporozoites infect the liver mul-

tiplying to produce hepatic schizonts, this phase taking between 6 and 16 days depending on the species of parasite. The schizont then releases several thousand merozoites into the circulation which invade erythrocytes and multiply intracellularly. The erythrocyte ruptures to release more merozoites and the cycle is repeated. Some merozoites, instead of undergoing schizogony inside the erythrocyte, mature into gametocytes which are taken up by another mosquito. In the stomach of the mosquito sexual reproduction takes place with the eventual production of sporozoites which make their way to the salivary gland, thus completing the life cycle. There is an important difference between *P. vivax* and *P. ovale* and the other two species in that the hepatic schizonts of these species do not all rupture at once but may persist for several years to give repeated attacks of disease.

TABLE 13–19.
The Serologic Diagnosis of Toxoplasmosis

Serologic Findings	Interpretation
1. IgG-negative	Toxoplasmosis is unlikely, but tests may be repeated in 2–4 wk if desired.
2. Seroconversion from negative to positive, or four-fold rise in IgG titer	Acute toxoplasmosis; may be confirmed by estimating IgM.
3. IgG-positive but IgM-negative	Acute toxoplasmosis unlikely; probably indicates past infection. However, a negative IgM does not exclude acute infection and the tests should be repeated in 2–4 wk, especially if the IgG is positive in high titer (>1,000). A stable or declining titer of IgG with negative IgM in the repeat specimen confirms past infection.
4. IgG-positive, IgM-positive	Acute toxoplasmosis is likely. May be confirmed by repeating tests in 2–4 wk when a rising titer will confirm acute infection.

TABLE 13–20.
Clinical Features of Malaria

1. Febrile paroxysm

Initial cold stage: shivering, rigors, peripheral vasoconstriction; duration about 1 hr

Hot stage: headache, nausea, vomiting; hot,
dry skin; pyrexia $\geq 40°C$; duration
2–6 hr

Sweating stage: fall in temperature plus profuse
sweating; fatigue leading to sleep;
duration 2–4 hr

These episodes may be periodic, occurring every 48
or 72 hr depending on the species of parasite, but
this is often not seen

**2. Complications (most likely to occur with
falciparum malaria)**

Hemolytic anemia

Hemoglobinuria (blackwater fever) due to intravascular hemolysis and leading to renal failure

Cerebral malaria leading to hemiplegia and other
neurologic deficit, hyperpyrexia, and coma

Hepatorenal syndrome

Splenic rupture

The different species of the parasite have a different geographic distribution[135] and this is of interest as the treatment given will depend to a certain extent on the infecting species. In Africa, *P. falciparum* predominates and *P. vivax* is rarely found. However, falciparum malaria is less common in the Indian subcontinent where *P. vivax* is the most common species, but both falciparum malaria and *P. vivax* infection are seen in South America. *Plasmodium ovale* is mainly restricted to Africa and *P. malariae* is found worldwide.

Almost all cases seen in the United States or United Kingdom will be in travelers or immigrants from abroad and the majority of these imported cases are due to *P. falciparum* and *P. vivax*.[136] It should be remembered that cases have been described in people living or working near international airports,[137] and transmission may also occur during blood transfusion and in intravenous drug abusers who share needles and syringes. It is not intended to discuss in detail the clinical presentation of malaria here and this is summarized in Table 13–20.

Malaria in pregnancy has a number of ntially serious consequences for both mother and fetus. There is an increased risk of clinical attacks of malaria in pregnant as opposed to nonpregnant women, even in the population of endemic areas where women are likely to be at least partially immune.[4] When malaria does occur it is more severe in pregnancy with a higher degree of parasitemia and this is especially evident in nonimmune women and in primigravidas.[135] This in turn leads to a greater risk of complications such as severe hemolysis.[4] The placenta may sequester large numbers of parasitized erythrocytes and this may lead to placental insufficiency resulting in preterm delivery, low-birth-weight infants, and possibly intrauterine death and abortion.[4] Severe, recurrent hypoglycemia is a complication of falciparum malaria which is most likely to be encountered in pregnant women and patients treated with quinine[4, 135, 138] which may induce inappropriate hyperinsulinemia. Congenital infection may also occur, particularly with *P. falciparum* and in nonimmune mothers.[4]

The diagnosis of malaria is confirmed by microscopy of peripheral blood films. Laboratory diagnosis is not difficult and the principle reason for delay in diagnosing malaria is a failure to think of it. The diagnosis must be considered in all febrile patients who have returned from an endemic area in the past 3 months, even if adequate prophylaxis was apparently taken.

The possible effects of malaria in pregnancy are sufficiently serious to outweigh the potential risks of treatment. The treatment of choice for all forms of malaria other than chloroquine-resistant *P. falciparum* is chloroquine. This agent, in the doses used for the prophylaxis and treatment of malaria, does not appear to pose a risk to the fetus.[138–140] In disease caused by *P. vivax* and *P. ovale* it is necessary to eradicate persisting hepatic schizonts with primaquine, but primaquine should not be given during pregnancy and treatment should be delayed until after delivery. Until then, chloroquine should be given once weekly to prevent relapses. Treatment regimens for malaria are presented in Table 13–21.

Chloroquine-resistant *P. falciparum* infec-

TABLE 13–21.
Treatment Regimens for Malaria During Pregnancy

1. All forms of malaria except chloroquine-resistant *Plasmodium falciparum* malaria*
   a. Initial dose of 600 mg chloroquine base; followed 6 hr later by 300 mg chloroquine base, then a single dose of 300 mg on the next 2 days
   b. In malaria due to *P. vivax* or *P. ovale* give 300 mg chloroquine base once weekly to prevent relapse; after delivery give primaquine base 15 mg daily for 14 days to eradicate persisting hepatic schizonts

2. Chloroquine-resistant *P. falciparum* infection*
   a. Quinine (as sulphate, hydrochloride, or bihydrochloride) 600 mg 3 times daily by mouth for 7 days followed by a single dose of 75 mg pyrimethamine† plus 1,500 mg sulfadoxine

*The nature and occurrence of chloroquine-resistant falciparum malaria are constantly changing and resistance is emerging to pyrimethamine and other agents. The reader is advised to consult a specialist reference center.
†See text.

tion poses a problem in the pregnant patient.[141] However, falciparum malaria is a potentially life-threatening condition and the use of agents such as quinine and pyrimethamine is justified, despite the (probably very small[132]) risk to the fetus resulting from the use of pyrimethamine. If this agent, a folic acid antagonist, is used, folinic acid supplements should be given to the mother.

With regard to prophylaxis, ideally the pregnant woman should refrain from traveling to endemic areas until after delivery. If this is not possible, chloroquine (300 mg base once weekly continuing for 6 weeks after return) is the agent of choice for all forms except for areas where chloroquine-resistant *P. falciparum* may be encountered. Recommendations for prophylaxis against this organism are constantly changing and the reader is advised to consult a reference center.

Helminth Infections

Infections with helminths are extremely common conditions with worldwide distribution. For example, it has been estimated that 1 billion people are infected with *Ascaris lumbricoides*. It is almost inevitable then that at some stage a physician may be called upon to consider treatment for such an infection in a pregnant woman. It is not possible in this chapter to discuss each infection in detail, and only the salient points will be mentioned. Table 13–17 presents details of the use of antihelminthic agents in pregnancy while Table 13–22 gives treatment regimens. Fortunately,

TABLE 13–22.
Treatment Regimens for Helminth Infection

Infection	Antihelminthic	Dose
Enterobiasis	Piperazine*	75 mg/kg body weight daily for 7 days; repeat after 2 wk
	Mebendazole*†	100-mg single dose; repeat after 2 wk
	Pyrantel†	11 mg/kg body weight (max. dose 1 g) as single dose; repeat after 2 wk
Ascariasis	Piperazine*	75mg/kg body weight daily for 2 days
	Mebendazole†	100 mg bid for 3 days
	Pyrantel*†	11 mg/kg body weight (max. dose 1 g) as single dose
Trichuriasis	Mebendazole†	100 mg bid for 3 days
Hookworm	Mebendazole†	100 mg bid for 3 days
	Pyrantel†	11 mg/kg body weight (max. dose 1 g) as single dose
Taenia (adult worm)	Niclosamide*	2-g single dose (plus an antiemetic when treating *T. solium* infection)

*See text and Table 13–17 for the safety of these agents in pregnancy.
†These agents are contraindicated in the pregnant patient.

in many cases of helminth infection treatment can be delayed until after delivery.

Enterobiasis (Threadworms, Pinworms)

This extremely common condition is due to *Enterobius vermicularis,* a nematode about 1 cm long. Infection is acquired by ingesting the infective ova; the adult worm hatches in the gut and the female worm emerges from the anus at night onto the perianal skin to deposit its ova. Ova may persist in linen and furniture for several weeks. Infection is seen most frequently in children but may occur at any age.

Symptoms of threadworm infection are due to the presence of the worm on the perianal skin causing irritation and pruritus. The diagnosis can be confirmed by obtaining ova from the perianal skin with a piece of adhesive transparent tape.

Although the infection is irritating treatment may be delayed until after delivery when mebendazole or pyrantel are the treatments of choice. These agents are not recommended in the pregnant woman.[142, 143] If treatment before delivery is essential, piperazine may be safe for use after the first trimester.[143] Other members of the family are likely to be infected even if asymptomatic and should be treated simultaneously.

Ascariasis

Ascaris lumbricoides is a nematode some 20 cm long. Infection is acquired by ingesting the ova; these hatch in the small gut and the larvae penetrate the wall of the gut and enter the circulation. In the lung the larvae cross over into the alveoli and are then brought up to the trachea by mucociliary action. The larvae are swallowed and mature in the small intestine.

Infection may be asymptomatic, but there are several possible clinical syndromes. The larval migration may lead to a hypersensitivity reaction with fever, bronchospasm, and eosinophilia. The adult worms may cause malabsorption and steatorrhea, or if there are large numbers of them, may obstruct the small ~~el~~. Finally, single worms may on occasion the biliary tree causing obstruction.

Diagnosis is made by examination of stool specimens for the characteristic ova. Mebendazole,[142] pyrantel,[143] and levamisole[144] are all effective agents for treatment, but are contraindicated in pregnancy. Piperazine may be given after the first trimester if treatment is essential.[143]

Trichuriasis (Whipworm)

Infection with the 3- to 5-cm nematode *Trichuris trichuria* is acquired by ingesting the ova which develop into the adult worm in the large bowel. There is usually an absence of symptoms although heavy worm loads may give rise to diarrhea and anemia.

The diagnosis is made by finding the characteristic ova in stool specimens. Treatment can usually be delayed until after delivery, and mebendazole is the agent of choice.

Hookworm

Hookworm infection is due to two small (1 cm) nematodes, *Necator americanus* and *Ancylostoma duodenale.* Infection is acquired when the larval worm penetrates the skin and enters the circulation. They then follow a similar course to *Ascaris* (see above), and ova are excreted in the feces. These then hatch in the soil to complete the life cycle. Since the ova require certain conditions of temperature and moisture to hatch, hookworm tends to be confined to tropical and subtropical areas where infection is extremely common.

Symptoms may result from the initial penetration of the skin leading to irritation and a rash, or from the migration of the larvae through the lungs. The adult worm feeds by ingesting blood, and a heavy worm load can lead to an iron deficiency anemia. This may be particularly apparent in pregnancy due to the increased iron requirements.

The characteristic ova of hookworm (the two species cannot be distinguished) are readily found in stool specimens. Iron deficiency will require appropriate management and the infection can be treated after delivery with mebendazole.

Tapeworm Infection

The tapeworms are the most primitive of

all the worms infecting humans, consisting of a head (scolex) plus a number of egg-producing segments (proglottids). The life cycle of these worms has two stages. Ingestion of ova by an appropriate intermediate host will result in migration of larvae to many organs where they encyst and develop into one or more viable scoleces. If the flesh of the intermediate host is eaten by the definitive host, the scolex is released and the adult worm develops in the intestine. These can be truly enormous animals with a length of up to 50 ft.

Man is the only definitive host for *Taenia saginata* (the beef tapeworm) and *T. solium* (the pork tapeworm) but may also act as the intermediate host for *T. solium* and *Echinococcus granulosus* (the dog tapeworm). Taeniasis is acquired by ingesting the undercooked meat of the intermediate host, while infection with the larval stage of *T. solium* is acquired by contact with the feces of an infected person. Autoinfection with the ova of *T. solium* may occur, usually through the transfer of ova to the mouth on the fingers. Echinococcosis (hydatid disease) is acquired by contact with dog feces containing the ova of the worm.

Adult-stage taeniasis is almost always asymptomatic despite the size of the worm. Infection is diagnosed by finding the characteristic ova in feces but it is impossible to distinguish the two species in this way. Proglottids are often present in feces and the two species can be differentiated by the morphology of these segments. This may be of importance in pregnancy since treatment of *T. saginata* infection can be delayed until after delivery but it may be more urgent to treat *T. solium* infection to prevent autoinfection with the larval stage leading to cysticercosis. This condition may affect any organ but often presents as a space-occupying lesion in the central nervous system. The treatment of choice for adult-stage taeniasis is niclosamide; although experience in pregnancy is limited there is no evidence of animal or human toxicity. In *T. solium* infection an antiemetic should be given at the same time to prevent regurgitation of ova and the development of cysticercosis.

Hydatid disease usually presents as a large space-occupying lesion, which may occur in many different organs but is most commonly seen in the liver. Treatment is usually surgical.

REFERENCES

1. Falkoff R: Maternal immunologic changes during pregnancy: A critical appraisal. *Clin Rev Allergy* 1987; 5:287–300.
2. Weinberg ED: Pregnancy-associated depression of cell-mediated immunity. *Rev Infect Dis* 1984; 6:814–831.
3. Nieman RE, Lorber B: Listeriosis in adults: A changing pattern. Report of eight cases and review of the literature, 1968–1978. *Rev Infect Dis* 1980; 2:207–227.
4. Lee RV: Parasites and pregnancy: The problems of malaria and toxoplasmosis. *Clin Perinatol* 1988; 15:351–363.
5. Wack EE, Ampel NM, Galgiani JN, et al: Coccidioidomycosis during pregnancy: An analysis of ten cases among 47,120 pregnancies. *Chest* 1988; 94:376–379.
6. Blanco JD, Gibbs RS: Immunizations in pregnancy. *Clin Obstet Gynecol* 1982; 25:611–617.
7. Immunization Practices Advisory Committee: General recommendations on immunization. *MMWR* 1989; 38:205–227.
8. Saballus MK, Lake KD, Wager GP: Immunizing the pregnant woman: Risks versus benefits. *Postgrad Med* 1987; 81:103–113.
9. Urinary tract infection during pregnancy (editorial). *Lancet* 1985; 2:190–192.
10. Hankins GDV, Whalley PJ: Acute urinary tract infections in pregnancy. *Clin Obstet Gynecol* 1985; 28:266–278.
11. Whalley PJ: Bacteriuria of pregnancy. *Am J Obstet Gynecol* 1967; 97:723–738.
12. Kass EH: Asymptomatic infections of the urinary tract. *Trans Assoc Am Physicians* 1956; 69:56–64.
13. Stamm WE, Counts GW, Running KR, et al: Diagnosis of coliform infection in acutely dysuric women. *N Engl J Med* 1982; 307:463–468.

14. Sobel JD, Kaye D: Host factors in the pathogenesis of urinary tract infections. *Am J Med* 1984; 765:122–130.

15. Orskov I, Ferencz A, Orskov F: Tamm-Horsfall protein or uromucoid is the normal urinary slime that traps type 1 fimbriated *Escherichia coli. Lancet* 1980; 1:887.

16. Buckley RM, McGuckin M, MacGregor RR: Urine bacterial counts following sexual intercourse. *N Engl J Med* 1978; 298:321–324.

17. Kelsey MC, Mead MG, Grunenberg RN, et al: Relationship between sexual intercourse and urinary tract infection in women attending a clinic for sexually transmitted diseases. *J Med Microbiol* 1979; 12:511–512.

18. Nicolle LE, Harding GKM, Preiksaitis J, et al: The association of urinary tract infection with sexual intercourse. *J Infect Dis* 1982; 146:579–583.

19. Kinane DF, Blackwell CC, Brettle RP, et al: ABO blood group, secretor state and susceptibility to recurrent urinary tract infection in women. *Br Med J* 1982; 285:7–9.

20. Lomberg H, Hanson LA, Jacobsson B, et al: Correlation of P blood group, vesicoureteral reflux, and bacterial attachment in patients with recurrent pyelonephritis. *N Engl J Med* 1983; 308:1189–1192.

21. Kunin CM: Genitourinary infections in the patient at risk: Extrinsic risk factors. *Am J Med* 1984; 76S:131–139.

22. Turck M, Goffe B, Petersdorf RG: The urethral catheter and urinary tract infection. *J Urol* 1962; 88:834–837.

23. Kunin CM, McCormack RD: Prevention of catheter-induced urinary tract infections by sterile closed drainage. *N Engl J Med* 1966; 274:1156–1161.

24. Harris RE, Gilstrap LC: Cystitis during pregnancy: A distinct clinical entity. *Obstet Gynecol* 1981; 57:578–580.

25. Ronald AR, Boutros P, Mourtarda H: Bacteriuria localisation and response to single-dose therapy in women. *JAMA* 1976; 235:1854–1856.

26. Leveno KJ, Harris RE, Gilstrap LC, et al: Bladder versus renal bacteriuria during pregnancy: Recurrence after treatment. *Am J Obstet Gynecol* 1981; 139:403–406.

27. Pedler SJ, Bint AJ: Comparative study of amoxycillin-clavulanic acid and cephalexin in the treatment of bacteriuria during pregnancy. *Antimicrob Agents Chemother* 1985; 27:508–510.

28. Jacobi P, Neiger R, Merzbach D, et al: Single dose antimicrobial therapy in the treatment of asymptomatic bacteriuria of pregnancy. *Am J Obstet Gynecol* 1987; 156:1148–1152.

29. Harris RE, Gilstrap LC, Pretty A: Single dose antimicrobial therapy for asymptomatic bacteriuria during pregnancy. *Obstet Gynecol* 1982; 59:546–549.

30. Pedler SJ, Bint AJ: Management of bacteriuria in pregnancy. *Drugs* 1987; 33:413–421.

31. Chng PK, Hall MH: Antenatal prediction of urinary tract infections in pregnancy. *Br J Obstet Gynaecol* 1982; 89:8–11.

32. Beydoun S: Morphologic changes in the renal tract in pregnancy. *Clin Obstet Gynecol* 1985; 28:249–256.

33. Gilstrap LC, Cunningham FG, Whalley PJ: Acute pyelonephritis in pregnancy: An anterospective study. *Obstet Gynecol* 1981; 57:409–413.

34. Cunningham FG, Morris GB, Mickal A: Acute pyelonephritis of pregnancy: A clinical review. *Obstet Gynecol* 1973; 42:112–117.

35. Cunningham FG: Urinary tract infections complicating pregnancy. *Bailliere Clin Obstet Gynaecol* 1987; 1:891–908.

36. Harris RE, Gilstrap LD: Prevention of recurrent pyelonephritis during pregnancy. *Obstet Gynecol* 1974; 44:637–641.

37. Lenke RR, Van Dorsten JP, Schifrin BS: Pyelonephritis in pregnancy: A prospective randomized trial to prevent recurrent disease evaluating suppressive therapy with nitrofurantoin and close surveillance. *Am J Obstet Gynecol* 1983; 146:953–957.

38. Gonik B: Septic shock in obstetrics. *Clin Perinatol* 1986; 13:741–754.

39. Blanco JD, Gibbs RS, Castaneda YS: Bacteremia in obstetrics: Clinical course. *Obstet Gynecol* 1981; 58:621–625.

40. Bryan CS, Reynolds KL, Moore EE: Bacteremia in obstetrics and gynecology. *Obstet Gynecol* 1984; 64:155–158.

41. Beller FK, Schmidt EH, Holzgreve W, et al: Septicemia during pregnancy: A study in different species of experimental animals. *Am J Obstet Gynecol* 1985; 151:967–975.

42. O'Brien WF, Golden SM, Davis SE, et al: Endotoxemia in the neonatal lamb. *Am J Obstet Gynecol* 1985; 151:671–674.

43. Morrison DC, Ryan JL: Endotoxins and disease mechanisms. *Annu Rev Med* 1987; 38:417–432.

44. Lee W, Clark SL, Cotton DB, et al: Septic shock during pregnancy. *Am J Obstet Gynecol* 1988; 159:410–416.

45. Ziegler EJ, McCutchan JA, Fierer J, et al: Treatment of gram-negative bacteremia and shock with human antiserum to a mutant *Escherichia coli. N Engl J Med* 1982; 307:1225–1230.

46. Lachman E, Pitsoe SB, Gaffin SL: Anti-lipopolysaccharide immunotherapy in management of septic shock of obstetric and gynaecological origin. *Lancet* 1984; 1:981–983.

47. Wolff LSM: The treatment of gram-negative bacteremia and shock. *N Engl J Med* 1982; 307:1267–1268.

48. Cohen J: Anti-endotoxin immunotherapy in septic shock. *J Antimicrob Chemother* 1986; 14:436–439.

49. Ziegler EJ: Protective antibody to endotoxin core: The emperor's new clothes? *J Infect Dis* 1988; 158:286–290.

50. Ledger WJ: Infections of the female pelvis, in Mandell GL, Douglas RG, Bennett JE (eds): *Principles and Practice of Infectious Diseases,* ed 2. New York, John Wiley & Sons, 1985, pp 738–745.

51. Eaton CJ, Peterson EP: Diagnosis and acute management of patients with advanced clostridial sepsis complicating abortion. *Am J Obstet Gynecol* 1971; 109:1162–1164.

52. Soper DE: Postpartum endometritis: Pathophysiology and prevention. *J Reprod Med* 1988; 33(suppl):97–100.

53. Gibbs RS: Clinical risk factors for puerperal infection. *Obstet Gynecol* 1980; 55(suppl):178S–183S.

54. Gibbs RS, Listwa HM, Read JA: The effect of internal fetal monitoring on maternal infection following cesarean section. *Obstet Gynecol* 1976; 48:653–658.

55. Hagen D: Maternal febrile morbidity associated with fetal monitoring and cesarean section. *Obstet Gynecol* 1975; 46:260–262.

56. Eschenbach DA, Rosene K, Tompkins LS, et al: Endometrial cultures obtained by a triple-lumen method from afebrile and febrile postpartum women. *J Infect Dis* 1986; 153:1038–1045.

57. Rosene K, Eschenbach DA, Tompkins LS, et al: Polymicrobial early postpartum endometritis with facultative and anaerobic bacteria, genital mycoplasmas, and *Chlamydia trachomatis:* Treatment with piperacillin or cefoxitin. *J Infect Dis* 1986; 153:1028–1037.

58. Duff P, Gibbs RS, Blanco JD, et al: Endometrial culture techniques in puerperal patients. *Obstet Gynecol* 1983; 61:217–222.

59. Fotunato SJ, Dodson MG: Therapeutic consideration in postpartum endometritis. *J Reprod Med* 1988; 33(suppl):101–106.

60. Hawrylyshyn PA, Bernstein P, Papsin FR: Short-term antibiotic prophylaxis in high-risk patients following cesarean section. *Am J Obstet Gynecol* 1983; 145:285–289.

61. Gonik B: Single- versus three-dose cefotaxime prophylaxis for cesarean section. *Obstet Gynecol* 1985; 65:189–193.

62. Department of Health and Social Security: *On the State of the Public Health,* 1987. London, Her Majesty's Stationery Office, 1988.

63. Centers for Disease Control: Summary of notifiable diseases: United States, 1987. *MMWR* 1988; 36:1–60.

64. Ewing CI, Roberts C, Davidson DC: Early congenital syphilis still occurs. *Arch Dis Child* 1985; 60:1128–1133.

65. Mascola L, Pelosi R, Blount JH, et al: Congenital syphilis revisited. *Am J Dis Child* 1985; 139:575–580.

66. Buttigieg G: Detection and management of syphilis in pregnancy. *Br J Hosp Med* 1985; 33:28–31.

67. Charles D: Syphilis. *Clin Obstet Gynecol* 1983; 26:125–137.

68. Tramont ED: *Treponema pallidum* (syphilis), in Mandell GL, Douglas RG, Bennett JE (eds): *Principles and Practice of Infectious Diseases,* ed 2. New York, John Wiley & Sons, 1985, pp 1323–1333.

69. Thornton JG, Foote GA, Page CE, et al: False positive results of tests for syphilis and outcome of pregnancy: A retrospective case-control study. *Br Med J* 1987; 295:355–356.

70. Fitzgerald TJ: *Treponema,* in Lennette EH, Balows A, Hausler WJ, et al (eds): *Manual*

of *Clinical Microbiology.* Washington, DC, American Society for Microbiology, 1985, pp 485–489.

71. Benenson AS: *Control of Communicable Diseases in Man,* ed 14. Washington, DC, American Public Health Association, 1985.

72. Centers for Disease Control: 1989 Sexually transmitted diseases: Treatment guidelines. *MMWR* 1989; 38(suppl 8):1–43.

73. Chow AW, Jewesson PJ: Pharmacokinetics and safety of antimicrobial agents during pregnancy. *Rev Infect Dis* 1985; 7:287–313.

74. Philipson A, Sabath LD, Charles D: Transplacental passage of erythromycin and clindamycin. *N Engl J Med* 1973; 288:1219–1221.

75. Ziaya PR, Hankins GDV, Gilstrap LC, et al: Intravenous penicillin desensitization and treatment during pregnancy. *JAMA* 1986; 256:2561–2562.

76. Kucers A, Bennett N McK: *The Use of Antibiotics,* ed 4. London, William Heinemann, 1987.

77. Easmon CSF, Ison CA: *Neisseria gonorrhoeae:* A versatile pathogen. *J Clin Pathol* 1987; 40:1088–1097.

78. Spence MR: Gonorrhea. *Clin Obstet Gynecol* 1983; 26:111–124.

79. Johnson AP: The pathogenesis of gonorrhoea. *J Infect* 1981; 3:299–308.

80. Hook EW, Holmes KK: Gonococcal infections. *Ann Intern Med* 1985; 102:229–243.

81. Blackwell AL, Eykyn SJ: Paediatric gonorrhoea: Non-venereal epidemic in a household. *Genitourin Med* 1986; 62:228–229.

82. Disseminated gonococcal infection (editorial). *Lancet* 1984; 1:832–833.

83. Bohnhoff M, Morello JA, Lerner SA: Auxotypes, penicillin susceptibility, and serogroups of *Neisseria gonorrhoeae* from disseminated and uncomplicated infections. *J Infect Dis* 1986; 154:225–230.

84. Adler MW, Belsey EM, Rogers JS: Sexually transmitted diseases in a defined population of women. *Br Med J* 1981; 283:29–32.

85. National Institutes of Health: Summary of a workshop on maternal genitourinary infections and the outcome of pregnancy. *J Infect Dis* 1983; 147:596–605.

86. Lacey CJN, Milne JD: Preterm labour in association with *Neisseria gonorrhoeae*: Case reports. *Br J Vener Dis* 1984; 60:123–124.

87. Dodson MG, Fortunato SJ: Microorganisms and premature labour. *J Reprod Med* 1988; 33(suppl):87–96.

88. Morello JA, Janda WM, Bohnhoff M: *Neisseria* and *Branhamella,* in Lennette EH, Balows A, Hausler WJ, et al (eds): *Manual of Clinical Microbiology,* ed 4. Washington, DC, American Society for Microbiology, 1985, pp 176–192.

89. Schachter J, McCormack WM, Smith RF, et al: Enzyme immunoassay for diagnosis of gonorrhea. *J Clin Microbiol* 1984; 19:57–59.

90. Ison CA, McLean K, Gedney J, et al: Evaluation of a direct immunofluorescence test for diagnosing gonorrhoea. *J Clin Pathol* 1985; 38:1142–1145.

91. Totten PA, Holmes KK, Handsfield HH, et al: DNA hybridization technique for the detection of *Neisseria gonorrhoeae* in men with urethritis. *J Infect Dis* 1983; 148:462–471.

92. Rice RJ, Thompson SE: Treatment of uncomplicated infections due to *Neisseria gonorrhoeae:* A review of clinical efficacy and in vitro susceptibility studies from 1982 through 1985. *JAMA* 1986; 255:1739–1746.

93. Centers for Disease Control: Antibiotic-resistant strains of *Neisseria gonorrhoeae*: Policy guidelines for detection, management and control. *MMWR* 1987; 36:(suppl 5S):1S–18S.

94. Washington AE: Update on treatment recommendations for gonococcal infections. *Rev Infect Dis* 1982; 4(suppl):S758–S771.

95. Thompson SE, Dretler RH: Epidemiology and treatment of chlamydial infections in pregnant women and infants. *Rev Infect Dis* 1982; 4(suppl):S747–S757.

96. Sweet RL, Schachter J, Landers DV: Chlamydial infections in obstetrics and gynecology. *Clin Obstet Gynecol* 1983; 26:143–164.

97. Schachter J: Chlamydiae (psittacosis-lymphogranuloma venereum-trachoma group), in Lennette EH, Balows A, Hausler WJ, et al (eds): *Manual of Clinical Microbiology,* ed 4. Washington, DC, American Society for Microbiology, 1985, pp 856–862.

98. Schmid GP, Blount JH: Chancroid in the United States: Reestablishment of an old disease. *JAMA* 1987; 258:3265–3268.

99. Schwarz RH: Chancroid and granuloma

inguinale. *Clin Obstet Gynecol* 1983; 26:138–142.

100. Hart G: *Calymmatobacterium granulomatis* (donovanosis, granuloma inguinale), in Mandell GL, Douglas RG, Bennett JE (eds): *Principles and Practice of Infectious Diseases,* ed 2. New York, John Wiley & Sons, 1985, pp 1379–1381.

101. Fleming HA: Antibiotic prophylaxis against infective endocarditis after delivery. *Lancet* 1977; 1:144–145.

102. Sugrue D, Blake S, MacDonald D: Pregnancy complicated by maternal heart disease at the National Maternity Hospital, Dublin, Ireland. *Am J Obstet Gynecol* 1981; 139:1–6.

103. Sugrue D, Blake S, Troy P, et al: Antibiotic prophylaxis against infective endocarditis after normal delivery—is it necessary? *Br Heart J* 1980; 44:499–502.

104. Durack DT: Prophylaxis of infective endocarditis, in Mandell GL, Douglas RG, Bennett JE (eds): *Principles and Practice of Infectious Diseases.* ed 2. New York, John Wiley & Sons, 1985, pp 539–544.

105. Report of a Working Party of the British Society for Antimicrobial Chemotherapy: The antibiotic prophylaxis of infective endocarditis. *Lancet* 1982; 2:1323–1326.

106. Acheson D: Listeriosis and food. Department of Health and Social Security, PL/CMO(89)3, Feb 16, 1989.

107. Barza M: Listeriosis and milk. *N Engl J Med* 1985; 312:438–440.

108. Schlech WF, Lavigne PM, Bortolussi RA, et al: Epidemic listeriosis—evidence for transmission by food. *N Engl J Med* 1983; 308:203–206.

109. Listeriosis (editorial). *Lancet* 1989; 1:83–84.

110. Kerr K, Dealler SF, Lacy RW: Listeria in cook-chill food. *Lancet* 1988; 2:37–38.

111. Gill P: Is listeriosis often foodborne illness? *J Infect* 1988; 17:1–5.

112. Gellin BG, Broome CV: Listeriosis. *JAMA* 1989; 261:1313–1320.

113. Cruikshank DP, Warenski JD: First-trimester maternal *Listeria monocytogenes* sepsis and chorioamnionitis with normal neonatal outcome. *Obstet Gynecol* 1989; 73:469–471.

114. Wise R: Prescribing in pregnancy: Antibiotics. *Br Med J* 1987; 294:42–46.

115. Millstein LG: FDA's "pregnancy categories". *N Engl J Med* 1980; 303:706.

116. Briggs GG, Freeman RK, Yaffe SJ: *Drugs in Pregnancy and Lactation: A Reference Guide to Fetal and Neonatal Risk,* ed 2. Baltimore, Williams & Wilkins Co, 1986.

117. Holt RJ: The imidazoles, in Speller DCE (ed): *Antifungal Chemotherapy.* Chichester, England, John Wiley & Sons, 1980, pp 107–147.

118. Patterson RM: Vulvovaginitis in pregnancy, in Pauerstein CJ (ed): *Clinical Obstetrics.* New York, John Wiley & Sons, 1987, pp 549–553.

119. Warnock DW: Antifungal drugs. *Curr Opin Infect Dis* 1989; 2:362–366.

120. Philpot CR, Lo D: Cryptococcal meningitis in pregnancy. *Med J Aust* 1972; 2:1005–1007.

121. Byrne WR, Wajszczuk CP: Cryptococcal meningitis in the acquired immunodeficiency syndrome (AIDS): Successful treatment with fluconazole after failure of amphotericin B. *Ann Intern Med* 1988; 108:384–385.

122. Stern JJ, Hartman BJ, Sharkey P, et al: Oral fluconazole therapy for patients with acquired immunodeficiency syndrome and cryptococcosis: Experience with 22 patients. *Am J Med* 1988; 85:477–480.

123. Sugar AM, Saunders C: Oral fluconazole as suppressive therapy of disseminated cryptococcosis in patients with acquired immunodeficiency syndrome. *Am J Med* 1988; 85:481–489.

124. Wright SG, Tomkins AM, Ridley DS: Giardiasis: clinical and therapeutic aspects. *Gut* 1977; 18:343–350.

125. Haddock DWR: Treatment of parasitic infestations and exotic disease in pregnancy. *Clin Exp Obstet Gynaecol* 1986; 13:168–172.

126. Lewis EA, Antia AU: Amoebic colitis: Review of 295 cases. *Trans R Soc Trop Med Hyg* 1969; 63:633–638.

127. Armon PJ: Amoebiasis in pregnancy and the puerperium. *Br J Obstet Gynaecol* 1978; 85:264–269.

128. Wolfe MS: The treatment of intestinal protozoan infections. *Med Clin North Am* 1982; 66:707–720.

129. McCabe R, Remington JS: Toxoplasmosis: The time has come. *N Engl J Med* 1988; 318:313–315.

130. Sever JL, Ellenberg JH Ley AC, et al: Toxoplasmosis: Maternal and pediatric findings in 23,000 pregnancies. *Pediatrics*

1988; 82:181–192.

131. Desmonts G, Couvreur J: Congenital toxoplasmosis: A prospective study of 378 pregnancies. *N Engl J Med* 1974; 290:1110–1116.

132. Pyrimethamine combinations in pregnancy (editorial). *Lancet* 1983,2:1005–1007.

133. Daffos F, Forestier F, Capella-Pavlovsky M, et al: Prenatal management of 746 pregnancies at risk for congenital toxoplasmosis. *N Engl J Med* 1988; 318:271–275.

134. Foulon W, Naessens A, Lauwers S, et al: Impact of primary prevention on the incidence of toxoplasmosis during pregnancy. *Obstet Gynecol* 1988; 72:363–366.

135. Manson-Bahr PEC, Bell DR: *Manson's Tropical Diseases,* ed 19. London, Bailliere Tindall, 1987.

136. Phillips-Howard PA, Bradley DJ, Blaze M, et al: Malaria in Britain: 1977–86. *Br Med J* 1988; 296:245–248.

137. Whitfield D, Curtis CF, White GB, et al: Two cases of falciparum malaria acquired in Britain. *Br Med J* 1984; 289:1607–1609.

138. White NJ, Warrell DA, Chanthavanich P, et al: Severe hypoglycemia nad hyperinsulinemia in falciparum malaria. *N Engl J Med* 1983; 309:61–66.

139. Public Health Laboratory Service Malaria Reference Laboratory: Prevention of malaria in pregnancy and early childhood. *Br Med J* 1984; 189:1296–1297.

140. Wolfe MS, Cordero JP: Safety of chloroquine in chemosuppression of malaria during pregnancy. *Br Med J* 1985; 290:1466–1467.

141. Main EK, Main DM, Krogstad DJ: Treatment of chloroquine-resistant malaria during pregnancy. *JAMA* 1983; 249:3207–3209.

142. Keystone JS, Murdoch JK: Mebendazole. *Ann Intern Med* 1979; 91:582–586.

143. Cline BL: Current drug regimens for the treatment of intestinal helminth infections. *Med Clin North Am* 1982; 66:721–742.

144. Glover SC: Drug treatment of helminthic infections. *Br J Hosp Med* 1983; 30:169–174.

145. Appendix II: Adverse effects of antiparasitic drugs on the mother and fetus, in MacLeod CL (ed): *Parasitic Infections in Pregnancy and the Newborn.* Oxford, England, Oxford University Press, 1988, pp 284–297.

146. Ledger WJ: Antibiotics in pregnancy. *Clin Obstet Gynecol* 1977; 20:411–421.

147. Landers DV, Green JR, Sweet RL: Antibiotic use during pregnancy and the postpartum period. *Clin Obstet Gynecol* 1983; 26:391–406.

148. Philipson A: Pharmacokinetics of ampicillin during pregnancy. *J Infect Dis* 1977; 136:370–376.

149. MacAulay MA, Charles D: Placental transfer of cephalothin. *Am J Obstet Gynecol* 1968; 100:940–946.

150. Morrow S, Palmisano P, Cassady G: The placental transfer of cephalothin. *J Pediatr* 1968; 73:262–264.

151. Creatsas G, Pavlatos M, Lolis D, et al: A study of the kinetics of cephapirin and cephalexin in pregnancy. *Curr Med Res Opin* 1980; 7:43–46.

152. Goodspeed AH: Cephalexin in special cases. *J Antimicrob Chemother* 1975; 1(suppl):105.

153. Craft I, Mullinger BM, Kennedy MRK: Placental transfer of cefuroxime. *Br J Obstet Gynaecol* 1981; 88:141–145.

154. Bousfield P, Browning AK, Mullinger BM, et al: Cefuroxime: Potential use in pregnant women at term. *Br J Obstet Gynaecol* 1981; 88:146–149.

155. Yoshioka H, Monma T, Matsuda S: Placental transfer of gentamicin. *J Pediatr* 1972; 80:121–123.

156. Weinstein AJ, Gibbs RS, Gallagher M: Placental transfer of clindamycin and gentamicin in term pregnancy. *Am J Obstet Gynecol* 1976; 124:688–691.

157. Bernard B, Garcia-Cazares SJ, Ballard CA, et al: Tobramycin: Maternal-fetal pharmacology. *Antimicrob Agents Chemother* 1977; 2:688–694.

158. Bernard B, Abate M, Thielen PF, et al: Maternal-fetal pharmacological activity of amikacin. *J Infect Dis* 1977; 135:925–932.

159. Mazzei T, Paradiso M, Nicoletti I, et al: Amikacin in obstetric, gynecologic, and neonatal infections: Laboratory and clinical studies. *J Infect Dis* 1976; 134(suppl):S374–S379.

160. Scott WC, Warner RF: Placental transfer of chloramphenicol (Chloromycetin). *JAMA* 1950; 142:1331–1335.

161. Schluter G: Ciprofloxacin: Review of potential toxicologic effects. *Am J Med* 1987; 82(suppl 4A):91–93.

162. McCormack WM, George H, Donner A, et al: Hepatotoxicity of erythromycin estolate during pregnancy. *Antimicrob Agents Chemother* 1977; 12:630–635.

163. Murray EDS: Nalidixic acid in pregnancy. *Br Med J* 1981; 282:224.

164. Hailey FJ, Fort H, Williams JC, et al: Foetal safety of nitrofurantoin macrocrystals therapy during pregnancy: a retrospective analysis. *J Int Med Res* 1983; 11:364–369.

165. Greene GR: Tetracycline in pregnancy. *N Engl J Med* 1976; 295:512–513.

166. Whalley PJ, Adams RH, Combes B: Tetracycline toxicity in pregnancy. *JAMA* 1964; 189:357–362.

167. Kunelis CT, Peters JL, Edmondson HA: Fatty liver of pregnancy and its relationship to tetracycline therapy. *Am J Med* 1965; 38:359–377.

168. Kline AH, Blattner RJ, Lunin M: Transplacental effect of tetracyclines on teeth. *JAMA* 1964; 188:178–180.

169. Tetracyclines in pregnancy (editorial). *Br Med J* 1965; 1:743–744.

170. Reid DWJ, Caille G, Kaufmann NR: Maternal and transplacental kinetics of trimethoprim and sulfamethoxazole, separately and in combination. *Can Med Assoc J* 1975; 112:67S–72S.

171. Ismail MA, Lerner SA: Disseminated blastomycosis in a pregnant woman: Review of amphotericin B usage during pregnancy. *Am Rev Respir Dis* 1982; 126:350–353.

172. Schonebeck J, Segerbrand E: *Candida albicans* septicaemia during first half of pregnancy successfully treated with 5-fluorocytosine. *Br Med J* 1973; 4:337–338.

173. Scholer HJ: Flucytosine, in Speller DCE (ed): *Antifungal Chemotherapy*. Chichester, England, John Wiley & Sons, 1980, pp 35–106.

174. Rubin A, Dvornik D: Placental transfer of griseofulvin. *Am J Obstet Gynecol* 1965; 92:882–893.

175. Davies RR: Griseofulvin, in Speller DCE (ed): *Antifungal Chemotherapy*. Chichester, England, John Wiley & Sons, 1980, pp 149–182.

176. Daneshmend TK: Systemic absorption of miconazole from the vagina. *J Antimicrob Chemother* 1986; 18:507–511.

177. Visser AA, Hundt HKL: The pharmacokinetics of a single intravenous dose of metronidazole in pregnant patients. *J Antimicrob Chemother* 1984; 13:279–283.

178. Rodin P, Hass G: Metronidazole and pregnancy. *Br J Vener Dis* 1966; 42:210–212.

179. Peterson WF, Stauch JE, Ryder CD: Metronidazole in pregnancy. *Am J Obstet Gynecol* 1966; 94:343–349.

180. Shepard TH, Fantel AG: Is metronidazole teratogenic? *JAMA* 1977; 237:1617.

CHAPTER 14

Viral Infections

J. S. M. Peiris
C. R. Madeley

Viruses are obligate intracellular parasites. They replicate inside the cells of the body, taking over the cell's functions to do so, sometimes damaging the cell lethally in the process. Hence, any viral infection has the potential to damage the host. However, virus infections in (nonpregnant) adults usually leave no permanent sequelae unless they involve tissues which are not repaired (such as the central nervous system [CNS]) or unless death occurs at the acute stage following a fulminant infection. This does not mean that no damage is done, only that the resultant cell death is repairable. When virus infection occurs in a pregnant woman, the actively growing and developing fetus is also at risk, and is particularly vulnerable. The consequences range from no detectable fetal damage to fetal death. The former presents no problem to the woman or her physician. The latter may not be recognized at all if it occurs before pregnancy is diagnosed (much of the fetal wastage is undiagnosed), or at worst, results in a short-term though sharp anguish. The real challenge for the clinician arises from the minority of instances where fetal organogenesis is irrecoverably interfered with, resulting in an individual with a permanent handicap for the rest of his life. The problem for the diagnostic virologist, therefore, is to provide the information on which the would-

be parents and their medical advisers can base a decision on whether to continue with the pregnancy. The necessary information will include the chances of fetal damage, its likely nature, and whether it can be repaired postnatally. A complete answer is rarely possible because assessments of risk are statistical, and provide only probability, not certainty, with regard to an individual patient. Nonetheless, there is a demand for available relevant information on which such decisions can be based, and one goal of this chapter is an attempt to provide it. The effects of viral infections on the fetus and neonate are summarized in Tables 14–1 and 14–2.

Pregnancy—by and large—has minimal effects on the severity of viral infections in the woman. The exceptions include polio; feco-orally transmitted non-A, non-B hepatitis, and, possibly, varicella-zoster. Polio is more likely to lead to paralytic disease in pregnancy[1]; feco-orally transmitted non-A, non-B hepatitis may carry a 10% to 20% mortality in the third trimester of pregnancy,[2] and it is suggested, though not proven, that varicella is more severe in pregnant women (see below).

Finally, the likelihood of a particular virus infection occurring during pregnancy depends upon (1) the proportion of women of childbearing age who are susceptible to the virus, (2) the level of virus activity in the com-

TABLE 14–1.
Effects of Maternal Infection on the Fetus and Neonate

Virus	Abortion/ Stillbirth	Prematurity/Low Birth Weight	Intrauterine Infection	Congenital Malformation	Perinatal Infection Acquired From Mother
Rubella	+	+	+	++*	+
Cytomegalovirus	?	−	+	++*	+
Herpes simplex	+	+	(+)†	−	++‡
Varicella-zoster	−	+	(+)	(+)§	++
Epstein-Barr	?	?	(+)	−	−
Human immunodeficiency virus	?	+	+	NK	++
Parvovirus	+	NK	+	?¶	NK
Measles	?	+	?	−	+
Mumps	+	−	(+)	−	−
Influenza	+	NK	(+)	−	+
Poliovirus	+	?	(+)	−	+
Coxsackievirus	−	−	(+)	?	+
ECHO	−	−	−	−	+
Papillomavirus	−	−	(+)	−	+
Polyomavirus (BK, JC)	NK	?	?	−	−

+ = association well documented; + + = association well documented, occurrence frequent enough to cause clinical concern; ? = contradictory reports, uncertain; (+) = probable association, occurrence very rare; − = no association documented, occasional case reports may be present in literature; NK = not known.
*The risk of congenital defects in the baby may be significant enough to consider advisability of termination of pregnancy. See text.
†Occasional occurrence following infections late in pregnancy.
‡Risk from neonatal herpes simplex may be high enough to consider cesarean delivery if active infection is documented at delivery. See text.
§Fetal varicella syndrome is documented, but is a rare occurrence. Not an indication for termination of pregnancy.
¶One case reported in an aborted fetus. Not an indication for termination of pregnancy.

TABLE 14–2.
Clinical Features of Babies Born With Some Common Congenital or Perinatal Viral Infections

	Impact of Defect on Long-Term Development	Congenital Rubella	Congenital Cytomegalovirus	Herpes Simplex (Neonatal Infection)	Varicella-Zoster Fetal Varicella Syndrome	Varicella-Zoster Neonatal Varicella
CNS						
Hearing defects	R	+	+	-	(+)	
Intellectual defects	P	+	+	+		
Gross mental retardation	P	+	+	+	+	
Paralysis	P	-	+*	+	+	
Microcephaly	P	-	+*	+	+	
Intracranial calcification	T,P	-	+*	-		
Meningoencephalitis		+	+	+		
Heart						
Congenital defects	R	+	-	-	-	-
Myocarditis	T	+	-	-	-	-
Eye						
Cataracts	R	+	-	+	+	
Glaucoma	T	+*	-	-	-	
Optic atrophy	P	-	+	-	-	
Chorioretinitis/retinopathy	P	+*	+	+	+	
Micropthalmia	P	+	-	-	+	
Conjunctivitis/keratoconjunctivitis	T	-	-	+*	-	
Skin						
Petichiae/purpura	T	+	+	+	-	
Vesicles	T	-	+	+*†	-	
Maculopapular rash	T	-	-	+	-	+
Cicatricial lesions with dermatomal distribution	P,R	-	-	-	+*	
Other						

Feature					
Hepatosplenomegaly	T	+	+		+
Jaundice	T	+	+		+
Pneumonitis	T	+‡	+		+
Bone lesion	T	+	−	−	+§
Adenopathy	T	+	−	−	
Laboratory features					
Laboratory virus isolation		+¶	+¶	+‖	+**
IgM in cord neonate blood		+	+	?	?
Persisting antibody in baby and/or higher titer than mother		(+)	(+)	(+)	(+)

R = repairable or treatable; P = permanent; T = transient.
*Characteristic lesion(s) associated with congenital infection.
†Characteristic, but may be absent in up to 50% of infected babies.
‡Radiologic abnormalities of long bones.
§Skeletal deformities.
¶From throat and urine.
‖From throat, urine, skin, eyes, vesicular lesions, CSF.
**From vesicles.

munity at large, (3) the infectivity and means of transmission of the virus, and (4) contact (by the woman) with the segments of the population that usually maintain the virus in the community. For example, in the case of rubella—an infection occurring most commonly in childhood—multiparous pregnant women had an attack rate 2.5 times that in primigravidas,[3] a factor reflecting the increased risk from close contact with young children.

The spectrum and approximate frequency of the different viral illnesses complicating pregnancy was documented by Sever and White.[4] In over 30,000 pregnancies they recorded 1,600 clinically diagnosed viral infections (excluding the common cold).

PATHOGENESIS OF FETAL INFECTION

The consequence of maternal viral infection on the fetus depends on the virus type, the virulence of the virus strain, the age of the fetus when exposed to the virus, and the defense mechanisms of the fetus.

Maternal viral infections can affect the fetus directly, or indirectly through the systemic effects of the maternal illness such as high fever or associated metabolic derangements. The latter is documented in varicella, variola, and measles.[5] Fetal infection most often follows maternal viremia and placental infection, or less commonly may be the result of ascending infection from the lower genital tract. Placental infection can lead to infective emboli being released into the fetal circulation, thereby resulting in fetal infection. Alternatively, it can infect the fetus via the involvement of the fetal membranes, infection of the amniotic fluid, and aspiration into the fetal respiratory tract. It should, however, be noted that placental infection does not invariably result in the infection of the fetus. Maternal placentitis without fetal involvement has been documented in rubella[6] and cytomegalovirus (CMV).[7] The unpredictability of the consequences of maternal infection on the fetus is exemplified by reports of binovular

twin pregnancies in which one infant was congenitally damaged while the other had no detectable abnormalities.[5]

Iatrogenic CMV infection of the fetus following intrauterine transfusion has been recorded[8] and transmission of infection via invasive methods of investigation remains a theoretical possibility. The use of fetal scalp monitors during delivery can result in the infection of the fetus with viruses present in the genital tract of the mother, e.g., herpes simplex virus.

LABORATORY DIAGNOSIS OF VIRAL INFECTIONS IN PREGNANCY

The effective use of the laboratory is indispensable to the good management of viral infection, but the consequences of a missed or incorrect diagnosis are particularly important in pregnancy.

Different viruses cause different problems for the virologist, and how they are investigated and managed is discussed individually in later sections of this chapter. Here it is necessary only to outline briefly the various principles of diagnosis used by the staff of the virology laboratory to investigate and diagnose infections, with an emphasis on those viruses likely to provide particular difficulties in pregnancy.

The laboratory diagnosis of virus infections is based on the demonstration of (in order of rapidity) (1) the virus by (a) visualization of typical virus particles by electron microscopy; (b) the detection of viral antigens, viral inclusions, or viral nucleic acids; (c) culture; and/or (2) a host immune response (almost always serum antibody) to the virus. With some slow-growing or fragile viruses an antibody response may be faster or more reliable than culture, and (a) or (b) are not available for all viruses.[9-15]

The specimens to be collected for laboratory diagnosis of the viral infections and clinical syndromes of relevance in pregnancy are summarized in Tables 14–3 and 14–4. This assumes a laboratory using the full range of diagnostic techniques. The tests available

TABLE 14–3.
Specimens to Be Collected From the Pregnant Woman and Congenitally/Perinatally Infected Neonate

Virus	Mother	Infant
Rubella	S, PS	S, U, TS
Cytomegalovirus	S, PS, U, TS	S, U, TS
Herpes simplex	Lesion scrape/swab* Vesicle fluid†	Lesion scrape/swab* Vesicle fluid† TS, NPS, CSF
Varicella-zoster	Lesion scrape/swab* Vesicle fluid† PS	Lesion scrape/swab* Vesicle fluid† PS
Epstein-Barr	S	S
Human immunodeficiency virus	S	S
Parvoviruses	S	S
Measles	TS, NPS, PS	NPS, TS, S
Mumps	TS, PS	TS, S
Influenza	TS, NPS, PS	NPS, TS, PS
Enteroviruses	TS, PS, stool‡	TS, PS, stool‡
Hepatitis B	S	S
Hepatitis A	S	S

S = Single serum. Collect without anticoagulant. Store at 4°C until it arrives at laboratory (see text).
PS = Paired sera. As for single serum (see text).
TS = Throat swab. Swab broken into virus transport medium. Transport to laboratory on wet ice.
U = Urine. Collect into sterile container. Transport on wet ice.
NPS = Nasopharyngeal aspirate. Nasopharyngeal secretions are collected by aspiration into a mucus trap. Transport to laboratory in this container, on wet ice.
*As for throat swab.
†Collect in 1-mL syringe with fine needle. Recap and send to laboratory without delay.
‡Collect into sterile container.

TABLE 14–4.
Specimens to Be Collected for the Investigation of Viral "Syndromes" in the Pregnant Woman and/or Contact (When Available)

Clinical Syndrome	Possible Viruses	Specimens to Be Collected*
1a. Fever and maculopapular rash	Rubella, measles, enteroviruses, parvoviruses, others	S, PS, TS, stool
b. Fever and arthralgia	Rubella, parvoviruses, enteroviruses (arboviruses)	S, PS, TS, stool
c. Fever, undifferentiated	Rubella, measles, enteroviruses, parvoviruses, influenza, EBV, CMV, others	S, PS, TS, stool, U
2. Vesicular rash	Varicella-zoster, herpes simplex; enteroviruses	Lesion scape, vesicle fluid, vesicle swab, stool
3. Genital ulcers	Herpes simplex	Lesion scrape, lesion swab, vesicle fluid
4. Hepatitis	Hepatitis A, B, C, non A, non B, EBV, CMV	S, PS
5. Mononucleosis-like illness	EBV, CMV, HIV	S, PS, U
6. Patient with opportunistic infections; High risk for HIV (AIDS)	HIV	S

EBV = Epstein-Barr virus; CMV = cytomegalovirus; HIV = human immunodeficiency virus; AIDS = human immunodeficiency syndrome.
*For codes for specimens to be collected, see Table 14–3.

for the investigation of any particular problem may vary from laboratory to laboratory, and it is essential that the local laboratory be contacted for advice on the nature of the specimens to be collected and, because viruses are fragile, the appropriate means for transporting them.

Specimen transport is crucial if the laboratory is to be able to identify the causative agent. In general, specimens for virus isolation must be carefully handled. Where appropriate (see Table 14–3), they should be put into *virus* transport medium. They should be transported on wet ice (4°C) and arrive at the laboratory as soon as possible. Serum or blood samples for serologic investigation are less fastidious, but are best kept cool (4°C) until sent to the laboratory. Lesion scrapes for immunofluorescence can be prepared by spreading the material from the scalpel blade used to scrape the lesion in a drop of saline placed on a glass slide. The material on the slide should be fixed by air-drying and is then relatively stable and may be sent by ordinary first-class mail to the laboratory.[9] For more details on the techniques used in the diagnosis of viral infections, the reader is referred to the text by Lennette, et al.[15]

RUBELLA

Rubella was the first virus demonstrated to have teratogenic potential.[16] In unvaccinated communities rubella is primarily an infection of school-age children, seroepidemiologic studies showing that approximately half of 9- to 11-year-olds have evidence of past infection, this proportion rising to 80% to 85% in women of childbearing age. This pattern is broadly consistent in most parts of the world where such studies have been carried out, though there are occasional reports of lower seroprevalences, e.g., in some cities of Japan, Hawaii, and India.[17, 18]

Effects of Infection on the Pregnant Woman

Pregnancy does not alter the severity of illness in the mother. The incubation pe-

riod of rubella is approximately 16 to 17 days (range 13–20 days). Up to 25% of infections can be subclinical. The clinical features of the infection in the pregnant woman are protean and include fever, a maculopapular rash, lymphadenopathy (occipital, cervical, or generalized) and arthralgia (or even frank arthritis). Often it is not possible to be certain of a clinical diagnosis. On the one hand, other viruses (e.g., enteroviruses, parvovirus B19, arboviruses) can present with very similar clinical features[19]; and on the other, atypical clinical presentations of rubella can be mistaken for undifferentiated viral fevers of diverse etiology or indeed remain unrecognized. Of children diagnosed to have congenital rubella, only 45% of their mothers gave a history of an illness with a rash during pregnancy, and 25% were unaware of any illness throughout the pregnancy.[20] If the question of rubella enters the mind of a clinician caring for a pregnant woman, that is sufficient indication to investigate the illness virologically, and the illness should be "rubella" until proved otherwise.

Effects of Maternal Infection on the Fetus and Newborn

The effect of maternal infection on the fetus depends on (1) the stage of fetal development at the time of maternal viremia, and (2) the mother's immune status vis-à-vis rubella. Infection of the fetus can occur following both apparent and inapparent maternal rubella infections.[21]

Infection in the first 2 months of pregnancy resulted in spontaneous abortion in approximately 20% of cases and in an increase in babies that were small for dates.[3, 22, 23] The early clinical studies (with no virologic confirmation of the diagnosis) indicated that the risk of congenital defects following rubella in pregnancy was 15% in women infected during the first month; 24% in the second month; 17% during the third month, and 6% in the fourth month of gestation (reviewed by Hanshaw et al.[17]). Miller et al.[3] reported recent studies on the consequences of virologically confirmed symptomatic maternal rubella on

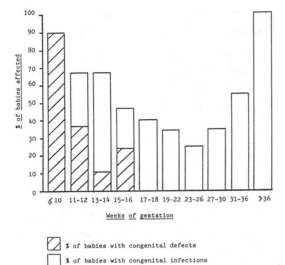

Weeks of gestation

◻⟋ % of babies with congenital defects
◻ % of babies with congenital infections

FIG 14–1.
Consequences of rubella at different stages of pregnancy. (Based on data from Miller et al.[3])

fetal infection and congenital disease (2-year follow-up after birth). Congenital *infection* rates declined from 90% in mothers infected during the first 10 weeks of pregnancy, to 25% at 23 to 36 weeks' gestation (Fig 14–1). The risk of congenital infection again rose to 60% between 31 and 36 weeks and all eight mothers developing rubella in the last month of pregnancy gave birth to infected infants. Comparable results were reported by Cradock-Watson et al.[24] in a study of rubella in the fourth to ninth months of pregnancy, and these authors also confirmed the increase in risk of congenital infection in the last month of pregnancy. The latter may reflect perinatal transmission of the virus at partus or via breast milk.

Data from the limited numbers of children followed up for evaluation of congenital *damage* indicated[3] that the estimated overall risk was 90% following rubella in the first 10 weeks of pregnancy, 20% between 11 and 16 weeks, and nil after the 17th week of gestation (see Fig 14–1). However, there are reports that maternal infection in the 17th and 18th weeks of pregnancy can occasionally give rise to congenital deafness.[25, 26]

Periconceptional rubella in the mother does not appear to result in fetal infection provided the illness occurs earlier than 12 days after the last menstrual period.[27] This probably indicates that infection of the fetus occurs only if maternal viremia occurs at or after conception.

The spectrum of clinical manifestations observed in children with congenital rubella correlates with the timing of the maternal infection.[3, 28] This is presumably related to the fetal organs actively developing at different periods of gestation, and whether damage to the target organ can be repaired or compensated. The occurrence of all defects progressively decreased (as expected) when rubella occurred later in pregnancy. Deafness and neurologic defects became the dominant clinical manifestations of congenital rubella when maternal infection occurred after the second month of gestation (Table 14–5). The clinical features of the congenital rubella syndrome are extensively reviewed by Hanshaw et al.[17] They have been classified into transient, permanent, and developmental.[22] Developmental defects are those that are not apparent at birth, but manifest later in life, either because the defect becomes clinically detectable (e.g., intellectual impairment, sensorineural deafness), or because the pathology is progressive (e.g., sensorineural deafness, diabetes mellitus). The transient manifestations such as thrombocytopenic purpura, hepatitis,

TABLE 14–5.
Clinical Manifestations of Congenital Rubella in Relation to Timing of Maternal Infection*

Congenital Defects	Timing of Maternal Rubella in Pregnancy		
	1st and 2nd Months	3rd Month	4th Month
	n = 166	n = 82	n = 43
Heart disease	57%[†]	21%	5%
Cataract/ glaucoma	37%	7%	0%
Neonatal purpura	34%	9%	5%
Deafness	76%	67%	49%
Neurologic deficit	58%	27%	26%

*Based on data from Cooper et al.[28]
†Percentage of infants affected.

and hemolytic anaemia clear spontaneously, but reflect extensive infection, and are associated with a higher rate of permanent sequelae and mortality. In severely affected infants, the virus can be found in virtually every organ of the body.[22] The final quality of life in a baby with the congenital rubella syndrome is related to the permanence and severity of the defects, and also whether the defects are correctable (see Table 14–2).

Rubella Reinfection

While solid and long-lasting immunity to rubella usually follows natural infection or vaccination, reinfection can occur with detectable boosts of antibody response. Two to three percent of seropositive (naturally immune) persons exposed during a rubella epidemic demonstrated booster antibody responses.[29] While in the past it was assumed that reinfections did not induce detectable rubella IgM, there is now evidence that a virus-specific IgM response can occur.[30, 31]

Asymptomatic rubella reinfection in early pregnancy has been documented in 41 women without fetal infection or ill effect.[30, 31] However, Best and her colleagues[32] have recently documented transfer of rubella virus to the fetus in five asymptomatic pregnancies in previously seropositive women. In three of the mothers rubella-specific IgM was recorded (it was not sought in the other two). Two of the pregnancies were terminated and rubella virus isolated from the conceptus. The remaining three went to term, and all had congenital defects. There are other well-documented instances where fetal infection and damage have followed rubella reinfection.[33, 34] These reports, which document reinfection, albeit rare, suggest that contact with "rubella" even in the "immune" should be investigated thoroughly. It is not possible at present, however, to give a reliable assessment of the risk of fetal damage in any given instance of rubella reinfection in pregnancy, other than to say that it is an "uncommon" occurrence.

Risks From Inadvertent Rubella Immunization During Pregnancy

Use of rubella vaccine—being a live attenuated vaccine, and given the known teratogenicity of the wild virus—is *not* recommended in pregnant women. *Women vaccinated for rubella should be advised to avoid pregnancy for 3 months postimmunization.* Still, it is comforting to note that data from women inadvertently vaccinated with rubella during pregnancy and going on to term have shown that, while the vaccine virus can cross the placenta and give rise to fetal infection in approximately 2% of instances, in no case was the vaccine associated with the congenital rubella syndrome.[23, 35, 36] On the basis of the number of cases studied, the maximum theoretical risk of congenital damage has been calculated to be 1.4% (on the basis of confidence intervals inherent in the small sample size). Thus inadvertent immunization of a pregnant woman with rubella vaccine is not by itself an indication for the termination of the pregnancy. The data suggest that the risk of fetal infection may be lower following RA27/3 vaccine than the Cendehill or HPV77 vaccines.[35, 36]

Laboratory Diagnosis

Virologic diagnosis of rubella is based on serology. While rubella virus can be cultured in vitro, it is both a fragile and a slow-growing virus. Virus culture is neither sufficiently rapid nor reliable enough to be of help in the management of a pregnant woman exposed to rubella or to establish the diagnosis in a contact. Virus culture from the urine and the throat is, however, useful in the diagnosis of a congenitally infected baby.

Antibody titers to the virus are usually measured by hemagglutination inhibition (HI), complement fixation (CF), or immunoassay techniques. The antibody response as detected by these serologic techniques is shown in Figure 14–2. In postnatal rubella, antibodies detectable by HI and IgM immunoassays usually appear with the onset of the rash, and increase in titer over the next week or two. Complement-fixing antibody (and that detected by single radial hemolysis) appears 6 to 8 days later, and the former was used (before IgM tests became widely available) in situations where the first available serum from a pregnant woman was taken too late in the illness to demonstrate a rising HI titer. A rise in titer by CF may yet be demonstrable.

Serologic diagnosis is now most commonly established by demonstrating rising antibody titers by HI tests or by the demonstration of rubella-specific IgM-class antibodies. While detection of IgM antibodies to rubella indicates recent infection, it should be noted that the duration of detectable IgM antibody depends on the sensitivity of the test used.[37] Using very sensitive techniques (e.g., radioimmunoassay), IgM antibody can be demonstrated for at least 1 year, and may be

irrelevant to the present pregnancy. Thus it is vital that the results of serology are interpreted in the context of the test used. Secondly, a low nonspecific "broad" IgM response can be a rare consequence of infectious mononucleosis, parvovirus B19 infection, and cytomegalovirus infection.[38] Finally, rubella reinfection can give rise to transient and low levels of IgM.

If there is evidence of rubella-specific IgM in a woman in whom rubella antibodies have been documented in the past, the possibility of reinfection has to be considered. A single serologic report documenting rubella antibodies sometime in the past, in a woman with evidence of rubella IgM during her present pregnancy, does not necessarily carry conviction. Possibilities of laboratory or clerical errors cannot be discounted. If the previous serum is available for retesting, or if there are

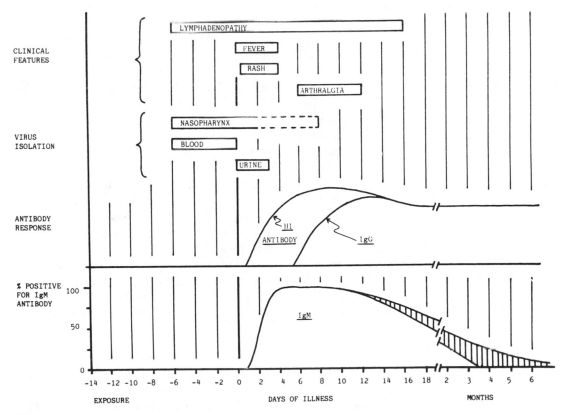

FIG 14–2.
Serologic diagnosis of rubella. Antibody response as measured by hemagglutination inhibition (HI) and IgG and IgM immunoassays.

multiple reports documenting seropositivity, the diagnosis of a rubella reinfection is more certain. A past history of immunization by itself is *not* evidence of past immunity because an immune response is not invariable. If there is any reason to doubt the validity of previous seropositivity, rubella IgM in a pregnant woman should be considered to be due to a primary rubella infection, and managed as such. If convincing evidence of prior immunity is present, however (i.e., a rubella reinfection), the risk to the fetus is much lower, but cannot be entirely discounted (see above). At present there are no data on which such a risk assessment can be based.

The implications of asymptomatic *rein*fection in early pregnancy to the health of the fetus are quite different from the risk of damage from primary infection (discussed above), the latter being a possible indication for terminating the pregnancy, while the former may not be.[38] There have been attempts to develop methods (based upon the avidity of the serum antibody produced) that could resolve this dilemma, though they are still under evaluation.[39]

The immune status of women can also be assessed by serology. The level of "long-term" antibody measured by HI, single radial hemolysis (SRH), or an IgG-specific immunoassay correlates with resistance to infection. The rubella status in pregnancy is usually assessed on a sample of blood taken at the first prenatal visit. Occasionally, high titers of rubella antibody are found during such screening, and may be an indication of recent infection. Demonstration of rubella-specific IgM in such sera will confirm a diagnosis of congenital rubella infection.

A serologic diagnosis of congenital rubella infection in an infant can be established by (1) demonstrating rubella-specific IgM; (2) testing sera, one from the mother and one from the baby in parallel and demonstrating a significantly higher titer of antibody in the baby; or (3) demonstrating the persistence of antibody in the baby beyond that expected from passively transferred maternal immunity (testing sera from the baby at intervals

of 2–3 months, and demonstrating no fall in antibody).

Management of the Pregnant Woman Having a Rubella-like Illness or in Contact With Rubella

Sources of rubella infection for pregnant women include children or adults with postnatally acquired rubella or babies with congenital rubella infection. In the former, the period of infectivity ranges from the week prior to the onset of the rash to the few days immediately after. Respiratory secretions are the likely source of infection. In congenital rubella, on the other hand, high-titer virus is shed for months in the urine, and is a significant source of infection[17] as well as the respiratory secretions. Although as many as a third of congenitally infected children continue to shed virus in the urine after the fourth month of life, the risk of transmitting infection is low by the time the baby has reached 3 months.[17] This is probably because the titer of virus in body secretions has fallen with increasing age. Whatever the source of infection, the probability of transmitting rubella is highest if contact has been close, prolonged, and indoors (e.g., household contact). Wherever possible, it is worth attempting to confirm a virologic diagnosis of rubella in the contact by demonstrating rubella-specific IgM or a rising titer of antibody in the blood.

Information on the date and type of exposure, past history of rubella immunization, and past rubella immune status (if known) should be obtained from past records if available. This may help in interpreting the laboratory investigations although patient recall in matters like rubella vaccination and immune status is fallible. In the end, only current and laboratory-proven facts matter; history by or about the patient is too unreliable as a basis for action.

Figure 14–3 shows an algorithm for laboratory investigation and interpretation of results. This is based on the following: (1) The incubation period of rubella can range from 13 to 20 days. Thus (a) rubella antibody (HI,

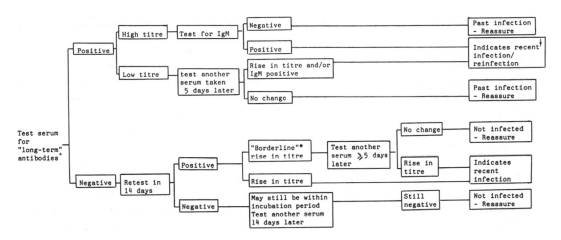

* Tests that detect "long-term" antibodies and which can be used to document rise in antibody titre includes HI tests and IgG immunoassays.

* "Borderline" rise in titre: changes in antibody titre that are insufficient to be conclusive, but leave room for suspicion.

† Risk to fetus depends on stage of pregnancy

FIG 14–3.
Management of rubella in pregnancy: an outline.

SRH, CF tests; IgG immunoassays) detected within the first 2 weeks after exposure is almost certainly due to previous immunity; (b) if infection has occurred, antibody should be detectable by 5 weeks after exposure at the latest. (2) Rubella-specific IgM and/or a significant rise in antibody titer between paired sera is indicative of recent infection (or reinfection).

If recent rubella (primary infection) in a pregnant woman has been established serologically, the risk to the fetus depends on the stage of gestation at which maternal viremia would have occurred, that is, the week before seroconversion or the appearance of the rash. As already discussed (see above), the risk of fetal *damage* (as contrasted to infection) is low after 16 weeks of gestation. The risks to the baby should be discussed with the parents, and they should be helped to decide whether to continue or terminate the pregnancy. Assessment of the risk posed by rubella (primary or reinfection) in pregnancy is by its nature statistical, and cannot predict with certainty the fate of a *particular* fetus. Direct evidence of fetal *damage* would be desirable, if such evi-

dence could be obtained, but there is no test at present. However, methods to establish fetal *infection* have been under investigation, and include attempts at isolating virus from the amniotic fluid (too slow a process to be useful, and a negative result could not be used to exclude infection); detecting virus-specific IgM in fetal blood obtained by fetoscopy[40]; and the use of nucleic acid probes on fetal samples to demonstrate virus.[41] Fetal IgM cannot be detected reliably until the 22nd week of gestation, when the fetal immune response has developed sufficiently. In addition, false-negatives are known to occur. DNA hybridization methods[41] have been assessed only in animal models as yet, but these and other newer methods may well be useful in future.

Screening for rubella immune status should be a routine part of the first prenatal examination of a pregnant woman during *every* pregnancy. If the laboratory keeps the serum for long enough, this will provide a first serum for investigating any subsequent infection (rubella or otherwise) during the pregnancy. Seronegativity should alert the clinician to the need for postpartum immunization.

CYTOMEGALOVIRUS

Cytomegalovirus (CMV) is one of the six (a seventh is now being characterized) herpesviruses infecting man. The virus has a single serotype although some strain heterogeneity can be demonstrated by sensitive neutralization tests and restriction-endonuclease analysis of the viral DNA.[42, 43] It shares with other members of the herpes family the propensity to remain latent within the host after primary infection, and to reactivate periodically. While reactivation is common in the immunosuppressed host, the stimuli triggering it in immunocompetent individuals are unknown. The biology and epidemiology of the virus has been reviewed by Ho.[43]

The virus can be transmitted (1) horizontally by droplet infection and direct contact via infected saliva and urine (particularly from congenitally infected babies); (2) venereally through infected cervical secretions and semen; and (3) vertically (from mother to child) in utero or perinatally, via infected maternal genital secretions bathing the child at birth and/or breast milk.[43–45] The virus can be transmitted iatrogenically via blood transfusions and via transplants of infected organs.[43]

Populations in Europe, North America, and Australia have a seropositivity of 40% to 50% by adolescence, and this figure increases by roughly 1% annually thereafter.[43, 46] In general, populations in the less developed areas of the world (e.g., Uganda, Morocco, Philippines) acquire infection earlier in life, but neither climate nor economic affluence are the decisive factors in determining the prevalence of the infection. The Japanese (96%) and the Eskimos (81%) also have high seroprevalences.[43] The observed geographic differences in virus prevalence are probably due to complex and as yet undefined sociologic factors.

CMV is not a highly infectious virus. However, given the prolonged period of virus excretion (in saliva and urine) from infected individuals, up to 50% of susceptible family members will seroconvert within 6 months of the index case.[47]

Effect of Infection on the Pregnant Woman

In developed countries, where approximately half the young female population are CMV-seronegative, the risk of primary infection (seroconversion in seronegatives) during pregnancy is approximately 1%.[48]

From examples of iatrogenic and perinatal transmission, the incubation period appears to be 4 to 8 weeks.[49] Asymptomatic infection is common. Virus shedding in the cervical secretions in the last trimester of pregnancy is comparable (at 11.3%) to that in the nonpregnant woman. Paradoxically, however, the percentage of women shedding virus is much lower in the first trimester of pregnancy (1.6%).[50]

The symptoms of CMV infection are pyrexia, lymphadenopathy, sore throat, polyarthropathy, or a Paul-Bunnell-Davidsohn test negative mononucleosis-like syndrome. Biochemical evidence of liver dysfunction is common, though clinical hepatitis is seen less often.[51] Pregnancy does not seem to increase the severity of the disease.

Effects of Maternal Infection on the Fetus and Newborn

The association of CMV in pregnancy with abortion (following infection early in pregnancy) has not been unequivocally established[17] though Altshuler[52] reported spontaneous abortion, associated with a placentitis and a specific fetal immune response, following CMV early in pregnancy.

CMV is the commonest congenital infection known at present, with an incidence between 0.2% and 2.2% of all live births. The risk of congenital infection was higher in lower income groups and can follow either primary or recurrent infection during pregnancy.[53]

Babies with congenital CMV infection may vary between being asymptomatic at birth (90%–95%) to having cytomegalic inclusion disease, permanent disability, or death. Those symptomatic were usually born to mothers whose primary infection was acquired during pregnancy. However, there are documented instances of congenitally damaged infants being born to mothers who were CMV-seropositive before conception.[54, 55] Congenital defects (CNS defects; hepatosplenomegaly) can follow primary infection at any stage of pregnancy.[53, 56] Congenitally infected babies who are apparently well at birth are not necessarily spared from the consequences of CMV. Ten to twenty percent of these congenitally infected babies will develop late neurologic sequelae. Moreover, such long-term morbidity can follow recurrent as well as primary CMV in pregnancy.[53, 56–58] The clinical findings in babies born with symptomatic congenital CMV are listed in Table 14–2, and are reviewed by Hanshaw and colleagues.[17]

CMV infection of the pregnant woman in late pregnancy results in perinatal infection through infected maternal genital secretions bathing the baby at birth, or via breast milk. The rate of virus shedding in cervical secretions apparently correlates with the rates of perinatal infection. In the United States, as well as in the United Kingdom, approximately 10% of young adult women shed the virus in their genital secretions,[50] resulting in 2% to 10% of children being infected by the age of 6 months.[59] Perinatal infection is thus very frequent, but does not appear to pose a significant threat to the baby although it may occasionally cause interstitial pneumonitis in the neonate. However, when neonates born to seronegative mothers acquired infection postnatally (e.g., through transfusions or other nosocomial sources), severe and even fatal disease can result.[60, 61] Thus CMV acquired perinatally from the mother is probably modulated by the passive maternal immunity transferred.

Laboratory Diagnosis

A laboratory diagnosis of postnatal CMV can be made by culturing the virus from throat swabs and urine. Conventional culture techniques which depend on the development of a viral cytopathic effect can take up to 2 to 4 weeks. However, using shell vial cultures and monoclonal antibodies to demonstrate the presence of the early antigens of CMV, a diagnosis can frequently be made within 48 hours—the DEAFF test (detection of early antigens by fluorescent foci).[12] Virus isolation cannot differentiate between primary and recrudescent CMV.

Primary CMV is associated with a rise in antibody titer to the virus and a virus-specific IgM response. Using a radioimmunoassay technique, specific IgM can be demonstrated in about 90% of primary infections,[62] the antibody being detectable for 3 to 4 months depending on the laboratory technique used. Recrudescent CMV is usually not associated with IgM antibodies, and thus rising antibody titers without an IgM response is very suggestive of a nonprimary infection. However, complement-fixing CMV antibody titers can fluctuate in apparently healthy individuals, and this must be kept in mind when interpreting CMV serology.[63]

Diagnosis of congenital CMV infection in the child can be best established by virus isolation, and in a proportion of cases by IgM detection in the cord or neonatal blood. In the case of the former, only virus isolated from specimens collected early in the neonatal period (within the first 3 weeks) will indicate congenital infection. The isolation of CMV *later in infancy* may be due to perinatal or postnatal infection and have no relevance to the defect observed. Indeed, over 10% of infants aged 6 months of age excrete the virus in their urine, much of this following perinatally acquired infection. The virus can be demonstrated by the electron microscopy of an ultracentrifuged deposit from urine, especially within the first 6 months of life in children with congenital CMV.[64]

The detection of virus-specific IgM in cord blood at birth, and in the infant's blood subsequently (first weeks of life) is useful, but about one fourth of congenital infections have no detectable IgM.

There is no reliable marker for the direct demonstration of infection of the fetus while still in utero. Culture of amniotic fluid has been used successfully, but is probably not sensitive enough to be used routinely. Preliminary data suggest that a defect in maternal cell-mediated immunity to CMV has been associated with congenital infection of the fetus.[65] Lange et al.[66] reported the detection of IgM antibodies in cord serum obtained via fetoscopy at 25 weeks' gestation in a fetus subsequently proved to have been infected in vitro.

Newer techniques such as the polymerase chain reaction have been applied to the detection of CMV in urine of congenitally infected children and may prove to be useful in the future for the demonstration of the virus in utero.[11]

It is difficult to differentiate between primary and recurrent infections in a pregnant woman with CMV. This distinction can only be made with certainty if pre-conception serum specimens are available for antibody testing. As mentioned above, rising antibody titers or virus isolation combined with a lack of an IgM response would probably be indicative of recurrent infection.

Management and Counseling of Women With Cytomegalovirus Infection in Pregnancy

Maternal infection with CMV is rarely diagnosed in pregnancy, because it is usually asymptomatic. The problem may arise following a mononucleosis-like illness in pregnancy, or following the exposure of a pregnant woman (most commonly health care personnel) to a baby known to be shedding the virus. In the latter instance it is worth remembering that CMV is not commonly transmitted by casual and brief contact. If primary CMV is confirmed in a pregnant woman, the course of action to be advised (given our present state of knowledge) is far from clear and needs to be tailored to each patient. The risks of congenital disease and long-term sequelae following CMV in pregnancy are summarized in Figure 14–4. While it is clear that congenital CMV infection will occur in 40% to 50% of the children, the risks of having a child with gross cytomegalic inclusion disease is low (probably less than 5% of first-trimester primary CMV infections). Some of these severely affected children will die in early infancy, and not add to the numbers of long-term mentally handicapped. This potential for long-term handicap in the baby has to be contrasted with the "background" risk of 2% to 3% congenital abnormalities seen in pregnancies with no evidence of viral infection. It has therefore been argued[49] that there is no indication for termination of pregnancy on the grounds of risk to the fetus. However, it is clear that more subtle development deficits (hearing and intellectual defects) do occur more often (up to 5% of babies born to mothers with primary CMV in pregnancy) (see above), and the mother may well find this risk unacceptable.

Recurrent (nonprimary) CMV in pregnancy appears to pose less of a risk of overt neonatal disease, but may still cause developmental defects developing later in life. The magnitude of this risk is still not well defined.

The dilemma faced by the clinician is illustrated by two instances of pregnant medical staff exposed to patients with CMV. The pregnant women were documented to have acquired primary CMV, and their pregnancies were terminated. CMV was recovered from the products of conception, and was compared by restriction enzyme analysis with that isolated from the index case and the mother. In both patients, the virus isolated from the index case was different from that isolated from the mother and fetus (cited by Griffiths[49]). Thus the congenital infection in these women would have occurred undetected if not for the totally unconnected episode of contact with CMV.

HERPES SIMPLEX VIRUS

Herpes simplex virus (HSV, *Herpesvirus hominis*) is subdivided into types 1 and 2, which have distinct but overlapping epidemiologic patterns. It shares with the other herpesviruses the characteristic of virus persistence. The primary infection is usually mucosal, but even though the clinical lesions heal, the virus persists in the sensory root ganglia, most frequently in the trigeminal (HSV-1) or the sacral (HSV-2) ganglia. The virus probably persists for life with periodic reactivation in the form of "cold sores" (usually at the mucocutaneous junctions of the face or genitalia). The frequency of reactivation declines with age. The virus is recovered readily from the lesions but may also be detected in throat or genital swabs from asymptomatic individuals, particularly those on immunosuppressive regimens.

HSV-1 is a common infection, and usually gives rise to lesions of the mouth, eyes, fingers (e.g., of the pulp space, a herpetic whitlow), and occasionally the CNS. HSV-2 typically causes genital and neonatal herpes infections. However, in recent years, 20% to 40% of genital herpes in some regions has been caused by HSV-1[67, 68] and about one fifth of neonatal herpes infections are due to HSV-1.[69, 70]

Herpes simplex infections can be primary or recrudescent, and the virologic and clinical course of the infection is affected by this. A primary infection is defined as the first infection with either HSV-1 or HSV-2, whether or not the episode is clinically overt. The first clinically or virologically apparent infection at a particular anatomic site in a person with serologic or historical evidence of previous HSV at a different site is termed an *initial* or a *first infection*. Recurrent infections occur at an anatomic site where there has been previous clinical or virologic evidence of HSV.[67] While most of these infections are due to recrudescence of latent virus (recrudescent infection), "reinfection" with exogenous virus has been documented.[71]

The definitive method of establishing that an infection is a true primary infection is by determining the serologic status to HSV-1 and -2 prior to or early in the acute stage of an infection. A past history of orolabial herpes does exclude a first-episode genital infection being a true primary infection, but the lack of such a history does not confirm it, since asymptomatic HSV infections occur frequently, particularly in childhood.

The incubation period of HSV ranges from 1 to 26 days (median 6–8 days). In primary infections, virus shedding may occur for many days before the onset, and persists for around 2 weeks (up to 1 month) after the onset of clinical illness. In recrudescent infections the duration of virus shedding and the duration and severity of clinical lesions

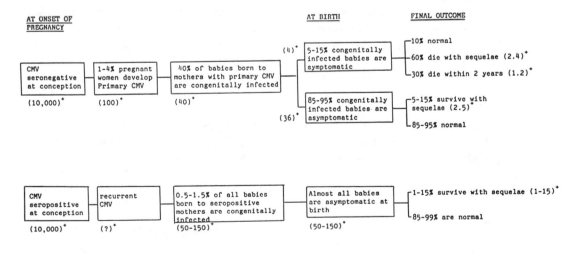

* If 10,000 pregnant women (seropositive and seronegative respectively) are followed up, the estimated number of babies affected is shown.

FIG 14–4.
Consequences of cytomegalovirus (CMV) infection during pregnancy.

are markedly reduced. The clinical features of herpes infections of different anatomic sites is reviewed elsewhere,[67, 72] but that of genital herpes in the woman will be briefly dealt with here.

Genital herpes may be asymptomatic, a fact that has been alluded to before. Symptomatic primary genital herpes is characterized by fever, headache, myalgias, and malaise. Local symptoms of pain, itching, or a "tingling" sensation are followed by the appearance of short-lived discrete vesicular lesions which rapidly ulcerate and become confluent. Regional lymph nodes are enlarged, and secondary infection with bacterial or fungal agents is common. The lesions are usually bilateral and affect the external genitalia, but involvement of the cervix and urethra (associated with urethral discharge and dysuria) is often found. Occasionally endometritis and salpingitis occur in nonpregnant women. Rectal or perianal lesions may be seen, usually with a history of rectal intercourse. Lesions can last from 6 to 30 days before healing occurs.[72]

Recurrences of genital herpes is common if the infecting virus is HSV-2 (with mean monthly recurrences of 0.33), but is tenfold less common in HSV-1 genital infections.[73] Recrudescent infections typically have little systemic manifestations, and the durations of the local lesions are short-lived (mean time to healing is 15 days).

Serologic studies indicate that as many as 20% of pregnant women have evidence of past HSV-2 infection, though only one fifth of the seropositives are aware that they have had genital herpes.[74] The prevalence of seropositivity is higher in blacks than in the white racial groups.

HSV-1 infection is relevant in pregnancy in that some genital and neonatal infections can be due to this virus (see above), and also because previous HSV-1 infection can influence the outcome of subsequent HSV-2 exposure. In the developed industrialized world, seroepidemiologic studies indicate that about 40% of young adults are infected with HSV-1, and the antibody prevalence increases by about 1.5% annually up to the age of 50 years.[75] Seroprevalence is lower in the upper socioeconomic groups, and overall seroprevalence has been falling over the last few decades with improvement in general living standards.[68] The prevalence of herpes simplex isolation from the oral cavity in healthy adult staff in a hospital at any given time is of the order of 2%, and approximately half of them have clinically overt nongenital herpetic disease in any given week.[76, 77]

Transmission of the virus (both HSV-1 and -2) occurs by infected body secretions coming into contact with mucosal surfaces. Under exceptional circumstances, the virus can enter directly via the skin, e.g., in sports with body contact, or via the needle puncture site on the scalp when fetal monitors are used during the pregnancy of a woman shedding HSV in her genital tract.

The titers of HSV from lesions is 100 to 1,000 times higher than that found in asymptomatic excretors of the virus. Thus the risk of transmission from asymptomatic infection is likely to be lower than that from clinically overt infections.[72]

Effect of Infection on the Pregnant Woman

In the vast majority of cases, the clinical course of overt infection is no different from that in nonpregnant women. The disease symptoms may, however, be less easily recognized in the midst of the other physiologic changes associated with pregnancy. There have, however, been rare instances of disseminated herpes infection in pregnancy, and if untreated, such disease is associated with both maternal and fetal mortality rates of 50%.[74]

The use of specific antivirals in the treatment of herpes infections in pregnancy is, however, affected by the fact that the antivirals available for use (acyclovir, vidarabine [both FDA category C], idoxuridine [topical use only in the United States] and foscarnet [investigational use only in the United States as of 1990]) are nucleoside analogues with potential adverse effects on the fetus. However, there have been no reports of teratogenic effects yet reported with acyclovir, and it should be used in any life-threatening HSV infection in a pregnant woman (e.g., HSV encephalitis or disseminated herpes). The use of antiviral chemotherapy in pregnancy is further discussed under Management of Varicella in Pregnancy.

Effects of Maternal Infection on the Fetus and Newborn

Genital herpes in late pregnancy can result in neonatally infected babies and premature birth, while infection in early pregnancy can result in an increased rate of abortion.[17, 69] There are occasional reports of congenital malformations associated with herpes simplex infection in utero but causality is as yet unproven.[17, 69]

Neonatal herpes simplex is a rare but potentially life-threatening infection. The incidence of neonatal HSV in the United States has been estimated to be 1 in 2,000 deliveries,[69] and the incidence appears to be increasing.[79, 80] This parallels the dramatic increase in genital herpes: estimates by the Centers for Disease Control of the number of clinical consultations for genital herpes indicate a ninefold increase, from 3.4 per 100,000 in 1966 to 29.2 per 100,000 in 1979.[81] While the increase in genital herpes is also seen in the United Kingdom, the problem of neonatal herpes appears to be rare in Britain. Of 6 million births in England and Wales between 1976 and 1985, only 18 neonatal deaths attributable to HSV and 111 laboratory isolations of the virus from neonates have been reported.[82] Whether this difference is a real one or a question of underrecognition or underreporting or both remains to be established.

It is accepted that symptomatic or asymptomatic herpes simplex in the mother around the time of partus can result in infection of a vaginally delivered baby. This occurs intrapartum, as the baby is bathed with the infected genital secretions of the mother. The virus enters the baby via the exposed mucosal surfaces, and also through the abraded skin. Babies born by vertex delivery not uncom-

monly have lesions on the scalp, while breech deliveries manifest lesions on the buttocks. Lesions can also occur at the site of scalp needles introduced for fetal monitoring during labor.[69]

Infection of the baby from primary maternal lesions appears to carry a worse prognosis than infection from recurrent or nonprimary initial infections. This may be because there is more virus in primary lesions, virus shedding is of longer duration, the cervix is more likely to be involved, and there is a lack of passively transferred maternal antibody to protect the fetus/neonate.

The question of perinatal infection due to intrauterine infection is more perplexing. It is undisputed that occasionally babies are born with evidence (clinical and laboratory) of HSV infection already present at the time of birth. The virus has been isolated from the placenta, though the possibility of contamination during vaginal delivery cannot be excluded. Though some of these intrauterine infections may be explained by ascending infection from the cervix following premature rupture of membranes, not all such case reports can be explained by this means.[69] At least 19 cases of neonatal herpes have occurred following cesarean delivery before rupture of membranes.[83] Thus infection does appear occasionally to take place in utero, even if the route is obscure.

Clinical evidence of neonatal herpes usually presents between the 5th and 17th day of life and though skin vesicles are characteristic of the disease, about 20 of infected neonates never have them.[69] About half the neonatal infections are generalized (hepatitis, pneumonitis, intravascular coagulopathy) with or without the involvement of the CNS, and these have a uniformly poor prognosis, less than 12% surviving without apparent sequelae. Of the localized neonatal herpes infections, those involving the eye, skin, or oral cavity leave over 60% of children surviving without sequelae, though localized infections involving the CNS have a poor prognosis. However, if untreated, 80% of children with localized disease will progress to disseminated disease, or CNS or eye involvement.[69]

The clinical presentation of neonatal infection is not dealt with in detail here; it is reviewed well by Nahmias and his colleagues.[69] The possibility of a herpes infection must be considered in any baby that "fails to thrive" during the first week, particularly if it is febrile. Specimens for virologic diagnosis must be taken, and prompt treatment with acyclovir begun where the diagnosis is likely. The mortality in disseminated disease is high (70%), even with early treatment.

Laboratory Diagnosis

Symptomatic Genital Infection in Pregnancy.—Vesicular fluid, scrapings of cells from the base of an active lesion, and a swab from the base of an ulcer broken off into virus transport medium and sent to the laboratory on wet ice, are the most productive specimens.

Vesicular fluid aspirated into a 1-mL syringe with a 26-gauge needle (it is not necessary for the amount of fluid within the syringe to be visible) should be sent to the laboratory with the needle recapped. Electron microscopy can demonstrate the presence of a herpesvirus within minutes. This technique is unable to distinguish readily between herpes simplex and varicella-zoster, but this may not be essential.

Scrapings from the base of the ulcers should be spread in a drop of saline over a well on a Teflon-coated slide and allowed to air-dry. This preparation is relatively stable and can be mailed to the laboratory, if need be, without loss of specimen quality. However, fixation of the air-dried slide in ice-cold acetone for 10 minutes is desirable prior to transport. It improves the stability of viral antigens during transit, and inactivates most pathogens. The preparation will be used for immunofluorescent diagnosis, and a positive result obtained within 1 to 2 hours.

A swab from the base of the ulcer, broken into transport medium and taken to the laboratory on ice, can be used for viral culture. Herpes simplex is a fast-growing virus, and usually a positive culture is apparent within

2 to 3 days. Using the shell vial assay, however, a reliable diagnosis can be established within 24 hours.[84] Cytologic techniques are reported to be useful, have a sensitivity of 60% to 75%, and can be done rapidly.[69]

Serologic diagnosis is of limited applicability except in cases of primary herpes infections. The antibody response is often poor, and many persons have preexisting antibody levels which may or may not change following recrudescent infection.

Asymptomatic Infection in Pregnancy.—Virus culture is the only reliable method of detecting asymptomatic virus shedding. High vaginal and/or cervical swabs taken carefully under direct vision should be sent in virus transport medium, on ice, to the laboratory. Immunofluorescence on direct specimens has not been adequately evaluated in asymptomatic herpes simplex infections. Cytologic investigations are useful, but the inclusion bodies can be detected for weeks after viral shedding has ceased,[79] and may not indicate active virus replication.

Neonatal Herpes Simplex.—The virus can be detected in vesicular lesions (if any) as described above. The virus may also be isolated from swabs from the conjunctiva, throat, skin, umbilicus, nasopharyngeal secretions, from the cerebrospinal fluid (CSF) (if CNS involvement has occurred), urine, and blood (in disseminated infections).

Management of Genital Herpes Infection in Pregnancy

The risk of congenital deformity in the baby following genital herpes in early pregnancy, though reported, is so rare that termination of pregnancy would not usually be considered. The clinical challenge posed by genital herpes in pregnancy is the assessment of the risk of transmission of the virus to the neonate, so that interventions to minimize this risk can be made.

The management of the pregnant woman with genital herpes simplex infection is con-

TABLE 14–6.
Management of Genital Herpes Infection in
Pregnancy

Clinical Category	Action Recommended
1. Clinically overt genital herpes at labor (primary or recurrent infection)	Cesarean delivery (prior to rupture of membranes if possible)
2. Clinically overt genital herpes earlier in pregnancy (primary or recurrent)	Confirm diagnosis virologically; do weekly cultures for herpes simplex virus (HSV) from 32nd wk of gestation to exclude continuing virus activity; if HSV isolated within 1 wk of labor, deliver by cesarean section; if negative, give a trial of vaginal delivery and consider cesarean if labor is prolonged
3. Past history of genital herpes but no clinical episode during present pregnancy	Examine genitalia and cervix at onset of labor for evidence of active herpetic lesions; if present, confirm diagnosis rapidly and virologically; if positive, deliver by cesarean section; if no evidence of overt lesions, allow vaginal delivery
4. No previous or present history of genital herpes	As above (3)

troversial. The majority (80%)—but not all—of neonatal herpes infections are acquired from the maternal genital tract at or around the time of delivery.[70] The presence of herpes simplex virus in the maternal genital tract (with or without symptoms) during a vaginal delivery predisposes to infection of the neonate. Cesarean delivery can reduce the risk of neonatal infection if undertaken before, or as soon as possible after (within 4 hours but even up to 24 hours), the rupture of membranes.[69] However, cesarean section carries a significant morbidity and mortality of its own to both mother and child, and in addition, it increases the cost of peripartum care.[85] Thus it is a question of balancing risks, but it is clear that cesarean section is not invariably the best decision.[82, 86]

Our suggestions for the management of genital herpes in pregnancy are summarized in Table 14–6, and are based on the following observations.

A baby born through a genital tract awash with herpes simplex virus is at risk of being infected (see Table 14–6, category 1). This risk is greater (50%) following primary maternal infection than following reactivation (less than 8%).[69, 87, 88] All women—symptomatic or asymptomatic—admitted for childbirth should be examined clinically for evidence of genital herpes lesions when they present at the labor room. If lesions are suspected, the diagnosis should be virologically confirmed (within a few hours; see above), and a cesarean delivery undertaken. In a rapidly progressing labor, the decision may have to be clinically based (but these may present less of a risk to the neonate). Recognition of genital herpes may pose problems in situations where the delivery is carried out outside hospitals, and by nonmedical staff.

If genital herpes has occurred earlier in the pregnancy (see Table 14–6, category 2), it is advisable to establish that viral shedding has ceased prior to partus. This is particularly so in primary herpetic infections where the duration of viral shedding is likely to be longer and asymptomatic recrudescence of the virus is more likely (this occurs in 33%).[89] Thus weekly virus cultures from the cervix and external genitalia from these patients are advisable from weeks 32 to 34 onward until delivery. If the woman is culture-negative in consecutive cultures leading up to childbirth, a vaginal delivery can be carried out.

While symptomatic genital herpes infection in the mother can be diagnosed by an alert clinician, asymptomatic virus shedding also poses a threat to the fetus and is more difficult to recognize. Prober and colleagues[88] (investigating a population with mixed socioeconomic background) found that 0.2% of asymptomatic women yielded positive HSV cultures from the external genitalia or cervix, or both, at the time of labor. In fact, the majority of neonatal herpes infections occur via asymptomatic infection of the mother.[70]

In response to this dilemma, some practitioners have recommended that women with a past history of recurrent genital herpes (see Table 14–6, category 3) be monitored by weekly viral cultures from week 32 of gestation onward, and cesarean delivery done if virus culture has been positive within a week of the woman going into labor.[69] If monitoring is to be carried out, it has to be done from the 32nd to 34th week or so, as premature labor is not uncommon in women with genital herpes in pregnancy. However, this recommendation cannot be substantiated on the available evidence.[82, 89] Yeager and Arvin[70] analyzed 31 consecutive cases of neonatal herpes infections and found that less than 10% of the mothers gave a typical history of previous recurrent genital herpes. Prober et al.[88] also found that limiting the screening to those with a previous history of recurrent genital herpes will result in more than 90% of babies exposed to the virus at birth being missed.

Virus shedding in recurrent infection is very transient.[90] Thus information on virus excretion a week prior to labor is *not* predictive of the situation at labor.[91] It is apparent from these studies that the only way in which the majority of babies exposed to asymptomatic HSV can be detected is by screening *all* women at the onset of labor. In order to influence the management of the pregnancy, the virologic culture results will have to be available within hours. There is at present no routinely available rapid (within a few hours) technique that is capable of detecting *asymptomatic* virus shedding. Therefore we do not believe that weekly viral cultures on women with a past history of genital herpes (except when this occurred during the present pregnancy) achieves anything, other than for medicolegal defense. It is more relevant to look for clinical evidence of active infection in *all* women, backed up by determined and rapid virologic diagnosis. At the present time, we have no means of detecting asymptomatic viral shedding in the intrapartum period, and until a rapid and inexpensive test for this purpose is developed, it is meaningless to pretend that we can.[82, 89]

A proportion of neonatal herpes infec-tions are acquired postnatally. Yeager and Arvin[70] reported that 10% of the neonates with herpes simplex infections were thought to have been infected from maternal orolabial herpes, and an equal proportion acquired their infections post partum, from sources other than the mother. Therefore mothers who have primary nongenital herpes simplex during the first month after partus need to be educated about the possibility of transmission of the infection to the baby. The lesions should be covered as far as possible, and there may be a place for using antivirals on the mother, to reduce the duration of virus shedding. The baby should be monitored carefully with rapid diagnosis and treatment employed at the first sign of infection. Finally, it is advisable that babies born to mothers with active herpes simplex infection be nursed in rooms separate from other patients, in order to reduce the risk of nosocomial infection.

VARICELLA-ZOSTER VIRUS

Varicella-zoster virus (VZV) is the etiological agent of chickenpox (varicella). Being a herpesvirus, it remains latent in the dorsal root ganglia after primary infection, and may be reactivated many years later as shingles (herpes zoster). This is caused by the virus traveling down the relevant sensory nerve to produce skin lesions with a characteristic dermatomal distribution.

In temperate countries, chickenpox—together with the other exanthems—is primarily a disease of childhood. Given that over 90% of women of childbearing age in the temperate zones are immune to VZV,[92] chickenpox in pregnancy is rare. A minimum frequency for the incidence of chickenpox in pregnancy was estimated to be 5 per 10,000 pregnancies.[4]

This may not be true everywhere in the world. In parts of Asia, varicella is predominantly a disease of young adults,[92] and the potential for varicella complicating pregnancy is correspondingly higher.

It is one of the more communicable infective diseases, though less so than measles. Attack rates in susceptible persons following household exposure to chickenpox is around 80%. However, the attack rate is lower (35%–65%) following community exposure, unlike measles, which is almost equally infectious in either setting. Transmission of the virus is imperfectly understood as yet, respiratory droplet spread from the oropharynx and direct contact with vesicular fluid (a rich source of infectious virus) being the most likely routes of spread. Patients are infectious during the prodromal illness 2 to 3 days before the rash appears, and communicability lasts up to 5 days after the onset of the rash.

Herpes zoster is usually an illness of older people or the immunocompromised, and is exceedingly uncommon in pregnancy.

Effect of Varicella Infection on the Pregnant Woman

The incubation period averages approximately 13 to 17 days, with a range of 10 to 20 days. Subclinical infection, particularly in adults, is uncommon and varicella in adults is generally more severe than it is in children. A review of the available reports of gestational varicella by Young and Gershon[93] suggested that it is more severe in pregnancy with a 29% (22/77) incidence of varicella pneumonia, and a 13% mortality. Paryani and Arvin[94] reported that 4 of 43 (9%) women with varicella in pregnancy developed varicella pneumonia, one with a fatal outcome. As there is a bias toward reporting the more severe cases, the validity of the contention that VZV is a more lethal illness in pregnancy (as compared with nonpregnant adults) remains unproven (see also Chap. 6, p. 216).

While herpes zoster is more frequent and more severe in immunosuppressed patients (e.g., leukemics under treatment or those who have had a recent organ transplant), there is no evidence that its course is any different in pregnant women as compared with nonpregnant healthy women of comparable age.

Effects of Maternal Infection on the Fetus and Newborn

Varicella in pregnancy can precipitate premature delivery.[94] It may also result in congenital or perinatal infection of the baby, the latter being the more frequent clinical problem.

The Fetal Varicella Syndrome.—In an 8-year follow-up study of 190,000 pregnancies, Siegal[95] found that babies born to mothers who had varicella in pregnancy had no higher incidence of congenital defects (3%) than children born to uninfected mothers. Similar results have been obtained in other studies. However, a characteristic constellation of congenital anomalies—the fetal varicella syndrome—becomes apparent when individual case reports of babies exposed to maternal varicella are reviewed.[93, 96] Limb deformities (hypoplasia, talipes, rudimentary digits), severe skin contractures localized to a dermatomal distribution, mental retardation, bulbar palsy, and ocular defects (optic atrophy, nystagmus, chorioretinitis, cataracts, microphthalmia, Horner's syndrome) have been reported, mostly following infections in the first 20 weeks of pregnancy. Less than half the babies born with the fetal varicella syndrome survive to their second birthday.

Congenital infection with VZV can occur, with the baby born apparently healthy. In such cases, the only indication of intrauterine infection may be an immune response to the virus or the occurrence of herpes zoster (without prior chickenpox) within the first year of life.[94]

Varicella-zoster virus induces chromosomal aberrations in cells in tissue culture. Long-term surveillance of children born to 270 women with chickenpox during pregnancy showed that two children subsequently died of leukemia.[97] The authors concluded that, statistically, this was more than would be expected, and postulate that varicella in pregnancy predisposed to malignancy in later life, a contention that requires confirmation.

Perinatal Varicella.—The more common clinical problem is that posed by perinatal chickenpox infection. This could be due to postnatal exposure or a result of transplacentally transmitted virus. Since the incubation period of postnatally acquired chickenpox ranges from 10 to 20 days, a baby developing a varicelliform rash within the first 10 days of life has probably been infected in utero. The incubation period of varicella acquired in utero is, however, shorter than that for postnatally acquired infection, the usual period being between 9 and 15 days, though it may occasionally range from 1 to 16 days.[93, 98]

Table 14–7 shows the consequences of maternal disease occurring around the time of partus.[99] Maternal infection occurring 5 days or more ante partum results in neonatal infection in one third of neonates, but even when infection occurs the prognosis is uniformly good. On the other hand, maternal varicella occurring less than 4 days ante partum or 2 days post partum results in perinatal varicella in 16% of the babies; 31% of these (i.e., 5% of all babies exposed to varicella in the mother during this period) die. This has been thought to be due to the lack of maternally derived passive immunity in the baby, probably because there is not enough time for an immune response to be mounted.[100] When maternal varicella occurred 7 days or more ante partum, all the neonates were born with passive antibody; if maternal infection occurred within 2 days of birth, none of the infants were antibody-positive.[98] In the intervening period (i.e., 3–7 days ante partum), the proportion of neonates without passive antibody ranged from 46% to 64%. Miller and colleagues[98] suggest therefore that the

"risk" period for neonates developing severe disease should include babies born to mothers with varicella during the week prior to partus.

Since the timing of maternal varicella is related to the timing of lesions appearing in the neonate, neonatal varicella in which the lesions appear within 4 days of birth carries a good prognosis, while if the lesions appear 5 to 10 days after birth, the disease will be fatal in 20% of the babies.

Illness occurring more than 10 days after birth is likely to have been acquired postnatally, and carries a good prognosis.[93, 99]

Laboratory Diagnosis

A rapid (2–4 hours) and accurate virologic diagnosis can be made by examining a scraping obtained from the base of a vesicle ulcer by fluorescent antibody staining using an appropriately specific antiserum.[9, 13] Electron microscopy of vesicular fluid will document the presence of a herpesvirus within minutes, but cannot differentiate VZV from HSV. VZV can be isolated from vesicular fluid or from swabs of the base of vesicle ulcers. Conventional culture can take weeks to give a positive result, but the use of the shell vial assay allows more rapid diagnosis (2–4 days).

Serologic evidence for recent VZV (both varicella and shingles) infection can be obtained by the demonstration of rising antibody titers, usually by the complement fixation (CF) test. CF antibodies are usually short-lived, and may be undetectable within a year of infection. It is therefore not a sensitive or reliable indicator of immunity to chickenpox through past infection, for which purpose im-

TABLE 14–7.
Consequences of Varicella Infection in Late Pregnancy*

Onset of Rash in Mother	% (No.) of Babies With Perinatal Varicella†	% (No.) Mortality in Cases With Perinatal Varicella†
4 days ante partum to 2 days post partum	16%(4/24)	31%(4/13)
≥5 days ante partum	32%(7/22)	0%(0/23)

*Based on data from Meyers.[99]
†Number of babies affected/number of babies studied.

munoassays or fluorescent antibody to membrane antigen (FAMA) tests are used.

Virologic diagnosis of VZV in a congenitally deformed infant is more difficult. Virus cannot usually be isolated from the baby at birth, as the infection may have occurred in early pregnancy many months previously. Serologic demonstration of (1) IgM in the cord blood or neonatal blood, (2) significantly higher titers of antibody in the baby as compared to the mother (excludes mere passive transfer of immunity), and (3) documenting that antibody levels in the baby do not fall in the subsequent months are diagnostic of congenital infection. However, serologic confirmation of congenital infection is not invariable.[94]

Management of Varicella in Pregnancy

Whether varicella is more severe in the pregnant woman than in nonpregnant adults is controversial (discussed above). There is no doubt, however, that it is a more serious illness in adults (pregnant or otherwise) than it is in children, varicella pneumonia being the major complication. There is good reason, therefore, to be more aggressive in the use of preventive or therapeutic interventions.

It is advisable to offer varicella-zoster immune globulin (VZIG) to a pregnant woman in close (e.g., within the family) contact with a patient with varicella, provided she has no previous history of chickenpox. As VZIG is a scarce resource, it is best if serologic evidence of susceptibility can be obtained (see above). It is most likely to be of benefit when administered as soon as possible, but may still be effective for up to 96 hours after exposure. The dose recommended is 125 units/10 kg body weight given intramuscularly.[101] VZIG may only modify the severity of the illness, and not prevent it completely. There is no guarantee, therefore, that fetal infection will be prevented (see below).[101]

Varicella pneumonia, or particularly severe episodes of adult varicella, should be treated with acyclovir (10 mg/kg every 8 hours) (see also Chap. 6, p. 216). The theoret-ical risk (yet unproven) of damage to the fetus has to be balanced against the risks to the mother. No teratogenic effects of acyclovir have yet been documented.[102] Though there is as yet insufficient evidence to recommend the routine use of acyclovir for minor herpes virus infections in pregnancy, its use may well be justified in situations such as varicella in pregnancy where the alternative can be much worse. In severe cases of varicella pneumonia, assisted ventilation may be required. It has been reported that regular or recent smokers are more likely to have pulmonary complications following varicella in adulthood.[103] If this finding is confirmed, this would be a subpopulation that can be identified for early antiviral therapy.

The management of fetal or neonatal problems arising from varicella during pregnancy are summarized in Table 14–8. It is based upon the following:

1. Though varicella in early stages of gestation does carry some risk of a congenitally deformed baby, this risk appears to be exceedingly small. Following first-trimester exposure, the risk of congenital deformity has been estimated to be 5%,[94] and even lower than this following exposure later in pregnancy. Thus varicella is not by itself a strong reason to recommend termination.

2. Babies born to mothers developing varicella 5 days or more before delivery are not in need of VZIG or prophylactic acyclovir. Since some of these children may develop mild varicella infection and become infectious, they should be kept away from other babies (and susceptible staff, if known), and discharged from hospital as soon as possible. Treatment of the baby with acyclovir may be considered if the illness is unusually severe.

3. Maternal varicella in late gestation is a threat to the newborn if it occurs less than 5 days before or 2 days after partus. Passive immunization of the baby by intramuscular VZIG is indicated. However, protection is by no means assured, and even repeated doses have failed to prevent neonatal varicella in the baby.[98] Miller and her colleagues[98] sug-

TABLE 14–8.
Management of Varicella Zoster Infections in Pregnancy: A Summary

	Risk	Action
1. Varicella or zoster in early pregnancy	Minimal risk to fetus	Discuss with parents-to-be; no indication for recommending termination
2. Maternal Varicella 5–20 days antepartum	Risk of neonatal varicella but prognosis good; baby potentially infectious even if no lesions present at birth	a. No VZIG for baby indicated b. ACV if neonatal illness severe c. Baby and mother nursed in "isolation"† and discharged from hospital as soon as possible
3. Maternal Varicella <5(7)* days before partus *or* <2 days after partus	Risk of neonatal varicella; 5% risk of fatality in baby; baby potentially infectious (see above)	a. Administer VZIG to neonate at birth b. Watch for neonatal varicella and treat with ACV c. ? Prophylactic ACV for neonate ? ACV for mother d. Nurse mother and baby in "isolation"†
4. Mother exposed to VZV 6–20 days antepartum; no past history of VZV; no clinical CP yet	Mother may develop varicella and give rise to neonatal varicella (item 3 above); mother and baby may be infectious	a. If mother seronegative, give VZIG to mother b. Nurse mother and baby in "isolation"†
5. Maternal zoster in late pregnancy	Minimal risk to fetus or newborn; potentially infectious to others	a. Confirm virological diagnosis b. Nurse mother and baby in "isolation"† c. No VZIG required for neonate d. No need to isolate baby from mother
6. Neonate exposed to postnatal varicella (nonmaternal)	Severe disease uncommon; however, advisable to use VZIG to prevent neonatal infection if mother is seronegative	a. If mother seronegative, give VZIG to neonate

*Recent data suggest that infection occurring up to 7 days before delivery can have serious consequences for the baby.
†"Isolation" nursing: Separate cubicles; handwashing; limit visitors and nursing staff to those with immunity to VZV, wherever possible. When lesions appear, the mother or baby is infective until no new lesions have appeared for 72 hours; all lesions are crusting; usually 5 days after onset of rash. In baby or mother exposed to VZV, the period of infectivity should cover known incubation period, i.e., 20 days from exposure.

gest that VZIG does little to prevent infection or illness, but that it may reduce the severity of neonatal disease. They found no difference (in preventing neonatal infection or illness) between dosages ranging from 100 to 250 mg of VZIG. There were no fatalities in 91 VZIG-treated seronegative neonates that were infected by their mothers during the 2-week period centered on delivery. However, since a controlled trial to study the efficacy of VZIG in this context is now unethical, evidence for the efficacy of VZIG prophylaxis in this study must rest on historical controls.

The early use of acyclovir therapeutically, at a dosage of 5 to 10 mg/kg every 8 hours intravenously, has been recommended.[94, 104] However, antiviral treatment begun after the onset of neonatal varicella is not always lifesaving. Intravenous acyclovir prophylaxis in conjunction with VZIG has been used in these "high-risk" patients though the numbers are too small to evaluate the results.[105] Acyclovir treatment of the mother before delivery (in addition to the treatment of the neonate as described above), with the aim of reducing maternal viremia and the risk of transmission to the fetus, is theoretically valid. Acyclovir administered to the mother does cross the placenta, and therapeutically active levels are found in the fetus.[106] In the absence of conclusive data at present, there is no widely agreed strategy for therapeutic management of this situation. (The above recommendation on the use of VZIG in pregnancy is that of the American Immunization Practices Advisory Committee,[101] but the recent study by Miller and her colleagues[98] suggests that maternal varicella in the 7 days up to delivery should be regarded as having a high risk of leading to severe neonatal illness. They recommend therefore that VZIG prophylaxis be extended to neonates born to mothers developing varicella up to 7 days prior to delivery.)

4. Passive immunization can be considered for a pregnant woman exposed to VZV infection (see above) provided she is seronegative to VZV. The record of VZIG in protecting susceptible contacts completely is not impressive, but it may moderate the infection and may confer some benefit on the baby, though there is no evidence to substantiate this. Administration of VZIG to the mother *does not* remove the necessity of giving VZIG to the newborn if it is born less than 5 days prior to, or within 2 days after, the onset of maternal varicella.

It is important to watch for the signs of varicella in both the mother and the baby, even if VZIG has been given, so that appropriate measures for early treatment and prevention of nosocomial spread are taken. If maternal chickenpox develops just before or up to 5 days after delivery, separating the mother from the baby until she is no longer infectious may be considered. There is no evidence that the virus is transmitted via breast milk and the risks of serious consequence have to be balanced against the interruption of normal bond formation. The mother will be infectious for 5 days after the skin lesions appear.

Pregnancy Complicated by Herpes Zoster

Pregnancy complicated by shingles is a rare occurrence and only a handful of cases have been reported to date.[17, 94, 107] Though case reports of congenital abnormalities following maternal zoster exist, their significance in relation to patient management is yet unclear.

Zoster in late pregnancy does not pose perinatal problems for the newborn.[98] The baby is protected by maternal antibody, and there is no need for the use of VZIG (Table 14–8). It is important, however, that the diagnosis be confirmed virologically, particularly in patients with zosteriform rashes in the lumbosacral area. Herpes simplex can present with a similar clinical picture, and this has quite different implications for patient management.

EPSTEIN-BARR VIRUS

Epstein-Barr virus (EBV) is a ubiquitous human herpesvirus commonly infecting children, usually with little or no clinical illness (e.g., mild pharyngitis). Infection in adolescence or adulthood typically results in infectious mononucleosis (the glandular fever syndrome). After primary infection the virus remains latent in the B lymphocytes of the host and can undergo reactivation. The clinical effects of reactivation are unremarkable (except in the immunocompromised) but could (in theory) give rise to infection of the fetus, as happens with CMV. The relevance of EBV infection to obstetrics depends, as it does with other herpes viruses, on (1) the proportion of women of childbearing age that are seronegative, (2) the frequency of EBV primary infections and reactivations in pregnancy, and (3) the frequency with which such infections in the mother cause infection and damage in the fetus.

The percentage of seronegative pregnant women in developed countries is very low (1%–4%), the proportion being greater in the higher socioeconomic groups than in the lower.[108, 109, 110] Prospective studies of EBV infections in pregnancy carried out on a total of over 12,000 pregnant women from the United States, Canada, and France have documented only three seroconversions.[108, 109, 110, 111] None of the infants born to these women had conclusive virologic evidence of intrauterine EBV infection (specific IgM or spontaneously transforming lymphocytes in the cord blood), though one of them had congenital heart disease. In developing countries, infection occurs even earlier in life, with over 90% being seropositive by the age of 2 years. Thus primary infection (and infectious mononucleosis) in women of childbearing age is even a rarer event in these countries.

Antibodies to the early antigen of EBV (indicative of recent infection or reactivation) were found more frequently (55%) in pregnant women as compared with nonpregnant controls matched for age and socioeconomic status (22%–32%).[110] These results were interpreted to indicate that reactivation of EBV was more frequent in pregnancy than in healthy nonpregnant women. However, there

was no evidence of an increase in small-for-dates babies, congenital abnormalities, or neonatal hepatitis in those with evidence of EBV early antibodies in their blood. There is one report, however, that documents a significantly higher (10% vs. 1%) incidence of congenital malformations (including low birth weight) in children born to mothers whose sera were positive for antibodies to EBV "early" antigens, both early and late in pregnancy.[108] This question requires further clarification.

Over 2,800 neonates have been studied for evidence of congenital infection by looking for spontaneous transformation of cord blood leukocytes and attempting virus isolation from nasopharyngeal secretions. Two neonates infected with the virus were documented, but neither had congenital defects (reviewed by Stagno and Whitley[112]).

The evidence implicating EBV in congenital damage (congenital heart disease, cataracts, multiple fetal malformations) is derived from case reports, and in the early ones the diagnosis of maternal infectious mononucleosis was based on clinical criteria, without virologic confirmation of an EBV infection.[113] Such data, of course, are inconclusive as an infectious mononucleosis–like illness can be caused by other etiologic agents, including CMV. However, there is at least one report[114] of an infant born with multiple congenital defects, with convincing virologic evidence for in utero EBV infection.

Laboratory Diagnosis

The virologic diagnosis of EBV infection can be established by detection of an IgM and IgG antibody response to different antigens of the virus. The most useful of these are the IgM and IgG antibodies to the virus capsid antigen (VCA). Recent infection is indicated by an IgM response or a rising IgG antibody titer. Static IgG titers are indicative of past infections. In addition to these two markers, antibodies to the early (EA) and nuclear (EBNA) antigens of the virus can be detected and help in the interpretation of the serology.[115]

The Paul-Bunnell-Davidsohn test is mainly of use as a screening test for a typical infectious mononucleosis illness.

Management and Counseling of Women With EBV Infection in Pregnancy

In summary, there are isolated case reports of EBV infections in pregnancy giving rise to intrauterine infections and congenital defects in the baby. However, the frequency of adverse consequences following maternal EBV infection cannot be assessed at this stage, because the latter is such a rare event. The patient would need to be counseled on the present state of ignorance on this question, and if she decides to go ahead with the pregnancy, the pregnancy and the baby should be carefully monitored for adverse effects. The etiology of the maternal infection and infection in utero in the neonate (cord blood) must be confirmed by EBV serologic markers. In this situation, EBV-specific serology is essential. Other tests (monospot or Paul-Bunnell-Davidsohn) are not reliable enough since they measure only heterophile antibodies and not specific ones to EBV.

HUMAN IMMUNODEFICIENCY VIRUS

Ten years ago infections with this virus were unrecognized. Since that time the rate of progress in understanding its effects on those it infects has been dramatic. It means also that any review may be outdated by rapidly emerging data before it is published. The full-blown disease is likely to be fatal and at present there is neither treatment nor prophylaxis to completely prevent its ravages.

Infection With HIV

There are three main routes of transmission of human immunodeficiency virus (HIV): (1) intimate physical (mainly sexual) contact, (2) "vertical" (perinatal) transmission, or (3) exposure to infected blood.

The chances of contracting the virus through sexual contact rises with the extent of contact—quantity, quality, and duration—and this probably accounts for the different patterns of infection in different parts of the world. Although the majority of infections still occur in homosexual or bisexual men, there has been an increase in female cases, particularly in Central Africa where up to 10% of pregnant women are infected. More recently, cases in women have been reported in the United States.[116] The majority of those infected are, at present, prostitutes or intravenous drug abusers, and it is still unclear how widely infection will spread outside these groups and into the general heterosexual population.

The virus may be transmitted by infected blood products. Intravenous drug abuse is the most obvious example, but transmission can arise wherever syringes and needles are reused. Batches of infected factor VIII or IX from paid donors transmitted the virus to a considerable number of hemophiliacs, although heat treatment has now reduced the chances of such transmission to negligible levels in most parts of the world.[117]

Estimates of transmissibility between sexual partners vary. Between 10% and 45% have seroconverted but only over several years.[118] Sensible, informed use of condoms ("safe" or, at least, saf*er* sex) will reduce the risk; however, abstention ("a foot of fresh air") is the only guarantee of safety. Frequent changes in sexual partners appears to increase the risks substantially, although whether for the obvious reason of sheer frequency or from the action of other factor(s) is not known.

Infection is followed 6 to 8 weeks later by a "flu-like" illness which is associated with the appearance of viral antigen in the blood. There is now some evidence[119] that the duration of this initial illness is related to the chances of developing more substantial disease later. In most cases, this is followed by a quiescent period which may last several years, during which only the presence of antibodies to the virus indicates that infection has taken place.

Progression to a state of generalized lymphadenopathy, which may be accompanied by personality changes, is often followed by a more general deterioration. Increasingly frequent opportunistic infections follow the decline in immunocompetence associated with loss of T4 (CD4-bearing) helper lymphocytes. This progression is often (but not invariably) heralded by the appearance of viral antigen in the blood. The patient's condition then gradually declines into fully developed acquired immunodeficiency syndrome (AIDS), and in about 70% of cases this has continued progressively until death. Whether the other 30% will survive is unclear at present but there are few grounds for optimism. Though antibodies are formed against a variety of antigens including the envelope glycoproteins (gp120 and gp41) and the stable core protein (p24), none appear to be protective.[117]

HIV-2

Although a considerable number of antigenic variants of HIV exist, there is now clearly a second and antigenically distinct virus: HIV-2. Originally described in West Africa, it is now being found, at lower frequency, in other parts of the world, including the United States, although most are imported cases. To date its epidemiology is uncertain, although there is no reason to suppose it behaves differently from HIV-1 in any respect. Tests for HIV-2 are much less widely available and, consequently, the data are scanty.[117] There is some cross-reactivity between HIV-1 and HIV-2. In serosurveys, some low-level positives are probably due to HIV-2 infection, and this virus may be more widespread than was first thought. The situation will become clearer in the next few years.

Laboratory Diagnosis

Diagnosis of HIV infection may be made by detecting circulating viral antigen, or antibodies to the envelope or core proteins. Tests for viral antigen are probably of limited value as the antigen is present in the blood only transiently during the initial flu-like illness and later during the course of the disease, when deterioration into AIDS and toward death has begun. Demonstration of antibodies to HIV (which appear within 2–4 weeks of infection) is therefore the common diagnostic test used.

Enzyme-linked immunosorbent assays (ELISA tests) are most often used as the screening test for detecting antibodies to HIV. Though earlier ELISA tests used HIV-infected cell extracts as the "target" for antibody detection, "new-generation" tests use recombinant DNA-derived (or synthetic peptide-based) antigens. The p24 core protein, the p31 polymerase protein, and the gp41 envelope protein are the antigens most often used, though the p24 core protein, being much less variable, is a particularly suitable candidate. Even the best screening tests give occasional false-positive results and therefore a positive ELISA test must be confirmed by a second test system, the possibilities being a Western blot or a different ELISA test.[15] Antibody positivity is not a reliable guide to prognosis or the state to which the infection has progressed. None of the above tests measure infectivity directly, although the presence of any markers (antigen or antibody) is taken as indicating infectiousness. This may be an overstatement, but it is the most practical interpretation at present.

HIV Infection During Pregnancy

In the earlier literature there was some evidence that pregnancy itself may hasten the development of AIDS in those infected with the virus, but this remains unclear.[120, 121, 121a] Nonetheless, pregnancy in a seropositive woman has consequences for both mother and child. If she is already aware of being positive, the mother-to-be will feel isolated because the infection will often be kept secret and she will often lack the support of others in a similar predicament. If she feels well she may be unwilling to accept the serologic findings and this may be followed by further pregnancies, despite an awareness of the possible consequences to the fetus.[122] Others may accept the situation and decide to terminate the pregnancy. Less than half will probably choose to abort,[123, 124] and some will become pregnant again. The role of the physician will be to help the woman face what will be a devastating situation, particularly if unexpected. It will affect her relation with her sexual partner, and have important implications for her future at a time when she is emotionally vulnerable. Handling this situation will require tact and sensitivity as well as an understanding of the infection. The present uncertainties concerning prognosis do not make this task easy.

At present no country has introduced routine testing of all pregnant women for evidence of infection, although this may yet be necessary and may solve some otherwise intractable problems of confidentiality. In its absence, deciding to test an individual is not easy. Because of the considerable current implications of finding an individual to be HIV-positive (in terms of future health, employability, eligibility for life insurance, and possibly even creditworthiness), testing at present is not justified without the patient's informed consent and is used mainly to diagnose manifestations of the disease. These include fever, poor weight gain (or even loss), cough, and diarrhea. These symptoms are nonspecific and not by themselves diagnostic. More severe opportunistic infections are later manifestations. Striking a balance between testing at every minor sign or symptom that might be due to HIV and missing florid AIDS requires judgment, and there are no simple tests (other than those for HIV) to help. For the time being, routine testing is likely to be confined to those who are found to be at high risk of having been exposed to the virus. Clues on drug abuse and prostitution can usually be obtained by careful questioning, and consent for testing obtained. If the results of tests are negative, repeat testing during pregnancy will be necessary for the sake of the baby at least. This will be difficult to do while maintaining confidentiality, and is but one example where care for the patient may conflict with confidentiality.

The possibility that someone may be infected is of enormous interest to everyone else and dealing with this requires clear thinking with regard to whose interests are being served. Testing should not be undertaken lightly and adequate counseling offered immediately in the event of a positive test.

Present information suggests that approximately one third of babies born to antibody-positive mothers will develop a detectable HIV infection,[124] but data are still being collected. In their recent study in France, Blanche and her colleagues[125] monitored 308 infants born to seropositive women, 62% of whom were intravenous drug abusers. Persistence of maternal antibody made early interpretation difficult, but of 117 babies evaluated at the age of 18 months, 26 were alive and seropositive and 6 had died of AIDS. While 76 were seronegative and normal, 9 were seronegative but had symptoms suggestive of HIV infection. The long-term outlook for these babies is unclear, but the evidence does offer some hope. Not all babies are necessarily infected and the majority, though initially seropositive, will become negative as they lose maternal antibody.[126] Whether prognostic markers, too, will emerge remains to be seen, but in the study done by Blanche and her co-workers,[125] the babies who became seropositive were no different from the others in birth weight, height, head circumference, or rate of malformations.

In the United Kingdom, the serious consequences of maternal-child transmission mean that seropositivity is an adequate justification for termination under the 1967 Abortion Act. Hence it is considered appropriate to inform a pregnant woman that she *may* be positive before complete confirmation is available. Since this may take a week or two and the risks of termination increase with time, the Royal College of Obstetricians and Gynaecologists in the United Kingdom consider that termination may be offered before final confirmation is available, but following full appropriate counseling.[127]

Management of labor in HIV-positive women is outside the scope of this book. It is not yet clear what proportion of babies will become infected from their mothers nor the exact mechanism by which transmission occurs. Even if it were much less than the current estimate of about one third, the possibility must be taken seriously. It is clear that prostitution and drug abuse are predisposing factors.[123]

The Use of Antiviral Chemotherapy

There is good evidence that drugs such as azidothymidine (zidovudine, formerly AZT), dideoxycytidine (DDC), and acyclovir (ACV) can interfere with the replication of HIV.[128] They are now being used, or considered for use, in treating asymptomatic patients infected with HIV as well as those with AIDS.[128a]

Their use in pregnant women is not, at present, recommended, due to the potential danger of damage to the fetus, although studies in pregnant rats have not shown any teratogenicity. They act by becoming incorporated into viral DNA and causing either termination of new DNA or nonsense coding. There is a real possibility of their being similarly incorporated into fetal DNA with resultant damage. Even ACV, which is generally very safe, would be used only in life-threatening herpes simplex or varicella-zoster infections in pregnancy, viruses against which its efficacy is well proven. Its value alone, or in combination with zidovudine, in AIDS or HIV infection is less clear-cut, with a correspondingly reduced indication for use.

Whether to take a woman already on zidovudine for HIV infection off the drug should she become pregnant is not likely to be an easy decision. There is not yet enough experience with its use for the answer to be clear and each case will have to be assessed individually. It is in areas such as these that new information will appear most frequently, and the reader is advised to monitor recent literature.

Opportunistic Infections

As of 1990 there have been few reports of opportunistic infectious complications of HIV infection in pregnant women[129] and recent evidence suggests that such problems are unusual in women without advanced HIV-related disease at the time of conception.[121]

Pneumocystis carinii pneumonia (PCP) is the most frequent life-threatening opportunistic infection in patients with HIV, and several fatal cases have been reported in pregnant women.[130] The few cases are insufficient to determine whether morbidity and mortality from PCP is altered during gestation and we are unaware of any data to suggest that early delivery will improve the prognosis. Nonetheless, the life-threatening nature of this infection makes early diagnosis essential, followed by treatment similar to that used in nonpregnant populations. Therefore, the treatment of choice for the pregnant patient with PCP is 3 weeks of trimethoprim-sulfamethoxazole (FDA category C; D if used near term) (trimethoprim: 15–20 mg/kg/day orally; sulfamethoxazole: 75–100 mg/kg/day orally or intravenously) despite the theoretical risk of administering a folate antagonist and a sulfa drug during gestation. If this is unsuccessful or cannot be tolerated, pentamidine (FDA category C) (4 mg/kg/day intravenously for 3 weeks) should not be withheld despite the lack of experience with this drug in pregnancy.

The United States Public Health Service has recently recommended prophylaxis with aerosolized pentamidine or oral trimethoprim-sulfamethoxazole for pneumocystis pneumonia in HIV-infected nonpregnant patients with a prior episode of PCP and in those with a CD4$^+$ lymphocyte count of less than 200/mm^3 or if such cells constitute less than 20% of total lymphocytes.[131] Prophylaxis was deemed "inadvisable" for pregnant women because of the lack of data concerning safety of these drugs during pregnancy. Nonetheless, the cumulative incidence of PCP over a 9-month period in HIV-infected nonpregnant populations with CD4$^+$ cell counts of less than 200/mm^3 is 10% to 15%[131] and therefore the physician should be vigilant for this life-threatening pulmonary complication in gravid patients with depressed T helper lymphocyte counts.

Nosocomial Risk

Those infected with HIV are not highly infectious. Where attendants, medical or nursing, have acquired the disease it is often because other known risk factors were involved.[132] In the absence of such factors, there seems very little risk from social contact or routine nursing care. Recent data suggest that the amount of infectious virus in the blood of HIV-infected patients is small and only about 0.5% of nearly 1,000 needle stick or lacerating injuries involving antibody-positive blood have been followed by seroconversion.[133] How many of those who seroconverted will later develop AIDS remains to be seen; however, there is no reason to believe the infection will behave differently from that acquired by other routes where the vast majority ultimately do progress to AIDS.

The virus is an enveloped one which survives poorly outside the body. It may survive better in dried body fluids but this can be prevented by early adequate swabbing down with household bleach while any spillage is still wet. Transmission through cutlery, crockery, and fomites has not been described, and no environmental transmission has been documented. Even kissing appears to be a low-risk activity.[134] For any procedures involving the patient's blood or body fluids, any open cuts or other lesions should be covered with a waterproof dressing and a pair of good quality, well-fitting surgical latex gloves should be worn.

Breast-Feeding and HIV

The route of perinatal transmission from mother to infant is not known and evidence for both prenatal[135] and postnatal[136, 137] transmission has been obtained. Since prenatal transmission can only be prevented with certainty by termination, we are concerned here only with postnatal transmission. HIV has been isolated from breast milk[138] and this opportunity to infect has led the government in the United Kingdom to advise HIV-positive mothers *not* to breast-feed. As Bradbeer[139] has pointed out, this may be too late to prevent infection in an infant already infected prior to delivery. However, evidence from Zambia shows that the babies of some mothers that were seronegative at delivery and who converted later became infected, presumably via breast-feeding. It is not clear whether the advice not to breast-feed will prevent transmission.

Hence the risk of transmission by breast-feeding (as the sole route) may be greatest in mothers who seroconvert postnatally. The additional risk of breast-feeding to the infant born to a previously seropositive mother has to be weighed against the benefits (transfer of immunity to other organisms, bonding, and, in some parts of the world, no realistic alternative). As stated by Bradbeer,[139] whether to breast-feed is the mother's decision. The physician's role is to advise on the basis of available evidence.

PARVOVIRUSES

Parvoviruses are DNA viruses that replicate in rapidly proliferating cells. A number of animal parvoviruses are known to cause intrauterine death and congenital disease. Of the parvoviruses that infect man (parvovirus B19, the "enteric" parvoviruses, and RA1), parvovirus B19 is relevant to pregnancy. It is the etiological agent of erythema infectiosum (fifth disease, slapped cheek disease),[140] and also causes aplastic crises and neutropenic episodes in patients with hemolytic anemias[141] and in the immunosuppressed.[142] The clinical features of B19 infections include a bright red macular rash, primarily affecting the face ("slapped cheek") but which may appear as a lacy reticular rash in other parts of the body. Children with the disease usually feel well, though a prodrome of low-grade fever, coryza, or gastrointestinal symptoms may be present. In adults, particularly women, a peripheral and symmetric polyarthralgia may be the dominant manifestation and may easily be confused clinically with rubella.[19] Asymptomatic infection also occurs. Serologic studies indicated that 28% to 46% of women of childbearing age in two European cities were susceptible to B19 infection.[143] Infection in the pregnant woman is no more severe than in nonpregnant adults.

Virologically confirmed B19 infection has been documented to cause fetal loss and hydrops fetalis.[144] Reviews of the case reports in the literature led to an estimate of fetal loss or hydrops occurring in 26% (16/60) of pregnancies complicated by B19 infection.[145] The adverse consequences mostly followed maternal infection in the first half of pregnancy, but there are reports of infection as late as the 39th week of gestation causing a stillbirth.[146] However, congenital abnormality associated with B19 has been reported only once so far, in the fetus of a mother who had had the infection in the sixth week of gestation. The pregnancy was terminated for other reasons and ocular abnormalities were noted in the products of conception.[147] Whether this fetus would have survived to term and resulted in a congenitally affected baby is impossible to say. Mortimer and others[143] studied sera taken within 4 months (mostly within 1 month) of birth from 253 babies with congenital abnormalities. Rubella- and CMV-positive specimens were excluded, but neither B19 DNA nor virus-specific IgM were detectable in the remainder. However, if B19 acts on the fetus in a "hit-and-run" fashion (unlike rubella and CMV, which cause persistent infections), maternal infections early on in the pregnancy may not leave virus DNA or virus-specific IgM at detectable levels at birth.

More accurate estimates of the risk of B19 to the fetus require a prospective longitudinal study of pregnant women infected with the virus. This study is now in progress in the United Kingdom, and preliminary data from this continuing study indicate that there is an increased fetal loss (up to 13% in the second trimester) associated with B19 infection in pregnancy. The majority (four fifths) of infected women that go to term appear to have normal babies (unpublished data, cited by Brown[145]). However, the long-term effects of this virus on intellectual development, for example, is not yet known. An apparently healthy baby can be born with evidence (anti-B19 IgM antibody in the cord blood) of intrauterine infection[148] and the demonstration of B19 virus DNA in myocardial cells indicates that the erythropoietic system is not the only potential target for this virus.[149]

At present B19 infection during pregnancy does not provide sufficient reason for advising termination of pregnancy. There is some risk of fetal loss, but there is nothing that can be done to avoid this, and there is no indication that recurrent fetal loss is any more likely. Given the risk of hydrops fetalis following B19 infection, it is logical to monitor the pregnancy for this complication by ultrasound and serum alpha fetoprotein levels, and to evaluate the role of exchange transfusion in the infants most severely affected.[145, 150] More detailed information obtained by prospective long-term follow-up of women acquiring B19 during pregnancy is required and will help to devise rational strategies for management.

Virologic diagnosis of parvovirus B19 infection can be made by demonstrating virus-specific IgM and/or virus DNA in the blood. Virus DNA is detectable (by dot blot DNA hybridization) in the blood for a few days during the prodromal stage of the illness. It is no longer detectable after the onset of the rash and the appearance of antibody. IgM antibodies persist for 2 to 3 months after infection. Postmortem tissues or the products of conception may be investigated by DNA probes for virus DNA, and by electron microscopy for the presence of large numbers of 22-nm spherical virus particles. IgG antibodies, demonstrated by immunoassay, are useful indicators of past infection, and can also indicate seroconversion.[151] Parvovirus diagnosis is available so far in only a few reference centers. This is mainly because the virus cannot be grown in vitro. The source of antigens used in serologic assays has therefore to be painstakingly sought in the serum of patients infected with the virus. It is probable that genetically engineered antigen will make B19 diagnosis more widely available in the future.

MEASLES

Measles is rare in pregnancy, with approximately 90% of adults acquiring immunity in childhood, either via natural infection or, in recent years, by vaccination. Prior to the widespread use of measles vaccine, the minimum incidence of measles in pregnancy was estimated to be between 4 and 6 per 100,000 pregnancies.[4, 152] The estimated incidence of measles in nonpregnant adults in the United States in recent years is 6 per 100,000 in the 15- to 19-year age group, declining to 0.3 per 100,000 in those over 25 years old.[153]

There are conflicting reports on the severity of measles in the pregnant mother. Young and Gershon[93] reviewed existing data and concluded that measles may be marginally more severe in pregnancy; pneumonia, left ventricular failure, and pulmonary edema are the most commonly reported complications.

Gestational measles has effects on the fetus, with an increase in prematurity and low-birth-weight babies (17% vs. 3% in controls).[152] An increase in the rate of abortion was not demonstrated in this study, though a retrospective study of the "virgin soil" epidemics in Greenland suggests that fetal loss is increased.[154] Given the rarity of gestational measles, the occurrence or absence of congenital defects has been hard to establish. In one controlled prospective study, there was no difference in the incidence of congenital malformations in the measles group (1 of 60 babies) when compared to controls.[95] A random collection of congenital defects said to be associated with measles are reported in the literature,[154] but there has been no characteristic constellation of defects associated with measles in pregnancy (reviewed by Young and Gershon[93]).

Gestational measles occurring in the last weeks of pregnancy can result in intrauterine or postnatal transmission of the virus to the baby. Given the incubation period of 13 to 14 days, measles occurring in the first 10 days of life is regarded as due to intrauterine trans-

mission, and that occurring after 14 days is regarded as postnatal infection. The latter is no more severe than measles later in childhood. Intrauterine transmission can result in measles in the baby with an incubation period of 2 to 10 days. This presumably indicates that a large amount of virus is transmitted across the placenta, causing disease in the baby, without the large buildup of virus required before symptoms appear in the adult. Not all babies exposed to the virus in utero develop the disease (only one third in one report), and the fatality rate appears to be higher in babies born prematurely (56%) as compared to those born at term (20%).[93]

On the basis of available evidence, measles in pregnancy does not appear to be a cause of fetal defects, and therefore is not a reason for considering terminating the pregnancy. The chances of abortion or stillbirth may be increased, but there is little that can be done to intervene in this process.

Pregnant women or neonates exposed to measles can be protected by normal human gamma globulin or immune globulin (750 mg in 5 mL by deep IM injection), ideally given as soon as possible, but it can be effective up to 72 hours after exposure. It may still be useful up to 7 days.

Measles vaccine (including measles-mumps-rubella [MMR] vaccine) is, like other live virus vaccines, contraindicated in pregnancy.

MUMPS

Mumps is less infectious than the other common childhood infections—measles and varicella. By the age of 10 years 75% of the population of the United States have been infected, the figure rising to 95% by the age of 20 years.[155] The incidence of mumps in the prevaccination era was 80 to 100 cases per 100,000 pregnancies, greater than the incidence of measles or varicella.[4]

Mumps in pregnancy is no more severe than in other nonpregnant adult women, nor is the ratio of subclinical to overt illness any different.[156]

Mumps virus can cross the placenta and give rise to intrauterine infection of the placenta and fetus,[157] but does not always do so.[158] Attenuated mumps virus has also been isolated from the placenta following vaccination of the mother.[159]

Siegal and Fuerst[152] found that mumps in the first trimester was associated with an increased risk of fetal loss (double that for controls). There was no increase in the risk of premature births. There are (as for measles) a number of case reports of congenital malformations following gestational mumps, but there is no clear pattern of defects associated with the illness (reviewed by Young and Gershon[93]). A controlled prospective study failed to show an association of congenital defects in the baby with mumps during gestation.[95] However, an association between mumps in pregnancy and endocardial fibroelastosis in the baby has been argued for some time, but so far unconvincingly.[93]

Perinatal mumps acquired either transplacentally (following maternal infection around partus) or postnatally appears to be a rare occurrence. It is not thought to present a significant clinical problem.[93]

Laboratory confirmation of a diagnosis of mumps is usually made serologically. Rising titers to the V and S antigens of mumps virus are usually demonstrable with the complement fixation test, and indicate recent infection. As antibody to the S antigen usually appears early and is short-lasting, its presence in high titer in a single serum is suggestive of recent infection. Isolation of the virus can be made from throat swabs or saliva, but is usually slow and can be unreliable.

In summary, mumps in pregnancy does not pose a serious threat to the normality of the fetus, and is not an indication for termination of pregnancy.

INFLUENZA

Influenza is usually a self-limiting illness except in those persons with underlying debilitating, respiratory, or cardiac illnesses and in the aged. The morbidity and mortality following influenza is not significantly altered by pregnancy, although earlier studies had indicated otherwise.[160] This topic, including the use of influenza vaccine, is detailed in Chap. 6, p. 216.

ENTEROVIRUSES

The human enteroviruses include poliovirus (3 serotypes), coxsackievirus groups A (23 serotypes) and B (6 serotypes), ECHO virus (32 serotypes), and the enteroviruses 68–71.

The manifestations of the nonpolio enterovirus infections are protean, and range from subclinical infections, undifferentiated fevers with or without a rash (rubelliform, vesicular), to respiratory infection, aseptic meningitis, myocarditis, conjunctivitis, herpangina, and hand-foot-and-mouth disease. The majority of enteroviral infections are subclinical—both in pregnant[161] and in nonpregnant adults. Enteroviruses (ECHO viruses in particular) may give rise to a rubelliform rash and cause concern in pregnancy because they are mistaken for rubella. Polio in pregnancy is thought to be a more severe illness than in nonpregnant women, with a higher incidence of paralytic complications.[1] Other enterovirus infections are not thought to be more serious in the pregnant woman, though atypical complications (e.g., disseminated peritoneal infection and uterine atony after cesarean section) have been reported.[162]

There is less evidence to document transplacental transmission of these viruses to the fetus following maternal infection in early pregnancy. Occasional case reports have described transplacental transmission of polio and coxsackieviruses following maternal infections early in gestation, though others have failed to observe infection in the fetus following coxsackievirus B5 infection in the first 6 months of pregnancy. The incidence of abortion is increased following gestational polio early in pregnancy. There is no evidence for increased abortion following coxsackie or ECHO virus infections.[163]

Brown and Karunas[161] compared 630 mothers of children with congenital defects of various types with 1,164 mothers chosen to serve as matched controls. Their serologic status to coxsackie B1–6; coxsackie A9: and ECHO 6 and 9 viruses were compared on paired sera collected in early and late pregnancy. The results show a statistical association between coxsackie B infections and urogenital and congenital heart disorders, and associate coxsackie A9 with developmental abnormalities of the gastrointestinal tract. However, the estimated increase in risk for congenital heart disease, for example, was from 0.5% to 0.9%. Even if the associations reported in this study are valid, the increase in risk is too small to justify an offer to terminate the pregnancy. In addition, the authors did not note any seasonality in the congenital defects observed, whereas enteroviruses have a seasonal increase in activity, usually with a summer peak. This is difficult to explain, and raises doubts whether enteroviruses did indeed contribute to the congenital defects. In any case, congenital developmental defects have not been associated with the polio or ECHO viruses.

Polio and coxsackievirus infection of the mother *late* in pregnancy does result in perinatal infection of the fetus and the newborn. Neonatal poliomyelitis carries a 25% mortality.[164] Nosocomial enterovirus infection in neonatal nurseries can also give cause for concern, though this is not covered in this chapter.[163, 165]

Live attenuated vaccines, including the oral polio vaccine, are best avoided in pregnancy. Whether the attenuated vaccine virus crosses the placenta following inadvertent administration of oral polio vaccine to a pregnant mother is unclear. But as viremia has been documented following oral polio vaccine, the possibility cannot be discounted. However, there is no direct evidence of adverse consequences to the fetus resulting from oral polio vaccination during pregnancy.[163, 166]

Virologic diagnosis of enterovirus infection can be made by the isolation of the virus

from stools, throat swabs, and other target organs affected (e.g., CSF; pericardial fluid, etc.). Serologic diagnosis is usually attempted only with the polio and coxsackie B viruses, as otherwise the large number of serotypes makes routine serology impractical.

GENITAL WARTS

Genital warts are predominantly venereally transmitted infections caused by the human papillomaviruses (HPV). The HPV types most often causing genital warts are types 6 and 11. The prevalence of the disease in adults is roughly on the order of 1%, though the asymptomatic infection rate with HPV 6 or 11 is around 5% in healthy adult populations.[167] Its incidence in pregnancy is unknown; only the larger warts give concern and are noted in pregnancy, the smaller lesions pass unrecorded.

The alterations in the immune system and the generalized increase in vascularity that occurs in pregnancy contribute to the proliferation of genital warts. Previously unnoticed warts may become noticeable, and minor lesions may become a major discomfort or even a physical impediment to vaginal delivery. Large warts may give rise to dystocia and severe hemorrhage if vaginal delivery is allowed. They may also provide foci for secondary bacterial infection which can adversely affect the fetus (chorioamnionitis, intrapartum fetal infections).[168]

The virus can be transmitted to the baby as it is born through an infected birth canal or, less commonly, can be transmitted to the fetus in utero. As a result, genital warts may occur in the baby at birth (congenital transmission) or may develop at varying periods after birth.[169] The risk of transmission from a mother with genital lesions is not known. One study found HPV DNA in 3 of 70 (4%) foreskins from unselected male babies undergoing circumcision.[170]

Genital warts in the baby may be a minor problem, but because genital warts are usually transmitted venereally and pediatric genital warts are considered potential indicators of child sex abuse,[171] the frequency of vertical transmission of the virus and the duration of its incubation period are relevant questions for which we have no answers to date.

The other consequence of vertical HPV infection is the occurrence of respiratory papillomatosis in the child.[172] There may be a long latent period lasting many years before the lesions are noticeable. Most commonly they affect the larynx and less commonly spread to the trachea and the rest of the respiratory tract. These papillomas can cause respiratory obstruction with lifelong morbidity. There is no reliable cure.

The management of genital warts should aim to ablate the lesions effectively early in the pregnancy. Trichloroacetic acid applications (50%–85%) and carbon dioxide laser therapy[173] are effective, while electrocoagulation, electrodessication, and cryotherapy can be used for smaller lesions. Podophyllin is contraindicated in pregnancy, and surgical excision can cause hemorrhage (reviewed by Kashima and Shah[172]). Intralesional interferon-α_{2b} has been reported to be effective, though painful, in nonpregnant adults, and it remains to be seen if these results will be confirmed.[174] The selection of the particular method would depend on the size, situation, and number of the warts. Success, however, cannot be guaranteed.

The use of cesarean section is indicated only if the size and location of lesions may obstruct delivery mechanically or cause dystocia. The risk of respiratory papillomatosis in a baby born to a mother with genital warts is very low (estimated to be about 1:1,000),[172] and does not by itself justify cesarean section. The effective treatment of genital warts early in pregnancy should reduce the virus load, and thereby reduce the risk for the baby even further.

POLYOMAVIRUSES

The human polyomaviruses BK and JC are common human infections, with 80% to 90% and 50%, respectively, of persons being infected by the time they reach adulthood.[175] Serologic evidence of virus reactivation is found in around 25% of pregnant women, with viruria being documented in 3% to 7%. Most of these infections are presumably reactivations; definite evidence of primary infection in pregnancy has yet to be found. No obvious disease in the pregnant woman has been associated with virus reactivation.[176, 177] Seventeen children with a range of congenital abnormalities (prematurity, hyperbilirubinemia, seizures, cerebral defects) were found to have IgM antibody to BK virus early in life (3–90 days old), and the virus was isolated from the urine of one.[178] Babies born to mothers excreting polyomavirus in the urine were more likely to be premature or jaundiced. However, unequivocal evidence of congenital infection has yet to be documented.[179]

IMMUNIZATION DURING PREGNANCY

No substance should be administered without good reason and particularly during pregnancy. This includes vaccines. Theoretically, inactivated vaccines pose no risk to the fetus, and the indications for the use of rabies (diploid cell) vaccine are unaltered by pregnancy. Hepatitis B vaccine is probably safe in pregnancy, but routine immunization of health care workers, for example, is best delayed until after the pregnancy is completed, provided this does not place the woman at excessive risk. The use of hepatitis B vaccine in postexposure prophylaxis is not contraindicated by pregnancy. Influenza A immunization is indicated in pregnancy only if underlying diseases make the woman more susceptible to influenza morbidity (i.e., the indications are the same as in the nonpregnant).

On the other hand, the use of live attenuated vaccines during pregnancy carries the theoretical risk of infecting the fetus and if the virus in question is potentially teratogenic, there is a possibility that fetal damage may occur. *As such, live vaccines are best avoided in pregnancy, and a woman immunized with one of these agents should be advised to avoid pregnancy for 3 months.* However, follow-up of pregnant women inadvertently vaccinated with the widely used live attenuated virus vaccines (i.e., polio, measles, rubella, mumps) has uncovered no evidence of damage to the fetus.[180, 181] The evidence is reviewed more completely under the individual viruses (see above). Oral polio[166] and yellow fever vaccines can be used in pregnant women who are at substantial risk of exposure to these viruses, for example, through travel or through exposure to an epidemic, although wherever possible it is advisable to give the vaccine as late in pregnancy as possible. In the case of polio, the inactivated vaccine is a preferable alternative if available. The risk of inadvertent immunization with any of these agents (measles, mumps, rubella, polio) during pregnancy does not appear to be sufficient to consider termination.

Persons given rubella, mumps, and measles vaccines can shed the viruses but do not usually transmit them. Thus vaccination of children need not be postponed because of pregnancy in the mother. Though oral polio vaccine is transmitted from the vaccinee to other contacts, polio vaccine virus is innocuous in pregnancy and therefore there is no hazard in immunizing the household contacts of a pregnant woman. The rare complication of vaccine-induced paralytic disease is more frequently seen in adults than in children. Therefore, if a pregnant woman has never been immunized against polio, it would be advisable to immunize her with the killed polio vaccine (if available), while her children receive the live oral vaccine. Other live attenuated vaccines, however, are documented to cause fetal damage; the TA-83 vaccine for Venezuelan equine encephalitis[182] and, in the past, smallpox immunization with vaccinia were associated with adverse sequelae for the fetus.[181] Proposals to use vaccinia virus as a vector for other genetically engineered vaccines will have to recognize hazards to pregnant women.

Gamma globulins, immune or pooled, are not hazardous to the pregnant woman, and the indications for their use are unaltered.

The immediate postpartum period is one where the mother (and child for that matter) are accessible to the health care system, and efforts should be made to immunize all rubella-seronegative women in order that subsequent pregnancies are protected.

The consequences of, and indications for,

TABLE 14–9.
Use of Vaccines in Pregnancy

| Vaccine | Risk to Fetus From Immunization | | Indications for Immunization in Pregnancy |
	Fetal Infection	Fetal Damage	
Live attenuated vaccines			
Rubella	Yes	No	None
Measles	?	No	None
Mumps	Yes	No	None
Polio	?	No	If high risk of exposure (e.g., travel or epidemic); use killed polio vaccine if available
Yellow fever	?	No	If high risk of exposure (e.g., travel or epidemic)
Varicella-zoster	?	?	None—still an investigational agent
Inactivated vaccines			
Rabies	No	No	As in nonpregnancy
Hepatitis B	No	No	Postexposure prophylaxis
Influenza A	No	No	If pregnancy complicated by serious underlying disease that increases morbidity from influenza

the use of vaccines in pregnant women are summarized in Table 14–9. Other reviews on the question of vaccination in pregnancy include those by Amstey[183] and Blanco and Gibbs.[184]

REFERENCES

References are arranged under the headings indicated, as they appear in the text. References cited in more than one section appear only under the heading of the section in which they are first cited.

Pathogenesis of Fetal Infection
1. Siegel M, Greenberg M: Incidence of poliomyelitis in pregnancy, its relation to maternal age, parity and gestational period. *N Engl J Med* 1955; 253:841–847.
2. Purcell RH, Ticehurst JR: Enterically transmitted non-A non-B hepatitis: Epidemiology and clinical characteristics, in Zuckermann AZ (ed): *Viral Hepatitis and Liver Disease.* New York, Alan Liss, 1988, pp 131–137.
3. Miller E, Cradock-Watson JE, Pollock TM: Consequences of confirmed maternal rubella at successive stages of pregnancy. *Lancet* 1982; 2:781–784.
4. Sever J, White LR: Intrauterine viral infections. *Annu Rev Med* 1968; 19:471–486.
5. Klein JO, Remington JS, Marcy SM: Current concepts of infections of the fetus and the newborn infant, in Remington JS, Klein JO (eds): *Infectious Diseases of the Fetus and the Newborn Infant,* ed 2. Philadelphia, WB Saunders Co, 1983, pp 1–26.
6. Alford CA, Neva FA, Weller TA: Virologic and serologic studies on human products of conception after maternal rubella. *N Engl J Med* 1964; 271:1275–1281.
7. Hayes K, Gilas H: Placental cytomegalovirus infections without fetal involvement following primary infection in pregnancy. *J Pediatr* 1961; 79:401–405.
8. King-Lewis PA, Gardner SD: Congenital cytomegalovirus infection following intrauterine transfusion. *Br Med J* 1969; 2:603–605.

Laboratory Diagnosis of Viral Infections in Pregnancy
9. Gardner PS, McQuillin J: *Rapid Viral Diagnosis: Application of Immunofluorescence,* ed 2.

London, Butterworths, 1980, p 317.
10. Arstila P, Halonen P: Direct antigen detection, in Lennette EH, Halonen P, Murphy FA (eds): *Laboratory Diagnosis of Infectious Diseases,* vol 2. New York, Springer-Verlag, 1988, pp 60–75.
11. Demmler GJ, Buffone GJ, Schimber CM, et al: Detection of cytomegalovirus in urine from newborns by using the polymerase chain reaction DNA amplification. *J Infect Dis* 1988; 158:1177–1184.
12. Griffiths PD, Panjwani DD, Stirk PR, et al: Rapid diagnosis of cytomegalovirus infection in immunocompromised patients by detection of early antigen fluorescent foci. *Lancet* 1984; 2:1242–1245.
13. Schirm J, Meulenberg JM, Pastoor GW, et al: Rapid detection of varicella-zoster virus in clinical specimens using monoclonal antibodies on shell vials and smears. *J Med Virol* 1989; 28:1–6.
14. Griffiths PD, Kangro HO: A user's guide to the indirect solid phase immunoassay for the detection of cytomegalovirus specific IgM antibodies. *J Virol Methods* 1984; 8:271–282.
15. Lennette EH, Halonen P, Murphey FA (eds): *Laboratory Diagnosis of Infectious Diseases. Principles and Practice. Vol 2: Viral Rickettsial and Chlamydial Diseases.* New York, Springer-Verlag, 1988, p 961.

Rubella
16. Gregg NM: Congenital cataract following German measles in the mother. *Trans Ophthalmol Soc Aust* 1941; 3:35.
17. Hanshaw JB, Dudgeon JA, Marshall WC: *Viral Disease of the Fetus and Newborn,* ed 2. Philadelphia, WB Saunders Co, 1985.
18. Assaad F, Ljungars-Esteves K: Rubella—World impact. *Rev Infect Dis* 1985; 7(Suppl 1):S29–S36.
19. Shirley JA, Revill S, Cohen BJ, et al: Serological study of rubella like illness. *J Med Virol* 1987; 21:369–379.
20. Sheppard S, Smithells RW, Peckham CS, et al: National congenital rubella surveillance 1971–75. *Health Trends* 1977; 9:38–41.
21. Cradock-Watson JE, Ridehalgh MKS, Anderson MJ, et al: Outcome of asymptomatic infections with rubella virus during pregnancy. *J Hyg (Camb)* 1981; 87:147–154.

22. Cooper LZ, Green RH, Krugman S, et al: Neonatal thrombocytopenic purpura and other manifestations of rubella contracted in utero. *Am J Dis Child* 1965; 110:416–428.

23. Best JM, Banatvala JE: Rubella, in Zuckerman AJ, Banatvala JE, Pattison JR (eds): *Principles and Practice of Clinical Virology.* Chichester, England, John Wiley & Sons, 1987, pp 315–353.

24. Cradock-Watson JE, Ridehalgh MKS, Anderson MJ, et al: Fetal infection resulting from maternal rubella after the first trimester of pregnancy. *J Hyg (Camb)* 1980; 85:381–391.

25. Grillner L, Forsgren M, Barr B, et al: Outcome of rubella during pregnancy with special reference to the 17th-24th weeks of gestation. *Scand J Infect Dis* 1983; 15:321–325.

26. Ueda K, Nishida Y, Oshima K, et al: Congenital rubella syndrome: Correlation of gestational age at time of maternal rubella with type of defect. *J Pediatr* 1979; 94:763–765.

27. Enders G, Wickerl-Packer U, Miller E, et al: Outcome of confirmed periconceptional maternal rubella. *Lancet* 1988; 1:1445–1447.

28. Cooper LZ, Ziring PR, Okerse AB, et al: Rubella: Clinical manifestations and management. *Am J Dis Child* 1969; 118:18–29.

29. Horstmann DM, Liebhaber H, Le Bouvier G, et al: Rubella reinfection of vaccinated and naturally immune persons exposed to an epidemic. *N Engl J Med* 1970; 283:771–776.

30. Cradock-Watson JE, Ridehalgh MKS, Anderson MJ, et al: Rubella reinfection and the fetus. *Lancet* 1985; 1:1039.

31. Morgan-Capner P, Hodgson J, Hambling MH, et al: Detection of rubella specific IgM in subclinical rubella reinfections in pregnancy. *Lancet* 1985; 1:244–246.

32. Best JM, Banatvala JE, Morgan-Capner P, et al: Fetal infection after maternal reinfection with rubella: Criteria for defining reinfection. *Br Med J* 1989; 299:773–775.

33. Enders G, Calm A, Schaub J: Rubella embryopathy after previous maternal rubella vaccination. *Infection* 1984; 12:96–98.

34. Forsgren M, Soren L: Subclinical rubella infection in vaccinated women with rubella-specific IgM response during pregnancy and transmission of virus to the fetus. *Scand J Infect Dis* 1985; 17:337–341.

35. Rubella vaccination during pregnancy— United States, 1971–1986. *MMWR* 1987; 36:457–461.

36. Burke JP, Hinman AR, Krugman S: International symposium on the prevention of congenital rubella infection. *Rev Infect Dis* 1985; 7(suppl 1):215.

37. Enders G, Knotek F: Detection of IgM antibodies against rubella virus: Comparison of two indirect ELISAs and an anti-IgM capture immunoassay. *J Med Virol* 1986; 19:377–386.

38. Morgan-Capner P: Diagnosing rubella. *Br Med J* 1989; 299:338–339.

39. Thomas HIJ, Morgan-Capner P: Rubella specific IgG subclass avidity ELISA and its role in the differentiation between primary rubella and rubella reinfection. *Epidemiol Infect* 1988; 101:591–598.

40. Daffos E, Forestier F, Grangeot-Keros L, et al: Prenatal diagnosis of congenital rubella. *Lancet* 1984; 2:1–3.

41. Ho-Terry L, Terry GM, Londesborough P, et al: Diagnosis of fetal rubella infection by nucleic acid hybridization. *J Med Virol* 1988; 24:175–182.

Cytomegalovirus

42. Huang E, Alford CA, Reynolds DW, et al: Molecular epidemiology of CMV infections in women and their infants. *N Engl J Med* 1980; 303:958–962.

43. Ho M: *Cytomegaloviruses: Biology and Infection.* New York, Plenum Press, 1982, p 309.

44. Stagno S, Reynolds DW, Pass RF, et al: Breast milk and the risk of cytomegalovirus infection. *N Engl J Med* 1980; 302:1073–1074.

45. Pass RF, August AM, Dworsky M, et al: Cytomegalovirus infection in a day care center. *N Engl J Med* 1982; 307:477–478.

46. Griffiths PD, Baboonian C: A prospective study of primary cytomegalovirus infection during pregnancy: Final report. *Br J Obstet Gynaecol* 1984; 91:307–315.

47. Taber LH, Frank AL, Yow MD, et al: Acquisition of cytomegalovirus infections in families with young children: A serol-

ogical study. *J Infect Dis* 1985; 151:948–952.

48. Rudd P, Peckham C: Infection of the fetus and the newborn: Prevention, treatment and related handicap. *Bailière Clinical Obstet Gynaecol* 1988; 2:53–71.

49. Griffiths PD: Cytomegalovirus, in Zuckerman AJ, Banatvala JE, Pattison JE (eds): *Principles and Practice of Clinical Virology*. Chichester, England, John Wiley & Sons, 1987, pp 75–109.

50. Stagno S, Reynolds D, Tsiantos A, et al: Cervical cytomegalovirus excretion in pregnant and non-pregnant women: Suppression in early gestation. *J Infect Dis* 1975; 131:522–527.

51. Cytomegalovirus in adults. *Lancet* 1977; 2:541.

52. Altshuler G: Immunologic competence of the immature human fetus. Morphologic evidence from intrauterine cytomegalovirus infection. *Obstet Gynecol* 1974; 43:811–816.

53. Stagno S, Pass RF, Dworsky ME, et al: Congenital cytomegalovirus infection: The relative importance of primary and recurrent maternal infection. *N Engl J Med* 1982; 306:945–949.

54. Ahlfors K, Harris S, Ivarsson S, et al: Secondary maternal CMV infection causing symptomatic congenital infection. *N Engl J Med* 1981; 305:284.

55. Rutter D, Griffiths P, Trompeter RS: Cytomegalovirus inclusion disease after recurrent maternal infection. *Lancet* 1985; 2:1182.

56. Preece PM, Pearl KN, Peckham CS: Congenital cytomegalovirus infection. *Arch Dis Child* 1984; 59:1120–1126.

57. Saigal S, Lunyk O, Larke RPB, et al: The outcome in children with congenital cytomegalovirus infection. *Am J Dis Child* 1982; 136:896–901.

58. Stagno S, Reynolds DW, Amos CS, et al: Auditory and visual defects resulting from symptomatic and subclinical congenital cytomegalovirus and toxoplasma infection. *Pediatrics* 1977; 59:669–678.

59. Stagno S, Pass RF, Dworsky ME, et al: Congenital and perinatal cytomegalovirus infections. *Semin Perinatol* 1983; 7:31–42.

60. Ballard RA, Drew L, Hufnagel KG, et al: Acquired cytomegalovirus infection in preterm babies. *Am J Dis Child* 1979; 133:482–485.

61. Gurevich I, Cunha BA: Non parenteral transmission of cytomegalovirus in a neonatal intensive care unit. *Lancet* 1981; 2:222–224.

62. Griffiths PD, Stagno S, Pass RF, et al: Infection with cytomegalovirus during pregnancy: Specific IgM antibodies during pregnancy: Specific IgM antibodies as a marker for recent primary infection. *J Infect Dis* 1982; 145:647–653.

63. Waner J, Weller TH, Kevy SV: Patterns of CMV complement fixing antibody: A longitudinal study of blood donors. *Pediatr Res* 1973; 127:538–543.

64. Stagno S, Pass RF, Reynolds DW, et al: Comparative study of diagnostic procedures for congenital cytomegalovirus infection. *Pediatrics* 1985; 65:251–257.

65. Stern H, Harringnon G, Booth J, et al: An early marker of fetal infection after primary cytomegalovirus infection in pregnancy. *Br Med J* 1986; 292:718–720.

66. Lange I, Rodeck CH, Morgan-Capner P, et al: Prenatal serological diagnosis of intrauterine cytomegalovirus infection. *Br Med J* 1982; 284:1673–1674.

Herpes Simplex

67. Longson M: Herpes simplex, in Zuckerman AJ, Banatvala JE, Pattison JR (eds): *Principles and Practice of Clinical Virology*. Chichester, England, John Wiley & Sons, 1987, pp 3–49.

68. Herpes simplex: Changing patterns. *Lancet* 1981; 1:1025–1026.

69. Nahmias AJ, Keyserling HJ, Kerrick GM: Herpes simplex, in Remingtom JS, Klein JO (eds): *Infectious Diseases of the Fetus and Newborn Infant*, Philadelphia, WB Saunders Co, 1983, pp 636–678.

70. Yeager AS, Arvin AM: Reasons for the absence of a history of recurrent genital infections in mothers of neonates infected with herpes simplex virus. *Pediatrics* 1984; 73:188–193.

71. Buchman T, Roizman B, Nahmias A: Demonstration of exogenous genital reinfection with herpes simplex virus type 2 by restriction endonuclease fingerprinting of viral DNA. *J Infect Dis* 1979; 140:295–304.

72. Corey L, Spear PG: Infections with herpes simplex viruses. *N Engl J Med* 1986; 314:686–691, 749–757.

73. Lafferty WE, Coombs RW, Bennedetti J, et al: Recurrences after oral and genital herpes simplex virus infections: Influence of site of infection and viral type. *N Engl J Med* 1987; 316:1444–1449.

74. Sullender WM, Yasukawa LL, Schwartz M, et al: Type specific antibodies to herpes simplex type 2 (HSV-2) glycoprotein G in pregnant women, infants exposed to maternal HSV-2 infection at delivery, and infants with neonatal herpes. *J Infect Dis* 1988; 157:164–171.

75. Wentworth BB, Alexander ER: Seroepidemiology of infections due to members of the *Herpesvirus* group. *Am J Epidemiol* 1971; 94:496–507.

76. Hatherly LI, Hayes K, Hennessy EM, et al: Herpes virus in an obstetric hospital: I. Herpetic eruptions. *Med J Aust* 1980; 2:205–208.

77. Hatherly LI, Hayes K, Jack I: Herpes virus in an obstetric hospital: II. Asymptomatic excretion in staff members. *Med J Aust* 1980; 2:273–275.

78. Stagno S, Whitley RJ: Herpes virus infections of pregnancy: Part II: Herpes simplex and varicella-zoster virus infections. *N Engl J Med* 1985; 313:1327–1330.

79. Binkin NJ, Alexander ER: Neonatal herpes: How can it be prevented? *JAMA* 1983; 250:3093–3094.

80. Sullivan-Bolyai J, Hull HF, Wilson C: Neonatal herpes simplex virus infection in King County, Washington: Increasing incidence and epidemiologic correlates. *JAMA* 1983; 250:3059–3062.

81. Genital herpes infection: United States 1966–1979. *MMWR* 1982; 31:26.

82. Kelly J: Genital herpes in pregnancy. Routine virological screening is futile. *Br Med J* 1988; 297:1146–1147.

83. Stone KM: Current considerations in the obstetric and gynecologic management of herpes simplex virus infections. *J Reprod Med* 1986; 31:452.

84. New tissue culture—fluorescent method speeds detection of herpes simplex virus. *JAMA* 1983; 250:3045.

85. Binkin NJ, Koplan JP, Cates W: Preventing neonatal herpes: The value of weekly viral cultures in pregnant women with recurrent genital herpes. *JAMA* 1984; 251:2816–2821.

86. Madeley CR, Davison JM: Genital herpes during pregnancy. *Br Med J* 1988; 297:1539.

87. Prober CG, Sullender WM, Yasukawa LL, et al: Low risk of herpes simplex infection in neonates exposed to the virus at the time of vaginal delivery to mothers with recurrent genital herpes simplex infections. *N Engl J Med* 1987; 316:240–244.

88. Prober CG, Hensleigh PA, Boucher FD, et al: Use of routine viral culture at delivery to identify neonates exposed to herpes simplex virus. *N Engl J Med* 1988; 318:887–891.

89. Brown ZA, Berry S, Vontver LA: Genital herpes simplex infections complicating pregnancy. Natural history and peripartum management. *J Reprod Med* 1986; 31(suppl):420–425.

90. Harger JH, Pazin GJ, Armstrong JA, et al: Characteristics and management of pregnancy in women with genital herpes simplex virus infection. *Am J Obstet Gynecol* 1983; 145:784–791.

91. Arvin AM, Hensleigh PA, Prober CG, et al: Failure of antepartum cultures to predict the infants risk of exposure to herpes simplex at delivery. *N Engl J Med* 1986; 315:796–800.

Varicella-Zoster Virus

92. Heath RB: Varicella zoster, in Zuckerman AJ, Banatvala JE, Pattison JR (eds): *Principles and Practice of Clinical Virology.* Chichester, England, John Wiley & Sons, 1987, pp 51–73.

93. Young NA, Gershon AA: Chickenpox, measles and mumps, in Remington JS, Klein JO (eds): *Infectious Diseases of the Fetus and the Newborn Infant.* Philadelphia, WB Saunders Co, 1983, pp 375–427.

94. Paryani SG, Arvin AM: Intrauterine infection with varicella-zoster virus after maternal varicella. *N Engl J Med* 1986; 314:1542–1546.

95. Siegel M: Congenital malformations following chickenpox, measles, mumps, and hepatitis. Results of a cohort study. *JAMA* 1973; 226:1521–1524.

96. Alkalay AL, Pomerance JJ, Rimoin DL: Fetal varicella syndrome. *J Pediatr* 1987; 111:321–323.

97. Adlestein AM, Donovan JW: Malignant disease in children whose mothers had chickenpox, mumps, or rubella in pregnancy. *Br Med J* 1972; 4:629–631.

98. Miller E, Cradock-Watson JE, Ridehalgh MKS: Outcome in newborn babies given anti-varicella zoster immunoglobulin after perinatal maternal infection with varicella-zoster virus. *Lancet* 1989; 2:371–373.

99. Meyers JD: Congenital varicella in term infants: Risk reconsidered. *J Infect Dis* 1974; 129:215–217.

100. Brunell PA: Placental transfer of varicella-zoster antibody. *Pediatrics* 1966; 38:1034–1038.

101. Centers for Disease Control: Varicella zoster immune globulin for the prevention of chickenpox. *Ann Intern Med* 1984; 100:859–865.

102. Williams H, Latif A, Morgan J, et al: Acyclovir treatment of neonatal varicella. *J Infect* 1987; 15:65–67.

103. Carter PE, Duffy P, Lloyd DJ: Neonatal varicella infection. *Lancet* 1986; 2:1459–1460.

104. Haddad J, Simeoni U, Messer J, et al: Transplacental passage of acyclovir. *J Pediatr* 1987; 110:164–165.

105. Brown ZA, Baker DA: Acyclovir therapy during pregnancy. *Obstet Gynecol* 1989; 73:526–531.

106. Ellis ME, Neal KR, Webb AK: Is smoking a risk factor for pneumonia in adults with chicken pox. *Br Med J* 1987; 294:1002.

107. Eyal A, Friedman M, Peretz Ba, et al: Pregnancy complicated by herpes zoster. *J Reprod Med* 1983; 28:600.

Epstein-Barr Virus

108. Icart J, Didier J, Dalens M, et al: Prospective study of Epstein Barr virus infection during pregnancy. *Biomedicine* 1981; 34:1579.

109. Le CT, Chang S, Lysson MH: Epstein Barr virus infections in pregnancy. A prospective study and a review of the literature. *Am J Dis Child* 1983; 137:466–468.

110. Fleisher GR, Bolognese R: Epstein-Barr virus infections in pregnancy: A prospective study. *J Pediatr* 1984; 104:374–379.

111. Hunter K, Stagno S, Capps E, et al: Prenatal screening of pregnant women for infections caused by cytomegalovirus, Epstein-Barr virus, herpesvirus, rubella, and *Toxoplasma gondii*. *Am J Obstet Gynecol* 1983; 145:269–273.

112. Stagno S, Whitley RJ: Cytomegalovirus infections of pregnancy: Part I. Cytomegalovirus and Epstein-Barr virus infections. *N Engl J Med* 1985; 313:1270–1274.

113. Leary DC, Welt LG, Beckett RS: Infectious mononucleosis complicating pregnancy with fatal congenital anomaly of infants. *Am J Obstet Gynecol* 1949; 56:381–384.

114. Goldberg GN, Fulginiti VA, Ray CG, et al: In utero Epstein-Barr virus (infectious mononucleosis) infection. *JAMA* 1981; 246:1576.

115. Fields BN: *Virology*. New York, Raven Press, 1985, p 1614.

Human Immunodeficiency Virus

116. Curran JW: Epidemiology and prevention of AIDS and HIV infection in the United States. Presented at the Third International Conference on AIDS, Washington, DC, June 1–5, 1987.

117. Moss AR, Bacchetti P: Natural history of HIV infection. *AIDS* 1989; 3:55–61.

118. Van der Graaf M, Diepersloot RJA: Transmission of human immunodeficiency virus (HIV/HTLVIII/LAV): A review. *Infection* 1986; 14:203–211.

119. Pedersen C, Lindhardt BO, Jensen BL, et al: Clinical course of primary HIV infection: Consequences for the subsequent course of the infection. Presented at the Fifth International Conference on AIDS, Montreal, June 4–9, 1989, abstract TAO 30.

120. HIV infection: Obstetric and perinatal issues. *Lancet* 1988; 1:806–807.

121. Selwyn PA, Schoenbaum EE, Davenny K, et al: Prospective study of human immunodeficiency virus infection and pregnancy outcomes in intravenous drug abusers. *JAMA* 1989; 261:1289–1294.

121a. Biggar RJ, Pahwa S, Minkoff H, et al: Immunosuppression in pregnant women infected with human immunodeficiency virus. *Am J Obstet Gynecol* 1989; 161:1239–1244.

122. Scott CB, Fischl MA, Klimas N, et al: Mothers of infants with the acquired immunodeficiency syndrome: Evidence for both symptomatic and asymptomatic carriers. *JAMA* 1985; 253:363–366.

123. Wofsy CB: Human immunodeficiency virus infection in women. *JAMA* 1987; 256:2074–2076.

124. Selwyn PA, Carter RJ, Schoenbaum EE, et al: Knowledge of HIV antibody status and decisions to continue or terminate pregnancy among intravenous drug users. *JAMA* 1989; 261:3567–3571.

125. Blanche S, Rouzieux C, Guihard Moscato M-L, et al: A prospective study of infants born to women seropositive for human immunodeficiency virus type 1. *N Engl J Med* 1989; 320:1643–1648.

126. Mok JYQ, Hague RA, Taylor RF, et al: The management of children born to human immunodeficiency virus seropositive women. *J Infect* 1989; 18:119–124.

127. Royal College of Obstetricians and Gynaecologists: *Report of the RCOG—Committee on Problems Associated with AIDS in Relation to Obstetrics and Gynaecology.* London, 1987.

128. Cameron JS: New developments in antiviral therapy, in Dimmock NJ, Griffiths PG, Madeley CR (eds): *Control of Virus Diseases.* Society for General Microbiology Symposium No. 45, Cambridge, England, Cambridge University Press, 1990, pp 341–373.

128a. Volberding PA, Lagakos SW, Koch MA, et al: Zidovudine in asymptomatic human immunodeficiency virus infection. A controlled trial in persons with fewer than 500 CD4-positive cells per cubic millimeter. *N Engl J Med* 1990; pp 941–949.

129. Dinsmoor MJ: HIV infection and pregnancy. *Med Clin North Am* 1989; 73:701–711.

130. Minkoff H, de Regt RH, Landesman S, et al: *Pneumocystis carinii* pneumonia associated with acquired immunodeficiency syndrome in pregnancy: A report of three maternal cases. *Obstet Gynecol* 1989; 67:284–287.

131. Centers for Disease Control: Guidelines for prophylaxis against *Pneumocystis carinii* pneumonia for persons infected with immunodeficiency virus. *MMWR* 1989; 38:1–9.

132. Update: Acquired immunodeficiency syndrome and human immunodeficiency virus infection among health-care workers. *MMWR* 1988; 26:229–239.

133. Marcus R, and the Cooperative Surveillance Group: Health care workers exposed to patients infected with human immunodeficiency virus (HIV), United States. Presented at the Fifth International Conference on AIDS, Montreal, June 4–9, 1989, abstract WAO 1.

134. Understanding AIDS: An information brochure being mailed to all US households. *MMWR* 1988; 37:261–269.

135. Vertical transmission of HIV. *Lancet* 1989; 2:1057–1058.

136. Lepage P, Van der Perre P, Cavael M, et al: Post-natal transmission of HIV from mother to child. *Lancet* 1987; 2:400.

137. Colebunders R, Kapita B, Nekwei W, et al: Breastfeeding and transmission of HIV. *Lancet* 1988; 2:147.

138. Thiry L, Sprecher-Goldberger S, Jonckheer T, et al: Isolation of AIDS virus from cell-free breast milk of three healthy virus carriers. *Lancet* 1985; 2:891–892.

139. Bradbeer CS: Mothers with HIV (editorial). *Br Med J* 1989; 299:806–807.

Parvoviruses

140. Anderson MJ, Jones SE, Fisher-Hoch S, et al: Human parvovirus, the cause of erythema infectiosum (fifth disease)? *Lancet* 1983; 1:1378.

141. Pattison JR, Jones SE, Hodgson J, et al: Parvovirus infections and hypoplastic crisis in sickle cell anaemia. *Lancet* 1981; 1:664–665.

142. Kurtzman GJ, Cohen BJ, Meyers P, et al: Persistent parvovirus infection as a cause of severe chronic anemia in children with acute lymphocytic leukaemia. *Lancet* 1988; 2:1159–1162.

143. Mortimer PP, Cohen BJ, Buckley MM, et al: Human parvovirus and the fetus. *Lancet* 1985; 2:1012.

144. Pattison JR: B19 infections in pregnancy, in Pattison JR (ed): *Parvoviruses and Hu-*

man Disease. Boca Raton, Fla, CRC Press, 1988, pp 133–137.

145. Brown KE: What threat is human parvovirus B19 to the fetus? A review. *Br J Obstet Gynaecol* 1989; 96:764–767.

146. Knott PD, Welpy GAC, Anderson MJ: Serologically proved intrauterine infection with parvovirus. *Br Med J* 1984; 289:1660.

147. Weiland HT, Vermy-Keers C, Salimans MMM, et al: Parvovirus B19 associated with fetal abnormality. *Lancet* 1987; 1:628–683.

148. Woernle CH, Anderson LT, Tattersall P, et al: Human parvovirus B19 infection during pregnancy. *J Infect Dis* 1987; 156:17–20.

149. Porter HJ, Quantrill AM, Fleming KA: B19 parvovirus infection of myocardial cells. *Lancet* 1988; 1:535–536.

150. Schwartz TF, Roggendorf MM, Hottentrager B, et al: Human parvovirus B19 in pregnancy. *Lancet* 1988; 2:566–567.

151. Cohen BJ: Laboratory tests for the diagnosis of infection with B19 virus, in Pattison JR (ed): *Parvoviruses and Human Disease.* Boca Raton, Fla, CRC Press, 1988, pp 69–83.

Measles

152. Siegel M, Fuerst HT: Low birth weight and maternal virus diseases. A prospective study of rubella, measles, mumps, chickenpox and hepatitis. *JAMA* 1966; 197:88–92.

153. Measles in the US. *MMWR* 1987; 36:457–461.

154. Jespersen CS, Littauer J, Sagild U: Measles as a cause of fetal defects. *Acta Pediatr Scand* 1977; 66:367–372.

Mumps

155. Feldman HA: Mumps, in Evans AS (ed): *Viral Infections of Humans. Epidemiology and Control.* New York, Plenum Medical Book Co, 1982, pp 419–435.

156. Philip RN, Reinhard KR, Lackman DB: Observations of a mumps epidemic in a virgin population. *Am J Epidemiol* 1959; 69:91.

157. Kurtz JB, Tomlinson AH, Pearson J: Mumps virus isolated from a fetus. *Br Med J* 1982; 284:471.

158. Chiba Y, Ogra PA, Nakano T: Transplacental mumps infection. *Am J Obstet Gynecol* 1975; 122:904–905.

159. Yamauchi T, Wilson C, St Geme JW: Transmission of live attenuated mumps to the human placenta. *N Engl J Med* 1974; 290:710–712.

Influenza

160. Prevention and control of influenza. *MMWR* 1985; 34:262.

Enteroviruses

161. Brown GC, Karunas RS: Relationship of congenital anomalies and maternal infection with selected enteroviruses. *Am J Epidemiol* 1972; 95:207.

162. Feldman RG, Bryant J, Ives KN, et al: A novel presentation of coxsackie B2 virus infection during pregnancy. *J Infect* 1987; 15:73–76.

163. Cherry JD: Enteroviruses, in Remington JS, Klein JO (eds): *Infectious Diseases in the Fetus and Newborn.* Philadelphia, WB Saunders Co, 1983, pp 290–334.

164. Pugh RCB, Dudgeon JA: Fatal neonatal poliomyelitis. *Arch Dis Child* 1954; 29:381–384.

165. Isaacs D, Dobson SRM, Wilkinson AR, et al: Conservative management of an ECHO virus 11 outbreak in a neonatal unit. *Lancet* 1989; 1:543.

166. Harjolehto T, Aro T, Hovi T, et al: Congenital malformations and oral polio vaccination during pregnancy. *Lancet* 1989; 1:771–772.

Genital Warts

167. Loryncz A, Temple GF, Patterson JA, et al: Correlation of cellular atypia and human papillomavirus DNA sequences in exfoliated cells of the uterine cervix. *Obstet Gynecol* 1986; 68:508–512.

168. Young RL, Acosta AA, Kaufman RH: The treatment of large condylomata complicating pregnancy. *Obstet Gynecol* 1973; 41:65–73.

169. Schwartz DB, Greenberg MD, Daoud Y, et al: The management of genital condylomas in pregnant women. *Obstet Gynecol Clin North Am* 1987; 14:589–599.

170. Roman A, Fife K: Human papillomavirus DNA associated with foreskin of nor-

mal newborns. *J Infect Dis* 1986; 153:855–861.

171. Genital warts and sexual abuse in children. *Am J Acad Dermatol* 1984; 11:529–530.

172. Kashima HK, Shah K: Recurrent respiratory papillomatosis. *Obstet Gynecol Clin North Am* 1987; 14:581–588.

173. Reid R: Superficial laser vulvectomy. III. A new surgical technique for appendage conserving ablation of refractory condylomas and vulvar intraepithelial neoplasia. *Am J Obstet Gynecol* 1985; 152:540–549.

174. Eron LJ, Judson F, Tucker S, et al: Interferon therapy for condyloma acuminata. *N Engl J Med* 1986; 315:1059–1963.

Polyomaviruses

175. McCance DJ, Gardner SD: Papovaviruses: Papillomaviruses and polyomaviurses, in Zuckerman AJ, Banatvala JE, Pattison JR (eds): *Principles and Practice of Clinical Virology.* Chichester, England, John Wiley & Sons, 1987, pp 479–506.

176. Coleman DV, Gardner SD, Mulholland C, et al: Human polyomaviruses in pregnancy. A model for the study of defence mechanisms to virus reactivation. *Clin Exp Immunol* 1983; 53:289–296.

177. Gibson PE, Field AM, Gardner SD, et al: Occurrence of IgM antibodies against BK and JC polyomaviruses during pregnancy. *J Clin Pathol* 1981; 34:674–679.

178. Rziha HJ, Belohradsky BH, Schneider U, et al: BK virus II: Serologic studies in children with congenital disease and parents with malignant tumors and immunodeficiencies. *Med Microbiol Immunol* 1978; 165:83–92.

179. Coleman DV: Recent developments in the papovaviruses: The human polyoma viruses (BK and JC virus), in Waterson AP (ed): *Recent Advances in Clinical Virology,* ed 2. Edinburgh, Churchill Livingstone, 1980, pp 89–110.

Immunization During Pregnancy

180. General recommendations on immunization. *MMWR* 1989; 38:205–227.

181. Levine MM, Edsall G, Bruce-Chwatt LJ: Live virus vaccines in pregnancy—risks and recommendations. *Lancet* 1974; 2:34–38.

182. Casamassima AC, Hess LW, Marty A: TC-83 Venezuelan equine encephalitis vaccine exposure during pregnancy. *Teratology* 1987; 36:287–289.

183. Amstey MS: Vaccination in pregnancy. *Clin Obstet Gynecol* 1983; 10:13–22.

184. Blanco JD, Gibbs RS: Immunization in pregnancy. *Clin Obstet Gynecol* 1982; 25:611–617.

CHAPTER 15

Neurologic Disorders

N. E. F. Cartlidge

The increasing involvement of internists in the management of pregnant women requires knowledge of the interaction of specific disorders with gestation. Among the medical disorders that afflict women of childbearing age are the common neurologic conditions. Migraine, epilepsy, and multiple sclerosis are the commonest neurologic disorders seen in this age group and each poses special problems. Furthermore, it is not unusual for the busy practitioner to encounter one cerebral bleed and manage a brain tumor during the course of a year. For these and many other reasons it is appropriate to review neurologic disorders and pregnancy. Two books devoted to these topics have appeared within the past few years[1, 2] and recently there has been a review of neurosurgical problems in pregnancy.[3]

For the purposes of this chapter I have adopted a disease-oriented classification. For each disorder the following topics are considered: (1) general discussion; (2) effect of pregnancy on the disease; (3) the effect of the disease on pregnancy; (4) the effect of the disease on the fetus and neonate; and (5) management, including prepregnancy counseling, prenatal management, delivery post partum, and breast-feeding.

The interaction between pregnancy and neurologic disorders occurs as a result of a number of differing pathophysiologic mechanisms.

1. Conditions which result from the physiologic or pathologic changes during pregnancy
2. Conditions which are merely aggravated by the physiologic changes during pregnancy
3. Conditions which result from the procedures or therapy given during pregnancy or at the time of birth

Reference to each of these mechanisms will be made where relevant.

ECLAMPSIA

This is one of the most frightening neurologic problems to be seen in pregnancy and at the same time one of the most serious. For details regarding this condition, see Chap. 1).

VASCULAR DISORDERS

Cerebrovascular disorders are common, occurring either on the basis of vascular occlusion or hemorrhage. Serious neurologic deficits may result from vascular disorders, which are a common cause of death and morbidity in older age groups. Stroke in women of childbearing age is uncommon but when it

TABLE 15–1.
Causes of Spontaneous Subarachnoid Hemorrhage During Pregnancy

Arterial aneurysm
Arteriovenous malformation
Hematologic disorders
    Anticoagulant therapy
    Abruptio placentae with disseminated intravascular
      coagulation
Mycotic aneurysm from subacute bacterial
    endocarditis
Vasculitis (lupus erythematosus)
Metastatic choriocarcinoma
Eclampsia
    Early—hypertensive intracerebral hematomas
    Late—cerebral infarction and multiple petechial
      hemorrhages
Postpartum cerebral phlebothrombosis
Rupture of spinal cord arteriovenous malformation
Ectopic endometriosis

occurs it often results from conditions which in other age groups are unusual.

Under the age of 35 years the annual stroke incidence rate for women is 4.1 per 100,000 and this increases considerably—to 25.7 per 100,000 for ages 35 to 44.[4] Better control of hypertension has led to a decreased stroke mortality in recent years[5] but this will probably have little impact on the incidence of stroke in young women, since atherosclerosis, the development of which is exacerbated by hypertension, is rarely the cause of stroke in women of childbearing age.[6] Overall, it has been estimated that pregnancy increases the risk of ischemic infarction some 13-fold over the expected rate for young women.[7]

Management of the pregnant stroke patient requires first and foremost determination of the precise type of stroke and this will usually require computed tomographic (CT) examination of the head, which with proper abdominal shielding may be performed during pregnancy (see Chap. 18). Magnetic resonance imaging (MRI) of the head has the advantage of being often more sensitive in detecting small ischemic strokes than CT and probably poses less risk to the fetus than does CT scanning.

Spontaneous Subarachnoid Hemorrhage

Ten percent of all maternal deaths occurring to women during pregnancy and the 6 postpartum months are caused by intracranial hemorrhage[8] and subarachnoid hemorrhage is the third most common cause of nonobstetric maternal death.[9] Ninety percent of such deaths occur within a few days of onset of symptoms. The exact incidence during pregnancy is uncertain, but estimates range from 1 to 5 per 10,000 pregnancies. The clinical presentation is usually that of a sudden headache followed by vomiting and in many cases loss of consciousness. Focal neurologic signs may be present resulting from either hemorrhage within the brain or associated cerebral arterial vasospasm.

The management of the pregnant patient who has suffered a suspected subarachnoid hemorrhage should be the same as that of the nonpregnant individual. A CT scan without contrast enhancement should be obtained to try and identify subarachnoid and/or ventricular blood. If blood is not seen on the CT scan, a lumbar puncture should be performed. Once the diagnosis has been confirmed, the next stage is to consider the timing of angiography to outline any vascular pathology that might be present. In the majority of cases either an intracranial aneurysm or arteriovenous malformation will be found. Rarer causes of subarachnoid hemorrhage should be considered (Table 15–1).

The timing of angiography depends on many factors but should not be deferred because the patient is pregnant, as the abdomen can be shielded. Delay may create greater risk through rebleeding.

Intracranial Aneurysms

The risk of rupture of an intracranial aneurysm increases with each trimester of pregnancy. Aneurysms seldom rupture initially during delivery, but rebleeding may occur at that time. Occasionally the development of a subarachnoid hemorrhage from an aneurysm late in pregnancy may precipitate labor.

Once an aneurysm has been demonstrated in a pregnant woman who has suffered a subarachnoid hemorrhage, the best treatment is intracranial clipping. If multiple aneurysms are present, the one responsible for the subarachnoid hemorrhage should be clipped before childbirth. A patient whose aneurysm has been cured can be delivered vaginally with only the usual risks of childbirth.[10] Women with multiple aneurysms or inoperable aneurysms should be delivered by cesarean section. In the rare patient who suffers a ruptured intracranial aneurysm and who then goes into labor, an immediate cesarean section should be performed. There are reports of such cases having immediate intracranial surgery.[11, 12]

Some patients who suffer aneurysmal subarachnoid hemorrhage may die shortly after admission and a decision in such cases will have to be taken regarding removal of the fetus by cesarean section if it is considered appropriate.

Patients who are known to have inoperable intracranial aneurysms should probably avoid pregnancy because of the risk of rupture. The risks are difficult to quantify and each case will have to be treated on its own merits.

Arteriovenous Malformations

Although rare, arteriovenous malformations may cause problems during pregnancy because they tend to bleed during the second trimester and during childbirth. It is assumed that the increased risk of bleeding from malformations during pregnancy occurs either as a result of increasing their size or from increased shunting of blood through the malformation. The highest risk of bleeding is during delivery and this is almost certainly related to the strenuous Valsalva maneuver that labor pains commonly produce.

The best treatment for an intracranial arteriovenous malformation discovered during pregnancy as a result of subarachnoid hemorrhage is total excision. If the malformation is thought to be inoperable, most centers rec-

ommend elective cesarean section at 38 weeks' duration. In patients who suffer a subarachnoid hemorrhage from an arteriovenous malformation during the second trimester, when the intracranial operation might be complex and prolonged, it may be appropriate to defer the operation until after cesarean section.

Medical therapy of subarachnoid hemorrhage in nonpregnant patients includes the use of fibrinolytic and calcium channel blocking agents, the latter recently shown to have a beneficial effect.[13] There are few data concerning the use of aminocaproic acid in pregnancy. However, calcium channel blockers have been used without apparent adverse effect for the treatment of preterm labor[14] and hypertension (see Chap. 1, p. 29). Although the safety of these agents has not been proved, their use in the treatment of subarachnoid hemorrhage during pregnancy appears to be justified by the life-threatening nature of the disease.

Spontaneous Intracranial Hemorrhage

This is a disorder of the older age groups and is invariably associated with hypertension. The diagnosis is usually made by CT scan and the prognosis is poor with a mortality approaching 80%.[15] Primary intracranial hemorrhage is rarely seen during pregnancy. For a discussion of intracranial hemorrhage associated with preeclampsia, see Chapter 1, p. 8.

Ischemic Cerebrovascular Disease

The sudden onset of a hemiplegia without headache and with preserved consciousness is typical of cerebral infarction. Such events are infrequent in young women, but the risk increases with age, pregnancy, and the use of oral contraceptives. Most cases of cerebral infarction during pregnancy result from arterial occlusion rather than cerebral venous thrombosis.[16]

Various studies have suggested an incidence of 1 ischemic stroke per 3,000 pregnancies, at least 10 times the risk of stroke for young nonpregnant women.[17]

The majority of such strokes involve the carotid artery and in those in whom angiography has been performed, middle cerebral artery occlusions are twice as common in pregnancy-associated strokes compared with a nonpregnant cohort.[16] There are great uncertainties as to why vascular disease is more common in women who are pregnant or taking oral contraceptives and no attempt will be made to review the extensive literature on this topic. Suffice it to say that a stroke in a young pregnant woman warrants a full and detailed investigation looking for unusual causes (Table 15–2). In one fourth of cases no obvious cause will be found and only one fourth will be shown to have premature atherosclerosis with hypertension, diabetes, or hyperlipidemia. The remaining half will have an unusual condition and most of these may be diagnosed on the basis of a thorough history, physical examination, and noninvasive investigations. If an obvious answer is not found, a decision will have to be made regarding angiography. There are differing views regarding the use of this investigation in the nonpregnant patient with stroke and the author believes that this is rarely indicated in pregnancy.

Anticoagulation for young pregnant women who have suffered a stroke should, in general, be avoided. However, indications include stroke occurring in association with atrial fibrillation, peripartum cardiomyopathy, and hypercoagulable states. Heparin is the preferred anticoagulant as it does not cross the placental barrier. Subcutaneous heparin can be given throughout pregnancy (see Chap. 6).

The prognosis for young pregnant women who have suffered a stroke is usually good unless there is evidence of underlying serious disease. Women who have suffered a cerebral ischemic stroke during pregnancy for which no cause can be found have a low risk of further episodes during subsequent pregnancies. Oral contraceptives should probably be avoided in women who have suffered a cerebral ischemic stroke during pregnancy.

Cerebral Venous Thrombosis

This is now an uncommon form of cerebrovascular disease and is usually seen in children in association with dehydration, polycythemia, leukemia, sickle cell crisis, and paroxysmal nocturnal hemoglobinuria. In women of childbearing age it is most commonly seen in association with either pregnancy, the puerperium, or oral contraceptives.[18]

Puerperal cerebral venous thrombosis is estimated to occur in between 1 in 2,500 and 1 in 10,000 deliveries.[19] Most commonly it develops some 3 to 30 days after childbirth. Eighty percent of cases begin in the second

TABLE 15–2.
Unusual Causes of Ischemic Stroke in Pregnancy and the Puerperium

Blood vessel disorders
  Vasculitides
    Systemic lupus erythematosus
    Polyarteritis nodosa
    Syphilis
  Takayasu disease
  Fibromuscular dysplasia
  Arterial dissection
    Spontaneous
    Traumatic
  Moyamoya disease

Embolism
  Paradoxical embolus
  Nonbacterial thrombotic endocarditis
  Fat or air embolism
  Aminotic fluid embolism
  Mitral valve prolapse
  Valvular heart disease
  Infective endocarditis

Hematologic Disorders
  Sickle hemoglobinopathies
  Thrombotic thrombocytopenic purpura
  Paroxysmal nocturnal hemoglobinuria

Miscellaneous
  Migraine
  Alcohol intoxication
  Drug abuse
  Metastatic trophoblastic carcinoma
  Eclampsia

or third postpartum weeks, age and parity are not determining factors, and labor and delivery are characteristically normal. The reasons for the development of cerebral venous thrombosis are unknown. Higher concentrations of some of the clotting factors are found during pregnancy but the significance of these is uncertain.

The clinical features depend on the site of venous thrombosis and the commonest site is thought to be within the cortical venous system. Headache is often an early feature followed by focal or generalized seizures and then by focal neurologic deficits, impairment of consciousness, signs of raised intracranial pressure, and coma.

Mild fever and leukocytosis may be present and a CT scan should be performed, which will usually show evidence of cerebral infarction with or without associated hemorrhagic areas, the appearance known as hemorrhagic infarction. Angiography is rarely indicated though may show a diagnostic appearance in the venous phase.

Mortality in some series has been as high as 30%. Impairment of consciousness and rapid progression of neurologic signs are bad prognostic indicators. In those who survive, the prognosis for recovery of neurologic function is usually good.

Symptomatic treatment in the form of maintaining hydration and treating seizures is important and the major decision is in relation to the need for anticoagulation. It is essential that a CT scan be performed before a decision is made regarding anticoagulation. A normal scan or an appearance of cerebral infarction should lead to early treatment with intravenous heparin.[20] The presence of significant hemorrhage on CT scan is generally regarded as a contraindication to anticoagulation.

There is no information in the literature concerning the risk of recurrence of cortical venous thrombosis in subsequent pregnancies. Common sense would suggest that it would be wise to avoid further pregnancies and it also appears advisable to avoid the use of oral contraceptives.

Spontaneous Carotid-Cavernous Fistulas

These fistulas occur as a result of shunts developing and enlarging between the tiny meningeal branches of the internal carotid artery and the cavernous sinus. They also occur as a result of rupture of intracavernous carotid aneurysms. Patients present with unilateral headache in association with conjunctival hyperemia, exophthalmos, retinal venous distention, and oculomotor paresis; an orbital bruit may be present and occasionally there is impairment of vision.

At all ages women are affected more than men, by a 3:1 margin. Twenty-five percent of all affected women develop the syndrome during the second half of pregnancy or during the puerperium.[2] The diagnosis may be confirmed by carotid angiography. Spontaneous resolution may occur, though surgical treatment may be indicated.[21]

NEUROPATHIES

Mononeuropathies During Pregnancy

Idiopathic Facial Palsy (Bell's Palsy)

This is a common condition at any age associated with the sudden development of a unilateral facial weakness which is often discovered in the morning when the patient awakes to find one half of the face paralyzed. Loss of taste on the anterior two thirds of the tongue is lost if the lesion is proximal to the branch of the chorda tympani and hyperacusis is present if the nerve to the stapedius is involved. Pain in and around the ear may be present. The etiology is uncertain though there is some evidence to suggest that Bell's palsy in the younger age group may be a viral mononeuropathy, whereas in older age groups it may be a manifestation of vascular disturbances.[22]

The incidence of women of childbearing age is 17 per 100,000 per year whereas the frequency during pregnancy and the first 2 postpartum weeks is 57 per 100,000 per year.[23] Three fourths of cases during pregnancy occur in the third trimester and the early puerperium. Recurrence during subsequent pregnancies is recognized.[24] The prognosis for patients with a partial facial palsy is usually good. A short course of prednisone may improve the prognosis and is not contraindicated during pregnancy.[23] The author prefers to use a 6-day course of oral prednisolone beginning with 60 mg on the first day and reducing the dose by 10 mg/day. The development of Bell's palsy does not affect the course of pregnancy.

Carpal Tunnel Syndrome

This is the most common nerve compression syndrome and is particularly common in pregnancy. Typical symptoms are those of pain or paresthesia in the hands developing in the early morning and often the pain radiates into the forearm.

As many as 25% of pregnant women may suffer from symptoms of the carpal tunnel syndrome, which usually develops between the fourth and ninth months of gestation.[25] Edema within the carpal tunnel is thought to be the commonest factor precipitating symptoms. Resolution of symptoms occurs in over 80% of pregnant women, usually within 2 to 3 months postdelivery. Occasionally symptoms may resolve much earlier.

Because of the good prognosis, treatment should be symptomatic and often reassurance is all that is required. A lightweight splint worn at the wrist may be of value and occasionally a corticosteroid injection into the carpal tunnel may be indicated. Nerve conduction studies are rarely necessary to confirm the diagnosis during pregnancy. For those whose symptoms do not resolve, surgical decompression should be considered.

Meralgia Paraesthetica

This is a minor but sometimes bothersome disorder of pregnancy occurring as a result of compression of the lateral cutaneous nerve of the thigh under the ilioinguinal ligament. Numbness, tingling, and pain occurring over the lateral aspect of the thigh are typical symptoms. The symptoms are exaggerated by standing or extending the leg and are relieved by sitting or lying.

Symptoms usually begin about the 30th week of gestation and may be bilateral.[26] Resolution invariably occurs following delivery though symptoms may recur in subsequent pregnancies. Surgical decompression of the nerve is rarely required during pregnancy.

Other Mononeuropathies

Other mononeuropathies during pregnancy are uncommon. In one series 2% of pregnant women complained of symptoms of ulnar nerve compression but there is probably no clear association of this disorder with pregnancy.[25]

One study has suggested that compression of the posterior tibial nerve at the ankle is a common cause of leg cramps or burning feet in pregnant women.[27] This is the so-called tarsal tunnel syndrome. Generally speaking, this is thought to be a rare disorder and confirmation of this study is awaited with interest.

There are occasional cases recorded of intercostal neuralgia occurring during pregnancy.[28]

Polyneuropathy and Pregnancy

Genetically Determined Neuropathies

Charcot-Marie-Tooth Disease (hereditary motor and sensory neuropathy type 1).—This is an autosomal dominant neuropathy associated with slowly progressive symmetric muscle atrophy affecting the feet and legs and ultimately the hands and forearms. Peripheral sensory loss is often present. The muscular weakness is rarely of a degree to have any significant effect on pregnancy but there are reports of patients with the condition becoming worse during pregnancy.[29] Improvement following delivery occurred and there was no effect on the fetus. The 50% risk of the fetus developing the condition will need to be discussed with parents.

Acute Intermittent Porphyria.—This is an inborn error of metabolism which affects

TABLE 15–3.
Factors Thought to Precipitate an
Acute Crisis in Porphyria

1. Drugs
   Barbiturates
   Sulfonamides
   Griseofulvin
   Phenytoin
   Estrogens
   Progesterone
   Oral contraceptives
2. Fasting
3. Acute febrile illnesses
4. Surgical procedures
5. Pregnancy

females more than males and is inherited as an autosomal dominant. Typically the neuropathy develops acutely in association with preceding abdominal pain and psychiatric disturbances in the form of depression or psychosis.

For most women pregnancy has no ill effects upon acute intermittent porphyria though over 100 exacerbations during pregnancy have been reported.[2] Sixty percent of these relapses occur in early pregnancy and do not affect the eventual outcome of the pregnancy.

More serious are the 15% of relapses which occur during the second or third trimester. Prematurity and high maternal and fetal mortality rates are common problems. Postpartum cases account for the remaining 25%. The children of porphyric mothers are normal at birth regardless of genotype.

The best treatment is prevention and avoidance of precipitating factors (Table 15–3). Although pregnancy is a well-recognized precipitating factor there are insufficient grounds for recommending that patients with porphyria avoid pregnancy. Symptomatic treatment is important in the management of abdominal symptoms and a variety of specific treatments have been tried. Of these the use of an infusion of hematin appears to be the most successful.[30] It appears to be safe and may be used during pregnancy. The greatest risk for a pregnant woman occurs when the existence of acute intermittent porphyria is unknown and symptoms develop for the first time during the pregnancy.

Genetic counseling is important and should involve a biochemical screen of all members of the family; although the disease is transmitted as an autosomal dominant trait, not all affected individuals are symptomatic.

Oral contraceptives should be avoided in patients who have porphyria or in those who are first-degree relatives of affected individuals.

Acquired Polyneuropathy and Pregnancy

Guillain-Barré Syndrome.—This is an acute inflammatory polyneuropathy of rapid onset associated in most incidences with profound muscular weakness. The condition occurs in both sexes and in all age groups, though it is less common in the very young and the elderly. The simultaneous occurrence of Guillain-Barré syndrome and pregnancy is probably coincidental and approximately 30 cases have been reported in the obstetric literature over the past 70 years.[31, 32] There is no evidence that the pregnancy affects the severity of the syndrome and the pregnancy appears to be unaffected. Parturition is usually normal. As with other illnesses associated with muscular weakness, uterine contractility is not impaired but in cases with weakness in the abdominal muscles second-stage assistance may be necessary.

In the third trimester there is a risk of premature labor. Fetal prognosis is generally favorable and most infants born to mothers with the Guillain-Barré syndrome are normal. (See Chap. 7, p. 252, for management of pregnant patients on mechanical ventilators.)

Chronic Inflammatory Demyelinating Polyneuropathy.—This is a slowly progressive demyelinating peripheral neuropathy which presents with slowly progressive motor and sensory deficits. The condition may show relapses and remissions and some cases have been described where a relapse has occurred during the course of a pregnancy.[33]

Gestational Distal Polyneuropathy.—This syndrome has now virtually disappeared from the Western World as a result of proper prenatal care and maintenance of good nutrition in pregnant mothers. It is similar if not identical to alcoholic peripheral neuropathy and beriberi. The cause is deficiency of the vitamin B group, notably thiamine, and in some instances the peripheral neuropathy is associated with the Wernicke-Korsakoff syndrome.[34] Apart from malnutrition, other etiological factors include alcoholism, hyperemesis gravidarum, and fad diets.[35]

Mortality in affected cases may be high, as is the fetal death rate. Treatment is by vitamin B complex administration intravenously.

Leprosy.—This is the most common cause of neuropathy worldwide and may occur in pregnancy and the puerperium.[36] It is considered further in Chapter 16.

Other Disorders Possibly of Peripheral Nerve Origin

The Restless Leg Syndrome

In this syndrome patients develop vague aching symptoms in the legs which are most pronounced at night and which are associated with an irresistible urge to move the legs. Relief is obtained by standing up and walking and insomnia may result.

Similar symptoms occur in as many as from 10% to 30% of pregnancies.[37] Symptoms usually resolve after delivery. The phenothiazine drug Largactil (unavailable in the United States at time of this writing) or the benzodiazepine clonazepam (FDA risk C) are effective forms of treatment but should be reserved for the rare patient with intractable disabling symptoms.

Leg Cramps

Cramps in the calves occur in up to 30% of pregnant women[38] and the cramps may spread to the thighs and buttocks. The symptoms mostly occur at night and claims have been made for a variety of different treatments. No randomized controlled treatment trials have been done.

MYONEURAL JUNCTION DISORDERS

Myasthenia Gravis

This is a rare disorder characterized by muscle fatigability. Prevalence is of the order of 40 cases per million population[39] and females are affected twice as commonly as males. The peak incidence of the disease occurs in the third decade. The basic defect in myasthenia gravis is at the neuromuscular junction where it is believed that antibodies to the acetylcholine receptor block the effect of acetylcholine released from the presynaptic membrane.

There is now good evidence that myasthenia gravis is an autoimmune disease and antibodies to the acetylcholine receptor may be detected in the serum of 90% of patients with myasthenia gravis.[40] As many as 75% of myasthenic patients have thymic abnormalities, most commonly thymic hyperplasia and less commonly (10%–15%) thymic tumors (thymomas).[41]

Muscle fatigue is the cardinal symptom and typically this begins in the extraocular muscles and other bulbar muscles and then spreads to the arms, legs, and trunk. The anticholinesterase group of drugs produces symptomatic improvement, the most effective drug being pyridostigmine given every 4 hours.

Recently there has been interest in manipulating the immune system. Thymectomy, particularly in young women, may be associated with remission of symptoms and the use of corticosteroids and other immunosuppressive drugs have become more widespread in recent years.

Effect of Pregnancy on Myasthenia Gravis

Pregnancy has an unpredictable but often profound effect on myasthenia gravis. The disease may remain stable, undergo partial or complete remission, or exacerbate, and the effect may vary in different pregnancies.[42–45] The majority of relapses or remissions of the disease tend to be established during the first trimester of pregnancy.[46] There is some evidence to suggest that the greatest risk of death from myasthenia gravis during a pregnancy is in the first year of the disease and that the risk decreases considerably thereafter. It has therefore been suggested that postponement of pregnancy is justified in newly diagnosed cases of myasthenia gravis.[47] Although management may be difficult in a newly diagnosed patient with myasthenia gravis who is pregnant, early therapeutic abortion is probably not justified.

The effect of pregnancy on the thymic hyperplasia associated with myasthenia gravis is unknown. However, there is some evidence to suggest that pregnancy has an adverse effect upon malignant thymoma.[48]

Effect of Myasthenia Gravis on Pregnancy

The effect of myasthenia gravis on pregnancy is small and there is no effect on fertility. There is a small increase in the incidence of spontaneous abortion but no increase in the prematurity rate or in the risk of pre-eclampsia.[49]

Management

The basic scheme of management is to ensure adequate rest for the mother and there should be careful supervision of medication and regular consultation with a neurologist (Table 15–4). In general, the usual drug therapy may be maintained and there is no evidence that anticholinesterase medication has any adverse effect on the uterus or fetus. Patients already established on prednisone and/or azathioprine pose special problems because of the risks to the fetus of these drugs. The risks of prednisone are small, but there may be a significant teratogenic risk from aza-

TABLE 15–4.
Management of Myasthenia Gravis (MG) During Gestation

1. Suspect MG if bulbar muscle weakness or respiratory difficulty develops. Confirm diagnosis with electromyography (repetitive stimulation, single-fiber studies) and serum antiacetylcholine receptor antibody titer.

2. In patients with an established diagnosis of MG, assess efficacy of treatment regimen (evaluation of muscle strength and vital capacity after and between medication doses).

3. If oral medication cannot be tolerated early in pregnancy, switch to the parenteral route.

4. Treat all infections aggressively and promptly.

5. Medications	Dosage	Maternal Side Effects
Anticholinesterase drugs Pyridostigmine bromide [C]* (Mestinon)	Begin with 15–30 mg q3–4h and then titrate dosage; may use timed-release capsule (180 mg) at night	Abdominal cramps, flatulence, diarrhea, nausea, vomiting, excessive secretion
Immunosuppressive drugs Prednisone [B]*	60–80 mg/day until improvement occurs	Patient should be hospitalized, since weakness may initially become worse on steroids

6. *Drugs to be avoided*: sedatives; aminoglycoside antibiotics (streptomycin, gentamycin, kanamycin); other antibiotics (tetracycline, colistin, neomycin, polymyxin, lincomycin); quinidine; **magnesium sulphate**; penicillamine; lithium; propranolol.

7. At the first sign of any respiratory difficulties transfer patient to intensive care unit.

8. Medications should be given parenterally during labor. Assistance with low forceps may be required.

9. Observe infant for signs of neonatal myasthenia gravis.

*[ ] = FDA risk category. See Preface for description of FDA risk classification.

thioprine. It should be noted, however, that a large number of women with renal transplants have had successful pregnancy outcomes while taking prednisone and azathioprine (see Chap. 2). Nonetheless, myasthenic patients taking these drugs should consider delaying pregnancy until disease improvement permits discontinuation of immunosuppressive agents.

The development of myasthenia gravis during pregnancy may require aggressive treatment to manipulate the immune system. Plasmapheresis may be performed in pregnancy, and there are reports of thymectomy being performed with successful results.[50]

Obstetric Management.—Labor and delivery are normal although muscle weakness may affect the second stage, requiring appropriate intervention. Cesarean section is warranted for obstetric reasons only.

Anesthesia.—Regional anesthesia is preferred and because of possible precipitating respiratory compromise, narcotic analgesia is best avoided.

Postpartum Management.—Decompensation during the postpartum period occurs in as many as one third of patients and careful observation is necessary.[51] Particular attention should be paid to avoiding infections and rest should be encouraged. Breastfeeding is permitted as normally.

Neonatal Myasthenia

Transient muscle weakness occurs in 12% of the babies born to myasthenic mothers. The neuromuscular symptoms usually develop within the first few days of life, most within hours of birth. Symptoms persist for just a few weeks. The symptoms appear to be produced by the acetylcholine receptor antibody crossing the placental barrier and entering the fetal circulation.[52]

All newborn children of myasthenic mothers should be carefully observed for muscle weakness, such as difficulty with feeding, floppiness, a weak Moro reflex, a feeble cry,

or respiratory distress. There appears to be no relation between duration and severity of the disease in the mother and the development of myasthenia in the baby. Three fourths of affected infants require anticholinesterase drugs and the response is usually excellent.[53]

MUSCLE DISORDERS

Muscle disorders are termed *myopathies* and are conveniently divided into the genetically determined myopathies, which include the muscular dystrophies, and the acquired myopathies.

Myopathies are characterized by muscle weakness which usually begins in the proximal muscles affecting the shoulder and the pelvic girdles. The most common obstetric problem is that of a pregnancy occurring in a patient with established muscle disease. Occasionally, acquired myopathies may develop during pregnancy and these produce special problems.

Genetically Determined Myopathy

Myotonic Dystrophy

This form of muscular dystrophy, which is inherited as an autosomal dominant, is characterized by the phenomenon of myotonia, which is a slowness of muscular relaxation. The condition is progressive and is associated with muscular weakness, which rarely, until the later stages of the disease, causes severe incapacity. However, myotonic dystrophy shows considerable variation in the extent and severity of the neurologic problems. Common associated features of the condition are cataracts, mental retardation, premature balding, decreased fertility, and cardiomyopathy.

Pregnancy is thought to be relatively uncommon, but one study described the course and outcome of 23 pregnancies in six women affected by myotonic dystrophy.[54] A high rate of complications was noted including polyhydramnios, premature onset of labor, cesarean section, postpartum hemorrhage, and neonatal death. One problem is that the uterine muscles may be affected leading to problems during labor. Indeed, prolonged labor has been a consistent complication of pregnancy in myotonic dystrophy.[55] Failure of the emptied uterus to contract may cause profuse postpartum hemorrhage.

Maternal death may occur in pregnant patients with myotonic dystrophy as a result of either cardiac failure or pneumonia and this is more likely to occur in severely affected patients and in those patients who have a cardiomyopathy as a complication of the condition.

A regional anesthetic is preferred.[56] Depolarizing muscle relaxation causes severe spasms and hyperthermia, while nondepolarizing agents such as curare can be used safely.[57]

One manifestation of the variability of myotonic dystrophy is that mildly affected mothers may produce severely affected children. Indeed, the dystrophy may become clinically manifest in utero and at birth the child may have the characteristics of the so-called floppy baby.

Genetic counseling is important because of the dominant mode of inheritance. The gene is located on the proximal long arm of chromosome 19, tightly linked to apolipoprotein C-2 near the marker for secretor. By analyzing amniotic fluid for secretor or apolipoprotein C-2, a prenatal diagnosis can be established.[58]

Myotonia Congenita

This is a dominantly inherited muscle disorder characterized by myotonia and increased muscle development without muscle weakness. Symptoms, which include muscle cramps, may be present from childhood.

The myotonia tends to become worse during the second half of the pregnancy[59] and recovery occurs after childbirth. No obstetric problems are likely to be encountered. The infants may have difficulty in feeding due to myotonia of the tongue.

Other Forms of Muscular Dystrophy

Pregnancy in other forms of muscular dystrophy is rare. The two problems most likely to cause difficulty are muscle weakness, resulting in poor pushing during the second stage of labor, and the genetic implications for children.

Acquired Myopathies

Polymyositis and Related Disorders

This group of disorders can be regarded as falling into the category of the so-called connective tissue disorders. They are the commonest forms of acquired myopathy and are characterized by muscular weakness, often with associated muscle pain. Treatment is with corticosteroids in addition to cytotoxic immunosuppressive drugs such as azathioprine.

There is a variable effect on muscle weakness but there is a high infant mortality rate of between 40% and 50%.[60, 61] Continued treatment with corticosteroids during pregnancy is necessary and this does not appear to have any serious adverse effect. Use of cytotoxic immunosuppressives requires a careful analysis of maternal benefits and potential fetal risks (see also Chap. 11).

Other Acquired Myopathies

There are rare case reports of other forms of acquired myopathy occurring in pregnancy, for example, hypokalemic myopathy,[62] without adverse effect on mother or child.

SPINAL CORD DISORDERS

Spinal Cord Injury

The incidence of spinal cord injury is thought to be 30 to 50 per million population of whom over half are between the ages of 15 to 30 years.[63] Cervical and thoracic cord damage accounts for 90% of all such injuries and over one third result from automobile accidents.

There is an extensive literature to show that paraplegics and even quadriplegics can be successful mothers.[64–66] Sexual intercourse is possible and fertility is unaffected. Orgasm is absent if both spinothalamic tracts are severed.

The pregnant spinal cord–injured female is at risk for a number of special problems. Anemia is common and urinary tract infections are more of a problem. The treatment of both of these is important because they may predispose to bed sores. Constipation is often aggravated; management of this problem is discussed in Chapter 9. Most women are able to continue with their usual bladder management until late in pregnancy when it may be necessary to use indwelling urethral catheterization.

Labor Management

Uterine contractility is not usually affected after spinal cord damage and therefore delivery via the vagina is preferred. Patients with damage above the lower thoracic segments have painless labor and because there may be difficulty in gauging the onset of uterine contractions, precipitous labor may occur. It is generally recommended that the pregnant paraplegic should be admitted at 32 to 34 weeks and have daily examinations. Continuous epidural anesthesia is usually successful and may prevent autonomic hyperreflexia (see below). One interesting observation is that catgut stitches are poorly absorbed by paraplegics. Breast-feeding is usually successful.[66]

Autonomic Hyperreflexia

This is the result of overstimulation of the splanchnic nerves uninhibited by higher centers. It involves a sudden reflex sympathetic discharge below the level of the cord damage resulting in throbbing headache, facial flushing, dilated pupils, sweating, and paroxysmal hypertension. The reflex may be stimulated by bladder distention, rectal digital examination, genital stimulation, and labor. The higher the level of the cord damage the greater the severity of the reaction.

It is important to distinguish autonomic hyperreflexia from preeclampsia, the incidence of which is not increased in paraplegics.[65]

Treatment involves general measures such as elevation of the head and bladder drainage, and pharmacologic measures such as the use of antihypertensive drugs.

Spinal Cord Tumors

Coexistence of spinal cord tumors in pregnancy is rare but as with cerebral tumors (see below) there may be rapid worsening of the signs during pregnancy.[67]

If a spinal cord tumor is suspected during pregnancy all the necessary radiographic investigations should be done despite radiation risk to the fetus. Where available magnetic resonance image scanning is the investigation of choice because of its safety. Each condition will need to be treated on its own merits.

Backache and Lumbar Disc Disease

Back pain is an almost universal symptom of pregnancy occurring in at least 50% of pregnant women.[68] The pain is thought to be musculoskeletal in origin resulting from relaxation of spinal joints and extenuation of the lumbar lordosis. Pain may also occur as a result of dysfunction of the sacroiliac joints. Treatment involves restriction of activity, localized heat, simple analgesics, and the avoidance of high-heeled shoes.

Acute herniation of a lumbar disc is uncommon during pregnancy, occurring in approximately 1 in 10,000 pregnancies.[69] Pain radiating to the leg (sciatica) is typical and appropriate signs of nerve root compression may be found. Conservative measures in the form of bed rest and analgesics are the treatment of choice.

Maternal Obstetric Palsies

Damage to the lumbosacral plexus may occur as a result of either trauma from the fetal head or from the forceps. The incidence has been calculated at between 1 in 2,600 to 1 in 6,400 deliveries.[70, 71]

The most susceptible portion of the plexus is the anterior division composed of the fourth and fifth lumbar roots. Pain in the leg during delivery is the most common complaint. The

TABLE 15–5.
Central Nervous System Infections in Pregnancy

Bacterial
  Purulent meningitis
    Rare; treatment satisfactory[72]
  Tuberculous meningitis
    3rd trimester; treatment appears to be safe[73]
  Syphilis
    See Chapter 13
  Lyme disease
    Transplacental infection[74]
Viral
  Polio
    Acute: risk of abortion[75]
    Chronic: effect on delivery
  Encephalitis
    Herpes simplex; treatment appears to be safe[76]
Other
  Cryptococcal meningitis[77]

---

most common residual deficit is weakness of ankle dorsiflexion and footdrop. Less common is damage to the femoral, obturator, or sciatic nerve. Neurophysiologic investigations in the form of electromyography and nerve conduction studies may localize the site of damage.

Treatment involves the use of appropriate splints, physiotherapy, and reassurance. Prognosis is usually good and may be determined accurately on the basis of the neurophysiologic investigations. Prevention of intrapelvic entrapment neuropathies during subsequent pregnancies requires recognition of any underlying cephalopelvic disproportion.

Complications of Regional Anesthesia

Epidural anesthesia causes less than one neurologic complication per 15,000 to 20,000 epidural blocks, most of which are transient. The most serious acute complication is the misplaced injection of local anesthetic. Epidural hematomas and abscess are rare. Postlumbar headache is more common in women who have had a spinal anesthetic and the incidence of this may be reduced by using smaller-gauge needles.

INFECTIONS OF THE NERVOUS SYSTEM

Any organism that can infect the nonpregnant patient is capable of infecting the pregnant patient. In general, the treatment of the infection can proceed despite the pregnancy, though knowledge of the potential adverse fetal effects of the agents used should be obtained. Special problems arise when the infected agent crosses the placental barrier (see below).

Table 15–5 presents a summary of some of the infections that may be seen in pregnancy.

Chronic Viral Infections (Slow Viruses)

These include the agents responsible for subacute sclerosing panencephalitis, kuru, and acquired immunodeficiency syndrome (AIDS). Of these only the last-named is likely to be seen with any degree of regularity; this is discussed in Chapter 14, p. 489.

Chorea Gravidarum

There is debate as to whether this condition should be included under infections because of the known association between chorea and the use of oral contraceptives.[78] However, there is an even stronger link of the condition with rheumatic fever and many believe that chorea gravidarum should be regarded as a manifestation of "rheumatic brain disease."

The incidence of chorea gravidarum is less than 1 case per 3,000 deliveries[79] and the average age of the affected women is 22. Eighty percent of attacks occur during the first pregnancy and half start in the first trimester. Sixty percent of women have previously had rheumatic chorea. One third of cases improved prepartum with remission of symptoms in the remainder soon after delivery.

There is no evidence that the malformation or abortion rate is higher but one fourth of patients will have recurrence during subsequent pregnancies.[80] Oral contraceptives should be avoided by women who have suffered from chorea gravidarum.

MULTIPLE SCLEROSIS

This is the commonest of the so-called demyelinating disorders, the clinical effects resulting from multiple focal areas of damage to central nervous system myelinated pathways. Age of onset is usually between the ages of 20 and 40 with a female preponderance.

The condition is characterized by a relapsing remitting course with considerable variation in the severity and frequency of relapses. The etiology is unknown and no specific treatment consistently influences disease progression.

Fertility

There is no evidence that fertility is affected in multiple sclerosis, though women with multiple sclerosis probably have fewer children than expected. This may be because females remain unmarried, elect to have fewer children, or become divorced because of increasing and severe disability. Some women with severe disease who have severe spastic paralysis of the legs and indwelling catheters may be incapable of having normal sexual relations.[81]

Effect of Pregnancy on Multiple Sclerosis

It has often been thought that a pregnancy might have an adverse effect on the disease process of multiple sclerosis, but more recent studies have modified this viewpoint.[82-85] The problem is that multiple sclerosis shows marked variability from patient to patient and it has required considerable statistical ingenuity and analysis of many pregnant and nonpregnant multiple sclerosis patients to provide useful information. Some of the available data are presented in Table 15–6.

Table 15–6 is concerned with the *pregnancy year*, defined as the 9 months of pregnancy and the 3-month postpartum period. From this information it can be concluded that fewer relapses can be expected during the 9 months of pregnancy but that half of all relapses during the pregnancy year occur during the puerperium. There is considerable debate as to why relapses are more common during the puerperium, but this is unknown.

Effect of Multiple Sclerosis on Pregnancy

Uncomplicated multiple sclerosis has almost no effect on pregnancy and usually no change in the management of delivery need be made.[83] The rate of congenital malformations among infants of women with multiple sclerosis is no greater than expected.

Problems arise with the handicapped patient with multiple sclerosis during pregnancy. Fatigability may become more of a problem and patients with neurogenic bladder problems are more prone to develop infections. The patient who is paraplegic should be managed as above. Vaginal delivery is usually possible unless there are specific obstetric contraindications. There is some evidence to

TABLE 15–6.
Relapse Rate of Multiple Sclerosis During Pregnancy Year*

Study	No. of Patients	No. of Pregnancies	Relapse Overall	Pregnancy Year	9 Months	Puerperium
Muller[85]	15	15	0.22	0.18	—	—
McAlpine & Compston[86]	24	33	0.39	0.33	—	—
Millar[87]	70	170	0.10	0.27	0.04	0.95
Korn-Lubetski et al[84]	338	199	0.28	0.43	0.10	0.82
Ghezzi & Kaputo[88]	119	206	0.29	0.36	0.21	1.74

*Adapted from Goldstein PJ: *Neurological Disorders of Pregnancy.* New York, Futura Publishing Co, Inc, 1986.

suggest that spinal anesthesia should be avoided and if cesarean section is desirable on obstetric grounds, general anesthetics should be used.[83, 89]

Management

A number of factors need to be considered in counseling women with multiple sclerosis about pregnancy[90]:

1. *Risks to the mother*. Apart from severely incapacitated women with multiple sclerosis, pregnancy appears to be safe.
2. *Risks to the baby*. It is clear that the children and siblings of patients with multiple sclerosis have an increased risk of developing the disease.[91]
3. *Child rearing*. In a disease such as multiple sclerosis, which is progressive, it is important that this aspect be considered fully by physician, patient, and spouse. Clearly, the more severely affected the patient, the more carefully this will have to be considered.

The treatment of acute relapses of multiple sclerosis during pregnancy can be the same as that of nonpregnant women. A short course of steroids may be given with reasonable safety, as may adrenocorticotropic hormone (ACTH).

A previously healthy woman may present with her first clinical manifestation of multiple sclerosis during pregnancy and it may be necessary to image the central nervous system either by CT, myelography, or ideally, if available, by MRI scanning. Lumbar puncture may be safely performed during pregnancy and there is no contraindication to investigation by evoked response studies.

Breast-feeding can be allowed in patients with multiple sclerosis. The use of oral contraceptives in patients with multiple sclerosis should probably be avoided, though hard data to support this assertion are not readily available.

BRAIN TUMORS

There is no evidence that brain tumors occur more commonly or present more commonly during pregnancy. However, the physiologic changes that occur during pregnancy may predispose a preexisting tumor to present for the first time. This is particularly likely to occur with pituitary tumors (see Chap. 4). The enlargement of tumors in pregnancy is thought to occur as a result of changes in salt and water balance and patients may even present with symptoms of a brain tumor during pregnancy with subsequent resolution following delivery. It has been shown that there are estrogen receptors in some meningiomas[92] and the hormonal changes of pregnancy might thus stimulate growth of meningiomas.

It is difficult to lay down absolute rules for the management of a pregnancy of a woman with a brain tumor. Investigations such as CT and MRI may be performed and with current techniques of neurosurgery appropriate surgical attack should be possible.[93, 94] In patients near to term it may be appropriate to delay such surgery until after delivery because the tumor may shrink and make the operation that much easier. The most difficult decisions are those in women with malignant tumors.[95] Women with malignancies and those with partially resected benign tumors are best advised to avoid pregnancy because of the risk of deterioration.

The oral contraceptive preparations may be used in women with malignant tumors but should be avoided in those with meningiomas.

Benign Intracranial Hypertension (Pseudotumor Cerebri)

This condition is associated with raised intracranial pressure without evidence of local intracranial space-occupying lesion. The cause is unknown though it is thought to result from overproduction or underabsorption of cerebrospinal fluid (CSF). Headache is a cardinal symptom and most patients show papilledema but no focal neurologic signs. Visual impairment may result from the pap-

TABLE 15–7.
The International Classification of Epileptic Seizures

I. Partial (focal, local) seizures
  A. Simple partial seizures (consciousness not impaired)
    1. With motor signs
    2. With sensory symptoms
    3. With autonomic symptoms (e.g., epigastric sensation)
    4. With psychic symptoms (e.g., déjà vu, macropsia)
  B. Complex partial seizures (consciousness is impaired)
  C. Partial seizures evolving to secondarily generalized seizures
II. Generalized seizures
  A. (1) Absence seizures
    (2) Atypical absence seizures
  B. Myoclonic seizures
  C. Tonic seizures
  D. Tonic-clonic seizures
  E. Atonic seizures
III. Unclassified epileptic seizures (e.g., due to inadequate or incomplete data)

illedema and occasionally false localizing signs in the form of a lateral rectus palsy may be seen.

For the pregnant woman who presents with headaches and papilledema it is important that a firm diagnosis be established and this will usually require some form of imaging of the brain, either CT or MRI. Lumbar punctures may be difficult to perform in pregnancy but the CSF pressure in a suspected case of benign intracranial hypertension should always be measured to confirm the diagnosis. The CSF constituents are normal.

Reviews of benign intracranial hypertension in pregnancy[96–99] suggest that it tends to present between the second and fifth months of pregnancy with a tendency to be more common in women who are obese. The pathogenesis is uncertain though hormonal changes during pregnancy may be important. The condition is self-limited and tends to resolve after delivery.

Management involves the use of regular lumbar punctures to reduce the CSF pressure and in cases where there is gross papilledema with visual impairment, dexamethasone may produce rapid improvement. In cases where there is no resolution of symptoms and vision is threatened, lumboperitoneal shunting is an effective treatment. With current methods of management therapeutic abortion is now rarely indicated.

There is a low risk of recurrence in future pregnancies. Oral contraceptives should probably be avoided.

Maternal Hydrocephalus

An increasing number of women with indwelling CSF shunts for the treatment of hydrocephalus are now reaching maturity and becoming pregnant. In the cases reported thus far the outcome has been satisfactory and obstetric management can be continued with only one special precaution: Subarachnoid injection of anesthetic agents should be avoided.

Complication rates are fewer and less severe with ventriculoperitoneal shunts compared to ventriculoatrial shunts and these may be installed and revised during pregnancy. Prophylactic antibiotics should be given during childbirth to patients with shunts.

EPILEPSY

This is one of the most common neurologic disorders and certainly one of the most frequent neurologic conditions encountered in pregnancy.[100, 101]

Epilepsy is a disorder of the brain characterized by recurrent seizures. The classification (Table 15–7) of epileptic seizures has now been internationally agreed upon.[102] Partial seizures come in many different forms and one of the commonest manifestations of partial seizures is a secondary generalized seizure. Generalized seizures are less common and may take the form of a minor seizure, such as an absence seizure, or a major convulsion, such as tonic-clonic seizure.

The treatment of epilepsy with the modern anticonvulsants is very effective with as many as 50% of patients being completely seizure-free. Those who develop epilepsy in adult life have a much better chance of seizure control and as many as 70% to 80% of such patients may be seizure-free on appropriate medication.

Effects of Pregnancy on Epilepsy

Seizure Frequency

Pregnancy has a variable effect on seizure frequency.[103, 104] Recent reviews suggest that seizure frequency is unchanged in 50% of pregnant women, decreases in a small percentage in some, and increases in the remainder (Table 15–8). There is some suggestion that noncompliance with the drug regimen and maternal sleep deprivation are the principle factors increasing seizure frequency. Other factors that may be responsible for alteration in seizure frequency during a pregnancy are psychologic,[105] hormonal,[106] and metabolic.[107]

The more frequent the seizures prior to pregnancy the more likely that seizures will increase in frequency during the pregnancy.[108] However, there is no consistent correlation between seizure type and seizure frequency during pregnancy. Other factors which do not appear to materially affect seizure frequency during pregnancy are the cause of the seizures, the age of the patient, the age of seizure onset, and a family history of epilepsy.

Anticonvulsant levels tend to fall during pregnancy and there are a number of factors which contribute to this. Blood levels of anticonvulsants that are heavily protein-bound tend to fall during pregnancy (Table 15–9). Standard serum anticonvulsant levels determine the total amounts of drug, both free and protein-bound. Serum levels of anticonvulsants reflect mainly the levels of bound drug. However, the efficacy of these anticonvulsants actually depends more on the free than the bound or total serum level of a drug. Consequently, in pregnant women with reduced protein binding, standard anticonvulsant levels may not be as reliable as a measure of anticonvulsant effectiveness. Free anticonvulsant levels may prove useful and these can now be measured.[113] Other factors which reduce serum levels during pregnancy are impaired anticonvulsant absorption, hormonal induction of liver enzymes responsible for anticonvulsant metabolism, and noncompliance.

Gestational Epilepsy

A seizure disorder which only becomes manifest during pregnancy is referred to as gestational epilepsy. Almost half of patients whose seizures start during pregnancy have further seizures only during subsequent pregnancies. The susceptibility is said to be most marked in the sixth and seventh months of pregnancy.[108]

Effect of Epilepsy on Pregnancy

The course of pregnancy is unaffected by epilepsy for most women, and socioeconomic status, marital status, parity, and prenatal care are more important factors than maternal epilepsy. However, there is information to suggest that pregnant women with epilepsy have

TABLE 15–8.
Effect of Pregnancy on Seizure Frequency in Epilepsy*

Study	Pregnancies	Seizure Frequency (%)		
		Increased	No Change	Decreased
Burnett (1946)[109]	19	42	52	6
McClure (1955)[110]	20	55	25	20
Sabin & Ozorn (1956)[111]	55	33	52	15
Suter & Klingman (1957)[112]	120	61	33	6
Knight & Rhind (1975)[108]	84	45	50	5
Total pregnancies	298			
Weighted averages		50	42	8

*Adapted from Donaldson JO: *Neurology of Pregnancy*, ed 2. London, WB Saunders Co, 1989.

TABLE 15–9.
Protein Binding Characteristic of Major Antiepileptic Drugs*

Drug	Free Fraction (% unbound)
Carbamazepine	27–40
Ethosuximide	90–100
Phenobarbital	50–55
Phenytoin	7–13
Primidone	70–100
Valproic acid	
<500 μmol/L	8–10
>500 μmol/L	10–30

*From Levy RH, Schmidt D: *Epilepsia* 1985; 26:199–203. Used by permission.

twice the incidence of unfavorable outcomes as the general population (Table 15–10).[114] The more frequent the seizures the greater the risk.

Generalized tonic-clonic seizures, especially when prolonged, have severe cardiovascular and metabolic effects and may produce hypoxia in the fetus. This is thought to be one cause of impaired intrauterine fetal growth. Partial seizures or any form of nonconvulsive seizure probably does not have a similar adverse effect.

Anticonvulsant Teratogenicity

This is one of the commonest causes of concern of pregnant women or women with epilepsy who wish to become pregnant.[115] One problem in assessing information concerning this concern is that the risk of fetal malformation due to the severity of the maternal epilepsy cannot be distinguished from the risk due to treatment. There are certainly data that suggest that the risk of birth defects in women with epilepsy who do not take anticonvulsants is higher than in women without epilepsy.[116] On the other hand, the highest malformation rate occurs in the children of women taking multiple anticonvulsants.[117] There is also some information to suggest that the children of fathers who have epilepsy have an increased risk of congenital malformations.[116, 118]

In fact, no anticonvulsants are absolutely safe and totally free of a significant teratogenic risk. On current available information, it is difficult to recommend any single anticonvulsant as clearly superior to all others in pregnancy. However, phenobarbital may have less teratogenic risk than other agents. In addition, trimethadione and valproic acid have been associated with a high incidence of congenital malformations and should be avoided.[115] Table 15–11 lists some of the main problems of the anticonvulsants in standard use.

General Management

First and foremost it should be determined whether a woman of childbearing age requires anticonvulsant drug treatment, and as far as possible monotherapy should be the aim. In some instances a woman may wish to consider stopping anticonvulsants either because the seizures have been completely controlled for many years or because of infrequent seizures. Unfortunately, at the pres-

TABLE 15–10.
Frequency of Maternal Complications and Fetal Outcomes for Pregnancies of Women With Epilepsy in Norway*

Maternal and Fetal Complications	Epilepsy	No Epilepsy
Total pregnancies	371	125,423
Hyperemesis gravidarum	1–3%	0.8%
Vaginal hemorrhage	5.1%*	2.2%
Toxemia	7.5%*	4.7%
Birth by		
Cesarean section	3.2%*	1.1%
Forceps/vacuum extractor	6.3%*	2.4%
Gestation <37 wk	8.9%*	5.0%
Birth weight <2,500 g	7.4%*	3.7%
Hypoxia at birth	1.9%	0.7%
Any congenital malformation	4.5%	2.2%
Cleft lip or palate	1.1%	
Infant Mortality Rates (per 1,000 Births)		
Stillbirth	5.3	7.8
Perinatal	31.8†	14.6
Neonatal death	29.3†	8.0
Postnatal death	5.3	3.4

*Adapted from Bjerkedal T, Bahana SL: *Acta Obstet Gynecol Scand* 1973; 52:245–247.
†P value is less than 0.01.

TABLE 15–11.
Teratogenicity of the Main Anticonvulsants*

Phenobarbital
  Probably no increase in fetal malformation rate
Phenytoin
  Orofacial clefts—possible
  Congenital heart defects—uncertain
  Dysmorphic facial features—uncertain
  Fetal hydantoin syndrome[119]
Carbamazepine†
  Possibly teratogenic—increased incidence of
    craniofacial defects, fingernail hypoplasia, and
    developmental delay[120]
Valproic acid/valproate sodium[121–123]
  Neural tube defects including hydrocephalus—
    1%–2% risk

*All above agents are FDA risk category D. See Preface for
  full description of FDA classification.
†Based on data in Jones KL, Lacro RV, Johnson, KA: *N
  Engl J Med* 1989; 320:1661–1666.

ent time it is not possible to predict the likelihood of seizures occurring in any one individual who stops anticonvulsants. Clearly, because of the greater risk of major convulsions causing problems to the fetus, patients with this type of seizure disorder should probably remain on anticonvulsants.

In general, it is recommended that anticonvulsant levels be checked regularly during pregnancy and if at all possible the anticonvulsant drugs should not be changed if seizures are well controlled. High anticonvulsant levels should be avoided, particularly in the early stage of a pregnancy. There is some debate as to what should be done with the patient whose anticonvulsant levels are low but whose epilepsy is well controlled. In general, it is recommended that the doses be increased to bring levels within the therapeutic range though of course the doses will need to be decreased in the puerperium. Table 15–12 summarizes the management of epilepsy during pregnancy and the puerperium.

Folic acid depletion has been described in individuals taking anticonvulsants, notably phenytoin, and it is advisable to determine folate levels and provide folate replacement as appropriate.[124]

The development of status epilepticus in pregnancy is a medical emergency requiring immediate treatment with parenteral anticonvulsants. The benzodiazepines are the drugs of choice using either diazepam or clonazepam.

TABLE 15–12.
Management of Epilepsy During Pregnancy and Puerperium

1. Discuss with parents risk of congenital malformations.
2. Check anticonvulsant levels regularly. Urge mother to take drugs regularly.

3. Medications*	Dosage Range and Therapeutic Level	Maternal Side Effects
Carbamazepine (Tegretol) [D]	200–1,200 mg/day 4–8 μg/mL	Drowsiness, blurred vision, ataxia, GI upset
Phenobarbital [D]	30–200 mg/day 10–35 μg/mL	Drowsiness, ataxia, rash
Phenytoin (Dilantin) [D]	300–1,200 mg/day 10–20 μg/mL	Drowsiness, ataxia, gum hyperplasia, hypertrichosis
Ethosuximide (Zarontin) [D]	500–1,500 mg/day 40–100 μg/mL	GI upset, headache
Clonazepam (Clonopin) [C]	1.5–20 mg/day 0.01–0.07 μg/mL	Drowsiness, ataxia

4. Give 1 mg phytonadione IV to the newborn.
5. Observe infant for symptoms of the neonatal depression syndrome or the drug withdrawal syndrome.
6. Consider decreasing maternal anticonvulsant dosage after delivery.

*These agents are not listed in order of preference. The choice of drug should be based on the physician's assessment
  of the risks and benefits associated with treating the epileptic gravida. FDA risk category is given in brackets.

TABLE 15–13.
A Classification of Headaches

1. Vascular headaches
    Migraine
        Classical
        Common
        Complicated (hemiplegic and ophthalmoplegic
            cluster headaches, migrainous neuralgia)
    Hypertensive
2. Muscle contraction (tension) headaches
    Familial
    Idiopathic
    Secondary—cervical spondylosis; depression,
    other
        psychiatric disorders
3. Intracranial disorders
    Raised intracranial pressure
    Lowered intracranial pressure
    Meningeal irritation—meningitis, subarachnoid
        hemorrhage
4. Extracranial disorders
    Diseases of the eye, ear, nose, throat, teeth, and
        sinuses
    Cranial arteritis
    Cranial neuralgias
    Atypical facial pain
    Temporomandibular joint dysfunction

Delivery

Proper administration of anticonvulsant medications during labor and delivery is a common concern, particularly when there may be a need for a general anesthetic. Under these circumstances parenteral anticonvulsants may be given. Phenytoin may be given by slow intravenous infusion, but all anticonvulsants may be given rectally as they are absorbed well by this route.

Epilepsy and the Neonate

Several anticonvulsants are known to interfere with vitamin K metabolism which can result in a hemorrhagic disorder in the newborn. Vitamin K given in the last month of pregnancy may prevent this and after delivery the infant may be given vitamin K prophylactically.

Sedation, hypotonia, and poor suckling are occasionally seen in neonates of mothers on high anticonvulsant levels. Respiratory depression is also occasionally seen, but these problems are rare. Occasionally, withdrawal symptoms may be seen in the neonate, particularly in children of mothers who are taking barbiturates.

Breast-Feeding

Often, a major concern of the pregnant woman with epilepsy is worry about the presence of anticonvulsants in her breast milk. All anticonvulsants are excreted in breast milk but the levels are exceedingly low and not a cause for concern. Mothers are also often worried that they might have a seizure and drop the baby, but in the author's experience this is such a rare occurrence as to lead him to advise the mother that she can nurse and look after her baby in a manner similar to any other mother.

Prenatal Counseling

This is one of the commonest problems facing the physician dealing with a young female patient with epilepsy. Patients are most commonly worried about the risks of anticonvulsants to the fetus and these risks need to be discussed quite openly. A similar concern is the risk that the baby might develop epilepsy, and genetic counseling here is important.[125] In the absence of a family history of epilepsy the risk of a child of a woman with epilepsy developing the problem is low other than in clearly defined epileptic syndromes that are known to be genetically determined (for example, true absence epilepsy).

HEADACHE

Headache[126] is the most common neurologic symptom and for many people the most distressing. Many different types of headache exist and Table 15–13 lists a classification of the major types.

Migraine

This is the most common of the vascular headaches and typically occurs as a paroxysmal disorder with the headache lasting from 2 to 12 hours. Headaches are often unilateral and in classic migraine the headaches are preceded by visual disturbances, such as teichopsia; vomiting and photophobia often accompany the headache.

It is generally recognized that as many as three fourths of pregnant women show a considerable improvement in their migraine attacks during a pregnancy.[126, 127] As many as one third of patients may be completely free of migraine though up to one fourth may either fail to improve or become worse. In those who improve recurrence of headaches may occur within the first postpartum week.

Focal migraine or *complicated migraine* are terms for migraine in which the vasospasm predominates, often with little in the way of symptoms of vasodilation, such as headache. This condition may develop during pregnancy in a patient who previously has suffered from classic migraine.[128]

Treatment

The ergot alkaloids, which in years gone by were frequently used in migraine, have now fallen somewhat into disrepute and should certainly be avoided in pregnancy owing to their oxytocic effect. In general, the treatment of an acute attack of migraine revolves around the use of an analgesic, such as aspirin, and an antiemetic, such as metoclopramide.

Prophylactic agents may be used and the β-adrenergic blocking agents such as propranolol or atenolol are well tolerated and are not thought to have serious effects on the fetus or the pregnancy. There are isolated case reports of fetal abnormalities occurring where the mother has taken propranolol in combination with ergotamine.[129]

Muscle Contraction Headache (Tension Headaches)

This is the commonest type of headache seen in pregnant women.[130] Use of standard analgesics is all that is required.

Table 15–14 summarizes the use of drugs for headache and migraine during pregnancy.

DEGENERATIVE DISORDERS

These are a group of progressive neurologic disorders of uncertain etiology which tend to occur in the older age groups and therefore are rarely seen in pregnant women. They share in common the following features: (1) unknown etiology, (2) progressive nature until death, (3) no effective treatment.

Amyotrophic Lateral Sclerosis (Motor Neuron Disease)

This is a rare disorder associated with progressive paralysis leading to death usually within 3 to 5 years. Occasional cases are described of women who develop the condition during pregnancy.[131] Management of these

TABLE 15–14.

Drugs Used For Headache and Their Safety in Pregnancy

Acetylsalicylic acid [C]*†
  Avoid regular use
  May cause multiple problems including delayed onset of labor, increased perinatal mortality, and impaired neonatal hemostasis
Paracetamol (acetaminophen) [B]*
  Probably the safest simple analgesic; there are claims that it may cause some fetal malformations but this is not proven
More powerful analgesics [C]*
  In practice rarely required
  Codeine appears to be safe when used for brief period
Tricyclic antidepressants
  Amitriptyline [C]* and imipramine [C]* appear to be safe
Benzodiazepines
  Not recommended for regular use; some risk of teratogenicity; also may cause neonatal withdrawal syndrome
Ergot derivatives
  Should be avoided because of oxytocic effect
β-Adrenergic blocking agents
  Propranolol [C]* and atenolol [C]* appear to be reasonably safe, no definite teratogenicity; may cause neonatal bradycardia and should be used in minimal dosage, particularly when approaching delivery

*FDA risk category. See Preface for description of FDA classification.
†FDA risk category D when used in third trimester.

patients depends on the severity of the condition, the rapidity of progression, and the stage of the pregnancy.

Parkinson's Disease

Although this disorder usually begins to show itself after most women have borne their children, there are a number of case reports of pregnancies occurring in women after the onset of symptoms. The average age at conception was 35. Treatment with levodopa and bromocriptine (both FDA category C) seems to have no adverse effect on the pregnancy.[132]

Familial Degenerative Disorders

There are a wide variety of familial degenerative disorders, the most common group being the familial ataxias, such as Friedreich's ataxia.[133] Many of these conditions may begin in childhood and be well established by the time a woman reaches childbearing age. In all instances the conditions are progressive, though in some the progression may be slow. Decisions as to advice regarding childbirth will depend on the severity of the disorder, its rate of progression, and individual factors. Genetic counseling may be needed.

REFERENCES

1. Goldstein PJ: *Neurological Disorders of Pregnancy.* New York, Futura Publishing Co, Inc, 1986.
2. Donaldson JO: *Neurology of Pregnancy,* ed 2. London, WB Saunders Co, 1989.
3. Bray RS, Lynch R, Grossman RG, et al: Management of neurosurgical problems in pregnancy. *Clin Perinatol* 1987; 14:243–257.
4. Robins M, Baum HM: Incidence. *Stroke* 1981; 12(suppl 1):I-45–I-57.
5. Whisnant JP: The decline of stroke. *Stroke* 1984; 15:160–168.
6. Snyder BD, Ramirez-Lassepas M: Cerebral infarction in young adults: Long term prognosis. *Stroke* 1980; 11:149–153.
7. Wiebers DO: Ischemic cerebrovascular complications of pregnancy. *Arch Neurol* 1985; 42:1106–1113.
8. Barnes JE, Abbott KH: Cerebral complications incurred during pregnancy and the puerperium. *Am J Obstet Gynecol* 1961; 82:192–207.
9. Barno A, Freeman DW: Maternal deaths due to spontaneous subarachnoid hemorrhage. *Am J Obstet Gynecol* 1976; 125:384–392.
10. Minielly R, Yuzpe AA, Drake CG: Subarachnoid haemorrhage secondary to ruptured cerebral aneurysm in pregnancy. *Obstet Gynecol* 1979; 53:64–70.
11. Conklin KA, Herr G, Fung D: Anaesthesia for Caesarean [sic] section and cerebral aneurysm clipping. *Can Anaesth Soc J* 1984; 31:451–454.
12. Lennon RL, Sundt TM, Gronert GA: Combined cesarean section and clipping of intracerebral aneurysm. *Anesthesiology* 1984; 60:240–242.
13. Pickard JD, Murray GD, Illingworth R, et al: Effect of oral nimodipine on cerebral infarction and outcome after subarachnoid hemorrhage: British aneurysm nimodipine trial. *Br Med J* 1989; 298:636–642.
14. Read MD, Wellby DE: The use of calcium antagonist (nifedipine) to suppress preterm labour. *Br J Obstet Gynaecol* 1986; 93:933–937.
15. Richardson A: Spontaneous intracerebral hemorrhage, in Ross-Russell RN (ed): *Vascular Disease of the Central Nervous System,* ed 2. Edinburgh, Churchill Livingstone, 1983, pp 245–263.
16. Cross JH, Castro PO, Jennett WB: Cerebral strokes associated with pregnancy and the puerperium. *Br Med J* 1968; 3:214–218.
17. Wiebers DO, Whisnant JP: The incidence of stroke among pregnant women in Rochester, Minnesota, 1955 through 1979. *JAMA* 1985; 254:3055–3057.
18. Srinivasan K: Cerebral venous and arterial thrombosis in pregnancy and puerperium. *Angiology* 1983; 34:731–746.
19. Carroll JD, Leek D, Lee HA: Cerebral thrombophlebitis in pregnancy and the puerperium. *Q J Med* 1966; 35:347–368.
20. Halpern JP, Morris JGL, Driscoll GL: Anticoagulants and cerebral venous thrombosis. *Aust NZ J Med* 1984; 14:643–648.
21. Stern WE: Carotid-cavernous fistula, in

Vinken PJ, Bruyn GW (eds): *Handbook of Clinical Neurology,* vol 24. Amsterdam, North Holland Publishing Co, Inc, 1976, pp 399–439.

22. Adour KK: Diagnosis and management of facial paralysis. *N Engl J Med* 1982; 307:348–351.

23. Hilsinger RL Jr, Adour KK, Doty HE: Idiopathic facial paralysis, pregnancy, and the menstrual cycle. *Ann Otol Rhinol Laryngol* 1975; 84:433–442.

24. McGregor JA, Guberman A, Amer J, et al: Idiopathic facial nerve paralysis (Bell's palsy) in late pregnancy and the early puerperium. *Obstet Gynecol* 1987; 69:435–438.

25. Voitk AJ, Mueller JC, Farlinger DE, et al: Carpal tunnel syndrome in pregnancy. *Can Med Assoc J* 1983; 128:277–281.

26. Rhodes P: Meralgia paresthetica in pregnancy. *Lancet* 1957; 2:831–832.

27. Helm PA, Nepomuceno C, Crane CR: Tibial nerve dysfunction during pregnancy. *South Med J* 1971; 64:1493–1494.

28. Pleet AB, Massey EW: Intercostal neuralgia of pregnancy. *JAMA* 1980; 243:770–772.

29. Bellina JH, Deming B: Charcot-Marie-Tooth disease and pregnancy: Report of a case. *J La State Med Soc* 1973; 125:393–395.

30. Watson CJ, Dhar J, Bossenmaier I, et al: Effect of hematin in acute porphyric relapse. *Ann Intern Med* 1973; 79:80–83.

31. Bravo RH, Katz M, Inturrisi M, et al: Obstetric management of Landry-Guillain-Barré syndrome: A case report. *Am J Obstet Gynecol* 1982; 142(pt 1):714–715.

32. Ahlberg G, Ahlmark G: The Landry-Guillain-Barré syndrome and pregnancy. *Acta Obstet Gynecol Scand* 1978; 57:377–380.

33. Dalakas MC, Engel WK: Chronic relapsing (dysimmune) polyneuropathy: Pathogenesis and treatment. *Ann Neurol* 1981; 9(suppl):134–145.

34. Chaturachinda K, McGregor EM: Wernicke's encephalopathy and pregnancy. *J Obstet Gynaecol Br Commnw* 1968; 75:969–971.

35. Karjalainen AO: Neurological disorders in pregnancy: Multiple sclerosis, gestational polyneuritis and meningitis. *Ann Chir Gynaecol Fenn* 1965; 54:453–461.

36. Duncan ME, Pearson JMH: Neuritis in pregnancy and lactation. *Int J Lepr* 1982; 50:31–38.

37. Massey EW, Cefalo RC: Neuropathies of pregnancy. *Obstet Gynecol Surv* 1979; 34:489–492.

38. Hammar M, Larsson L, Tegler L: Calcium treatment of leg cramps in pregnancy. *Acta Obstet Gynecol Scand* 1981; 60:345–347.

39. Kurtzke JF: Epidemiology of myasthenia gravis. *Adv Neurol* 1978; 19:545–548.

40. Lindstrom JM, Seybold ME, Lennon VA, et al: Antibody to acetylcholine receptor in myasthenia gravis: Prevalence, clinical correlates, and diagnostic valve. *Neurology (Minneap)* 1976; 26:1054–1059.

41. Castleman B: The pathology of the thymus gland in myasthenia gravis. *Ann NY Acad Sci* 1966; 135:496–503.

42. Osserman KE: Pregnancy in myasthenia gravis and neonatal myasthenia gravis. *Am J Med* 1955; 19:718–721.

43. Viets HR, Schwab RS, Brazier MAB: The effect of pregnancy on the course of myasthenia gravis. *JAMA* 1942; 119:236–238.

44. Fraser D, Turner JWA: Myasthenia gravis and pregnancy. *Proc R Soc Med* 1963; 56:379–381.

45. Eden RD, Gall SA: Myasthenia gravis and pregnancy: A reappraisal of thymectomy. *Obstet Gynecol* 1983; 62:328–333.

46. Plauche WC: Myasthenia gravis in pregnancy. *Am J Obstet Gynecol* 1964; 88:404–406.

47. Scott JS: Immunologic diseases in pregnancy. *Prog Allergy* 1977; 23:371–373.

48. Goldman KP: Malignant thymoma in pregnancy. *Br J Dis Chest* 1974; 68:279–283.

49. Foldes FF, McWall PG: Myasthenia gravis: A guide for anesthesiologists. *Anesthesiology* 1967; 23:837–839.

50. Ip MS, So SY, Lam WK, et al: Thymectomy in myasthenia gravis during pregnancy. *Postgrad Med J* 1986; 62:473–474.

51. Rolbin SH, Levinson G, Shnider SM, et al: Anesthetic considerations for myasthenia gravis and pregnancy. *Anesth Analg* 1978; 57:441–447.

52. Provenzano C: Neonatal myasthenia gravis: Clinical and immunological study of seven mothers and their newborn infants. *J Neuroimmunol* 1986; 12:155–161.

53. Namba T, Brown SB, Grob D: Neonatal myasthenia gravis: Report of two cases and a review of the literature. *Pediatrics* 1970; 45:488–504.

54. Webb D, Muir I, Faulkner J, et al: Myotonia dystrophica: Obstetric complications. *Am J Obstet Gynecol* 1977; 132:265–270.

55. Shore RN: Myotonic dystrophy: Hazards of pregnancy and infancy. *Dev Med Child Neurol* 1975; 17:356–361.

56. Cope DK, Miller JN: Local and spinal anesthesia for cesarean section in a patient with myotonic dystrophy. *Anesth Analg* 1986; 65:687–690.

57. Mitchell MM, Ali HH, Savarese JJ: Myotonia and neuromuscular blocking agents. *Anesthesiology* 1978; 49:44–48.

58. Lunt PW, Meredith A, Harper PS: First-trimester prediction in fetus at risk for myotonic dystrophy. *Lancet* 1986; 2:350–351.

59. Hakim CA, Thomlinson J: Myotonia congenita in pregnancy. *J Obstet Gynaecol Br Commnw* 1969; 76:561–562.

60. Barnes AB, Link DA: Childhood dermatomyositis and pregnancy. *Am J Obstet Gynecol* 1983; 146:335–336.

61. Bauer KA, Siegler M, Lindheimer MA: Polymyositis complicating pregnancy. *Arch Intern Med* 1979; 139:449–452.

62. Houston BD, Turner T: Severe electrolyte abnormalities in a pregnant patient with a jejunoileal bypass. *Arch Intern Med* 1978; 138:1712–1713.

63. National Spinal Cord Injury Model Systems Project: Unpublished data. Rehabilitation Services Administration, US Department of Health, Education and Welfare, 1978.

64. Guttmann L, Frankel HL: Cardiac irregularities during labour in paraplegic women. *Paraplegia* 1965; 3:144–151.

65. Robertson DNS: Pregnancy and labour in the paraplegic. *Paraplegia* 1972; 10:209–211.

66. Robertson DNS, Guttmann L: The paraplegic patient in pregnancy and labour. *Proc R Soc Med* 1963; 56:381–382.

67. Divers WA, Hoxsey RJ, Dunnihoo DR: A spinal cord neurolemmona in pregnancy. *Obstet Gynecol* 1978; 52:47S–52S.

68. LaBan MM, Perrin JCS, Latimer Fr: Pregnancy and the herniated lumbar disc. *Arch Phys Med Rehabil* 1983; 64:319–321.

69. King AB: Neurologic conditions occurring as complications of pregnancy. *Arch Neurol Psychiatr* 1950; 63:611–643.

70. Cole JT: Maternal obstetric paralysis. *Am J Obstet Gynecol* 1946; 52:372–385.

71. Hill EC: Maternal obstetric paralysis. *Am J Obstet Gynecol* 1962; 83:1452–1454.

72. Sandberg T: Meningitis and septicemia due to *H. influenzae*, type B in pregnancy. *Br Med J* 1981; 282:946–948.

73. deMarch P: Tuberculosis and pregnancy. *Chest* 1975; 6:800–812.

74. Schlesinger PA, Duray PH, Burke BA, et al: Maternal-fetal transmission of the Lyme disease spirochete, *Borrelia burgdorferi. Ann Intern Med* 1985; 103:67–68.

75. McCord WJ, Alcock AJW, Hildes JA: Poliomyelitis in pregnancy. *Am J Obstet Gynecol* 1955; 69:265–276.

76. Roman-Campos G, Navarro-de-Roman LI, Toro G, et al: Herpes encephalitis in pregnancy. *Am J Obstet Gynecol* 1979; 135:158–160.

77. Philpot Cr: Cryptococcal meningitis in pregnancy. *Med J Aust* 1972; 2:1005–1008.

78. Nausieda PA, Koller WC, Weiner WJ, et al: Chorea induced by oral contraceptives. *Neurology* 1979; 29:1605–1609.

79. Zegart KN, Schwarz RH: Chorea gravidarum. *Obstet Gynecol* 1968; 32:24–27.

80. Willson P, Preece AA: Chorea gravidarum. *Arch Intern Med* 1932; 49:471–533, 671–697.

81. Poser S, Poser W: Multiple sclerosis and gestation. *Neurology* 1983; 33:1422–1427.

82. Poser S, Raun NE, Wikstrom J, et al: Pregnancy, oral contraceptives and multiple sclerosis. *Acta Neurol Scand* 1979; 59:108–118.

83. Birk K, Rudick R: Pregnancy and multiple sclerosis. *Arch Neurol* 1986; 43:719–726.

84. Korn-Lubetzki I, Kahana E, Cooper G, et al: Activity of multiple sclerosis during pregnancy and puerperium. *Ann Neurol* 1984; 16:229–231.

85. Muller R: Studies on disseminating sclerosis with special reference to symptomatology, course and prognosis. *Acta Med Scand [Suppl]* 1949; 133:222.

86. McAlpine D, Compston N: Some aspects of the natural history of disseminating sclerosis. *Q J Med* 1952; 21:135–147.

87. Millar JHD: The influence of pregnancy on multiple sclerosis. *Proc R Soc Med* 1961; 54:4–6.

88. Ghezzi A, Caputo D: Pregnancy: A factor influencing the course of multiple sclerosis. *Eur Neurol* 1981; 20:115–117.

89. Stenuit J, Marchand P: Les séquelles de rachis-anesthésie. *Acta Neurol Belg* 1968; 68:626–628.

90. Sadovnick AD, Baird PA: Reproductive counselling for multiple sclerosis patients. *Am J Med Genet* 1985; 20:349–354.

91. Mackay RP, Myrianthopoulos N: Multiple sclerosis in twins and their relatives. *Arch Neurol* 1966; 15:449–451.

92. Magdelenat H, Pertuiset BF, Poissom, et al: Steroid receptor status difference in recurrent intracranial meningioma and breast cancer in the same patient. *J Neurooncol* 1986; 4:155–157.

93. Allan J, Eldridge R, Koerber T: Acoustic neuroma in the last months of pregnancy. *Am J Obstet Gynecol* 1974; 119:516–520.

94. Roelvink NCA, Camphorst W, Van Alphen HSM, et al: Pregnancy related primary brain and spinal tumours. *Arch Neurol* 1987; 44:209–215.

95. Toakley G: Brain tumors in pregnancy. *Aust NZ J Surg* 1965; 35:148–154.

96. Powell JL: Pseudotumor cerebri and pregnancy. *Obstet Gynecol* 1972; 40:713–715.

97. Kassam SH, Hadi HA, Fadel HE, et al: Benign intracranial hypertension in pregnancy: Current diagnostic and therapeutic approach. *Obstet Gynecol Surv* 1983; 38:314–316.

98. Digre KB, Varner MW, Corbett JJ: Pseudotumor cerebri and pregnancy. *Neurology* 1984; 34:721–729.

99. Abouleish E, Vaseem A, Tang RA: Benign intracranial hypertension and anesthesia for cesarean section. *Anesthesiology* 1985; 63:705–707.

100. Janz D: The teratogenic risk of antiepileptic drugs. *Epilepsia* 1975; 16:159.

101. Hauser WA, Kurland LT: The epidemiology of epilepsy in Rochester, Minnesota 1935 through 1967. *Epilepsia* 1975; 16:1–16.

102. Commission on Classification and Terminology of the International League Against Epilepsy: Proposal for revised clinical and electroencephalographic classification of epileptic seizures. *Epilepsia* 1981; 22:501–506.

103. Schmidt D, Canger R, Avanzini G, et al:

Change of seizure frequency in pregnant epileptic women. *J Neurol Neurosurg Psychiatry* 1983; 46:751–753.

104. Gjerde IO, Strandjord RE, Ulstein M: The course of epilepsy during pregnancy: A study of 78 cases. *Acta Neurol Scand* 1988; 78:198–205.

105. Schmidt D: The effect of pregnancy on the natural history of epilepsy: Review of the literature, in Janz D, Dam M, Richens A, et al (eds): *Epilepsy, Pregnancy, and the Child.* New York, Raven Press, 1982, pp 3–14.

106. Mattson RH, Cramer JA: Epilepsy, sex hormones and antiepileptic drugs. *Epilepsia* 1985; 26(suppl 1):S40–46.

107. Levy RH, Yerby MS: Effects of pregnancy on antiepileptic drug utilization. *Epilepsia* 1985; 26(suppl 1):S52–58.

108. Knight AH, Rhind EG: Epilepsy and pregnancy: A study of 153 pregnancies in 59 patients. *Epilepsia* 1975; 16:99–105.

109. Burnett CWF: A survey of the relation between epilepsy and pregnancy. *J Obstet Gynaecol Br Emp* 1946; 53:539–556.

110. McClure JH: Idiopathic epilepsy in pregnancy. *Am J Obstet Gynecol* 1955; 70:296–301.

111. Sabin M, Ozorn H: Epilepsy and pregnancy. *Obstet Gynaecol* 1956; 7:175–179.

112. Suter C, Klingman WO: Seizure states and pregnancy. *Neurology* 1957; 7:105–118.

113. Levy RH, Schmidt D: Utility of free level monitoring of antiepileptic drugs. *Epilepsia* 1985; 26:199–203.

114. Bjerkedal T, Bahana SL: The course and outcome of pregnancy in women with epilepsy. *Acta Obstet Gynecol Scand* 1973; 52:245–247.

115. Dalessio DJ: Seizure disorders and pregnancy. *N Engl J Med* 1985; 312:559–562.

116. Nakane Y: Congenital malformations among infants of epileptic mothers treated during pregnancy. *Folia Psychiatr Neurol Jpn* 1979; 33:363–369.

117. Janz D: On major malformations and minor anomalies in the offspring of parents with epilepsy: Review of the literature, in Janz D, Dam M, Richens A, et al (eds): *Epilepsy, Pregnancy and the Child.* New York, Raven Press, 1982, pp 211–222.

118. Ottman R, Annegers JF, Hauser WA, et al: Higher risk of seizures in offspring of mothers than of fathers with epilepsy. *Am*

J Hum Genet 1988; 43:257–264.

119. Short Communication: Genetics and fetal hydantoin syndrome. *Acta Paediatr Scand* 1989; 78:125–126.

120. Jones KL, Lacro RV, Johnson KA, et al: Pattern of malformations in the children of women treated with carbamazepine during pregnancy. *N Engl J Med* 1989; 320:1661–1666.

121. Lammer EJ, Sever LE, Oakley GP: Teratogen update: Valproic acid. *Teratology* 1987; 35:465–473.

122. Winter RM, Donnai D, Burn J, et al: Fetal valproate syndrome: Is there a recognisable phenotype? *J Med Genet* 1987; 24:692–695.

123. Huot C, Gauthier M, Lebel M, et al: Congenital malformations associated with maternal use of valproic acid. *Can J Neurol Sci* 1987; 14:290–293.

124. Janz D: Antiepileptic drugs and pregnancy: Altered utilization patterns and teratogenesis. *Epilepsia* 1982; 23(suppl 1):S53.

125. Blandfort M, Tsuboi T, Vogel F: Genetic counseling in the epilepsies. *Hum Genet* 1987; 76:303–331.

126. Dalessio DJ: Classification and treatment of headache during pregnancy. *Clin Neuropharmacol* 1986; 9:121–131.

127. Graham JR: Migraine: Clinical aspects, in Vinken PJ, Bruyn GW (eds): *Handbook of Clinical Neurology,* vol 5. Amsterdam, North-Holland Publishing Co, 1968; pp 45–58.

128. Wright DS, Patel MK: Focal migraine and pregnancy. *Br Med J* 1986; 293:1557–1558.

129. Hughes HE, Goldstein DA: Birth defects following maternal exposure to ergotamine, beta blockers and caffeine. *J Med Genet* 1988; 25:396–399.

130. Lance JW: *Mechanisms and Management of Headache.* London, Butterworth Scientific Publishers, 1982.

131. Levine MS, Michels RM: Pregnancy and amyotrophic lateral sclerosis. *Ann Neurol* 1977; 1:408–410.

132. Cook DG, Klawans HL: Levodopa during pregnancy. *Clin Neuropharmacol* 1985; 8:93–95.

133. Myrianthopoulos NC: *Neurogenetic Directory.* Pt 1, in Vinken PJ, Bruyn GW (eds): *Handbook of Clinical Neurology,* vol 42. Amsterdam, North Holland Publishing Co, 1981.

CHAPTER 16

Dermatologic Diseases

Iris K. Aronson

Barbara Halaska

Gravidas are susceptible to the same skin disorders as are nonpregnant women, and in addition, pregnancy is accompanied by physiologic changes which may result in hyperpigmentation, hirsutism, hair loss, and a variety of cutaneous vascular changes. The physiologic and hormonal alterations of gestation may also affect certain tumors and other cutaneous diseases which predate conception. Finally, there are several pregnancy-specific skin disorders which are important to recognize as they may affect both fetal and maternal health. This chapter begins with a brief review of the physiologic changes in the skin during gestation. Detection and management is then discussed in three broad categories: the effect of pregnancy on cutaneous tumors, skin eruptions unique to gestation, and finally, cutaneous disorders which may be influenced by pregnancy.

PHYSIOLOGIC SKIN CHANGES IN PREGNANCY

Pigment Changes

Hyperpigmentation

Some degree of hyperpigmentation during pregnancy is a normal phenomenon, occurring in up to 90% of pregnancies.[1, 2] Women of dark complexion are more susceptible than are fair-skinned women. The hyperpigmentation may begin as early as the first trimester.[2] Typically, skin that is normally somewhat hyperpigmented, such as the areolae, becomes darker. In addition, darkening of nipples, umbilicus, vulva, and perianal skin may be seen and the normally hypopigmented linea alba becomes the hyperpigmented linea nigra. Ephelides (freckles), melanocytic nevi,[3] and recent scars may also darken during pregnancy. Hyperpigmentation may also occur on the face causing the so-called mask of pregnancy or melasma (or chloasma), seen in 50% to 73% of pregnancies.[4] *Melasma* is characterized by well-demarcated hyperpigmented macules and patches occurring in a centrofacial (most common), malar, or mandibular pattern. The pigmentation may appear light to dark brown, ash-gray, or blue, depending on the amount and distribution of melanin.

Melasma is a result of increased melanin deposition in the epidermis and/or dermal macrophages.[5] Increased melanin restricted to the epidermis produces light-brown pigmentation clinically, whereas melanin contained in the dermis appears gray-blue. The mixed type of hyperpigmentation appears dark brown.

The precise etiology of the hyperpigmentation is unclear. Elevated circulating levels of estrogen and progesterone[4, 6] and perhaps melanocyte-stimulating hormone (MSH)[7, 8] are thought to be responsible. Estrogen and progesterone are capable of directly stimulating melanogenesis.[9] Melasma is also seen in 5% to 34%[10] of women taking oral contraceptives, lending support for a causative role of estrogens and progestins. These women, in turn, are especially susceptible to developing melasma during pregnancy. Controversy exists as to the role MSH plays in producing hyperpigmentation. While some investigators[7] have found elevated serum and urine levels of MSH during pregnancy, others[11] have found normal plasma β-MSH levels in late pregnancy. Lastly, ultraviolet (UV) light plays a substantial exacerbating role in the development of melasma by virtue of its ability to stimulate melanogenesis.

The clinical appearance of melasma is characteristic but occasionally melasma may be confused with hyperpigmentation that can occur after any type of inflammation, i.e., postinflammatory hyperpigmentation. In addition, phototoxic reactions to cosmetics[12] must be considered as well as ingestion of certain substances known to cause hyperpigmentation, i.e., gold, silver, copper, bismuth, arsenic, iron, and quinacrine. Marked generalized hyperpigmentation is rare and when it occurs, hyperthyroidism should be excluded.[2, 13]

The management of melasma in pregnancy is limited to avoidance of excessive sun exposure. In addition, a broad-spectrum sunscreen (suncreen protection factor equal to or greater than 15) designed to block out both UVA and UVB rays should be used daily. Continued use of sunscreens is necessary post partum to avoid recurrence.

Post partum, hyperpigmentation will partially or completely resolve.[1, 5] Melasma likewise may completely disappear or regress significantly in the majority of women.[2, 3] However, one study found that 30% of women had persistent melasma for 10 years or longer.[2] For those individuals with residual melasma, depigmentation may be attempted post partum by topical application of 2% to 5% hy-

droquinone. Melasma of the epidermal type is most likely to respond to treatment. Broad-spectrum sunscreens during and after therapy is necessary; otherwise melasma may recur.

Hair Growth

Hirsutism.—Mild hirsutism, especially of the face, is not uncommon during pregnancy. Marked hirsutism, however, is very uncommon and may indicate the presence of a virilizing tumor[3, 14] or polycystic ovarian disease.[15] Increased hair growth is usually noted in the first trimester and may be most noticeable on the face, but the arms, legs, back, and abdomen may also be involved. Hairs may vary from fine to coarse.

As with other physiologic changes during pregnancy, hirsutism is primarily of endocrinologic origin. The proportion of anagen (growing) hair to telogen (resting) hairs is increased[16] during pregnancy accounting, at least in part, for the apparent hirsutism. Increased secretion of adrenocorticotropin hormone, adrenocorticosteroids, and ovarian androgens have been suggested as possible factors responsible for this change in the hair cycle.[17]

Mild hirsutism does not usually require treatment, since it usually disappears within 6 months after delivery.[1, 2] Coarse hairs, however, may persist. Patients with pronounced hirsutism should be studied for the presence of an arrhenoblastoma or bilateral ovarian enlargement, especially if other signs of virilization (e.g., acne, deepening voice) are present.[3]

Telogen Effluvium (Hair Loss).— Varying degrees of hair loss on the scalp are commonly seen in the postpartum period.[4, 5, 18] The term *telogen effluvium* refers to the abrupt loss of telogen hairs beginning 2 to 4 months post partum.[4] In the immediate postpartum period there is an abrupt conversion of hairs from anagen (growth phase) to telogen (resting phase) with subsequent shedding. This change is thought to be of endocrinologic origin. Estrogens have been noted to prolong the anagen phase.[4] Patients will typically complain of increased amounts of hair being shed, particularly after combing or shampooing, and the degree of hair loss may be substantial and alarming to the patient. It may be most marked in the frontal area. The hair loss is asymptomatic and there is no associated erythema, scaling, pruritus, or scarring.

No treatment other than reassurance is necessary for telogen effluvium. In general, the hair returns to its normal prepregnancy cycle and complete regrowth occurs in 6 to 15 months post partum.[12, 17] In rare circumstances the hair may never be as thick as it was prior to pregnancy.[4]

Striae Distensae

Striae distensae, appearing in the sixth to seventh month, are seen in up to 90% of pregnant women.[4] There may be genetic and racial predisposing factors. Striae appear as atrophic linear bands which are pink to purple in color. They typically develop on the abdomen, breasts, thighs, and inguinal region.

Two principal factors are thought to be involved in the production of striae. First, stretching or distention of the skin is necessary. However, distention alone will not necessarily produce striae. Hormonal factors, particularly adrenocorticosteroids and placental estrogens, are thought to promote tearing of collagen fibers and rupturing of elastic fibers in the dermis.[2] Histologically, fresh striae display breakage, retraction, and curling of elastic fibers,[4] in addition to dilatation of blood vessels. There is no available therapy at the present time for striae. Striae persist permanently; however, patients should be reassured that over months, the purplish color fades to a less apparent flesh color.

Vascular Changes

Some clinically recognizable evidence of vascular change occurs in the majority of pregnant women. High levels of circulating estrogens are thought to be responsible.[19] The changes consist of increased vascular permeability and proliferation. Clinically, these effects may be manifested as vascular spiders, palmar erythema, edema, and hemangiomas.

Spider Angiomas.—Spider angiomas consist of a central red arteriole with radiating tortuous branches resembling a spider. They are estimated to occur in approximately 70% of pregnant white females and in 10% of pregnant black females.[13] They appear on the face, neck, chest, and upper extremities between the second to ninth months.[4] The majority of spider angiomas disappear by 3 months post partum.[19] Remaining spiders may be lightly cauterized.

Palmar Erythema.—Palmar erythema may appear as early as the second month of pregnancy. The erythema may be localized to the midpalmar, hypothenar, and thenar areas or it may be diffuse with a mottled appearance. Systemic lupus erythematosus, hyperthyroidism, and hepatic cirrhosis may also cause palmar erythema.[3] Palmar erythema spontaneously fades post partum.

Edema.—Some evidence of increased vascular permeability occurs in 50% of pregnant women.[20] Edema of the eyelids, hands, and ankles is common.[20] Pregnancy-related edema must be differentiated from the edema of cardiac, renal, or hepatic origin.

Hemangiomas.—Small capillary hemangiomas may develop on the head and neck areas in 5% of pregnant women.[13] They appear as small 2- to 10-mm red papules that may or may not blanch with compression. The majority of these lesions will spontaneously involute after delivery. Persistent lesions may be treated surgically.

An outline of the physiologic skin changes in pregnancy is given in Table 16–1.

TABLE 16–1.
Physiologic Skin Changes in Pregnancy

I. Pigmentary changes
   1. Hyperpigmentation—of areola, nipples, umbilicus, vulva, and perineal skin; linea alba → linea nigra
   2. Melasma—hyperpigmented patches on face
II. Hair growth
   1. Hirsutism
   2. Hair loss (telogen effluvium)
III. Striae
IV. Vascular changes
   1. Spider angiomas
   2. Palmar erythema
   3. Edema—increased vascular permeability
   4. Hemangiomas

CUTANEOUS TUMORS AFFECTED BY PREGNANCY

In addition to hemangiomas, other cutaneous tumors also appear or enlarge with increased frequency during pregnancy. The most common include the so-called pregnancy tumor, molluscum gravidarum, and melanocytic nevi. The most controversial tumor that may be seen in pregnancy is malignant melanoma.

Pyogenic Granuloma of Pregnancy (Granuloma Gravidarum Pregnancy Tumor)

The so-called pregnancy tumor is a benign intraoral tumor histologically identical to the typical pyogenic granuloma. It has an alleged incidence of 2%,[5, 20] appearing usually between the second and the fifth months. This lesion appears as a soft, red-to-purple nodule, 2 mm to several centimeters in diameter.[20] Pregnancy tumors often arise from the gingival papillae, but may also develop on the buccal or lingual surface of the marginal gingiva.[20] They are often seen in association with extensive gingivitis,[20] which is thought to predispose to the development of the tumor. These lesions may remit spontaneously post partum.[5] Removal of local irritants may cause

the lesion to disappear entirely.[20] Lesions persisting post partum may be surgically excised.

Molluscum Gravidarum

Molluscum gravidarum are simply skin tags that develop during gestation. They are exceedingly common but no statistics are available on their exact incidence. They appear as small 1- to 4-mm skin-colored or slightly hyperpigmented soft pedunculated lesions typically over the sides of the neck, inframammary folds, and axillae. They often arise in the second half of pregnancy.

These skin tags are primarily of cosmetic concern. The lesions may disappear spontaneously post partum.[5, 21] Persistent lesions may be removed by simple scissors excision, level with the skin surface. Alternatively, they may be lightly electrodesiccated or frozen with liquid nitrogen.

Melanocytic Nevi

Melanocytic nevi are present in virtually all persons. The normal, benign nevus is easily recognized by its uniform color, small size (usually 6 mm or less), distinct borders, and symmetry. During pregnancy, nevi not uncommonly enlarge or darken, causing occasional diagnostic problems in distinguishing these lesions from a developing malignant melanoma clinically. Histologic examination of these nevi may reveal larger melanocytes, increased amounts of melanin, and even occasional atypical cells.[5, 22] There is no evidence, however, to indicate that nevi undergo malignant transformation with greater frequency during pregnancy.[23, 24] Any lesion clinically suspicious for melanoma should be subject to excisional biopsy without delay.

Malignant Melanoma

Despite nearly 40 years of study, the subject of malignant melanoma and pregnancy remains controversial. While there is general agreement that the prevalence of melanoma is no higher in pregnant women as compared to nonpregnant women,[25, 26] the prognostic impact that pregnancy has on melanoma is debated. The widespread impression that pregnancy has a negative influence on survival is supported by case reports of fatal courses of melanoma associated with pregnancy,[27, 28] and of rapidly growing melanomas,[29] sometimes followed by spontaneous regression, after pregnancy.[30–32] In addition, an early study of 32 women with associated pregnancy and melanoma found that almost half of the women died from melanoma within 3 years of diagnosis.[27] More recently, a retrospective analysis of 18 patients with initiation or stimulation of melanoma during pregnancy also found a higher-than-expected death rate from melanoma.[33] Moreover, multiple investigators have demonstrated the presence of estrogen receptor binding in some melanomas,[34–36] fueling the suspicion that melanoma is a hormonally responsive tumor.

Balanced against these findings, however, are multiple studies showing no decrease in survival[25, 37–41] or even an increased survival.[42] A consideration crucial to the issue of survival is the evidence that patients who present with melanoma during pregnancy tend to do so at a later stage of disease (i.e., stage II or beyond) than their nonpregnant counterparts[25, 26, 37] and with primary lesions on the trunk, a prognostically unfavorable site.[25, 27, 37] Whether these trends are a result of delayed diagnosis or of a hormonally mediated acceleration of tumor growth is unknown.[43] Shiu et al.[37] demonstrated no statistically significant difference in 5-year survival rates for stage I melanoma between nulliparous, parous nonpregnant, and pregnant women. However, pregnant patients with stage II disease had a significantly lower survival rate at 5 years than did nulliparous women. On the contrary, Houghton et al.[25] studied pregnant women with melanoma and found comparable 5-year survival rates for both stage I and II disease when these patients were matched with nonpregnant case controls by age, anatomic location of primary lesion, and stage of diagnosis. Thus it appears

that pregnant women who present with stage I melanoma experience no decrease in survival, whereas the prognosis for pregnant women with stage II disease is not entirely clear.

While reports of melanoma metastatic to the placenta[28] and subsequent fatal metastatic disease in the fetus itself[44] have been reported, these events are exceptionally rare.[27, 43] In the vast majority of cases, the fetus remains unaffected by maternal melanoma.[27, 43]

Management.—The management of melanoma in the pregnant patient is the same as for the nonpregnant patient.[43, 45] Wide excision with or without regional lymph node dissection is indicated.[43, 45] There is no evidence that maternal survival is improved by therapeutic abortion,[27, 43, 45] and therefore it need not be recommended.

Perhaps the most controversial issue is the advisability of future pregnancy after the diagnosis and treatment of melanoma has been made. It appears that women whose melanoma was not initiated or stimulated by pregnancy may subsequently become pregnant without experiencing a reactivation of their disease.[43] In the case of a woman whose melanoma was apparently activated by pregnancy, however, it has been recommended by some that she refrain from ever becoming pregnant again[43] or at least for 3 to 5 years and only if no evidence of persistent disease exists.[29, 43] Lastly, considering the possibly deleterious effects of estrogens, it seems advisable to also avoid hormonal means of contraception.[43, 45]

SKIN ERUPTION UNIQUE TO PREGNANCY

Pruritus Gravidarum (Cholestasis of Pregnancy)

Pruritus is a common problem during pregnancy and may be due to many causes.[1] *Pruritus gravidarum* (Table 16–2) is the term used to describe pregnancy-associated generalized pruritus which is found in the absence of any primary skin lesions but is associated with intrahepatic cholestasis and elevated serum bile acids (see also Chap. 10, p. 345). It is a milder, anicteric form of recurrent cholestatic jaundice of pregnancy.[46] The incidence of cholestasis of pregnancy varies from 0.02% to 2.4% worldwide but Chile (14%) and the Scandinavian countries (3.0%) report a higher incidence, suggesting the influence of genetic factors.[47] Pruritus gravidarum (PG) occurs most commonly in the third trimester, but symptoms may appear earlier in the second and also in the first trimester.

There are no primary skin lesions in PG, but excoriations due to scratching may be extensive. To make the diagnosis of PG, signs and symptoms of other hepatic diseases such as viral hepatitis, biliary colic, and exposure to drugs known to induce cholestasis must be excluded. Laboratory findings may show biochemical abnormalities suggesting intrahepatic cholestasis, and the most important feature that characterizes cholestasis is impaired biliary excretion of bile acids and their accumulation in the blood.[48] Though serum levels of bilirubin, alkaline phosphatase, and aminotransferases may be slightly elevated or normal, serum bile acids, particularly cholic acid, are most characteristically increased.[48] Liver biopsy shows mild nonspecific cholestasis without significant liver cell damage.[47]

Characteristically, PG disappears rapidly (from a few hours to days) post partum, and tends to recur in subsequent pregnancies though symptom-free pregnancies may intervene between cholestatic pregnancies.[49] The pruritus in PG and cholestasis has always been attributed to increased level of bile acids, and more specifically the bile acids in *skin* rather than serum,[50] since pruritus has been noted in patients with low levels of serum bile acids, and relief from pruritus may occur even in the presence of high serum bile acid levels.[51] More recent evidence indicates that bile acids may not be the pruritus-inducing factor, but rather the factor may be another constituent of bile that binds to cholestyramine and is photolabile.[51]

The increase in serum bile acids in pregnancy is related to decreased hepatic excretion of organic anions (bilirubin, bile acids). Estrogens and progestins appear to interfere with hepatic excretion of bile in genetically susceptible individuals.[47]

Cholestasis of pregnancy–PG is associated with increased risk of complications for both mother and fetus. There is a significantly increased incidence of premature deliveries,[49, 52–54] and low-birth-weight babies, intrapartum fetal distress,[52–54] unexplained stillbirths, and perinatal death.[52, 53]

The maternal complication seen with PG is an increased incidence of postpartum hemorrhage,[49, 52, 54] which may possibly be related to vitamin K deficiency.[52] These complications for both mother and child indicate that patients with PG need to be followed as a high-risk pregnancy with all the appropriate tests associated with that group.

Management.—Treatment of pruritus gravidarum with severe pruritus may present substantial difficulties. Topical therapy with moisturizers, antipruritics (such as calamine or emollient lotion with 0.25% menthol), or topical steroids may be tried, but generally offers little relief for those individuals with

TABLE 16–2.
Pruritus Gravidarum

Onset	Third trimester; but may appear earlier
Clinical appearance	Generalized excoriations due to scratching; pruritus may be intense
Distribution	Generalized
Histopathology	NA
Immunofluorescence	NA
Immunogenetic	—
Maternal complications	Pruritus; postpartum hemorrhage
Effect on fetus	Prematurity, low birth weight, intrapartum fetal distress, unexplained stillbirth and perinatal death
Recurrences	Yes
Treatment	Cholestyramine, UV light
NA = not applicable.	

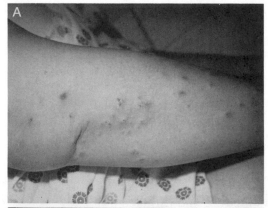

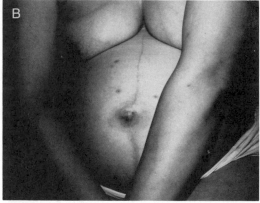

FIG 16–1.
A, papular eruption of pregnancy (prurigo of pregnancy). Multiple 1- to 3-mm pruritic excoriated papules grouped on extremities and trunk. **B,** papular dermatitis of pregnancy. Lesions are 3- to 5-mm pruritic, excoriated papules widely scattered without grouping.

more severe pruritus. Antihistamines have not been helpful in this process either. Oral cholestyramine resin (FDA category C), which forms a nonabsorbable complex with bile acids allowing for their fecal excretion (4 g one to three times daily), may alleviate pruritus in some patients.[54, 55] Phenobarbital (FDA category D) has been shown to increase bile excretion in hepatic cholestasis and has been helpful in improving the associated pruritus[51] but it has not been found to be particularly effective in PG in some studies,[54, 55] while successfully relieving the pruritus in half the cases in another study.[56] A new promising modality of treatment for the pruritus of cholestasis may be phototherapy with UV light, either UVA or UVB, although controlled studies in PG have not yet been published.[51]

Pruritic Folliculitis of Pregnancy

In the second or third trimester, some women develop a pruritic acnelike eruption which appears on the shoulders, upper back, arms, chest, and abdomen. The lesions consist of multiple 2- to 4-mm follicular papules or pustules and clinically resemble steroid acne. Histopathologic examination shows inflammation in the hair follicle and surrounding dermis.[57] Direct immunofluorescence examination is negative. The approach to treatment of pruritic folliculitis is similar to that of mild acne, with low-potency benzoyl peroxide lotion applied to lesions only. If pruritus is severe, 1% hydrocortisone cream may alleviate the symptoms, but response to any treatment may be minimal until the postpartum period.

Papular Eruptions During Pregnancy

The discussion of pruritic papular eruptions during pregnancy is marked by controversy regarding the suggestion that there are two types of pruritic papular eruption, one of them benign (prurigo gestationis, PGe),[58] the other associated with high fetal mortality (papular dermatitis of pregnancy, PDP).[59, 60] The controversy stems from the fact that except for two original reports[59, 60] there have been no other reported series of patients with papular dermatitis of pregnancy that substantiated the findings of high fetal mortality (27%) or abnormal biochemical findings.

The clinical evidence that purported to differentiate the two papular disorders, PGe and PDP, was that in PGe the lesions were small (1–3 mm), itchy, rapidly excoriated papules that were grouped on the extensor surfaces of the limbs and upper trunk (Fig 16–1, A) whereas in PDP the lesions were pruritic 3- to 5-mm papules, often excoriated, but, unlike PGe, widely scattered without grouping or a predilection for any area (Fig 16–1, B). Current assessment of these papular disorders is that the widespread distribution of the lesions in PDP does not indicate a separate disorder, but that it may simply represent a more widespread form of PGe.[61]

Another characteristic used to separate PDP from PGe was the biochemical finding of markedly elevated levels of urinary chorionic gonadotropin, reduced plasma cortisol, and low urinary estriol levels in PDP.[59, 60] These biochemical investigations have not been described in PGe nor have they all been repeated in another group of patients with PDP.

There are also a number of problems with the data used to draw the conclusion of unfavorable effect of papular dermatitis on the fetus. The authors did not indicate how many of the affected pregnancies ended in spontaneous abortion and how many with stillbirth and furthermore these studies did not include appropriate control populations. In addition, the 8 of 11 pregnancies which ended in fetal demise were not accompanied by a cutaneous eruption and were reported retrospectively. The one fetal demise in the group that occurred during the actual time of the study and which was accompanied by a rash was associated with a rapidly rising Rh titer. It is therefore difficult to attribute that death to papular dermatitis of pregnancy rather than Rh incompatibility.

The etiology and pathogenesis of these papular eruptions are unknown. Spangler and co-workers[59, 60] attributed PDP to abnormal placental function or hypersensitivity to placental tissue. Holmes and Black[61] have attributed the papular eruption in pregnancy to an atopic diathesis, categorizing it as a form of eczema.

The diagnosis of PDP must be based on the clinical appearance of a primary papular eruption. We have studied 16 patients with papular-type eruptions in pregnancy in whom liver functions and bile acids were measured to exclude cholestasis of pregnancy. We found no clinical or biochemical evidence to suggest that more than one disorder differentiated by distribution or extensiveness was represented. We found no evidence that papular eruption in pregnancy is a disorder with high risk for the fetus.[62]

Management.—The goals of treatment of any dermatoses of pregnancy, including the papular eruptions, are to make the mother more comfortable and to prevent fetal loss. Therapy with topical nonsteroidal antipruritics or steroid creams and ointments and systemic antihistamines is often adequate to control the pruritus. It is absolutely not necessary to administer high-dose systemic steroids for the papular dermatoses of pregnancy. Although this dermatosis may represent a form of underlying hypersensitivity reaction, there is no evidence at the present time to indicate that high-dose corticosteroids are necessary for delivery of a viable infant. Assessment of the intrauterine environment with appropriate fetal monitoring is a reasonable approach until more is known about the pathophysiology of the papular dermatoses.

Herpes Gestationis

Herpes gestationis (HG) (see Table 16–3) is a pruritic blistering eruption of pregnancy and the puerperium that has also been described in association with the trophoblastic tumor hydatiform mole and with choriocarcinoma. Although it is called "herpes" gestationis, it has nothing whatsoever to do with the herpesvirus. It is, as are some other bullous dermatoses, an autoimmune process in which an antibody directed against the basement membrane zone of the epidermis induces inflammation and blister formation.

The incidence of HG has been estimated at anywhere from 1 in 3,000 to 1 in 60,000, but an incidence of 1 in 50,000 is considered more accurate.[63, 64] Herpes gestationis most commonly begins in the second or third trimester, but may begin as early as 2 weeks of gestation or early in the postpartum period (from hours after delivery to 1 week post partum). The course of the disorder involves exacerbations and remissions with postpartum exacerbations being very common (75%–80%).[64] The average postpartum duration has been noted as 4 weeks for the bullous lesions and 60 weeks for the urticarial lesions,[59] but the frequent use of systemic steroids to treat HG may be changing these features.[64] Postpartum flares of HG are common and may occur either premenstrually or with ovula-

TABLE 16–3.
Differential Diagnosis of Herpes Gestationis (HG) and Pruritic Papules and Plaques of Pregnancy (PUPP)

	Herpes Gestationis	PUPPP*
Onset	2 wk gestation to 1 wk post partum	Most commonly 3rd trimester; some 2nd trimester and rarely earlier
Clinical appearance	Variable urticarial papules and plaques, polycylic or generalized erythema, vesicles, bullae	Erythematous papules, urticarial papules and plaques, patchy or generalized; erythema; small vesicles
Distribution	Abdomen, extremities, or generalized	Abdomen, thighs, buttocks, arms, or more widespread
Histopathology	Dermal edema and infiltrate of lymphocytes, histiocytes, and eosinophils Subepidermal blister	Perivascular lymphohistiocytic infiltrate with some eosinophils; some have epidermal edema or small vesicles
Immunofluorescence	Linear C3 deposition with or without IgG at basement membrane zone	Negative for any specific findings
Immunogenetic	High frequency of HLA antigens HLA-A1, -B8, -DR3, and combined HLA-DR3/DR4	—
Maternal complications	Pruritus, discomfort, secondary infections	Pruritus, discomfort
Effect on fetus	± ↑ Incidence of spontaneous abortion and stillbirth Increased frequency of low-birth-weight and small-for-date babies *Neonatal HG* 2%–5%, usually mild and transient	None known
Recurrence	Recurs in subsequent pregnancies, or with oral contraceptives	Possible, but not as a rule
Treatment	Mild cases—topical steroids More severe cases—systemic steroids	Topical corticosteroid creams

*PUPPP = pruritic urticarial papules and plaques of pregnancy.

tion,[65] and they also appear with the use of oral contraceptives.[65] Herpes gestationis is a recurrent disease process that appears earlier in gestation with subsequent pregnancies.[66]

Clinically, the features which characterize HG include pruritus, which is usually severe and may precede the cutaneous lesions. The eruption frequently begins in or around the umbilicus, but arms or legs may also be initial sites, and it then spreads to the abdomen and thighs (Plate 1, A and B). The back, breasts, palms, and soles are frequently affected, but face, scalp, and mucosa are involved infrequently (less than 10%).[59, 63, 64] The morphologic features of the eruption are erythematous urticarial papules, urticarial plaques, polycyclic or extensive erythema, and erythematous edematous plaques subsequently followed by vesicles and bullae. Vesicles and tense bullae appear at the margins of erythematous edematous plaques, on top of an erythematous edematous base, or in otherwise clinically uninvolved skin. Healing usually occurs without scarring if secondary infection does not intervene.

The histopathology of HG varies with the type of lesion biopsied. The classic HG blister is subepidermal; the urticarial lesion shows epidermal edema, and both show an edematous upper dermis which contains an infiltrate of lymphocytes, histiocytes, and eosinophils in varying proportions. Direct immunofluorescence of skin lesions (and perilesional skin) demonstrates linear deposition of complement (C3) in essentially all cases, and IgG in some (25%), at the basement membrane zone. A circulating serum factor called *herpes gestationis factor,* which fixes complement at the basement membrane of human skin in complement-binding studies, is present. This

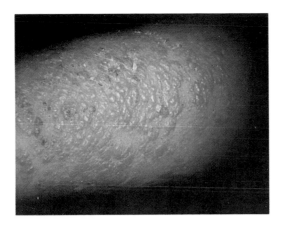

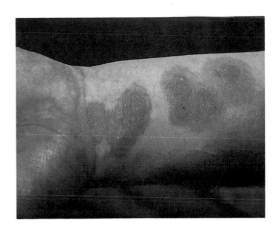

PLATE 1.
Herpes gestationis. Vesicular eruption on forearm.
Erythematous plaques were present on other sites.

PLATE 2.
Herpes gestationis. Targetlike lesions.
Bullae were present at other sites.

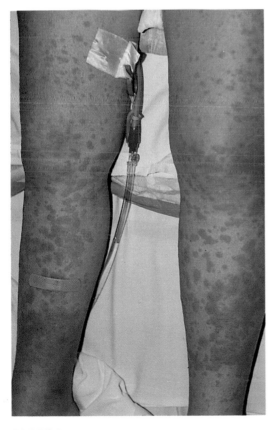

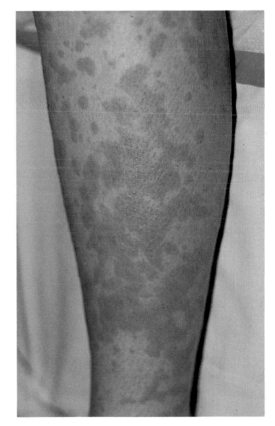

PLATE 3.
Pruritic urticarial papules and plaques of pregnancy
(PUPPP) on thighs and legs. Lesions were also present
on abdomen, buttocks, and arms.

PLATE 4.
Detail from Plate 3.

factor has been shown to be an IgG molecule capable of crossing the placenta and of activating complement pathways in the deposition of C3 at the basement membrane zone.[63, 64] This HG factor has also been shown to react with amniotic epithelial membrane,[67] supporting the proposal that HG factor may be induced by placental antigens and cross-reacts with skin antigens. Herpes gestationes factor has recently been found to react with a 180-kilodalton human epidermal antigen.[68]

The etiology of HG is not known, but there appears to be a genetic predisposition toward its development, similar to the genetic predisposition toward other immunologically mediated disease. HLA studies reveal an increase in HLA-A1, -B8, and -DR3 antigens.[64, 65] Sixty to eighty-five percent of patients with HG have HLA-DR-3 and 43% to 45% have the combination of HLA-DR3 and -DR4.[64, 65] An increased frequency in these HLA-DR antigens has been found in association with a number of diseases of immune origin including Graves' disease, thyroiditis, type I diabetes, Addison's disease, dermatitis herpetiformis, and systemic lupus erythematosus.[64] Disease association with HLA-DR3 and/or -DR4 may be the result of an HLA-DR3- and/or -DR-4-related immune response gene that confers increased immune responsiveness and predisposition to "autoimmune disease."[65, 66]

Herpes gestationis must be differentiated from diseases that occur coincidentally during pregnancy, including erythema multiforme, pemphigus, dermatitis herpetiformis, and bullous drug eruptions. But the important differential diagnosis of HG is distinguishing it from the more common pruritic urticarial papules and plaques of pregnancy (PUPPP), also called toxic erythema of pregnancy (TEP) or polymorphous eruption of pregnancy (PEP) (see Table 16–3). The distribution of PUPPP is similar to HG with edematous papules beginning on the abdomen and arms prior to becoming more generalized. In many HG patients the papular/urticarial lesions precede the bullous component by over a month, and in the prebullous stage differentiating HG from PUPPP may be very difficult. Some patients with HG may not develop bullae at all in their first pregnancy. Vesicles do occur in both HG and PUPPP, but vesicles in PUPPP are never larger than a few millimeters (1–2 mm), whereas they may progress to larger bullae in HG. PUPPP is commonly most severe in the last few weeks of pregnancy and almost always resolves within a few weeks of delivery, whereas HG is often quiescent at parturition but then commonly flares post partum. The one single means that definitively differentiates between HG and PUPPP is the direct immunofluorescence finding of a linear band of C3 at the basement membrane zone which is always positive in HG but consistently negative in PUPPP.[66]

The maternal morbidity associated with HG involves severe pruritus, the great discomfort associated with blistering eruptions, and the risk of secondary bacterial infections due to the blistering disruption of the cutaneous barrier as well as the use of systemic steroid therapy. There is no increase in maternal mortality.

The incidence of fetal morbidity and mortality in HG is controversial, with some studies reporting no increased incidence of stillbirth or spontaneous abortion[63, 69, 70] while another shows an increased risk of stillbirth (7.7% as compared with 1.3% in the general population) and prematurity (23% vs. 5%).[71] A recent study reported a significant increase in the frequency of low-birth-weight and "small-for-dates" infants associated with HG.[70] In this study, 44% of patients received systemic corticosteroid during the pregnancy and there were no great differences in birth weight and frequency of small-for-date infants between these patients and those who did not receive corticosteroids.[70]

Neonatal HG occurs infrequently (2%–5%)[63, 65] and is usually mild and transient, resolving within a month without specific treatment. The lesions in neonatal HG may be only erythematous papules or frank bullae,[72] associated with deposition of C3 at the basement membrane zone.[63, 72]

Management.—Treatment in the milder

cases of maternal HG may consist of topical steroids and antihistamines. More severely affected patients for whom topical steroids offer no relief are treated with systemic steroids. The majority of HG patients will respond to 40 mg prednisone daily, which can then be tapered to lower doses until the postpartum period, when exacerbation may necessitate increasing the dosage again. Success using plasmapheresis has been reported anecdotally in a few patients when very high prednisone doses did not control the process.[63, 73]

Patients with HG should be followed closely as in any pregnancy with potential high risk, including frequent fetal monitoring.[70] Once HG has occurred it will almost always recur in subsequent pregnancies, appear earlier in the pregnancy, tend to have a more severe course, and may have recurrence induced by oral contraceptives. Due to these findings oral contraceptives are best avoided in HG patients and subsequent pregnancies should be carefully monitored beginning early in gestation.

Pruritic Urticarial Papules and Plaques of Pregnancy (PUPPP)

This urticarial and erythematous eruption of pregnancy (see Table 16–3) has been described by a number of observers, each giving it another name,[58, 61, 74–78] thus leading to some confusion. There is still disagreement as to which name to use. Pruritic urticarial papules and plaques of pregnancy (PUPPP)[78] is the most commonly used term in the United States, but since it does not satisfactorily describe the clinical spectrum of this process, we will refer to it here as PUPPP/TEP (toxic erythema of pregnancy) where PUPPP describes the urticarial portion of the spectrum and TEP the erythematous patches and plaques, often with superimposed small papules and vesicles.

The reported incidence of PUPPP/TEP varies from 1 in 120[74] to 1 in 240.[77] The majority of cases begin in the third trimester, but it may also appear in the second trimester, and we have seen it in the first trimester as well (I.K.A., personal observation). PUPPP often begins with small papules in abdominal striae, and abdominal striae are prominent in a significant percentage of these patients. The eruption spreads with erythematous urticarial papules and plaques to the rest of the abdomen, thighs, buttocks, and arms (see Plate 1, C and D). Many patients will also have small erythematous papules surrounded by blanched halos on the legs. In the form of the eruption described as toxic erythema of pregnancy, the lesions are erythematous patches and plaques, not urticarial in appearance, that may be discrete or confluent and surmounted by tiny (1 mm) papules and vesicles which may be excoriated. This form will also often have the small papules surrounded by a blanched halo on the legs. The erythematous patches and plaques are often widespread, involving not only abdomen, thighs, buttocks, and legs, but also thorax, arms, feet (including palms and soles in some), and the face (personal observation of the authors).

Some patients have mainly the urticarial form of the dermatitis, others have mainly the erythematous pattern with papules and tiny vesicles, while others have a combination of the two. Some may even have targetlike lesions reminiscent of erythema multiforme. It is this spectrum of clinical appearances that led Holmes and Black[61] to suggest the name polymorphic eruption of pregnancy (PEP).

There are no laboratory abnormalities found in PUPPP/TEP. Histopathologically, light microscopy reveals a nonspecific perivascular lymphohistiocytic infiltrate with some eosinophils in the dermis. Some patients will also have edema or small vesicles in the epidermis. Immunofluorescence staining of lesional biopsies in these cases is consistently negative for a linear band of complement or immunoglobulins at the basement membrane, thus differentiating it from HG. However, some of the lesions do have deposits of C3 or IgM in blood vessel walls as well as granular deposits of C3 at the dermal epidermal junction[78, 79] (unpublished observations of authors). The significance of the presence of these immune reactants in some cases has not been elucidated.

The absence of linear deposit of complement at the basement membrane is the crucial determining test that can differentiate PUPPP/TEP from HG, in which a linear C3 band and sometimes a linear IgG band is found. Since there is significant clinical and histologic overlap between these two entities, it is prudent to have direct immunofluorescence biopsies done in these cases confirming the diagnosis. In addition to differentiating PUPPP/TEP from HG, the eruption must also be differentiated from pityriasis rosea occurring in pregnancy or from drug eruptions which can appear urticarial or as a generalized erythematous macular and papular eruption. We have seen at least four cases of PUPPP/TEP appear from 3 to 24 hours after terbutaline was given for premature labor. Whether the terbutaline or the premature labor had an etiologic role in the appearance of the eruption is not yet clear.

Management.—Maternal morbidity associated with PUPPP/TEP is simply the discomfort associated with the pruritus. The goal of therapy is to make the mother comfortable. While some patients may obtain adequate relief from pruritus with emollients alone, most patients will require topical applications of intermediate-potency steroid creams and ointments or lower-potency hydrocortisone creams for relief of the pruritus. In some patients oral antihistamines such as chlorpheniramine maleate (FDA category B) may be beneficial.

Although there are no known fetal complications with PUPPP/TEP, we recommend monitoring the fetus with weekly nonstress tests through the duration of the eruption. This recommendation is based on our experience with three patients in whom fetal monitoring produced a positive nonstress test which led to induction of labor. PUPPP/TEP generally resolves within 2 to 5 weeks if it occurs intrapartum early in the pregnancy, or 1 to 3 weeks post partum, if it begins late in the pregnancy.

Impetigo Herpetiformis

Impetigo herpetiformis (IH) is a rare pustular eruption occurring in pregnancy that is considered by many[3, 80, 81] to be a form of pustular psoriasis which happens to be triggered by pregnancy, and by others to be a distinct entity unrelated to psoriasis.[82, 83] It usually appears in the last 3 months of pregnancy and may appear earlier with subsequent pregnancies.[84]

The cutaneous lesions may consist of round, polycyclic, or irregular patches of erythema studded with superficial sterile pustules at the margins. It commonly begins in flexures and extends peripherally until the entire body may be covered. As the lesions extend pustules break down and become impetiginized, while the peripheral margin advances with new pustule formation. Pruritus is not usually a severe problem in IH. Flexural area lesions may develop vegetative characteristics resembling condylomata.[5] Mucous membranes, including the oral and respiratory tract, may be affected, and subungual pustules may cause oncholysis.[80]

Impetigo herpetiformis is commonly associated with severe systemic symptoms and signs including fever, chills, nausea, vomiting, and diarrhea. Hypoalbuminemia, hypocalcemia, and hypocalcemia-induced tetany, as well as hyperuricemia, may be present in IH. Of the original five patients reported by Hebra[85] in 1872, four died. The high mortality rate reported in IH was due to sepsis, hypocalcemic tetany, seizures,[85] hyperthermia, renal failure, or cardiac failure.[86] Laboratory findings in IH commonly show leukocytosis and elevated sedimentation rates; hypoalbuminemia, hypoparathyroidism, and hypocalcemia have been frequently reported.

The pustular lesions of IH are sterile until they rupture, at which time they may become secondarily infected. The histopathology of IH is basically indistinguishable from pustular psoriasis, showing a spongelike cavity in the epidermis which is filled with neutrophils and called the *spongiform pustule of Ko-*

goj. The microabscess enlarges and a clinically apparent intraepidermal pustule is formed. Impetigo herpetiformis must be differentiated from impetigo, HG, or pemphigus.

Management.—The treatment for IH is systemic steroids in doses varying from 40 to 80 mg to effectively control the process. This, in conjunction with antibiotics, has changed the maternal prognosis in this once-fatal disease. Impetigo herpetiformis tends to remit from a few weeks to a few months after pregnancy.[84] Although the maternal prognosis has changed with systemic steroids, antibiotics, and careful general medical monitoring, fetal prognosis is still poor with a high reported incidence of stillbirths despite cordicosteroid therapy.[83, 84] Careful monitoring of fetal well-being is recommended. If fetal pulmonary maturity is adequate, or should the maternal condition worsen or fetal well-being be questionable, termination of pregnancy has been recommended.[81]

The dermatoses specific to pregnancy are listed in Table 16–4.

SKIN DISEASES AFFECTED BY PREGNANCY

The endocrine and immunologic changes that occur during pregnancy may affect a variety of prexisting skin diseases ranging from acne to malignancies. Infections, including syphilis, and herpes simplex and herpes varicella/-l zoster, are discussed in Chapters 13 and 14, respectively. Immunologically mediated diseases such as lupus erythematosus, dermatomyositis, and scleroderma are discussed in Chapter 11.

Acne, psoriasis, and eczema, common dermatologic problems, may show no change, improve, or worsen during pregnancy.

Pemphigus vulgaris and *pemphigus foliaceus* have been reported to occur in pregnancy and may appear for the first time during, or be aggravated by, pregnancy.[87, 88] The clinical appearance of pemphigus may be similar to herpes gestationis so that skin biopsy and im-

munofluorescence examination are necessary to differentiate the two bullous dermatoses. Of the 29 reported cases of pemphigus in pregnancy, 4 resulted in stillbirth,[89] and therefore pregnancies in pemphigus patients must be considered a high risk for the fetus. Pemphigus is treated with dapsone or high-dose prednisone, the latter predisposing the mother to risk of infection.

Neurofibromatosis may be adversely affected by pregnancy with the initial appearance or increase in number and size of neurofibromas and café au lait spots.[90] Spontaneous hemothorax and renal artery rupture due to neurofibromas invading vessel walls have been reported.[91, 92] Hypertension is extremely common during pregnancy in patients with neurofibromatosis.[90]

Leprosy (Hansen's disease, HD) is a chronic granulomatous bacterial infection caused by *Mycobacterium leprae.*[93] It primarily affects the skin and peripheral nerves, but larynx, nose, and pharynx may be involved and complications include deformities of the hands and feet, amyloidosis, ulceration of the skin, perforation of the nasal septum, blindness, and laryngeal obstruction.[94] Leprosy is adversely affected by pregnancy in a number of ways. Pregnancy may precipitate the appearance of the disorder in women who have never shown clinical evidence of the disease.[95] Women who have completed the treatment period for the tuberculoid form of leprosy and are considered "cured" are liable to have a relapse during pregnancy or after parturition. The relapse may appear in the first, second, or even a later pregnancy after a cure.[95] Leprosy may show

TABLE 16–4.
Specific Dermatoses of Pregnancy

Pruritus gravidarum (cholestasis of pregnancy)
Pruritic folliculitis of pregnancy
Papular eruption of pregnancy (prurigo of pregnancy, papular dermatitis of pregnancy)
Herpes gestationis
Pruritic urticarial papules and plaques of pregnancy (PUPPP, toxic erythema of pregnancy, polymorphic eruption of pregnancy)
Impetigo herpetiformis

exacerbation of disease in pregnant women receiving apparently adequate treatment.[95] Patients may show transient worsening despite effective therapy, or significant deterioration caused by emergence of dapsone-resistant organisms. The immunosuppressive factors of pregnancy may permit drug-resistant *M. leprae* bacilli to increase and cause worsening of the disease.[95]

Worsening or exacerbation of leprosy is recognized by increases in the concentration or viability, or both, of bacilli in the skin smear, conversion of a negative bacillary index to positive, the appearance of new skin lesions, extension of existing lesions, or the appearance of erythema in tuberculoid lesions.[95] There may also be a "downgrading" or shift toward the lepromatous end of the leprosy spectrum.[96]

Pregnancy also affects the reactional states of leprosy. Type 1 lepra reactions are diagnosed by erythema and edema (and/or ulcerations) of skin lesions, tender enlargement of nerves with or without loss of nerve function, loss of nerve function without tender nerves (silent neuritis), or tenosynovitis.[95] These reactions increase in the first trimester, decrease until delivery, and then increase after delivery and during lactation, often continuing for many months.[95] The high incidence of this reactional state post partum is most likely due to the postpartum recovery of the cell-mediated immune system from its suppression during pregnancy.[95]

Type 2 lepra reactions are diagnosed by the appearance of crops of painful red nodules that are frequently associated with fevers, malaise, lymphadenopathy and tender enlarged peripheral nerves (erythema nodosum leprosum, ENL), iridocyclitis, or dactylitis. Type 2 lepra reactions increase during pregnancy and lactation, are associated with exacerbation of leprosy, and occur throughout pregnancy with peaks in the third trimester, slowly decreasing during first year of lactation.[95] This reaction is associated with suppressed cell-mediated immunity in pregnancy, and with increased numbers of bacilli.[95, 96]

In Duncan and Pearson's study[96], 15% of patients had ENL reactions almost continuously from the third trimester to 15 months post partum. This reaction involved the skin more frequently during the pregnancy, and the nerves more frequently post partum.[96]

The effect of the mother's leprosy on the baby included growth retardation, fetal distress, low birth weight, small placentas, and effects were most marked in mothers with the lepromatous form of the disorder.[97] Leprosy is uncommon in very young children, even in the presence of infectious family members, but transplacental transmission of *M. leprae* appears to be approximately 5%.[90]

Treatment of leprosy during pregnancy includes dapsone (FDA category C), the main therapeutic antibiotic used in this disease. Unfortunately, resistance to dapsone is not uncommon, especially during pregnancy, and additional therapy to decrease the risk of dapsone resistance may be necessary. Clofazimine (FDA category C) given after the first trimester for a period of 1 year would decrease the appearance of drug resistance and transient relapse and also would treat or prevent erythema nodosum leprosum.[96] However, since neonatal death and other neonatal abnormalities have been reported in association with the use of clofazimine,[94] these patients must be closely monitored.

REFERENCES

1. Fitzpatrick TB, Eisen AZ, Wolff K, et al: *Dermatology in General Medicine.* New York, McGraw-Hill Book Co, 1979, pp 1363–1370.
2. Wong RC, Ellis CN: Physiologic skin changes in pregnancy. *J Am Acad Dermatol* 1984; 10:929–940.
3. Braverman IM: *Skin Signs of Systemic Disease.* Philadelphia, WB Saunders Co, 1981, pp 761–776.
4. Wade TR, Wade SL, Jones HE: Skin changes and diseases associated with pregnancy. *Obstet Gynecol* 1978; 52:233–234.
5. Winton GB, Lewis CW: Dermatoses of pregnancy. *J Am Acad Dermatol* 1982; 6:977–978.
6. Snell RS, Bischitz PG: The effect of large doses of estrogen and progesterone on melanin pigmentation. *J Invest Dermatol* 1960; 35:73–82.

7. Shizume K, Lerner AB: Determination of melanocyte-stimulating hormone in urine and blood. *J Clin Endocrinol* 1954; 14:1491–1510.

8. McGuinness BW: Melanocyte-stimulating hormone: A clinical and laboratory study. *Ann NY Acad Sci* 1963; 100:640–657.

9. Snell RS, Turner R: Skin pigmentation in relation to the menstrual cycle. *J Invest Dermatol* 1966; 47:147–155.

10. McKenzie AW: Skin disorders in pregnancy. *Practioner* 1971; 206:773–780.

11. Thody AJ, Plummer NA, Burton JL, et al: Plasma beta-melanocyte stimulating hormone levels in pregnancy. *J Obstet Gynaecol Br Commnw* 1974; 81:875–877.

12. Fisher AA: *Contact Dermatitis.* Philadelphia, Lea & Febiger, 1986, pp 375–376.

13. Hellreich PD: The skin changes of pregnancy. *Cutis* 1974; 13:82–86.

14. Judd HL, Benirschke K, DeVane G, et al: Maternal virilization developing during a twin pregnancy: Demonstration of excess ovarian androgen production associated with theca lutein cysts. *N Engl J Med* 1973; 288:118–122.

15. Fayer JA, Bunch TR, Miller GL: Virilization in pregnancy associated with polycystic ovary disease. *Obstet Gynecol* 1974; 44:511–521.

16. Lynfield YL: Effect of pregnancy on the human hair cycle. *J Invest Dermatol* 1960; 35:323.

17. Benson RC: *Current Obstetric and Gynecologic Diagnosis and Treatment.* Los Altos, Calif, Lange Medical Publications, 1982, p 841.

18. Schiff BL, Kern AB: A study of postpartum alopecia. *Arch Dermatol* 1963; 87:609.

19. Bean WB, Cogswell R, Dexter M, et al: Vascular changes of the skin in pregnancy. *Surg Gynecol Obstet* 1949; 88:739–752.

20. Demis DJ: *Clinical Dermatology* vol 2. New York, Harper & Row Publishers, Inc, 1975, unit 12–25, pp 1–9.

21. Cummings K, Derbes VJ: Dermatoses associated with pregnancy. *Cutis* 1967; 3:120–125.

22. Foucar E, Bentley TJ, Laube DW, et al: A histopathologic evaluation of nevocellular nevi in pregnancy. *Arch Dermatol* 1985; 121:350–354.

23. Lerner AB, Nordlund JJ, Kirkwood JM: Effects of oral contraceptives and pregnancy on melanoma. *N Engl J Med* 1979; 301:47.

24. Ariel IM: Theories regarding the cause of malignant melanoma. *Surg Gynecol Obstet* 1980; 150:907–927.

25. Houghton AN, Flannery J, Viola MV: Malignant melanoma of the skin occurring during pregnancy. *Cancer* 1981; 48:407–410.

26. Danforth DN, Russell N, McBride CM: Hormonal status of patients with primary malignant melanoma: A review of 313 cases. *South Med J* 1982; 75:661–664.

27. Pack GT, Scharnagel IM: The prognosis for malignant melanoma in the pregnant woman. *Cancer* 1951; 4:324–334.

28. Moller D, Ipsen L, Asschenfeldt P: Fatal course of malignant melanoma during pregnancy with dissemination to the products of conception. *Acta Obstet Gynecol Scand* 1986; 65:501–502.

29. Riberti C, Marola G, Bertani A: Malignant melanoma: The adverse effect of pregnancy. *Br J Plast Surg* 1981; 34:338–339.

30. Allen EP: Malignant melanoma—spontaneous regression after pregnancy. *Br Med J* 1955; 2:1067.

31. Stewart H: A case of malignant melanoma and pregnancy. *Br Med J* 1955; 1:647–650.

32. Sumner WC: Spontaneous regression of melanoma—report of a case. *Cancer* 1953; 6:1040–1043.

33. Sutherland CM, Loutfi A, Mather FJ, et al: Effect of pregnancy upon malignant melanoma. *Surg Gynecol Obstet* 1983; 157:443–446.

34. Grill HJ, Benes P, Manz B, et al: Steroid hormone receptor analysis in human melanoma and non-malignant human skin. *Br J Dermatol* 1982; 107 (suppl):64–65.

35. Fisher RI, Neifeld JP, Lippman ME: Oestrogen receptors in human malignant melanoma. *Lancet* 1976; 2:337–339.

36. Chaudhuri PK, Walker MJ, Briele HA, et al: Incidence of estrogen receptor in benign nevi and human malignant melanoma. *JAMA* 1980; 244:791–793.

37. Shiu MH, Schottenfeld D, Maclean B, et al: Adverse effect of pregnancy on melanoma—a reappraisal. *Cancer* 1976; 37:181–187.

38. White LP, Linden G, Breslow L, et al: Studies on melanoma—the effect of pregnancy on survival in human melanoma. *JAMA* 1961; 177:235–238.

39. George PA, Fortner JG, Pack GT: Melanoma with pregnancy—report of 115 cases. *Cancer* 1960; 13:854–859.

40. Reintgen DS, McCarty KS, Vollmer R, et al: Malignant melanoma and pregnancy. *Cancer* 1985; 55:1340–1344.

41. Shaw JHF: Malignant melanoma in Auckland, New Zealand. *Surg Gynecol Obstet* 1988; 166:425–430.

42. Hersey P, Morgan G, Stone DE, et al: Previous pregnancy as a protective factor against death from melanoma. *Lancet* 1977; 1:451–452.

43. Winton GB: Skin diseases aggravated by pregnancy. *J Am Acad Dermatol* 1989; 20:1–13.

44. Weber FP, Scharwz E, Hellenschmied R: [co]ntaneous inoculation of melanotic sar[coma fr]om mother to foetus: report of a case. [Br Med J] 1930; 1:537–539.

45. [Gilli]an WL: Cancer and pregnancy. *Cancer* [19]3:194–214.

46. [Ha]ch RT: Jaundice in pregnancy— [.] *Am J Med* 1976; 61:367–373.

47. [Reye]s H, Gonzalez MC, Ribalta J, et al: [Prev]alence of intrahepatic cholestasis of [pregn]ancy in Chile. *Ann Intern Med* 1978; [89:48]7–493.

48. [L]aatikainen T, Ikonen E: Serum bile acids in cholestasis of pregnancy. *Obstet Gynecol* 1977; 50:313–318.

49. Johnston WG, Baskett TF: Obstetric cholestasis; A 14 year review. *Am J Obstet Gynecol* 1979; 133:299–301.

50. Varadi DP: Pruritus induced by crude bile and purified bile acids. *Arch Dermatol* 1974; 109:678–681.

51. Garden JM, Ostrow JD, Roenigk HH Jr: Pruritus in hepatic cholestasis, pathogenesis and therapy. *Arch Dermatol* 1985; 121:1415–1420.

52. Reid R, Ivey KJ, Rencoret RH, et al: Fetal complications of obstetric cholestasis. *Br Med J* 1976; 1:870–872.

53. Furhoff AK: Itching in pregnancy. *Acta Med Scand* 1974; 196:403–410.

54. Shaw P, Frohlich J, Wittmann BAK, et al: A prospective study of 18 patients with cholestasis of pregnancy. *Am J Obstet Gynecol* 1982; 142:621–625.

55. Laatikainen T: Effect of cholestyramine and phenobarbital on pruritus and serum bile acid levels in cholestasis of pregnancy. *Am J Obstet Gynecol* 1978; 132:501–506.

56. Heikkinen J, Mäentausta O, Ylöstalo P, et al: Serum bile acid levels in intrahepatic cholestasis of pregnancy during treatment with phenobarbital or cholestyramine. *Eur J Obstet Gynecol Reprod Biol* 1982; 14:153–162.

57. Zoberman E, Farmer E: Pruritic folliculitis of pregnancy. *Arch Dermatol* 1981; 117:20–22.

58. Nurse DS: Prurigo of pregnancy. *Aust J Dermatol* 1968; 9:258–267.

59. Spangler AS, Reddy W, Bardawil WA, et al: Papular dermatitis of pregnancy. A new clinical entity. *JAMA* 1962; 181:577–581.

60. Spangler AS, Emerson K Jr: Estrogen levels and estrogen therapy in papular dermatitis of pregnancy. *Am J Obstet Gynecol* 1971; 110:534–537.

61. Holmes RC, Black MM: The specific dermatoses of pregnancy. *J Am Acad Dermatol* 1983; 8:405–412.

62. Aronson IK, Halaska B, Bardawil W, et al: A study of papular dermatitis of pregnancy. *Clin Res* 1984; 32:569A.

63. Shornick JK, Bangert JL, Freeman RG, et al: Herpes gestationis: Clinical and histologic features of twenty-eight cases. *J Am Acad Dermatol* 1983; 8:214–224.

64. Shornick JK: Herpes gestationis. *J Am Acad Dermatol* 1987; 17:539–556.

65. Holmes RC, Black MM, Jurecka W, et al: Clues to the aetiology and pathogenesis of herpes gestationis. *Br J Dermatol* 1983; 109:131–139.

66. Holmes RC, Black MM: Herpes gestationis. *Dermatol Clin* 1983; 1:195–203.

67. Ortonne JP, Hsi BL, Verrando P, et al: Herpes gestationis factor reacts with the amniotic epithelial basement membrane. *Br J Dermatol* 1987; 117:147–154.

68. Morrison LH, Labib RS, Zone JJ, et al: Herpes gestationis autoantibodies recognize a 180-kd epidermal antigen. *J Clin Invest* 1988; 81:2023–2026.

69. Kolodny RC: Herpes gestationis. *Am J Obstet Gynecol* 1969; 104:39–45.

70. Holmes RC, Black MM: The fetal prognosis in pemphigoid gestationis (herpes gestationis) *Br J Dermatol* 84; 110:67–72.

71. Lawley TJ, Stingl G, Katz SI: Fetal and maternal risk factors in herpes gestationis. *Arch Dermatol* 1978; 114:552–555.

72. Bonifazi E, Meneghini CL: Herpes gestationis with transient bullous lesions in the newborn. *Pediatr Dermatol* 1984; 215–218.

73. Van De Weil A, Hart HC, Flinterman J, et al: Plasma exchange in herpes gestationis. *Br Med J* 1980; 281;1041–1042.

74. Bourne G: Toxaemic rash of pregnancy. *Proc R Soc Med* 1962; 55:462–464.

75. Cooper AJ, Fryer JA: Prurigo of late preg-

nancy. *Aust J Dermatol* 1980; 21:79–84.

76. Faber WR, VanJoost T, Hausman R, et al: Late prurigo of pregnancy. *Br J Dermatol* 1982; 106:511–516.

77. Holmes RC, Black MM, Dann J, et al: A comparative study of toxic erythema of pregnancy and herpes gestationis. *Br J Dermatol* 1982; 106:499–510.

78. Lawley TJ, Hertz KC, Wade TR, et al: Pruritic urticarial papules and plaques of pregnancy. *JAMA* 1979; 241:1696–1699.

79. Yancey KB, Hall RP, Lawley TJ: Pruritic urticarial papules and plaques of pregnancy. *J Am Acad Dermatol* 1984; 10:473–480.

80. Lawley TJ: Skin changes in pregnancy, in Fitzpatrick TB, Eisen AZ, Wolff K, et al (eds): *Dermatology in General Medicine,* ed 3. New York, McGraw-Hill Book Co, 1987, pp 2082–2088.

81. Oosterling RJ, Nobrega RE, DuBoeuff JA, et al: Impetigo herpetiformis or generalized pustular psoriasis. *Arch Dermatol* 1978; 114:1527–1529.

82. Pierard GE, Pierard-Franchimont C, de la Brassine M: Impetigo herpetiformis and pustular psoriasis during pregnancy. *Am J Dermatopathol* 1983; 5:215–220.

83. Lotem M, Katznelson V, Rotem A, et al: Impetigo herpetiformis: A variant of pustular psoriasis or a separate entity *J Am Acad Dermatol* 1989; 20:338–341.

84. Oumeish OY, Farraj SE, Bataineh AS: Some aspects of impetigo herpetiformis. *Arch Dermatol* 1982; 118:103–105.

85. Sasseville D, Wilkinson RD, Schnader JY: Dermatoses of pregnancy. *Int J Dermatol* 1981; 20:223–241.

86. Rook A, Wilkinson DS, Ebling FJG: *Textbook of Dermatology.* London, Blackwell Scientific Publications, 1979, pp 220–224, 1362.

87. Green D, Maize JC: Maternal pemphigus vulgaris with in-vivo bound antibodies in the stillborn fetus. *J Am Acad Dermatol* 1982; 7:388–392.

88. Moncada B, Kettelson S, Hernandez-Moctezuma JL, et al: Neonatal pemphigus vulgaris: Role of passively transferred pemphigus antibodies. *Br J Dermatol* 1982; 106:465–468.

89. Ross MG, Kant B, Frieder R, et al: Pemphigus in pregnancy: A reevaluation of fetal risk. *Am J Obstet Gynecol* 1986; 155:30–33.

90. Swapp GH, Main RA: Neurofibromat pregnancy. *Br J Dermatol* 1973; 80:4

91. Brade DB, Bolan JC: Neurofibrom spontaneous hemothorax in pregna case reports. *Obstet Gynecol* 1984; 63(suppl):35–38.

92. Tapp E, Hickling RS: Renal artery in a pregnant woman with neurofibr sis. *J Pathol* 1969; 97:398–402.

93. Maurus JN. Hansen's disease in pre *Obstet Gynecol* 1978; 52:22–25.

94. Farb H, West DP, Pedvis-Leftick A zamine in pregnancy complicated by lepro *Obstet Gynecol* 1982; 59:122–123.

95. Duncan ME, Pearson JMH, Ridley DS, et al: Pregnancy and leprosy: The consequences of alterations of cell-mediated and humoral immunity during pregnancy and lactation. *Int J Lepr* 1982; 50:425–435.

96. Duncan ME, Pearson JMH: The association of pregnancy and leprosy—III. Erythema nodosum leprosum in pregnancy and lactation. *Lepr Rev* 1984; 55:129–142.

97. Duncan ME: Babies of mothers with leprosy have small placentae, low birth weights and grow slowly. *Br J Obstet Gynecol* 1980; 87:471–479.

98. Duncan ME, Melsom R, Pearson JMH, et al: A clinical and immunological study of four babies of mothers with lepromatous leprosy, two of whom developed leprosy in infancy. *Int J Lepr* 1983; 51:7–17.

CHAPTER 17

Drug Abuse

Ira J. Chasnoff
Richard V. Lee

For the last decade drug use by women of childbearing age has escalated. While there has been a steady rate of alcohol, marijuana, and opiate use there has been a sharp rise in the use of cocaine by pregnant women. A recent survey found that 11% of all pregnant women delivered in 36 hospitals across the United States had used an illicit substance at some time during pregnancy.[1] The most common illicit drugs used were cocaine and marijuana followed at a distance by heroin, phencyclidine hydrochloride (PCP), and amphetamines. Drug use was alarming regardless of the area of the country in which the hospitals were located. At Jackson Memorial Hospital in Miami 12.5% of 300 consecutive women admitted to labor and delivery had a positive urine toxicology for cocaine. At Chicago Osteopathic Hospital 16% of 158 consecutively born infants had cocaine in their urine at the time of delivery. At the University of California Davis Hospital in Sacramento, 25% of 800 consecutive women admitted to labor and delivery had cocaine, amphetamines, or heroin found on toxicologic examination of the urine. These figures underscore the need of the physician to assess the use of licit and illicit substances as a part of the evaluation of every pregnant woman (Table 17–1).

Since substance abuse by pregnant women is common,[2] there is no place for complacency in medical practice. Unfortunately, there is a curious contemporary mentality that prompts many women to discontinue the use of prescribed medication because of fears of adverse effects upon the fetus, but to think nothing of occasionally using cocaine, or continuing to smoke, or to consume alcohol during their pregnancy. Medical staff must be curious, even suspicious, about drug use during pregnancy.

The impact of substance abuse can be divided into pharmacologic effects (dependence, withdrawal, overdosage, etc.) and environmental effects (infectious disease risks associated with needles, and sexual license, malnutrition, and social isolation) (Tables 17–2 and 17–3). The clinician needs to be alert to subtle, unusual, sometimes absurdly obvious, clues suggesting substance abuse; for example, crude tattoos to cover scars of old needle tracks.

Ideal management of substance-abusing mothers would remove both pharmacologic and environmental risks. However, not infrequently the clinician is able only to protect the patient and her fetus from some of the environmental risks. In some instances, as with heroin addiction, it is prudent to maintain the patient's addiction through a program of controlled substitution with methadone.

TABLE 17–1.
Pregnancy and Drugs of Abuse

Agent	How Used	Abstinence Syndrome		Teratogenic	Impaired Fetal Growth	Developmental Delay
		Maternal	Fetal/Neonatal			
Alcohol	Oral	Yes	Yes	Yes	Yes	Yes
Sedatives	Oral	Yes	Yes	Not proven	Yes	Not proven
Cocaine	Inhalation, IV	Yes	No	Probably	Yes	Yes
Narcotics	IV, inhalation	Yes	Yes	Not proven	Yes	Yes
Tobacco	Inhalation	Yes	Yes	Not proven	Yes	Not proven
Marijuana	Inhalation	Yes	Yes	Not proven	Yes	Yes
Amphetamines	Inhalation, oral, IV	Yes	Yes	Not proven	Yes	Yes
Hallucinogens (PCP, LSD, etc.)	Oral	No	No	Not proven	Yes	Not proven

PCP = phencyclidine hydrochloride; LSD = lysergic acid diethylamide.

TABLE 17–2.
Maternal Consequences of Substance Abuse

Pharmacologic Effects	Environmental Effects
Dependence/addiction	Inadequate prenatal care
Withdrawal	Malnutrition
Overdosage	Infection
Drug-specific effects	Social isolation
Premature labor	Trauma
	Premature labor

TABLE 17–3.
Fetal Consequences of Substance Abuse

Pharmacologic Effects	Environmental Effects
Teratogenesis	Transplacental infection
Dependence/addiction	Trauma
Withdrawal	Premature delivery
Premature delivery	Growth retardation
Growth retardation	
Teratogenesis	

IDENTIFICATION OF THE SUBSTANCE-ABUSING PREGNANT WOMAN

Substance-abusing pregnant women are often suspicious or frightened of a probing history and physical examination. Guilt, fear of legal or police involvement, and the self-deception and denial that so often accompany drug abuse may cause the patient to camouflage physical and historical evidence of her condition. Pregnancy can be converted into an opportunity to engage the patient, voluntarily, in therapy and drug rehabilitation. But many substance-abusing mothers are ambivalent about pregnancy and are trapped in the substance-abusing life (Table 17–4), so that they put off obstetric and medical care, sometimes until labor begins.

Use of multiple drugs is common. Tobacco and alcohol are almost constant companions of illicit substance abuse. The intensity of "highs" and "lows" has fostered the use of combinations, such as cocaine and opium, or the serial use of stimulants alternating with sedatives. The clinician may be confronted with a confusing combination of findings caused by multiple chemical dependencies.

Medical and Obstetric History

In the medical history (Table 17–5), a positive history of hepatitis, cirrhosis, bacterial endocarditis, cellulitis, pneumonia, or pancreatitis should call attention to the possibility of substance abuse. Twenty-five to 40% of the admissions to hospital general medical units and emergency services are related to the effects of chemical dependence, tobacco and alcohol being the most common agents.[3] Medical staff must explore specific questions regarding prior hospitalizations and must obtain appropriate medical records in order to document the patient's history. Regardless of the extent of the patient's self-disclosure, prior complications of pregnancy due to perinatal substance abuse require exploration and a request for past obstetric records.

Complications associated with drug use in previous pregnancies may include spontaneous abortion, premature labor, prema-

TABLE 17–4.
Substance Abuse: The Clinical Picture—Social Clues

Repetitive noncompliance, excessive appointment truancy
Inability to hold employment
Family disruption
Frequent legal and financial entanglements
Criminal behavior
Spouse or family member with substance abuse problems

TABLE 17–5.
Substance Abuse: The Clinical Picture—Medical Clues

Unusual and/or frequent requests for analgesics, stimulants, and/or sedatives
Use of multiple physicians and pharmacies to obtain prescriptions
History of multiple injuries
Frequent or unusual infections (skin infections, endocarditis, multiple sexually transmitted diseases)
Hepatitis B (past or present)
Human immunodeficiency virus (HIV) infection
Chronic liver disease
Pancreatitis
Insomnia, agitation, chronic pain syndromes
Blackout spells

TABLE 17–6.
Substance Abuse: The Clinical Picture—
Obstetric Clues

History of:
  Premature labor
  Premature rupture of membranes
  Intrauterine fetal death
  Habitual abortion
  Placental abruption
  Intrauterine growth retardation
  Neonatal withdrawal syndrome
Presence of:
  Malnutrition or weight loss
  Fetal tachycardia
  Fetal mortality
  Premature labor
  Premature rupture of membranes
  Placental abruption
  Intrauterine fetal death
  Intrauterine growth retardation

ture rupture of membranes, abruptio placentae, fetal death, meconium-stained amniotic fluid, or a low-birth-weight infant (Table 17–6). Pertinent findings in regard to the present pregnancy may include poor weight gain, spotting or vaginal bleeding, an inactive or hyperactive fetus, reports of early contractions. Obstetric history taking provides the interviewer with an opportunity to discuss the patient's emotional response to the current pregnancy. An inconsistent pattern of prenatal care may indicate apathy or ambivalence regarding the pregnancy. On the other hand, frequent emergency room visits may reveal extreme anxiety regarding the physical well-being of the fetus, and in this setting the interviewer can explore the patient's coping mechanism. A good question to introduce the substance abuse history would be asking how the woman handles stress. Questions about medications and other substances are a natural extension to discussing stress.

Drug use ought to be explored in a nonjudgmental manner. The patient's substance use history should begin with the earliest exposure to cigarettes, over-the-counter medications, prescribed medications, alcohol, marijuana and other illicit drugs, and continue along a time continuum to the present. The current substance abuse history should begin at least 1 month prior to the last normal

menstrual period; many substance-abusing women do not have a regular menstrual cycle, and often they are unaware of a pregnancy until late in gestation. It is important to look for substance abuse patterns during past pregnancies. Some women abstain from drugs during pregnancy while others curb drug use but return to drugs immediately post partum. There are women who have binges of substance abuse; others are addicted and use drugs continually regardless of their pregnancy. Some questions to be explored regarding past pregnancies are:

1. Did the patient experience any complications with the pregnancy, labor, or delivery?
2. Did the patient's pediatrician notice any physical or behavioral problems with the newborn?
3. How is the child doing now?
4. Does the patient notice any differences in behavior or growth patterns?

Physical Appearance and Laboratory Tests

The physical appearance of the patient may give subtle or overt clues to alert the interviewer to possible substance abuse. The following areas of concern should be noted:

1. Is the patient well oriented?
2. Does the patient appear physically exhausted?
3. Are the patient's pupils extremely dilated or constricted?
4. Does the appearance of the patient's pregnancy coincide with the stated gestational age?
5. Are there signs of needle track marks, abscesses, or edema in the upper or lower extremities?

The physical appearance and signs of chemical dependence and needle use are especially helpful in diagnosing the intravenous substance abuser. But pregnant women using oral drugs, not using needles, may have fewer overt physical signs of chemical dependence.

Urine toxicologic examination is essential for diagnosis, evaluation, and intervention. The physician should be certain as to what compounds are included in a screening toxicology and specifically request those drugs or metabolites not routinely included. Urine toxicology is a necessary part of the evaluation for substance abuse, but it should never replace a thorough history and physical examination as part of the screening procedure. Regardless of the type of evaluation and intervention procedure used, any woman with a history or evidence of substance use or abuse during the current pregnancy should be immediately referred for treatment, as any illicit drug use during pregnancy can have major ramifications for the unborn child.

GENERAL MANAGEMENT OF SUBSTANCE ABUSE DURING PREGNANCY

Intervention can include patient confrontation, education, and inpatient or community referral to chemical dependence treatment, or referral to a social worker or clinical nurse specialist for in-depth interviews and/or follow-up for treatment. Care of a woman who abuses drugs during pregnancy requires a multidisciplinary team. The group should include obstetricians and internists practiced in identifying and treating the medical problems frequently encountered among addicted women. Also invaluable are a psychologist or psychiatrist experienced in caring for persons addicted to drugs and a specially trained nurse or social worker qualified to provide guidance and support. Although members of the team often function individually, their efforts must be integrated and directed toward common goals that extend beyond the pregnancy.

Toxicology screens on maternal urine should be obtained at each visit. The patient should be tested on a random basis as well.

Any maternal or fetal infections, especially urinary tract infection, vaginitis, and sexually transmitted diseases, demand aggressive treatment. Every substance-abusing woman should be tested for human immunodeficiency virus (HIV) and hepatitis B infections. Attention to nutrition includes liberal vitamin and mineral supplementation.

Serial ultrasound examinations are needed to measure the biparietal diameter, head and abdominal circumference, fetal femur length, and to establish gestational age and the fetal growth pattern. Because menstrual irregularity is common in drug abusers, obtaining the growth-adjusted sonar age is essential.

Prenatal care of substance-abusing patients should include plans for delivery. Every effort should be made to deliver in an obstetric center that is equipped with a neonatal intensive care unit to manage the neonate and to manage any maternal complications that may arise.

Guidelines for managing labor are the same as for the nonaddicted patient. The physician should use whatever methods of anesthesia or analgesia are deemed necessary to provide pain relief for labor and delivery. Addicted women experience as much pain during labor as other women. It is unnecessary to withhold medications under the misapprehension that they will contribute to the addictive process.

Figure 17–1 and Table 17–7 provide steps and guidelines for the management of substance abuse during pregnancy.

ALCOHOL

It is estimated that 10% to 12% of pregnant women are problem drinkers.[4, 5] The effects of alcohol upon a woman's health are unaltered by pregnancy. Pregnant women get drunk, develop pancreatitis and alcoholic hepatitis, and suffer from alcohol withdrawal seizures and delirium tremens just like nonpregnant women. Alcohol can have devastating effects upon the fetus throughout gestation. It is alcohol's impact upon the fetus that makes detection, treatment, and rehabilitation of alcohol-abusing mothers so urgent and important.

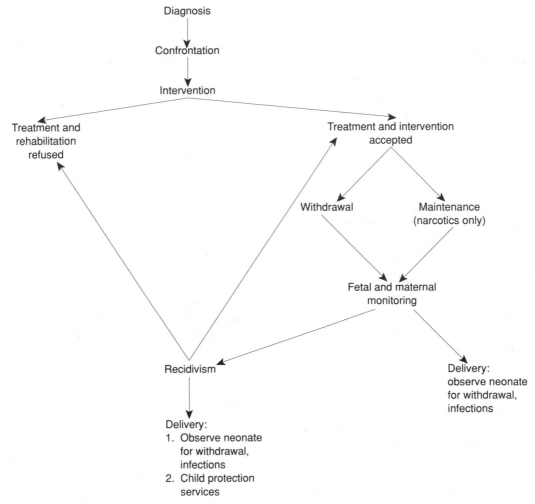

FIG 17–1.
Algorithm indicating steps in the management of gestational drug abuse.

TABLE 17–7.
Management Guidelines for the Pregnant Addict

	Remote From Term	Close to Term
Alcohol and barbiturates	Withdrawal with tapering sedation, i.e., benzodiazepines	Withdrawal; sedate to prevent seizures, delirium tremens
	Monitor fetal status	Monitor fetal status
		Observe newborn for withdrawal
Tobacco and marijuana	Withdrawal	Withdrawal
Narcotic analgesics	Methadone maintenance	Methadone maintenance
		Observe newborn for withdrawal
Cocaine, amphetamines	Sheltered withdrawal including long-term admission if necessary	Sheltered withdrawal
	Monitor fetal status	Monitor fetal status
		Observe newborn for neurological changes

TABLE 17–8.
Fetal Alcohol Syndrome

Eyes	Epicanthal folds, strabismus, ptosis, hypoplastic retinal vessels
Mouth	Poor suck, cleft lip, cleft palate
Ears	Deafness
Skeleton	Radioulnar synostosis, fusion of cervical vertebrae, retarded bone growth
Heart	Atrial and ventricular septal defects, tetralogy of Fallot, patent ductus arteriosus
Kidney	Renal hypoplasia, hydronephrosis, urogenital sinus
Liver	Extrahepatic biliary atresia, hepatic fibrosis
Immune system	Increased infections—otitis media, upper respiratory infections, immunodeficiencies
Tumors	Nonspecific neoplasms
Skin	Abnormal palmar creases, irregular hair whorls

The Fetal Alcohol Syndrome

A recent study revealed that fetal alcohol syndrome is currently the most common cause of mental retardation in the United States.[6] The notion that heavy maternal drinking is detrimental to offspring regained scientific status when Lemoine et al.[7] and Jones and Smith[8] observed a common pattern of malformations in offspring of chronic alcoholic women. Jones and Smith[8] coined the term *fetal alcohol syndrome* (FAS) to define a pattern of prenatal and postnatal growth deficiency, developmental delay or mental retardation, microcephaly, fine motor dysfunction, and a characteristic facial dysmorphology. The initial publications describing FAS stimulated case reports from around the world, which have been followed by thousands of clinical, epidemiologic, and experimental studies (Table 17–8).

In 1980 the fetal alcohol study group of the Research Society on Alcoholism agreed on the importance of standard minimal criteria for the diagnosis of FAS.[9, 10] They recommended that the diagnosis be made when there are signs in each of three categories.

1. Prenatal or postnatal growth retardation (weight, length, and/or head circumference below the 10th percentile).

2. Central nervous system (CNS) involvement (signs of neurologic abnormality, developmental delay, or intellectual impairment),

3. Characteristic facial dysmorphology with at least two of the following signs:
   a. Microcephaly.
   b. Microphthalmia and/or short palpebral fissures.
   c. Poorly developed philtrum, thin upper lip, or flattening of the maxillary area.

There is an increased incidence of major and minor anomalies among neonates of heavy drinkers. Some have estimated that approximately 5% of all congenital anomalies may be associated with prenatal alcohol exposure, making alcohol the third leading cause of birth defects and the most common teratogen.[11]

Clinical and experimental research findings point to multiple mechanisms which underlie alcohol's effects on fetal growth and development. Alcohol in high concentrations modifies cell functions throughout the body, affecting all organ systems. Direct and indirect actions have been observed on the maternal-placental-fetal system. Biochemical and pathophysiologic effects of ethanol and its metabolite, acetaldehyde, can alter fetal development by disrupting cell differentiation and growth. Alcohol-induced alterations in maternal physiology and in the intermediate metabolism of carbohydrates, proteins, and fats can alter the environment in which the fetus develops. Chronic exposure to high doses of alcohol can interfere with the passage of amino acids across the placenta and the incorporation of amino acids into proteins.

FAS results from the cumulative actions of high blood alcohol concentrations on the maternal-placental-fetal system throughout pregnancy. Variability occurs in the nature and extent of the abnormalities seen in children exposed to alcohol in utero. It has been estimated that 2% to 10% of pregnancies complicated by alcohol produced children with FAS; another 30% to 40% have some other adverse effects.[9–11] The differences are related to several factors, including dose levels, chronicity of alcohol use, gestational stage and duration of exposure, and sensitivity of fetal tissue.

Women consuming more than 1 oz of absolute alcohol per day are at greatest risk.[4] A patient taking 4 oz of 80 proof spirit or a liter of wine a day is at the threshold for probable adverse effects upon her fetus. Unfortunately there is no clear-cut threshold dosage or dose-response relationship for any of the adverse effects of alcohol upon the fetus. The American Medical Association recommends that pregnant women abstain from alcoholic beverages in any amount during pregnancy. As of 1989, United States law requires that all beer, wine, and spirits be labeled with warnings about birth defects. On the other hand, there is little to be gained by punishing or frightening pregnant patients who have consumed small amounts of alcohol on occasion.

Reduction of heavy drinking has been associated with improved neonatal outcomes as measured by growth parameters, somatic status, and/or CNS development in case reports and prospective studies.[12, 13] In a Seattle program, 80% of the women who drank heavily were able to modify their drinking patterns. Fetal alcohol effects occurred three times more often when mothers continued drinking than when mothers reduced drinking. The Atlanta program reported that 35% of the at-risk women stopped drinking heavily. Increased neurobehavioral alterations were found in infants of women who continued to drink during pregnancy as compared with abstainers and with women who discontinued use by midpregnancy. The observed benefits were attributed to cessation of drinking and not to maternal characteristics. The group of women who successfully abstained and the group who failed to respond to treatment were similar in demographic characteristics. No significant differences were found in patterns of alcohol consumption reported at the time of clinic registration. Among the women in the Atlanta study, there were no differences in the prevalence of alcohol-related pathology, although the group that continued to drink had begun drinking at an earlier age and were more likely to meet criteria for the diagnosis of alcohol dependence.

Greater understanding of the mechanisms of alcohol's effects on fetal development has put new demands on prenatal care providers.[14, 15] Identification and treatment of problem-drinking women represents an important challenge for the prevention of alcohol-related birth defects. Since alcohol has the capacity to adversely affect each stage of fetal development, the earlier in pregnancy that heavy drinking ceases, the greater is the potential for improved outcome.

Detecting Alcoholism During Pregnancy

Stereotypical ideas about the chronic alcoholic are inappropriate for obstetric practice. Women with alcoholic liver disease often have irregular menses and rarely conceive. Drinking pregnant women usually do not fit the stereotype of the chronic alcoholic since they are young and in the early stages of their alcohol dependence. Although women who drink heavily differ statistically from other pregnant women on a series of behavioral and demographic traits, these traits have low predictive power and are not effective as specific clinical markers.

A brief ten-question drinking history has been developed which can be administered routinely as part of every intake examination (Table 17–9). The reliability of the questionnaire has been tested by Larsson[16] who reported good agreement between two occasions of history taking.

Separate, direct questions are asked about the frequency, quantity, and variability of the consumption of beer, wine, and liquor. Va-

TABLE 17–9.
Ten-Question Drinking History

Beer:	How many times per week?
	How many cans each time?
	Ever drink more?
Wine:	How many times per week?
	How many glasses each time?
	Ever drink more?
Liquor:	How many times per week?
	How many drinks each time?
	Ever drink more?
Has your drinking changed during the past year?	

TABLE 17–10.
Maternal Complications of Alcohol Abuse

1. Malnutrition
   A. Folic acid deficiency
   B. Iron deficiency
   C. Thiamine deficiency (Wernicke's encephalopathy)
2. Bone marrow suppression
   A. Thrombocytopenia
3. Liver and pancreatic disease
4. Gastritis and ulcer disease
5. Acute intoxication
   A. Increased risk for trauma
   B. Alcoholic hallucinosis
6. Withdrawal syndromes
   A. Alcohol withdrawal seizures
   B. The "shakes"
   C. Delirium tremens

lidity of self-reports has been shown to improve when specific questions are asked about each beverage. Inquiry about quantity, frequency, and variability of use further improves the accuracy of self-reports. The first nine questions ascertain present drinking patterns. Alcohol use is assumed, thereby diminishing moral projections. The tenth question explores changes in drinking habits during the past year. This allows for discussion of previous patterns, which often provides validation of reports of current use.

When the ten questions are asked in a direct, nonjudgmental fashion, most patients will accept the clinician's concern and respond candidly. Simple introductory statements reassure the pregnant woman that the questions are being asked in an effort to improve pregnancy outcome. Patients who answer evasively should be calmly and firmly engaged in further discussion. Defensive reactions often indicate alcohol problems.

Administering the questionnaire requires less than 5 minutes when women are not drinking at risk levels. For women who are abusing alcohol, the questionnaire provides a basis for discussing alcohol use and initiating supportive counseling.

Maternal Effects of Alcoholism

Emphasis on the fetal effects of alcohol has probably obscured the important, adverse effects of alcohol on maternal health (Table 17–10). The relationship between alcohol and serious trauma from falls and vehicular accidents is well known; pregnant women are not spared. Acutely intoxicated pregnant women are just as susceptible to coma and hypothermia as nonpregnant alcoholics. Alcohol abuse is often accompanied by malnutrition.[17, 18] Alcoholics consume calories with their drink and suffer from nausea and anorexia associated with gastritis and pancreatitis. Folic acid deficiency, common in alcoholics, is exaggerated by the demands imposed by pregnancy. Alcohol is a bone marrow toxin so that increased mean corpuscular volume, despite normal serum levels of folic acid and vitamin B_{12} and thrombocytopenia may be observed in alcoholics. Thiamine deficiency is also common in alcoholics and may result in beriberi and/or Wernicke's encephalopathy. "Wet" beriberi, high-output congestive heart failure, and dilated cardiomyopathy may be exacerbated by the cardiovascular changes of pregnancy and can be confused with peripartum cardiomyopathy which is unique to the postpartum female. Wernicke's syndrome is characterized by confabulatory dementia, ophthalmoplegia, and ataxia. It is sometimes accompanied by peripheral neuropathies and a high-output cardiac state. Emergent administration of thiamine is vital.

Neurologic disorders related to alcohol withdrawal may cause obstetric consternation. Alcohol withdrawal seizures usually occur within 24 hours of stopping drinking and are most often single, grand mal events. A seizing pregnant woman with macrocytic anemia, thrombocytopenia, liver tenderness, and abnormal liver enzymes customarily means severe preeclampsia to obstetricians: a potent stimulus for prompt delivery, which may be inappropriate for the alcoholic mother and her fetus. Alcohol withdrawal seizures during pregnancy should be managed as in the nonpregnant patient. Delirium tremens, even in experienced tertiary care medical centers, is fatal in 5% to 10% of afflicted patients. A heavily drinking woman admitted for premature labor may become agitated at 24 to 48 hours and progress to visual hallucinations, confabulation, and hyperthermia before adequate sedation (mistakenly withheld because she is pregnant) is provided. Alcohol withdrawal syndromes may also occur in the neonates of alcoholic mothers. The alcohol-dependent gravida poses special problems for obstetric services; however, there is no difference from the management of withdrawal in nonpregnant alcoholics. Sedation with benzodiazepine drugs is desirable to reduce the risk of acute or severe withdrawal, but sedation has risks for the fetus, especially if delivery is imminent. An alert, oriented, manageable parturient is highly desirable for all concerned and maternal sedation may delay or reduce the severity of the fetal-neonatal withdrawal syndrome.

The benzodiazepines have replaced paraldehyde and chloral hydrate in the management of alcohol withdrawal because of their ease of administration and demonstrated utility.[17] The agents most widely used are diazepam, chlordiazepoxide, and lorazepam (FDA category C). They should be given in sufficient dose to produce sedation, a quantity which because of cross-tolerance induced by alcohol, may be stunningly large. Once sedation is achieved the dose should be tapered on a schedule appropriate for the clinical setting. Administration ad libitum or as needed should be avoided.

Heavy drinking is accompanied by an increase in obstetric complications.[4, 19] Alcoholics are twice as likely as non–alcohol abusers to have a history of habitual abortion or stillbirths.[20] The risks of amnionitis, placental abruption, and preterm delivery are greater.[21] First- and second-trimester bleeding is three times more common among heavy drinkers than among abstainers.[21]

COCAINE

Consonant with the increasing use of cocaine in the general population, increasing numbers of women are using cocaine during pregnancy.[22] Several reports have indicated that cocaine abuse during gestation is associated with a poor pregnancy and neonatal outcome.[23–25] Cocaine use in early pregnancy is associated with an increased incidence of spontaneous abortions, and continued use during pregnancy results in an increased rate of abruptio placentae, premature labor and delivery, and intrauterine growth retardation. The risks of adverse effects of cocaine upon pregnancy are difficult to estimate because the number of cocaine-using women and their frequency and pattern of use are no more than a crude estimate. However, the incidence of positive urine toxicology tests among women suffering premature labor and placental abruption ranges from 15% to 20%. One large urban health maintenance organization reported that cocaine was used by 1% to 2% of mothers of all livebirths.[26]

Smoking "crack" is the most prevalent contemporary method of using cocaine. It produces an intense, short-lived "high," and "binges" are common. Crack is extraordinarily addicting so that daily use is common. Nutrition, finances, and personal relationships suffer, setting the stage for thievery and prostitution; exposure to infections, especially HIV; risk of trauma; and social isolation. Of great concern is the advent of smokable synthetic amphetamines which may supplant cocaine as the inexpensive drug of choice. Cocaine continues to be extracted from the coca plant requiring a complicated chain of growing, processing, and transporting.

Diagnosis of cocaine abuse may be difficult. However, cocaine metabolites may be found in urine for 2 to 3 days and for weeks in hair.[27] As with all substance abuse, a suspicious clinician is the major component of successful management. Sheltered withdrawal is essential, with careful monitoring of both mother and fetus. Recidivism, despite pregnancy and despite intensive, compassionate prenatal care, is discouragingly high.

Fetal and Neonatal Effects of Cocaine

Neonates exposed to cocaine in utero

demonstrate neurobehavioral deficiencies with diminished interactive and responsive behaviors.[20] These infants also have an increased rate of seizures, and are at risk for malformations of the gastrointestinal, genitourinary, and central nervous systems.[28, 29] Cerebral infarctions in infants whose mothers took cocaine within 48 to 72 hours of the onset of labor, and necrotizing enterocolitis in a term newborn associated with maternal cocaine use, have also been reported.[30, 31] The cause of these complications is suspected to be related to the intense vasoconstriction produced by cocaine, which in turn produces an increase in maternal blood pressure and a concomitant decrease in placental blood flow.[32, 33] A study in pregnant ewes demonstrated that reductions in placental perfusion were dose-dependent and that hypoxemia developed in fetal lambs at all cocaine doses tested.[33]

Maternal Effects of Cocaine

In addition to the obstetric and infectious complications associated with substance abuse, cocaine's powerful sympathomimetic effects can produce acute medical emergencies in the pregnant woman (Table 17–11).

Cardiac complications of cocaine intoxication include myocardial ischemia, arrhythmias, and cardiomyopathies.[34–43] The initial cardiac effects are the result of catecholamine release and consist of tachycardia and hypertension.[39] Low doses of cocaine usually cause stimulation of the myocardium and higher doses always produce myocardial depression with decreases in both the rate and force of contraction.[39] Myocardial ischemia associated with cocaine use is produced by the direct effects of the drug on the heart and the indirect effects from vasoconstriction, all of which occur in a brief period of time. The vasoconstriction induced by cocaine affects the coronary and systemic circulation so that the patient can have hypertension with increased peripheral resistance and segmental coronary artery vasospasm.[32, 33, 39] Myocardial infarction may ensue because of the combination of ischemia and increased myocardial

work.[40, 41, 43] Individuals with an underlying anatomic defect are at increased risk as demonstrated by several patients who experienced acute myocardial infarction following cocaine use and subsequently were found to have fixed obstruction of the coronary arteries at cardiac catheterization.[41–43] There have also been reports of myocardial infarction in patients where no fixed obstruction was found.[32, 34, 40]

Arrhythmias represent a potentially fatal complication of cocaine intoxication. Arrhythmias that have been documented following cocaine intoxication include sinus tachycardia, ventricular fibrillation, and asystole.[44, 45]

Cases of dilated cardiomyopathy following chronic cocaine use have been recently reported in nonpregnant addicts.[46] Two cases of cardiac myopathies have occurred in the postpartum period in pregnant women enrolled in our program at Northwestern Memorial Hospital. It is hypothesized that the stress of pregnancy places the women at increased risk of cocaine's cardiac effects.

Sudden death due to rupture of the aorta following cocaine intoxication has been reported. Postmortem examination revealed an enlarged heart consistent with chronic hypertension.[47, 48]

TABLE 17–11.
Medical Complications of Cocaine Use

Cardiovascular
Myocardial ischemia
Arrhythmias
Cardiomyopathies
Hypertension
Central Nervous System
Seizures
Hyperpyrexia
Cerebrovascular accidents
Respiratory
Pneumothorax
Pulmonary dysfunction
Perforation of the nasal septum
Gastrointestinal
Ischemia of bowel with possible perforation
Hepatotoxicity
Renal
Rhabdomyolysis
Renal failure

Central nervous system complications following acute exposure to cocaine can also occur.[49–52] The most frequent complications are seizures, focal neurologic deficits, headaches, and transient loss of consciousness. There have been several reports of subarachnoid hemorrhage occurring shortly after cocaine use. The cause of the hemorrhages was felt to be due to the sudden increases in blood pressure associated with acute cocaine intoxication. In addition to hemorrhage, cerebral infarction has also been reported. In utero cerebral infarction has been documented in fetuses of cocaine-using pregnant women.[30]

Hyperpyrexia is frequently observed during acute cocaine intoxication and may be a leading cause of death.[53] Hyperpyrexia has also been documented as a cause of teratogenic effects, and thus in itself can pose a danger to the fetus.[54]

Inhalation of cocaine can be associated with respiratory complications related to acute, direct effects from the drug. While many of the pulmonary complications are the result of chronic cocaine abuse, acute intoxication can result in respiratory failure or pulmonary edema. Cocaine may damage the alveolar wall and thereby predispose patients to pneumothorax, pneumomediastinum, or pneumopericardium, especially when associated with a forced Valsalva maneuver used to intensify the euphoria that comes with cocaine smoking.[55, 56] Chronically inhaled cocaine can diminish gas exchange capabilities in the individual user, with these abnormalities persisting for several weeks after cessation of drug use.[57]

Perforation of the nasal septum due to the local vasoconstrictive effects of cocaine can occur after prolonged or frequent intranasal cocaine use.

The oral ingestion of cocaine can produce gastrointestinal ischemia with possible death from gram-negative sepsis.[58] Hepatotoxicity with elevated hepatic enzymes in as many as 80% of cocaine and heroin users and jaundice have been reported associated with cocaine intoxication.[59] Rhabdomyolysis with muscle weakness and myoglobinuria may produce profound weakness and transient renal impairment.[60–62]

Mother and fetus both suffer an abstinence syndrome marked by neuromuscular irritability and profoundly depressed mood. Fetal expulsion or death resulting from maternal cocaine withdrawal has not yet been reported. The greatest risk to the fetus seems to be active use of cocaine, especially crack binges. Withdrawal in a protective environment with careful maternal and fetal monitoring is recommended. Indeed, some women have been kept in jail, by request and by court order, so that they may stay drug-free. There is no cocaine "antagonist" approved for use during pregnancy. Recidivism is common. Child protection services should be regularly alerted.

NARCOTICS

The pharmacologic effects of narcotic analgesics abused during pregnancy include dependence in both mother and fetus, retardation of fetal growth, and the risk of overdosage.[63, 64] Withdrawal symptoms in both mother and fetus follow cessation of drug use. Some women use heroin irregularly. Because the concentrations of heroin in "street bags" is variable, these women may not develop tolerance or dependence. Such less tolerant users are especially susceptible to narcotic overdosage. Coma with pinpoint pupils, respiratory arrest, and pulmonary edema not responding to the usual measures are manifestations of narcotic overdosage. Naloxone, a narcotic antagonist with no respiratory depressant effects, should be given intravenously and promptly.

The use of narcotic antagonists can precipitate withdrawal or abstinence syndrome: mydriasis, piloerection, perspiration, rhinorrhea, lacrimation, yawning, and agitation. Prolonged abstinence in the addict may produce abdominal and uterine cramps, diarrhea, myalgias, and muscular irritability. Withdrawal is uncomfortable but rarely fatal for the mother. However, the fetus may be expelled when severe uterine contractions occur during the first trimester.[65] Maternal withdrawal symptoms are almost always accompanied by fetal withdrawal which produces hypoxia, hyperactivity, passage of meconium, and, occasionally, intrauterine fetal death.[66] It is because of the risk to the fetus that narcotic withdrawal ("cold turkey") is not encouraged during pregnancy. Similarly, the use of narcotic antagonists during pregnancy such as pentazocine (FDA category B when used for brief periods remote from term) and naloxone (FDA category B) should be undertaken with great caution.

The ecology of heroin addiction includes criminal behavior, sexual promiscuity, and dirty needles.[67] Sexually transmitted infections including HIV and hepatitis B are prominent scourges of people using narcotics and needles. Almost half of heroin-using mothers were reported to have had fever and skin or urinary tract infection and a third had evidence of infection of the placenta, chorion, and amnion.[63] Premature labor, low birth weight, abnormal bleeding, and preeclampsia all have been reported to occur more frequently in narcotic addicts.[63, 65]

Repetitive circulation of particulate materials, antigens, and microorganisms predisposes the needle using narcotic addict to serious infection, pulmonary granulomas, and hyperglobulinemia. Infectious endocarditis, involving both right-sided and left-sided cardiac valves, and uncommon pathogens such as fungi, exotic gram-negative bacteria, as well as the common *Staphylococcus aureas,* is one of the most serious of these problems. Infectious arteritis may culminate in the rupture of a mycotic aneurysm.

Although women account for only 7% of the total population of patients with the acquired immunodeficiency syndrome (AIDS) in the United States, the largest proportion of women with AIDS are intravenous drug abusers.[68] It has been estimated that approximately 75,000 intravenous drug–abusing women in the United States are currently infected with the HIV. Because asymptomatic HIV infection appears to have little or no effect on fertility, the population of HIV-infected pregnant women will very likely continue to grow. Counseling and screening for HIV antibodies should be offered to all substance-abusing women of childbearing age. Infected women should be advised to refrain from sharing needles or syringes or donating blood or organs (see also Chap. 14, p. 489 for discussion of HIV infection).

Women who are chronic carriers of hepatitis B virus (HBV) and those with acute HBV in the month before or after delivery are more likely to transmit the HBV to their offspring than those who have acute HBV infection in the first or second trimester and then recover.[69, 70] Any woman who is HBsAg-positive at the time of delivery has a high chance of infecting her infant. Proper immunoprophylaxis of the newborn infant is essential to all babies born to mothers with HBsAg. All mothers should be screened for hepatitis B (see also Chap. 10, p. 348).

Pregnant heroin addicts are best cared for in methadone maintenance programs.[71] Methadone is a synthetic, long-acting opiate which can be administered by mouth. Methadone blunts the euphoria produced by heroin and deflects the craving for shooting up. Methadone is not a narcotic antagonist: it produces tolerance and dependence, and abstinence results in withdrawal symptoms. Over 20 years of experience with methadone maintenance for pregnant narcotic addicts has convincingly demonstrated the value of reducing the pernicious effects of the needle ecology. Neonatal withdrawal symptoms in children of mothers maintained on methadone tends to be less severe, perhaps because such children are targeted for special neonatal surveillance and care. Despite conscientious prenatal care, one third of children born to methadone-maintained mothers are small-for-gestational-age, which implies a direct, negative effect of narcotics upon fetal growth.[71]

MARIJUANA

Marijuana (tetrahydrocannabinol) is one

TABLE 17–12.
Sedatives and Tranquilizers Which May Be
Abused and Overdosed During Pregnancy

Barbiturate sedatives
  Phenobarbital
  Secobarbital (Seconal)
  Butabarbital sodium (Butisol Sodium)
  Mephobarbital (Mebaral)
Nonbarbiturate sedatives
  Methyprylon (Noludar)
  Glutethimide (Doriden)
  Ethchlorvynol (Placidyl)
  Meprobamate (Miltown)
Benzodiazepines
  Chlordiazepoxide hydrochloride (Librium)
  Diazepam (Valium)
  Lorazepam (Ativan)
  Triazolam (Halcion)
  Temazepam (Restoril)
  Flurazepam hydrochloride (Dalmane)
  Chlorazepate dipotassium (Tranxene)
  Oxazepam (Serax)
  Alprazolam (Xanax)

of the most commonly used drugs, alone and in combination with other substances. Marijuana ("grass," "pot") is almost always smoked and its use carries all of the risks to health that accompany tobacco smoking. On the street, marijuana is used as an introduction to the substance abuse scene. Entry to substance abuse and conversion to more potent agents are made easier by the acceptance and wide use of tobacco cigarettes; smoking pot or crack can be regarded by some people as only an extension of smoking tobacco, not a new and highly dangerous activity.

Cannabis, in addition to euphoria and disorientation, has an antiemetic effect. Some women may use marijuana more frequently during early pregnancy as self-medication for nausea and vomiting.[72] Long-term, daily use can produce apathy, endocrine abnormalities, and chronic bronchitis.[73] Whether marijuana is addicting or can cause fetal anomalies are not clearly defined because marijuana is so often only one constituent in patterns of multiple drug use. Human studies report no increase in fetal abnormalities associated with maternal marijuana use.[74] Animal studies document a detrimental effect on fetal development.[75, 76] However, combined alcohol and marijuana use during pregnancy can result in a fivefold increase in the fetal alcohol syndrome.[77]

The clinician should regard marijuana as a marker for multiple substance abuse and as a potentiator to the effects of other drugs. A history of marijuana use should prompt a careful search for evidence of use of other substances. The ubiquity of marijuana means that every pregnant user, regardless of socioeconomic status, should be thoroughly tested and examined for multiple substance abuse.

SEDATIVES AND ANXIOLYTIC AGENTS

Barbiturates, nonbarbiturate sedatives, and so-called tranquilizers are commonly prescribed and commonly abused drugs (Table 17–12). Regular use of all of these drugs can lead to tolerance and dependence, with the risks of abstinence syndrome upon withdrawal, in both mother and fetus. Controlled medical use of sedatives and tranquilizers, such as treatment with phenobarbital to control seizure disorders, poses less risk to mother and fetus than illegal, surreptitious use. Because "downers" are so often a component of multiple substance abuse, it is hard to reliably ascribe adverse effects upon pregnancy or the neonate to any one drug. Attention to their negative effects upon general health has prompted federal and state restrictions upon their use. For example, in New York State benzodiazepine compounds can be prescribed using only triplicate prescription forms identical to those used for narcotic analgesics.

Sedatives and tranquilizers are an important part of a seesaw pattern of drug use: stimulation alternating with sedation. They are used to combat abstinence symptoms, as with alcohol or amphetamines. Overdosage in this setting is common. Stimulants are used to abort the depressive effects of sedation, establishing a dangerous, socially isolated cycle.

Phenobarbital and benzodiazepines have a less severe abstinence syndrome than the short-acting barbiturates.[78] However, overdosage with any of these agents may produce maternal coma, prolonged hypoxia, and fetal distress. Despite claims for the relative safety of the benzodiazepine compounds, overdosage during pregnancy carries a grave prognosis. Considerable concern about teratogenesis is evoked when sedatives and/or tranquilizers are used during pregnancy.[79–81] As with all medications the benefits of their use must clearly exceed the risks.

Short-acting barbiturate withdrawal in adults and in neonates, unlike cocaine and narcotic withdrawal, may have a fatal outcome if not recognized and treated.[82] Abstinent patients become restless and irritable with autonomic hyperactivity and can progress to delirium, psychosis, and seizures. Abrupt maternal withdrawal can be followed by intrauterine fetal withdrawal.[82] Controlled withdrawal from barbiturates during pregnancy should be accomplished in a hospital. Decremental doses of pentobarbital are used to safely withdraw the patient.

Inadequate prenatal care, maternal malnutrition, and infectious diseases characterize the condition of sedative-abusing mothers. Admission to hospital is frequently clinically useful since it allows attention to nutrition, detoxification from a variety of other drugs, and identification and treatment of infections.

REFERENCES

1. Finnegan LP (ed): *Drug Dependence in Pregnancy: Clinical Management of Mother and Child.* NIDA Services Research Monograph Series. Rockville, Md, US Government Printing Office, 1978, pp 33–35.
2. Chasnoff IJ: Drugs and women: Establishing a standard of care. *[Ann NY Acad Sci* (in press)].
3. Stark MJ, Nichols HG: Alcohol related admissions to a general hospital. *Alcohol Health Res World* 1977; 11–14.
4. Halmesmaki E, Raivio KO, Ylikorkala O: Patterns of alcohol consumption during pregnancy. *Obstet Gynecol* 1987; 69:594–597.
5. Rodgers BD: Substance abuse in pregnancy. *Med Clin North Am* 1989; 38:6865–6871.
6. Abel EL, Sokol RJ: Incidence of fetal alcohol syndrome and economic impact of FAS-related anomalies. *Drug Alcohol Depend* 1987; 19:51–70.
7. Lemoine P, Harousseau H, Borteyru JP, et al: Les enfants de parents alcooliques: Anomalies observées. A propos des 127 cas [Children of alcoholic parents: anomalies observed in 127 cases]. *Quest Med* 1968; 21:476–482.
8. Jones KL, Smith DW: Recognition of the fetal alcohol syndrome in early infancy. *Lancet* 1973; 2:999–1001.
9. Rosett HL, Weiner L: *Alcohol and the Fetus: A Clinical Perspective.* New York, Oxford University Press, 1984.
10. Rosett HL: A clinical perspective of the fetal alcohol syndrome. *Alcohol Clin Exp Res* 1980; 4:119–122.
11. Olegard R, Sabel KG, Aronsson M: Effects on the child of alcohol abuse during pregnancy; Retrospective and prospective studies. *Acta Paediatr Scand* [Suppl] 1979; 275:112–121.
12. Little RE, Young A, Streissguth AP, et al: Preventing fetal alcohol effects: Effectiveness of a demonstration project, in *Ciba Found Symp 105, Mechanisms of Alcohol Damage in Utero.* London, Pitman Press, 1984, pp 254–274.
13. Smith IE, Lancaster JS, Moss-Wells S: Identifying high-risk pregnant drinkers: biological and behavioral correlates of continuous heavy drinking during pregnancy. *J Stud Alcohol* 1987; 48:304–309.
14. Weiner L, Morse BA, Garrido P: FAS/FAE: Focusing prevention on women at risk. *Int J Addict* 1989; 24:385–395.
15. Weiner L, Rosett HL, Edelin KC: Behavioral evaluation of fetal alcohol education for physicians. *Alcohol Clin Exp Res* 1982; 6:230–233.
16. Larsson G: Prevention of fetal alcohol effects: An antenatal program for early detection of pregnancies at risk. *Acta Obstet Gynecol Scand* 1983; 62:171–178.
17. Turner RC, Lichstein PR, Peden JG, et al: Alcohol withdrawal syndromes: A review of pathophysiology, clinical presentation, and treatment. *J Gen Intern Med* 1989; 4:432–444.
18. Fisher SE, Atkinson M, Burnap JK, et al: Ethanol-associated selective fetal malnutrition: A contributing factor in the fetal alcohol syndrome. *Alcohol Clin Exp Res* 1982; 6:197–201.
19. Ylikorkala O, Halmesmaki E, Viinikka L: Urinary prostacyclin and thromboxane metabolites in drinking pregnant women and in their infants: Relations to the fetal alcohol

effects. *Obstet Gynecol* 1988; 71:61–66.

20. Kline J, Shrout P, Stein Z, et al: Drinking during pregnancy and spontaneous abortions. *Lancet* 1980; 2:176–180.

21. Sokol KJ, Miller SI, Reed G: Alcohol abuse during pregnancy: An epidemiologic study. *Alcohol Clin Exp Res* 1980; 4:135–145.

22. Zuckerman B, Amarro H, Cabral H: Validity of self-reporting of marijuana and cocaine use among pregnant adolescents. *J Pediatr* 1989; 115:812–815.

23. Chasnoff IJ, Burns WJ, Schnoll SH, et al: Cocaine use in pregnancy. *N Engl J Med* 1985; 313:666–669.

24. Chasnoff IJ, Griffith DR, MacGregor S, et al: Temporal patterns of cocaine use in pregnancy: Perinatal outcome. *JAMA* 1989; 261:1741–1744.

25. Doering PL, Davidson CL, LaFance L, et al: Effects of cocaine on the human fetus: A review of clinical studies. *Ann Pharmacother* 1989; 23:639–645.

26. Mark PM, St. Pierre A, McClearly M, et al: Drug abuse in pregnancy. *HMO Pract* 1989; 3:205–209.

27. Graham K, Koren G, Klein J, et al: Determination of gestational cocaine exposure by hair analysis. *JAMA* 1989; 262:3328–3330.

28. Chasnoff IJ, Chisum GM, Kaplan WE: Maternal cocaine use and genitourinary tract malformations. *Teratology* 1988; 37:201–204.

29. Bingol N, Fuchs M, Diaz V, et al: Teratogenicity of cocaine in humans. *J Pediatr* 1987; 110:93.

30. Chasnoff IJ, Bussey M, Savich R, et al: Perinatal cerebral infarction and maternal cocaine use. *J Pediatr* 1986; 108:456–459.

31. Telsey AM, Merrit TA, Dixon SD: Cocaine exposure in a term neonate: Necrotizing enterocolitis as a complication. *Clin Pediatr (Phila)* 1988; 27:547–550.

32. Isner JM, Choksi SK: Cocaine and vasospasm. *N Engl J Med* 1989; 321:1604–1606.

33. Woods JR, Plessinger MA, Clark KE: Effect of cocaine on uterine blood flow and fetal oxygenation. *JAMA* 1987; 257:957–961.

34. Lange RA, Ciggarroa RG, Yancy CW, et al: Cocaine-induced coronary artery vasoconstriction. *N Engl J Med* 1989; 321:1557–1562.

35. Karch SB, Billingham ME: The pathophysiology and etiology of cocaine-induced heart disease. *Arch Pathol Lab Med* 1988; 112:225–230.

36. Cregler LL, Mark H: Cardiovascular dangers of cocaine abuse. *Am J Cardiol* 1986; 57:1185–1186.

37. Lathers CM, Tyan LS, Spino MM, et al: Cocaine-induced seizures, arrhythmias and sudden death. *J Clin Pharmacol* 1988; 28:584–593.

38. Herman EH, Vick J: A study of direct effect of cocaine on the heart. *Fed Proc* 1987; 46:1146.

39. Isner JM, Estes NAM, Thompson PD, et al: Acute cardiac events temporally related to cocaine abuse. *N Engl J Med* 1986; 315:1438.

40. Pasternack PF, Colvin SB, Bauman GF: Cocaine induced angina pectoris and acute myocardial infarction in patients younger than 40 years old *Am J Cardiol* 1985; 55:847.

41. Cregler LL, Mark H: Relation of acute myocardial infarction to cocaine abuse. *Am J Cardiol* 1985; 56:794.

42. Cregler LL, Mark H: Medical complications of cocaine abuse. *N Engl J Med* 1986; 315:1495–1500.

43. Schachne JS, Roberts BH, Thompson PD: Coronary artery spasm and myocardial infarction associated with cocaine abuse. *N Engl J Med* 1984; 310:1665–1666.

44. Young D, Glauber JJ: Electrocardiographic changes resulting from acute cocaine intoxication. *Am Heart J* 1947; .pa 34:272.

45. Jonsson S, O'Meara M, Young JB: Acute cocaine poisoning. *Am J Med* 1983; 75:1061–1064.

46. Weiner RS, Lockhart JT, Schwartz RG: Dilated cardiomyopathy and cocaine abuse. *Am J Med* 1986; 81:699–700.

47. Barth CW, Bray M, Roberts WC: Rupture of the ascending aorta during cocaine intoxication. *Am J Cardiol* 1986; 57:496.

48. Mittleman RE, Wetli CV: Cocaine and sudden "natural" death. *J Forensic Sci* 1987; 32:11–19.

49. Lowenstein DH, Massa SM, Rowbotham MC, et al: Acute neurologic and psychiatric complications associated with cocaine abuse. *Am J Med* 1987; 83:841–846.

50. Myers JA, Earnest MP: Generalized seizures and cocaine abuse. *Neurology* 1984; 34:675–676.

51. Lichentfeld PJ, Rubin DB, Feldman RS: Subarachnoid hemorrhage precipitated by cocaine smoking. *Arch Neurol* 1984; 41:223–224.

52. Allred RJ, Ewer S: Fatal pulmonary edema following intravenous freebase cocaine. *Ann Emerg Med* 1981; 10:441–442.

53. Roberts JR, Quattrocchi E, Howland MA: Severe hyperthermia secondary to intravenous drug abuse. *Am J Emerg Med* 1984; 2:273.

54. Nilsen N: Vascular abnormalities due to hyperthermia in chick embryos. *Teratology* 1984; 30:237–251.

55. Luque MA, Cavallaro DL, Torres M, et al: Pneumomediastinum, pneumothorax, and subcutaneous emphysema after alternate cocaine inhalation and marijuana smoking. *Pediatr Emerg Care* 1988 3:107–109.

56. Adrouny A, Magnusson P: Pneumopericardium from cocaine inhalation. *N Engl J Med* 1985; 313:48–49.

57. Itkonen J, Schnoll S, Glassworth J: Pulmonary dysfunction in "freebase" cocaine users. *Arch Intern Med* 1984; 144:2195–2197.

58. Nalbaudian H, Sheth N, Dietrich R, et al: Intestinal ischemia caused by cocaine ingestion. *Surgery* 1985; 97:374–376.

59. Marks V, Chapple PAL: Hepatic dysfunction in heroin and cocaine users. *Br J Addict* 1967; 62:189–195.

60. Roth D, Alarcon JJ, Fernandez JA, et al: Acute rhabdomyolysis associated with cocaine intoxication. *N Engl J Med* 1988; 319:673–677.

61. Herzlich BC, Arsura EL, Pagala M, et al: Rhabdomyolysis related to cocaine abuse. *Ann Intern Med* 1988; 108:335–336.

62. Skluth HA, Clark JE, Ehringer GL: Rhabdomyolysis associated with cocaine intoxication. *Drug Intell Clin Pharm* 1988; 22:778–780.

63. Naeye RL, Blane W, Le Blanc W, et al: Fetal complications of maternal heroin addiction: Abnormal growth, infection, and episodes of stress. *J Pediatr* 1973; 83:1055–1062.

64. Rodgers BD, Lee RV: Drug abuse, in Burrow GN, Ferris TF (eds): *Medical Complications During Pregnancy*. Philadelphia, WB Saunders Co, 1988, pp 570–581.

65. Rementeria JL, Nunag NN: Narcotic withdrawal in pregnancy: Stillbirth incidence with a case report. *Am J Obstet Gynecol* 1973; 116:1152–1156.

66. Zuspan FP, Gumpel JA, Meijia-Zelaya A, et al: Fetal stress from methadone withdrawal. *Am J Obstet Gynecol* 1975; 122:43–46.

67. Louria DB, Hensle T, Rose J: The major medical complications of heroin addiction. *Ann Intern Med* 1967; 67:1–11.

68. Guinan ME, Hardy A: Epidemiology of AIDS in women in the United States. *JAMA* 1987; 257:2039–2042.

69. Stevens CE, Toy PT, Tong MJ, et al: Perinatal hepatitis B virus transmission in the United States. Prevention by passive-active immunization. *JAMA* 1985; 253:1940–1945.

70. Arevalo JA, Washington AE: Cost-effectiveness of prenatal screening and immunization for hepatitis B virus. *JAMA* 1988; 259:365–369.

71. Blinick G, Jerez E, Wallach RC: Methadone maintenance, pregnancy and progeny. *JAMA* 1973; 225:477–481.

72. Harclerode J: *The Effect of Marijuana on Reproduction and Development*. National Institute on Drug Abuse Monograph No. 31. Bethesda, Md, National Institute on Drug Abuse, 1980.

73. Walter CW, Johnson LJ, Buelke J, et al: Marijuana: An Annotated Bibliography. New York, Collier Macmillan, 1982.

74. Greeland S, Staisch KJ, Brown N, et al: the effects of marijuana use during pregnancy. A preliminary epidemiology study. *Am J Obstet Gynecol* 1982; 143:408–413.

75. Harbison R, Bernardo MP, Lubin D: Alteration of delta-9 tetrahydrocannabinol induced teratogenicity by stimulation and inhibition of its metabolism. *J Pharmacol Exp Ther* 1972; 202:455.

76. Sofia R, Strasbaugh J, Banerjee B: Teratologic evaluation of synthetic delta-9 tetrahydrocannabinol in rabbits. *Teratology* 1979; 19:361–366.

77. Hingson R, Alpert LL, Day N, et al: Effects of maternal drinking and marijuana use on fetal growth and development. *Pediatrics* 1982; 70:539–546.

78. Scanlon JW: Effect of benzodiazepines in neonates. *N Engl J Med* 1975; 292:649–650.

79. Milkovich L, Van den Berg BJ: Effects of prenatal meprobamate and chlordiazepoxide hydrochloride on human embryonic and fetal development. *N Engl J Med* 1974; 291:1268–1271.

80. Rosenberg L, Mitchell AA, Parsells JL, et al: Lack of relation of oral clefts to diazepam use during pregnancy. *N Engl J Med* 1983; 309:1282–1285.

81. Donaldson JO: *Neurology of Pregnancy*, ed 2. London, WB Saunders Co, 1989.

82. Desmond MM, Schwanecke RP, Wilson GS, et al: Maternal barbiturate utilization and neonatal withdrawal symptomatology. *J Pediatr* 1972; 80:190–197.

CHAPTER 18

The Effect of Embryonic and Fetal Exposure to X-ray, Microwaves, Ultrasound, Magnetic Resonance, and Isotopes*

Robert L. Brent

The effects of high-energy radiation (x-rays, gamma rays, particulate radiation) have been studied more extensively than has any other environmental hazard. In spite of the vast amount of knowledge available about ionizing radiation, many physicians are unfamiliar with the quantitative and qualitative effects of ionizing radiation.[1] In this respect our laboratory frequently is consulted when women of reproductive age are exposed to diagnostic x-rays. More often than not, the exposed women have received erroneous information without the benefit of a minimal collection of data. In one instance, a woman was advised to have an abortion following exposure to diathermy because of confusion about the difference between microwave and ultrasound energy. Actually, these three forms of energy have quite different biologic effects (Table 18–1).

It would be preferable from an educational viewpoint to limit the use of the term *radiation* to high-energy ionizing radiation. Radar, microwaves, short wave diathermy,

FM broadcast range, and radiofrequencies are various forms of long-wavelength electromagnetic waves that have little in common with x-rays and gamma rays, at least from a biologic standpoint. The use of radiation to describe ultrasound may even be more confusing and erroneous. In England, physicians refer to diagnostic ultrasound as sonography and consciously refrain from using the term *radiation* in conjunction with any aspect of the clinical use of ultrasound. It is best to limit the use of the term *radiation* in a clinical setting because of the connotations it may suggest.

Radiation is an anxiety-provoking term because of its association with the effects of ionizing radiation. These associations and effects follow.

1. The term *radiation* is related to the effects of the atomic bomb. In the minds of many, it is impossible to separate the effects of low-dose ionizing radiation from the psychologic, physical and radiation effects of the atomic bomb. The fact that the horrendous effects of the atomic and hydrogen bombs are at one end of a continuum of radiation effects

*The preparation of this chapter was supported by grants NIH HD 19165 and 5 RO1 HD 22386.

TABLE 18–1.
Comparative Aspects of Various Forms of Radiation

Type	Physical Characteristics	Biologic Effects
X-rays, gamma rays	Short wavelength: Electromagnetic waves, highly penetrating, with the capacity of producing ionization within tissues and subsequent electrochemical reactions.	Electrochemical reactions. Can result in tissue damage from high exposures that result in cell death, mutation, cancer, and developmental defects. These effects are dose-related.
Microwaves, radar, diathermy	Longer electromagnetic waves with variable ability to penetrate but no ability to produce ionization within tissues.	The primary biologic effect is hyperthermia, although the existence of nonthermal effects of these electromagnetic waves is still being investigated. Cataract development is the most widely known complication of extensive microwave or radar exposure.
Ultrasound	Sound waves with a frequency above the audible range that produce mechanical compressions and rarefactions in matter, with *no* capability of producing ionization.	If the energy is high enough, sound waves can cause tissue disruption by the production of cavitation and streaming as well as hyperthermia. None of these effects occurs with the energies utilized in diagnostic ultrasonography.

distorts to a greater or lesser extent the risks of all forms of energy labeled *radiation.*

2. Populations that have had high exposures to ionizing radiation have increased incidences of cancer. These populations include radium dial workers, uranium miners, patients receiving radiation therapy or isotope therapy for various diseases, and the persons who received the higher exposures in Hiroshima and Nagasaki following the atomic bomb detonation.[2] *Cancer* itself is also an anxiety-provoking term. In our culture it is a disease with which people are "afflicted," and it is a disease that is dreaded by a large segment of the population. Few persons are aware of the extremely small maximum risk for the occurrence of cancer in populations exposed to much lower doses of radiation.

3. The immense psychologic consequences of high-energy radiation exposure are extremely important and cannot be ignored when one considers the deleterious effects of radiation. A review of the 30-year study of the survivors of the Hiroshima and Nagasaki bombings revealed some interesting findings.[30]

Thirty years of study clearly showed that radiation effects are dose dependent. A survivor aware of the magnitude of the radiation dose can better understand the extent of his own risks. More than 90 per cent of survivors received much less than 10 rads from the A-bombs. With this knowledge, such survivors can realize that their fears of disease from A-bomb exposure may be exaggerated and that the possibility of their developing any such disease is no greater than those of nonexposed individuals. Those who received higher doses have greater risks. It is worth noting that, thus far, the life expectancy of the exposed population under study and of their offspring is at least equal to that for the population in the rest of Japan. Thirty years of study has not eradicated radiation damage but has yielded reasonable estimates of the risks involved.[3]

In spite of the fact that the results of the Atomic Bomb Casualty Commission data have been widely disseminated in Japan, the psychologic burden of radiation exposure is still prominent: "The parents of a man wishing to marry a woman known to be a survivor, or the daughter of a survivor, may object to or even attempt to prevent their marriage, fearing the woman's health may be adversely affected, or their children might have genetic defects."[3]

Granted that the risks from high-energy radiation exposure may be exaggerated or not well understood, there is no question that high-energy radiation can damage tissue and produce long-term effects. If the quantitative data pertaining to radiation effects are understood, the effects of radiation can be placed in better perspective. Radiation risks should be compared with spontaneous risks and risks produced by exposure to other environmental hazards.

Teratogenic and Carcinogenic Effects of In Utero Ionizing Radiation

There have been many experiments and observations about the effects of radiation on the developing embryo. Nevertheless, we have a great deal to learn about radiation teratogenesis and teratogenesis in general. The subject is summarized briefly here. For further details the reader is referred to more complete reviews.[4-9]

Prior to summarizing the effects of irradiation at different stages of gestation it is important to emphasize that all the effects described are produced at or above specific doses. Since the vast majority of embryopathologic effects are threshold phenomena, there are doses of ionizing radiation which will not produce these effects.

Before implantation, the embryo is a multicellular organism with a decreased sensitivity to the teratogenic and growth-retarding effects of radiation and a greater degree of sensitivity to the lethal effects of irradiation (Figs 18-1, 18-2, 18-3, Tables 18-2, 18-3).[10-12] This does not indicate that malformations cannot be produced but that the cytogenetic abnormalities and malformations, if produced, result in a high incidence of mortality. During early organogenesis the embryo is very sensitive to the growth-retarding, teratogenic, and lethal effects of irradiation but has the ability to recover somewhat from the growth-retarding effects in the postpartum period.[11, 13-15] During the early fetal period the fetus has diminished sensitivity to multiple organ teratogenesis but retains central nervous system (CNS) sensitivity; it is growth-

retarded at term and recovers poorly from the growth retardation in the postpartum period. During the later fetal stages, the embryo is not grossly deformed by radiation but can sustain permanent cell depletion of various organs and tissues if the radiation exposure is high enough.[7, 9]

One can postulate many mechanisms for the effects of irradiation, including cell death, mitotic delay, disturbances of cell migration, and others. Until we know more about the mechanisms involved in embryopathology, it is difficult to determine which mechanisms are most important in the process of radiation-induced embryopathologic disorders. Furthermore, the same pathogenic mechanisms may not be primarily operative at all stages of gestation. Radiation-induced cell death may be minimally important at one stage of gestation because of the embryo's ability to replace the killed cells. At another stage of gestation, cell death may be a primary factor because the embryo has lost the ability to replace dead cells and the fetus may be permanently cell-depleted.

Other radiation-induced effects that have been invoked to explain embryopathologic conditions are cytogenetic abnormalities and somatic mutations.[16, 17] Cytogenetic abnormalities may be responsible for preimplantation death in the irradiated mammalian zygote,[10, 17, 18] but point mutations are less likely to be a contributing factor to abnormal morphogenesis. If one uses the known radiation mutation rate in mammalian cells (as determined by Russell and colleagues[11, 14, 19] in the mouse) for estimating potential teratogenicity, it becomes perfectly obvious that radiation-induced point mutation could not account for even a small proportion of radiation-induced teratogenicity unless it simply involved cell death. Of course, neither phenomenon has been studied adequately at every stage of mammalian gestation.

Radiation effects may appear at once and result in cell death, embryonic death, or teratogenesis. Other effects may not be obvious immediately and can be measured or ascertained only in the postpartum or adult period.

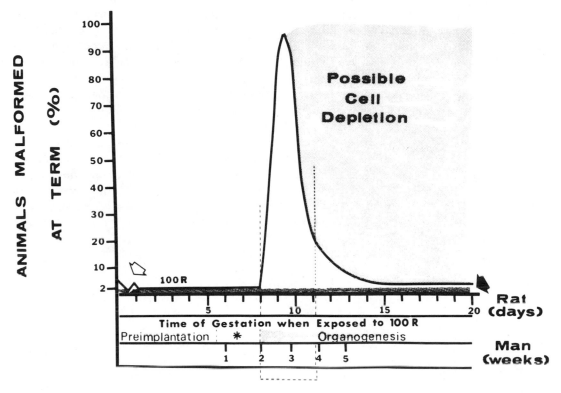

FIG 18–1.
This graph depicts the relative incidence of gross congenital malformations in the rat following an exposure of 100 rad. The *solid arrow* on the right side of the ordinate points to the 2% control incidence of congenital malformations seen in this species. The incidence of malformations before the ninth day is the same as in the controls. The *open arrow* on the left side of the ordinate points to a slight increase in malformations on the first day. (This was inserted because of the work of Russell and Saylors[17] in a particular strain of mice.) A very large increase in malformations occurs during the early organogenetic period. Note that this corresponds to the third and fourth weeks of human pregnancy. This high incidence of gross malformations falls off rapidly as organogenesis diminishes. Note that organogenesis to some degree (central nervous system) continues to term. Also note that although gross malformations may not be produced during the late fetal stages with 100 rad, an irreversible cell loss occurs. The significance of these cell losses is under study. The asterisk (*) is placed at the stage of implantation to indicate that although malformations are not readily produced at this stage, growth retardation can be induced.

Neuronal depletion, infertility, tissue hypoplasia, neoplasia, or shortening of life span are phenomena the significance of which can be evaluated only in the postpartum or adult organism.[4, 9, 20–25]

The neurophysiologic and behavioral changes in adult organisms that have been irradiated in utero are the most difficult to evaluate. The difficulties arise for several reasons: (1) It is not easy to eliminate postnatal environmental effects as contributing factors; (2) reported findings are frequently not reproducible and are not dose-related; (3) behavioral changes may not be able to be cor-

related with the neuroanatomic changes; and (4) animal behavior tests may have minimal application to the human situation. This subject has been reviewed.[6, 26] Except for the work of Piontkovskii,[27, 28] all behavioral studies of animals or human beings exposed to radiation during gestation do not exhibit any measurable changes if exposure was below the 20- to 25-rad range (0.2–0.25 Gy).

Human Radiation Teratogenesis

The classic effects of radiation on the developing mammal are gross congenital malformations, intrauterine growth retardation (IUGR), and embryonic death. Each of these effects has a dose-response relationship, and a threshold exposure below which there is no difference between the irradiated and the control populations. Because human pregnancies predominantly consist of a single embryo, it would be unusual to see the classic triad of effects; although it is conceivable that if the dose and timing were appropriate, a stillborn growth-retarded, malformed embryo could result.

Growth retardation and CNS effects, such as microcephaly or eye malformations, are the cardinal manifestations of intrauterine radiation effects in humans. The occurrence of microcephaly is such a significant component of the effects of intrauterine radiation that a "teratogen update" has been written about this subject.[29] The reports of Zappert,[30] Goldstein and Murphy,[31–33] Dekaban,[34] Miller,[35] Wood et al.,[36, 37] Plummer,[38] and Yamazaki et al.[39] indicate that microcephaly is the most common malformation observed in human beings randomly exposed to high doses of radiation during pregnancy. In Goldstein and Murphy's reports,[31–33] 19 of 75 irradiated embryos became microcephalic or hydrocephalic

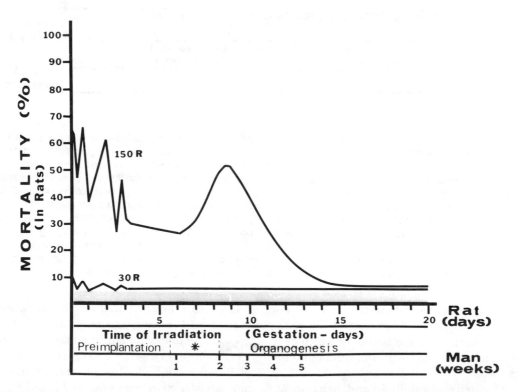

FIG 18–2.
The lethal effect of radiation in rats is greater on the first day. It appears that the LD_{50} shifts at different times of the day during early gestation, possibly because the cells are dividing synchronously; therefore, the zygote will vary in its radiosensitivity, depending on the stage of the cell cycle. Note that the embryo becomes somewhat resistant in the implantation stage and then becomes sensitive to the lethal effect of radiation during early organogenesis. A 30-rad dose apparently does increase the resorption rate when radiation takes place on the first day. The superimposition of the lethality curve for rats onto the human embryonic development timetable may not be appropriate and is for purposes of comparison only, but it allows one to estimate roughly the stages at which the human embryo might be most readily killed by high doses of radiation.

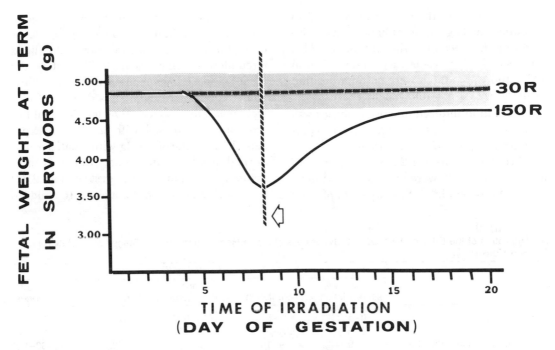

FIG 18–3.

The *fetal weight* in the Wistar colony of rats in our laboratory averages 4.8 g on the 22nd day when delivered by cesarean section that morning. Note that 150 rad causes growth retardation just after implantation but before the stage is sensitive to teratogenesis (*arrow* pointing to vertical line). From the time of implantation until term, 150 rad produced some degree of growth retardation. Note that 30 rad does not appear to produce significant deviations in growth, although it may be that all experimental groups are too small to show differences in weight at this low dose.

children, having received an estimated dose of greater than 100 rad as a minimum. Almost all the microcephalic children were mentally retarded. The following malformations also were reported: two children with hypoplastic genitalia, one child with cleft palate, one child with hypospadias, an abnormality of the large toe, and an abnormality of the ear. Many of the children had intrauterine growth retardation, and three had various abnormalities of the eyes, including microphthalmia, cataracts, strabismus, retinal degeneration, and optic atrophy. The unique finding was that no visceral, limb, or other malformations were found unless the child exhibited intrauterine growth retardation, microcephaly (congenital malformations of the brain), or readily apparent eye malformations. Dekaban[34] reported that 22 infants exposed between the 3rd to 20th weeks of human gestation were microcephalic, mentally retarded, or both (Fig 18–4). The estimated protracted exposure was 250 rad (2.5 Gy), and all of the malformed infants exhibited growth retardation. The most frequent abnormalities were (1) small size at birth and stunted growth, (2) microcephaly, (3) mental retardation, (4) microphthalmia, (5) pigmentary changes in the retina, (6) genital and skeletal malformations, and (7) cataracts (see Fig 18–4). All of the embryos reported by Dekaban received hundreds of rads. The patients were treated with radiation for various reasons, including dysmenorrhea, menorrhagia, myomata, arthritis or tuberculosis of the sacroiliac joint, and malignant tumor of the uterus or cervix. In several instances, radiation was initiated without knowing the patients were pregnant.

It is of interest to note that in one of the case reports[40] a typical camptomelic dwarf was reported, and the cause was believed to be radiation. High-dose radiation was delivered from the second to the fifth month. This rare recessive syndrome was not described in 1930, and the authors were not in a position to recognize its possible genetic cause.[40]

Radiation-induced microcephaly, growth retardation, and microphthalmia are represented in Figures 18–5 and 18–6.

From a sample of 1,265 subjects in utero at Hiroshima, 182 were analyzed by Miller[35] and by Wood et al.[36, 37] Seventy-eight of these fetuses were younger than 16 weeks of age at the time of irradiation; 105 were 16 weeks or older. Of the 78, 25 were microcephalic (head circumference more than 2 SD below the mean), and 11 were mentally deficient. Of the 105, 7 were microcephalic as defined, and 4 were mentally deficient. The incidence of microcephaly increased with increasing exposure. In 14 of the offspring with smaller-than-normal head circumference who were also mentally deficient, 10 were greater than 2 SD below the mean height for age. In 16 children

TABLE 18–2.

A Compilation of the Effects of 10 rad (0.1 Gy) or Less of Acute Radiation in Various Stages of Gestation in Rat and Mouse*

	Stage of Gestation (Days)				
	Preimplantation	Implantation	Early Organogenesis	Late Organogenesis	Fetus Stages
Mouse	0–4$\frac{1}{2}$	4$\frac{1}{2}$–6$\frac{1}{2}$	6$\frac{1}{2}$–8$\frac{1}{2}$	8$\frac{1}{2}$–12	12–18
Rat	0–5$\frac{1}{2}$	5$\frac{1}{2}$–8	8–10	10–13	13–22
Corresponding human gestation period	0–9	9–14	15–28	28–50	50–280
Lethality	+[†]				
Growth retardation at term	−	−	−	−	−
Growth retardation as adult	−	−	−	−	−
Gross malformations (aplasia, hyperplasia, absence or overgrowth of organs or tissues)	±[‡]	−	−	−	−
Cell depletions, minimal but measurable tissue hypoplasia	−	−	−	−	−
Sterility	−	−	−	−	−
Significant increase in germ cell mutations[¶]	±	±	±	±	±
Cytogenetic abnormalities	−	−	−	−	−
Neuropathology[§]	−[‡]	−	−	−	−
Tumor induction[§, ‖]	−	−	±	±	±
Behavior disorders**	−	−	−	−	−
Reduction in life span[§]	−	−	−	−	−

− = indicates no observed effect; ± = questionable but reported or suggested effect; + = demonstrated effect; + + = readily apparent effect; + + + = occurs in high incidence.
*Dose fractionation or protraction effectively reduces the biologic result of all the pathologic effects reported in this table.
†At this stage the murine embryo is most sensitive to the lethal effects of irradiation. With 10 rad in the mouse, Rugh reports a slight decrease in litter size in the mouse.[7]
‡Rugh reports a 1% incidence of exencephalia in a strain of mice given 15 and 25 rad. Others have not been able to repeat these results.[10]
§Recent reevaluation of the atomic bomb victims data suggests the possibility that mental retardation is a risk in the 10- to 20-rad range. This is not supported by most other data.
¶The potential for mutation induction exists in the embryonic term cells or their precursors. Several long-term studies indicate that considerably greater doses in mice and rats do not affect longevity, tumor incidence, incidence of congenital malformations, litter size, growth rate, or fertility.
‖Stewart and colleagues and others have reported that 2 rad increases the incidence of malignancy by 50% in the offspring. See text for discussion.
**Piontkovskii reports behavioral changes in the rat after 1-rad daily irradiation.[27, 28] This work has not been reproduced. See text for discussion.

TABLE 18–3.

A Compilation of the Effects of 100 rad (1 Gy) of Acute Radiation on Embryonic Development at Various Stages of Gestation in Rat and Mouse*

Feature	Preimplantation	Implantation	Early Organogenesis	Late Organogenesis	Fetal Stages
			Stage of Gestation (Days)*		
Mouse	$0–4\frac{1}{2}$	$4\frac{1}{2}–6\frac{1}{2}$	$6\frac{1}{2}–8\frac{1}{2}$	$8\frac{1}{2}–12$	12–18
Rat	$0–5\frac{1}{2}$	$5\frac{1}{2}–8$	8–10	10–13	13–22
Corresponding human gestation period	0–9	9–14	18–36	36–50	50–280
Lethality	+ + +[†]	+	+ +	±	−
Growth retardation at term	−	+	+ + +	+ +	+
Growth retardation as adult	−	+	+ +	+ + +	+ +
Gross malformations (aplasia, hypoplasia, absence or overgrowth of organs or tissues)	−	−	+ + +	±[‡]	−[‡]
Cell depletions, minimal but measurable tissue hypoplasia	−	−	±	+ +	+[§]
Sterility[¶]		−	±	−	+ +[¶]
Significant increase in germ cell mutations[‖]	±	±	±	±	±
Cytogenetic abnormalities**	±			+*	+*
Cataracts	−	−	+	I	+
Neuropathology[§, ‡‡]		−	+ + +	+ + +	+ +
Tumor induction[††]	−	−	±	±	±
Behavior disorders[§, ‡‡]	−	−	+	+ + +	+
Reduction in life span[§§] (in nonmalformed embryos)	−	−	−	−	−

   − = no observed effect; ± = questionable but reported or suggested effect; + = demonstrated effect; + + = readily apparent effect; + + + = occurs in high incidence.

*Dose fractionation or protraction effectively reduced the biologic result of all the pathologic effects reported in this table.

[†]Russell et al. reported that 200 rad increased the incidence of XO aneuploidy in 2% to 5% of offspring in mice with a spontaneous incidence of 1%. A dose of 100 rad kills substantial numbers of mouse and rat embryos at this stage, but the survivors appear and develop normally.

[‡]One hundred rad produce changes in the irradiated fetus that are subtle and necessitate detailed examination and comparison with comparable controls.

[§]There is a consensus that the brain maintains a marked sensitivity to radiation throughout all of gestation. Mental retardation is a serious risk at this dose.

[¶]The male gonad in the rat can be made extremely hypoplastic by irradiation in the fetal stages with 15 rad. In the mouse the newborn female is most sensitive to the sterilizing effects of radiation. Much of this research on other animals cannot be applied to the human.

[‖]The potential for mutation induction exists in embryonic germ cells or their precursors. The relative sensitivity of the embryonic germ cells when compared to adult germ cells is not known. Several long-term studies in animals do not indicate any exceptional differences.

**Footnote * refers to the aneuploidy produced in a strain of mice with a 1% incidence of spontaneous XO to aneuploidy. Bloom has reported a much higher percentage of chromosome breaks in human embryos receiving 100 to 200 rad in utero than in adults receiving the same dose of irradiation. As yet there have been no diseases associated with this increase in frequency of chromosome breaks.

[††]Animal experiments and the data from Hiroshima and Nagasaki do not support the concept that in utero irradiation is much more tumorigenic than extrauterine irradiation. On the other hand, Stewart and colleagues and many others report that irradiation from pelvimetry (2 rad) increases the incidence of leukemia and other tumors.

[‡‡]A statistically significant increase in the percentage of mental retardation occurs with this dose of radiation. On the other hand, normal intelligence has been found in children receiving much higher doses in utero.

[§§]Animal experiments indicate that survivors of in utero irradiation have a life span that is longer than that of groups of animals given the same dose of radiation during their extrauterine life and the same life expectancy as nonirradiated controls.

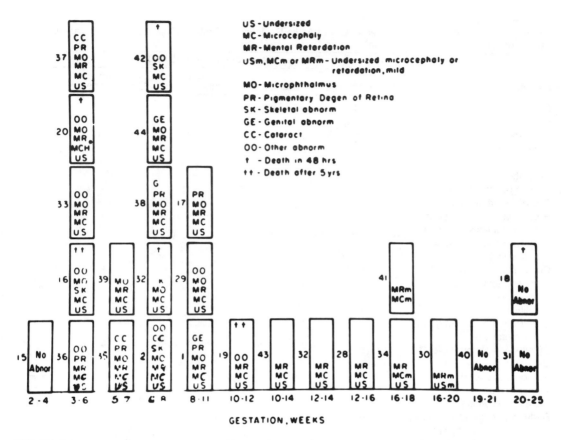

FIG 18–4.
The spectrum of malformations in 26 human infants in utero. Note that all infants receiving therapeutic doses of radiation are growth-retarded if they were irradiated between 3 and 20 weeks of gestation. Note that in no instance is there an associated malformation in structures other than the nervous system without either microcephaly or mental retardation. (From Dekaban AS: *J Nucl Med* 1968;9:471–477. Used by permission.)

with small heads who were not mentally deficient, there was no marked reduction in stature. Tables 18–4 and 18–5 summarize some of the characteristics of the patients exposed in utero before the 16th week of gestation. Severe mental retardation was not observed in any patient that received less than 50 rad while in utero. In a summary of the data on microcephaly Blot[41, 42] noted that although there was no increased risk for microcephaly in the population exposed to less than 150 rad in Nagasaki, there was an increased risk in the population exposed to much lower doses in Hiroshima (see Table 18–5). There is a possibility that the decreased head size observed at the lower doses was unrelated to the radiation exposure in Hiroshima but was instead due to other causes. It also should be pointed out that 10 to 20 rad of low linear energy transfer (LET) radiation will not increase the incidence of microcephaly in experimental animals.[7] Although Otake and Schull[42a] report some mental retardation at very low exposures the allegation is not biologically plausible and is not supported by animal experiments, the known histopathological effects of radiation, or other human studies.

Analysis of the human data reveals some interesting and important facts. Growth retardation, microcephaly, and mental retardation are predominant observable effects following acute exposures to greater than 50 rad (low LET radiation). No report of a bona

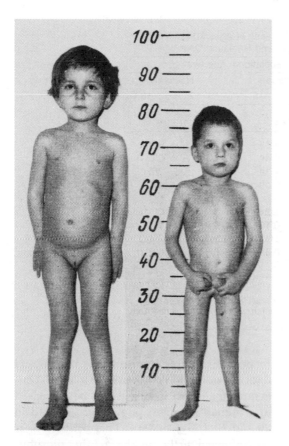

FIG 18–5.
The smaller child received in utero radiation during the third to fourth months of gestation. The skin dose of the abdomen was 900 rad and was delivered for the purpose of sterilization of the mother because she had metastatic carcinoma of the breast. The child was full-term but weighed only 1,900 g. He had microcephaly and cerebral atrophy. Growth retardation persisted into childhood, as evidenced by comparison with a child the same age who is in the 50th percentile. There was shortening of the left tibia. The eyes had decreased vessel size and pallor of the left disk. There were abnormal motor movements, weakness, and severe mental retardation.

fida, radiation-induced morphologic malformation has been reported in a human being who has not exhibited growth retardation or a CNS abnormality. One might question why the CNS seems to be more sensitive in humans than in experimental animals, in which many organ systems are malformed by irradiation. The explanation for this apparent discrepancy is that the CNS maintains its sen-

sitivity to radiation throughout gestation and into the neonatal period, whereas the other organ systems have much narrower periods during which obvious morphologic alterations can be produced (see Fig 18–1). Secondly, the period of exquisite sensitivity to multiple system malformations is proportionately quite small in humans (the 2nd through the 5th week from conception) when compared with the rat (the 9th to the 11th day). In humans, all organ systems can be readily malformed by high doses of radiation during 5% of pregnancy, whereas in the rat, radiation can produce gross malformations during 20% of pregnancy. Thirdly, human exposures have occurred at random during pregnancy, and the exposure is controlled for purposes of therapeutic irradiation (hundreds of rads) or not controlled, as at Hiroshima and Nagasaki. Therefore, the exposures that occur in humans during the period of maximum sensitivity will be infrequent and/or will result in a high incidence of abortions, whereas the great majority of exposures will occur during the fetal stages when the CNS is still sensitive

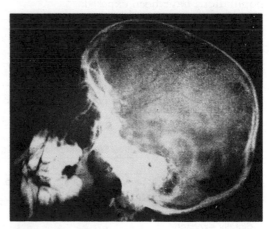

FIG 18–6.
Lateral view of the skull of the patient in Figure 18–5. The encephalogram revealed microcephaly and porencephaly. The mother received 900 rad of radiation to the abdomen. Based on the kilovoltage of the x-ray machine and the filtration, the estimated exposure to the embryo was 200 to 300 rad. The embryo could have been as young as 9 weeks or as old as 20 weeks at the time of irradiation on the basis of the meager history that is available.

TABLE 18–4.
Frequency of Small Head Circumference at Ages 10–19 Years According to City, Gestational Age, and Radiation Dose*†

	Gestational Age (wk)			
	Hiroshima		Nagasaki	
Dose (rad)	0–17	18+	0–17	18+
Not in City or Distally Exposed	31/764		10/246	
0–9	4(1)/63+	4/65+	0/1	0/9
10–19	6(1)/54	0/44	0/7	0/6
20–29	6/24	1/14	0/5	2/7
30–39	4/8	0/10	2/4	0/6
40–49	3/11	0/6	0/6	0/3
50–59	9(2)/20	2/24	0/9	0/11
100–149	2/4	0/10	0/2	1/5
150+	5(5)/13	1(1)8+	8(3)9	2(1)9
Unknown	1/7	0/3	0/0	0/0
Total (in city)	40(9)/204	8(1)/184	10(3)/43	5(1)/56

*From Blot W: *J Radiat Res (Tokyo)* 1975; 16 (suppl): 82–88. Used by permission.
†Cases in parentheses give number with small head circumference and mental retardation. Plus (+) indicates one person with mental retardation without small head circumference.

to radiation-induced damage. Thus, the nature of radiation effects in the human and the apparent discrepancies with animal data can be explained by the manner in which human populations have been exposed.

Irradiation of the human fetus from diagnostic exposures of less than 5 rad (0.05 Gy) have not been observed to cause congenital malformations or growth retardation,[43–47] but not all such epidemiologic studies are negative.[48] These are extremely difficult studies

to perform, and it appears that the animal data support the contention that gross congenital malformations will not be increased in a human pregnant population exposed to 20 rad (0.2 Gy) or less. This contention is strengthened further by the fact that most human exposures to extensive diagnostic radiation studies are fractionated and/or protracted. This type of exposure is likely to be less effective in producing malformations than is an acute exposure of low LET radiation.[49, 50]

TABLE 18–5.
Number of Cases and Relative Risk of Mental Retardation According to Dose Category*

	Hiroshima				Nagasaki			
Dose (rad)	Sample Size	Cases†	Relative Risk‡		Sample Size	Cases	Relative Risk	
Not in city or distally exposed	830	5(2)	1.0	(1.0)	246	4(2)	1.0	(1.0)
0–9	145	3(1)	3.4	(3.8)	11	0		—
10–49	189	2(1)	1.8	(1.5)	45	0		—
50–99	47	3(1)	10.6	(11.8)	20	0		—
100–199	29	4(1)	22.9	(28.6)	13	0		—
200–299	8	3	66.3	(104)	5	1(1)	12.3	
300	6	2	55.3	(92.2)	7	3	26.4	(52.7)

*From Blot W: *J Radiat Res (Tokyo)* 1975; 16 (suppl): 82–88. Used by permission.
†Numbers in parentheses are numbers of cases (included in the totals) whose mental retardation was apparently due to causes other than intrauterine radiation.
‡Numbers in parentheses are relative risks, excluding cases whose mental retardation was apparently due to nonradiation causes.

TABLE 18–6.
Risk of Leukemia in Various Groups with Specific Epidemiologic and Pathologic
Characteristics in Populations Followed for 10 to 30 Years*

Group	Approximate Risk	Increased Risk Over Control Population	Occurrence
Identical twin of leukemia twin	1/3	1,000	Weeks to months
Irradiation-treated polycythemia vera	1/6	500	10–15 yr
Bloom syndrome	1/8	375	<30 yr old
Hiroshima survivors who were within 1,000 m of the hypocenter	1/60	50	Average, 12 yr
Down's syndrome	1/95	30	<10 yr old
Irradiation-treated patients with ankylosing spondylitis	1/270	10	15 yr
Siblings of leukemic children	1/720	4.0	To 10 yr
Children exposed to pelvimetry in utero (gestational exposure)	1/2,000	1.5	<10 yr
US white children <15 yr	1/2,800	1.0	To 10 yr

*Modified from Miller RW: Epidemiologic conclusions from radiation toxicity studies, in Fry RJM, Grahn D, Griem ML (eds): *Late Effects of Radiation*. London, Taylor & Francis, 1970, pp 245–256.

Although the animal and human data support the contention that exposures in the 5-rad (0.05 Gy) range would not be expected to increase the incidence of anatomic malformations, growth retardation, mental retardation, or abortion, there is the theoretical possibility that functional or biochemical changes may be produced at low levels with low incidence. We have investigated a number of these functional and biochemical parameters, such as thyroid function, liver function, and fertility, and have not found them to be more sensitive to radiation than the above-mentioned parameters. That does not mean, however, that some other parameter, still unstudied, would not be permanently altered by low-level radiation.

There are three stochastic phenomena that must be evaluated when one is considering prenatal radiation: (1) mutagenesis, (2) abortion during the preimplantation period, and (3) oncogenesis (see Table 18–6 to 18–9): The risk estimates for the mutagenic effects of radiation for germ cell mutations or somatic mutations listed in Tables 18–8 and 18–9 are based on the mutation rates derived from adult animal radiation experiments. Although there is a threshold effect for the induction of abortion during and after early organogenesis (>25 rad; see Table 18–8), there is a possibility that abortion in the preimplantation period may be a stochastic phenomenon. Exposures of 10 rad on the first day of mammalian development produced no apparent increase in abortions, but these experiments involved only hundreds of embryos. It would not be possible to examine whether a dose of 10 rad had increased the spontaneous risk of abortion by 1.0% or 0.1% unless the experimental groups were considerably increased. Similarly, it would be even more difficult to evaluate the effects of a 1-rad exposure on the spontaneous abortion rate. There are data neither to support nor to refute the theory that radiation-induced abortion during the preimplantation period is a stochastic phenomenon.

Besides the production of congenital malformations, abortion, or intrauterine growth retardation, it has been suggested that prenatal irradiation is more oncogenic than the same exposures in the child or the adult.

Oncogenic Effect of Prenatal Radiation

Stewart and her colleagues[65–69] suggested that the human embryo was more sensitive to the leukemogenic effects of radiation, and

TABLE 18–7.
Reported Effects of Low Exposures of Radiation on the Embryo When Administered Throughout Pregnancy

Study	Organism	Source	Approximate Exposure Rate per Minute (rad)	Exposure per Day	Exposure per Pregnancy	Comments	Effects
Russell et al[19]	Mouse	^{137}Cs	0.0086	12.4 rad	171.0 rad	Days 1–18	None except shortened breeding period in female
Ronnback[51]	Mouse	^{137}Cs		8.4 rad	170.0 rad	During gestation and in some instances 20 days post partum	None
Vorisek[52]	Rat	^{60}Co	0.0017	2.5 rad		Daily during pregnancy	None
Stadler & Gowen[53]	Mouse		0.0015	2.2 rad		Continuous through 10 generations	None
Coppenger & Brown[54]	Rat	^{60}Co	0.0014	2.0 rad		Continuous through 10 generations	None
Konerman[55]	Mice	^{60}Co	0.0017	10 rad / 20 rad / 20 rad	180.0 rad / 360.0 rad	Days 1–18 / Days 1–18 / Days 6–13 only	None / Growth retardation / None
Wesley[56]	Humans	Background		0.3 mrad	0.1 rad	Variation in background radiation	Increased congenital malformations
Gentry et al[57]	Humans	Background		0.3 mrad	0.1 rad	Variation in background radiation	Increased malformations
Grahn & Kratchman[58]	Humans	Background		0.3 mrad	0.1 rad	Variation in background radiation	Background radiation not a factor in incidence of congenital malformations
Segall et al[59]	Humans	Background		0.3 mrad	0.1 rad	Background radiation	Background radiation level not a factor in incidence of congenital malformations
Kriegal & Langendorff[60]	Mouse	X-ray		2.5 rad / 5.0 rad / 10 rad / 20 rad		Acute dose given daily	No influence / No influence / No influence / Malformations, resorptions, growth retardations
Piontkovskii[28]	Rat	X-ray		1 rad	20.0 rad	Acute dose given daily	Functional changes in behavior and motor activity (questionable)
Laskey et al[61]	Rat	HTO	Continuous 0.01–10 µCi HTO mL of body water	0.003–3.0 rad/day	0.066–66.0	Tritiated water, continuous exposure	Male testes reduced 10 µCi; no growth or reproductive impairment in F$_1$; F$_2$ generation had reduced weight

TABLE 18–8.
Estimation of the Risks of Radiation in the Human Embryo Based on Human Epidemiologic Studies and Mouse and Rat Radiation Embryologic Studies

Embryonic Age (Days)	Minimal Lethal Dose (rad)	Approximate LD_{50} (rad)	Minimum Dose (rad) for Permanent Growth Retardation in the Adult	Increased Incidence of Mental Retardation	Minimum Dose for Recognized Gross Anatomic Malformation (rad)	Minimum Dose for Induction of Genetic, Carcinogenic, and Minimal Cell Depletion Phenomena (rad)
1–5	10	<100	No effect in survivors			Unknown
18–28	25–50	140	20–50	20–50 Severe CNS anatomic malformations more likely than mental retardation	20	Unknown
36–50	50	200	25–50	50*	50	Unknown
50–150	>50	>100	25–50	50*	—†	Unknown
To term	>100	Same as mother	>50	100	—	Unknown

*Recent information to be published by Otake and Schull[2a] suggest an increased risk at lower exposures.
†Anatomic malformations of a severe type cannot be produced this late in gestation except in the genitourinary system and tissue hypoplasia in specific organ systems, such as the brain and testes.

TABLE 18–9.
Estimate of Risks of 1-Rad Exposure (Low LET) to the Developing Human Embryo

Age (Days)	Mutagenic Effect[*][†][‡]	Childhood Carcinogenic Effect (Stewart et al.[§])	Maximum Childhood Carcinogenic Effect (ABCC)[¶][†]	Gross Congenital Malformations, Death, Growth Retardation	Permanent Cell Depletion
1	No data	No data	No data	?[‖]	No Effect
18–28	10^{-7} per locus	3.2×10^{-4}	5×10^{-6} 5×10^{-6}	Same as controls	?
50		3.2×10^{-4}	5×10^{-6}		
Late fetus to term		3.2×10^{-4}	5×10^{-6}		

LET = linear energy transfer; ABCC = Atomic Bomb Casualty Commission.
*Based on an estimated doubling dose for mutagenesis of 100 rad, assuming a linear dose-response curve and no threshold for mutagenic effects.
†The mutagenic effects have not been studied in the preimplantation period; the surviving embryos are not reduced in size even when the dose is very high, although at this stage the embryo is very sensitive to the lethal effects of radiation.
‡The estimate is assumed to be adult risk because there was no increased carcinogenic effect in the population of exposed fetuses in Hiroshima and Nagasaki.
§The data of Stewart et al. would indicate that the embryo is more sensitive to the carcinogenic effect of radiation than the adult. This is a controversial matter, and others[7, 8, 62–64] feel that this association may be other than a radiation effect.
¶Atomic Bomb Casualty Commission data on carcinogenesis do not indicate that the embryo and fetus are at increased risk. The risk presented is the same carcinogenic risk attributed to adults, assuming maximal effect at low doses, namely, a linear dose-response curve, and no threshold for carcinogenic effects.[79, 80, 81, 87]
‖Radiation-induced embryonic death might possibly be a stochastic effect in the first few days of gestation, although the present data involving hundreds of embryos indicate no effect at 5 to 10 rad.

in later publications they have concluded that other cancers also occur more frequently in persons exposed in utero to diagnostic radiologic procedures (primarily pelvimetry). The present estimate is that a 1- to 2-rad, in utero radiation exposure increases the chance of leukemia developing in the offspring by a factor of 1.5 to 2.0 over the natural incidence. This incidence is considerably greater than the increase resulting from 2 rad delivered to an adult. In fact, a 2-rad dose delivered to an adult population would not make a perceptible change in the incidence of leukemia even for very large population groups.[70, 71] Lilienfeld[72] reviewed the epidemiologic considerations with respect to leukemogenesis. The results of Lilienfeld,[72] McMahon and Hutchinson,[73] Graham et al.,[74] Polhemus and Koch,[75] Yamazaki et al.,[39] Ager et al.,[76] and Ford and Patterson[77] support the thesis that diagnostic radiation absorbed in utero is associated with increases in risk of leukemia. Six of nine studies reported in Lilienfeld's paper indicate an increase in leukemia risk of 1.3- to 1.8-fold following diagnostic radiation exposure in utero. Lilienfeld states: "When one considers the variety of control groups used and the sampling variability, the results

are remarkably consistent in showing an excess frequency of leukemia among children of radiation-exposed pregnant mothers."[72] Diamond et al.[62] have extended the studies of Lilienfeld and have corroborated their early finding of a higher incidence of leukemia (threefold) in children exposed to diagnostic radiation in utero. They also report that this effect did not occur in the black population.

There are a number of interesting associations in these data that should be pointed out. In the studies of Stewart and colleagues[68, 69] there was a higher incidence of previous abortion in the mothers receiving pelvimetry, and also the children in the pelvimetry group had a higher incidence of upper respiratory infections prior to the development of leukemia. Others have reported that infants from families with a strong family history of allergy are also more susceptible to radiation-induced leukemia when exposed to diagnostic radiation in utero.[78] The problem with these data is that in some instances patients with an allergic history and no preconception radiation had a higher frequency of leukemia than did some groups that had received irradiation in utero. Tabuchi[45] reported no increase in leukemia following diagnostic radiologic procedures. In some of the studies that did not report an increased risk of leukemia, the number of patients was small. Of the 86 persons exposed in utero at Nagasaki, none developed leukemia.[79] These persons received considerably higher doses of radiation than did those patients in the previous studies. Kato[80] studied 1,300 people, some of whom were exposed to the atomic bomb while in utero, and observed no increased evidence of malignancy in the first 24 years of follow-up, although there was an increased mortality in the first year of life and after 10 years of age.

It is of interest that Graham et al.[74] reported an increased risk of leukemia that was identical whether a mother had received radiation from diagnostic procedures shortly before or after conception. Hoshino et al.[81] reported no increase in leukemia in a study of 17,000 children of parents who had received radiation before conception. The question arises as to what extent the same biases that contribute to the increased risk of leukemia in the cases of radiation exposure before conception also affect the in utero radiation cases. Graham et al.[74] pointed out that children of mothers with a history of abortion or stillbirth also had children with a higher risk of leukemia. Neutel and Buck[82] found that childhood malignancy occurred more often in offspring of mothers who smoked. Fasal et al.[83] reported that infants who were heavier at birth were more likely to get leukemia. It appears that whenever one looks for the association of an event with the occurrence of leukemia, it can be readily found.

At present, it is not clear whether radiation exposure during the preconception or postconception cases is a causative or associative factor in the increased incidence of leukemia. Miller[64] and others[9, 63, 84] dissent from the conclusions of Stewart and colleagues and all the reports that support their hypothesis. Miller writes:

> Minimal doses of x-ray are equally oncogenic whether exposure occurred before conception or during pregnancy, whether the neoplasm studied was leukemia or any other

major cancer of childhood, and whether the study was based on interviews which may be biased, or on hospital records. Taken in aggregate, the similarity of results, in the absence of a dose-response effect or of supporting data from animal experimentation, raises a question about biologic plausibility of a causal relationship.[64]

Furthermore, Miller points out that siblings of leukemic children have an incidence of leukemia of 1 in 720 per 10 years, which is greater than the 1:2,000 risk of leukemia following pelvimetry exposure and the 1:3,000 probability of leukemia in the general population of children followed for 10 years (see Table 18–6). Stewart and Kneale's[67] publication on this subject reinforces the contention that radiation may not be the etiologic factor responsible for the induction of malignancy because the unirradiated siblings of the irradiated patient population with a higher incidence of leukemia also had a higher incidence of malignancy. The incidence was greater than in control siblings and in control patients. This observation certainly would indicate that genetic or other environmental factors may be of more importance in the production of leukemia than is prenatal diagnostic radiation.

Rugh et al.[85] irradiated mice with 100 rad on each day of gestation and observed the incidence of tumors in the offspring. There was no statistical increase in the incidence of tumors in adult animals from irradiation in utero on any day. Brent and Bolden[20, 86] exposed pregnant mice to doses of 30, 60, and 90 rad after $1/2$, $7^1/_2$, $8^1/_2$, $12^1/_2$, and $16^1/_2$ days of gestation. They also did not observe an increase in the incidence of tumors.

At present, a number of investigators believe that in utero exposure to small amounts of radiation increases the risk of leukemia and other malignancies, whereas other investigators seriously question that the embryo is markedly more sensitive to the leukemogenic effects of irradiation when compared to the child or adult. Until the mechanism is understood, there always will be doubt concerning the magnitude of the role of in utero radiation in leukemia induction. The increased incidence of cancer in children exposed in utero to diagnostic radiation has to be clarified in view of the fact that much higher doses of radiation to animal embryos and to the children exposed in utero at Hiroshima and Nagasaki have not resulted in a marked increase in the incidence of cancers from high doses of radiation, which one would expect if the embryo were as sensitive to the carcinogenic effects of radiation as Stewart and colleagues suggest.[35, 36, 80] One cannot overemphasize either the importance of the multiplicity of factors involved or the difficulties in their identification and control. Even laboratory experiments concerned with tumor production are difficult to interpret. For example, Ross and Bras[88] reported that the incidence of spontaneous tumors varied with the diet and weight of the animals. Heavier animals on high-protein diets had a higher incidence of tumors than did the lighter rats on low-protein diets. Hence, there are many unanswered questions concerning the relationship between leukemia and malignancy and in utero radiation exposure.

Recently published results of the occurrence of cancer in adults who were irradiated in utero in Hiroshima and Nagasaki indicate that there is an increase in the incidence of cancer in the exposed population and that the cancers occur earlier than usual during adult life. Thus, the long-term study in Hiroshima and Nagasaki does not support the increased incidence in childhood malignancies suggested by Stewart and colleagues and the incidence of cancer in the adults does not support the markedly increased sensitivity of the fetus to radiation-induced cancer as suggested by those authors. There is little disagreement with the concept that low doses of radiation present a carcinogenic risk to the embryo and adult, and that there may be different risks per rad at different stages of development. The concept that is difficult to explain from a basic science viewpoint is, why would a proliferating embryonic cell be several orders of magnitude more sensitive to the carcinogenic effect

of radiation than a proliferating child's or adult's cell.

Although it is our opinion that a dose of less than 10 rad to the implanted embryo does not result in a significant increase in the incidence of congenital malformations, growth retardation, or fetal death, low-risk tumorigenic or genetic hazards cannot be ruled out. Even if one believed that the tumorigenic (leukemogenic) effects of low-level radiation were real, let us examine how difficult it would be to use this information in counseling a patient who has received a dose of perhaps 2 rad during her pregnancy. According to Stewart and colleagues, the risk of leukemia following this exposure in utero is 1:2,000 versus 1:3,000 in unexposed controls over a 10-year period (see Table 18–6). If one were inclined to recommend therapeutic abortion for this embryo because the probability of developing leukemia is 50% greater than controls, one would perform abortions in 1,999 exposed nonleukemic subjects for every leukemic subject "saved." It is one thing to avoid radiation because of a potential or conjectured hazard, but it is another matter to recommend therapeutic abortion on this basis. If a physician were inclined to accept this increased probability (1:2,000) as a risk great enough to recommend therapeutic abortion, he or she would be placed in a serious dilemma because there are other epidemiologic situations in which the risk of leukemia is greater. In fact, the hypothetic incremental risk for 2 rad of in utero radiation is 1:6,000 over a 10-year period. It is the combination of the control risk plus the incremental radiation risk that results in a 1:2,000 risk for these patients. If one examines Table 18–6, it is obvious that the risk of leukemia is greater in "unirradiated" siblings of leukemics (1:720) than in patients subjected to diagnostic radiation (1:2,000), according to the data of Stewart and colleagues.

Certainly, the position that all future pregnancies of parents with one leukemic child should be aborted would be untenable. One can carry this argument to its ridiculous ex-

TABLE 18–10.
Risk of 0.5 rem (Maximum Permissible Exposure for Women Radiation Workers With Reproductive Potential)

	0 rem	Additional Risk of 0.5 rem
Risk of spontaneous abortion	150,000/10^6	0
Risk of major congenital malformations	30,000/10^6	0
Risk of severe mental retardation	5,000/10^6	0
Risk of childhood malignancy/10-yr period	7,000/10^6/10 yr	166/10^6/10 yr[67–69]
		or
		2.5/10^6/10 yr (ABCC data)
Risk of early- or late-onset genetic disease	100,000/10^6	Risk in next generation is negligible
Total risk (using Stewart data[67–69])	285,700/10^6	166/10^6 [67–69]
Ratio of total risk to additional risk of radiation		1721/1
Total risk (using ABCC)	285,700/10^6	2.5/10^6 (ABCC)
Ratio of total additional risk of radiation		114,280/1

ABCC = Atomic Bomb Casualty Commission.

treme by advocating that all pregnancies should be aborted because the risk of malformation is approximately 40 to 60 per 1,000 deliveries, and this does not include the probability of postnatal diseases occurring in these offspring. Some may interpret this as a facetious discussion, but the clinician and the patient must recognize that "spontaneous" risks of pregnancy are two orders of magnitude greater than the theoretical risks of diagnostic radiation (Table 18–10).

Counseling the Pregnant Woman Exposed to Radiation: Estimating the Risks

It is appropriate to utilize the results of radiation studies in pregnant animals as part of the data on which you estimate the reproductive risks of embryonic radiation.

Radiation effects in various mammalian embryos are more similar than the effects of most other teratogens or embryopathic agents because radiation has a direct effect on the developing embryo.[10, 16, 63, 86–88] Variations in placental transport and maternal metabolism do not alter significantly the extrapolation of results of radiation experiments with pregnant mammals to humans as do those of experiments using any teratogen.

Table 18–7 lists the effects of low exposures to developing mammalian embryos. The

data indicate that continuous exposures below 2,000 mrad/day to pregnant animals have no effect on numerous parameters such as fertility, growth, mortality, or the incidence of congenital malformations.

The biologic effects of embryonic radiation are summarized for exposures of 10 rad in Table 18–2 and 100 rad in Table 18–3 for various species and different stages of gestation. Table 18–8 lists the estimated median lethal dose (LD_{50}), the minimal malforming dose, the minimal lethal dose, the minimal dose producing growth retardation, and other parameters for the human embryo, based on extrapolations from animal data.

The hazards of exposures in the range of diagnostic roentgenology (20–5,000 mrad) present an extremely low risk to the embryo, when compared with spontaneous mishaps that can befall humans (see Tables 18–8 and 18–10). Approximately 30% to 50% of human embryos abort spontaneously. Many patients abort before pregnancy is diagnosed or recognized. Human infants have a 2.75% major malformation rate at term, which rises to approximately 6% to 10% once all malformations and genetic diseases become manifest. In spite of the fact that doses of 1 to 3 rad can produce cellular effects and the fact that diagnostic exposure during pregnancy has been associated with malignancy in childhood, the maximum theoretical risk to the human embryos exposed to doses of 5 rad or less is extremely small (see Tables 18–9 and 18–10). In my experience, when the data and risks are explained to the patient, the family with a wanted pregnancy invariably continues with the pregnancy. The difficulty that frequently arises is that the radiation risk from diagnostic radiation is often evaluated without consideration of the significant normal risks of pregnancy, and the physician giving advice may be very concerned about radiation effects, especially if he or she has a poor background in radiation biology.[6] We have records in our files of patients advised to terminate pregnancy despite the fact that exposure was well below 5 rad, and/or the fact that exposure took place prior to conception. Such problems can be avoided if physicians try to become more familiar with radiation biology, or if they consult with the appropriate specialist when questions arise.

The physician will never be able to guarantee the outcome of a pregnancy, but the basic logic of the practice of medicine would be undermined if some of its practitioners recommended therapeutic abortion for risks with probabilities of occurrence far below the expected spontaneous incidence in the embryo and infant. When counseling parents concerning the risks to the embryo of a particular exposure to radiation, the biologic knowledge is only one facet to be considered. The risk of radiation damage is based on the estimated dose and the stage of gestation.

The parental interpretation of this risk depends on the age of the parents, the number of children in the family, the religious and ethnic background of the family, and the options available to the family based on the state laws regarding therapeutic interruptions of pregnancy. There is also important information to be gathered, more difficult to acquire, on the emotional maturity of the family and whether the pregnancy was planned or unplanned. The following information should be obtained:

- Stage of pregnancy of the exposure

- Menstrual history
- Previous pregnancy history
- History of congenital malformations
- Other potential harmful environmental factors during the pregnancy
- Age of the mother and father
- Type of radiation study; dates and number of studies performed
- Calculation of the embryonic exposure by a medical physicist or competent radiologist (Table 18–11)
- Status of the pregnancy: wanted or unwanted

An evaluation should be made of this information, with both patient and counselor arriving at a decision. The physician should place in the medical record a summary of this information, that the patient has been informed, that every pregnancy has a significant risk of problems, and that the decision to continue the pregnancy does not mean that the counselor is guaranteeing the outcome of the pregnancy.

Diagnostic Radiation Exposures

Our experience has taught us that there are many variables involved in the evaluation

TABLE 18–11.
Estimated Embryonic and Fetal Dose During Diagnostic Radiological Examinations*

Examination	Dose (mrad)[†]
Upper extremity	1
Lower extremity	1
Skull film	4
Chest	
Radiography	8
Fluoroscopy	70
Cholecystography	200
Abdomen	290
Intravenous pyelography	400
Upper gastrointestinal series	560
Barium enema	800

*Modified from Brent RL: Irradiation in pregnancy, in Sciarra JJ (ed): *Davis' Gynecology and Obstetrics,* vol 2. New York, Harper & Row, 1972, pp 1–32.
[†]These are estimated means, but reported ranges vary substantially and may change with progressing gestation. Thus each case should be assessed individually and consultation with a radiologist or radiation physicist is advisable when decisions have to be made.

of a radiation exposure to a pregnant or potentially pregnant woman. Therefore, it is impossible to provide the same routine response for every patient. The following examples are some typical cases of radiation exposure in which evaluation and counseling were provided.

A 19-year old unmarried secretary went to her physician because of abdominal pain. She told him her menstrual periods were regular and the pain was periumbilical and persistent. An upper gastrointestinal series was performed but was unsatisfactory because the young girl had eaten breakfast before the study. When the second study was performed, she mentioned that she was 2 weeks past her scheduled menstrual period and that she could be pregnant. The father of the child was married. The radiation therapist at the hospital recommended a therapeutic abortion because of radiation hazards to the embryo. The estimated dose to the embryo over a period of 3 days was 1.6 rad.

Our laboratory was called and informed of the case history and recommendation. Our conclusion was that this dose of radiation would not result in embryonic malformation, growth retardation, or death, and that the nonexistent radiation hazard should not be used to obtain a therapeutic abortion for "social" reasons. The laws of that state, at that time, did not permit therapeutic abortions; so the girl flew to another state, where the therapeutic abortion was performed.

Case histories similar to this are transmitted to our laboratory frequently. In most instances, the dose to the embryo is less than 5 rad (0.05 Gy) and frequently less than 1 rad (0.01 Gy). Unfortunately, variations in the approach of the physician in charge depend on many factors: (1) whether the pregnant woman is married, (2) whether the pregnancy was planned, (3) the mental status of the mother and/or father, and (4) the abortion laws of the state, rather than the knowledge of the physician regarding radiation hazards to the embryo.

We believe the specter of radiation hazards should not be invoked to circumvent a social or legal problem. If the abortion laws are archaic or unfair, physicians should work together to change them. They should not create an implied serious radiation hazard that is not justified by the facts to solve social, psychologic, or legal problems.

A 29-year-old housewife (gravida 1, para 0, abortus 0) presented in her sixth month of pregnancy with the history that she had been to her dentist the week before and had one radiograph of her left upper first molar. She was anxious and very worried about the effect of radiation on her baby. She was reassured, but called back six times asking new questions. The estimated dose to the embryo was below 1 mrem (10 nGy). She continued to be anxious and hyperactive. She delivered a 3,100-g baby boy with minimal syndactyly of the fourth and fifth fingers of the left hand, who was otherwise normal. A legal suit was almost instituted in this case.

A surprising number of cases are evaluated or brought to trial in which the only radiation exposure of the mother was to the head, the neck, or the chest, and yet there is both clinical and basic science information that indicates that embryopathologic conditions are only a consequence of direct embryonic exposure. High doses of radiation to the mother, while shielding the embryo, result in offspring who have the same incidence of congenital malformation as do control embryos.[89–92]

There were many instances in the past in which a radiologist recommended a therapeutic abortion for a patient whose embryo received a fractionated dose of 0 to 5 rad during the first trimester of pregnancy, because of the possibility that the embryo might be malformed. Frequently, this recommendation was made for unmarried women, primarily to assist them in eliminating unwanted pregnancies. It is this type of recommendation that will reap retribution when that same radiologist attempts to defend himself or herself against the contention that a series of diagnostic radiologic examinations caused a particular malformation.

Exposure From Radiation Therapy

There is ample evidence to indicate that radiation therapy in the region of the abdomen can result in doses of radiation that will affect the fetus deleteriously. In such a case, it is important to consult with either the radiotherapist or a qualified medical physicist to determine the total dose delivered to the embryo. If the fetus absorbs 50 rad (0.5 Gy) or more at any time during gestation, there is a significant possibility that the fetus may be damaged. Of course, there are instances in which human fetuses have survived greater doses[33, 93] and appeared normal, but at this dose the probability of CNS damage or other malformations is real, and the parents should be so informed. If the dose absorbed by the embryo during the early organogenetic period amounts to several hundred rads, there is reasonable possibility that the embryo may abort. As one proceeds into the second and third trimesters, the chance of abortion and malformation declines, but irreparable damage to the CNS can occur. The risk of 100-rad (1 Gy) acute radiation from the 8th to 15th weeks of gestation presents a substantial risk for mental retardation to the surviving fetus.[34, 39, 64, 71]

When the radiation therapist fails to investigate the possibility of pregnancy or fails to record all the information regarding the pregnancy and the steps taken in arriving at a decision, the therapist places himself or herself in double jeopardy. He or she may be accused of poor medical practice in a suit over a malformed infant and thereby may be more likely to lose the case even when the radiation could not have been responsible for the abnormal embryonic development.[94] Let us examine some representative cases.

A 31-year-old woman was in her sixth month of pregnancy when her physician noted an enlarged lymph node in the anterior cervical region. A diagnosis of Hodgkin's disease was made, and she received approximately 3,200 rad to the anterior cervical region and adjacent areas over a period of 4 weeks. The fetus was viable at the time of the diagnosis, and the family wanted the baby. The dose of radiation to the fetus was approximately 25 rad (0.25 Gy). The mother delivered a full-term baby who appeared to be normal.

In this case, the counselor told the family that he could not say that the fetus was not at increased risk. The mother's question was somewhat different: namely, was it very likely that the fetus would be severely affected? Of course the answer was that while the risks were increased there was a greater chance that the embryo would not be seriously affected at this stage of gestation. Since the family was not certain of the mother's prognosis and, therefore, whether future children were a possibility, they elected to go through with the pregnancy.

A 36-year-old woman (gravida 6, para 4, abortus 1) was 1 week past her menstrual period, which usually was regular. Examination revealed a moderate-sized lesion of the cervix. The pregnancy test was positive. A biopsy of the cervix revealed a carcinoma of the cervix that had invaded the muscle layer. Dilatation and curettage was performed, and the patient was treated with the instillation of radium.

In this case, the options were presented to the family before the biopsy, and the above-mentioned course was taken.

The Use of Diagnostic or Therapeutic Radiation in Women of Reproductive Age When the Ovaries or Uterus Will Be Exposed

In a woman of reproductive age, it is important for the patient and physician to be aware of the pregnancy status of the patient before any type of abdominal x-ray exposure is planned. If the embryonic exposure will be 5 rad (0.05 Gy) or less, the radiation risks to the embryo are minuscule when compared with the spontaneous risks. The patient will accept the information if it is offered as part of the preparation for the x-ray studies at a time when both the physician and patient are aware that a pregnancy exists.

The pregnancy status of the patient can be determined by several means: (1) The x-ray referral slip can request the date of the last menstrual period (LMP) and the previous menstrual period (PMP) and whether the patient possibly could be pregnant; (2) if the patient is uncertain about her pregnancy status, a pregnancy test should be performed; (3) pregnancy tests could be performed on all hospital admissions of women of reproductive age.

Because the risks of 5-rad (0.05 Gy) fetal irradiation are so small, the immediate medical care of the mother should take priority over the risks of diagnostic radiation exposure of the embryo. X-ray studies that are essential for optimal medical care of the mother and evaluation of medical problems that need to be diagnosed or treated should not be postponed (see Table 18–11). Elective procedures such as employment examinations or follow-up examinations, once a diagnosis has been made, need not be performed on a pregnant woman even though the risk to the embryo is very small. If other procedures (e.g., ultrasound) can provide adequate information without exposing the embryo to ionizing radiation, then of course they should be used. There is an initial period when a pregnancy test may be negative and the patient can still be pregnant. Furthermore, the menstrual history will be of little use in this circumstance, but the risks of 5 rad or less of radiation are extremely small during this period of gestation. The patient will benefit from knowing that the diagnostic study was indicated and should be performed in spite of the fact that she may be pregnant.

In those instances in which elective x-ray studies need to be scheduled, it is difficult to know whether to schedule them during the first half of the menstrual cycle before ovulation or during the second half of the menstrual cycle, when most women will not be pregnant. The risk of diagnostic exposures to the oocyte or the preimplanted embryo is extremely small, and there are meager data with which to compare the relative risk of 5 rad to the oocyte or the preimplanted embryo.[4, 9, 86] If the diagnostic study is performed in the first 14 days of the menstrual cycle, should the patient be advised to defer conception for

several months, based on the assumption that the deleterious effect of radiation to the ovaries decreases with increasing time between radiation exposure and a subsequent ovulation? The physician is in a quandary because he or she is warning the patient about a very-low-risk phenomenon. On the other hand, avoiding conception for several months is not an insurmountable hardship. This potential hazard is quite speculative for man, as indicated by the report of the National Council on Radiation Protection (NCRP) dealing with preconception radiation:

> It is not known whether the interval between irradiation of the gonads and conception has a marked effect on the frequency of congenital changes in human offspring, as has been demonstrated in the female mouse. Nevertheless, it may be advisable for patients receiving high doses to the gonads (>25 rad) to wait for several months after such exposures before conceiving additional offspring.[95]

During diagnostic radiologic procedures the patients absorb considerably less than 25 rad; therefore the recommendation made here may be unnecessary, but it involves no hardship to the patient or physician. Because both the NCRP and International Council on Radiation Protection have previously recommended that elective radiologic examinations of the abdomen and pelvis be performed during the first part of the menstrual cycle to protect the zygote from possible but largely conjectural hazards, a recommendation to reduce another possible hazard by avoiding fertilization of recently irradiated ova perhaps should merit equal attention.

If a women is exposed to more than 5 rad of radiation and then is found to be pregnant, a determination of the merits of continuing the pregnancy must be made by the physician, the patient, and an expert in radiation. A decision to terminate the pregnancy will depend on (1) the nonradiation-related hazard of the pregnancy to the expectant mother, (2) the extent and type of radiation hazard to the embryo or fetus, (3) the ethnic and religious background of the family, (4) the laws of the state pertaining to legal abortion, and (5) any other relevant consideration.

If exposures of less than 5 rad to the pelvis do not measurably affect the exposed embryos, and others[9] recommend performing diagnostic procedures at any time of the menstrual cycle for the medical care of the patient, why is there so much effort and energy in determining the pregnancy status of the patient? There are several reasons why the physician should have the burden of determining the pregnancy status before an x-ray or nuclear medicine procedure is performed. First, if the physician is forced to include the possibility of pregnancy in the differential diagnosis, a small percentage of diagnostic studies may no longer be considered necessary. Early symptoms of pregnancy may mimic certain types of gastrointestinal or genitourinary disease. Second if the physician and patient are both aware that pregnancy is a possibility and the procedure is still performed, it is much less likely that the patient will be upset if she subsequently proves to be pregnant. Third, the careful evaluation of the reproductive status of women undergoing diagnostic procedures will prevent many unnecessary lawsuits. Many lawsuits are stimulated by the factor of surprise and won on the basis of the double jeopardy of the defendant.[96] In some instances the jury is not concerned with cause and effect but with the fact that something was not done properly by the physician. In this day and age, failure to communicate adequately can be interpreted as less-than-adequate medical care. Both these factors are eliminated if the patient's pregnancy status has been evaluated properly and the situation discussed adequately with the patient. Physicians are going to have to learn that practicing good technical medicine may not be enough in a litigation-prone society. Even more important, the patient will have more confidence if the decision to continue the pregnancy is made before the medical x-ray procedure is performed, because the necessity of the procedure would have been determined with the knowledge that the patient may be pregnant.

MICROWAVE AND ULTRASOUND

The physical and biologic characteristics of microwave and ultrasound energy are summarized in Table 18–1. These two forms of energy have characteristics much different from x-ray and gamma rays because they do not produce ionization.[1, 7]

Maximum permissible levels for occupational and medical exposure have been suggested for both these forms of energy. Persons working near FM radio stations, radar, and microwave ovens are not exposed to the maximum permissible level. A microwave oven generates 2,450-MHz microwaves. This wavelength can produce hyperthermia above the 24 mW level with a penetration of several centimeters. There is no way to receive exposure from a microwave oven without bypassing several safety interlocks, and it is very easy to shield microwaves; a proper screen or thin metal foil is 100% effective in shielding all radiation.

Theoretically, if a microwave oven had a door leak, one could expose herself by placing a part of her body in direct contact with the area. In this way, it is conceivable that after several hours one might receive a measurable exposure. On the other hand, the flux of electromagnetic waves is diminished in relation to the square root of the distance of the object from the source. It is obvious that a leaking microwave oven would have no consequences several meters away unless it interfered with some electronic device that was sensitive to that wavelength of electromagnetic radiation.

Radar, microwaves, radiowaves, FM, and diathermy all involve electromagnetic waves ranging in frequency from 27.5 MHz (diathermy, 26,500 vibrations per second) to 10^4 to 10^5 MHz (microwave communications). Diathermy electromagnetic waves have great penetration and can readily heat a human torso. Microwaves of 2,450 MHz or 915 MHz have less penetration but also can produce significant hyperthermia. Microwaves with frequencies above 10,000 MHz have less organ penetration but could produce significant hyperthermia at the skin level if the energy were high enough.

Although a nonthermal effect has not been clearly demonstrated for these forms of electromagnetic irradiation, the matter of nonthermal effects still is being investigated. The organs most vulnerable to the thermal effects of microwave radiation are the eye and developing embryo because these structures have the least capacity to dissipate heat. There is no indication that these forms of electromagnetic energy have the capacity to produce mutations or malignancy; therefore, the clinician can reassure patients that microwave ovens properly handled are reasonably safe.

The use of diagnostic ultrasound has increased dramatically in the past 10 years. Although there are still ongoing studies dealing with the effects of ultrasound, this form of energy appears to be relatively safe.[7, 8, 97] Because ultrasound does not produce tissue ionization, the use of diagnostic ultrasound should reduce the necessity for many x-ray procedures.

The use of ultrasound for fetal monitoring and fetal diagnosis is rapidly expanding. Epidemiologic studies have so far indicated that diagnostic ultrasound does not have any measurable or significant biologic effects. Of course, studies on the biologic effects of ultrasound are continuing. Furthermore, epidemiologic studies of infants who are exposed in utero are continuing. There are some data on the biologic effects of ultrasound involving DNA repair, cytogenetic alterations, and teratogenesis. At the present time, the results would indicate that low exposure to ultrasound presents either minimal risks or none at all to the developing embryo and the benefits far outweigh the risks.

MAGNETIC RESONANCE IMAGING

There has been a dramatic revolution in diagnostic imaging in the past two decades with the introduction of computed tomography, (CT scans), ultrasonography, and magnetic resonance imaging (MRI). The last two use energy forms that do not result in tissue ionization and therefore have a much lower risk of producing mutagenesis and carcinogenesis. Furthermore, these last two procedures have replaced many routine diagnostic radiographic procedures. While there is a general consensus that ultrasound and MRI present "less of a risk" at diagnostic exposure levels than diagnostic radiographic procedures, much less is known about the reproductive effects of these newer modalities.

Any physical or chemical agent can become a significant risk if the quantitative exposure is high enough. Literally, there is no chemical, drug, or physical agent that is safe at any dose.

We will examine the available experimental and clinical data pertaining to MRI. These techniques have gained rapid acceptance and for some diagnostic studies, have become the procedure of choice. The exposure fields of MRI techniques consist of several forms:

1. Powerful static magnetic fields.
2. RF (radiofrequency) fields.
3. Varying magnetic fields.

Thus MRI exposes the embryo to a complex set of electromagnetic fields.

1. What are the reproductive risks of exposing embryos to these fields?
2. How does the sensitivity of the embryo vary with the embryonic or fetal stage?
3. Do we have enough information to perform a rational risk-benefit analysis?

Although it would appear that in 1987 there was meager information on the biologic effects, a National Institutes of Health (NIH) Consensus Development Conference recommended that women in their *first trimester* of pregnancy should avoid MRI procedures unless the clinical condition could not be managed utilizing other diagnostic techniques.[98] The shortsightedness of this decision relates to the fact that the developing CNS is still sensitive to embryotoxic agents in the *second trimester* and at that time the fetal CNS has poor repairability.

MRI procedures, as mentioned previously, utilize three forms of electromagnetic fields: static magnetic fields, pulsed magnetic fields that vary, and signal-producing RF radiations. The patient is placed in a powerful magnetic field. Unlike the CT scan or diagnostic radiography the embryo cannot be readily shielded or avoided. Thus, most procedures involving examination of the torso will expose the embryo in a pregnant woman.

The image is produced by placing the patient in the very strong static magnetic field, which aligns the hydrogen nuclei of water and other charged nuclei with the magnetic field to produce a net magnetic moment. The subject is then exposed to RF energy, which is absorbed by certain protons in the patient depending on the magnetic field in particular areas and the RF frequency. When the RF frequency is turned off the protons that were excited return to their ground state by radiating their absorbed RF energies which are collated and reconstructed into an interpretable image.[99]

In evaluating the reproductive effects of this procedure, one has to be concerned that varying effects may occur at different RF frequencies (3.5–100 MHz) and various magnetic field strengths (0.08–2.0 tesla [T]).[100, 101]

The purpose of this chapter is not to discuss the entire field of the bioeffects of MRI but to concentrate on its reproductive risks. Obviously, some effects observed in adults may be important for the embryo and fetus, but such things as electrocardiographic abnormalities,[102] visual light flashes,[103] and magnetic field disturbances that affect orientation[104, 105] are probably of minimal concern. Other reported effects could effect embryonic development depending on the magnitude of the effect—such as hyperthermia, loss of ionized calcium from nerve membranes, altered permeability of endothelial cells, altered blood-brain barrier, and interference with nerve conduction. While these effects may not be deleterious to children or adults they may effect embryonic development.

Reproductive Effects in Experimental Animals

A number of investigators have exposed chick embryos to electromagnetic fields with variable results. Significant harmful effects were observed in chick embryos with electromagnetic fields with pulse durations of 0.5 ms and pulse repetition rates of 10 to 1000 Hz.[106–109] But in other instances there was no difference between the sham-irradiated eggs and those exposed to the magnetic fields.[110, 111] In other experiments with the chick embryo both positive and negative findings were reported with regard to embryotoxicity depending on the embryonic stage when the embryos were exposed to the pulsed electromagnetic fields, the earliest stages being the most sensitive.

Juutilainen and Liimatainen[112] exposed salmonella to electromagnetic fields that were dosimetrically compared to experiments which produced malformations in chick embryos and were unable to demonstrate any mutagenic effect.

Very frequently the chick embryo is sensitive to a teratogenic milieu to which the mammalian embryo is resistant. This is particularly true of agents that produce hyperthermia, as an example, because of the marked differences in temperature control and heat dissipation between the chick and mammal. Not surprisingly, the mammalian embryo has also been reported to be sensitive or resistant to the effects of the physical environment created by MRI techniques. Ozil and Modlinski[113] exposed two cell rabbit embryos to electric fields which resulted in normal surviving embryos, but this is a stage which is more susceptible to the lethal effects of environmental agents rather than the teratogenic effects. Stuchly et al.[114] exposed pregnant rats to alternating magnetic fields with a sawtooth waveform similar to that produced by video display terminals for 7 hr/day. The magnetic field intensities were 5.7, 23, or

66 μT. Although there was a slight drop in the maternal lymphocyte count there were no reproductive effects. Sikov et al.[115] found no increase in the malformation rate in mice exposed to field strengths of 0.1 to 1.0 T. A gradient magnetic field of 2.7 T/min with a 1.0-T uniform static field resulted in no increase in malformations in the products of exposed animals. Sikov and coworkers[116] exposed miniature swine and rats to chronic exposures of 60-Hz electric fields. The pregnant swine were exposed 20 hr/day in 30-kV/m electric fields. Although there was some increase in the malformation rates in the exposed groups the results were inconsistent and equivocal. The pregnant rats were exposed 19 hr/day to 100-kV/m unperturbed electric fields. The fertility rate of the exposed female rats was decreased and the malformation rate was increased in one experimental group but not in another.

Microwave radiation, which also consists of electric fields and electromagnetic waves in the RF range, can produce hyperthermia, which is the key explanation for its reproductive toxic and teratogenic effects.[117] It appears that frequencies in the "old" diathermy range have the greatest potential for producing hyperthermia and reproductive toxic effects.[118]

It is really not the purpose here, for several reasons, to analyze the effects of microwave radiation or the hazards of video terminals. Since the MRI RF energies do not produce increases in temperature, the studies dealing with microwaves may have little meaning in predicting the risks of MRI to the fetus. MRI devices have a limited power deposition rate and it is estimated that the temperature of an exposed uterus will not rise more than 0.2°C, which would have no biologic effect on the developing embryo or fetus. Video terminal studies are even less relevant to the study of MRI risks because the magnitude of the electromagnetic field strength is so much smaller. Thus negative results in exposed pregnant women to video display terminals could only represent that low exposures to magnetic fields are not reproductively toxic.

At this stage of our knowledge we have meager information concerning the reproductive risks of MRI to the pregnant woman and her offspring.[98, 119, 120] Heinricks, et al.[119, 121] exposed pregnant mice during early organogenesis to 0.35-T static fields, an RF of 15 MHz, and the associated gradient magnetic field. While there were no induced skeletal anomalies, the primary focus of the project, significant reduction in length, was reported after 16 hours of exposure at higher field strengths (2.3 T; RF 100 MHz). Studies which attempted to separate magnetic field effects from RF radiation suggest that the combination is more effective, but this is only a preliminary finding.[119] Lengthy exposures over hours or days have little relevance to the usual utilization of MRI techniques in humans.

Studies involving pregnant goats reported no teratogenic effects.[120, 122] These studies were performed during midgestation and therefore would be unlikely to produce malformations, but could have been used to evaluate the effects on the fetal brain.

Clinical Application of the Biologic Effect Data

Obviously the clinician faces a dilemma, in that the risks of MRI have not been completely evaluated. The NIH has suggested a conservative approach to utilization of MRI.[119] This places the physician in an untenable position and may inhibit appropriate utilization of these techniques. On the other hand there are reports of MRI use during known pregnancies for the evaluation of the status of congenital malformations.[123] There really are not enough data for the clinician to be able to do a risk-benefit analysis.

The more difficult scenario will occur when both the patient and physician are surprised following an MRI to find out that the patient was pregnant. In the case of ionizing radiation we have vast amounts of quantitative animal and human data on which to estimate the risk. Furthermore, we usually can estimate the embryonic exposure in roentgen equivalents (rem) or grays (Gy).

With MRI exposure we have minimal and controversial animal data following long exposures and minimal ability to estimate exposure except within broad ranges. The minimal data available would indicate the following:

1. We need more and better animal data.
2. We need to be cautious in the use of MRI during pregnancy.
3. With an inadvertent exposure in a *wanted* pregnancy the present accumulated data would not warrant an interruption of pregnancy, although more careful monitoring, counseling, and support of the patient and her pregnancy would be appropriate.

ISOTOPES AND THE EMBRYO

Effects of Medically Administered Radioisotopes

The effects of various radioisotopes administered to the pregnant mammal have been studied less well than the effects of external irradiation. It is difficult to generalize about the effect of radioisotopes because (a) they may have specific target organs, (b) they may or may not cross the placenta, (c) the distribution of irradiation may be nonrandom, (d) the metabolism of radioactive elements or compounds may vary with individual biologic differences or disease states, and (e) the radiation dose rate decreases exponentially with time.

The precise estimation of the hazards of a particular isotope depends on accurate dosimetry, i.e., determination with greater or lesser precision of the total dose absorbed by the fetus or a particular fetal tissue, and the dose rate.

The use of particular radioisotopes (and their frequency of utilization) has changed considerably. For example, the frequency of various radioisotope procedures performed in a division of nuclear medicine at a 700-bed hospital has changed dramatically in the past

four decades. A total of 13,136 studies were performed on 7,682 patients during 1983–1984. In 1970 the same hospital performed 3,134 studies on 2,641 patients. Over the past 3 years the number of nuclear medicine procedures has remained constant. Over the past 15 years a number of procedures have been introduced and others have been eliminated. Of interest to the obstetric patient is the elimination of nuclear medicine procedures to localize the placenta. In the earlier days isotopes other than technetium (^{99m}Tc) were utilized and they could deliver a measurable dose to the embryo. Although ^{99m}Tc placentography delivers a very low dose to the embryo (<10 mrem), ultrasonography has eliminated the need for placental localization with isotopes. Table 18–12 lists the various procedures in which radiopharmaceuticals are utilized.

Table 18–13 lists the commonly utilized radioisotope and the embryonic exposure in rads per millicurie of administered isotope. Table 18–14 lists the estimated dose to the fetal thyroid in rads per microcurie of iodine 131 (^{131}I) administered at different stages of gestation.

It is obvious that most procedures will result in extremely low fetal exposures. In the case of iodine this may not be the case, especially if the patient is being treated for thyroid malignancy or hyperthyroidism. It is extremely important that a competent expert calculate the fetal dose once the question of fetal or embryonic exposure has been raised.

Radioactive Iodine

Radioactive iodine is a frequently used isotope, its usual forms being ^{123}I, ^{125}I, and ^{131}I. ^{131}I is used predominantly for uptake studies and radioactive scanning. The isotope may be administered as the inorganic ion or may be bound to protein through its affinity for the tyrosine molecule. Radioactive serum albumin (RISA) can be utilized for determining blood volume, protein leakage, placental localization, position of brain tumors, and other studies. Radioactive ^{125}I has been used to label nanogram doses of hormones for

TABLE 18–12.

Clinical Radiopharmaceutical Procedures*

Radiopharmaceutical	Study	Adult Administered Activity
^{32}P sodium phosphate	Therapy, polycythemia vera	2.3 mCi/m²
^{51}Cr albumin	Gastrointestinal protein loss	50 µCi IV
^{51}Cr chromate	Red cell survival	160 µCi IV
^{51}Cr chromate	Red cell mass	25 µCi IV
^{51}Cr chromate	Red cell in vivo	160 µCi IV
^{51}Cr chromate red blood cells	Spleen imaging	200 µCi IV
^{57}Co vitamin B$_{12}$	Vitamin B$_{12}$ absorption	0.5 µCi po
^{60}Co vitamin B$_{12}$	Vitamin B$_{12}$ absorption	0.5 µCi po
^{59}Fe citrate	Iron absorption	5 µCi po (700 µg ferrous ammonium sulfate, 300 mg ascorbic acid)
^{59}Fe citrate	In vivo counting for effective hematopoiesis	20 µCi IV
^{59}Fe citrate	Iron plasma clearance and turnover	20 µCi IV
^{59}Fe citrate	Iron red blood cell uptake	20 µCi IV
^{67}Ga citrate	Tumor imaging	3–4 mCi IV
^{67}Ga citrate	Abscess imaging	3–4 mCi IV
^{75}Se selenomethionine	Pancreas imaging	250 µCi IV or 4 µCi/kg whichever is less
^{99m}Tc diphosphonate	Myocardial imaging	15 mCi IV
^{99m}Tc disphophonate or pyrophospate	Bone imaging	15 mCi IV
^{99m}Tc-DTPA	Brain imaging	15–20 mCi IV (no perchlorate)
^{99m}Tc-DTPA	Kidney imaging	15 mCi IV
^{99m}Tc DTPA iron ascorbate	Kidney imaging	15 mCi IV
^{99m}Tc human serum albumin	Pericardial imaging	10 mCi IV
^{99m}Tc human albumin microspheres	Lung perfusion study	3 mCi IV
^{99m}Tc human serum albumin	Placenta imaging	1–2 mCi IV
^{99m}Tc macroaggregated albumin	Lung perfusion study	3 mCi IV
^{99m}Tc macroaggregates	Venous imaging for thrombosis	6 mCi IV
^{99m}Tc pertechnetate	Vascular flow	20 mCi IV
^{99m}Tc pertechnetate	Thyroid uptake when uptake is low, organification blocked	1–3 mCi IV
^{99m}Tc pertechnetate	Ectopic gastric tissue (e.g., Meckel's diverticulum)	100 µCi/kg
^{99m}Tc pertechnetate	Brain imaging	15–20 mCi IV (200 mg potassium percholorate orally prior to examination)
^{99m}Tc pertechnetate	Carotid or cerebral hemisphere flow studies	20 mCi IV
^{99m}Tc sulfur colloid	Bone marrow imaging	10 mCi IV
^{99m}Tc sulfur colloid	Spleen imaging	3 mCi IV
^{99m}Tc sulfur colloid	Liver imaging	3 mCi IV
^{111}In DTPA	Cerebrospinal fluid rhinorrhea	0.5 mCi i.t.
^{111}In DTPA	Normal-pressure hydrocephalus	0.5 mCi i.t.
^{123}I iodide	Thyroid uptake	100 µCi po
^{123}I iodide	TSH thyroid uptake study	100 µCi po (10 units thyrotropin [Thytropar] IM × 3 days prior to test)
^{123}I iodide	T$_3$ suppression	100 µCi po (25 µg liothyronine sodium (Cytomel) TID × 7 days prior to test)

(Continued)

TABLE 18–12. *(cont.)*

[123]I iodide	Thyroid imaging	100 μCi po
[123]I iodohippurate	Kidney function	1–2 mCi IV
[123]I iodohippurate	Kidney imaging	1–2 mCi IV
[125]I human serum albumin	Plasma volume	4 μCi IV
[131]I fibrinogen	Venous imaging for thrombosis	100 μCi
[131]I iodide	Thyroid uptake	10 μCi po
[131]I iodide	TSH uptake study	10 μCi po (10 units thyrotropin IM × 3 days prior to test)
[131]I iodide	T3 suppression	10 μCi po (25 μg liothyronine sodium TID × 7 days prior to test)

DTPA = diethylenetriamine pentaacetic acid; TSH = thyroid-stimulating hormone; T$_3$ = triiodothyronine; i.t. = intrathecal.
*Data from references 124–126.

TABLE 18–13.
Dose Estimated to Embryo From Radiopharmaceutical*

Radiopharmaceutical	Embryo dose (rad/mCi Administered)
[99m]Tc human serum albumin	0.018
[99m]Tc lung aggregate	0.035
[99m]Tc polyphosphate	0.036
[99m]Tc sodium pertechnetate	0.037
[99m]Tc stannous glucoheptonate	0.040
[99m]Tc sulfur colloid	0.032
[123]I sodium iodide (15% uptake)	0.032
[131]I sodium iodide (15% uptake)	0.100
[123]I rose bengal	0.130
[131]I rose bengal	0.680

*From Saenger EL: *Protocol Book.* Radioisotope Laboratory, University of Cincinnati Medical Center, 1976.

in vivo and in vitro assays. A reasonable estimate of the exposure of the fetal and maternal tissues for a given dose of radioactive iodine can be made (see Table 18–14).

The fetal thyroid absorbs and incorporates iodides readily by the tenth week of gestation and continues to do so thereafter. Fetal thyroid activity for iodides is greater than maternal thyroid activity.[127, 128] Inorganic iodides readily cross the placenta; however, even in the case of bound iodides that do not cross the placenta, in time, a substantial amount of iodide released from the binding molecule becomes available to the fetus. There probably is no form of radioactively labeled iodide compound that does not release some radioactivity that may reach the fetus.

Reported fetal effects from therapeutic (ablative) doses of ^{131}I administered to pregnant women include total fetal thyroid destruction. Although there are no reports of immediate deleterious fetal effects from tracer doses of radioactive iodine, a theoretical concern about the induction of thyroid cancer cannot be disregarded. The use of radioactive iodine should be avoided during pregnancy, unless its utilization is essential for the medical care of the mother and there is no substitute. Even if administered during the first 5 to 6 weeks of human gestation, when the fetal thyroid has not yet developed, the total dose to the embryo should be estimated. Ordinarily, the whole-body dose to the embryo from ^{131}I is insignificant when compared with the thyroid dose, because the whole-body dose primarily is due to gamma irradiation, while the thyroid dose is due to beta particles as well as gamma rays emitted from iodides concentrated in the thyroid tissue. But if large

TABLE 18–14.
Thyroidal Radioiodine Dose to the Fetus*

Gestation Period	Fetal/Maternal Ratio (Thyroid Gland)	Dose to Thyroid (Fetus) (rad/μCi)†
10–12 wk	—	0.001 (precursors)
12–13 wk	1.2	0.7
2nd trimester	1.8	6.0
3rd trimester	7.5	—
Birth imminent	—	8.0

*From Book S, Goldman M: *Health Phys* 1975; 29:874. Used by permission.
†Dose of ^{131}I ingested by mother.

doses of ^{131}I are administered, significant embryonic or fetal exposure can occur because of the accumulation of ^{131}I in the bladder adjacent to the uterus.

Other Isotopes

Inorganic radioactive potassium, sodium, phosphorus, cesium, thallium, selenium, chromium, iron, and strontium cross the placenta readily. Experiments in animals with radioactive phosphorus and strontium indicate that if the dose is large enough, embryonic abnormality and death can result.[129, 141] These isotopes are used in less than 1% of procedures; only radioactive phosphorus or gold may be utilized therapeutically, e.g., in the treatment of polycythemia or management of malignancies involving peritoneal surfaces. Most new isotope agents are bound to some complex macromolecule or macroaggregate. The one most commonly used is ^{99m}Tc pertechnetate. These newer agents cross the placenta in minuscule amounts and deliver extremely low doses to the embryo.

^{99m}Tc offers many advantages in diagnostic procedures. Total body dose is considerably lower with ^{99m}Tc bound to macromolecules than with protein labeled with ^{131}I, and there can be less concern about the fetal thyroid as a target organ.

For each procedure, the dose to the embryo must be calculated individually and is dependent on the form of the isotope, the site of administration, and the nature of the disease. Estimates of approximate fetal and maternal exposure for standard doses and procedures have been published (see Tables 19–13 and 19–14). Often, the embryonic dose will be less than the maternal dose because the nature of the isotope preparation prevents its transfer across the placenta. Even in procedures in which the fetal thyroid absorbs significant dosage (e.g., >5 rad) total fetal body exposure is quite low. Localization of the placenta with ^{99m}Tc results in approximately 1% of the radiation dose that would be absorbed from soft x-ray radiographic placentography. Of course neither procedure has been necessary since the advent of ultrasonography.

Rarely is a pregnant women given a radioactive isotope after it is known that she is pregnant. It is much more common for a woman to be exposed to diagnostic radiographic procedures before the pregnancy becomes known. This is due to the fact that (a) diagnostic radiographic procedures are more frequently performed, (b) radiologists are more sensitized to question patients about pregnancy before the use of isotopes, (c) therapeutic doses of radioactive isotopes are primarily utilized in patients with malignancies, i.e., in an older population in whom pregnancy is less likely, and (d) vague symptoms associated with pregnancy may simulate intraabdominal disease and warrant diagnostic radiographic procedures. In any event, the actual problem created by the use of isotopes during pregnancy is insignificant compared to the anxiety, chaos, and medicolegal suits resulting from exposure of pregnant women to diagnostic radiographic procedures.[94, 96, 130] When radioisotopes are to be utilized in a woman of childbearing age, the following procedure is recommended if the procedure is necessary for the benefit of the patient and the risk is estimated to be very small.

1. Record the date of the LMP and determine whether the woman could be pregnant.
2. If pregnancy is a possibility, determine the stage of gestation and the estimated dose to the fetus or fetal target organs.
3. Communicate this information to the patient or a responsible member of the family, and record this information, the time and place of the communication, and an informed consent in the patient's record.

Let us examine some typical cases:

A 34-year-old pregnant woman was admitted to the hospital on the 42nd day of gestation with fever of 38.4°C and pain and swelling of the right leg. There was extreme tenderness in the femoral region and a diagnosis of thrombophlebitis was suggested. The obstetrician requested an ^{131}I-labeled fibrinogen imaging to diagnose the problem and locate the extent of the thrombus. The radiologist canceled the procedure because the patient was pregnant.

The obstetrician called our laboratory to determine whether a significant risk was present, and if there was not a risk, whether we would convince the radiologist to perform the study. The radiologist was primarily concerned about fetal thyroid irradiation, not the whole-body radiation exposure. Both, of course, have to be considered with isotopes of iodine. In this particular patient the embryo's thyroid had not yet differentiated to the point of being able to concentrate iodine and therefore the only exposure that needs to be considered is the whole-body exposure from [131]I. Since the amount of ^{131}I-labeled fibrinogen utilized in this procedure was 100 μCi, the embryo would receive approximately 10 mrad as its total dose. This is less than the 9-month dose of background radiation that the embryo will receive. Therefore, the radiologist was in error in refusing to do the procedure—at least on the basis of concern about a radiation risk.

A 27-year-old woman was evaluated for a thyroid nodule. Thyroid imaging with 100 μCi of ^{131}I iodide revealed active uptake in the nodules and areas outside the thyroid. A biopsy revealed a thyroid carcinoma. Seventy-five millicuries of ^{131}I iodide was administered orally. It was discovered 1 week later that the patient had missed her menstrual period and was 36 days postconception when she received the radioactive iodine.

Although the thyroid is not yet developed in the embryo at this stage of gestation, at least with regard to concentrating iodine, the embryo could receive a significant exposure, depending on the thyroid uptake of the mother. This could range between 2.5 and 7.5 rad. Since the counselors use 5 rad as the dose cutoff for advising continuation of pregnancy, at least with regard to risk, this was a difficult problem. Because the exposure is protracted, the patient was advised that if there was an increased risk, it was small compared with the spontaneous risk. She elected to continue the pregnancy and she delivered a normal baby weighing 3,300 g. The baby developed normally.

A 16-year-old pregnant girl was administered 20 mCi of ^{131}I iodide for the treatment of hyperthyroidism at a small community hospital. The administration of the radioactive iodine occurred with the knowledge that the girl was pregnant. She was referred to the nearest medical center for evaluation.

It was determined that the isotope was administered at approximately the 116th day of gestation. At this stage the fetal thyroid would receive a substantial dose of radiation. Using the figures in Table 18–13 and 18–14, one can estimate a dose of 120,000 rad to the fetal thyroid. This is an exposure that should ablate the fetal thyroid and produce hypothyroidism in the newborn. The risk was presented to the prospective mother who elected to continue the pregnancy. The obstetricians discussed whether thyroid hormone should be periodically instilled in the amniotic cavity, but this was rejected. After 40 weeks of gestation the mother delivered a normal baby that was euthyroid. The results were never resolved, but it is possible that the original treatment was miscalculated since the patient's hyperthyroidism had to be brought under control by other medical means.

If a dose of irradiation large enough to represent a significant hazard to the embryo already has been administered, the physician and patient must decide on the relative merits of interrupting the pregnancy. This decision will depend on the risk of the pregnancy for the mother, the extent of the radiation hazard to the fetus, the ethnic and religious background of the family, the laws of the state pertaining to abortion, and other individual considerations. In the vast majority of instances a careful analysis will reveal that the exposure is too low to present a significant risk to the embryo.[131] (See Chapter 6, p. 220, for discussion of the use of radionuclide ventilation-perfusion lung scanning in the diagnosis of pulmonary embolism.)

SUMMARY

The term *radiation* evokes emotional responses both from laypersons and professionals. Many spokespersons are unfamiliar with radiation biology or the quantitative nature of the risks. Frequently, microwave, magnetic fields, ultrasound, and ionizing radiation risks are confused.

Although it is impossible to prove no risk for any environmental hazard, it appears that exposure to microwave radiation below the maximal permissible levels presents no measurable risk to the embryo. Ultrasound exposure from diagnostic ultrasonographic imaging equipment also is quite innocuous.[132] It is true that continued surveillance and research into potential risks of these low level exposures should continue, but at present ultrasound not only improves obstetric care but also reduces the necessity of diagnostic x-ray procedures.

The data with regard to the reproductive risks of MRI exposures in pregnant women are scant. There are conflicting and minimal animal data. With the usual clinical exposures, it would appear that we do not have enough data to infer that there is a substantial risk to the embryo. Wanted pregnancies should, therefore, be continued with inadvertent exposures.

Embryonic and fetal exposures to isotopes present variable risks, depending on the isotope and the exposure, and have to be individually assessed. The calculations and risk assessment are frequently quite complicated.

In the field of ionizing radiation, we have a better comprehension of the biologic effects and the quantitative maximum risks than for any other environmental hazard. Although the animal and human data support the conclusion that there is a threshold dose for the production of congenital malformations, namely, that no increases in the incidence of gross congenital malformations, intrauterine growth retardation, or abortion will occur with exposures less than 5 rad, that does not mean that there are definitely no risks to the embryo exposed to lower doses of radiation. Whether there exists a linear or exponential dose-response relationship or threshold exposure for genetic, carcinogenic, cell-depleting, and life-shortening effects has not been determined. In establishing maximum permissible levels for the embryo at low exposures, refer to Tables 18–4, 18–5, 18–6, 18–8, and 18–9. It is obvious that the risks of 1-rad (0.010 Gy) or 5-rad (0.05 Gy) acute exposure are far below the spontaneous risks of the developing embryo because 15% of human embryos abort, 2.7% to 3.0% of human embryos have major malformations, 4% have intrauterine growth retardation, and 8% to 10% have early- or late-onset genetic disease. The maximal risk attributed to a 1-rad exposure, approximately 0.003%, is thousands of times smaller than the spontaneous risks of malformations, abortion, or genetic disease. Thus, the present maximal permissible occupational exposures of 0.5 rem for pregnant women (see Table 18–10) and 5.0 rem for medical exposure, are extremely conservative. Medically indicated diagnostic roentgenograms are appropriate for pregnant women, and there is no medical justification for terminating a pregnancy in women exposed to 5 rad or less because of a radiation exposure. On the other hand, diagnostic x-ray studies that can be replaced by ultrasound or other procedures should be avoided simply because the unnecessary use of x-ray procedures is not good medical practice. Counseling women of reproductive age should be based on sound information about the risks of radiation exposure.

REFERENCES

1. Brent RL: X-ray, microwave, and ultrasound: The real and unreal hazards. *Pediatr Ann* 1980;9:43–47.
2. *Proceedings of the Symposium on the Late Effects of Ionizing Radiation, March 13–17, 1978.* Vienna, International Atomic Energy Agency, vol 1, 1978.
3. Okada S, Hamilton JB, Egami N, et al: A review of thirty-year study of Hiroshima and Nagasaki atomic bomb survivors. *J Radiat Res (Tokyo)* 1975;16(suppl):1–164.

4. Brent RL: Effects of radiation on the foetus, newborn and child, in Frym RJM, Grahn D, Griem ML, et al (eds): *Late Effects of Radiation.* London, Taylor & Francis, 1970, pp 23–60.

5. Brent RL: Irradiation in pregnancy, in Sciarra JJ (ed): *Davis' Gynecology and Obstetrics,* vol 2. New York, Harper & Row, 1972, pp 1–32.

6. Brent RL: Environmental factors: Radiation, in Brent RL, Harris MI (eds): *Prevention of Embryonic, Fetal, and Perinatal Disease,* vol 3. Bethesda, Fogarty International Center Series on Preventive Medicine, US Department of Health, Education, and Welfare, DHEW Publication No (NIH) 76-853, 1976M 00, 179–197.

7. Brent RL: Radiations and other physical agents, in Wilson JG, Frasers FC (eds): *Handbook of Teratology,* vol 1. New York, Plenum Press, 1977, pp 153–223.

8. Brent RL: Radiation teratogenesis. *Teratology* 1980;21:281–298.

9. Brent RL, Gorson RO: Radiation exposure in pregnancy, in Moseley RD, Baker DH, Gorson RO, et al (eds): *Current Problems in Radiology,* vol 2. Chicago, Year Book Medical Publishers, Inc, 1972, pp 1–48.

10. Brent RL, Bolden BT: The indirect effect of irradiation on embryonic development. III. The contribution of ovarian irradiation, oviduct irradiation, and zygote irradiation to fetal mortality and growth retardation in the rat. *Radiat Res* 1967;30:759–773.

11. Russell LB: X-ray-induced developmental abnormalities in the mouse and their use in analysis of embryological patterns. I. External and gross visceral changes. *J Exp Zool* 1950;114:545–602.

12. Russell LB, Russell WL: The effects of radiation on the preimplantation stages of the mouse embryo. *Anat Res* 1950;108:521.

13. Rugh R: Major radiobiological concepts and ionizing radiation on the fetus, in Nokkentred K (ed): *Effect of Radiation Upon the Human Fetus,* Copenhagen, Munksgaard, 1968, pp 228.

14. Russell LB: X-ray-induced developmental abnormalities in the mouse and their use in analysis of embryological patterns. II. Abnormalities of the vertebral column and thorax. *J Exp Zool* 1956;131:329–395.

15. Russell LB, Russell WL: An analysis of the changing radiation response of the developing mouse embryo. *J Cell Comp Physiol* 1954;43:103–149.

16. Russell LB, Major MH: Radiation-induced presumed somatic mutations in the house mouse. *Genetics* 1957;42:161–175.

17. Russell LB, Saylors CL: The relative sensitivity of various germ-cell stages of the mouse to radiation-induced nondysjunction, chromosome losses and deficiencies, in Sobel (ed): *Repair From Genetic Radiation.* New York, Pergamon Press, 1963, pp 313–342.

18. Rugh R: Effect of ionizing radiations, including radioisotopes, on the placenta and embryo. *Birth Defects* 1965;1:64–73.

19. Russell LB, Badgett SK, Saylors CL: Comparison of the effects of acute, continuous and fractionated irradiation during embryonic development, in Sobel (ed): *Repair From Genetic Radiation.* New York, Pergamon Press, 1963, pp 333–342.

20. Brent RL, Bolden BT: The long-term effects of low-dosage embryonic irradiation. *Radiat Res* 1961;14:453–454.

21. Cowen D, Geller LM: Long-term pathological effects of prenatal x-irradiation on the central nervous system of the rat. *J Neuropathol Exp Neurol* 1968;19:488–527.

22. Hicks SP, D'Amato CJ: Effects of ionizing radiation on mammalian development, Woolam DHM (ed): *Advances in Teratology,* vol 1. London, Logos Press, 1966, pp 196–243.

23. Murphree R, Pace H: The effects of prenatal radiation on postnatal development in the rat. *Radiat Res* 1960;12:495–504.

24. Rugh R, Wohlfromm M: X-irradiation sterilization of the premature female mouse. *Atompraxis* 1964;10:511–518.

25. Rugh R, Wohlfromm M: Can x-irradiation prior to sexual maturity affect the fertility of the male mammal (mouse)? *Atompraxis* 1964;10:33–42.

26. Furchgott E: Behavioral effects of ionizing radiations, 1955–1961. *Psychol Bull* 1963;60:157–200.

27. Piontkovskii IA: Certain properties of the higher nervous activity in adult animals irradiated prenatally by ionizing radiations: The problem of the effect of ionizing irradiation on offspring [in Russian]. *Bull Exp Biol Med* 1958;46:77–80.

28. Piontkovskii IA: Some peculiarities of

higher nervous activity in adult animals subjected to radiation in utero, pt 3 [in Russian]. *Bull Exp Biol Med* 1961;51:24–31.

29. Miller RW, Mulvihill JJ: Small head size after atomic irradiation. Teratogen update. *Teratology* 1976;14:355–358.

30. Zappert J: Über roentgenogene fetale Microcephalie. *Monatsschr Kinderheilkd* 1926;34:490–493.

31. Goldstein L, Murphy DP: Microcephalic idiocy following radium therapy for uterine cancer during pregnancy. *Am J Obstet Gynecol* 1929;18:189–195; 281–283.

32. Goldstein L, Murphy DPL: Etiology of ill health in children born after maternal pelvic irradiation. II. Defective children born after postconceptional maternal irradiation. *Am J Roentgenol* 1929;22:322–331.

33. Murphy DP, Goldstein L: Micromelia in a child irradiated in utero. *Surg Gynecol Obstet* 1930;40:79–80.

34. Dekaban AS: Abnormalities in children exposed to x-irradiation during various stages of gestation: Tentative timetable of radiation injury to the human fetus. *J Nucl Med* 1968;9:471–477.

35. Miller RW: Delayed radiation effects in atomic bomb survivors. *Science* 1969;166:569–574.

36. Wood JW, Johnson KG, Omori Y: In utero exposure to Hiroshima atomic bomb. An evaluation of head size and mental retardation-twenty years later. *Pediatrics* 1967;39:385–392.

37. Wood J, Johnson K, Omari Y, et al: Mental retardation in children exposed in utero to the atomic bombs in Hiroshima and Nagasaki. *Am J Public Health* 1967;57:1381–1390.

38. Plummer G: Anomalies occurring in children exposed in utero to the atomic bomb in Hiroshima. *Pediatrics* 1952;10:687–692.

39. Yamazaki J, Wright S, Wright P: Outcome of pregnancy in women exposed to the atomic bomb in Nagasaki. *Am J Dis Child* 1954;87:448–463.

40. Marotcaux P, Sprangcr J, Opitz JM, et al: Le syndrome camptomelique. *Presse Med* 1971;22:157–1162.

41. Blot W: Growth and development following prenatal and childhood exposure to atomic radiation. *J Radiat Res (Tokyo)* 1975; 16(suppl):82–88.

42. Blot WJ, Miller RW: Mental retardation following in utero exposure to the atomic bombs of Hiroshima and Nagasaki. *Radiology* 1973;106:617–619.

42a. Otake M, Schull WJ: In utero exposure to A-bomb radiation and mental retardation: A reassessment. *Br J Radiol* 1984;57:409–414.

43. Kinlen LJ, Acheson FD: Diagnostic irradiation, congenital malformations, and spontaneous abortion. *Br J Radiol* 1968;41:648–654.

44. Nokkentred K: *Effect of Radiation Upon the Human Fetus.* Copenhagen, Munksgaard, 1968.

45. Tabuchi A: Fetal disorders due to ionizing radiation. *Hiroshima J Med Sci* 1964;13:125–173.

46. Tabuchi A, Nakagawa S, Hirai T, et al: Fetal hazards due to x-ray diagnosis during pregnancy. *Hiroshima J Med Sci* 1967;16:49–66.

47. Vilumsen A: *Environmental Factors in Congenital Malformations.* Copenhagen, FDAL's Forlag, 1970.

48. Jacobsen L, Mellemgaard L: Anomalies of the eyes in descendants of women irradiated with small x-ray doses during age of fertility. *Acta Ophthalmol (Copenh)* 1968; 46:352–354.

49. Brent RL: The response of the 9–1/2 day-old rat embryo to variations in dose rate of 150 R X-irradiation. *Radiat Res* 1971;45:127–136.

50. Brizzee KR, Brannon RB: Cell recovery in foetal brain after ionizing radiation. *Int J Radiat Biol* 1972;21:375–378.

51. Ronnback C: Effects of continuous irradiation during gestation and suckling period of mice. *Acta Radiol Ther* 1965;3:169–176.

52. Vorisek P: Einfluss der kontinuierlichen intrauterinen Bestrahlung auf die perinatale Mortalität der Frucht. *Strahlentherapie* 1965;127:112–120.

53. Stadler J, Gowen JW: Observations on the effects of continuous irradiation over 10 generations on reproductivities of different strains of mice, in Carlson WD, Gassner FX (eds): *Proceedings of an International Symposium on the Effects of Ionizing Radiation on Reproductive Systems.* New York, Pergamon Press, 1964.

54. Coppenger CJ, Brown SO: The gross manifestations of continuous gamma irradiation on the prenatal rat. *Radiat Res* 1967;31:230–242.

55. Konerman G: Die Keimesentwicklung der Maus nach Einwirkung kontinuierlicher ^{60}Co Gammabestrahlung während der Blastogenese, der Organogenese und der fetalen Periode. *Strahlentherapie* 1969;137:451–466.

56. Wesley JP: Background radiation as a cause of congenital malformations. *Int J Radiat Biol* 1960;2:97–118.

57. Gentry J, Parkhurst E, Bulin G: An epidemiological study of congenital malformations in New York State. *Am J Public Health* 1959;49:497.

58. Grahn D, Kratchman J: Variation in neonatal death rate and birth rate in the United States and possible relations to environmental radiation, geology and altitude. *Am J Hum Genet* 1963;15:329–352.

59. Segall A, MacMahon B, Hannigan M: Congenital malformations and background radiation in northern New England. *J Chron Dis* 1964;17:915–932.

60. Kriegal H, Langendorff H: Wirkung einer fraktionierten Roentgenbestrahlung auf die Embryonalentwicklung der Maus. *Strahlentherapie* 1964;123:429–437.

61. Laskey JW, Parrish JL, Cahill DF: Some effects of lifetime parental exposure to low levels of tritium on the F_2 generation. *Radiat Res* 1973;56:171–179.

62. Diamond EL, Schmerler H, Lilienfeld AM: The relationship of intrauterine radiation to subsequent mortality and development of leukemia in children. A prospective study. *Am J Epidemiol* 1973;97:283–313.

63. Jablon S: Comments. *Health Phys* 1973;24:257–258.

64. Miller RW: Epidemiological conclusions from radiation toxicity studies, in Fry RJM, Grahn D, Griem ML, et al (eds): *Late Effects of Radiation*. London, Taylor & Francis, 1970, pp 242–256.

65. Stewart AM: Myeloid leukaemia and cot deaths. *Br Med J* 1972;4:423.

66. Stewart A: The carcinogenic effects of low-level radiation: A reappraisal of epidemiologists methods and observations. *Health Phys* 1973;24:223–240.

67. Stewart A, Kneale GW: Radiation dose effects in relation to obstetric X-rays and childhood cancers. *Lancet* 1970;1:1185–1188.

68. Stewart A, Webb D, Giles D, et al: Malignant disease in childhood and diagnostic irradiation in utero. *Lancet* 1956;2:447.

69. Stewart A, Webb D, Hewitt D: A survey of childhood malignancies. *Br Med J* 1958;1:1495–1508.

70. Lewis EB: Leukemia and ionizing radiation. *Science* 1957;125:865–972.

71. *The Effects on Populations of Exposure to Low Levels of Ionizing Radiation*. Report of the Advisory Committee on the Biological Effects of Ionizing Radiations, Division of Medical Sciences, National Academy of Sciences, National Research Council, Washington, DC, 1972.

72. Lilienfeld AM: Epidemiological studies of the leukemogenic effects of radiation. *Yale J Biol Med* 1966;39:143–164.

73. McMahon B, Hutchinson GB: Prenatal x-ray and childhood: A review. *Acta Union Int Contra Cancrum* 1964;20:1172–1174.

74. Graham S, Levin MI, Lilienfeld AM, et al: Preconception, intrauterine and postnatal irradiation as related to leukemia. *Natl Cancer Inst Monogr* 1966;19:347–371.

75. Polhemus D, Koch R: Leukemia and medical irradiation. *Pediatrics* 1969;23:453–461.

76. Ager E, Schuman L, Wallace H, et al: An epidemiologic study of childhood leukemia. *J Chron Dis* 1965;18:113–132.

77. Ford D, Patterson T: Fetal exposure to diagnostic X-rays and leukemia and other malignant diseases in childhood. *JNCI* 1959;22:1093–1104.

78. Natarajan N, Bross IDJ: Preconception radiation and leukemia. *J Med* 1973;4:276–281.

79. Burrow G, Hamilton H, Hrubec Z, et al: Study of adolescents exposed in utero to the atomic bomb. Nagasaki, Japan. I. General aspects: Clinical laboratory data. *Yale J Biol Med* 1964;36:430–444.

80. Kato H: Mortality in children exposed to the A-bombs while in utero. *Am J Epidemiol* 1971;93:435–442.

81. Hoshino T, Itoga T, Kato H: Leukemia in the offspring of parents exposed to the atomic bomb at Hiroshima and Nagasaki. Presented at Japanese Association of Hematology, March 28–30, 1965.

82. Neutel CI, Buck C: Effect of smoking dur-

ing pregnancy on the risk of cancer in children. *JNCI* 1971;47:59–64.

83. Fasal E, Jackson EW, Klauber MR: Birth characteristics and leukemia in children. *JNCI* 1971;47:501–509.

84. Wright FW: Diagnostic radiology and the fetus. *Br Med J* 1973;3:693–694.

85. Rugh R, Duhamel L, Skaredoff L: Relation of embryonic and fetal X-irradiation to life-time average weights and tumor incidence in mice. *Proc Soc Exp Biol Med* 1966;121:714–718.

86. Brent RL, Bolden BT: Indirect effect on x-irradiation on embryonic development. V. Utilization of high doses of material irradiation on the first day of gestation. *Radiat Res* 1968;36:563–570.

87. Wood J, Keehn R, Kawamoto S, et al: The growth and development of children exposed in utero to the atomic bombs in Hiroshima and Nagasaki. *Am J Public Health* 1967;57:1374–1380.

88. Ross MH, Bras G: Tumor incidence patterns and nutrition in the rat. *J Nutr* 1965;87:245–260.

89. Brent RL: The indirect effect of irradiation on embryonic development. II. Irradiation of the placenta. *Am J Dis Child* 1960;100:103–108.

90. Brent RL, Bolden BT: The indirect effect of irradiation on embryonic development. The lethal effects of maternal irradiation on the first day of gestation in the rat. *Proc Soc Exp Biol Med* 1967;125:709–712.

91. Brent RL, McLaughlin MM: The indirect effect of irradiation on embryonic development. I. Irradiation of the mother while shielding the embryonic site. *Am J Dis Child* 1960;100:94–102.

92. Neifakh AA: Role of the maternal organism in the irradiation illness of fetal mice. *Dokl Akad Nauk BSS* 1957;116:821–824.

93. Ronderos A: Fetal tolerance to radiation. *Radiology* 1961;76:454–456.

94. Brent RL: Medicolegal aspects of teratology. *J Pediatr* 1967;71:288–289.

95. National Council on Radiation Protection and Measurements: *Basic Radiation Criteria,* NCRP Report No. 39. Washington, DC 1971.

96. Brent RL: Litigation-produced pain, disease and suffering: An experience with congenital malformation lawsuit. *Teratology,* 1977;16:1–13.

97. *Antenatal Diagnosis: Report of a Consensus Development Conference (Sponsored by the National Institute of Child Health and Human Development).* Bethesda, Md, National Institutes of Health, NIH Publication No. 79–1973, 1979.

98. Marx JL: Imaging technique passes muster. *Science* 1987;238:888–889.

99. Damadian R: US patent 3,789,832 filed March 17, 1972.

100. Bottomley PA: NMR imaging techniques and applications: A review. *Rev Sci Instrum* 1982;59:1319.

101. Fullerton GD: Basic concepts for nuclear magnetic resonance imaging. *Magn Reson Imaging* 1982;1:39.

102. Tenforde TS, Faffey CT, Moyer BR, et al: Cardiovascular alterations in Macaca monkeys exposed to stationary magnetic fields: Experimental observations and theoretical analysis. *Bioelectromagnetics* 1983;4:1–9.

103. Lovsund P, Nilsson SEG, Reuter T, et al: Magnetophosphenes: A quantitative analysis of thresholds. *Med Biol Eng Comput* 1982;20:243–248.

104. Frankel RB: Magnetic guidance or organisms. *Annu Rev Biophys Bioeng* 1985;13:85–100.

105. Kalmijn AJ: Biophysics of geomagnetic field detection. *IEEE Trans Magn* 1981;17:1113–1115.

106. Delgado JMR, Monteagudo JL, Gracia MQ, et al: Teratogenic effects of weak magnetic fields. *IRCS Med Sci* 1981;9:392.

107. Juutilainen J, Saali K: Development of chick embryos in 1 Hz and 100 kHz magnetic fields. *Radiat Environ Biophys* 1986;25:135–140.

108. Juutilainen J, Harri M, Saali K, et al: Effects of 100-Hz magnetic fields with various waveforms on the development of chick embryos. *Radiat Environ Biophys* 1986;25:65–74.

109. Ubeda A, Leal J, Trillo MA, et al: Pulse shape of magnetic fields influences chick embryogenesis. *J Anat* 1983;137:513–536.

110. Maffeo S, Miller MW, Carstensen EL: Lack of effect of weak low frequency electromagnetic fields on chick embryogenesis. *J Anat* 1984;139:613–618.

111. Maffeo S, Brayman AA, Miller MW, et al: Weak low frequency electromagnetic fields and chick embryogenesis: Failure to repro-

duce positive findings. *J Anat* 1988;157:101–104.

112. Juutilainen J, Liimatainen A: Mutation frequency in Salmonella exposed to weak 100-Hz magnetic fields. *Hereditas* 1986;104:145–147.

113. Ozil J, Modlinski JA: Effects of electric field on fusion rate and survival of 2-cell rabbit embryos. *J Embryol Exp Morphol* 1986;96:211–228.

114. Stuchly MA, Ruddick J, Villeneuve D, et al: Teratological assessment of exposure to time-varying magnetic field. *Teratology* 1988;38:461–466.

115. Sikov MR, Mahlum DD, Montgomery LD, et al: Development of mice after intrauterine exposure to direct current magnetic fields, in Phillips RD, Gillis MF, Kaune WT, et al (eds): *Biological Effects of Extremely Low Frequency Electromagnetic Fields.* Washington, DC, US Department of Energy, 1978, pp 462–473.

116. Sikov MR, Rommereim DN, Beamer JL, et al: Developmental studies of Hanford miniature swine exposed to 60-Hz electric fields. *Bioelectromagnetics* 1987;8:229–242.

117. Lary JM, Conover DL, Foley ED, et al: Teratogenic effects of 27.12-MHz radiofrequency radiation in rats. *Teratology* 1982;26:299–309.

118. Dietzel F, Kern W: Fehlgeburt nach Kurzwellenbehandlung-tierexperimentelle Untersuchungen. *Arch Gynecol* 1970;209:237–255.

119. Heinricks WL, Heinrichs S, Flannery M, et al: Magnetic resonance spectroscopy (MRS): Embryotoxicity in balb/c pregnant mice (abstracted). Presented at the Society for Gynecologic Investigation 33rd Annual Meeting, Toronto, 1986, p 146.

120. Foster MA, Knight CH, Rimmington JE, et al: Fetal imaging by nuclear magnetic resonance: A study in goats. *Radiology* 1983;149:193–195.

121. Heinricks WL, Fong P, Flannery M, et al: Midgestational exposure of pregnant BALB/C mice to magnetic resonance imaging conditions. *Magn Reson Imaging* 1988;6:305–314.

122. Smith FW, MacLennan F: NMR imaging in human pregnancy: A preliminary study. *Magn Reson Imaging* 1984;2:57–64.

123. Turner RJ, Hankins GDV, Weinreb JC, et al: Magnetic resonance imaging and ultrasonography in the antenatal evaluation of conjoined twins. *Am J Obstet Gynecol* 1986;155:645–649.

124. Kereiakes JG, Feller PA, Ascoi FA, et al: Pediatric radiopharmaceutical dosimetry, in *Radiopharmaceutical Dosimetry Symposium.* Rockville, Md, US Department of Health, Education, and Welfare, HEW Publication No. (FDA) 76–8044, Bureau of Radiological Health, Food and Drug Administration, 1976.

125. Roedler HD, Kaul A, Hine GJ: *Internal Radiation Dose in Diagnostic Nuclear Medicine.* Berlin, Verlag H Hoffman, 1978.

126. Saenger EL: *Protocol Book.* Radioisotope Laboratory, University of Cincinnati Medical Center, 1976.

127. Book S, Goldman M: Thyroidal radioiodine exposure of the fetus. *Health Phys* 1975;29:874.

128. Jacobson AG, Brent RL: Radioiodine concentration by the fetal mouse thyroid. *Endocrinology* 1959;65:408–416.

129. Sikov MR, Noonan TR: Anomalous development induced in embryonic rat by the maternal administration of radiophosphorus. *Am J Anat* 1958;103:137.

130. Brent RL: The effect of embryonic and fetal exposure to x-ray, microwaves, and ultrasound: Counseling the pregnant and nonpregnant patient about these risks. *Semin Oncol* 1989;16:347–369.

131. Brent RL: The effects of ionizing radiation, microwaves and ultrasound in the developing embryo: Clinical interpretations and applications of the data, vol 14. Year Book Medical Publishers, Inc, Chicago, 1984, pp 1–87.

132. Brent RL: Ultrasonography in fetal diagnosis. *Pediatr Ann* 1981;10:49–60.

CHAPTER 19

Psychiatric Issues

Nada L. Stotland

Psychiatric issues in pregnancy include frank psychologic illness as well as psychiatric factors affecting compliance with obstetric care, life adjustment, patient satisfaction, and the ability to cope with medical complications. Pregnancy presents somatic and psychosocial challenge to the organism. Optimally, the response to the challenge results in a new, higher level of organization and maturity.[1] Health care professionals aware of the challenges can promote these optimal outcomes by fostering communication and active engagement with normal anxieties and dilemmas.

The stress of pregnancy and the postpartum period disturbs the fragile equilibrium of some women at medical and/or psychosocial risk. Among them are patients with peripartum medical complications. Informed and timely diagnosis and treatment can improve perinatal outcome,[2] and make the difference between long-term or chronic maladjustment, with impaired self-esteem, and the satisfaction of mastering a developmental task. Lastly, a small subgroup of women suffer serious psychiatric disorders during and after pregnancy. Appropriate interventions in these cases can prevent major morbidity and mortality.

This chapter begins with a brief review of the history of the literature on psychiatric illness during pregnancy and proceeds to a discussion of the emotional concomitants of normal pregnancy, effects of recent social changes on the psychologic experience of pregnancy and perinatal medical care, and signs and symptoms of major peripartum psychiatric illnesses. The chapter concludes with a practical clinical section addressing issues vital to the medical consultant: the detection of psychiatric complications during regular or high-risk prenatal care, emotional reactions to medical complications of pregnancy, office, and bedside management; indications for, and technique of, psychiatric referral; and the use of psychoactive drugs during pregnancy and lactation.

BACKGROUND

Almost all of the premodern literature on peripartum psychiatric complications concerns postpartum psychoses. A puerperal delirium beginning with sleeplessness and agitation on the 6th postpartum day, progressing to delirium on the 11th, and resulting in death on the 17th, was described by Hippocrates in the fourth century B.C.[3] Pathophysiology was ascribed to the redirection of suppressed lochial discharge toward the brain.

Hundreds of papers on the subject were published during the nineteenth century. A woman in Essex, England, was acquitted of murdering her child by reason of insanity secondary to puerperal mania—as early as 1848.[4] A popular and comprehensive text was published by Marcé in 1858, *Traité de la folie des femmes enceintes*,[5] and its influence was such that the currently active medical society devoted entirely to peripartum psychiatric illness is called The Marcé Society.

The Importance of Psychological Well-Being to Gestation

Attention to psychologic concomitants and complications of pregnancy, mentioned above, can enhance normal adaptation and the coping of expectant mothers whose psychosocial stability is marginal. In addition, understanding and addressing a patient's emotional conflicts is often the only successful way to elicit compliance with either routine, preventive prenatal care, or active monitoring and intervention for patients at increased obstetric risk. An interrelated set of factors is the relationship between the patient and the members of the obstetric care team. A history of sexual abuse, current domestic violence, and/or traumatic experiences with medical-obstetric care, inhibit the patient's sense of trust and resultant compliance. Recent social developments, to be discussed below, have had a major impact on the doctor-patient relationship.

The current obstetric experience will shape the patient's attitude about her body and its functioning and about medical care. As women in most families are responsible for the health care not only of children but of male adults as well, these attitudes will have an impact on the health care of the entire family. Her state of psychologic health is a major determinant of functioning of the family unit.

Psychological issues have a direct relationship with obstetric outcome.[6] Researchers studying prepared childbirth were surprised to find that normal patients who had attended Lamaze classes had fewer complications of labor than matched controls.[7] Frank psychiatric illness is probably associated with an adverse intrauterine environment for the fetus; psychotic and depressed gravidas eat, sleep, and care for themselves poorly. Clinically, intrauterine growth retardation may be reversed by inpatient treatment of women with severe psychiatric illness. Such patients are also at risk for injurious behaviors such as drug overdoses and self-inflicted abdominal stab wounds. Psychiatric symptoms may be the first indications of a space-occupying intracranial lesion, infection, metabolic derangement, or acquired immunodeficiency syndrome (AIDS). New psychotic ideation or major behavioral change requires the appropriate medical investigation.

Influence of Social Change

A number of cultural conditions directly and indirectly affect the experience, climate, and psychiatric complications of pregnancy. One is the demographics of the childbearing population. Both older patients who have delayed pregnancy for career or other reasons, and adolescents, have special, and different, stresses, needs, and biopsychologic complications. An increasing percentage of pregnant patients are unmarried. In the clinical setting, as in this chapter, the term and concept of "husband" cannot be used generically for the father of the unborn child.

Major social movements, feminism and consumerism, have been associated with changes in the relationship between obstetric care providers and pregnant women. These movements encourage information gathering, comparison shopping for medical opinions, and skepticism about the expertise of authorities. The current malpractice climate engenders wariness on both sides of the doctor-patient relationship. In addition, while standards of care continue to rise, society in the United States, unlike many other developed countries,[8] increasingly fails to provide financial support for the care of the many uninsured patients at risk for medical and psychosocial complications. But social changes can also foster informed decision making, respectful mutual collaboration between patients and physicians, increased responsibility of patients for their own behavior and care, and better patient preparation for obstetric experiences and complications.

TABLE 19–1.
Psychological Issues in Successive Trimesters of
Pregnancy and Post Partum

First Trimester
    Accepting reality of pregnancy—patient and
       family, discomforts of nausea, vomiting, urinary
       frequency
    Awaiting results of prenatal diagnostic tests

Second Trimester
    Increasing girth and quickening make fetus
       tangible
    Lowest incidence of physical and emotional
       problems

Third trimester
    Ungainliness
    Distortion of body image; fears of loss of
       attractiveness
    Plans for child care and changed life style of
       couple and family
    Preoccupation with and preparation for risk and
       pain of childbirth

Post partum
    Acceptance of realities of childbirth
       Physiological events and experiences
       Behavior of self and significant others
       Obstetric care
    Acceptance of infant: gender, appearance,
       behavior
    Exhaustion
    Adjustments in life style and relationships
    Resumption of sexual activity; family planning
    Breast-feeding

"Prepared childbirth" has become the standard for prenatal care. Classes provide information about the process of pregnancy and delivery, techniques for relaxation, collaboration, and distraction, and the opportunity to share experiences and concerns with others in a similar situation. Since there is some evidence (see above) that preparation improves outcome, it is useful for the care provider to identify small (eight couples or less), well-taught classes in his or her area, develop a working relationship with the teacher, and become familiar enough with the techniques practiced so that they can be supported during labor.

Preparation must take into account the fact that the experiences of labor and medical complications often make women feel depen-dent and overwhelmed and are unpredicta-ble. At least one author has described a small series of patients in whom psychiatric symptoms were attributed by the patients to disappointment or "failure" in the experience of delivery after childbirth education classes.[9]

Patients with medical complictions of pregnancy may be unable to attend classes. Arrangements for bedside instruction can often be made and are reassuring and normalizing. These patients are more likely to need intensive monitoring during labor and to undergo surgical delivery. They can be encouraged to focus on the usefulness of information and relaxation, rather than the importance of spontaneous birth. It is important to discuss these difficulties with patients, in advance if possible, in order to forestall unnecessary guilt and dissatisfaction with care.

PSYCHOLOGY OF NORMAL PREGNANCY

The psychology of pregnancy is often conceptualized in terms of trimesters (Table 19–1). The psychologic task of the first trimester is to accept the reality of pregnancy. From the moment conception is confirmed, the pregnant woman is a mother. In our culture, she and her medical care providers are held responsible for the well-being of the unborn child. Although medically and psychologically healthy women are usually proud, excited, and joyful, conflicting feelings are inevitable. The woman's life has been changed forever. Her behaviors are constrained by the need to provide a safe and nurturing intra-uterine environment for the developing embryo. She faces predictable and unpredictable bodily alterations and symptoms.

In the older psychoanalytic literature, nausea and vomiting of pregnancy were char-acterized as manifestations of extreme am-bivalence, immaturity, and fear of feminin-ity. These studies were methodologically flawed by today's standard. It may well be that the unpleasantness of physiologically based symptoms arouses emotional neediness and negative feelings about the pregnancy.

Hyperemesis gravidarum may be severely debilitating and is frequently associated with psychologic problems. It is likely that emotional and hormonal factors are neurobiologically interrelated. Supportive psychotherapy is indicated and helpful in these cases.[10] (Table 19–2) (see also Chap. 9 and 10).

The possibility of prenatal diagnosis of fetal defects is both a reassurance and a source of anxiety.[11] Both amniocentesis and chorionic villi sampling are invasive and somewhat uncomfortable procedures. The former, much more widely practiced than the latter, does not yield results until the second trimester. This delay can interfere with the normal attachment to the unborn child. Even without prenatal diagnostic procedures, awareness of the frequency of spontaneous abortion in the first trimester, which is increased in high-risk pregnancy, makes women wary of making definite plans and informing people outside their most intimate circles.

Within that circle, relationships with members of the immediate family are tested by the need to adapt to the forthcoming changes in roles. Is the father of the expected baby excited and supportive, or frightened and avoidant? Does the woman's mother promote her self-confidence, or, frightened by the evidence of her own aging, compete and denigrate? Obstetric screening and care can include questions about the progress of the family's adaptation to the pregnancy. Family members in conflict with the patient can be invited to participate in office visits for education and counseling if the patient wishes.

During the second trimester, most women are gratified by the end of morning sickness and the realities of maternity clothes and fetal movement. Psychologic stress is lowest in this trimester. Increasing abdominal girth and pressure on abdominal and thoracic viscera make women feel ungainly and uncomfortable during the third trimester. This is the time when parental plans ranging from names and layettes to child care arrangements are solidified. Whenever possible, a woman's plans for returning to work should be flexible. Especially in the presence of medical compli-

cations, it is impossible to predict how she will feel physically and emotionally after delivery.

Preparations and fears concerning childbirth are also heightened during the last trimester. As mentioned above, prospective discussion between expectant parents and care providers about wishes, expectations, and techniques of delivery, allowing for considerable adaptation to circumstances, tends to decrease later disappointment and anger. However, it is never possible to fully anticipate the realities of labor.

APPROACH TO PSYCHIATRIC DISORDERS DURING PREGNANCY

The literature on psychiatric disorders during pregnancy is very sparse, especially when compared with studies of postpartum psychiatric illness. Of Marcé's 1858 case series of peripartum mental disease, only 9%

TABLE 19–2.
Approach to Hyperemesis Gravidarum

1. Medical assessment
    Vital signs
    Electrolytes
    Hydration
    Fetal health and development
2. Psychologic assessment
    History
        Psychiatric illness
        Psychiatric complications of pregnancy
        Family history of complications of pregnancy
    Premorbid and lifetime level of function
        Past history of somatization in response to stress
    Current function
    Relations with significant others
    Current psychiatric illness
3. Management
    Hospitalization
    Antiemetics
    Medical support
        Hydration, nutrition, electrolyte repletion
    Psychologic support
        Reassurance
        Family and individual counseling
        Reduction of demands and stimulation

occurred before birth. In the latter half of the twentieth century as well, pregnant women seem to account for a disproportionately low number of psychiatric hospital admissions.[12] It is not at all clear whether the explanation is hormonal, psychologic, or sociocultural. Certainly the psychosocial demands on a pregnant woman are less than those on a new mother, and our emphasis on prenatal care offers more support to the former than to the latter. Currently, many psychiatric hospitals are loathe to admit pregnant patients otherwise eligible for inpatient treatment because of medical-legal and clinical concerns about the availability of adequate obstetric back-up.

There is no particular constellation of psychiatric illnesses associated with pregnancy. Rational and irrational thought content of psychiatrically disordered pregnant women often centers on the fetus. Pseudocyesis is by definition not a psychiatric complication of pregnancy, but an unconsciously psychologically motivated simulation of, or belief in, a nonexistent pregnancy. This poorly understood and probably heterogeneous disorder was described as early as Hippocrates, but its incidence and prognosis are not known.[13] Patients, who range in age from prepubertal to postmenopausal, believe they are pregnant and manifest signs and symptoms of pregnancy, including not only abdominal distention, subjective experience of fetal movement and weight gain, but also nausea and vomiting, breast and cervical changes, and amenorrhea. A persistent corpus luteum may be involved; prolactin, luteinizing hormone, and gonadotropins have been found to be elevated in some cases. The patients have no other delusions, hallucinations, or psychotic manifestations. While the symptoms are not consciously simulated to manipulate the environment, multiple unconscious psychodynamic motivations can often be discerned: for example, the desire to hold the interest of a mate or physician, to assert one's femininity and fertility.

Negative results of pregnancy tests and ultrasound can be nonjudgmentally shared with the patient. Forceful confrontation may succeed only in inducing her to begin the process again within another health care setting. Psychiatric referral and psychotherapy within the team context of obstetric follow-up offers the optimal opportunity for understanding and helping the patient, and not incidentally, increasing our knowledge about this obscure and fascinating condition. In some cases a primary symptom is the denial of a confirmed pregnancy. These patients are at risk for unattended delivery and neonatal neglect and/or murder.[10] Emergency psychiatric evaluation is indicated; involuntary hospitalization for the protection of the fetus raises difficult ethical questions, but may be rationalized in the case of psychosis by the fact that harm befalling the unborn child would be a major psychologic trauma to the mother.

Pregnant patients may suffer remissions or exacerbations of any preexisting psychiatric illness, and the onset of new ones, including anxiety disorders, somatization, psychosis, affective illness (mania and depression), personality disturbances, and acute situational reactions. Women who have physically abusive partners are at increased risk of abuse during pregnancy. Specific diagnostic and management issues related to psychiatric illness are discussed below. It cannot be said too often, however, that a few simple screening questions in even the most routine obstetric history can identify these problems in many cases, facilitating effective early intervention. The questions are:

- Have you ever had a psychiatric illness or trouble with your nerves?
- Have you ever been treated by a psychiatrist or counselor, or been admitted to a psychiatric hospital?
- Do arguments in your family sometimes get physically violent?

Table 19–3 is an outline of psychiatric data optimally obtained at the first prenatal visit while Table 19–4 indicates criteria for psychiatric referral.

TABLE 19–3.
The First Prenatal Visit: Psychiatric Data

I. Physical/sexual abuse
   A. Past/childhood
   B. Current
II. Medical/obstetric experiences
   A. Complications
   B. Frightening and/or frustrating interactions
      with medical staff
III. History of psychiatric illness
   A. Family history
   B. Personal history
     1. Symptomatic episodes and relationship to
       pregnancy
       a. Depression/mania
       b. Psychosis
       c. Anxiety
       d. Other
     2. Outpatient psychiatric treatment*
       a. Name of therapist
       b. Mode(s) of treatment
       c. Outcome
       d. Current relationship
     3. Psychiatric hospitalization*
       a. Where
       b. When
IV. Recent/current psychosocial stress
V. Level of function
   A. Highest attained
   B. Current
VI. Current signs and symptoms
   A. Depression
     1. Decreased sleep, appetite, mood, con-
       centration, interest, hope
     2. Suicidality
   B. Mania
     Increased energy, activity, speech; sleep-
     lessness, grandiosity
   C. Psychosis
     Hallucinations, delusions
   D. Substance abuse
   E. Anxiety interfering with role performance
   F. Somatization
     1. Generalized anxiety
     2. Panic attacks
     3. Phobic behavior

*Obtain signed release from patient and send for records.

POSTPARTUM PSYCHIATRIC ILLNESS

This spectrum of illness is mentioned here, though outside the term of pregnancy, because it is the best-known category of peripartum psychiatric disturbance. Terms including *postpartum psychosis* and *postpartum de-*

pression tend to be used in an undifferentiated manner, to refer to severe psychobehavioral disease. The time of onset, too, may be unspecified or may range from days to 6 months or a year post partum. There is also confusion with the much more common "baby blues." Occurring in up to 60% or 70% of new American mothers, this clinical picture includes emotional lability with unexplained weeping, sadness, and feelings of inadequacy.[14] Whether blues, psychosis, and depression post partum are points on a biopsychologic continuum, or distinct entities, is a hotly debated topic. There seems to be a real clustering of admissions to psychiatric units post partum. It is not clear whether these patients suffer from a specific clinical entity related to childbearing, or from episodes of a variety of diseases.[15] One possible etiologic factor that may be exacerbated in the patient who suffered medical complications of pregnancy is the loss of the intense involvement and monitoring of the medical-obstetric team.

PSYCHOLOGIC RAMIFICATIONS OF MEDICALLY COMPLICATED PREGNANCY

Background

The occurrence of medical complications, as mentioned above, is a significant added psychologic stress in pregnancy, and results in psychiatric symptoms in many cases. For example, in a prospective study of pregnant diabetic women, two thirds exhibited psychopathology; specific common syndromes were anxiety and depression.[16] In another con-

TABLE 19–4.
Indications for Psychiatric Consultation

1. Active psychosis
2. Active mood disorder
3. Suicidality/homicidality
4. Unusually poor and/or decreasing level of function
5. Physical symptoms or concerns without discernible basis
6. Psychologic factors interfering with compliance
7. Anxiety interfering with function or comfort
8. Medication assessment and management

trolled, prospective study, preeclamptic women were more depressed and less verbal than healthy women, and their husbands were found to be less supportive.[17]

Medical complications exacerbate the usual psychologic tasks and conflicts of pregnancy. These include concerns about the capacity for effective mothering; fears about loss of control; bodily pain and damage, and damage to the unborn child; ambivalence about the continuation of pregnancy; feelings of guilt and shame about behaviors or conditions which may (or are imagined to) have contributed to the complications; grief and disappointment at the loss of the idealized pregnancy experience; demands on loved ones for additional emotional and practical support; inability to fulfill accustomed roles and perform necessary and/or enjoyable tasks; intolerance for physical discomforts; and the need to work out relationships with obstetric care providers.

As reproduction and parenting are central tasks and roles in human development, their successful performance confers an important sense of mastery and maturity.[18] When there are complications, the woman generally feels she has failed her mate, her family, and her fetus. She also feels cheated of the idealized experience she would like and which she imagines that other pregnant women enjoy. The dangers to which her complications expose the fetus make her feel burdened, vulnerable, and guilty.

Responsibility and Decision Making

If the medical condition was preexisting, the patient may have been counseled to avoid pregnancy. She often has to face, as soon as the pregnancy is confirmed, a weighty decision about whether to undergo therapeutic abortion. Painful questions ensue. Will she ever have another chance to become a mother? Is it fair, or moral, to bring a child into a situation in which its mother is ill? Is it moral to terminate the pregnancy because of the danger to the mother? Not infrequently, direct comments and innuendoes of friends, rela-

tives, and medical personnel increase the sense of guilt and helplessness: "It isn't right for a person in your condition to bring a child into the world." "We will have to monitor you carefully; your condition could result in damage to your baby." "If you don't relax, your blood pressure will get even higher."

Effects of Medical Management

Psychologic reactions to medical complications of pregnancy are also affected by the diagnostic and therapeutic maneuvers required for clinical management. In addition to fear and guilt, the patient has to suffer uncomfortable or even painful interventions, such as prolonged fetal monitoring, repeated amniocenteses, venipunctures, etc.[19] A prominent side effect of tocolytic agents is significant dysphoria. Bed rest, hospitalization, frequent clinic visits, and other nonintrusive modalities, in addition to making a woman feel like a useless burden, make it almost impossible for her to distract herself from a morbid preoccupation with the details of her medical-obstetric condition.[10] Seemingly thoughtless noncompliance may reflect an incapacity to delegate her usual duties to others, and to rely upon them for her care. Sometimes there is no one she can call on.

Religious Issues

Religious beliefs are an important component of many women's experiences. When the tenets of the denomination of the woman and/or her family are at variance with her wishes and/or the advice of her physicians, the psychologic conflict can be exacerbated to the point of symptom formation and interference with her decision making. On the other hand, a strong religious belief can give a woman the strength to carry her through a difficult situation.

Consultation with a religious leader who is experienced with this sort of problem, psychologically sensitive, and flexible, is valuable, as is contact with a health professional familiar and comfortable with the particular

TABLE 19–5.
Psychologic Management of Spontaneous Abortion/Stillbirth

I. Introduce and explain roles of relevant care providers
II. Explain what has happened
   Indicate availability for repeated and expanded explanations
III. Offer options and elicit patient preferences
   A. Location in hospital—pre- or post-partum or gynecology unit
   B. Opportunity to view, handle, photograph* products of conception
      1. With expert care provider
      2. With significant other(s)
   C. Disposition of remains
      1. Autopsy
      2. Burial
      3. Hospital disposal
   D. Religious personnel and rituals
   E. Visits by friends and family—offer to inform them
   F. Presence of staff
IV. Express acceptance of wide range of emotions
V. Counsel bereaved parents—separately and together
   A. Foster communication
   B. Arrange follow-up visits—2, 6, 12, and 26 weeks post partum
      1. Convey autopsy results
      2. Assess function of family unit—refer if distress and dysfunction not resolving

*Take photographs routinely for later referral.

religious system in question. Neither may be necessary if the involved staff are able to allow the patient to ventilate, able to listen and try to understand her conflict, and, with her family as appropriate, to support her working it through. Sometimes it is the staff who are most pained by a clinical situation, as when a Jehovah's Witness refuses a medically imperative blood transfusion. In that case, it is the staff who need information, ventilation, collaboration, and support, in order to formulate and carry out a coherent and benign approach to the patient.

Perinatal Loss: The Role of Nonpsychiatric Medical Staff

Religious support is often useful to patients whose complications result in fetal wastage, stillbirth, or neonatal death (Table 19–5). Again, both medical and religious personnel can be involved. They can ask the patient whether she is a religious person, and how her religious beliefs are affecting her response to the loss. Bereaved parents frequently feel conflicted, frustrated, and sinful because they feel angry at God for inflicting this pain on them and their innocent offspring, while other people become parents without even appreciating or desiring it.

Being enraged at God, they feel they can no longer find solace in faith. They are often very relieved to hear that God made people the way they are and understands that they get mad when they suffer pain for reasons they can't comprehend. Religious families also benefit from the opportunity to make arrangements for some sort of memorial service or funeral, for any but the earliest spontaneous abortion.[20]

In addition to allowing for ventilation and enhancing religious support, there are other psychosocial interventions helpful to women experiencing the loss of a pregnancy or neonate. The opportunity to observe and hold the fetus or stillborn infant allows the parents and other relatives to accept the reality of the death, say good-by, and feel that they have physically communicated their parental love to the dead child. When the child is damaged or deformed, the parents' fantasies are almost invariably worse than the reality. The body can be wrapped in a blanket as aesthetically as possible, and the parents can hold and examine it as they feel comfortable, in the presence of a knowledgeable and sensitive professional who can explain the abnormalities and point out the normal features.

Staff are often at a loss whether to leave the mother alone or to remain with her, whether to leave her in the prenatal or postnatal unit or transfer her (to the gynecology floor, for example), whether to talk or remain silent.[21] The best approach is to offer these choices to the patient, allow her some time to consider, and explain that it is fine if she changes her mind. Tell her that she will experience denial, shock, anger, and sadness, not necessarily in that order, and that the staff consider all of these feelings perfectly appropriate. Offer to help with arrangements and to mediate so that persons comforting to the patient are allowed access to her whenever she wishes and others are excluded. Friends and relatives generally accept the dictates of hospital staff much more easily than those of the patient, and refusing to see certain people is too difficult for most patients.

Bereaved parents benefit enormously from careful medical explanations of the sequence of events leading up to the fetal death and the medical care undertaken in an attempt to prevent it. An outpatient session to review autopsy findings when they become available is an opportunity to increase the information communicated, repeat explanations necessarily forgotten in the midst of the acute situation, and monitor the state of the patient and family as they react to the loss.[22] These parents often feel that no one who has not suffered the loss of a child can possibly understand or help, and appreciate referral to a family that has recovered from its grief.[23]

RECOMMENDATIONS FOR THE PRIMARY PHYSICIAN: DIAGNOSIS, MANAGEMENT, AND REFERRAL

Suggestions for the handling of some specific clinical situations have been introduced in the relevant sections above. The major general issues are screening, differential diagnosis, support and management by the primary team, the use of psychotropic drugs during pregnancy, indications and techniques for referral and the choice of mental health professional. Screening questions for psychiatric illness and violence were outlined above. Screening for psychosocial stress, domestic violence, and psychiatric illness is indicated as part of routine prenatal care and particularly important in the presence of medical complications. It is as easily accomplished as screening for other conditions, which is routinely performed even though they may be less prevalent.

If there is a printed form for the chart, questions about abuse and psychiatric history should be added, and the review of systems should include symptoms of anxiety, difficulty in functioning, and mood changes. The examiner should determine what the essential nature of the patient's living situation is: how many people in the home, who they are, economic state and stability, major tensions in relationships. These straightforward inquiries serve two purposes: They elicit some information immediately, and they indicate to the patient the fact that these subjects are legitimate ones to bring up with the health care team when she feels able and/or when problems arise.

A brief follow-up can be part of each prenatal visit. It is often difficult for patients to bring up personal problems. Therefore, ask the questions as though problems were to be expected: For example, What problems have come up at home since your last visit? rather than, Do you have problems at home? If a recitation of problems is elicited, ask the patient whether she feels she can cope or needs help.

Diagnosis

How does the physician primarily responsible for a pregnant patient decide whether she has a significant psychiatric illness? These illnesses are not esoteric; clinicians using the current diagnostic system in psychiatry do not have to detect unconscious motivations and hidden conflicts, but rather to catalogue signs and symptoms (DSM-III-R).[24] For example, a patient is diagnosed as *depressed* if she manifests, for 2 weeks or more, five of the following symptoms:

- Loss of appetite
- Loss of libido
- Decreased energy
- Decreased ability to concentrate
- Sad mood
- Thoughts of death or suicide
- Inability to enjoy previously pleasurable activities
- Difficulty sleeping

Patients with serious thoughts of suicide or homicide require emergency psychiatric evaluation. If the patient expresses intentions or plans for these behaviors, do not leave her alone until a psychiatrist has seen her.

Mania is characterized by an excess of energy; the patient sleeps little, makes impetuous and rash decisions typically involving the profligate expenditure of money, and has little interest in eating or other bodily necessities. She may be either euphoric or irritable, and her thoughts, speech, and behaviors race. Before effective treatments were available, some patients died of exhaustion.

The diagnosis of *somatization disorder* requires that the patient have suffered from many somatic symptoms, with onset by adolescence, and that they have caused her to seek medical advice and/or compromised her performance of her responsibilities. *Panic disorder* is characterized by palpitations, hyperventilation, subjective sense of dyspnea, and a terrible feeling of dread and impending death. *Generalized anxiety disorder* may manifest physically, through somatic symptoms, or directly, with nervousness interfering with ordinary activities. Significant anxiety is a common complication of high-risk pregnancy.

Psychotic patients suffer from *delusions* (irrational beliefs other than those common to a cultural group), *hallucinations* (sensory experiences not produced by external stimuli), and *thought disorders* (loosening of the normal associative links). In common parlance, they cannot distinguish the unreal from the real. They may dress, look, or behave in a bizarre manner. However, even disorders as severe as these can be missed during routine obstetric visits in the absence of specific screening.

Psychotic symptoms are obstetrically significant, as mentioned above, because they may interfere with medical compliance, the ability to recognize and appropriately react to signs and symptoms of labor and/or complications, general self-care, and the ability to get along with other persons, including supportive friends and family and medical staff. The patient may be taking, or require, anti-psychotic medication. In some states, psychiatrists are forbidden by law to communicate to anyone, including other physicians, the fact that a patient is under psychiatric care. This reality underscores the need for screening in the obstetric setting.

Substance abuse, which is discussed in Chapter 17, is another psychiatric disorder with a high prevalence in the population, including the population of pregnant women, and with significant deleterious effects on obstetric outcome. It is not limited to a particular socioeconomic class.[25] The diagnosis can be made by asking the relevant questions directly, unapologetically, and nonjudgmentally.

* Tell me all the medications you are taking which have been prescribed by a doctor.
* Are you taking any drugs which are not prescribed?
* Do you drink alcohol every day? Get drunk at intervals? Feel you need alcohol to get through the day? Does drinking ever interfere with your ability to do your work, at home or outside?

The possibility of substance abuse, intoxication, and withdrawal should be part of the diagnostic thinking in every case. Physicians should be aware that patients can obtain substances of abuse in the hospital setting, as well. Substance abuse generally requires both the intervention of a specialist and participation in a specific support and treatment group.[26]

Psychiatric Referral

Once a psychiatric disorder or symptom complex has been identified, how should the patient be managed? There is no essential difference between preexisting psychiatric disorders and those which first manifest during pregnancy. Patients at risk of damage to themselves or others, and psychotic patients, should be referred to a psychiatrist immediately (Table 19–6). If there is the slightest doubt about the patient's safety, do not leave her alone, even to make a call. Request a psychiatric consultation in the obstetric setting, or see that the patient is conducted—again, without being left alone, even in the bathroom—to an emergency psychiatric facility.

In the absence of an acute emergency, indications for referral include the following: a history of previous major psychiatric hospitalization, worsening symptoms further complicating the medical condition, interference with compliance, the patient's wish for psychologic help, and unresolved diagnostic questions. The primary team may also have questions about the patient's capacity to comply with outpatient treatment, or to consent to or refuse recommended interventions.[27] When the problem is one of situational stress, is stable or beginning to resolve, or relatively mild, the primary physician can decide, on the basis of available resources, his or her own talents, interests, and expertise, and the wishes of the patient, whether to refer or treat.

Technique of Psychiatric Referral.— The referral of a patient to a psychiatrist, or informing a patient that a psychiatric consultant will be called, is perceived as difficult by most nonpsychiatrists. Here are some suggestions (see Table 19–6): Always tell the patient; do not attempt to pass the consultation off in a disguised way, nor let the task fall to the consultant. Ground the explanation and goals in the observed realities of the situation: "We are not sure what is causing your loss of energy," or "Your taking tranquilizers has gotten out of hand," or "We want to make sure you are able to make a clear decision about the treatment we have recommended."

Explain that the psychiatrist is part of the team and staff. Psychiatric referral early, rather than late and desperate, in the clinical course facilitates patient acceptance and effective collaboration. Make it clear that the psychiatric consultation does not imply abandonment or disinterest by the original care providers by indicating that you will ask the patient afterward how the consultation went

and will discuss the case with the psychiatric consultant. In some cases, the patient may want portions of her communications to the psychiatrist kept confidential; the best response is that the content can be kept confidential unless there is danger to the patient's safety. Make another appointment to see the patient at the same time you make the psychiatric referral. When psychosis is not a serious diagnostic consideration, you might want to reassure the patient that no one thinks she is crazy; this concern is what frightens and alienates some patients.[28]

The choice of mental health professional may be a consideration. In some settings, nonpsychiatrists such as psychologists, social workers, pastoral counselors, and/or nurse/ clinicians may be a part of the team working with high-risk or other patients. Interdisciplinary collaboration allows for adequate medical participation in the differential diagnosis and management of psychiatric signs and symptoms. Psychiatric emergencies and the need to consider psychiatric hospitalization and/or the use of psychotropic medications absolutely require management by a psychiatrist, that is to say, a physician specializing in disorders of emotion and behavior. In intermediate cases, the availability of specialists of various disciplines and the need for medical expertise must be weighed in each clinical situation.

Prognosis

In general, the patient's premorbid adjustment and the length of the current psy-

TABLE 19–6.
How to Make a Psychiatric Referral

1. Consider and discuss psychiatric involvement earlier, rather than later, in workup and treatment
2. Stress ongoing and future involvement of referring physician
3. Introduce psychiatrist as a member of the medical team
4. Ground the explanation in observable data—the patient's own symptoms and the distress they cause her

chosocial disturbance are the most useful prognostic signs. A physician who works with a patient over a number of years may become familiar with her pattern of relative de- and recompensation, and knowledgeable about the interventions which facilitate recovery. For example, she may do well once relatives are alerted and come to help out for a few weeks. A physically or emotionally abusive member of the household may have to be arrested by the police or otherwise relocated. In these situations, the opinion of a physician treating a pregnant patient often carries some weight with the family and community, and can facilitate the necessary intervention.

Office Management

Effective office or bedside counseling by the primary physician is focused on the precipitants of the acute situation.[29] It sometimes takes considerable effort for the patient and physician to realize what events or feelings triggered the current episode, but after this work is accomplished, the resolution of the problem is often obvious and relatively easy. Occasionally, the source of the patient's distress is her misinterpretation of the obstetric findings or prognosis, or the recognition that the anticipated complications and management will severely tax her psychosocial resources. Discussions with hospital staff and with other patients who have managed to cope can allay these anxieties.

Another useful principle is to explore with the patient her usual methods of coping with stress and to support them. For example, the patient may usually dispel tension by activity; the curtailment of activity by obstetric complications leads to mood changes and/or morbid somatic preoccupations. She and her care providers might think creatively about constructive projects she can carry out without moving around a good deal.

For a patient who is used to being in control, reading about her condition and participating in record keeping and decision making can relieve symptoms. While some patients thrive on dependency, many women find it almost unbearable to be unable to take care of their families and jobs. The care provider can remind these patients that it is valuable for her family to take care of her at times. They can devise ways for her to stay in touch, as with charts of family activities.

PSYCHOTROPIC MEDICATIONS IN PREGNANCY

Decisions about psychoactive medications play a part in the management of patients with psychiatric symptoms (Table 19–7). The absence of knowledge about long-term effects on the fetus and neonate and the implications of psychiatric illness for the outcome of pregnancy complicate the pharmacologic treatment of obstetric patients. A psychiatrist should first consider psychosocial interventions, such as frequent medical visits, provision of home support services, and hospitalization. The known and unknown risks of pharmacologic treatments should be weighed carefully against the risks of the psychiatric illness and the other resources available for its management. The patient must collaborate in this decision-making process, and her "significant others" should be strongly encouraged to participate constructively—with her permission. The whole process should be documented in the chart for both clinical and medical-legal reasons.

Methodologic and ethical problems have made the accumulation of an adequate database about psychotropic drug use in pregnancy extremely difficult. Information about the obstetric and psychiatric outcomes of major psychiatric illness in pregnancy *not* pharmacologically treated is likewise lacking. Psychotic patients suffer from acute and chronic stress and their physiologic concomitants. In one unpublished study, pregnancies of actively psychotic patients were complicated by intrauterine growth retardation and other conditions which were reversed after psychiatric hospitalization and multimodal treatment as indicated.[30]

There are no specific guidelines for psy-

TABLE 19–7.
Psychotropic Drug Use in Pregnancy: Selected Agents*

Drug	Major Psychiatric Indication(s)	FDA Risk Factor[†]	Comments
Lithium	Manic-depressive illness	D	Fetal Ebstein's anomaly; other cardiovascular malformations; toxicity in newborn
Amitriptyline	Depression, panic disorder	D	Rare malformations; neonatal withdrawal?
Imipramine	Depression, panic disorder	D	Rare malformations; neonatal withdrawal
Phenelzine	Depression	C	?Malformations; monoamine oxidase inhibitor
Diazepam	Anxiety	D	Cleft lip/palate; neonatal complications; benzodiazepine
Chlorpromazine	Psychosis, manic excitement	C	Low-potency neuroleptic; avoid near term—associated with maternal hypotension
Haloperidol	Psychosis, manic excitement	C	Reported use during labor without adverse effects

*Adapted from Briggs GB, Freeman RK, Yaffe SJ: *Drugs in Pregnancy and Lactation*, ed 2. Baltimore: Williams & Wilkins Co, 1986.
[†]See Preface for description of FDA risk classification.

chotropic drug dosages during pregnancy, delivery, or lactation. All psychotropic drugs require titration to the response and sometimes blood level measurements for each patient. Doses should be chosen with the aim of preventing florid recurrence rather than eliminating as many symptoms as possible. The management of such cases without psychiatric collaboration is inadvisable, and the following data are offered as scientific information and to inform the clinician practicing in an area where psychiatric consultation is unavailable. The diagnosis of pregnancy may be delayed in patients with major psychotic illness. Treatment with antipsychotics, antidepressants, or antianxiety agents may have proceeded into or through the first trimester, leading to concern about teratogenicity. Treatment perinatally raises questions about effects on labor and on the physiologic functioning of the neonate. In some cases, patients on psychoative agents ask for advice before deciding to conceive and/or breast-feed.[31]

Lithium carbonate, used for mania and/or depression, is associated with an increased risk of cardiovascular anomalies in the neonate whose mother has therapeutic blood levels at the time of birth. It also appears in breast milk at up to half the concentration in the maternal serum, and is associated with cyanosis, hypotonia, and hypothermia in some of the nursing infants.[32] Alternative pharmacologic agents with apparently lower risk of teratogenicity include carbamazepine, clonazepam, and the major tranquilizers and tricyclic antidepressants.

For the mother, the use of lithium requires meticulous dosing and monitoring because of the renal changes of pregnancy. If at all possible, the drug should be gradually discontinued in the weeks before the due date; if this is not possible, dosage should be decreased by 50% just prior to labor, to allow for the fluid shifts associated with parturition.

Tricyclic antidepressants can be used to manage depression and anxiety/panic disorders in the pregnant patient. No significant morphologic teratogenicity has been identified; neurobehavioral sequelae are being studied.[33] The safety of monoamine oxidase inhibitors is more questionable, and they should not be prescribed. Anticholinergic side effects are a potential problem for both mother and infant. These are lowest in association with secondary amines such as nortriptyline or desipramine, which also allow for clinically useful plasma level measurement.[31] A major disadvantage in the use of tricyclic antidepressants in the depressed patient is their lethal potential in the event of overdose. Again, close collaboration with a psychiatrist is mandatory.

There is a growing body of evidence on the adverse affects of benzodiazepines on the embryo and fetus. These agents are of particular concern for two reasons: the fact that they are used for conditions which themselves have no major sequelae, and the fact that they are the most commonly prescribed agents in the United States. A recent paper describes eight children suffering from characteristic dysmorphic features, growth aberrations, and central nervous system abnormalities.[34] Anxious patients should be assessed to determine the source(s) of anxiety, and then offered explanations, reassurance, support, and psychotherapy, in that order. True panic disorders are best treated with tricyclics, as mentioned above. Major tranquilizers can also be used.

Neuroleptic agents are used to treat symptoms of psychosis and agitation. The choice of agent depends on the patient's known responsiveness, and on the side effects to be particularly avoided or sought in the individual case. Low-potency agents are more sedating, but may be more teratogenic.[31] Anticholinergic effects, lowering of the seizure threshold, and parkinsonian signs and symptoms are all factors to be considered. These agents are found in the breast milk of treated mothers, and can result in sedation or significant extrapyramidal complications in breast-feeding infants.[35] The reader should consult comprehensive sources[32, 36] for further data on the use of drugs during pregnancy or lactation.

CONCLUSION

The detection and management of psychiatric complications of pregnancy represent a particular challenge when medical disorders are also present. The stakes are high, and too little is known about therapeutic agents and conditions which can have a major impact on the outcome of pregnancy. Uncooperative patients and those with inadequate social support represent a major challenge to the clinician's time, energy, and resourcefulness. A careful psychiatric history and mental status examination are essential to identify psychiatric illness, forestall emergencies, and facilitate timely referral for expert collaborative management. These diagnostic and preventive measures can, surprisingly often, redeem a difficult situation and contribute to a positive obstetric outcome.

REFERENCES

1. Nadelson CC: "Normal" and "special" aspects of pregnancy: a psychological approach, in *The Woman Patient: Medical and Psychological Interfaces,* vol 1, in Nadelson CC, Notman MT (eds): *Sexual and Reproductive Aspects of Women's Health Care.* New York, Plenum Press, 1978.
2. Levin JS, DeFrank RS: Maternal stress and pregnancy outcomes: A review of the psychosocial literature. *J Psychosom Obstet Gynecol* 1988;9:3–16.
3. Jones WHS: *Hippocrates,* with English translation, vol. 1. London, William Heinemann, 1923.
4. Karnosh LJ, Hope JM: Puerperal psychoses and their sequelae. *Am J Psychiatry* 1937;94:537–550.
5. Marcé LV: *Traité de la folie des femmes enceintes des nouvelles accouchées et des nourrices.* Paris, JB Baillière et Fils, 1858.
6. Charles AG, Norr KL, Block CR, et al: Obstetric and psychological effects of psychoprophylactic preparation for childbirth. *Am J Obstet Gynecol* 1978;131:44–52.
7. Hughey M: Complications of labor in prepared and unprepared primiparae. *Am J Obstet Gynecol* 1976;21:62–69.
8. Sundstrom-Feigenberg K: Reproductive health and reproductive freedom: Maternal health care and family planning in the Swedish health system: *Women Health* 1988;13:35–55.
9. Stewart DE: Psychiatric symptoms following attempted natural childbirth. *Can Med Assoc J* 1982;127:713–716.
10. Gise LH: Psychiatric implications of pregnancy, in Cherry SH, Berkowitz RL, Kase NG (eds): *Rovinsky and Guttmacher's Medical, Surgical, and Gynecological Complications of Pregnancy.* Baltimore, Williams & Wilkins Co, 1985, pp.

11. Notman MT: Reproduction and pregnancy: a psychodynamic developmental perspective, in Stotland N (ed): *Psychiatric Aspects of the New Reproductive Technologies.* Washington, DC, American Psychiatric Press, 1990.

12. Hamilton JA: *Postpartum Psychiatric Problems.* St Louis, CV Mosby Co, 1962.

13. Murray JG, Abraham GE: Pseudocyesis: A review. *Obstet Gynecol* 1978;51:627–631.

14. Dix C: *The New Mother Syndrome.* Garden City, NY, Doubleday, 1985.

15. Youngs DD, Lucas MJ: Postpartum depression: hormonal versus alternative perspectives, in Youngs DD, Erhardt AA (eds): *Psychosomatic Obstetrics and Gynecology.* New York, Appleton-Century-Crofts, 1980, pp 30–38.

16. Barglow P, Hatcher R, Wolston J, et al: Psychiatric risk factor in the pregnant diabetic patient. *Am J Obstet Gynecol* 1981;140:46–52.

17. Pilowsky I, Sharp J: Psychological aspects of pre-eclamptic toxemia: A prospective study. *J Psychosom Res* 1971;15:193–197.

18. Seiden A: The sense of mastery in the childbirth experience, in *The Woman Patient: Medical and Psychological Interfaces,* vol 1, in Nadelson CC, Notman MT (eds): *Sexual and Reproductive Aspects of Women's Health Care.* New York, Plenum Press, 1978

19. Jackson JD: Psychological aspects of fetal monitoring: Maternal reactions to the monitor and staff behavior. *J Psychosom Obstet Gynecol* 1983;2:97–101.

20. Case R: When birth is also a funeral. *J Pastoral Care* 1978;32:6–21.

21. Knapp RJ, Peppers LG: Doctor-patient relationships in fetal/infant death encounters. *J Med Educ* 1979;54:775–780.

22. Kennell JH, Slyter J, Klaus MH: The mourning responses of parents to the death of a newborn infant. *N Engl J Med* 1970;283:344–349.

23. Schiff HS: *The Bereaved Parent.* New York, Crown Publishers, 1977.

24. American Psychiatric Association: *Diagnostic and Statistical Manual of Mental Disorders,* ed 3, revised [DSM-III-R]. Washington, DC, American Psychiatric Association, 1987.

25. Hackett TP: Alcoholism: acute and chronic states, in Hackett TP, Cassem NH (eds): *Massachusetts General Hospital Handbook of General Hospital Psychiatry,* ed 2. Littleton, Mass, PSG Publishing Co, 1987, pp 15–28.

26. Renner JA: Drug addiction, in Hackett TP, Cassem NH (eds): *Massachusetts General Hospital Handbook of General Hospital Psychiatry,* ed 2. Littleton, Mass, PSG Publishing Co, 1987, pp.

27. Groves JE, Vaccarino JM: Legal aspects of consultation, in Hackett TP, Cassem NH (eds): *Massachusetts General Hospital Handbook of General Hospital Psychiatry,* ed 2. Littleton, Mass, PSG Publishing Co, 1987, pp.

28. Stotland NL, Garrick TR: *Manual of Psychiatric Consultation.* Washington, DC, American Psychiatric Press, Inc, 1990.

29. Bellak L, Small L: *Emergency Psychotherapy and Brief Psychotherapy.* New York, Grune & Stratton, Inc, 1965.

30. Carrano M: Personal communication, 1985

31. Cohen LS, Heller VL, Rosenbaum JF: Treatment good for psychotropic drug use in pregnancy. *Psychosom Med* 1989;30:25–33.

32. Berkowitz RL, Coustan DR, Mochizuki TK: *Handbook for Prescribing Medications During Pregnancy,* ed 2. Boston, Little, Brown & Co, 1986.

33. Coyle LR: Changes in developing behavior following pre-natal administration of imipramine. *Pharmacol Biochem Behav* 1975;3:799–807.

34. Laegreid L, Olegard R, Walstroom J, et al: Teratogenic effects of benzodiazepine use during pregnancy. *J Pediatr* 1989;114:126–131.

35. Dubovsky SL: Psychiatric approach to high-risk obstetrics, in Abrams RS, Wexler P (eds): *Medical Care of the Pregnant Patient.* Boston, Little, Brown & Co, 1983, pp 373–384.

36. Robinson GE, Stewart DE, Flak E: The rational use of psychotropic drugs in pregnancy and postpartum. *Can J Psychiatry* 1986;31:183–190.

APPENDIX

A Guide to Laboratory Values in Pregnant Women

As is stressed throughout this volume, physiological adaptations to gestation affect virtually every organ system and alter the normal range of many laboratory determinations. Cognizance of these changes will help the clinician avoid diagnostic errors, lead to earlier awareness of disease states, and reduce futile investigation of what appears to be an abnormal laboratory value.

Unfortunately, tables listing normal ranges for laboratory data in pregnant women are difficult to construct and easily misinterpreted. This is because values may change throughout the course of gestation, alterations may be dependent on local population characteristics, and there is a paucity of data in the literature concerning changes in some parameters. Thus, we have chosen to provide the following "where-to-find-it" guide, which directs the reader to the specific text page(s) where information about changes in key laboratory values may be found.

INDEX